HYPERTENSION
A Companion to Braunwald's Heart Disease

THIRD EDITION

HYPERTENSION
A Companion to Braunwald's Heart Disease

George L. Bakris, MD, FAHA, FASN, FASH
Professor of Medicine
Director, ASH Comprehensive Hypertension Center
Section of Endocrinology, Diabetes and Metabolism
University of Chicago Medicine
Chicago, Illinois

Matthew J. Sorrentino, MD, FACC, FASH
Professor of Medicine
Section of Cardiology
University of Chicago Medicine
Chicago, Illinois

ELSEVIER

ELSEVIER

1600 John F. Kennedy Blvd.
Ste 1800
Philadelphia, PA 19103-2899

HYPERTENSION: A COMPANION TO BRAUNWALD'S HEART DISEASE,
THIRD EDITION

ISBN: 978-0-323-42973-3

Notices

Knowledge and best practice in this field are constantly changing. As new research and experience broaden our understanding, changes in research methods, professional practices, or medical treatment may become necessary.

Practitioners and researchers must always rely on their own experience and knowledge in evaluating and using any information, methods, compounds, or experiments described herein. In using such information or methods they should be mindful of their own safety and the safety of others, including parties for whom they have a professional responsibility.

With respect to any drug or pharmaceutical products identified, readers are advised to check the most current information provided (i) on procedures featured or (ii) by the manufacturer of each product to be administered, to verify the recommended dose or formula, the method and duration of administration, and contraindications. It is the responsibility of practitioners, relying on their own experience and knowledge of their patients, to make diagnoses, to determine dosages and the best treatment for each individual patient, and to take all appropriate safety precautions.

To the fullest extent of the law, neither the Publisher nor the authors, contributors, or editors, assume any liability for any injury and/or damage to persons or property as a matter of products liability, negligence or otherwise, or from any use or operation of any methods, products, instructions, or ideas contained in the material herein.

Previous editions copyrighted 2013 and 2007.

Library of Congress Cataloging-in-Publication Data

Names: Bakris, George L., 1952- editor. | Sorrentino, Matthew J., editor.
Title: Hypertension : a companion to Braunwald's heart disease / [edited by]
 George L. Bakris, Matthew J. Sorrentino.
Other titles: Hypertension (Black) | Complemented by (expression):
 Braunwald's heart disease. 10th edition.
Description: Third edition. | Philadelphia, PA : Elsevier, [2018] |
 Complemented by: Braunwald's heart disease / edited by Douglas L. Mann,
 Douglas P. Zipes, Peter Libby, Robert O. Bonow, Eugene Braunwald. 10th
 edition. 2015. | Includes bibliographical references and index.
Identifiers: LCCN 2016054229 | ISBN 9780323429733 (hardcover : alk. paper)
Subjects: | MESH: Hypertension
Classification: LCC RC681 | NLM WG 340 | DDC 616.1/2–dc23
LC record available at https://lccn.loc.gov/2016054229

Content Strategist: Dolores Meloni
Senior Content Development Specialist: Marybeth Thiel
Publishing Services Manager: Catherine Jackson
Senior Project Manager: Daniel Fitzgerald
Designer: Renee Duenow

Printed in China.

Last digit is the print number: 9 8 7 6 5 4 3 2 1

Working together
to grow libraries in
developing countries

www.elsevier.com • www.bookaid.org

Contributors

Ailia W. Ali, MD
Fellow, Sleep Medicine, Division of Pulmonary, Allergy, and
Critical Care Medicine, University of Pittsburgh, Pittsburgh,
Pennsylvania, United States

Radica Z. Alicic, MD, FHM
Associate Director for Research, Providence Health Care,
Clinical Associate Professor of Medicine, University of
Washington School of Medicine, Spokane, Washington,
United States

Laurence Amar, MD, PhD
Hypertension Unit, Hôpital Européen Georges Pompidou,
Assistance Publique-Hôpitaux de Paris, Paris-Descartes
University, Paris, France

Saif Anwaruddin, MD
Assistant Professor of Medicine and Co-Director,
Transcatheter Valve Program, Cardiovascular Medicine,
University of Pennsylvania School of Medicine, Philadelphia,
Pennsylvania, United States

Lawrence J. Appel, MD, MPH
C. David Molina Professor of Medicine, Johns Hopkins
University School of Medicine; Director, Welch Center for
Prevention, Epidemiology and Clinical Research, Johns
Hopkins University, Baltimore, Maryland, United States

Phyllis August, MD, MPH
Ralph A. Baer MD Professor of Research in Medicine,
Nephrology and Hypertension, New York Presbyterian/Weill
Cornell Medicine, New York, New York, United States

Michel Azizi, MD, PhD
Hypertension Unit, Hôpital Européen Georges Pompidou,
Assistance Publique-Hôpitaux de Paris, Paris-Descartes
University, Paris, France

George L. Bakris, MD, FAHA, FASN, FASH
Professor of Medicine, Director, ASH Comprehensive
Hypertension Center, Section of Endocrinology, Diabetes
and Metabolism, University of Chicago Medicine, Chicago,
Illinois, United States

José R. Banegas, MD
Professor of Preventive Medicine and Public Health,
Universidad Autónoma de Madrid-IdiPAZ–CIBERESP, Madrid,
Spain

Robert L. Bard, MA
Research Associate, Division of Cardiovascular Medicine,
University of Michigan, Ann Arbor, Michigan, United States

Orit Barrett, MD
Senior Resident, Department of Medicine D, Soroka
University Medical Center, Faculty of Health Sciences,
Ben-Gurion University of the Negev, Beer Sheva, Israel

Athanase Benetos, MD, PhD
Head, Geriatric Medicine, Université de Lorraine, Nancy,
France

Kenneth E. Bernstein
Director of Experimental Pathology, Professor of Biomedical
Sciences, Pathology and Laboratory Medicine, Cedars-Sinai
Medical Center, Los Angeles, California, United States

Deepak L. Bhatt, MD, MPH
Executive Director of Interventional Cardiovascular
Programs, Brigham and Women's Hospital Heart and Vascular
Center; Senior Physician, Brigham and Women's Hospital;
Senior Investigator, TIMI Study Group, Professor of Medicine,
Harvard Medical School, Boston, Massachusetts,
United States

Italo Biaggioni, MD
Professor of Medicine and Pharmacology, Associate Director,
Clinical Research Center, Vanderbilt Autonomic Dysfunction
Center, Division of Clinical Pharmacology, Vanderbilt
University School of Medicine, Nashville, Tennessee,
United States

Roger S. Blumenthal, MD
Kenneth Jay Pollin Professor of Cardiology and Director,
Johns Hopkins University School of Medicine and Ciccarone
Center for the Prevention of Heart Disease, Baltimore,
Maryland, United States

Guillaume Bobrie, MD
Hypertension Unit, Hôpital Européen Georges Pompidou,
Assistance Publique-Hôpitaux de Paris, Paris, France

Robert D. Brook, MD
Professor of Internal Medicine, Division of Cardiovascular
Medicine; Director, ASH Comprehensive Hypertension Center,
University of Michigan, Ann Arbor, Michigan, United States

J. Brian Byrd, MD, MS
Assistant Professor of Medicine, Division of Cardiovascular
Medicine, University of Michigan, Ann Arbor, Michigan,
United States

Barry L. Carter, PharmD, FCCP, FAHA, FASH, FAPHA
Patrick E. Keefe Professor of Pharmacy, Department of
Pharmacy Practice and Science, College of Pharmacy;
Professor, Department of Family Medicine, College of
Medicine, University of Iowa, Iowa City, Iowa, United States

Debbie L. Cohen, MD
Associate Professor of Medicine, Perelman School of
Medicine—Renal, Electrolyte and Hypertension Division,
University of Pennsylvania, Philadelphia, Pennsylvania,
United States

Contributors

William C. Cushman, MD
Chief, Preventive Medicine, Medical Service, Veterans Affairs Medical Center; Professor, Preventive Medicine, Medicine, and Physiology, University of Tennessee Health Science Center, Memphis, Tennessee, United States

Peter Wilhelmus De Leeuw, MD, PhD
Professor of Medicine, Department of Medicine, Maastricht University Medical Center, Maastricht, Netherlands; Department of Medicine, Zuyderland Medical Center, Geleen/Heerlen, The Netherlands

Georg B. Ehret, MD
Médecin Adjoint Agrégé et Chargé de Cours, Cardiology, Department of Specialities of Medicine, Geneva University Hospitals, Geneva, Switzerland; Research Associate, McKusick-Nathans Institute of Genetic Medicine, Johns Hopkins University School of Medicine, Baltimore, Maryland, United States

William J. Elliott, MD, PhD
Professor of Preventive Medicine, Internal Medicine and Pharmacology, Pacific Northwest University of Health Sciences, Chair, Department of Biomedical Sciences; Chief, Division of Pharmacology, Pacific Northwest University of Health Sciences, Yakima, Washington, United States

Michael E. Ernst, PharmD, FCCP
Professor, Department of Pharmacy Practice and Science, College of Pharmacy; Professor, Department of Family Medicine, College of Medicine, University of Iowa, Iowa City, Iowa, United States

Muhammad U. Farooq, MD, FACP, FAHA
Division of Stroke and Vascular Neurology, Mercy Health Hauenstein Neurosciences, Grand Rapids, Michigan, United States

Anne-Laure Faucon, MD
Hypertension Unit, Hôpital Européen Georges Pompidou, Assistance Publique-Hôpitaux de Paris, Paris-Descartes University, Paris, France

Lauren Fishbein, MD, PhD
Assistant Professor of Medicine, University of Colorado School of Medicine, Department of Medicine, Division of Endocrinology, Metabolism and Diabetes, Aurora, Colorado, United States

Joseph T. Flynn, MD, MS
Chief, Division of Nephrology, Seattle Children's Hospital; Professor, Department of Pediatrics, University of Washington School of Medicine, Seattle, Washington, United States

Toshiro Fujita, MD, PhD
Chief, Division of Clinical Epigenetics, Research Center for Advanced Science and Technology, The University of Tokyo, Emeritus Professor, The University of Tokyo, Tokyo, Japan

Mary G. George, MD, MSPH, FACS
Senior Medical Officer and Deputy Associate Director for Science, Division for Heart Disease and Stroke Prevention, Centers for Disease Control and Prevention, Atlanta, Georgia, United States

Philip B. Gorelick, MD, MPH, FACP, FAAN, FANA, FAHA
Medical Director, Mercy Health Hauenstein Neurosciences; Professor, Department Translational Science & Molecular Medicine, Michigan State University College of Human Medicine, Grand Rapids, Michigan, United States

Elvira O. Gosmanova, MD
Nephrology Section Chief, Medical Service, Samuel S Stratton VA Medical Center, Associate Professor of Medicine, Division of Nephrology, Department of Medicine, Albany Medical College, Albany, New York, United States

Carlene M. Grim, BSN, MSN, SpDN
Founder and President, Shared Care Research and Education Consulting, Inc., Stateline, Nevada, United States

Clarence E. Grim, MS, MD, FACP, FAHA, FASH
Owner, High Blood Pressure Consulting, Stateline, Nevada; Senior Consult, Shared Care Research and Education Consulting, Inc., Stateline, Nevada; Retired (Semi) Professor of Medicine, Medical College of Wisconsin, UCLA, and Indiana U.; Board Certified Internal Medicine, Geriatrics, Hypertension Specialist, United States

Rajeev Gupta, MD, PhD
Chairman, Preventive Cardiology & Internal Medicine, Eternal Heart Care Centre and Research Institute, Jaipur, India

John E. Hall, PhD
Arthur C. Guyton Professor and Chair, Department of Physiology and Biophysics; Director, Mississippi Center of Obesity Research, University of Mississippi Medical Center, Jackson, Mississippi, United States

Michael E. Hall, MD, MS
Assistant Professor of Medicine, Division of Cardiology, Department of Medicine, University of Mississippi Medical Center, Jackson, Mississippi, United States

Coral D. Hanevold, MD
Clinical Professor of Pediatrics, University of Washington, Seattle Children's Hospital, Division of Nephrology, Seattle, Washington, United States

David G. Harrison, MD
Betty and Jack Bailey Professor of Medicine, Clinical Pharmacology, Department of Medicine, Vanderbilt University, Nashville, Tennessee, United States

Qi-Fang Huang, MD, PhD
Research Associate, The Shanghai Institute of Hypertension, Shanghai, China

Alun Hughes, BSc, MB, BS, PhD
Professor of Cardiovascular Physiology and Pharmacology, Institute of Cardiovascular Science, Faculty of Pop Health Sciences, University College London, London, United Kingdom

Philip Joseph, MD
Assistant Professor of Medicine, McMaster University, Hamilton, Ontario, Canada; Investigator, Population Health Research Institute, Hamilton Health Sciences & McMaster University, Hamilton, Ontario, Canada

vii

Contributors

Kazuomi Kario, MD, PhD
Professor & Chairman, Division of Cardiovascular Medicine,
Department of Medicine, Jichi Medical University School
of Medicine, Tochigi, Japan

Kunal N. Karmali, MD, MS
Clinical Instructor, Department of Medicine, Division of
Cardiology, Northwestern University Feinberg School of
Medicine, Chicago, Illinois, United States

Anastasios Kollias, MD, PhD
National and Kapodistrian University of Athens Clinical
Fellow, Hypertension Center STRIDE-7, National and
Kapodistrian University of Athens, Third Department of
Medicine, Sotiria Hospital, Athens, Greece

Luke J. Laffin, MD
Cardiology Fellow, Department of Medicine, The University
of Chicago, Medicine & Biological Sciences, Chicago, Illinois,
United States

Lewis Landsberg, MD
Irving S. Cutter Professor of Medicine, Northwestern
University, Feinberg School of Medicine, Chicago, Illinois,
United States

Donald M. Lloyd-Jones, MD, ScM, FACC FAHA
Chair and Eileen M. Foell Professor, Preventive Medicine,
Northwestern University Feinberg School of Medicine,
Senior Associate Dean for Clinical & Translational Research,
Northwestern University Feinberg School of Medicine,
Chicago, Illinois, United States

Anne-Marie Madjalian, MD
Hypertension Unit, Hôpital Européen Georges Pompidou,
Assistance Publique-Hôpitaux de Paris, Paris-Descartes
University, Paris, France

Line Malha, MD
Instructor in Medicine, Nephrology, Hypertension, and
Transplantation Medicine, Weill Cornell Medicine,
New York, New York, United States

Giuseppe Mancia, MD
Emeritus Professor of Medicine, University of
Milano-Bicocca, Milano, Italy

John W. McEvoy, MB BCh BAO, MHS
Assistant Professor, Division of Cardiology, Johns Hopkins
University School of Medicine and Ciccarone Center for
the Prevention of Heart Disease, Baltimore, Maryland,
United States

George A. Mensah, MD, FACC, FCP(SA) Hon
Director, Center for Translation Research and
Implementation Science, NIH/National Heart, Lung, and
Blood Institute, Acting Director, Division of Cardiovascular
Sciences, NIH/National Heart, Lung, and Blood Institute,
Bethesda, Maryland, United States

Ross Milner, MD, FACS
Professor of Surgery, Department of Surgery, Director,
Center for Aortic Diseases, Section of Vascular Surgery and
Endovascular Therapy, The University of Chicago, Chicago,
Illinois, United States

Jiangyong Min, MD PhD
Division of Stroke and Vascular Neurology, Mercy Health
Hauenstein Neurosciences, Grand Rapids, Michigan,
United States

Juan Eugenio Ochoa, MD, PhD
Researcher, Department of Cardiovascular, Neural and
Metabolic Sciences, S. Luca Hospital, IRCCS, Istituto
Auxologico Italiano, Milan, Italy

Takeyoshi Ota, MD, PhD
Associate Professor of Surgery, Department of Surgery;
Co-Director, Center for Aortic Diseases, Section of Cardiac
& Thoracic Surgery, The University of Chicago, Chicago,
Illinois, United States

Christian Ott, MD
Assistant Professor, Department of Nephrology and
Hypertension, Friedrich-Alexander University
Erlangen-Nürnberg, Erlangen, Germany

Gianfranco Parati, MD
Professor of Cardiovascular Medicine, Department of
Medicine and Surgery, University of Milano-Bicocca; Head,
Department of Cardiovascular, Neural and Metabolic
Sciences, S. Luca Hospital, IRCCS, Istituto Auxologico
Italiano, Milano, Italy

Carl J. Pepine, MD
Professor of Medicine, Division of Cardiovascular Medicine,
University of Florida College of Medicine, Gainesville, Florida,
United States

Vlado Perkovic, MBBS, PhD, FRACP, FASN
Executive Director, George Institute, University of Sydney,
Sydney, Australia

Tiina Podymow, BSc, MDCM
Associate Professor, Department of Nephrology, McGill
University, Montreal, Canada

Kazem Rahimi, FRCP, DM, MSc, FESC
Associate Professor of Cardiovascular Medicine, University
of Oxford; Deputy Director, The George Institute for Global
Health, James Martin Fellow in Healthcare Innovation, Oxford
Martin School; Honorary Consultant Cardiologist, Oxford
University Hospitals NHS Trust, The George Institute for
Global Health, Oxford Martin School, University of Oxford,
Oxford, United Kingdom

Luis Miguel Ruilope, MD, PhD
Chief of Hypertension and Cardiovascular Risk Group,
Institute of Research i+12, Hospital 12 de Octubre,
Madrid-28009; Professor of Public Health & Preventive
Medicine, Public Health, Universidad Autonoma, Madrid,
Spain

Gema Ruiz-Hurtado, PhD
Laboratory Head of Hypertension and Cardiovascular
Risk Group, Hypertension Unit, Institute of Research i+12,
Hypertension and Cardiovascular Risk Group, Hospital
Universitario 12 de Octubre, Madrid, Spain

Roland E. Schmieder, MD
Professor of Medicine, Department of Nephrology and
Hypertension, Friedrich-Alexander University
Erlangen-Nürnberg, Erlangen, Germany

Shigeru Shibata, MD, PhD
Associate Professor, Division of Nephrology, Department of
Internal Medicine, Teikyo University, School of Medicine;
Project Lecturer, Division of Clinical Epigenetics, Research
Center for Advanced Science and Technology, The University
of Tokyo, Tokyo, Japan

Steven M. Smith, PharmD, MPH, BCPS
Assistant Professor of Pharmacy and Medicine, Departments of Pharmacotherapy & Translational Research and Community Health & Family Medicine, Colleges of Pharmacy and Medicine, University of Florida, Gainesville, Florida, United States

Matthew J. Sorrentino, MD, FACC, FASH
Professor of Medicine, Section of Cardiology, University of Chicago Medicine, Chicago, Illinois, United States

George S. Stergiou, MD, FRCP
Professor of Medicine and Hypertension, Hypertension Center STRIDE-7, National and Kapodistrian University of Athens, Third Department of Medicine, Sotiria Hospital, Athens, Greece

Hillel Sternlicht, MD
Fellow in Hypertension, ASH Comprehensive Hypertension Center, The University of Chicago Medicine and Biological Sciences, Chicago, Illinois, United States

Patrick J. Strollo, Jr., MD, FACP, FCCP, FAASM
Professor of Medicine and Clinical and Translational Science; Chairman of Medicine VA Pittsburgh Health System; Vice Chair of Medicine for Veterans Affairs, University of Pittsburgh School of Medicine, Pittsburgh, Pennsylvania, United States

Sandra J. Taler, MD
Professor of Medicine, Division of Nephrology and Hypertension, Mayo Clinic, Rochester, Minnesota, United States

Akiko Tanaka, MD, PhD
Aortic Fellow, Department of Cardiothoracic and Vascular Surgery, The University of Texas, Austin, Texas, United States

Stephen C. Textor, MD
Professor of Medicine, Division of Nephrology and Hypertension, Mayo Clinic, Rochester, Minnesota, United States

Raymond R. Townsend, MD
Professor of Medicine, Perelman School of Medicine, University of Pennsylvania, Philadelphia, Pennsylvania, United States

Katherine R. Tuttle, MD, FASN, FACP
Executive Director for Research, Providence Health Care, Regional Principal Investigator and Clinical Professor of Medicine, Institute of Translational Health Sciences, University of Washington School of Medicine, Spokane, Washington, United States

Ji-Guang Wang, MD, PhD
Director, Centre for Epidemiological Studies and Clinical Trials; Professor, Shanghai Key Laboratory of Hypertension; Director, The Shanghai Institute of Hypertension; Director, Department of Hypertension; Professor, Ruijin Hospital; Professor, Shanghai Jiaotong University School of Medicine, Shanghai, China

Seamus P. Whelton, MD, MPH
Pollin Cardiology Fellow in Preventive Cardiology, Johns Hopkins University School of Medicine and Ciccarone Center for the Prevention of Heart Disease, Baltimore, Maryland, United States

William B. White, MD
Professor of Medicine and Division Chief, Division of Hypertension and Clinical Pharmacology, Calhoun Cardiology Center, University of Connecticut School of Medicine, Farmington, Connecticut, United States

Bryan Williams, MD
Department of Medicine, Institute of Cardiovascular Sciences, University College London, London, United Kingdom

Talya Wolak, MD
Head of Hypertension Services, Soroka University Medical Center, Faculty of Health Sciences, Ben-Gurion University of the Negev, Beer Sheva, Israel

Hala Yamout, MD
Department of Internal Medicine (Nephrology), Saint Louis University, John Cochran Division, Veterans Affairs St. Louis Health Care System, St. Louis, Missouri, United States

Clyde W. Yancy, MD, MSc, MACC, FAHA, MACP, FHFSA
Vice Dean, Diversity & Inclusion, Magerstadt Professor of Medicine, Professor of Medical Social Sciences; Chief, Division of Cardiology, Northwestern University, Feinberg School of Medicine; Associate Director, Bluhm Cardiovascular Institute, Northwestern Memorial Hospital; Deputy Editor, JAMA Cardiology, Chicago, Illinois, United States

William F. Young, Jr., MD, MSc
Tyson Family Endocrinology Clinical Professor, Professor of Medicine, Mayo Clinic College of Medicine, Division of Endocrinology, Diabetes, Metabolism, and Nutrition, Mayo Clinic, Rochester, Minnesota, United States

Salim Yusuf, DPhil, FRCPC, FRSC, OC
Professor of Medicine, McMaster University, Hamilton, Ontario, Canada; Executive Director, Population Health Research Institute, Hamilton Health Sciences & McMaster University, Hamilton, Ontario, Canada

Foreword

Hypertension has been recognized as an important cardiovascular disorder since the dawn of the 20th century, when Riva-Rocci and then Korotkoff described the sphygmomanometric method of measuring arterial pressure. Despite intense study since then, hypertension currently presents an extraordinary opportunity and challenge for investigators, teachers, health officials, and clinicians in the field. Hypertension has spread to the developing world and is reaching pandemic proportions. More inclusive definitions as well as more accurate and detailed measurements of blood pressure indicate that the prevalence and health threat of hypertension worldwide are even greater than previously thought.

The *Companions to Heart Disease: A Textbook of Cardiovascular Medicine* aim to provide cardiologists and trainees with important additional information in critically important segments of cardiology that go beyond what is contained in the "mother book," thereby creating an extensive cardiovascular information system. The first two editions of *Hypertension,* edited by Drs. Henry R. Black and William J. Elliott, clearly accomplished this goal.

Drs. George Bakris and Matthew Sorrentino have accepted the baton and have brilliantly edited the third edition. They have selected internationally recognized authorities as authors, who have summarized the important research carried out in the last 5 years. This edition also includes rigorous comparisons among the classes of antihypertensive drugs. The volume also presents revised practice guidelines that synthesize much useful information for clinical practice. This comprehensive book will be of great value and interest to clinicians, investigators, and trainees in this important subspecialty of cardiology.

Eugene Braunwald
Douglas P. Zipes
Peter Libby
Robert O. Bonow
Douglas L. Mann
Gordon F. Tomaselli

Preface

There have been many books published dealing with the topic of hypertension across a spectrum of diseases. However, it is rare to find one source that has an encyclopedic and timely spectrum of topics across the disease spectrum with a focus on hypertension. This third edition of *Hypertension* has expanded the topic variety from previous editions and presents novel topics of emerging areas of hypertension. Examples include a chapter dealing with hypertension as an immune disease with a pathophysiology based on immune changes relating to inflammation rather than hemodynamic changes. There is also a focused chapter dealing with sleep disorders, not just sleep apnea, as a major cause of hypertension. Lastly, there is a novel chapter on environmental pollution and its contribution to endothelial dysfunction. In addition to these new chapters, all other chapters have been consolidated and updated with the latest information sourced from basic science to clinical trials and guidelines so that information is applicable to the clinician.

Although there are now more than 125 different antihypertensive medications, blood pressure control rates around the world vary from as low as 15% in some Southeast Asian countries to over 50% in North America. Clearly, this does not relate to the price of medication but rather to individual patients, understanding, attitudes, and behaviors toward quelling a silent killer, hypertension. There are chapters in the book that address some of these issues, but the only real solution is a multipronged approach involving governmental policy makers, the pharmaceutical industry, payers, and the medical professionals. We hope you will find the book a valuable resource to address a spectrum of questions surrounding the disease of hypertension.

The book is divided into multiple parts including epidemiology, mechanisms of hypertension, pathophysiology of disease, pharmacology of antihypertensive drugs, clinical outcome trials, and guideline discussions focusing on process rather than what was produced.

ACKNOWLEDGMENTS

We would like to thank our families and our wives especially for being supportive through this editing and writing process. We are especially thankful to all the authors that contributed time and effort and produced excellent chapters for your reading knowledge and pleasure.

George L. Bakris, MD, FASN, FAHA, FASH
Matthew J. Sorrentino, MD, FACC, FASH

Contents

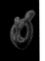

Contents

Braunwald's Heart Disease Family of Books

BRAUNWALD'S HEART DISEASE COMPANIONS

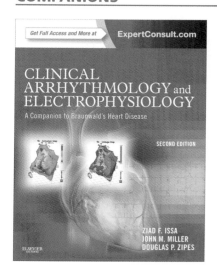

ISSA, MILLER, AND ZIPES
Clinical Arrhythmology and Electrophysiology

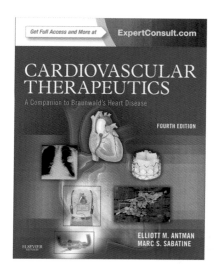

ANTMAN AND SABATINE
Cardiovascular Therapeutics

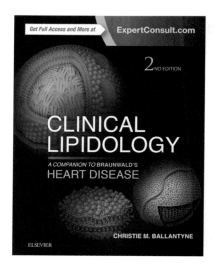

BALLANTYNE
Clinical Lipidology

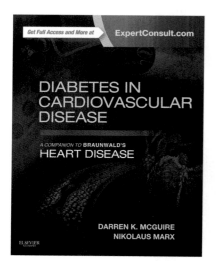

MCGUIRE AND MARX
Diabetes in Cardiovascular Disease

Braunwald's Heart Disease Family of Books

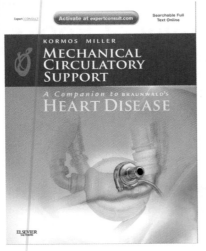

KORMOS AND MILLER
Mechanical Circulatory Support

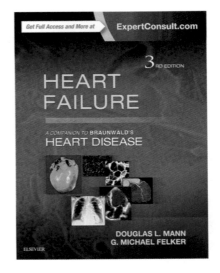

MANN AND FELKER
Heart Failure

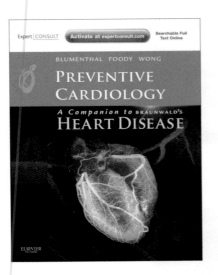

BLUMENTHAL, FOODY, AND WONG
Preventive Cardiology

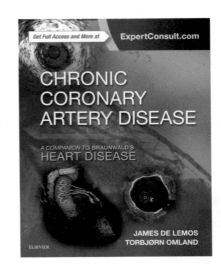

DE LEMOS AND OMLAND
Chronic Coronary Artery Disease

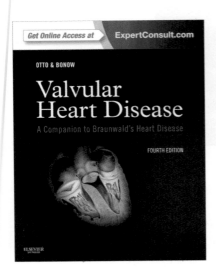

OTTO AND BONOW
Valvular Heart Disease

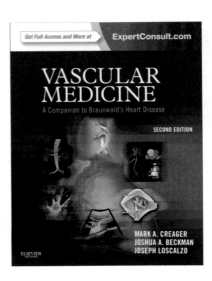

CREAGER, BECKMAN, AND LOSCALZO
Vascular Medicine

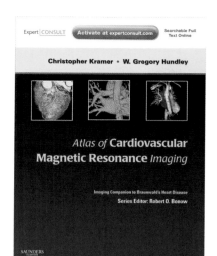

KRAMER AND HUNDLEY
Atlas of Cardiovascular Magnetic Resonance Imaging

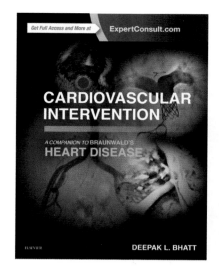

BHATT
Cardiovascular Intervention

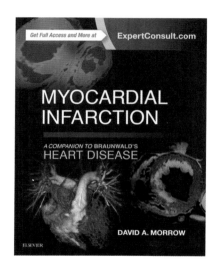

MORROW
Myocardial Infarction

BRAUNWALD'S HEART DISEASE REVIEW AND ASSESSMENT

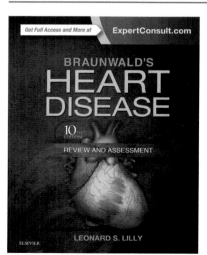

LILLY
Braunwald's Heart Disease Review and Assessment

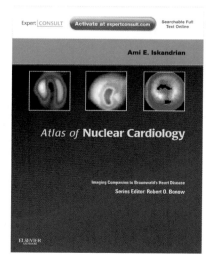

ISKANDRIAN AND GARCIA
Atlas of Nuclear Cardiology

BRAUNWALD'S HEART DISEASE IMAGING COMPANIONS

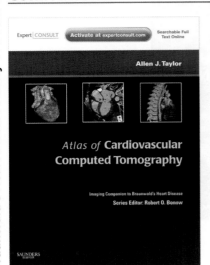

TAYLOR
Atlas of Cardiovascular Computer Tomography

COMING SOON!

SOLOMON
Essential Echocardiography

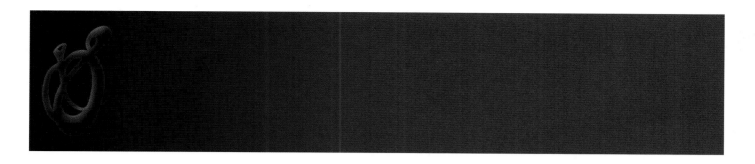

HYPERTENSION
A Companion to Braunwald's Heart Disease

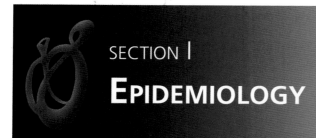

1

General Population and Global Cardiovascular Risk Prediction

Donald M. Lloyd-Jones

Systemic arterial hypertension is the condition of persistent, nonphysiologic elevation of systemic blood pressure (BP). It is typically defined as a resting systolic BP (SBP) 140 mm Hg or higher, or diastolic BP (DBP) 90 mm Hg or higher, or receiving therapy for the indication of BP-lowering.[1] Hypertension afflicts a substantial proportion of the adult population worldwide, and a growing number of children. Numerous genetic, environmental, and behavioral factors influence the development of hypertension. In turn, hypertension has been identified as one of the major causal risk factors for cardiovascular disease (CVD), including heart disease, peripheral vascular disease and stroke, as well as renal disease. An understanding of the basic epidemiology of hypertension is essential for effective public health and clinical efforts to prevent, detect, treat, and control this common condition.

EPIDEMIOLOGY AND RISK FACTORS

An epidemiologic association between a proposed risk factor and a disease is likely to be causal if it fulfills the following criteria: (1) exposure to the proposed risk factor precedes the onset of disease; (2) there is a strong association between exposure and incidence of disease; (3) the association is dose-dependent; (4) exposure is consistently predictive of disease in a variety of populations; (5) the association is independent of other risk factors; and (6) the association is biologically and pathogenetically plausible, and is supported by animal experiments and clinical investigation.[2] In addition, more definitive support for a causal association between a proposed risk factor and disease may arise from clinical trials in which intervention to modify or abolish the risk factor (by behavioral or therapeutic means) is associated with a decreased incidence of the disease. As discussed later, hypertension fulfills all of these criteria, and represents an important target for intervention in reducing the population and individual burden of CVD and renal disease.

PREVALENCE AND SECULAR TRENDS

Data from recent United States National Health and Nutrition Examination Surveys (NHANES) from 2011 to 2014 indicated that the prevalence of hypertension among adults 18 years of age and older in the U.S. was 29%, or nearly one in three adults, with 30% of men and 28.1% of women affected.[3] In the context of the entire population, approximately 80 million U.S. adults are estimated to have hypertension. Despite significant advances in our understanding of the risk factors, pathogenesis, and sequelae of hypertension, and multiple trials over the past 5 decades indicating the benefits of antihypertensive therapy, hypertension remains a significant public health problem. Although there were steady and significant reductions over the last 4 decades in population levels of BP and prevalence of hypertension in the U.S., recent data indicate a plateau in these favorable trends. Between the late 1970s and the mid-1990s, the prevalence of hypertension in the U.S. declined from about 32% to 25%.[4,5] However, more recent survey data indicate that there was an increase in prevalence between 1988 to 1994 and 1999 to 2002. The prevalence appears to have been stable from 1999 to 2014, however, at approximately 29%.[3,6] The current pandemic of obesity and aging of the population are likely to increase rates of hypertension substantially over the next decades.

Huffman et al examined trends in SBP levels in the U.S. from 1991 to 2008.[7] They observed that SBP levels declined in US adults during this time period. However, there were significant differences noted when stratified by age group in men and women. In the overall population, SBP declined significantly only in those older than 60 years of age, from an average of 139 to 133 mm Hg, whereas in younger and middle-aged individuals, SBP levels were essentially unchanged. Patterns were similar among untreated individuals, with untreated men over age 60 years experiencing an 11 mm Hg decline and women a 6 mm Hg decline in mean SBP from 1991 to 2008, and stable mean SBP in younger individuals. Among treated individuals, mean SBP levels declined from 1991 to 2008 in men and women of all age groups.[7]

African Americans, and especially African-American women, have a prevalence of hypertension that is among the highest in the world. Currently, it is estimated that 41.2% of non-Hispanic African-American adults have hypertension (including 40.8% of men and 41.5% of women), compared with

TABLE 1.1 Trends in Prevalence, Awareness, Treatment and Control of Hypertension in the United States, From the National Health and Nutrition Examination Surveys

	NHANES II 1976-1980	NHANES III 1988-1991	NHANES III 1991-1994	NHANES 1999-2000	NHANES 2007-2008	NHANES 2011-2012
Prevalence	31.8%	25.0%	24.5%	28.7%	29.6%	29.1%
Awareness	51%	73%	68%	69%	80.6%	82.7%
Treatment	31%	55%	54%	60%	73.7%	75.6%
Control to <140/ <90 mm Hg	10%	29%	27%	30%	48.4%	51.8%

NHANES, National Health and Nutrition Examination Surveys.

28% of non-Hispanic whites, 24.9% of non-Hispanic Asians, and 25.9% of Hispanic Americans.[3] Asian Americans and most other ethnic groups tend to have similar BP levels and hypertension prevalence as whites. Trends in the prevalence of hypertension have followed a similar pattern in all ethnicities from the 1990s to the present.[5] Prevalence rates are similar between men and women, but they increase dramatically with age, from 7.3 to 32.2 to 64.9% among those aged 18 to 39, 40 to 59 and 60 years or older, respectively.[3]

There have been substantial improvements in awareness, treatment, and control of hypertension over the last 2 decades, but the number of hypertensive individuals who are aware of their hypertension, receiving treatment, or treated and controlled remains well below optimal levels (Table 1.1). Data from NHANES 2011 to 2012 indicate that 82.7% of hypertensive individuals were aware of their elevated BP, 75.6% of them were receiving antihypertensive therapy, but only 51.8% had a BP of less than 140/90 mm Hg, the level considered to be "controlled" or at goal.[8] These data reflect a significant increase in treatment and control rates from approximately 60% and 30%, respectively, in 2000, to the current levels of treatment and control. Nonetheless, extrapolating these data to the current estimate of 80 million Americans with hypertension,[9] there are still over 38 million hypertensive individuals who are unaware of their diagnosis, aware but untreated, or treated but uncontrolled (Fig. 1.1).

Rates of awareness, treatment, and control of BP tend to differ by age, sex, and race/ethnicity. After years of relative stagnation, trends in awareness, treatment, and control have shown remarkable progress in the last decade among all age, sex, and race groups.[6] Overall, awareness of elevated BP increased significantly from 69.6% to 80.6% between 1999 and 2008, with women and non-Hispanic black adults being more likely to be aware, and Mexican Americans being the least likely to be aware of their hypertension.[6] Currently, women are somewhat more likely than men to be aware of their hypertension, to receive treatment with antihypertensive drug therapy, and to be at goal BP (Table 1.2). Individuals with hypertension aged 18 to 39 years are far less likely to be aware, treated, or controlled compared with middle-aged and older individuals. Compared with other race/ethnic groups, non-Hispanic Asians are significantly less likely to be aware of their hypertension or to have it treated, but control rates are similar across all race/ethnic groups (see Table 1.2).[8]

There is also substantial geographic variation in the epidemiology of hypertension in the U.S. Prevalence of hypertension is highest in the southeastern U.S., but so are awareness, treatment and control of hypertension. Areas of the southwestern U.S. in New Mexico, Colorado, and Texas have some of the lowest rates of awareness, treatment and control.[10]

Global Burden of Hypertension

International data indicate that hypertension is even more prevalent in other countries, including developed countries. Hypertension is also the leading single cause of global burden

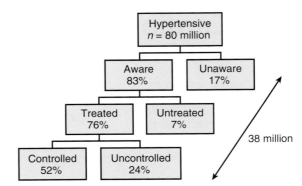

FIG. 1.1 Number and percentage of Americans who are aware of their hypertension, treated, and controlled to goal levels from the National Health and Nutrition Examination Surveys 2007-2008. *(Data from references 6, 8, 27)*

TABLE 1.2 Awareness, Treatment and Control of Hypertension in the United States, 2011-12, by Sex and Race/Ethnicity

	AWARENESS OF HYPERTENSION	PREVALENCE OF ANTIHYPERTENSIVE TREATMENT	CONTROL TO <140/ <90 MM HG
Men	80.2%	70.9%	49.3%
Women	85.4%	80.6%[a]	55.2%[a]
Age 18-39 years	61.8%	44.5%	34.4%
Age 40-59 years	83.0%[b]	73.7%[b]	57.8%[b]
Age ≥60 years	86.1%[b]	82.2%[b]	50.5%[b]
Non-Hispanic white	82.7%	76.7%	53.9%
Non-Hispanic black	85.7%	77.4%	49.5%
Non-Hispanic Asian	72.8%[c]	65.2%[c]	46.0%
Hispanic-American	82.2%	73.5%	46.5%

[a]Significantly different compared with men
[b]Significantly different compared with ages 18-39 years
[c]Significantly different compared with all other race/ethnic groups
Data from Nwankwo T, Yoon SS, Burt V, Gu Q. Hypertension among adults in the United States: National Health and Nutrition Examination Survey, 2011–2012. NCHS data brief, no 133. Hyattsville, MD: National Center for Health Statistics;2013.

of diseases.[11,12] Fig. 1.2 reveals the estimated proportion of deaths attributable to high systolic blood pressure by country across the globe. There is substantial variation globally and regionally, with the lowest proportion of deaths attributable to high systolic blood pressure in Chad, at 3.8%, and the highest in Georgia, at 40.4%.[13]

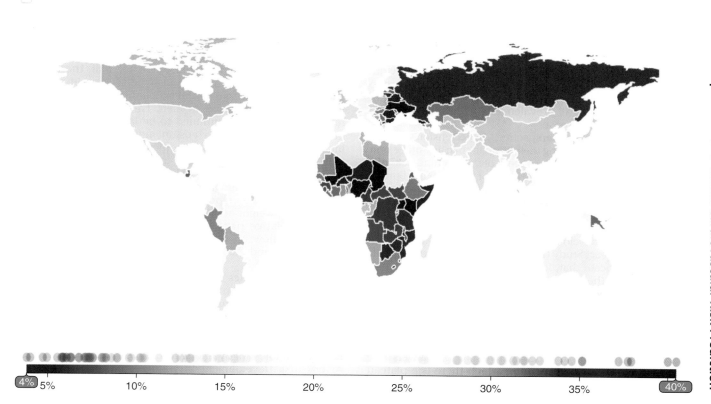

FIG. 1.2 Percentage of deaths attributable to high systolic blood pressure worldwide for both sexes and all ages. Global Burden of Diseases study 2013. *(Data from Institute for Health Metrics and Evaluation [IHME]. GBD Compare. Seattle, WA: IHME, University of Washington, 2015. Available from http://vizhub.healthdata.org/gbd-compare/. Accessed April 20, 2016.)*

Although data from low-income and middle-income countries around the world had been sparse, in recent years the scope and trends in the global burden of hypertension have become clearer. Danaei and colleagues[14] described the current levels and trends in SBP for adults 25 years and older in 199 countries using data from published and unpublished health examination surveys and epidemiologic studies including 5.4 million participants. In 2008, age-standardized mean SBP worldwide was 128.1 mm Hg in men and 124.4 mm Hg in women. The investigators estimated that between 1980 and 2008, global SBP decreased by 0.8 mm Hg per decade in men and 1.0 mm Hg per decade in women. There was significant regional variation in SBP trends over time. Female SBP decreased by 3.5 mm Hg or more per decade in Western Europe and Australasia. Male SBP fell most, by 2.8 mm Hg per decade in high-income North America. SBP rose in Oceania, East Africa, and South and Southeast Asia for both sexes, and in West Africa for women. Female SBP was highest in some East and West African countries, with means of 135 mm Hg or greater. Male SBP was highest in Baltic and East and West African countries, at 138 mm Hg or more. Men and women in Western Europe had the highest SBP in high-income regions. SBP is currently highest in low-income and middle-income countries overall, creating a substantial burden of disease in these countries.[14]

Surveys of the prevalence of hypertension indicate a growing global burden. Using data from the 1990s, the prevalence of hypertension in adults aged 35 to 74 years in Canada has generally been similar to that of the U.S. (at approximately 28%), and concurrent data from six European countries revealed an overall prevalence of 44%.[15] In Europe, clinical practice guidelines have typically recommended higher BP thresholds before initiation of drug therapy, causing even lower rates of treatment and control of BP.[14,16] Of the European countries studied, Italy had the lowest prevalence (38%), whereas Germany had the highest (55%).[15] The increase in BP and in prevalence of hypertension with age has been steeper in European countries compared with the U.S. and Canada. The correlation between hypertension prevalence and stroke mortality rates is very strong (r = 0.78), with a stroke mortality rate of 27.6 per 100,000 in North America and 41.2 per 100,000 in European countries.[15] Furthermore, treatment rates in Europe have been substantially lower, in association with higher BP thresholds for treatment in clinical practice guidelines promulgated in Europe and Canada until recently. Among 35- to 64-year-old hypertensives, over half (53%) were treated in the U.S., compared with 36% in Canada and 25% to 32% in European countries. The associated differences in levels of BP control were dramatic, with 66% of U.S., 49% of Canadian, and 23% to 38% of European hypertensives controlled to BP levels of less than 160/95 mm Hg, and 29%, 17%, and 10% or lower, respectively, controlled to levels of less than 140/90 mm Hg.[16]

RISK FACTORS FOR HYPERTENSION

Hypertension is a complex phenotype with multiple genetic and environmental risk factors, as well as important gene-environment interactions. Age, with its concomitant changes in the vasculature, and demographic and socioeconomic variables are among the strongest risk factors for hypertension.

Age

The prevalence of hypertension increases sharply with advancing age: although only 8.6% of men and 6.2% of women ages 20 to 34 years are affected, 76.4% of men and 79.9% of women aged 75 years and over have hypertension (Fig. 1.3).[9] Thus, in older patients, hypertension is by far the most prevalent risk factor for CVD. About 81% of hypertensive individuals in the U.S. are aged 45 years and older, although this group comprises only 46% of the U.S. population.[17] With the aging of the population, the overall prevalence of hypertension in the population is sure to increase.

Viewed from another perspective, hypertension already affects more individuals during their lifespan than any other trait or disease studied to date. The concept of the "lifetime risk" of a given disease provides a useful measure of the absolute burden and public health impact of a disease, as well as providing an average risk for an individual during his or her lifetime. Lifetime risk estimates account for the risk of developing disease during the remaining lifespan and the competing risk of death from other causes before developing the disease of interest. Data from the Framingham Heart Study (FHS), a longstanding study of CVD epidemiology, indicate that, for men and women free of hypertension at age 55, the remaining lifetime risks for development of hypertension through age 80 are 93% and 91%, respectively. In other words, more than 9 out of 10 older adults will develop hypertension before they die. Even those who reach age 65 free of hypertension still have a remaining lifetime risk of 90%.[18]

In Western societies, SBP tends to rise monotonically and inexorably with advancing age. Conversely, DBP levels rise until about age 50 to 55 years, after which there is a plateau for several years and then a steady decline to the end of the usual lifespan.[15,19,20] A variety of factors, particularly related to changes in arterial compliance and stiffness,[21,22] contribute to the development of systolic hypertension and to decreasing DBP with age. Both of these phenomena contribute to a marked increase in pulse pressure (PP), defined as SBP minus DBP, after age 50 years. Thus, hypertension, and particularly systolic hypertension, is a nearly universal condition of aging, and few individuals escape its development. Only in societies where salt intake is low, physical activity levels are very high, and obesity is rare, are age-related increases in SBP avoided.

Weight

Increasing weight is one of the major determinants of increasing BP. In recent NHANES surveys, the prevalence of hypertension among obese individuals, with a body mass index (BMI) 30 kg/m² or higher, is 42.5%, compared with 27.8% for overweight individuals (25 to 29.9 kg/m²), and 15.3% for individuals with BMI less than 25 kg/m².[23] Comparing NHANES 1988-1994 with NHANES 1999-2004, Cutler et al found an overall increase in the prevalence of hypertension by 13% in men and 24% in women. After adjustment for BMI, there was no statistically significant change in hypertension in men, indicating that the increase in BMI accounted for nearly all of the increase in hypertension in men. For women, after adjustment for BMI, there continued to be large relative increases in the prevalence of hypertension, indicating that some of the increases in hypertension in women were attributable to factors other than their increases in BMI in the recent NHANES period.

Data from Framingham also reveal marked increases in risk for development of hypertension with higher BMI. Compared with normal weight adult men and women, the multivariable-adjusted relative risks for development of hypertension in long-term follow up were 1.48 and 1.70 for overweight men and women, and 2.23 and 2.63 for obese men and women, respectively.[24]

Numerous studies have also demonstrated the important role of weight gain in BP elevation and weight reduction in BP lowering. As discussed above, SBP and DBP tend to rise with age beginning at around age 25 years in most adults.[19,20] However, recent data indicate that these "age-related" increases in SBP and DBP may be avoided in young adults who maintain stable BMI over long-term follow up. In the Coronary Artery Risk Development In young Adults (CARDIA) study, those who maintained a stable BMI at all six examinations over 15 years had no significant changes in either SBP or DBP, whereas those who had an increase in their BMI of 2 kg/m² or more had substantial increases in BP.[25]

The influence of weight gain on BP, and the benefits of maintaining stable weight or losing weight extend down even to young children. One large birth cohort study of children examined BMI at ages 5 and 14 and the association with SBP and DBP at age 14. Children who were overweight at age 5 but had normal BMI at age 14 had similar mean systolic and diastolic BP to those who had a normal BMI at both time points. Conversely, children who were overweight at both ages, or who had a normal BMI at age 5 and were overweight at age 14, had higher systolic and diastolic BP at age 14 than those who had a normal BMI at both ages, even after adjustment for potential confounders.[26]

Other Risk Factors

As discussed above, sex influences the prevalence of hypertension in an age-dependent fashion. Until about the sixth decade of life, men have a higher prevalence, after which women predominate increasingly (Fig. 1.3). Overall, more women than men are affected by hypertension, in part because of their longer life expectancy.

Race/ethnicity has also been shown to be significantly associated with hypertension. Although non-Hispanic white persons make up about two-thirds of the U.S. adult hypertensive population, this is consistent with their representation in the overall population. African Americans are disproportionately affected, and have among the highest rates of hypertension in the world, with mean systolic BP levels approximately 5 mm Hg higher than whites, and prevalence rates at least 10% higher than whites.[27,28] Other racial/ethnic groups in the U.S., including Hispanic Americans, have a prevalence of hypertension similar to whites.[17,19,27-29] Education status also influences rates of hypertension, with lower education levels being strongly associated with hypertension. However, much of this inverse association of education with BP appears to be explained by differences in

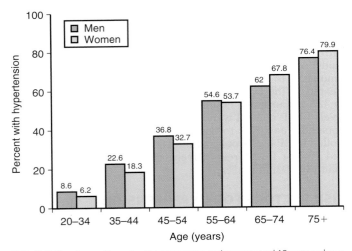

FIG. 1.3 Prevalence of hypertension among men and women aged 18 years and over, from National Health and Nutrition Examination Surveys 2005-2008. (Data from Mozaffarian D, Benjamin EJ, Go AS, et al. Heart disease and stroke statistics—2016 update: A report from the American Heart Association. Circulation. 2016;133:e38-60.)

diet and in BMI between less educated and more educated individuals.[30]

Among dietary influences on BP level, high dietary sodium intake has consistently been related to rates of hypertension in numerous populations and cohort studies. Conversely, higher potassium, calcium, and magnesium intakes appear to be associated with lower rates of hypertension in various populations.[31] Patients with omnivorous diets have higher BP levels than those who are vegetarian, but the types of dietary fat do not appear to influence BP levels directly (with the possible exception of mild lowering by omega-3 fatty acids). The evidence linking heavy alcohol intake to hypertension is unequivocal. More than 50 epidemiologic studies have demonstrated an association between intake of 3 or more drinks per day and hypertension, although regular alcohol intake is associated with a lower risk of atherothrombotic CVD events.

Genetic Factors

Numerous studies have examined potential genetic susceptibilities for hypertension. Data consistently indicate that BP levels are heritable. Using data from the multigenerational FHS cohorts, Levy et al estimated that heritability for single-examination measures were 0.42 for SBP and 0.39 for DBP. Using data from multiple examinations, long-term systolic and diastolic BP phenotypes had high heritability estimates, at 0.57 and 0.56, respectively.[32]

The availability of high-throughput technology has recently allowed for genome-wide association studies to be performed in large pooled cohorts to assess for linkage between identified areas of the genome and BP levels. A large consortium of studies[33] tested 2.5 million genotyped and imputed single-nucleotide polymorphisms (SNPs) across the genome for association with systolic and diastolic BP levels in 34,433 subjects of European ancestry and followed up findings with direct genotyping in 71,225 participants of European ancestry and 12,889 of Indian Asian ancestry. They also performed *in silico* comparison in another large consortium ($n = 29,136$). This group identified associations between systolic or diastolic BP and common variants in eight genomic regions near a number of potential genes of interest: *CYP17A1* ($p = 7 \times 10^{-24}$), *CYP1A2* ($p = 1 \times 10^{-23}$), *FGF5* ($p = 1 \times 10^{-21}$), *SH2B3* ($p = 3 \times 10^{-18}$), *MTHFR* ($p = 2 \times 10^{-13}$), *c10orf107* ($p = 1 \times 10^{-9}$), *ZNF652* ($p = 5 \times 10^{-9}$) and *PLCD3* ($p = 1 \times 10^{-8}$) genes. All variants associated with continuous BP were associated with the phenotype of dichotomous hypertension as well. The authors concluded that these associations between common variants and BP and hypertension could offer mechanistic insights into the regulation of BP and may point to novel targets for interventions to prevent cardiovascular disease.[33]

Updates to these genome-wide association studies continue to appear with the addition of more cohorts and refined genotyping methods.[34] To date, more than 60 loci (many in novel or unexpected genes) have now been associated with blood pressure phenotypes or the diagnosis of hypertension, with similarities noted in diverse race/ethnic groups.[34] Similarly, rare inherited genetic syndromes are associated with hypertension, including Liddle syndrome and 11β-hydroxylase and 17α-hydroxylase deficiencies. However, because hypertension is a complex phenotype, and BP levels are determined by the complex interactions of multiple neurologic, renal, endocrinologic, cardiac and vascular processes, as well as environmental and behavioral factors, there have not been any single-gene polymorphisms discovered that explain more than a small fraction of hypertension alone or jointly in the population at large. The study of rare and low-frequency genetic polymorphisms, gene-gene interactions, gene-environment interactions and epigenetics is likely to lead to novel insights on blood pressure regulation, and may provide potential future targets for prevention or treatment of hypertension.

CLASSIFICATION OF BLOOD PRESSURE

Formal classification of BP stages by consensus panels began to take shape in the early 1970s with the first National Conference on High Blood Pressure Education. The first report of the Joint National Committee (JNC) was published in 1977 and has been followed by six subsequent reports in 1980, 1984, 1988, 1993, 1997, and 2003. The seventh report (JNC 7, published in 2003)[1,35] was the clinical standard for the prevention, detection, evaluation and treatment of hypertension in the U.S. until recently. Current U.S. and international guidelines still use the same classification system. JNC 7 recognized several important concepts that have evolved in our understanding of hypertension over the past decades. First, systolic hypertension confers at least as much, and usually greater, risk for adverse events as diastolic hypertension, which was not fully appreciated in the first four JNC reports. Thus, the JNC report recommends that for middle-aged and older hypertensives (who represent the vast majority of hypertensives in the population), SBP should be the primary target for staging of BP and initiation of therapy. Second, hypertension rarely occurs in isolation, and is usually present in the context of one or more other CVD risk factors. Therefore, in recommending treatment for hypertension, the JNC 7 report recommended some consideration of global risk for CVD.

It has long been recognized that BP confers risk for CVD beginning at levels well within the clinically "normal" range, with risk increasing in a continuous, graded fashion to the highest levels, as discussed in detail later. Thus, although clinical practice guidelines impose certain thresholds for considering individuals to be hypertensive, and for initiation of therapy, this conception is an artificial construct designed to assist clinicians and patients with treatment decisions.

The current scheme for classifying BP stages is shown in Table 1.3. Although BP lower than 120/80 had previously been termed "optimal," it is now termed "normal." A category of "prehypertension" is defined, including individuals with untreated SBP 120 to 139 or DBP of 80 to 89 mm Hg. The prior classification of Stage 3 hypertension was dropped because of its relatively uncommon occurrence, and all individuals with SBP 160 mm Hg or higher or DBP 100 mm Hg or higher are now classified as having Stage 2 hypertension.[1]

Individuals are classified into their BP stages on the basis of both systolic and diastolic BP levels. When a disparity exists between SBP and DBP stages, patients are classified into the higher stage. Several studies[36-38] have examined this phenomenon of "upstaging" based on disparate systolic and diastolic BP levels. In one study,[36] 64.6% of subjects had congruent stages of systolic and diastolic BP, 31.6% were upstaged on the basis of SBP, and only 3.8% on the basis of DBP. Thus, among

TABLE 1.3 **Blood Pressure Staging System of the Seventh Report of the Joint National Committee on Prevention, Detection, Evaluation, and Treatment of High Blood Pressure**

JNC 7 BLOOD PRESSURE STAGE	BLOOD PRESSURE RANGE
Normal	Untreated SBP <120 *and* DBP <80 mm Hg
Prehypertension	Untreated SBP 120-139 *or* DBP 80-89 mm Hg
Stage 1 hypertension	SBP 140-159 *or* DBP 90-99 mm Hg
Stage 2 hypertension	SBP ≥160 *or* DBP ≥100 mm Hg

DBP, Diastolic blood pressure; *JNC,* Joint National Committee; *SBP,* systolic blood pressure.
Reused with permission from Chobanian AV, Bakris GL, Black HR, et al. Seventh Report of the Joint National Committee on Prevention, Detection, Evaluation, and Treatment of High Blood Pressure. Hypertension. 2003;42:1206-1252.

all participants, 96% were correctly classified by knowledge of their SBP alone, whereas only 68% were correctly classified by knowledge of the DBP alone. Thus, SBP elevation out of proportion to DBP is common in middle-aged and older persons, and SBP appears to play a greater role in the determination of BP stage and eligibility for therapy.[36] Among younger individuals, upstaging because of DBP is somewhat more common. However, after the age of 50 years, which includes the vast majority of hypertensives, upstaging because of SBP clearly occurs for an overwhelming proportion of the population and determines hypertensive status and/or eligibility for therapy.[38]

Isolated systolic hypertension in older people reflects progressive large artery stiffening seen with aging. In younger hypertensive patients, isolated diastolic hypertension (SBP <140 and DBP ≥90 mm Hg) and systolic-diastolic hypertension (SBP ≥140 and DBP ≥90 mm Hg) tend to predominate, whereas beyond age 50, isolated systolic hypertension (ISH, SBP ≥140 and DBP <90 mm Hg) predominates. ISH is the most common form of hypertension over age 60, being present in more than 80% of untreated hypertensive men and women.[38]

These observations, coupled with data on risks of systolic hypertension and the benefits of treating systolic hypertension, prompted the National High Blood Pressure Education Program's Advisory Panel to recommend a major paradigm shift in 2000 in urging that SBP become the major criterion for the diagnosis, staging, and therapeutic management of hypertension, particularly in middle-aged and older Americans.[22] This recommendation was incorporated into the staging system and treatment guidelines for JNC 7 and subsequent guidelines.[1,35]

SEQUELAE AND OUTCOMES WITH HYPERTENSION

Hypertension is a major risk factor for atherosclerotic CVD (ASCVD), and almost all other manifestations of CVD. Higher BP levels generally increase risk in a continuous and graded fashion for total mortality, CVD mortality, coronary heart disease (CHD) mortality, myocardial infarction (MI), heart failure (HF), left ventricular hypertrophy (LVH), atrial fibrillation, stroke/transient ischemic attack, peripheral vascular disease, and renal failure. For many of these endpoints, there is effect modification by sex, with male hypertensives being at higher absolute risk for CVD events than female hypertensives (HF being a notable exception). There is also substantial effect modification by age, with older hypertensives being at similar relative risk but at much greater absolute risk than younger ones.[39] As discussed later, hypertension rarely occurs in isolation, and it confers increased risk for CVD across the spectrum of overall risk factor burden, but with increasing importance in the setting of other risk factors.[40]

Absolute levels of risk for ASCVD increase substantially with increasing risk factor burden, and are augmented still further by elevations in BP (Fig. 1.4). As shown by the arrows in Fig. 1.4, the slope of increasing ASCVD risk is greater with increasing BP levels when the burden of other risk factors is greater. Thus, BP levels, and the risk they confer, must always be considered in the context of other risk factors and the patient's global risk for ASCVD. For example, because the combination of hypertension and diabetes (DM) is particularly dangerous, JNC 7 recommended lower goal BP levels for patients with DM (<130/<80 mm Hg) than for those without DM (<140/<90 mm Hg).[1]

Individuals with hypertension have a two-fold to three-fold increased relative risk for CVD events compared with age-matched normotensives. Hypertension increases relative risks for all manifestations of CVD, but its *relative* impact is greatest for stroke and HF (Fig. 1.5). Because CHD incidence is greater than incidence of stroke and HF, however, the *absolute* impact of hypertension on CHD is greater than for other manifestations of CVD, as demonstrated by the excess risks shown in Fig. 1.5.

To illustrate the importance of hypertension as a risk factor, let us consider the case of HF. Between 75% and 91% of individuals who develop HF have antecedent hypertension.[41,42] In a study from the FHS, hypertension conferred a hazard ratio for the development of HF of approximately 2 for men and 3 for women over the ensuing 18 years.[42] As shown in Fig. 1.6, the hazard ratios for HF associated with hypertension (2 to 3) were far lower than the hazard ratios for HF associated with MI, which were greater than 6 for both men and women. However, the population prevalence of hypertension was 60%, compared with approximately 6% for myocardial infarction. Therefore, the population-attributable risk (PAR) of HF, that is, the fraction of HF in this population that was because of hypertension, was 59% in women and 39% in men. The PARs for MI were 13% and 34% for women and men, respectively.[42]

Investigators from the comprehensive Olmsted County cohort in Minnesota have also estimated PARs for various HF risk factors. In that study, the relative risks for HF were again high for CHD and DM, with odds ratios of 3.05 and 2.65, respectively, whereas the odds ratio associated with hypertension was 1.44. However, hypertension was prevalent in two-thirds of the cohort. The PAR was highest for CHD and hypertension; each accounted for 20% of (HF) cases in the population overall, although CHD accounted for the greatest proportion of cases in men (PAR 23% for CHD versus 13% for hypertension) and hypertension was of greatest importance in women (PAR 28% for hypertension versus 6% for CHD).[43]

Importance of Systolic Blood Pressure

It has been recognized for 4 decades that elevated SBP confers at least as great, and, in most groups studied, substantially greater risk for CVD as an elevated DBP.[44] However, translation of this knowledge into clinical guidelines and clinical practice was slow to evolve. In numerous studies, increasing SBP has consistently been associated with higher risk for adverse events than increasing DBP, whether these BP variables are considered separately or together, and whether they are treated as linear covariates or in quintiles, deciles, or JNC stages. For example, in the Cardiovascular Health Study of older Americans (Table 1.4), a one standard deviation increment in SBP was associated with higher adjusted risk for CHD and stroke than was a one standard deviation increment in DBP (or PP). In models with SBP and DBP together or SBP and PP together, SBP consistently dominated as the greater risk factor.[45] When men who were screened for inclusion in the Multiple Risk Factor Intervention Trial (MRFIT) were stratified into quintiles of SBP or DBP, risks for each SBP quintile were the same or higher than for the corresponding quintile of DBP (Fig. 1.7A).[46] Similar findings were observed when MRFIT screenees were stratified into deciles of SBP and DBP; at every level, SBP was consistently associated with higher risk for CHD mortality than the corresponding decile of DBP (Fig. 1.7B).[47] Finally, when men were stratified by JNC level of SBP and DBP, SBP was associated with greater risk for CHD mortality than DBP in each JNC BP stage.[47]

In fact, when DBP is considered in the context of the SBP level, an inverse association for DBP and CHD risk has been observed. Franklin et al demonstrated that, at any specified level of SBP, relative risks for CHD decreased with increasing

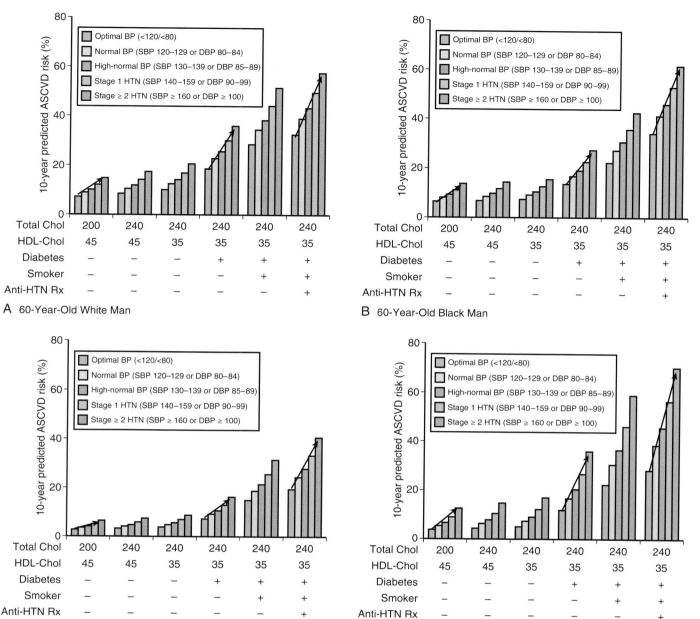

FIG. 1.4 Predicted 10-year risk for atherosclerotic cardiovascular disease by increasing burden of risk factors and systolic blood pressure, in a 60-year-old white man (Panel **A**), African-American man (Panel **B**), white woman (Panel **C**), and African-American woman (Panel **D**), based on the Pooled Cohort Equations.[66] *ASCVD,* Atherosclerotic cardiovascular disease; *BP,* blood pressure; *DBP,* diastolic blood pressure; *HDL-Chol,* high-density lipoprotein cholesterol; *HTN,* hypertension; *SBP,* systolic blood pressure.

DBP. For example, at an SBP of 150 mm Hg, the estimated hazards ratio for CHD was 1.8 if the DBP was 70 mm Hg, but only approximately 1.3 if the DBP was 95 mm Hg. The higher the SBP level, the steeper the decline in CHD risk with increasing DBP.[48] These data provide some compelling evidence for the importance of PP as a measure of risk, because PP represents the difference between SBP and DBP, and higher risk was observed in this study when the PP widened.[48] Pulse pressure will be discussed in greater detail later.

The increased risks associated with SBP are clear. When it is also appreciated that systolic hypertension out of proportion to diastolic elevation is by far the most common form of hypertension, as discussed earlier, it becomes clear that

the PAR for CVD conferred by SBP vastly outweighs the PAR for DBP. Finally, lack of control to goal BP in the community appears to be overwhelmingly because of lack of SBP control to less than 140 mm Hg.[38,49,50]

In national samples, significant cross-sectional predictors of lack of BP control among those who are aware of their hypertension include age 65 years or older, male sex, and no visits to a physician in the preceding 12 months.[50] Age and the presence of LVH likely represent higher initial SBP before initiation of therapy and longer duration of hypertension, both of which can contribute to greater difficulty in achieving lower BP levels. In addition, it appears likely that clinicians are reluctant to treat older hypertensive individuals to lower BP goals,

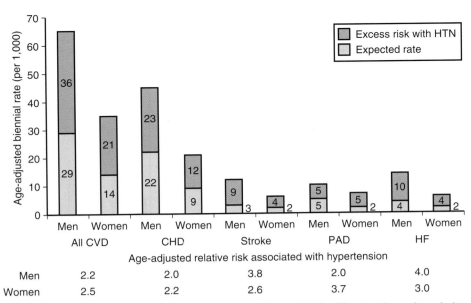

FIG. 1.5 Age-adjusted biennial rates, relative risks and absolute excess risks associated with hypertension for different cardiovascular endpoints: Framingham Study, 36-Year follow-up, persons aged 35-64 years. *CVD,* Cardiovascular disease; *CHD,* coronary heart disease; *HF,* heart failure; *HTN,* hypertension; *PAD,* peripheral arterial disease.

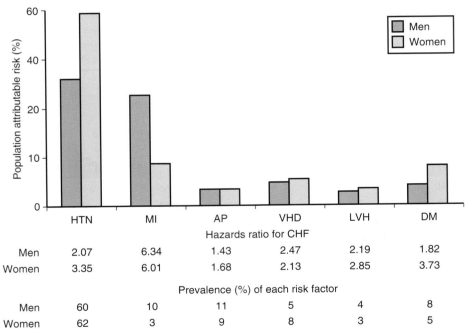

FIG. 1.6 Hazards ratios for congestive heart failure associated with selected risk factors, prevalence of each risk factor, and population-attributable risk for each factor in congestive heart failure. *AP,* Angina pectoris; *DM,* diabetes mellitus; *HTN,* hypertension; *LVH,* electrocardiographic left ventricular hypertrophy; *MI,* myocardial infarction; *VHD,* valvular heart disease. (*Data from Levy D, Larson MG, Vasan RS, Kannel WB, Ho KK. The progression from hypertension to congestive heart failure. JAMA. 1996;275:1557-1562.*)

TABLE 1.4 **Risks for Cardiovascular Disease Associated With Different Components of Blood Pressure in the Cardiovascular Health Study**

	1 STANDARD DEVIATION	ADJUSTED HAZARDS RATIO (95% CI)	
		Myocardial Infarction	**Stroke**
Systolic Blood Pressure	21.4 mm Hg	1.24 (1.15-1.35)	1.34 (1.21-1.47)
Diastolic Blood Pressure	11.2 mm Hg	1.13 (1.04-1.22)	1.29 (1.17-1.42)
Pulse Pressure	18.5 mm Hg	1.21 (1.12-1.31)	1.21 (1.10-1.34)

CI, Confidence interval.
Data from Psaty BM, Furberg CD, Kuller LH, et al. Association between blood pressure level and the risk of myocardial infarction, stroke, and total mortality. Arch Intern Med. 2001;161:1183-1192.

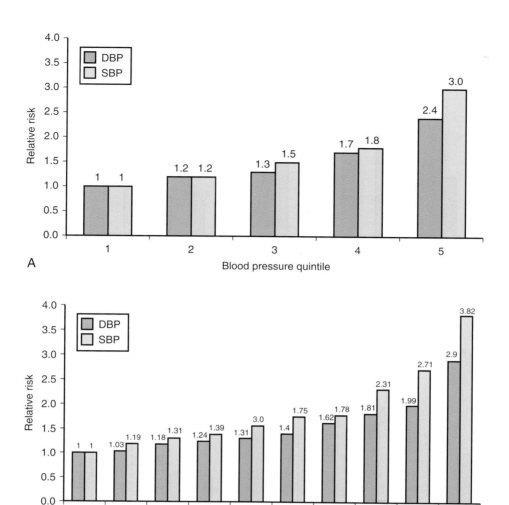

FIG. 1.7 Relative risks for coronary heart disease mortality among men screened for the Multiple Risk Factor Intervention Trial, by quintiles (Panel **A**) or deciles (Panel **B**) of systolic and diastolic blood pressure. *DBP*, Diastolic blood pressure; *SBP*, systolic blood pressure.

perhaps as a result of concerns over orthostasis and risk for falls, polypharmacy, or the controversial observation that there may be an increase in CVD events and mortality among the oldest hypertensives when DBP is lowered below 60 or 65 mm Hg (the J-shaped curve phenomenon).[51]

ISH has been clearly demonstrated as a risk factor for adverse CVD outcomes in older individuals, but there has been some debate as to its importance in younger adults, in whom it was felt to represent measurement artifact or labile blood pressure without significant consequences. Yano et al[52] recently examined 31-year follow up of 27,000 men and women aged 18 to 49 years in the Chicago Heart Association Detection Project in Industry. They observed that, compared with those who had normal BP levels, men with ISH had significant 23% and 28% higher hazards for CVD and CHD mortality. In women with ISH, hazard ratios were 1.55 (95% confidence interval 1.18 to 2.05) and 2.12 (1.49 to 3.01), respectively.[52] These data may cause guidelines to change their approach to ISH in the young.

Risk Across the Spectrum of Blood Pressure and the Importance of Stage 1 Hypertension

As noted above, increasing BP is associated with increasing risks for CVD, beginning at levels well within the so-called "normal" range. The Prospective Studies Collaboration, a pooling study of around 1,000,000 men and women in a number of large epidemiologic cohorts, and including data on more than 56,000 decedents, demonstrated that risks for CVD death increase steadily beginning at least at levels as low as an SBP of 115 mm Hg and DBP of 75 mm Hg. When considered in isolation, for each 20 mm Hg higher SBP and each 10 mm Hg higher DBP, there is approximately a doubling of risk for stroke death and ischemic heart disease death for both men and women.[39]

Similarly, the large data set of more than 347,000 men aged 35 to 57 years screened for the MRFIT provides a precise estimate of incremental CVD risk beginning at lower BPs. The data from the MRFIT screenees, shown in Fig. 1.8A, confirm a continuous, graded influence of SBP on multivariable-adjusted relative risk for CHD mortality beginning at BP levels well below 140 mm Hg.[53] Men with SBP of 150 to 159 mm Hg have over three times the risk and men with SBP greater than 180 mm Hg nearly six times the risk of men with SBP less than 100 mm Hg. These data also make an important point about BP levels in the population at which the majority of CVD events occur. In Fig. 1.8B, the numbers above each bar indicate the number of men in that stratum of SBP at baseline. Taking into account the number of men in each stratum and the expected rates of CHD death, the CHD death rates observed in the MRFIT screenee cohort indicate excess CHD deaths occurring at the rates indicated by the line in Fig. 1.8C. The proportion of excess CHD deaths by SBP stratum is indicated in Fig. 1.8D. As shown, nearly two-thirds of excess CHD deaths occurred in

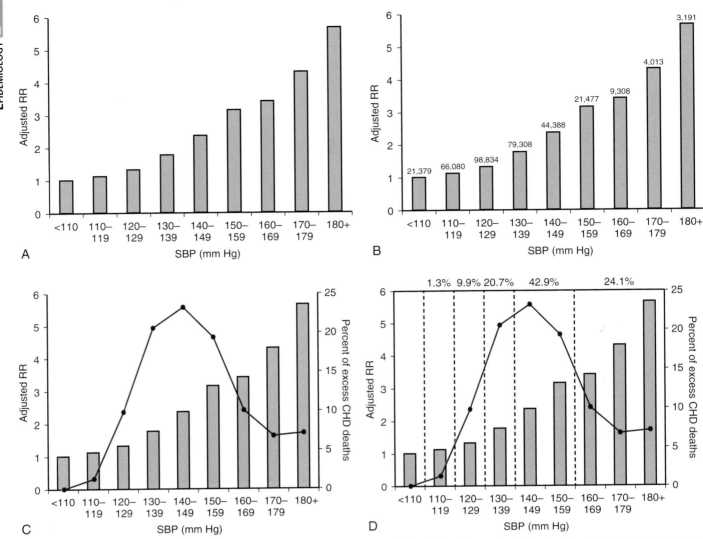

FIG. 1.8 Relative risks for coronary heart disease (CHD) mortality among screenees for the Multiple Risk Factor Intervention Trial by level of systolic blood pressure (SBP; Panel **A**), with: number of men in each stratum of SBP (Panel **B**); distribution of excess CHD deaths by SBP stratum (Panel **C**); and distribution of excess CHD deaths by Joint National Committee stage (Panel **D**).

men with SBP between 130 and 159 mm Hg, relatively "mild" levels of elevated BP. These findings were recently replicated in the more contemporary Framingham and Atherosclerosis Risk in Communities cohorts.[54]

Data from the FHS also indicate that the risk associated with BPs in the range of 130 to 139 mm Hg systolic or 85 to 89 mm Hg diastolic are substantial, despite the fact that these levels are not classified as "hypertension." These levels of BP are associated with significantly elevated multivariable-adjusted relative risks for CVD of 2.5 in women and 1.6 in men.[55] Likewise, individuals with SBP between 120 and 139 mm Hg or DBP between 80 and 89 mm Hg have a high likelihood of progressing to definite hypertension over the next 4 years, especially if they are age 65 or older.[56]

Pulse Pressure and Risks for Cardiovascular Disease

Pulse pressure is defined as the systolic minus the diastolic BP. In recent years there has been intense interest in PP as a risk factor for CVD. However, various investigators have struggled with how best to "anchor" the PP. For example, a patient with a BP of 120/60 has the same PP (60 mm Hg) as a patient with a BP of 150/90, although the latter patient is clearly at higher risk for adverse events. Different investigators have anchored the PP to

the DBP, the mean arterial pressure, and the SBP. As discussed earlier, Franklin et al demonstrated that increasing PP was associated with marked increases in hazard of CHD for subjects with the same SBP.[48] Chae et al also found that PP was an independent predictor of HF in an elderly cohort, even after adjustment for mean arterial pressure, prevalent CHD, and other HF risk factors.[57] In another study, Haider and colleagues observed that SBP and PP conferred similar risk for HF.[58] However, other studies have found that SBP confers greater risk than PP, when SBP and PP are considered separately or as covariates in the same multivariable model.[45] The aforementioned Prospective Studies Collaboration, which pooled data from 61 large epidemiologic studies and around 1,000,000 men and women, found that the best measure of BP for prediction of CVD events was the mean of SBP and DBP, which predicted better than SBP or DBP alone, and much better than the PP.[39] The recommendation of JNC 7 was that clinical focus should remain on the SBP in determining need for therapy and achieving goal BP.[1]

Mosley and colleagues compared the predictive utility of PP and other BP measures for diverse CVD outcomes (including hospitalizations and mortality from stroke, MI and HF) using long-term follow-up data from the Chicago Heart Association Detection Project in Industry.[59] Baseline BP measures were assessed for predictive utility for fatal and nonfatal events over 33 years. Among 36,314 participants, who were a mean age of 39 years, 43.4% were women. In univariate analyses, hazards ratios for stroke death per one standard deviation of PP, SBP, and DBP, respectively, were 1.49, 1.75, and 1.71. Multiple metrics all indicated better predictive utility for SBP and DBP compared with PP. Results for CHD or HF death, and stroke, MI, or HF hospitalization outcomes were similar. PP had weaker predictive utility at all ages, but particularly for those younger than 50 years of age. Overall then, in this large cohort study, PP had predictive utility for CV events that was inferior to SBP or DBP. These findings tend to support the approach of current guidelines in the use of SBP and DBP to assess risk and the need for treatment.[59]

Renal Disease

Hypertension is also a major risk factor for renal disease. Of the estimated 93,000 cases of incident end-stage renal disease (ESRD) diagnosed annually, it is estimated that over 25% are because of hypertension, and more than 40% because of DM.[60] However, these numbers may substantially underestimate the contribution of BP to the increasing incidence of renal disease, because these data provide only a single diagnostic cause, and hypertension is present in the vast majority of those with DM. African Americans have approximately four times the risk of whites of developing ESRD, in part because of their significantly higher prevalence of hypertension.[41] In addition to its contribution to ESRD, elevated BP also occurs in and exacerbates milder forms of chronic kidney disease and worsens proteinuria.

Cognitive Function

An association between higher baseline BP levels, typically measured at a single time point, and lower cognitive function has been well established.[61] Nontraditional components of BP, such as the variability in BP from visit-to-visit (so-called long-term BP variability) have also been associated with cognitive function in older individuals. However, long-term BP variability throughout young adulthood to middle age has only recently been examined as a potential predictor of cognitive function in middle age. Investigators from the CARDIA study examined BP variability in 2326 participants across eight serial examinations over 25 years and the association with cognitive function at an average age of 50 years. Long-term BP variability over 25 years beginning in young adulthood was associated with worse psychomotor speed and verbal memory tests in midlife, independent of cumulative exposure to BP during follow up.[61] In a parallel study, the investigators used data from ambulatory blood pressure monitoring performed at an average age of 35 years and linked it to the same cognitive function testing in midlife.[62] In this analysis, less nocturnal SBP dipping and higher nocturnal diastolic BP levels were associated with lower executive function in midlife, independent of multiple measures of office BP during long-term follow up. Nocturnal BP was not associated with psychomotor speed and verbal memory, suggesting that different aspects of BP exposure over the lifespan may affect regions of the brain differentially.[62]

Competing Outcomes With Hypertension

Individuals with hypertension are at risk for multiple potential outcomes simultaneously, including non-CVD death, CHD, stroke, HF, and other causes of CVD death. Traditional survival analysis methods typically only evaluate each of these outcomes independently, without understanding their joint probabilities of occurring. A recent analysis used novel methodology to explore these competing risks among all FHS subjects who had new-onset hypertension and were initially free of CVD. There were 645 men and 702 women with new-onset hypertension (mean age 57 years). Compared with matched nonhypertensive controls, subjects with new-onset hypertension were significantly more likely to experience a CVD event first rather than non-CVD death. Among new-onset hypertensives, the 12-year competing

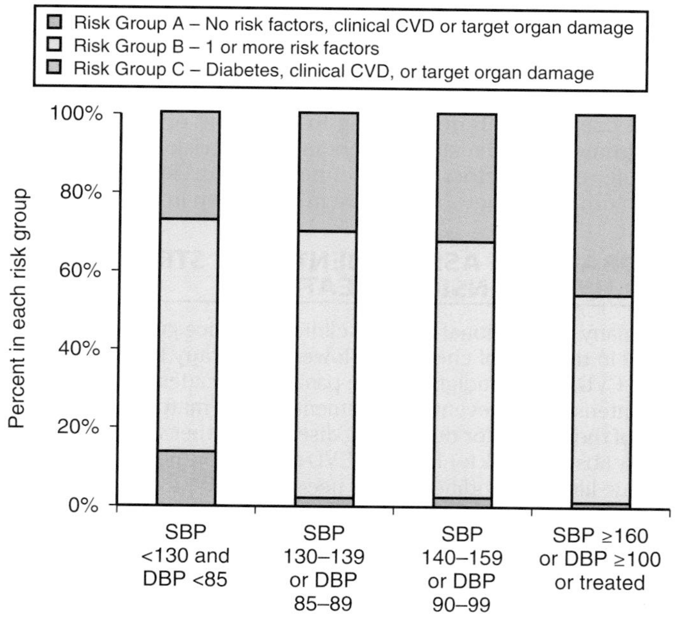

FIG. 1.9 Cross-classification of risk groups and blood pressure stages among 4962 Framingham Heart Study subjects. *CVD,* Cardiovascular disease; *DBP,* diastolic blood pressure; *SBP,* systolic blood pressure. *(Data from Lloyd-Jones DM, Evans JC, Larson MG, O'Donnell CJ, Wilson PW, Levy D. Cross-classification of JNC VI blood pressure stages and risk groups in the Framingham Heart Study.* Arch Int Med. *1999;159:2206-2212.)*

cumulative incidence of any CVD endpoint as a first event in men was 24.7%, compared with 9.8% for non-CVD death (hazard ratio, 2.53; 95% confidence interval, 1.83 to 3.50); in women, the competing incidences were 16.0% versus 10.1%, respectively (hazard ratio 1.58; 1.13 to 2.20). The most common first major CVD events among those with new-onset hypertension were CHD death or nonfatal MI (8.2%) in men and stroke (5.2%) in women. Type and incidence of first CV events varied by age, sex and severity of hypertension at onset, with stroke predominating among older men and women at all ages with new-onset hypertension.[63] These results represent a novel approach to understanding the complications of hypertension and could help target therapies for patients with new-onset hypertension to optimize prevention strategies. For example, an older individual (>60 years) with new-onset hypertension is at greatest risk for stroke as a first event; BP lowering would likely be of paramount importance to prevent this. However, a younger man with new-onset hypertension is most likely to have a major CHD event first, so aspirin and statin therapy, in addition to BP lowering, might be emphasized.

RISK FACTOR CLUSTERING

Hypertension occurs in isolation very infrequently. Data from 4962 FHS subjects were used to assess the cross-classification of JNC VI BP stages and risk groups (Fig. 1.9) in a middle-aged and older community-based population.[64] In this study, higher BP stages were associated with higher mean number of risk factors and higher rates of clinical CVD and/or target organ damage. Overall, among those with high-normal BP or hypertension, only 2.4% had no associated risk factors, whereas 59.3% had at least one associated risk factor, and 38.2% had target organ damage, clinical CVD or (DM).[64]

The current epidemic of obesity among Western societies has led to a greater understanding of the phenomenon of risk factor clustering, and of the pathophysiologic links between hypertension, obesity, DM and CVD risk. The cluster of risk factors including central obesity, atherogenic dyslipidemia (with low HDL-cholesterol, high triglycerides, and small, dense LDL-cholesterol particles), impaired glucose metabolism, vascular inflammation, proatherogenic milieu, and elevated BP has been termed the "metabolic syndrome." Visceral adiposity and insulin resistance appear to play central roles in the development of MS and elevated BP is a key diagnostic feature.[65] In some ethnicities, such as African Americans, elevated BP is the most common criterion leading to diagnosis of the metabolic syndrome. Hypertension confers increased risk for CVD in the absence of risk factors, but absolute risk increases dramatically when other risk factors are present, as shown in Fig. 1.4.

GLOBAL RISK ASSESSMENT AS A STRATEGY FOR HYPERTENSION TREATMENT

For many international and U.S. clinical practice guidelines, especially in the area of cholesterol-lowering therapy to prevent incident CVD, the paradigm for the past two decades has been that the intensity of preventive treatment should match the absolute risk of the patient for developing disease. In other words, patients at low absolute risk for having a CVD event in the near term should pursue lifestyle modification as needed, but typically should not be treated with drug therapy, given the concomitant costs and potential side effects. Patients at high enough risk should pursue both lifestyle modification and drug therapy when their risk is above the threshold where net clinical benefit has been demonstrated and could be expected to accrue to the patient. In this paradigm, guidelines use multivariable equations to predict the 10-year risk for CVD to estimate the risk for a given patient and aid in decision making. In the U.S., recent cholesterol guidelines in 2002 and 2013 adopted multivariable risk scores as decision aids. The 2013 American College of Cardiology/American Heart Association prevention guidelines developed and promulgated the Pooled Cohort Equations, based on data from 25,000 white and African-American men and women aged 40 to 79 years, to predict 10-year risks for CHD death, nonfatal myocardial infarction, or fatal or nonfatal stroke.[66] These equations form the basis of the data presented in Fig. 1.4, in which it is clear that BP levels (and the requirement for antihypertensive therapy) contribute significantly to the prediction of CVD risk. Gaziano and colleagues[67] have also promulgated a risk score that does not require the use of laboratory-based data, such as total cholesterol levels, instead using all clinic-based values to predict CVD risk. In those equations, which have shown good predictive utility in a variety of international settings, body mass index is substituted for cholesterol with good maintenance of predictive utility.

BP guidelines have generally not adopted this approach, instead continuing to use absolute BP levels, rather than absolute levels of CVD risk, as thresholds for initiation of drug therapy. However, increasing data suggest that risk-based treatment approaches may have a role for BP management as well. Sundstrom et al recently used data from the large Blood Pressure Lowering Treatment Trialists' Collaboration to examine the relative and absolute risk reductions associated with antihypertensive therapy across strata of baseline absolute predicted 5-year CVD risk. In 51,917 participants from 11 trials 4167 (8%) had a cardiovascular event during a median of 4.0 years (interquartile range 3.4–4.4) of follow up. The mean estimated baseline levels of 5-year cardiovascular risk for each of four increasing risk strata were 6.0%, 12.1%, 17.7%, and 26.8%. In each consecutive higher risk group, blood pressure-lowering treatment reduced the relative risk of cardiovascular events by 18% (95% CI 7–27), 15% (4–25), 13% (2–22), and 15% (5–24), respectively ($p = 0.30$ for trend). However, in terms of absolute risk reduction, treatment was more efficient for higher risk than lower risk individuals. Treating 1000 patients in each group with blood pressure-lowering treatment for 5 years would prevent 14 (95% CI 8–21), 20 (8–31), 24 (8–40), and 38 (16–61) cardiovascular events, respectively ($p = 0.04$ for trend). Similarly, Eddy et al used simulation modeling to estimate that risk-based approaches to treatment of hypertension would be far more efficient than current BP threshold-based decisions, treating fewer patients to prevent the same number of CVD events, or preventing more CVD events for the same cost as guideline-directed BP thresholds.[68]

IMPORTANCE OF PREVENTING THE DEVELOPMENT OF ELEVATED BLOOD PRESSURE

As noted earlier, BP levels tend to rise from young adulthood to the end of life. Once hypertension has been diagnosed, many effective lifestyle interventions and drug therapies can lower blood pressure, with dramatic reduction in CVD risk. However, it has been an open question as to whether treatment to lower BP once hypertension is diagnosed could fully reduce risk for CVD events to the low levels observed in individuals whose blood pressure always remained low. Liu et al[69] recently used data from the Multi-Ethnic Study of Atherosclerosis (MESA) to examine this issue. Outcomes were compared between participants without or with antihypertensive treatment at three BP levels: less than 120/80 mm Hg, systolic BP 120 mm Hg to 139 mm Hg or diastolic BP 80 mm Hg to 89 mm Hg, and systolic BP 140 mm Hg or higher or diastolic BP 90 mm Hg or higher (systolic BP ≥130 or diastolic BP ≥80 mm Hg for participants with diabetes). Among MESA participants aged 50 years or over at baseline, those with BP lower than 120/80 mm Hg on treatment had higher left ventricular mass index, prevalence of estimated glomerular filtration rate less than 60 mL/min per 1.73 m², prevalence of coronary calcium score greater than 100, and twice the incident cardiovascular disease rate over 9.5 years of follow up than those with BP lower than 120/80 mm Hg without treatment. At higher levels of BP, those who were treated to a given BP level also tended to be at greater risk for CVD compared with those whose BP was at the same level without treatment (Table 1.5).[69]

TABLE 1.5 Multivariable–Adjusted Hazard Ratios for all Cardiovascular Disease, Coronary Heart Disease, Heart Failure and Stroke, Stratified by Baseline Blood Pressure and Antihypertensive Treatment Status in 5798 Multi-Ethnic Study of Atherosclerosis Participants

OUTCOME	NO. OF EVENTS	MULTIVARIABLE-ADJUSTED HAZARD RATIO (95% CI)					
		BP <120/<80 MM HG AT BASELINE		SBP 120-139 OR DBP 80-89 MM HG AT BASELINE		SBP ≥140 OR DBP ≥90 MM HG AT BASELINE	
		Untreated	Treated and Well Controlled	Untreated	Treated and Controlled	Untreated	Treated and Uncontrolled
CVD	603	1.0 (ref)	2.19 (1.56, 3.07)	1.42 (1.03, 1.95)	2.21 (1.60, 3.05)	2.76 (2.04, 3.72)	2.96 (2.20, 3.97)
CHD	423	1.0 (ref)	2.02 (1.37, 2.97)	1.29 (0.89, 1.86)	2.09 (1.45, 3.03)	2.28 (1.60, 3.25)	2.52 (1.79, 3.55)
HF	226	1.0 (ref)	1.70 (0.92, 3.12)	1.41 (0.80, 2.51)	2.42 (1.40, 4.19)	2.43 (1.42, 4.15)	3.04 (1.83, 5.04)
Stroke	171	1.0 (ref)	2.56 (1.25, 5.28)	1.76 (0.90, 3.45)	3.13 (1.62, 6.09)	4.20 (2.27, 7.76)	4.67 (2.55, 8.56)

BP, Blood pressure; CHD, coronary heart disease; CI, confidence interval; CVD, cardiovascular disease; DBP, diastolic blood pressure; HF, heart failure; SBP, systolic blood pressure. Data from Liu K, Colangelo LA, Daviglus ML, et al. Can antihypertensive treatment restore the risk of cardiovascular disease to ideal levels? The Coronary Artery Risk Development in Young Adults (CARDIA) Study and the Multi–Ethnic Study of Atherosclerosis (MESA). J Am Heart Assoc. 2015;4: e002275.

The data suggest that, based on the current approach, antihypertensive treatment that is begun after significant BP elevation (typically to 140 mm Hg systolic) does not restore cardiovascular disease risk to ideal levels. Emphasis should therefore be placed on primordial prevention of BP increases to further reduce cardiovascular disease morbidity and mortality.

SUMMARY

Hypertension is the most prevalent major risk factor for all forms of CVD and renal disease. Risk factors for development of hypertension are well-understood, and numerous dietary and personal habits, as well as societal issues, must be addressed if we are to lower population levels of BP and to control individual patients' BPs, particularly SBP. Major public health and clinical efforts are needed to improve prevention of hypertension, especially through better control of weight. Newer research understanding the genetic underpinnings of hypertension and important gene-environment interactions may help to point the way for novel means of prevention. Although the benefits of antihypertensive therapy are substantial, too few patients achieve optimal BP reduction, and so do not realize the potential reductions in risk for CVD and renal disease. More widespread treatment and control are needed, but a greater focus on primordial prevention of hypertension would be a far more effective means for reducing the population impact of elevated BP on healthy longevity.

References

1. Chobanian AV, Bakris GL, Black HR, et al. Seventh Report of the Joint National Committee on Prevention, Detection, Evaluation, and Treatment of High Blood Pressure. *Hypertension*. 2003;42:1206-1252.
2. Hill AB. The environment and disease: association or causation? *Proc R Soc Med*. 1965;58: 295-300.
3. Yoon SS, Fryar CD, Carroll MD. *Hypertension prevalence and control among adults: United States, 2011-2014. NCHS data brief, no 220*. Hyattsville, MD: National Center for Health Statistics; 2015.
4. Burt VL, Culter JA, Higgins M, et al. Trends in the prevalence, awareness, treatment, and control of hypertension in the adult US population. Data from the health examination surveys, 1960 to 1991. *Hypertension*. 1995;26:60-69.
5. Hajjar I, Kotchen TA. Trends in prevalence, awareness, treatment, and control of hypertension in the United States, 1988-2000. *JAMA*. 2003;290:199-206.
6. Yoon S, Otschega Y, Louis T. *Recent trends in the prevalence of high blood pressure and its treatment and control, 1999-2008*. Hyattsville, MD: National Center for Health Statistics; 2010.
7. Huffman MD, Capewell S, Ning H, Shay CM, Ford ES, Lloyd-Jones DM. Cardiovascular Health Behavior and Health Factor Changes (1988–2008) and Projections to 2020: results from the National Health and Nutrition Examination Surveys. *Circulation*. 2012;125:2595-2602.
8. Nwankwo T, Yoon SS, Burt V, Gu Q. *Hypertension among adults in the United States: National Health and Nutrition Examination Survey, 2011–2012. NCHS data brief, no 133*. Hyattsville, MD: National Center for Health Statistics; 2013.
9. Mozaffarian D, Benjamin EJ, Go AS, et al. Heart Disease and Stroke Statistics—2016 update: a report from the American Heart Association. *Circulation*. 2016;133:e38-60.
10. Olives C, Myerson R, Mokdad AH, Murray CJL, Lim SS. Prevalence, Awareness, Treatment, and Control of Hypertension in United States Counties, 2001-2009. *PLoS ONE*. 2013; 8: e60308.
11. Forouzanfar MH, Alexander L, Anderson HR, et al. Global, regional, and national comparative risk assessment of 79 behavioural, environmental and occupational, and metabolic risks or clusters of risks in 188 countries, 1990-2013: a systematic analysis for the Global Burden of Disease Study. *Lancet*. 2013;386:2287-2323.
12. Lim SS, Vos T, Flaxman AD, et al. A comparative risk assessment of burden of disease and injury attributable to 67 risk factors and risk factor clusters in 21 regions, 1990-2010: a systematic analysis for the Global Burden of Disease Study. *Lancet*. 2010;380:2224-2260.
13. *Evaluation IfHMa. GBD 2013*; 2013. http://vizhub.healthdata.org/gbd-compare/. Accessed April 20, 2016.
14. Danaei G, Finucane MM, Lin JK, et al. National, regional, and global trends in systolic blood pressure since 1980: systematic analysis of health examination surveys and epidemiological studies with 786 country-years and 5.4 million participants. *Lancet*. 2011;377:568-577.
15. Wolf-Maier K, Cooper RS, Banegas JR, et al. Hypertension prevalence and blood pressure levels in 6 European countries, Canada, and the United States. *JAMA*. 2003;289:2363-2369.
16. Wolf-Maier K, Cooper RS, Kramer H, et al. Hypertension treatment and control in five European countries, Canada, and the United States. *Hypertension*. 2004;43:10-17.
17. Fields LE, Burt VL, Cutler JA, Hughes J, Roccella EJ, Sorlie P. The burden of adult hypertension in the United States 1999 to 2000. A rising tide. *Hypertension*. 2004;44:398-404.
18. Vasan RS, Beiser A, Seshadri S, et al. Residual lifetime risk for developing hypertension in middle-aged women and men: The Framingham Heart Study. *JAMA*. 2002;287:1003-1010.
19. Burt VL, Whelton P, Roccella EJ, et al. Prevalence of hypertension in the US adult population: results from the Third National Health and Nutrition Examination Survey, 1988-1991. *Hypertension*. 1995;25:305-313.
20. Franklin SS, Gustin W, Wong ND, et al. Hemodynamic patterns of age-related changes in blood pressure. The Framingham Heart Study. *Circulation*. 1997;96:308-315.
21. Lakatta EG, Levy D. Arterial and cardiac aging: major shareholders in cardiovascular disease enterprises: Part I: aging arteries: a "set up" for vascular disease. *Circulation*. 2003;107:139-146.
22. Izzo JL, Levy D, Black HR. Importance of systolic blood pressure in older Americans. *Hypertension*. 2000;35:1021-1024.
23. Wang Y, Wang QJ. The prevalence of prehypertension and hypertension among US adults according to the new Joint National Committee guidelines. *Arch Intern Med*. 2004;164:2126-2134.
24. Wilson PWF, D'Agostino RB, Sullivan L, Parise H, Kannel WB. Overweight and obesity as determinants of cardiovascular risk: the Framingham experience. *Arch Intern Med*. 2002;162:1867-1872.
25. Lloyd-Jones DM, Liu K, Colangelo LA, et al. Consistently stable or decreased body mass index in young adulthood and longitudinal changes in metabolic syndrome components: the Coronary Artery Risk Development in Young Adults Study. *Circulation*. 2007;115:1004-1011.
26. Mamun AA, Lawlor DA, O'Callaghan MJ, Williams GM, Najman JM. Effect of body mass index changes between ages 5 and 14 on blood pressure at age 14: findings from a birth cohort study. *Hypertension*. 2005;45:1083-1087.
27. Roger VL, Go AS, Lloyd-Jones DM, et al. Heart Disease and Stroke Statistics–2011 Update: a Report from the American Heart Association. *Circulation*. 2011;123:e18-209.
28. Cutler JA, Sorlie PD, Wolz M, Thom T, Fields LE, Roccella EJ. Trends in hypertension prevalence, awareness, treatment, and control rates in United States adults between 1988-1994 and 1999-2004. *Hypertension*. 2008;52:818-827.
29. *CDC Health Disparities and Inequalities Report—United States, 2013*. Atlanta, GA: Centers for Disease Control & Prevention; 2013.
30. Stamler J, Elliott P, Appel L, et al. Higher blood pressure in middle-aged American adults with less education-role of multiple dietary factors: the INTERMAP study. *J Hum Hypertens*. 2003;17:655-775.
31. Stamler J, Rose G, Elliott P, et al. Findings of the International Cooperative INTERSALT Study. *Hypertension*. 1991;17(Suppl 1):I9-I15.
32. Levy D, DeStefano AL, Larson MG, et al. Evidence for a gene influencing blood pressure on chromosome 17. Genome scan linkage results for longitudinal blood pressure phenotypes in subjects from the framingham heart study. *Hypertension*. 2000;36:477-483.
33. Newton-Cheh C, Johnson T, Gateva V, et al. Genome-wide association study identifies eight loci associated with blood pressure. *Nat Genet*. 2009;41:666-676.
34. Zheng J, Rao DC, Shi G. An update on genome-wide association studies of hypertension. *Applied Informatics*. 2015;2:1-20.
35. The Seventh Report of the Joint National Committee on Prevention, Detection, Evaluation, and Treatment of High Blood Pressure: The JNC 7 Report. *JAMA*. 2003;289:2560-2571.
36. Lloyd-Jones DM, Evans JC, Larson MG, O'Donnell CJ, Levy D. Differential impact of systolic and diastolic blood pressure level on JNC-VI staging. *Hypertension*. 1999;34:381-385.
37. Pogue VA, Ellis C, Michel J, Francis CK. New staging system of the fifth Joint National Committee report on the detection, evaluation, and treatment of high blood pressure (JNC-V) alters assessment of the severity and treatment of hypertension [see comments]. *Hypertension*. 1996;28:713-718.
38. Franklin SS, Jacobs MJ, Wong ND, L'Italien GJ, Lapuerta P. Predominance of isolated systolic hypertension among middle-aged and elderly US hypertensives. *Hypertension*. 2001;37:869-874.
39. Collaboration PS. Age-specific relevance of usual blood pressure to vascular mortality: a meta-analysis of individual data for one million adults in 61 prospective studies. *Lancet*. 2002;360:1903-1913.
40. Wilson PW, D'Agostino RB, Levy D, Belanger AM, Silbershatz H, Kannel WB. Prediction of coronary heart disease using risk factor categories. *Circulation*. 1998;97:1837-1847.
41. Association AH. *Heart disease and stroke statistics—2005 update*. Dallas, TX: American Heart Association; 2004.
42. Levy D, Larson MG, Vasan RS, Kannel WB, Ho KK. The progression from hypertension to congestive heart failure. *JAMA*. 1996;275:1557-1562.
43. Dunlay SM, Weston SA, Jacobsen SJ, Roger VL. Risk factors for heart failure: a population-based case-control study. *Am J Med*. 2009;122:1023-1028.
44. Kannel WB, Gordon T, Schwartz MJ. Systolic versus diastolic blood pressure and risk of coronary heart disease. The Framingham Study. *Am J Cardiol*. 1971;27:335-345.
45. Psaty BM, Furberg CD, Kuller LH, et al. Association between blood pressure level and the risk of myocardial infarction, stroke, and total mortality. *Arch Intern Med*. 2001;161:1183-1192.
46. Neaton JD, Wentworth DN. Serum cholesterol, blood pressure, cigarette smoking, and death from coronary heart disease: overall findings and differences by age for 316,099 white men. *Arch Intern Med*. 1992;152:56-64.
47. Neaton JD, Kuller L, Stamler J, Wentworth DN. Impact of systolic and diastolic blood pressure on cardiovascular mortality. In: Laragh JH, Brenner BM, eds. *Hypertension: Pathophysiology, Diagnosis, and Management*. 2nd ed. New York: Raven Press; 1995:127-144.
48. Franklin SS, Khan SA, Wong ND, Larson MG, Levy D. Is pulse pressure useful in predicting risk for coronary heart disease? The Framingham Heart Study. *Circulation*. 1999;100:354-360.
49. Lloyd-Jones DM, Evans JC, Larson MG, O'Donnell CJ, Roccella EJ, Levy D. Differential control of systolic and diastolic blood pressure: factors associated with lack of blood pressure control in the community. *Hypertension*. 2000;36:594-599.
50. Hyman DJ, Pavlik VN. Characteristics of patients with uncontrolled hypertension in the United States. *N Engl J Med*. 2001;345:479-486.
51. Somes GW, Pahor M, Shorr RI, Cushman WC, Applegate WB. The role of diastolic blood pressure when treating isolated systolic hypertension. *Arch Intern Med*. 1999;159:2004-2009.
52. Yano Y, Stamler J, Garside DB, et al. Isolated Systolic Hypertension in Young and Middle-Aged Adults and 31-Year Risk for Cardiovascular Mortality: The Chicago Heart Association Detection Project in Industry Study. *J Am Coll Cardiol*. 2015;65:327-335.
53. Stamler J, Stamler R, Neaton JD. Blood pressure, systolic and diastolic, and cardiovascular risks. US population data. *Arch Intern Med*. 1993;153:598-615.
54. Karmali KN, Ning H, Goff DC, Lloyd-Jones DM. Identifying individuals at risk for cardiovascular events across the spectrum of blood pressure levels. *J Am Heart Assoc*. 2015; 4: e002126.
55. Vasan RS, Larson MG, Leip EP, et al. Impact of high-normal blood pressure on the risk of cardiovascular disease. *N Engl J Med*. 2001;345:1291-1297.
56. Vasan RS, Larson MG, Leip EP, Kannel WB, Levy D. Assessment of frequency of progression to hypertension in non-hypertensive participants in the Framingham Heart Study: a cohort study [comment]. *Lancet*. 2001;358:1682-1686.
57. Chae CU, Pfeffer MA, Glynn RJ, Mitchell GF, Taylor JO, Hennekens CH. Increased pulse pressure and risk of heart failure in the elderly. *JAMA*. 1999;281:634-639.
58. Haider AW, Larson MG, Franklin SS, Levy D. Systolic blood pressure, diastolic blood pressure, and pulse pressure as predictors of risk for congestive heart failure in the Framingham Heart Study. *Ann Intern Med*. 2003;138:10-16.
59. Mosley WJ, Greenland P, Garside DB, Lloyd-Jones DM. Predictive utility of pulse pressure and other blood pressure measures for cardiovascular outcomes. *Hypertension*. 2007;49:1256-1264.
60. System USRD. *USRDS 2003 Annual Data Report*. Bethesda, MD: National Institute of Diabetes and Digestive and Kidney Diseases, National Institutes of Health (NIH), DHHS; 2003.

61. Yano Y, Ning H, Allen N, et al. Long-term blood pressure variability throughout young adulthood and cognitive function in midlife: the Coronary Artery Risk Development in Young Adults (CARDIA) Study. *Hypertension.* 2014;64:983-988.

62. Yano Y, Ning H, Muntner P, et al. Nocturnal blood pressure in young adults and cognitive function in midlife: the Coronary Artery Risk Development in Young Adults (CARDIA) Study. *Am J Hypertens.* 2015;28:1240-1247.

63. Lloyd-Jones DM, Leip EP, Larson MG, Vasan RS, Levy D. Novel approach to examining first cardiovascular events after hypertension onset. *Hypertension.* 2005;45:39-45.

64. Lloyd-Jones DM, Evans JC, Larson MG, O'Donnell CJ, Wilson PW, Levy D. Cross-classification of JNC VI blood pressure stages and risk groups in the Framingham Heart Study. *Arch Intern Med.* 1999;159:2206-2212.

65. Third Report of the National Cholesterol Education Program (NCEP) Expert Panel on Detection, Evaluation, and Treatment of High Blood Cholesterol in Adults (Adult Treatment Panel III) Final Report. *Circulation.* 2002;106:3143-3421.

66. Goff DC, Lloyd-Jones DM, Bennett G, et al. 2013 ACC/AHA Guideline on the Assessment of Cardiovascular Risk: a Report of the American College of Cardiology/American Heart Association Task Force on Practice Guidelines. *Circulation.* 2014;129(25 suppl 2):S49-S73.

67. Gaziano TA, Young CR, Fitzmaurice G, Atwood S, Gaziano JM. Laboratory-based versus non-laboratory-based method for assessment of cardiovascular disease risk: the NHANES I Follow-up Study cohort. *Lancet.* 2008;371:923–931.

68. Eddy DM, Adler J, Patterson B, Lucas D, Smith KA, Morris M. Individualized guidelines: the potential for increasing quality and reducing costs. *Ann Int Med.* 2011;154:627-634.

69. Liu K, Colangelo LA, Daviglus ML, et al. Can antihypertensive treatment restore the risk of cardiovascular disease to ideal levels? The Coronary Artery Risk Development in Young Adults (CARDIA) Study and the Multi-Ethnic Study of Atherosclerosis (MESA). *J Am Heart Assoc.* 2015:4: e002275.

2 Hypertension in Latin/Hispanic Population

Luis Miguel Ruilope, José R. Banegas, and Gema Ruiz-Hurtado

The term Hispanic or Latino refers to a person of Cuban, Mexican, Puerto Rican, South or Central American, or other Spanish culture or origin regardless of race according to the definition of the United States Census Bureau published in 2010. The term includes a very relevant part of the population of Latin American and Caribbean (LAC) region to which around 50 million (16%) of the U.S. population has to be added. Brazil, French Guyana, and a few Caribbean islands are also included in the term LAC region.

The LAC region is extremely diverse but exists as a continent with historic entity and cultural, linguistic, and religious liaisons among the different countries.[1] The territory exceeds 21 million square miles and the population approaches 600 million inhabitants. Marked health care disparities within countries exist related to striking economic differences that lead to important changes in health risk coverage and outcomes between the different countries. In fact the demographic, economic and social changes observed in LAC in recent years are the main contributors to explain the growing epidemic of cardiovascular disease (CVD) in this region.[2] At the same time, all these facts explain why the literature related to cardiovascular (CV) risk and arterial hypertension in particular in the LAC region is both sparse and confusing. In this chapter we will review the most recent literature dealing with CV risk and arterial hypertension in Latin/Hispanic population both in LAC region and in the U.S.

CARDIOVASCULAR DISEASE IN LATIN/HISPANIC POPULATION

Cardiovascular diseases account for around 30% of deaths in LAC (1.6 million) and is the leading cause of death in all countries including the lowest-income countries (Haiti, Bolivia, and Nicaragua)[3] and around half a million deaths take place in people younger than 70 years. One-third of premature deaths arising from CVD occurs in the poorest quintile of the population whereas only 13% are in the richest one.[4] The prevalence of CVD among Latin/Hispanic population living in the U.S. is alarming and also represents the most important cause of death in this population accounting for 31% of the total.[5] This can be explained by a higher prevalence of obesity, diabetes mellitus, hypertension, and dyslipidemia in Latin/Hispanic than in Caucasians.[5] As previously commented LAC region is characterized by an extreme diversity, but the great majority of countries are in the group of low to middle income countries where the CVD risk is the highest.[6]

Table 2.1 contains the ten "level 3" risks in terms of disability-adjusted life years (DALYs) for both sexes for the following locations: global, U.S., and the LAC region.[7] The last is divided into Andean Latin America (Bolivia, Ecuador, Peru), Caribbean (Antigua and Barbuda, Barbados, Belize, Cuba, Dominica, Dominican Republic, Grenada Guyana, Haiti, Jamaica, Saint Lucia, Saint Vincent and the Grenadines, Suriname, the Bahamas, Trinidad and Tobago), Central Latin America (Colombia, Costa Rica, El Salvador, Guatemala,

Honduras, Mexico, Nicaragua, Panama, Venezuela), Tropical Latin America (Brazil, Paraguay) and Southern Latin America (Argentina, Chile, Uruguay). As can be seen, increased levels of blood pressure (BP), body mass index and fasting plasma glucose, in agreement with global data, are the three most frequent risk factors for CVD in the Latin/Hispanic population both in the U.S. and LAC. Unlike in global data, the presence of low glomerular filtration rate (GFR) appears as a risk factor in LAC and the U.S. occupying positions from the fifth to the eighth in LAC region and the tenth in the U.S. It is well known that arterial hypertension, obesity and diabetes facilitate together with CVD the development of chronic kidney disease (CKD).[8]

Global prevalence of death attributed to CVD is increasing as a consequence of population growth, the aging of populations, and epidemiologic changes in diseases.[9] Table 2.2 contains the six different patterns of demographic and epidemiologic changes in cardiovascular mortality. As can be seen there are significant differences among the different areas in the LAC region and in the U.S. The worst prognosis for the near future corresponds to the Caribbean with a continuous increase in the number of CVD deaths. Relative increases because of population growth and aging are expected in Central, Tropical, and Andean Latin America. Large declines in CVD death rates led to a small decline in mortality.

ARTERIAL HYPERTENSION IN THE LATIN AMERICAN AND CARIBBEAN REGION AND THE UNITED STATES

Arterial hypertension is one of the main risk factors for ischemic heart disease and the leading determinant of cerebrovascular disease, and it affects between 20% and 40% of adults in the LAC region.[10-13] The increase in CVD mortality in most LAC region countries is facilitated by the frequent and growing presence of arterial hypertension; in fact, the rising incidence of high BP could contribute to explain why in LAC countries, where rates of CVD death have declined, the trend has been considerably lower than that seen in the U.S.[14] However, recently published data[15] reflecting that globally high BP is number one cause of deaths and burden of disease, show that the participation of the LAC region in both parameters is smaller than that observed in high-income regions, Central Asia and Eastern Europe, East and Southeast Asia and Oceania and South Asia, being comparable to the contribution of Middle East and North Africa and Sub-Saharan Africa (Fig. 2.1). This relatively smaller contribution could be related to the fact that total population in LAC region represents only around 8% of the global.

In the U.S., recent surveys indicate that the prevalence of arterial hypertension that increased continuously until 2000 has remained unchanged afterwards.[16-18] This is shown in Table 2.3 illustrating the evolution since the early 2000s for optimal BP, prehypertension, stage 1 and stage 2 hypertension in the U.S. for white non-Hispanic, black non-Hispanic, and Mexican Americans, the latter group representing 66% of the

TABLE 2.1 The Ten Leading Level 3 Risks in 2013 in Terms of Disability-Adjusted Life Years by Location for Both Sexes Combined in Latin American and Caribbean Region and United States

RISK	1	2	3	4	5	6	7	8	9	10
Global	Blood Pressure	Smoking	Body mass index	Childhood undernutrition	Fasting plasma glucose	Alcohol use	Household air pollution	Unsafe water	Unsafe sex	Fruit
United States	Body mass index	Smoking	Blood Pressure	Fasting plasma glucose	Alcohol use	Total cholesterol	Physical activity	Drug use	Fruit	Glomerular filtration
South Latin America	Smoking	Body mass index	Blood Pressure	Alcohol use	Fasting plasma glucose	Glomerular filtration	Total cholesterol	Fruit	Vegetables	Drug use
Latin America & Caribbean	Body mass index	Blood Pressure	Fasting plasma glucose	Alcohol use	Smoking	Glomerular filtration	Total cholesterol	Whole grains	Physical activity	Fruit
Andean Latin American	Alcohol use	Body mass index	Blood Pressure	Fasting plasma glucose	Glomerular filtration	Smoking	Childhood undernutrition	Iron deficiency	Total cholesterol	Unsafe sex
Caribbean	Blood Pressure	Body mass index	Fasting plasma glucose	Smoking	Unsafe sex	Childhood undernutrition	Alcohol use	Glomerular filtration	Physical activity	Whole grains
Central Latin America	Body mass index	Fasting plasma glucose	Blood Pressure	Alcohol use	Glomerular filtration	Smoking	Processed meat	Total cholesterol	Whole grains	Sweetened beverages
Tropical Latin America	Blood Pressure	Body mass index	Alcohol use	Fasting plasma glucose	Smoking	Total cholesterol	Sodium	Glomerular filtration	Fruit	Whole grains

Modified from Forouzanfar MH, Alexander L, Anderson HR, et al. Global, regional, and national comparative risk assessment of 79 behavioural, environmental and occupational, and metabolic risks or clusters of risks in 188 countries, 1990-2013: a systematic analysis for the Global Burden of Disease Study 2013. Lancet. 2015;386:2287-2323.

TABLE 2.2 Patterns of Demographic and Epidemiologic Change in Cardiovascular Mortality in Latin American and Caribbean Region and United States

Category	CHANGE IN CARDIOVASCULAR DEATHS, 1990-2013	EFFECT OF POPULATION GROWTH	EFFECT OF POPULATION AGING	EFFECT OF AGE-SPECIFIC CARDIOVASCULAR DEATH RATE	REGIONS LATIN AMERICAN AND CARIBBEAN & UNITED STATES
1. **Population growth and aging:** regions with large and continuous increases in the number of cardiovascular deaths because of population growth or aging but little change in age-specific rates of death	Increase	Large (≥20%)	Large (>30%)	Small (decline <30%)	Caribbean
2. **Population growth:** regions with increases in deaths mostly because of population growth	Increase	Large (>80%)	Small (<10%)	Small (decline <30%)	—
3. **Population aging:** regions in which cardiovascular deaths rose and then fell during preceding 20 years, resulting in a net increase in deaths because of population aging and only small decrease in age-specific rates of cardiovascular death	Increase then decrease	Very small (<20%)	Moderate (>20%)	Very small (decline <15%)	—
4. **Improved health moderating effect of population aging:** regions in which large increases in the number of cardiovascular deaths because of population aging were moderated by a fall in age-specific rates of death	Increase	Small (<30%)	Very large (>70%)	Large (decline >30%)	—
5. **Improved health moderating effect of population growth and aging:** regions with large relative increases in the number of cardiovascular deaths because of both population growth and aging that were moderated by a fall in age-specific rates of death	Increase	Large (>30%)	Large (>30%)	Large (decline >30%)	Central Latin America Tropical Latin America Andean Latin America
6. **Improved health exceeding effect of population growth and aging:** regions in which large declines in age-specific cardiovascular death rates have led to only small increases or even a decline in the number of cardiovascular deaths despite the large effects of an aging population	Small increase or decrease	Small (<40%)	Large (>30%)	Large (decline >30%)	Southern Latin America North America

Modified from Roth GA, Forouzanfar MH, Moran AE, et al. Demographic and epidemiologic drivers of global cardiovascular mortality. N Engl J Med. 2015;372:1333-1341.

Latin/Hispanic population in the U.S.[19] As can be seen, there is generally an increase after the year 2000 in the prevalence of optimal BP and prehypertension whereas in stage 1 and stage 2 hypertension changes occurred in the opposite direction albeit were less clear. Importantly, the current prevalence of prehypertension amounted to one-third of the Mexican American population, and the prevalence of hypertension affected over half of the population.

Table 2.4 contains the degree of awareness and control in a series of urban settings in LAC regions. As can be seen a relevant percentage of hypertensive patients remains unaware of their high blood pressure (and the accompanying risk), and an adequate control is attained at the most in only one third of patients. A comparison of prevalence and control performed in Mexico and in immigrant Mexicans and U.S.-born Mexicans showed that hypertension was more common in Mexico than among Mexican immigrants in the U.S.[20] The most widely used drugs are diuretics, beta-blockers, angiotensin converting enzyme inhibitors, angiotensin receptor blockers, and calcium channel blockers alone or in combination,[1] and the low percentage of good BP control indicate, as in other regions in the world, the need for an earlier start of combination therapy.[21] In any case the response of Latin/Hispanic population to the most widely used combinations (components ×2 or ×3 angiotensin-converting-enzyme inhibitor/angiotensin-receptor blocker

[ACEi/ARB], calcium channel blocker [CCB] and diuretic) is totally adequate.[22] Table 2.5 contains data of prevalence, awareness, treatment and control in a series of countries from Europe, Asia, Africa, as well as Australia and Canada, to compare with the situation in LAC and Latin Hispanic in the U.S. As can be seen, there is a big variation among countries and continents. The situation in Latin/Hispanic in the U.S. compares with several European countries and is above Asia and Africa, but still far from Canada. Data from the LAC region show variable data with countries similar to the U.S. and other in lower values of control but still above Asia and Africa. In any case, there is still a long way before attaining a global control of arterial hypertension.

On the other hand, a significant deficit in treatment and control of hypertension among Latin/Hispanic population in the U.S. has also been described particularly in those without health insurance.[19,23] However, the recent situation of awareness (80.2%), treatment (71.5%) and control (45.3%) in the U.S. for the Latin/Hispanic population is significantly better than in LAC regions, albeit adequate control of hypertension is lower than in non-Hispanic whites and non-Hispanic blacks.[24] The use of antihypertensive medication and in particular of single pill and multiple pill combinations has increased significantly in the U.S. contributing importantly to the improvement in BP control, including Latinos.[25]

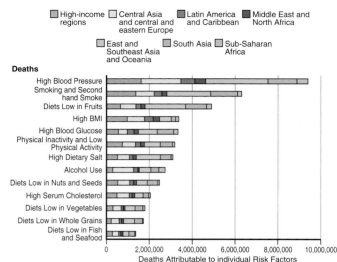

Legend: High-income regions; Central Asia and central and eastern Europe; Latin America and Caribbean; Middle East and North Africa; East and Southeast Asia and Oceania; South Asia; Sub-Saharan Africa

Deaths

High Blood Pressure
Smoking and Second hand Smoke
Diets Low in Fruits
High BMI
High Blood Glucose
Physical Inactivity and Low Physical Activity
High Dietary Salt
Alcohol Use
Diets Low in Nuts and Seeds
High Serum Cholesterol
Diets Low in Vegetables
Diets Low in Whole Grains
Diets Low in Fish and Seafood

Deaths Attributable to individual Risk Factors

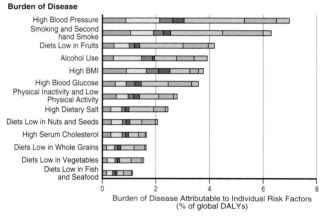

Burden of Disease

High Blood Pressure
Smoking and Second hand Smoke
Diets Low in Fruits
Alcohol Use
High BMI
High Blood Glucose
Physical Inactivity and Low Physical Activity
High Dietary Salt
Diets Low in Nuts and Seeds
High Serum Cholesterol
Diets Low in Whole Grains
Diets Low in Vegetables
Diets Low in Fish and Seafood

Burden of Disease Attributable to Individual Risk Factors (% of global DALYs)

FIG. 2.1 Deaths and burden of disease attributable to selected behavioral and dietary risk factors in 2010 and the metabolic and physiologic mediators of their hazardous effects. *BMI*, Body mass index. *(Reprinted with permission from Ezzati M, Riboli E. Behavioral and dietary risk factors for noncommunicable diseases. N Engl J Med. 2013;369:954-964.)*

Finally, it is worth mentioning that some organization such as the Pan American Health Organization (PAHO) is prioritizing the prevention and control of hypertension in LAC countries through a series of systematic interventions and strong partnerships.[1,3] Enhanced surveillance methods will assess the impact of health promotion and clinical interventions. Efforts to promote physical activity and healthy diets (especially lowering dietary salt) aim to reduce the prevalence of hypertension and improve control. The program has already developed a mechanism to make antihypertensive drugs more available and affordable within the Americas as a key short-term success. Assisting countries implement chronic care models focusing on hypertension control using simplified approaches is also an ongoing focus as are efforts to incorporate risk assessment into routine hypertension management. It is thus hoped that the PAHO effort will achieve and surpass the United Nations target of a 25% decrease in uncontrolled hypertension and provide global best practices.

SUMMARY AND CONCLUSIONS

Cardiovascular disease constitutes an epidemic among the Latin/Hispanic population in both the LAC region and U.S. populations. The prognosis of patients is however different with a better awareness, treatment and control of hypertension among Latin/Hispanics in the U.S. Table 2.6 summarizes the key points favoring this epidemic in LAC region and in the U.S. and lists the corrections to improve the prognosis of Latin/Hispanic population both in LAC region and the U.S.[13,15,19,26-31]

Complete information for those interested in current hypertension guidelines in Latin America is included in reference number 1.

ACKNOWLEDGMENTS

This work was supported by PI14/01841 grant from Instituto de Salud Carlos III and FONDOS FEDER.

TABLE 2.3 Age-Adjusted Percentage of Hypertensives With Optimal Blood Pressure, Prehypertension, Stage 1 Hypertension and Stage 2 Hypertension Levels in White Non-Hispanic, Black Non-Hispanic and Mexican Americans

	2003-2004, % (SE) n = 1664	2005-2006, % (SE) n = 1518	2007-2008, % (SE) n = 2113	2009-2010, % (SE) n = 2116	2011-2012, % (SE) n = 1844
Optimal Blood Pressure					
White non-Hispanic	13.4 (1.2)	15.3 (1.1)	18.4 (1.6)	22.8 (1.4)	20.3 (2.2)[a]
Black non-Hispanic	13.3 (1.9)	13.3 (1.1)	18.1 (1.5)	19.6 (1.7)	14.6 (1.9)
Mexican Americans	10.6 (1.6)	11.5 (4.1)	14.4 (1.6)	11.6 (1.1)	13.9 (2.2)
Prehypertensive Level					
White non-Hispanic	27.3 (2.0)	29.1 (2.0)	32.5 (1.3)	33.3 (1.9)	33.6 (2.0)[a]
Black non-Hispanic	24.4 (2.6)	29.5 (1.7)	26.8 (1.5)	28.0 (2.1)	34.8 (1.6)[a]
Mexican Americans	23.7 (2.8)	27.3 (2.3)	26.8 (2.3)	24.1 (2.5)	31.4 (5.2)
Stage 1 Hypertension					
White non-Hispanic	43.9 (2.7)	41.5 (1.7)	38.9 (1.8)	35.1 (2.3)	36.0 (3.1)[a]
Black non-Hispanic	37.1 (2.2)	39.9 (2.5)	36.9 (2.1)	38.4 (2.6)	33.3 (1.6)
Mexican Americans	40.6 (2.6)	42.9 (4.6)	41.0 (3.3)	46.2 (3.7)	39.7 (5.6)
Stage 2 Hypertension					
White non-Hispanic	15.4 (1.2)	14.1 (1.2)	10.2 (1.0)	8.9 (0.9)	10.1 (1.9)[a]
Black non-Hispanic	25.2 (2.8)	17.2 (1.4)	18.2 (1.5)	14.0 (2.3)	17.4 (1.8)[a]
Mexican Americans	25.1 (2.6)	22.0 (2.7)	17.8 (2.3)	18.1 (2.8)	15.0 (6.8)[b]

[a]P-trend <0.05.
[b]relative SE is >30%.
SE, Standard error.
Modified from Yoon SS, Gu Q, Nwankwo T, Wright JD, Hong Y, Burt V. Trends in blood pressure among adults with hypertension: United States, 2003 to 2012. Hypertension. 2015;65:54-61.

TABLE 2.4 Hypertension Awareness and Control Estimates of Diverse Urban Settings in Latin American and Caribbean Regions (2001-2010)

COUNTRY	AGE (YEARS)	N	AWARENESS (%)	CONTROL (%)
Argentina	25-64	1482	64.1	18
Brazil	≥18	1717	74.4	34.3
Chile	25-64	1655	60.1	20.3
Colombia	25-64	1553	68.8	30.6
Ecuador	25-64	1638	67.6	28
Mexico	25-64	1720	75.7	41
Peru	25-64	1652	53.1	12
Venezuela	25-64	1848	72.0	20.7

From Burroughs Peña MS, Mendes Abdala CV, Silva LC, Ordúñez P. Usefulness for surveillance of hypertension prevalence studies in Latin America and the Caribbean: the past 10 years. Rev Panam Salud Publica. 2012;32:15-21.

TABLE 2.5 Awareness, Treatment and Control of Hypertension in a Series of Countries From Europe, Asia, Africa, as well as Australia and Canada

COUNTRY/YEAR	PREVALENCE (%)	AWARENESS (%)	TREATMENT (%)	CONTROL (%)	REFERENCE
Australia/2005-2010	25	60	35	51	32
Canada/2012-2013	23[a]	84	80	68	33
Spain/2008-2010	33	59	79	49	34
Portugal/2011-2012	42	77	75	43	35
Finland/1982-2007	40	65	55	40	36
Italy/2013-2014	55	67	35	58	37
Germany/2008-2011	32	82	72	51	38
England/2011	32	71	58	37	39
Japan/1986-2002	39	—	44	50	40
China/2003-2012	27	45	35	11	41
India/1950-2013 (urban data)	30	42	38	20	42
India/1950-2013 (rural data)	30	25	25	11	
Egypt/1995	26	38	24	8	43
Guinea/2009	30	24	35	16	44
South Africa/2011	39	—	31	13	45

[a]Represents the number of treated patients.

TABLE 2.6 Factors Favoring the Epidemic of Hypertension and Cardiovascular Disease in Latin American and Caribbean Region and in the United States

COMMON TO LATIN AMERICAN AND CARIBBEAN AND UNITED STATES	
Factor	Correction
Lack of access to health care (absence of treatment)	Providing medical insurance[a]
Low socioeconomic status (insurance)	Providing medical insurance[a]
Degree of acculturation (understanding the risk)	Education about cardiovascular diseases and their treatment
Poor doctor-patient communication (compliance)	Time devoted by doctors and nurses
Metabolic syndrome, obesity and diabetes	Specific drugs
Sugar-sweetened beverages and salt sensitivity	Life style changes
Dyslipidemia	Access to statins
Absence of adequate outcome studies	Design of specific trials for Latin/Hispanic

Obtained from 13, 15, 19, 26-31.
[a]Paid by the state or private system.

References

1. Alcocer L, Meaney E, Hernandez-Hernandez H. Applicability of the current hypertension guidelines in Latin America. *Ther Adv Cardiovasc Dis.* 2015;9:118-126.
2. Fernando L, Pamela S, Alejandra L. Cardiovascular disease in Latin America: the growing epidemic. *Prog Cardiovasc Dis.* 2014;57:262-267.
3. Ordunez P, Martinez R, Niebylski ML, Campbell NR. Hypertension Prevention and Control in Latin America and the Caribbean. *J Clin Hypertens (Greenwich).* 2015;17:499-502.
4. Rodríguez T, Malvezzi M, Chatenoud L, Bosetti C, Levi F, Negri E, et al. Trends in mortality from coronary heart and cerebrovascular diseases in the Americas: 1970-2000. *Heart.* 2006;92:453-460.
5. Heart disease and stroke statistics-2010 update: a report from the American Heart Association. (2010). Dallas, TX. http://my.americanheart.org/idc/groups/ahamah-public/@wcm/@sop/documents/downloadable/ucm_319689.
6. Yusuf S, Rangarajan S, Teo K, Islam S, Li W, Liu L, et al. Cardiovascular risk and events in 17 low-, middle-, and high-income countries. *N Engl J Med.* 2014;371:818-827.
7. Forouzanfar MH, Alexander L, Anderson HR, Bachman VF, Biryukov S, Brauer M, et al. Global, regional, and national comparative risk assessment of 79 behavioural, environmental and occupational, and metabolic risks or clusters of risks in 188 countries, 1990-2013: a systematic analysis for the Global Burden of Disease Study 2013. *Lancet.* 2015;386:2287-2323.
8. Ruiz-Hurtado G, Ruilope LM. Does cardiovascular protection translate into renal protection? *Nat Rev Cardiol.* 2014;11:742-746.
9. Roth GA, Forouzanfar MH, Moran AE, Barber R, Nguyen G, Feigin VL, et al. Demographic and epidemiologic drivers of global cardiovascular mortality. *N Engl J Med.* 2015;372:1333-1341.
10. Schargrodsky H, Hernández-Hernández R, Champagne BM, Silva H, Vinueza R, Silva Ayçaguer LC, et al. CARMELA: assessment of cardiovascular risk in seven Latin American cities. *Am J Med.* 2008;121:58-65.
11. Burroughs Peña MS, Mendes Abdala CV, Silva LC, Ordúñez P. Usefulness for surveillance of hypertension prevalence studies in Latin America and the Caribbean: the past 10 years. *Rev Panam Salud Publica.* 2012;32:15-21.

12. Rivera-Andrade A, Luna MA. Trends and heterogeneity of cardiovascular disease and risk factors across Latin American and Caribbean countries. *Prog Cardiovasc Dis.* 2014;57:276-285.

13. Avezum Á, Costa-Filho FF, Pieri A, Martins SO, Marin-Neto JA. Stroke in Latin America: Burden of Disease and Opportunities for Prevention. *Glob Heart.* 2015;10:323-331.

14. Rasolt D. Rising hypertension, cardiovascular disease, in Latin America (2014). Madeira Beach, FL: Defeat Diabetes Foundation. http://www.defeatdiabetes.org/rising-hypertension-cardiovascular-disease-latin-america/#sthas.KyhrN4Qg.wPYHEO01.dpuf.

15. Ezzati M, Riboli E. Behavioral and dietary risk factors for noncommunicable diseases. *N Engl J Med.* 2013;369:954-964.

16. Egan BM, Zhao Y, Axon RN. US trends in prevalence, awareness, treatment, and control of hypertension, 1988-2008. *JAMA.* 2010;303:2043-2050.

17. Yoon SS, Ostchega Y, Louis T. Recent trends in the prevalence of high blood pressure and its treatment and control, 1999-2008. *NCHS Data Brief.* 2010:1-8.

18. Yoon SS, Burt V, Louis T, Carroll MD. Hypertension among adults in the United States, 2009-2010. *NCHS Data Brief.* 2012:1-8.

19. Ventura H, Piña IL, Lavie CJ. Hypertension and antihypertensive therapy in Hispanics and Mexican Americans living in the United States. *Postgrad Med.* 2011;123:46-57.

20. Barquera S, Durazo-Arvizu RA, Luke A, Cao G, Cooper RS. Hypertension in Mexico and among Mexican Americans: prevalence and treatment patterns. *J Hum Hypertens.* 2008;22:617-626.

21. Ruilope LM. Current challenges in the clinical management of hypertension. *Nat Rev Cardiol.* 2012;9:267-275.

22. Lewin AJ, Kereiakes DJ, Chrysant SG, Izzo JL, Oparil S, Lee J, et al. Triple-combination treatment with olmesartan medoxomil/amlodipine/hydrochlorothiazide in Hispanic/Latino patients with hypertension: the TRINITY study. *Ethn Dis.* 2014;24:41-47.

23. Sorlie PD, Allison MA, Avilés-Santa ML, Cai J, Daviglus ML, Howard AG, et al. Prevalence of hypertension, awareness, treatment, and control in the Hispanic Community Health Study/Study of Latinos. *Am J Hypertens.* 2014;27:793-800.

24. Yoon SS, Gu Q, Nwankwo T, Wright JD, Hong Y, Burt V. Trends in blood pressure among adults with hypertension: United States, 2003 to 2012. *Hypertension.* 2015;65:54-61.

25. Gu Q, Burt VL, Dillon CF, Yoon S. Trends in antihypertensive medication use and blood pressure control among United States adults with hypertension: the National Health And Nutrition Examination Survey, 2001 to 2010. *Circulation.* 2012;126:2105-2114.

26. Campbell PT, Krim SR, Lavie CJ, Ventura HO. Clinical characteristics, treatment patterns and outcomes of Hispanic hypertensive patients. *Prog Cardiovasc Dis.* 2014;57:244-252.

27. Daviglus ML, Talavera GA, Avilés-Santa ML, Allison M, Cai J, Criqui MH, et al. Prevalence of major cardiovascular risk factors and cardiovascular diseases among Hispanic/Latino individuals of diverse backgrounds in the United States. *JAMA.* 2012;308:1775-1784.

28. Rodriguez CJ, Daviglus ML, Swett K, González HM, Gallo LC, Wassertheil-Smoller S, et al. Dyslipidemia patterns among Hispanics/Latinos of diverse background in the United States. *Am J Med.* 2014;127:1186-1194.e1.

29. Perez A. Acculturation, health literacy, and illness perceptions of hypertension among Hispanic adults. *J Transcult Nurs.* 2015;26:386-394.

30. Richardson SI, Freedman BI, Ellison DH, Rodriguez CJ. Salt sensitivity: a review with a focus on non-Hispanic blacks and Hispanics. *J Am Soc Hypertens.* 2013;7:170-179.

31. Heiss G, Snyder ML, Teng Y, Schneiderman N, Llabre MM, Cowie C, et al. Prevalence of metabolic syndrome among Hispanics/Latinos of diverse background: the Hispanic Community Health Study/Study of Latinos. *Diabetes Care.* 2014;37:2391-2399.

32. Carrington MJ, Jennings GL, Stewart S. Pressure points in primary care: blood pressure and management of hypertension in 532050 patients from 2005 to 2010. *J Hypertens.* 2013;31:1265-1271.

33. Padwal RS, Bienek A, McAlister FA, Campbell NR. ORTF of the CHE program. Epidemiology of Hypertension in Canada: an Update. *Can J Cardiol.* 2016;32:687-694.

34. Banegas JR, Graciani A, de la Cruz-Troca JJ, León-Muñoz LM, Guallar-Castillón P, Coca A, et al. Achievement of cardiometabolic goals in aware hypertensive patients in Spain: a nationwide population-based study. *Hypertension.* 2012;60:898-905.

35. Polonia J, Martins L, Pinto F, Nazare J. Prevalence, awareness, treatment and control of hypertension and salt intake in Portugal: changes over a decade. The PHYSA study. *J Hypertens.* 2014;32:1211-1221.

36. Kastarinen M, Antikainen R, Peltonen M, Laatikainen T, Barengo NC, Jula A, et al. Prevalence, awareness and treatment of hypertension in Finland during 1982-2007. *J Hypertens.* 2009;27:1552-1559.

37. Tocci G, Muiesan ML, Parati G, Agabiti Rosei E, Ferri C, Virdis A, et al. Trends in prevalence, awareness, treatment, and control of blood pressure recorded from 2004 to 2014 during World Hypertension Day in Italy. *J Clin Hypertens (Greenwich).* 2016;18:551-556.

38. Neuhauser HK, Adler C, Rosario AS, Diederichs C, Ellert U. Hypertension prevalence, awareness, treatment and control in Germany 1998 and 2008-11. *J Hum Hypertens.* 2015;29:247-253.

39. Falaschetti E, Mindell J, Knott C, Poulter N. Hypertension management in England: a serial cross-sectional study from 1994 to 2011. *Lancet.* 2014;383:1912-1919.

40. Ikeda N, Gakidou E, Hasegawa T, Murray CJ. Understanding the decline of mean systolic blood pressure in Japan: an analysis of pooled data from the National Nutrition Survey, 1986-2002. *Bull World Health Organ.* 2008;86:978-988.

41. Li D, Lv J, Liu F, Liu P, Yang X, Feng Y, et al. Hypertension burden and control in mainland China: analysis of nationwide data 2003-2012. *Int J Cardiol.* 2015;184:637-644.

42. Anchala R, Kannuri NK, Pant H, Khan H, Franco OH, Di Angelantonio E, et al. Hypertension in India: a systematic review and meta-analysis of prevalence, awareness, and control of hypertension. *J Hypertens.* 2014;32:1170-1177.

43. Ibrahim MM, Rizk H, Appel LJ, el Aroussy W, Helmy S, Sharaf Y, et al. Hypertension prevalence, awareness, treatment, and control in Egypt. Results from the Egyptian National Hypertension Project (NHP). NHP Investigative Team. *Hypertension.* 1995;26(6 Pt 1):886-890.

44. Camara A, Baldé NM, Diakité M, Sylla D, Baldé EH, Kengne AP, et al. High prevalence, low awareness, treatment and control rates of hypertension in Guinea: results from a population-based STEPS survey. *J Hum Hypertens.* 2016;30:237-244.

45. Seedat YK. Control of hypertension in South Africa: time for action. *S Afr Med J.* 2012;102:25-26.

3 Hypertension in East Asians and Native Hawaiians

Ji-Guang Wang and Qi-Fang Huang

With the changes in lifestyle and increasing longevity, the prevalence of hypertension increases worldwide. However, several classes of efficacious antihypertensive drugs are readily available for the management of hypertension in most countries or regions. In the past several decades, several national or regional epidemiologic studies on hypertension and outcome trials on the management of hypertension were conducted in East Asians and native Hawaiians. In this chapter, we review the literature of epidemiology and outcome trials on hypertension in this region.

EPIDEMIOLOGY OF HYPERTENSION IN EAST ASIANS AND NATIVE HAWAIIANS

Prevalence of Hypertension

After World War II, the prevalence of hypertension increased substantially in most countries and regions in East Asia and Hawaii. If the case of China would be taken as an example, the prevalence of hypertension increased from less than 10% before 1980[1,2] to approximately 25% in the latest nationwide survey in 2012 (Fig. 3.1).[3,4] This increase can to some extent be attributable to the increased number of elderly people over the years. However, the Westernized lifestyle characterized by high salt, high fat, high sugar and high calorie diet and physical inactivity could be a major risk factor for the increasing prevalence of hypertension in these populations.

When the most recent data from East Asians and native Hawaiians were compared across countries or regions, the prevalence of hypertension ranged from about 25% in Chinese living either in the mainland[4] or in Taiwan[5] and Koreans[6] to approximately 40% in Mongolians[7] and Native Hawaiians (Table 3.1).[8,9] The overall prevalence of hypertension was not reported in the most recent Japanese national blood pressure survey in 2010. The age-specific data suggested that the prevalence of hypertension in Japanese was high.[10] The prevalence of hypertension in persons aged 60 to 69 years was more than 60% in both men and women,[10] much higher than the 49.1% of prevalence in Chinese aged 60 years or older in 2002.[4]

Awareness, Treatment, and Control of Hypertension

There is not much high quality data on the management of hypertension except for the national blood pressure surveys in China[4] and Korea.[5] According to the currently available data, Koreans[6] and Japanese[10] seemed to have higher awareness, treatment, and control rates of hypertension than other East Asian populations[4,5,7] and native Hawaiians (Table 3.1).[9] The control rate of hypertension was about 35% in Koreans[6] and Japanese,[7] 24% in Mongolians,[7] and less than 10% in Chinese.[4]

OUTCOME TRIALS IN HYPERTENSION IN EAST ASIANS AND NATIVE HAWAIIANS

Placebo-Controlled Trials

Since the late 1980s, several placebo-controlled outcome trials were conducted in China to investigate whether antihypertensive therapy would prevent cardiovascular complications in hypertensive patients (Table 3.2).[11-14]

The Systolic Hypertension in China (Syst-China) trial investigated whether active antihypertensive treatment would prevent fatal and nonfatal stroke in 2394 elderly (≥60 years) patients with isolated systolic hypertension (systolic blood pressure ≥160 mm Hg and diastolic blood pressure <95 mm Hg). Active antihypertensive treatment was initiated by nitrendipine, with the possible addition of captopril and hydrochlorothiazide, to achieve the goal systolic blood pressure of 150 mm Hg or lower. At 2 years of follow up, active treatment (n = 1253), compared with placebo (n = 1141), reduced systolic/diastolic blood pressure by 9.1/3.2 mm Hg. During a median follow up of 3 years, active treatment reduced the incidence rate of fatal and nonfatal stroke by 38%. Active treatment also significantly reduced all-cause mortality, cardiovascular mortality, stroke mortality and all fatal and nonfatal cardiovascular endpoints by 39%, 39%, 58%, and 37%, respectively.[11]

The Shanghai Trial of Nifedipine in the Elderly (STONE) was a single-blind study in 1632 elderly (60 to 79 years) patients with hypertension (systolic blood pressure 160 to 219 mm Hg or diastolic blood pressure 96 to 124 mm Hg), alternatively allocated to either nifedipine (n = 817) or placebo (n = 815). During a mean follow up of 30 months, nifedipine treatment reduced systolic/diastolic blood pressure by 9.3/5.5 mm Hg, and the incidence of fatal and nonfatal

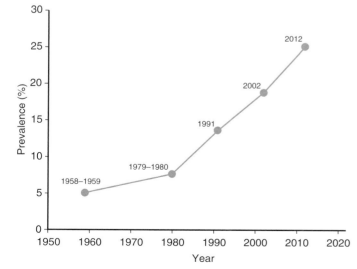

FIG. 3.1 Prevalence of hypertension in five China national surveys from 1958 to 2012. Data on the 2012 survey was only available in a governmental brief.

TABLE 3.1 Characteristics of Epidemiologic Studies on Hypertension in East Asians and Native Hawaiians

COUNTRY OR REGION AND YEAR	AGE RANGE, YEARS	NUMBER OF SUBJECTS	PREVALENCE, %	AWARENESS, %	TREATMENT, %	AWARE AND TREATED, %	CONTROL, %	TREATED AND CONTROLLED, %
China								
1991[3]	≥15	950,356	11.3	26.6	12.1	45.5	2.8	23.1
2002[4]	≥18	141,892	18.8	30.2	24.7	81.8	6.1	25.0
2002[4]	≥60	NR	49.1	37.6	36.2	96.3	7.6	24.1
Japan[10]								
2010	30-39	NR	Men 20; Women 5.6	—	—	—	—	—
2010	40-49	NR	Men 29.9; Women 12.6	—	—	—	—	—
2010	50-59	NR	Men 63.2; Women 38.4	—	Men 43.4; Women 31.2	—	Men 32.1; Women 44.1	—
2010	60-69	NR	Men 65.6; Women 62.3	—	Men 50.6; Women 68.8	—	Men 29.9; Women 40.9	—
2010	70-79	NR	Men 80.8; Women 71.2	—	Men 29.9; Women 12.6	—	Men 33.3; Women 40.5	—
Korea[6]								
2008	≥30	9146	24.9	60.6	52.2	86.2	36.7	70.3
Mongolia[7]								
2009	15-64	4502	36.5	65.8	35.9	54.6%	24.1	67.1
Native Hawaiians[9]								
1985	20-59	257	25	—	—	—	—	—
Taiwan[5]								
1993-1996	≥19	6,479	23.5	—	—	—	—	—

NR, Not reported.

TABLE 3.2 Characteristics of Trials

TRIAL	MASKING	NUMBER OF PATIENTS	ANTIHYPERTENSIVE TREATMENT (MG)	AGE, YEARS Entry Criteria	AGE, YEARS Mean (SD)	Entry Criteria	SBP/DBP, MM HG Mean (SD) at Baseline	Difference During FU	FU TIME	FAVORABLE RESULTS
Active treatment vs. placebo or no treatment										
FEVER[13]	Double	9800	HCTZ (12.5)+felodipine (5-10) vs. HCTZ (12.5)+placebo	50-79	61.5 (7.2)	140-180/90-100 on HCTZ (12.5 mg)	154.3/91.2 (17.5/9.6)	4.2/2.1	40 m	Felodipine
PATS[14]	Double	5665	Indapamide (2.5) vs. placebo	None	60 (8)	None	154/93 (23/13)	5/2	2 y	Indapamide
STONE[12]	Single	1632	Nifedipine vs. placebo	60-79			168.5/97.7 (—/—)	9.4/5.5	30 m	Nifedipine
Syst-China[11]	Double	2394	Nitrendipine (10-40)+captopril (12.5-50)+HCTZ (12.5-50) vs. placebo	≥60	66.5 (5.5)	160-219/<95	170.5/86.0 (11.1/6.8)	9.1/3.2	3.0 y	Active treatment
Actively controlled trials										
CASE-J[17]	Open	4728	Amlodipine (2.5-10) vs. Candesartan (4-8)	None	63.8 (10.5)	140-179/90-109 (<70 y) or 160-179/90-109 (≥70 y)	162.8/91.7 (14.2/11.2)	1.7/0.6	3.2 y	Neutral
COPE[18]	Open	3293 (3501)[a]	Benidipine (4)+ARB vs. Benidipine (4)+α-blocker vs. Benidipine (4)+diuretic	40-85	63.1 (10.7)	140-199/90-119 on/off treatment	153.9/88.8 (11.6/9.7)	0.8/0.6	3.61 y	Neutral
JMIC-B[16]	Open	1650	Nifedipine Retard (20-40) vs. ACE inhibitors	<75	64.5 (8.5)	≥150/90-120 or treated	146/82 (19.5/11.5)	4/1	36 m	Neutral
NICS-EH[15]	Double	414	Nicardipine SR (40-80) vs. Trichlormethiazide (2-4)	≥60	69.8 (6.5)	160-220/<115	172.3/93.8 (11.9/10.2)	−1/−1	3 y	Neutral
Intensive vs. less intensive										
JATOS[22]	Open	4418 (4508)[a]	<140 vs. 140-159 mm Hg	65-85	73.6 (5.3)	≥160/	171.6/89.1 (9.8/9.5)	9.7/3.3	2 y	Neutral
VALISH[23]	Open	3260	<140 vs. 140-149 mm Hg	70-84	76.1 (4.1)	160-199/–	169.5/81.5	5.4/1.7	3.07	Neutral
Subgroup of multinational trials										
HYVET[26]	Double	3845 (1526)[b]	Indapamide (1.5)+perindopril (2-4) vs. placebo	≥80	83.6 (3.2)	160-199/<110	173.0/90.8 (8.5/8.5)	15.0/6.1	1.8 y	Active treatment
PROGRESS[24]	Double	6105 (2352)[b]	Perindopril (4)+indapamide (2.5) vs. placebo	None	64 (10)	<180/<110	147/86 (19/11)	9/4	3.9 y	Active treatment

[a]The number of patients analyzed was reported together with the number of randomized patients in the parentheses.
[b]In the parentheses was the number of patients recruited in China for the HYVET trial and in China and Japan for the PROGRESS trial.
FU, Follow-up; HCTZ, hydrochlorothiazide; SBP/DBP, systolic/diastolic blood pressure; SD, standard deviation; SR, sustained release.
Acronyms of trials are explained in a separate section of this article.

stroke by 58%. Nifedipine also significantly reduced the incidence of all fatal and nonfatal cardiovascular events by 60%.[12]

The Felodipine Event Reduction (FEVER) trial compared felodipine (5 mg daily) with placebo in 9800 patients (50 to 79 years of age) with a systolic/diastolic blood pressure in the range of 140 to 180/90 to 100 mm Hg after six weeks of treatment with hydrochlorothiazide (12.5 mg per day). During a mean follow up of 3.3 years, felodipine, compared with placebo, reduced systolic/diastolic blood pressure by 4.2/2.1 mm Hg, and the primary endpoint (fatal and nonfatal stroke) by 27%. Felodipine also significantly reduced all cardiovascular events, all cardiac events, all-cause mortality, coronary events, heart failure, cardiovascular death, and cancer by 27%, 35%, 31%, 32%, 30%, 33%, and 36%, respectively.[13]

The Post-stroke Antihypertensive Treatment Study (PATS) was a double-blind blood pressure lowering trial with indapamide (2.5 mg daily) in hypertensive and nonhypertensive patients with a history of stroke or transient ischemic attack. During a median follow up of 2 years, indapamide reduced systolic/diastolic blood pressure by 5/2 mm Hg, and the incidence of recurrent stroke by 29%. Indapamide also significantly reduced the incidence of all fatal and nonfatal cardiovascular endpoints by 23%.[14]

Actively Controlled Trials

Since 1990 several actively controlled outcome trials were conducted in Japan to compare various classes or combinations of antihypertensive drugs as initial therapy for the prevention of cardiovascular complications (Table 3.2).[15-18] All these trials had an open design, except for the double-dummy National Intervention Cooperative Study in Elderly Hypertensives (NICS-EH),[15] and had a relatively small sample size in the detection of a modest or moderate difference between antihypertensive drug classes.

NICS-EH compared two outdated antihypertensive drugs (sustained-release nicardipine [n = 204] versus trichlormethiazide [n = 210]) in 414 elderly (≥60 years) patients with hypertension (systolic blood pressure 160 to 220 mm Hg and diastolic blood pressure <115 mm Hg). During 5 years of follow up, nicardipine was slightly less efficacious than trichlormethiazide in lowering systolic/diastolic blood pressure (−1/−1 mm Hg). During follow-up, a total of 39 events occurred in the two groups combined, and no significant difference was observed in any outcome between the two treatment groups.[15]

The Japan Multicenter Investigation for Cardiovascular Diseases-B (JMIC-B) trial compared nifedipine retard with angiotensin-converting enzyme inhibitors (enalapril 5 to 10 mg, imidapril 5 to 10 mg, or lisinopril 10 to 20 mg, once daily) in 1650 patients with both hypertension and coronary heart disease, diagnosed according to coronary angiography (stenosis ≥75%), a history of angina pectoris (>2 episodes per week), or ST-segment depression of at least 1 mm during the treadmill exercise test. During a mean follow up of 36 months, blood pressure reductions were greater in the nifedipine group than the angiotensin converting enzyme (ACE) inhibitors group (−4/−1 mm Hg): The incidence rate of the primary endpoint (cardiac events: cardiac death or sudden death, myocardial infarction, hospitalization for angina pectoris or heart failure, serious arrhythmia, and coronary interventions) was similar in the nifedipine (116 events, 14.0%) and angiotensin converting enzyme inhibitors (106 events, 12.9%) groups (+5%; p = 0.75).[16]

The Candesartan Antihypertensive Survival Evaluation in Japan (CASE-J) trial compared amlodipine- with candesartan-based antihypertensive regimens in 4728 high risk hypertensive patients. To achieve the goal blood pressure

of 140/90 mm Hg or below, diuretics, α-blockers, β-blockers, and/or αβ-blockers could be added. During a mean follow up of 3.2 years, systolic/diastolic blood pressures were 1.7/0.6 lower in the amlodipine group than the candesartan group, despite the fact that more patients in the candesartan group required addition of other antihypertensive drugs (54.5% versus 42.7%; p < 0.0001). The incidence rates of the primary (sudden death and cerebrovascular, cardiac, renal, and vascular events) and secondary endpoints were not statistically different between the two treatment groups. The risk of stroke was slightly but not significantly lower in the amlodipine group than the candesartan group (−23%; p = 0.28).[17]

The Combination Therapy of Hypertension to Prevent Cardiovascular Events (COPE) trial was designed to compare three combinations of antihypertensive drugs in the prevention of cardiovascular events in 3501 patients 40 to 85 years old and with uncontrolled hypertension (systolic/diastolic blood pressure ≥ 140/90 mm Hg) by calcium channel blocker benidipine 4 mg per day. Patients were randomly assigned to receive angiotensin receptor blocker (n = 1167), β-blocker (n = 1166), or thiazide diuretic (n = 1168) in addition to benidipine. During a median follow up of 3.61 years, blood pressure was reduced similarly in the three groups, with a control rate of 64.1%, 66.9%, and 66.0% at the end of treatment in the benidipine-angiotensin receptor blocker, benidipine-β-blocker, and benidipine-thiazide groups, respectively. The cardiovascular composite endpoint occurred in 41 (3.7%), 48 (4.4%), and 32 (2.9%) patients, respectively, with a hazard ratio of 1.26 (p = 0.35) in the benidipine-angiotensin receptor blocker and 1.54 (p = 0.06) in the benidipine-β-blocker groups compared with the benidipine-thiazide group.[18]

None of these trials had sufficient power to detect a modest or moderate but clinically relevant difference between various classes of antihypertensive drugs. However, if the results of these trials would be pooled with that of studies in other populations, there could be significant difference between different drug classes. For instance, if the CASE-J trial[17] was combined with the Valsartan Antihypertensive Long-term Use Evaluation (VALUE)[19] and Irbesartan Diabetic Nephropathy Trial (IDNT),[20] trials that also compared amlodipine with an angiotensin receptor blocker, amlodipine provided superior protection against stroke and myocardial infarction by 16% and 17%, respectively.[21]

Intensive Versus Less Intensive Blood Pressure Control

Two Japanese trials compared intensive with less intensive blood pressure control in elderly hypertensive patients.[22,23] These two trials again had a relatively small sample size and hence inadequate power in the detection of a modest or moderate difference between different levels of blood pressure control.

The Japanese Trial to Assess Optimal Systolic Blood Pressure in Elderly Hypertensive Patients (JATOS) compared two-year effect of intensive (systolic blood pressure <140 mm Hg, n = 2212) versus less intensive treatment (systolic blood pressure 140 to 159 mm Hg, n = 2206) in 4418 elderly (65 to 85 years) patients with essential hypertension (pretreatment systolic blood pressure ≥160 mm Hg). The first line drug was a long-acting calcium channel blocker, efonidipine. At the last clinic visit, systolic/diastolic blood pressures were significantly lower in the intensive than the less intensive-treatment group (135.9/74.8 versus 145.6/78.1 mm Hg), with a between group difference of 9.7/3.3 mm Hg. However, no significant difference between the two treatment groups was observed for the incidence of the primary endpoint (combination of cardiovascular disease and renal failure, 86 patients in each group; *p* = 0.99) and for total mortality (54 in the intensive-treatment group versus 42 in the less intensive-treatment group, *p* = 0.22). In a post-hoc analysis, however, there was interaction between age and treatment for the primary endpoint (*p* = 0.03). Intensive blood pressure control tended to confer benefit in younger elderly (65 to 74 years) but harm in older elderly (≥75 years).[22]

The Valsartan in Elderly Isolated Systolic Hypertension (VALISH) Study compared intensive (systolic blood pressure ≤140 mm Hg, n = 1545) with less intensive blood pressure control (systolic blood pressure 140 to 150 mm Hg, n = 1534) in the prevention of cardiovascular mortality and morbidity in 3260 elderly patients (70 to 84 years) with isolated systolic hypertension (systolic blood pressure 160 to 199 mm Hg). At baseline, age averaged 76.1 years, and systolic/diastolic blood pressures were 169.5/81.5 mm Hg. At 3 years of follow up, systolic/diastolic blood pressures were 136.6/74.8 mm Hg and 142.0/76.5 mm Hg, respectively, with a between-group difference of 5.4/1.7 mm Hg. During a median follow-up of 3.07 years, the overall rate of the primary composite endpoint was slightly lower in the intensive (10.6/1000 patient-years) than the less intensive blood pressure control group (12.0/1000 patient-years, hazard ratio 0.89; 95% CI 0.60 to 1.34; *p* = 0.38). However, none of the differences between the two groups reached statistical significance for any outcome.[23]

Subgroups of Multinational Trials

Since 1990, several multinational trials in blood pressure lowering treatment involved East Asians, such as the perindopril PROtection aGainst REcurrent Stroke Study (PROGRESS)[24] and the HYpertension in the Very Elderly Trial (HYVET).[25]

The PROGRESS trial was designed to determine the effects of a blood-pressure lowering regimen in 6105 hypertensive and nonhypertensive patients with a history of stroke or transient ischemic attack, recruited from 172 centers in Asia, Australasia, and Europe. Over 4 years of follow up, active treatment (perindopril 4 mg daily with the possible addition of indapamide, n = 3051), compared with placebo (n = 3054), reduced blood pressure by 9/4 mm Hg, and the incidence of fatal and nonfatal stroke by 28%. Active treatment also significantly reduced the risk of total major vascular events by 26%.[24] Of particular note, the PROGRESS trial included 2335 Asians, either Chinese or Japanese. Active treatment reduced systolic/diastolic blood pressure by 10.3/4.6 mm Hg in Asians and by 8.1/3.6 mm Hg in Western participants. The risk reduction also tended to be greater in Asians for stroke (39% versus 22%, *p* for homogeneity = 0.10) and major vascular events (38% versus 20%, *p* for homogeneity = 0.06).[26]

The HYVET trial investigated whether or not antihypertensive treatment would reduce the risk of stroke in 3845 very elderly (≥80 years) patients with hypertension (systolic blood pressure ≥160 mm Hg and diastolic blood pressure <110), recruited from Australasia, China, Europe, and Tunisia. Active treatment was started by indapamide (sustained release, 1.5 mg) with the possible addition of perindopril 2 or 4 mg. At 2 years of follow up, active treatment (n = 1933), compared with placebo (n = 1912), reduced systolic/diastolic blood pressure by 15.0/6.1 mm Hg. During a median follow up of 1.8 years, active treatment reduced the incidence of fatal and nonfatal stroke by 30%, stroke mortality by 39%, all-cause mortality by 21%, cardiovascular mortality by 23%, and heart failure by 64%.[25] The HYVET trial included 1526 patients from China. Although the outcome results in Chinese were not published separately, the overall results should apply for the Chinese people of 80 years or older.[27]

SUMMARY

There is some but insufficient epidemiologic and outcome trial data from patients of East Asian and native Hawaiian origin. Nonetheless, the currently available data suggested that the prevalence of hypertension was high and antihypertensive treatment was highly efficacious in the prevention of cardiovascular complications especially stroke. The trials that compared intensive with less intensive antihypertensive therapy did not prove to be superior in lowering blood pressure to a level below 140 mm Hg in elderly Japanese. These trials had a relatively small sample size and short duration of follow up, and therefore probably had inadequate power to detect modest or moderate benefit. There is still apparently a need for high quality epidemiologic studies and outcome trials in East Asians and native Hawaiians.

CONFLICTS OF INTEREST

Dr. Wang reports receiving lecture and consulting fees from MSD, Novartis, Pfizer, Sankyo, Sanofi, and Servier. Dr. Huang declares no conflict of interest.

ACRONYMS OF TRIALS

CASE-J (Candesartan Antihypertensive Survival Evaluation in Japan Trial); **COPE** (The Combination Therapy of Hypertension to Prevent Cardiovascular Events); **FEVER** (Felodipine Event Reduction Study); **HYVET** (Hypertension in the Very Elderly Trial); **IDNT** (Irbesartan Diabetic Nephropathy Trial); **JATOS** (The Japanese Trial to Assess Optimal Systolic Blood Pressure in Elderly Hypertensive Patients); **JMIC-B** (Japan Multicenter Investigation for Cardiovascular Diseases-B); **NICS-EH** (National Intervention Cooperative Study in Elderly Hypertensives); **PATS** (Post-stroke Antihypertensive Treatment Study); **PROGRESS** (Perindopril PrOtection Against Recurrent Stroke Study); **STONE** (Shanghai Trial of Nifedipine in the Elderly); **Syst-China** (Systolic Hypertension in China trial); **VALISH** (The Valsartan in Elderly Isolated Systolic Hypertension); and **VALUE** (Valsartan Antihypertensive Long-term Use Evaluation (VALUE).

References

1. Wu YK, Lu CQ, Gao RC, Yu JS, Liu GC. Nation-wide hypertension screening in China during 1979-1980. *Chin Med J (Engl)*. 1982;95:101-108.
2. Wu YK, Wu ZS, Yao CH. Epidemiologic studies of cardiovascular diseases in China. *Chin Med J (Engl)*. 1983;96:201-205.
3. Wu X, Duan X, Gu D, Hao J, Tao S, Fan D. Prevalence of hypertension and its trends in Chinese populations. *Int J Cardiol*. 1995;52:39-44.
4. Li LM, Rao KQ, Kong LZ, Yao CH, Xiang HD, Zhai FY, Ma GS, Yang XG and the Technical Working Group of China National Nutrition and Health Survey. A description on the Chinese national nutrition and health survey in 2002. *Chin J Epidemiol*. 2005;26:478-484 (Chinese).
5. Pan WH, Chang HY, Yeh WT, Hsiao SY, Hung YT. Prevalence, awareness, treatment and control of hypertension in Taiwan: results of Nutrition and Health Survey in Taiwan (NAHSIT) 1993-1996. *J Hum Hypertens*. 2001;15:793-798.
6. Lee HS, Lee SS, Hwang IY, et al. Prevalence, awareness, treatment and control of hypertension in adults with diagnosed diabetes: the Fourth Korea National Health and Nutrition Examination Survey (KNHANES IV). *J Hum Hypertens*. 2013;27:381-387.
7. Otgontuya D, Oum S, Palam E, Rani M, Buckley BS. Individual-based primary prevention of cardiovascular disease in Cambodia and Mongolia: early identification and management of hypertension and diabetes mellitus. *BMC Public Health*. 2012;12:254.
8. Kaholokula JK, Iwane MK, Nacapoy AH. Effects of perceived racism and acculturation on hypertension in Native Hawaiians. *Hawaii Med J*. 2010;69(Suppl 2):11-15.
9. Curb JD, Aluli NE, Huang BJ, et al. Hypertension in elderly Japanese Americans and adult native Hawaiians. *Public Health Rep*. 1996;111(Suppl 2):53-55.
10. Miura K, Nagai M, Ohkubo T. Epidemiology of hypertension in Japan: where are we now? *Circ J*. 2013;77:2226-2231.
11. Liu L, Wang JG, Gong L, Liu G, Staessen JA, for the Systolic Hypertension in China (Syst-China) Collaborative Group. Comparison of active treatment and placebo for older Chinese patients with isolated systolic hypertension. *J Hypertens*. 1998;16:1823-1829.
12. Gong L, Zhang W, Zhu Y, et al. Shanghai trial of nifedipine in the elderly (STONE). *J Hypertens*. 1996;14:1237-1245.
13. Liu L, Zhang Y, Liu G, Li W, Zhang X, Zanchetti A. FEVER Study Group: The Felodipine Event Reduction (FEVER) Study: a randomized long-term placebo-controlled trial in Chinese hypertensive patients. *J Hypertens*. 2005;23:2157-2172.
14. PATS Collaborative Group. Post-stroke antihypertensive treatment study: A preliminary result. *Chin Med J*. 1995;108:710-717.
15. National Intervention Cooperative Study in Elderly Hypertensives Study Group. Randomized double-blind comparison of a calcium antagonist and a diuretic in elderly hypertensives. *Hypertension*. 1999;34:1129-1133.

16. Yui Y, Sumiyoshi T, Kodama K, et al. Comparison of nifedipine retard with angiotensin converting enzyme inhibitors in Japanese hypertensive patients with coronary artery disease: the Japan Multicenter Investigation for Cardiovascular Diseases-B (JMIC-B) randomized trial. *Hypertens Res*. 2004;27:181-191.

17. Ogihara T, Nakao K, Fukui T, et al. Effects of candesartan compared with amlodipine in hypertensive patients with high cardiovascular risks: candesartan antihypertensive survival evaluation in Japan trial. *Hypertension*. 2008;51:393-398.

18. Matsuzaki M, Ogihara T, Umemoto S, et al. Prevention of cardiovascular events with calcium channel blocker-based combination therapies in patients with hypertension: a randomized controlled trial. *J Hypertens*. 2011;29:1649-1659.

19. Julius S, Kjeldsen SE, Weber M, et al. Outcomes in hypertensive patients at high cardiovascular risk treated with regimens based on valsartan or amlodipine: the VALUE randomised trial. *Lancet*. 2004;363:2022-2031.

20. Lewis EJ, Hunsicker LG, Clarke WR, et al. Renoprotective effect of the angiotensin-receptor antagonist irbesartan in patients with nephropathy due to type 2 diabetes. *N Engl J Med*. 2001;345:851-860.

21. Wang JG, Li Y, Franklin S, Safar M. Prevention of stroke and myocardial infarction by amlodipine and angiotensin receptor blockers: a quantitative overview. *Hypertension*. 2007;50:181-188.

22. JATOS Study Group. Principal results of the Japanese trial to assess optimal systolic blood pressure in elderly hypertensive patients (JATOS). *Hypertens Res*. 2008;31:2115-2127.

23. Ogihara T, Saruta T, Rakugi H, et al. Target blood pressure for treatment of isolated systolic hypertension in the elderly: valsartan in elderly isolated systolic hypertension study. *Hypertension*. 2010;56:196-202.

24. PROGRESS Collaborative Group: Randomised trial of a perindopril-based blood pressure lowering regimen among 6105 individuals with prior stroke or transient ischaemic attack. *Lancet*. 2001;358:1033-1041.

25. Arima H, Anderson C, Omae T, et al. Perindopril-based blood pressure lowering reduces major vascular events in Asian and Western participants with cerebrovascular disease: the PROGRESS trial. *J Hypertens*. 2010;28:395-400.

26. Beckett NS, Peters R, Fletcher AE, et al. Treatment of hypertension in patients 80 years of age or older. *N Engl J Med*. 2008;358:1887-1898.

27. Liu L, Wang JG, Ma SP, et al. Chinese subjects entered in the Hypertension in the Very Elderly Trial (HYVET). *Chin Med J*. 2008;121:1509-1512.

4 Hypertension in South Asians

Philip Joseph, Rajeev Gupta, and Salim Yusuf

Elevated blood pressure (BP) is a growing health problem in South Asia, where it is the second largest risk factor for disability-adjusted life years lost, predominantly because of its strong relationship with cardiovascular disease (CVD) development. Within India, it has been estimated that hypertension accounts for 57% of all stroke related deaths and 24% of coronary artery disease related deaths. Thus, a significant proportion of death and disability in the region can be reduced by improving BP control.[1]

In South Asia, there has been a steady rise in both the age- and sex-adjusted mean population BP, and the prevalence of hypertension, over the past two decades.[2] Significant gaps in hypertension management are also present across South Asia, with less than half of individuals with high BP aware of it, and poor control in more than 80% with high BP. If left unaddressed, these trends will substantially increase CVD morbidity and mortality related to elevated BP. This chapter will focus on the epidemiology of hypertension and its management in South Asian populations. First we will examine the prevalence of hypertension, and its variation across South Asia. Next, we will examine the major modifiable and genetic risk factors associated with hypertension incidence in South Asians, and finally, we will summarize current gaps in hypertension management that need to be addressed in the region.

PREVALENCE OF HYPERTENSION IN SOUTH ASIAN POPULATIONS

Definition of Hypertension in the South Asian Population

It has been recommended that some CVD risk factors in South Asians (e.g., obesity) warrant lower thresholds to define risk when compared with other ethnic groups. This is because of evidence that CVD in South Asians occurs at lower age and risk factor thresholds. Studies also suggest that certain physiologic BP parameters (e.g., pulse pressure, postexercise BP) differ, and that BP may have a stronger association with stroke risk in South Asians compared with white Europeans.[3,4] However, there is no definitive evidence that, for a given BP, South Asian populations are at a higher CVD risk, and a systolic blood pressure (SBP) greater than 140 mm Hg and/or diastolic blood pressure (DBP) greater than 90 mm Hg remains the currently accepted threshold to diagnose hypertension in South Asian populations.

Prevalence of Hypertension in South Asia

Estimates of hypertension vary substantially across countries in South Asia, which is partly due to demographic differences between the populations studied. For example, in a systematic review of 33 observational studies (of 220,539 participants, with a mean age of 43.7 years) from seven countries in South Asia, the prevalence of hypertension was approximately 27%, ranging from 17.9% in Bangladesh to 33.8% in Nepal.[5] By contrast, in the Prospective Urban Rural Epidemiology (PURE) study, which studied a slightly older population cohort of 33,000 participants (mean age 48.5 years, age range 35 to 70

years) from India, Pakistan, and Bangladesh, hypertension was diagnosed in one-third of individuals, with the highest prevalence in Bangladesh (39.3%), followed by Pakistan (33.3%), and lowest in India (30.7%).[6] Despite these observed differences between studies, the prevalence of hypertension has been consistently shown to be higher in men compared with women, and in urban compared with rural areas.[5]

In fact, transition from the rural to urban environment is a key societal factor driving the increasing prevalence of hypertension. In India, the prevalence of hypertension has increased dramatically over the past several decades with a higher burden reported in urban areas.[1] In a systematic review of 142 studies conducted in India, it was estimated that 29.8% of adults had hypertension; and in urban areas, where extensive changes in health-related behaviors have already occurred, the prevalence of hypertension was higher (33.8%) compared with rural areas (27.6%) (Fig. 4.1). Furthermore, the prevalence of hypertension varied substantially in rural areas (which was not observed in urban areas) likely reflecting the different stages of economic development, urbanization and transitions in health-related behaviors occurring across rural environments in India.[7]

Prevalence of Hypertension in South Asians Who Have Migrated to North America or Europe

Compared with other ethnic groups living in the same macroenvironment, South Asians have a unique cardiovascular risk profile, characterized by a higher risk of diabetes, higher percent body fat, and lower high density lipoprotein concentration compared with other ethnic groups. Some studies suggest that the risk of hypertension is also modestly increased in South Asians compared with Caucasians living in the same country. In a systematic review of 13 hypertension prevalence studies (n ≈ 650,000 individuals) in Canada, the risk of hypertension was slightly higher in South Asians compared with Caucasians (odds ratio [OR] 1.11, 95% confidence interval [CI] 1.02 to 1.22, p = 0.02).[8] However, this association has not been consistently observed among South Asian populations residing in Europe.[9] Also, while the prevalence of some cardiovascular risk factors (e.g., obesity) appear to be steadily increasing in these South Asian populations over time, whether such a trend is also occurring with the prevalence of hypertension is not clearly established.[10]

RISK FACTORS FOR HYPERTENSION IN SOUTH ASIAN POPULATIONS

Genetic Factors

Although it is estimated that 30% to 70% of the phenotypic variance of BP is heritable, at the population level, only a small fraction of this variance has been explained by common genetic polymorphisms through genome wide association studies (GWAS).

GWAS have identified approximately 70 single nucleotide polymorphisms (SNPs) associated with BP. Although most of these were identified in white European populations,

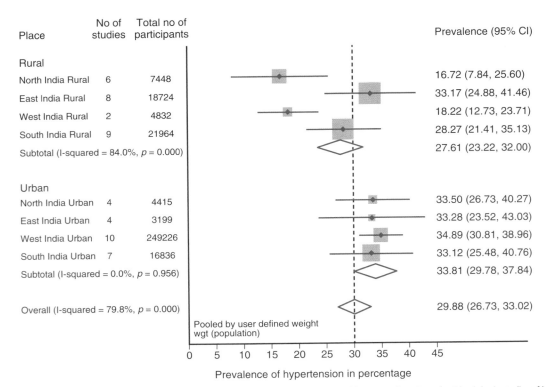

FIG. 4.1 Variations in hypertension prevalence in India by urban-rural area and geographic locations. In this systematic review of epidemiologic studies of hypertension in India, significant variation in the prevalence of hypertension was observed across different geographic region in rural areas, whereas urban areas had a similar hypertension prevalence. Overall, hypertension prevalence was higher in urban areas compared with rural areas. *wgt,* Weight. *(From Anchala R et al. Hypertension in India: A systematic review and meta-analysis of prevalence, awareness, and control of hypertension.* J Hypertens. *2014;32:1170-1177).*

approximately one-fifth appear to be shared in South Asians. Metaanalysis of 28 GWAS studies in 69,395 participants of European ancestry identified 28 independent loci significantly associated with either SBP or DBP of which six were also significantly associated with BP in 23,977 participants of South Asian ancestry.[11] Also, a recent transethnic metaanalysis of 320,251 participants of European, South Asian, and East Asian origins identified polymorphisms from 12 independent loci associated with BP traits, with consistent effects across all three ethnic groups.[12] These studies suggest that South Asians share a similar genetic predisposition to hypertension compared with other ethnic groups. However, GWAS have thus far failed to identify polymorphisms unique to South Asians that impact BP; although this may be because of methodologic factors, such as the relatively small sample sizes (and limited power) of current GWAS performed in South Asians, the limited power of GWAS to identify significant effects associated with rare polymorphisms, and differences in linkage disequilibrium between ethnic groups. Some genetic associations may be further impacted by gene-environment interactions, which could result in different genetic effects between ethnic groups when patterns of health-related behaviors also differ.

Modifiable Risk Factors for Hypertension

Risk factors for hypertension development are examined in detail in Section III of this book. Of these, several are of particular importance in South Asian populations because of their high prevalence or increasing burden within the region.

Overweight and obese: It is estimated that the risk of hypertension increases by 20% for each 5% gain in weight, and in South Asian populations obesity (commonly defined as body mass index ≥25 kg/m^2 for this group) is a common risk factor for both hypertension development, and poor hypertension control.[7,13,14] In the past two decades, the prevalence

of obesity has increased across the region; and in India, approximately 9% of men and 13% of women now meet clinical criteria for obesity, with a higher prevalence in South India, in urban areas and among women.[13]

Diabetes is associated with a three-fold to four-fold increase in the risk of hypertension in South Asian populations; and its prevalence in South Asia is now among the highest in the world.[7] In India, between 5% and 15% of individuals have diabetes depending on geographic location, with a similar prevalence reported among men and women, and a higher prevalence in urban areas.[15-17]

Smoking and alcohol consumption are each associated with a 1.5-fold to two-fold increase in hypertension risk in South Asian populations.[7] Both are substantially more common in men compared with women. National survey data from India report that 29% of men currently smoke, as compared with only 2% of women.[18] Similarly, regular alcohol use has been reported in 8% of males compared with only 1% of females.[19]

The **nutrition transition** in India as a consequence of urbanization and economic development has resulted in *lower consumption of fruits, vegetables and fiber; higher consumption of saturated fats/meat products;* and *higher sodium consumption.*[20] Although there is limited evidence examining how diet impacts BP in South Asians, available data in this population suggest that low fruit and vegetable consumption, higher fat consumption, and higher discretionary sodium consumption are associated with hypertension. Mean sodium consumption in the South Asian population is currently estimated between 3.5 and 4 g/day, a range where there is no clear impact on CVD risk.[21] However, in individuals who consume higher amounts of sodium (e.g., >5 g/day), counselling on dietary sodium reduction should occur.

In individuals without hypertension, **regular physical activity** modestly reduces BP.[22] However, epidemiologic data suggest that 54% of adults in India are physically inactive, with lower levels of physical activity occurring in urban areas, and among men. Furthermore, 85% of individuals do not engage in any recreational physical activities.[23] Although this may be partly counterbalanced by obligatory physical activity (e.g., occupational activities), a greater public health emphasis on policies that promote physical activity is still needed.

MANAGEMENT OF HYPERTENSION IN SOUTH ASIANS

Lifestyle and Behavioral Modification

Adopting healthy behaviors is an important component for both preventing hypertension and reducing BP in patients with established hypertension. Particular emphasis should be placed on weight loss in overweight or obese individuals, reducing sodium consumption in those with high sodium intake (e.g., >5 g/day), increasing fruit and vegetable intake, and reducing saturated fat intake. Smoking avoidance or cessation, and limiting alcohol consumption should be promoted in all individuals, with a particular focus on men, where the prevalence of both is substantially higher compared with women. Increasing physical activity can reduce BP both directly and indirectly through weight loss. In patients with hypertension, these lifestyle changes have each been shown to have small to moderate effects on BP reduction (ranging between 2 and 3 mm Hg for SBP), but the promotion of a healthy lifestyle also reduces CVD risk independent of BP lowering, and should be encouraged in all individuals with and without hypertension.[24]

Initiation of Antihypertensive Therapy and Treatment Targets

Most patients with hypertension will require both lifestyle modification and pharmacologic therapy to control BP. There is no consistent evidence to suggest that BP targets should differ in South Asian populations compared with other ethnic groups. Clinical outcome studies have consistently observed that in patients with stage 2 hypertension (defined as SBP of 160 to 179 mm Hg or DBP >100 to 109 mm Hg by the International Society of Hypertension), pharmacologically lowering BP is associated with a reduction in adverse cardiovascular events. Proportionally larger reductions in CVD adverse events also occur with greater reductions in BP, with no clear overall differences in outcomes based on the particular pharmacologic agent used.[25] In the SPRINT trial, which enrolled older subjects with CVD or at high CVD risk and an SBP between 130 mm Hg and 180 mm Hg (with mean enrollment BP of approximately 140/78 mm Hg), intensive BP treatment (to a target SBP <120 mm Hg) reduced cardiovascular events compared with standard BP treatment to an SBP of less than 140 mm Hg. Mean SBP was 122 mm Hg in the intensive-treatment group compared with 134 mm Hg in the standard-treatment group, and although intensive treatment was associated with better cardiovascular outcomes, this required an average of three different drugs in these individuals, and there were more side effects (including acute kidney injury and syncope).[26] The large benefits observed in SPRINT are somewhat tempered by results of other studies, such as the ACCORD study in diabetics, where similar reductions in BP with intensive treatment compared with standard management (119 mm Hg versus 134 mm Hg) resulted in a 41% reduction in stroke risk, but not in overall adverse CV events.[27] Furthermore, the recent HOPE-3 study found that in intermediate CVD risk individuals, pharmacologic blood pressure lowering only reduced major CVD events in those with a baseline systolic BP > 143 mm Hg, with no benefit in lower BP ranges.[28]

Based on current data, antihypertensive therapy should be strongly recommended for those with stage 1 or 2 hypertension (e.g., a BP > 140/90 mm Hg). In patients at otherwise

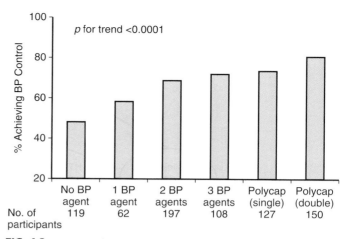

FIG. 4.2 Proportion of participants with baseline hypertension achieving adequate blood pressure control (defined as a systolic blood pressure <140 mm Hg) in TIPS-1 and TIPS-2. *BP*, Blood pressure. *(From Mente A, et al. The Role of the Polypill in Hypertension.* Special Issues in Hypertension, *2012, with permission of Springer.)*

low cardiovascular risk, a BP of less than 140/90 mm Hg is an acceptable target with pharmacologic therapy. In patients with diabetes, lower treatment targets (e.g., <130/80 mm Hg) may be considered because of its potential benefit for reducing stroke risk; and in patients with established CVD or at high risk of CVD development, intensive BP treatment to an SBP target of 120 mm Hg can be considered if the therapies are well tolerated.

Choice of Pharmacotherapy

In some ethnic groups it has been shown that certain antihypertensive agents are less efficacious (e.g., angiotensin converting enzyme inhibitors in Africans), however there are no studies that report different pharmacologic effects in South Asians. Therefore, any first line antihypertensive drugs can be considered for the treatment of hypertension. Greater BP reduction is achievable using low doses of combinations of two or three antihypertensive agents compared with standard doses of a single agent, and should be the preferred approach in most individuals when initiating pharmacologic therapy.[29]

Two studies in Indian participants have evaluated combination BP and cholesterol reduction using fixed dose combination therapy with a polypill (ie, Polycap) containing hydrochlorothiazide (12.5 mg), atenolol (25 mg), Ramipril (5 mg), simvastatin (20 mg) and aspirin (75 mg). In a 12-week, multiple comparison, randomized control trial comparing once-daily Polycap with its individual pharmacologic components it was reported that Polycap reduced SBP by 7.4 mm Hg and DBP by 5.6 mm Hg. This was significantly larger than the effects of any one BP lowering drug, and similar to the effect of all three BP lowering drugs given separately. In fact, in participants with baseline hypertension, the number of antihypertensive pills taken was significantly associated with the achievement of better BP control (Fig. 4.2). Side-effects and discontinuation rates were similar to groups that received only one of the component drugs.[30] A second clinical trial compared low dose with high-dose Polycap in 518 South Asian participants, and found that the high dose regimen further reduced BP by 25%, with similar discontinuation rates.[31] The use of a polypill has several potential benefits for hypertension management in low- and lower-middle-income countries. Firstly, larger BP reductions are achievable using combination antihypertensive treatment, which will result in a greater proportion of patients with hypertension achieving adequate BP control. Secondly, reductions in both BP and serum cholesterol can be achieved with a single pill, allowing

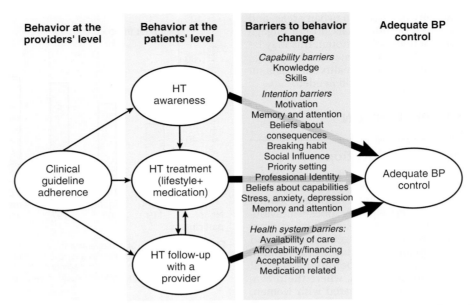

FIG. 4.3 The influence of patient and provider/health system barriers on hypertension control. *BP,* Blood pressure; *HT,* hypertension. *(From Khatib R, Schwalm JD, Yusuf S et al. Patient and healthcare provider barriers to hypertension awareness, treatment and follow up: A systematic review and meta-analysis of qualitative and quantitative studies. PloS One. 2014;9:e84238)*

for better optimization of vascular risk factors with a simplified regimen that can be applied to a broad range of socioeconomic settings. Finally, using inexpensive components, a polypill can be marketed at a very low cost, which is of particular benefit in countries (including those in South Asia) where affordability remains a significant barrier to medication use.

Overcoming the Barriers to Hypertension Management in South Asia

The PURE study has reported that hypertension management is subpar across South Asia, with only 40% of individuals with hypertension aware of the diagnosis, 32% of those with hypertension treated, and 13% controlled.[6] Consistent results were observed in a recent systematic review of 142 observational studies within India, with even poorer hypertension management in rural areas of India; where 42% of patients with hypertension were aware of the diagnosis in urban areas compared with only 25% in rural areas; 35% received treatment in urban areas compared with 20% in rural areas; and 20% achieved BP control in urban areas compared with 11% in rural areas.[7]

The factors resulting in poor hypertension treatment are complex, and include barriers to care at the patient level, in addition to "upstream" barriers at the health care provider and health systems levels (Fig. 4.3).[32] To overcome these barriers, innovative and multifaceted policies and interventions are needed to address these care gaps. Key public health policies should include reducing smoking and alcohol consumption, promoting physical activity, reducing saturated and transunsaturated fat intake, and national guidance on the appropriate levels of sodium consumption for the population.

Greater promotion of hypertension education is needed at the patient level. Many patients with hypertension are asymptomatic, and may be reluctant to make lifestyle changes or start pharmacologic treatments if they are feeling well. It is necessary to increase awareness of hypertension and its consequences, promote available resources for hypertension screening and treatment, and provide counselling on the importance of lifestyle changes that reduce BP. It is also necessary to emphasize the benefits of medication adherence

to patients; provide adequate knowledge of medication side effects so patients can recognize problems and seek necessary changes to their antihypertensive regimen; and provide simplified dosing regimens, such as with single-pill combination therapy.[32]

At the provider and health system levels, opportunistic BP evaluations at each physician health encounter can significantly increase hypertension detection, as can *task sharing* of hypertension screening to include nonphysician health workers (NPHWs) (e.g., pharmacists, nurses, and skilled community health workers). In rural India, community based screening using a NPHW has been shown to improve the detection of CVD. In the Rural Andhra Pradesh Cardiovascular Prevention Study (RAFCAPS), community screening using NPHWs resulted in a 12% increase in CVD detection compared with usual care.[33] It is possible that similar NPHW initiated community based programs can improve hypertension detection, and such programs are currently being evaluated. It has also been shown that allowing pharmacists or nurses to treat BP can further improve control, and consideration should be given to restructuring health care systems in the region to allow for a broader number of health personnel to prescribe simple to administer and well-tolerated antihypertensive medications (which currently occurs in several high- and middle-income countries).[34]

Both the affordability and availability of CVD medications significantly impact their use, and the affordability of basic medications is low in middle- and low-income countries.[35] In India, although most cardiovascular disease medications are available as generics they are not affordable.[35] In this situation, greater use of low-cost fixed-dose therapies may be particularly useful for improving hypertension control and optimizing overall vascular risk. In addition to medication costs, systematic methods to reduce additional health care provider costs to patients (e.g., affordable health insurance) also need to be addressed. Additional barriers that may need to be overcome include difficulty with transportation to health facilities, absent or inaccessible facilities, shortage of physicians, inability to easily obtain medication refills, and the time-consuming nature of clinic visits.[32] A summary of key strategies to improve hypertension detection, treatment and control is provided in Table 4.1.[36]

TABLE 4.1 Strategies to Improve Hypertension Management in South Asia

Public education and health promotion	• Increasing public knowledge that hypertension is a major risk factor for stroke, heart disease and death • Increasing knowledge for the need for hypertension screening • Promoting population level public health policies that reduce BP (smoking cessation, limiting alcohol use, dietary changes and increasing physical activity)
Hypertension screening	• Greater access to hypertension screening, particularly in rural areas. • Opportunistic physician screening • "Task-shifting" of hypertension screening to NPHW both in clinics and in the community (e.g., pharmacies, outreach programs) • Simplifying the initiation of pharmacotherapy by treating individuals with BP >160/>100 mm Hg on repeated measures at a single visit with at least a combination of two antihypertensive drugs.
Patient education and empowerment	• Emphasizing simple approaches to lifestyle changes, focusing on: moderate weight loss, smoking cessation, reducing alcohol consumption, increasing fruit and vegetable intake, and reducing sodium intake if high • Importance of adhering to pharmacologic antihypertensive treatments • Self-monitoring blood pressure • E-health/mobile-health reminders to monitor BP and adhere to treatment
Pharmacologic treatment	**System or provider level initiatives:** • Task sharing of pharmacologic management • Education of health professionals/update of hypertension guidelines • Use of clinical support systems, audit-feedback mechanisms and incentives for achieving hypertension control • Ensure priority pharmacologic therapies are available at the community level **Choice of pharmacologic therapies:** • Use affordable low-cost, antihypertensive pharmacologic drugs • Early use of combination antihypertensive therapy and simplified treatment regimens (e.g., FDC therapy) • Add lipid lowering with a statin to further reduce the risk of CVD events in conjunction with antihypertensive drugs.

Adapted from Gupta & Yusuf. Towards better hypertension management in India. Indian J Med Res. *2014;139:657-660.*
BP, Blood pressure; CVD, cardiovascular disease; FDC, fixed-dose combination; NPHW, nonphysician health workers.

CONCLUSIONS

Elevated BP is substantially contributing to the growing burden of CVD in South Asia, and its control is contingent on several factors. First, health-related behaviors (e.g., diet, physical activity, alcohol consumption) and other modifiable risk factors for hypertension (e.g., obesity, diabetes) have increased dramatically as a consequence of urbanization and economic development, and public health strategies are needed to address them. Second, there are major gaps in the detection, treatment, and control of hypertension in this region; and comprehensive policies are needed targeting system-level, provider-level, and patient-level barriers that are limiting hypertension management. These include strategies to improve access to health care resources and health providers to better manage BP (e.g., regular BP being checked at routine visits to health care providers, task sharing) and the greater use of simplified, low-cost combination pharmacologic treatments to control BP. It is expected that through such innovative strategies, the burden of hypertension and related cardiovascular complications in the region can be greatly reduced.

References

1. Gupta R. Trends in hypertension epidemiology in India. *J Hum Hypertens.* 2004;18:73-78.
2. Danaei G, Finucane MM, Lin JK, et al. National, regional, and global trends in systolic blood pressure since 1980: systematic analysis of health examination surveys and epidemiological studies with 786 country-years and 5.4 million participants. *Lancet.* 2011;377:568-577.
3. Chaturvedi N, Bathula R, Shore AC, et al. South Asians have elevated postexercise blood pressure and myocardial oxygen consumption compared to Europeans despite equivalent resting pressure. *J Am Heart Assoc.* 2012;1:e000281.
4. Eastwood SV, Tillin T, Chaturvedi N, et al. Ethnic differences in associations between blood pressure and stroke in south Asian and European men. *Hypertension.* 2015;66:481-488.
5. Neupane D, McLachlan CS, Sharma R, et al. Prevalence of hypertension in member countries of south Asian association for regional cooperation (saarc): systematic review and meta-analysis. *Medicine.* 2014;93:e74.
6. Chow CK, Teo KK, Rangarajan S, et al. Prevalence, awareness, treatment, and control of hypertension in rural and urban communities in high-, middle-, and low-income countries. *JAMA.* 2013;310:959-968.
7. Anchala R, Kannuri NK, Pant H, et al. Hypertension in India: a systematic review and meta-analysis of prevalence, awareness, and control of hypertension. *J Hypertens.* 2014;32:1170-1177.
8. Rana A, de Souza RJ, Kandasamy S, et al. Cardiovascular risk among south Asians living in Canada: a systematic review and meta-analysis. *CMAJ open.* 2014;2:E183-E191.
9. Agyemang C, Bhopal RS. Is the blood pressure of south Asian adults in the UK higher or lower than that in European white adults? A review of cross-sectional data. *J Hum Hypertens.* 2002;16:739-751.
10. Chiu M, Maclagan LC, Tu JV, et al. Temporal trends in cardiovascular disease risk factors among white, south Asian, Chinese and black groups in Ontario, Canada, 2001 to 2012: a population-based study. *BMJ open.* 2015;5:e007232.
11. Ehret GB, Munroe PB, Rice KM, et al. Genetic variants in novel pathways influence blood pressure and cardiovascular disease risk. *Nature.* 2011;478:103-109.
12. Kato N, Loh M, Takeuchi F, et al. Trans-ancestry genome-wide association study identifies 12 genetic loci influencing blood pressure and implicates a role for DNA methylation. *Nat Genet.* 2015;47:1282-1293.
13. Jayawardena R, Byrne NM, Soares MJ, et al. Prevalence, trends and associated socio-economic factors of obesity in south Asia. *Obesity Facts.* 2013;6:405-414.
14. Vasan RS, Larson MG, Leip EP, et al. Assessment of frequency of progression to hypertension in non-hypertensive participants in the Framingham heart study: a cohort study. *Lancet.* 2001;358:1682-1686.
15. Ramachandran A, Snehalatha C, Kapur A, et al. High prevalence of diabetes and impaired glucose tolerance in India: National urban diabetes survey. *Diabetologia.* 2001;44:1094-1101.
16. Mohan V, Deepa M, Deepa R, et al. Secular trends in the prevalence of diabetes and impaired glucose tolerance in urban south India—the Chennai urban rural epidemiology study (cures-17). *Diabetologia.* 2006;49:1175-1178.
17. Anjana RM, Pradeepa R, Deepa M, et al. Prevalence of diabetes and prediabetes (impaired fasting glucose and/or impaired glucose tolerance) in urban and rural India: phase I results of the Indian council of medical research-India diabetes (ICMR-INDIAB) study. *Diabetologia.* 2011;54:3022-3027.
18. Rani M, Bonu S, Jha P, et al. Tobacco use in India: prevalence and predictors of smoking and chewing in a national cross sectional household survey. *Tob Control.* 2003;12:e4.
19. Neufeld KJ, Peters DH, Rani M, et al. Regular use of alcohol and tobacco in India and its association with age, gender, and poverty. *Drug Alcohol Depend.* 2005;77:283-291.
20. Misra A, Singhal N, Sivakumar B, et al. Nutrition transition in India: secular trends in dietary intake and their relationship to diet-related non-communicable diseases. *J Diabetes.* 2011;3:278-292.
21. Powles J, Fahimi S, Micha R, et al. Global, regional and national sodium intakes in 1990 and 2010: A systematic analysis of 24 h urinary sodium excretion and dietary surveys worldwide. *BMJ open.* 2013;3:e003733.
22. Cox KL, Burke V, Morton AR, et al. Long-term effects of exercise on blood pressure and lipids in healthy women aged 40-65 years: the sedentary women exercise adherence trial (sweat). *J Hypertens.* 2001;19:1733-1743.
23. Anjana RM, Pradeepa R, Das AK, et al. Physical activity and inactivity patterns in India—results from the icmr-indiab study (phase-1) [ICMR-INDIAB-5]. *Int J Behav Nutr Phys Act.* 2014;11:26.
24. Dickinson HO, Mason JM, Nicolson DJ, et al. Lifestyle interventions to reduce raised blood pressure: a systematic review of randomized controlled trials. *J Hypertens.* 2006;24:215-233.
25. Blood Pressure Lowering Treatment Trialists Collaboration. Effects of different blood-pressure-lowering regimens on major cardiovascular events: results of prospectively-designed overviews of randomised trials. *Lancet.* 2003;362:1527-1535.
26. Wright Jr JT, Williamson JD, Whelton PK, et al. A randomized trial of intensive versus standard blood pressure control. *New Engl J Med.* 2015;373:2103-2116.
27. Cushman WC, Evans GW, Byington RP, et al. Effects of intensive blood-pressure control in type 2 diabetes mellitus. *New Engl J Med.* 2010;362:1575-1585.
28. Lonn E, Bosch J, Lopez-Jaramillo P, et al. Blood-Pressure Lowering in Intermediate-Risk Persons without Cardiovascular Disease. *New Engl J Med.* 2016;374:2009-2020.
29. Wald DS, Law M, Morris JK, et al. Combination therapy versus monotherapy in reducing blood pressure: meta-analysis on 11,000 participants from 42 trials. *Am J Med.* 2009;122:290-300.
30. Yusuf S, Pais P, Afzal R, et al. Effects of a polypill (polycap) on risk factors in middle-aged individuals without cardiovascular disease (tips): a phase ii, double-blind, randomised trial. *Lancet.* 2009;373:1341-1351.
31. Yusuf S, Pais P, Sigamani A, et al. Comparison of risk factor reduction and tolerability of a full-dose polypill (with potassium) versus low-dose polypill (polycap) in individuals at high risk of cardiovascular diseases: the second Indian polycap study (tips-2) investigators. *Circ Cardiovasc Qual Outcomes.* 2012;5:463-471.
32. Khatib R, Schwalm JD, Yusuf S, et al. Patient and healthcare provider barriers to hypertension awareness, treatment and follow up: a systematic review and meta-analysis of qualitative and quantitative studies. *PloS one.* 2014;9:e84238.
33. Joshi R, Chow CK, Raju PK, et al. The rural Andhra Pradesh cardiovascular prevention study (rapcaps): a cluster randomized trial. *J Am Coll Cardiol.* 2012;59:1188-1196.
34. Carter BL, Rogers M, Daly J, et al. The potency of team-based care interventions for hypertension: a meta-analysis. *Arch Intern Med.* 2009;169:1748-1755.
35. Khatib R, McKee M, Shannon H, et al. Availability and affordability of cardiovascular disease medicines and their effect on use in low-income, middle-income, and low-income countries: an analysis of the pure study data. *Lancet.* 2015.
36. Gupta R, Yusuf S. Towards better hypertension management in India. *Indian J Med Res.* 2014;139:657-660.

SECTION II
Pathophysiology

5 Pathogenesis of Hypertension

Michael E. Hall and John E. Hall

Primary (essential) hypertension accounts for the vast majority (>90%) of human hypertension and involves complex interactions of multiple organ systems and neurohormonal controllers of blood pressure (BP) as well as local tissue control systems. Although primary hypertension is a heterogeneous disorder, overweight and obesity account for as much as 65% to 75% of the risk for increased BP in these patients.[1,2] Genetics and other factors such as increased dietary sodium intake, sedentary lifestyle, and excess alcohol consumption may also contribute to primary hypertension. Activation of neurohormonal systems such as the sympathetic nervous system (SNS) and renin-angiotensin-aldosterone system (RAAS) also play an important role in the pathogenesis of hypertension. Many of these contributors to primary hypertension ultimately cause kidney dysfunction which initiates or sustains increased BP.[3]

In this chapter we discuss short-term and long-term BP control systems and how multiple organ systems interact to maintain tissue blood flow, salt and water balance, and overall homeostasis. We also briefly review various factors that influence activities of the SNS and RAAS, endothelial function, and oxidative stress that ultimately influence BP through effects on cardiac output (CO), vascular resistance, and renal salt and water excretion.

CONTROL OF BLOOD PRESSURE, BLOOD FLOW, AND CARDIAC OUTPUT

Effective circulatory regulation involves complex interactions of neurohormonal and local control systems that regulate BP and tissue blood flow. According to the well-known formula, BP is the product of CO and total peripheral vascular resistance (TPR): mean arterial BP = CO × TPR. This equation directs attention to factors that affect cardiac and vascular function and is adequate for describing short-term

Acknowledgments: The authors' research was supported by grants from the National Heart, Lung and Blood Institute (PO1 HL51971), National Institute of General Medical Sciences (P20 GM104357), National Institute of Diabetes and Digestive and Kidney Diseases (1K08DK099415-01A1), and the American Heart Association. We thank Stephanie Lucas for expert assistance in preparing this chapter.

BP control. However, chronic BP regulation is more complex and involves additional systems that regulate circulatory volume in relation to vascular capacitance (sometimes called "effective blood volume"); these systems may adjust BP to satisfy other critical homeostatic needs, such as the requirement to maintain balance between intake and output of salt and water.

CO represents the total blood flow of the circulation and is often described as the product of stroke volume and heart rate. Stroke volume, in turn, is determined by cardiac pumping ability and by peripheral circulatory factors that influence venous return to the heart. The heart normally pumps the amount of blood returned to it (ie, venous return) which is the sum of all blood flows returning from the tissues. Venous return and CO are therefore equal, except for momentary differences, and are determined by multiple factors that influence tissue blood flow, especially the metabolic demands of the tissues. For example, normal growth of the tissues is associated with increases in CO whereas loss of tissue mass (eg, loss of muscle mass that may occur with aging or with amputation of a limb) leads to decreases in CO.

Even without changes in tissue mass, metabolic rate greatly influences tissue blood flow and therefore CO. When metabolic rate increases during exercise or hyperthyroidism, for example, tissue blood flow and CO also increase to meet the higher metabolic needs of the tissues. In most cases, average daily CO remains relatively constant unless tissue mass or metabolism is altered. Even with conditions that cause marked sodium retention and increased blood volume, such as primary aldosteronism and sodium loading in subjects with impaired kidney function, CO remains relatively constant after initial transient changes that generally last only a few days.[4] This is because most tissues autoregulate their blood flow over a wide range of BP according to their specific needs.[5] Thus, although many patients with chronic hypertension have increased TPR, blood flows in most tissues are maintained at relatively normal levels as a result of local autoregulatory mechanisms. For example, increased BP and vascular stretch activates myogenic vasoconstriction, a response that can be observed even in isolated blood vessels.[6] Also, when blood flow increases above that required to meet metabolic requirements, local vasoconstrictor mechanisms are activated in most tissues. With chronic increases in BP, there are structural changes in the blood vessels, such as thickening of vessel walls and decreased numbers of capillaries (rarefaction), which ensure relatively normal tissue blood flow despite increased perfusion pressure. Therefore, TPR often changes in parallel with BP, helping to maintain normal tissue blood flow and attenuating changes in vascular stretch.

In some instances, increased TPR and elevated BP are associated with high levels of vasoconstrictors, such as angiotensin II (Ang II) or endothelin, although it has been challenging to identify abnormally elevated levels of specific vasoconstrictors in most patients with primary hypertension. Even in cases where high levels of vasoconstrictors are found, tissue perfusion is usually maintained at a level that is appropriate for the metabolic requirements.[7] However, blood flow "reserve" and the ability to increase tissue blood flow in response to increased metabolic requirements (eg, during exercise) may be impaired in some hypertensive subjects.

Although adequate BP is obviously required to maintain blood flow and nutrient supply to the tissues, blood flow and CO can be regulated independently of perfusion pressure when BP is elevated above normal. Moreover, BP is regulated by factors that may not be directly related to blood flow to most peripheral tissues, except for the kidneys which require a BP that maintains urinary excretion of water and electrolytes at a level equal to intake. As discussed later, chronic hypertension may represent a "trade off" that permits the kidneys to excrete normal amounts of salt and water, equal to intake, in the face of disturbances that impair renal function.[3] For example, constriction of the renal arteries or aortic coarctation above the renal arteries initiates compensatory increases in systemic arterial pressure that eventually restore renal perfusion and excretion of salt and water to normal levels. In contrast, reducing perfusion pressure to nonrenal tissues such as skeletal muscle (eg, by aortic coarctation below the renal arteries) does not lead to chronic hypertension. Although insufficient blood flow to the brain may initiate emergency mechanisms (eg, sympathetic activation) that acutely raise BP, the importance of cerebral perfusion in long-term BP regulation is still unclear.

LONG-TERM BLOOD PRESSURE CONTROL: ROLE OF RENAL PRESSURE NATRIURESIS

In contrast to the mechanisms that rapidly adjust vascular and cardiac function for moment-to-moment BP regulation, long-term regulation of average daily BP is closely linked with salt and water homeostasis. Fig. 5.1 shows a conceptual framework for integrating chronic control of BP and body fluid volumes. A key element of this feedback system is the effect of increased BP to raise renal sodium/water excretion, often called renal-pressure natriuresis/diuresis. Even temporary imbalances between intake and output will change extracellular fluid volume (ECFV) and potentially BP if cardiac and vascular functions are adequate. In some cases, increased BP serves to maintain salt and water balance, via pressure natriuresis, in the face of abnormalities that tend to cause salt/water retention. Although temporary imbalances between intake and output of salt and water occur routinely in daily life and excess sodium can be stored in tissues such as skin, independent of volume retention,[8] balance between average intake and output must eventually be achieved; otherwise, continued expansion or contraction of body fluids would occur and ultimately lead to circulatory failure.

The kidneys have powerful intrarenal and neurohormonal systems that help maintain salt and water balance, often with minimal changes in extracellular fluid volume or BP over a wide range of salt and water intakes. For example, when salt intake is increased in persons who have normal kidney and neurohormonal functions, minimal changes in BP occur and these individuals are called "salt-resistant." However, in "salt-sensitive" individuals with impaired kidney function, because of abnormal neurohormonal control or because of intrinsic kidney abnormalities (eg, kidney injury), increased BP and subsequent pressure natriuresis/diuresis provide another means of maintaining salt/water balance.[4,9] In some circumstances, renal-pressure natriuresis may play a critical role in maintaining balance between intake and output of salt and water and in preventing excessive fluid retention.[4]

Some investigators have argued that pressure natriuresis has minimal role in long-term BP regulation because the kidneys can adapt to elevated BP.[10] However, considerable evidence indicates that renal perfusion pressure has a sustained

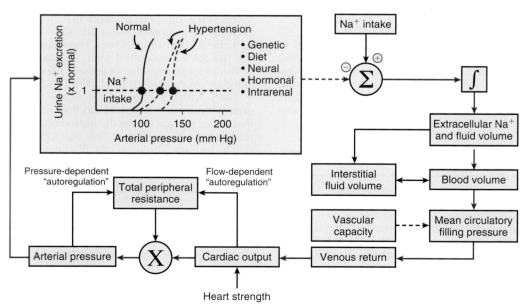

FIG. 5.1 Basic renal-body fluid feedback mechanism for long-term blood pressure regulation. A key component of this feedback is the effect of arterial pressure and urine sodium excretion, called renal-pressure natriuresis/diuresis. The *dashed* pressure natriuresis *lines* show impaired pressure natriuresis in salt-sensitive and salt-insensitive hypertension. Increased arterial pressure may cause secondary increases in total peripheral resistance via pressure-dependent or flow-dependent "autoregulation" in various tissues. Increased vascular capacity tends to reduce mean circulatory filling pressure.

effect on salt and water excretion and plays a critical role in chronic BP regulation.[11-13] For example, using a split-bladder preparation to collect urine separately from each kidney and servo-controlling renal perfusion pressure in each of the two kidneys independently, we found that small changes in BP cause large alterations in NaCl/water excretion that persisted as long as pressure was altered (12 days)[14] (Fig. 5.2). We also tested the importance of pressure natriuresis in maintaining NaCl/volume balance in several forms of experimental hypertension, including Ang II, aldosterone, deoxycorticosterone acetate (DOC)-salt, norepinephrine, adrenocorticotropic hormone plus norepinephrine, and vasopressin hypertension.[15-20] In each case, increases in renal perfusion pressure played a key role in maintaining salt and water balance; when renal artery pressure was servo-controlled at the normal level during development of hypertension, there was progressive sodium/water retention as well as continued increases in ECFV and systemic arterial pressure. In some cases, extreme salt/volume retention occurred when pressure natriuresis was prevented during development of hypertension, leading to circulatory congestion and pulmonary edema in a few days.

An important implication of the fact that renal perfusion pressure has a long-term effect on salt and water excretion is that chronic hypertension cannot be sustained unless pressure natriuresis is shifted to a higher BP. If pressure natriuresis was not reset, the elevated BP would increase sodium excretion and decrease ECFV and CO until BP returned to normal levels[13] (Fig. 5.3). Thus, chronic hypertension cannot be sustained by nonrenal vasoconstriction or increased CO unless there is also resetting of renal-pressure natriuresis.

Renal-pressure natriuresis is affected by many neurohormonal systems that can augment or blunt the effects of BP on salt and water balance. As discussed previously, high salt intake normally causes reductions in antinatriuretic hormones (Ang II and aldosterone) and increased formation of natriuretic hormones which together enhance the effects of pressure natriuresis, allowing the kidneys to maintain sodium balance with minimal changes in BP. However, excessive activation of antinatriuretic systems (eg, RAAS or SNS) reduces the effectiveness of pressure natriuresis, requiring a higher BP to maintain sodium balance.

In all forms of experimental or human hypertension studied thus far, there is a shift of pressure natriuresis to higher BP.[11,12,21] This shift may be because of neurohormonal or intrarenal disorders that either reduce glomerular filtration rate (GFR) or increase renal tubular salt or water reabsorption. The increased BP, in turn, helps to return salt and water excretion to normal, via pressure natriuresis, despite kidney dysfunction.

Sodium Retention Does Not Always Cause Hypertension

Although impaired pressure natriuresis is required for chronic hypertension to be sustained, sodium retention does not always elevate BP.[22] In pathophysiologic conditions such as chronic heart failure and cirrhosis, salt and water retention occur without hypertension. In these cases, salt and water retention occurs as a compensation for inadequate cardiac or vascular functions which tend to reduce BP. In heart failure, salt and water retention tend to increase ECFV which may raise cardiac filling pressures sufficiently to return CO and BP toward normal if cardiac dysfunction is not too severe. In cirrhosis there is loss of fluid from the circulation into the interstitial spaces and/or increased vascular capacitance and pooling of blood in the portal circulation because of liver fibrosis. This also leads to activation of various antinatriuretic systems which cause salt and water retention, helping to sustain normal BP.

Impaired Renal-Pressure Natriuresis Does Not Always Cause Sodium Retention or Increases in Blood Volume and Cardiac Output

Although ECFV and blood volume are key components of long-term BP regulation, via the renal-body fluid feedback

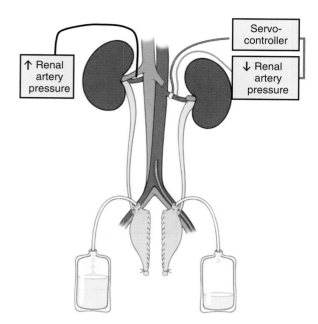

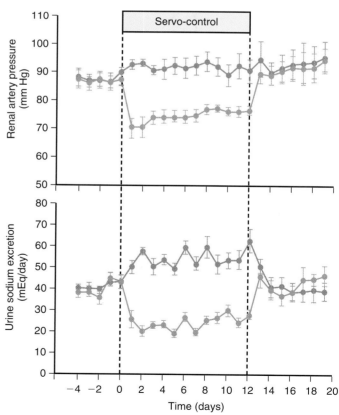

FIG. 5.2 Renal artery pressure and urine sodium excretion, collected separately from each kidney using a split bladder method from kidneys of the same dogs in which pressure of one kidney was servo-controlled at a level about 10 to 12 mm Hg below control *(dashed lines)* whereas pressure in the contralateral kidney increased about 4 to 5 mm Hg above control *(solid lines)*. Data are shown for 4 days of control measurements, 12 days of servo-controlling renal perfusion pressure, and 7 days of recovery. *(Data from Mizelle HL, Montani JP, Hester RL, et al. Role of pressure natriuresis in long-term control of renal electrolyte excretion. Hypertension. 1993;22:102-110.)*

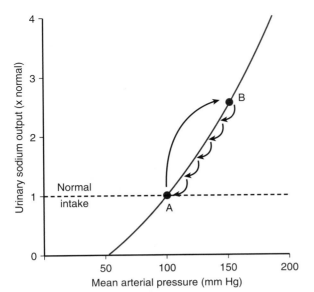

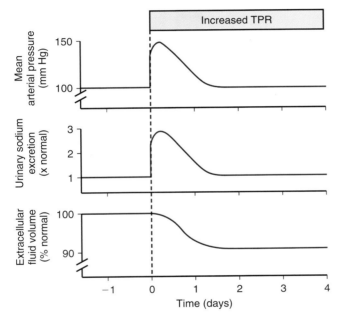

FIG. 5.3 Long-term effects of increased total peripheral resistance (TPR), such as that caused by closure of a large arteriovenous fistula, with no change in the renal-pressure natriuresis relationship. Blood pressure (BP) is initially increased from point A to point B, but elevated BP cannot be sustained because sodium excretion exceeds intake, reducing extracellular fluid volume until blood pressure returns to normal and sodium balance is reestablished. *(From Hall JE. The kidney, hypertension, and obesity.* Hypertension. *2003;41:625-633.)*

TABLE 5.1 Examples of Experimental Kidney-Specific Disorders and Monogenic Human Disorders That Cause Salt-Sensitive Increases in Blood Pressure

Experimental Kidney-Specific Disorders	• Surgical reduction of kidney mass • Partial kidney infarction/nephron loss • 2-kidney, 1-clip Goldblatt hypertension • Hydronephrosis • Uninephrectomy at a young age • Kidney tubulointerstitial inflammation • Glomerulonephritis, IgA nephropathy • Adenine-induced kidney injury • Collecting duct-specific deletion of NOS1 • Collecting duct-specific deletion of endothelin B receptors • Collecting duct-specific overexpression of renin • Increased renal medullary-specific oxidative stress
Monogenic Human Disorders	• Liddle syndrome • Activating MR mutation exacerbated by pregnancy • Apparent mineralocorticoid excess (AME) • Gordon syndrome • Glucocorticoid remediable aldosteronism (GRA) • Congenital adrenal hyperplasia (CAH) • Familial hyperaldosteronism not remediable by glucocorticoids (FH-III and FH-IV)

IgA, Immunoglobulin A; *MR,* mineralocorticoid receptor, *NOS1,* nitric oxide synthase 1.
Note: This is only a partial list of the many kidney-specific disorders that have been shown to cause salt-sensitive blood pressure (see Hall[4] for more extensive discussion).

renal-pressure natriuresis is necessary for the hypertension to be sustained.

SALT SENSITIVITY AND HYPERTENSION

Because excess salt intake increases the risk for hypertension, moderation of salt intake is an important strategy for prevention of cardiovascular and kidney disease, especially in salt-sensitive subjects.[24,25] Although there is significant heterogeneity of BP responses to high salt intake over several days,[9,26] BP salt sensitivity may worsen with chronic exposure to excessive salt intake.[4] Salt sensitivity may also increase with aging or with various pathophysiologic conditions that cause kidney dysfunction, such as diabetes, hypertension, and various types of kidney disease.[4,9] Gene mutations or neurohormonal changes that increase renal tubule sodium reabsorption may also increase BP salt sensitivity.[27,28] Salt sensitivity also occurs more frequently in blacks than whites. Despite the seemingly disparate causes of salt sensitivity, all individuals with salt-induced chronic increases in BP have the common characteristic of impaired renal-pressure natriuresis and maintenance of salt balance at the expense of increased BP.

Experimental and clinical studies indicate that several types of kidney-specific disorders increase BP salt sensitivity (Table 5.1): (1) kidney injuries that cause loss of functional nephrons or decreased glomerular capillary filtration coefficient; (2) patchy (nonhomogeneous) increases in preglomerular resistance; (3) inability to modulate the RAAS appropriately; and (4) acquired or genetic disorders that directly or indirectly increase renal NaCl reabsorption, especially in the distal and collecting tubules. The various types of kidney dysfunction that induce salt-sensitive hypertension are distinct from those that cause salt-resistant hypertension.[4]

Loss of Nephrons and Kidney Injury Cause Salt Sensitivity

Although surgical removal of up to 70% of kidney mass does not generally cause marked hypertension, it does greatly

mechanism, BP is not a function of blood volume *per se* but of blood volume in relation to vascular capacity. This concept is sometimes referred to as "effective blood volume."[23] When vascular capacity increases (eg, large varicose veins), greater blood volume is needed to maintain normal BP. Conversely, less volume is required to maintain normal BP with vasoconstriction. When high concentrations of strong vasoconstrictors such a norepinephrine and Ang II are present, the kidneys may actually undergo pressure-induced natriuresis and ECFV may decrease even though these vasoconstrictors also have important antinatriuretic effects which maintain the hypertension.[3,18] Thus, in some forms of hypertension associated with marked peripheral vasoconstriction (eg, pheochromocytoma or renin secreting tumor) there may be reduced blood volume even though impaired

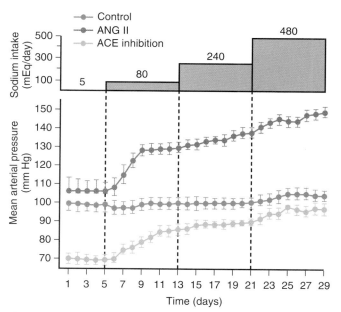

FIG. 5.4 Changes in mean arterial pressure during chronic changes in sodium intake in normal control dogs, after angiotensin-converting enzyme (ACE) inhibition, or after angiotensin II (Ang II) infusion (5 ng/kg/min) to prevent Ang II from being suppressed when sodium intake was raised. *(Data from Hall JE, Guyton AC, Smith MJ, Jr., et al. Blood pressure and renal function during chronic changes in sodium intake: role of angiotensin. Am J Physiol. 1980;239:F271-F280.)*

enhance BP salt sensitivity.[29] Partial kidney infarction, tubulointerstitial inflammation, immune cell infiltration of the kidneys, immunoglobulin A (IgA) nephropathy, hydronephrosis, and many other types of renal insults also increase BP salt sensitivity.[4] In patients with chronic kidney disease, BP salt sensitivity increases exponentially as creatinine clearance decreases.[30] Thus, acquired renal injuries attributed to aging, diabetes, hypertension, and various types of acute and chronic kidney injury, even when they are subtle, usually increase BP salt sensitivity.[31]

Loss of functional nephrons or renal injury also makes the kidneys more susceptible to additional insults that impair their function or to additional challenges of sodium homeostasis. Thus, hypertension associated with excess mineralocorticoids is more severe after reducing kidney mass.[4] Moreover, loss of substantial numbers of nephrons may initiate compensatory vasodilation and hyperfiltration of the surviving nephrons that eventually cause further nephron loss, greater salt sensitivity, higher BPs, and ultimately kidney failure in some patients.[4]

Inability to Effectively Modulate the Renin-Angiotensin-Aldosterone System Causes Salt Sensitivity

When the RAAS is fully functional, sodium balance can be achieved over a wide range of intakes with minimal BP changes[32] (Fig. 5.4). However, excessive activity of the RAAS or fixed low activity of the RAAS increases BP salt sensitivity.[33] As discussed later, one of the major functions of the RAAS is to permit wide variations in intake and excretion of sodium without large fluctuations in BP that would otherwise be needed to maintain the sodium balance.

Focal nephrosclerosis or patchy constriction of preglomerular blood vessels, as occurs with renal infarction, leads to increased renin secretion in ischemic nephrons and low levels of renin release by overperfused nephrons. Thus, the ischemic as well as overperfused nephrons are unable to adequately suppress renin secretion during high salt intake and BP becomes salt sensitive.[3]

Another cause of decreased responsiveness of the RAAS is increased distal and collecting tubular sodium reabsorption, as occurs with mineralocorticoid excess or gene mutations that increase distal and collecting tubule reabsorption (eg, Liddle syndrome, apparent mineralocorticoid excess, Gordon syndrome, and glucocorticoid-remediable aldosteronism).[27,28] In these conditions, excess sodium retention causes almost complete suppression of renin secretion, resulting in an inability to further decrease renin release and Ang II formation during high sodium intake. Consequently, BP becomes highly salt-sensitive.

Blockade of the RAAS, with angiotensin-converting enzyme (ACE) inhibitors, Ang II receptor blockers (ARBs), or mineralocorticoid receptor (MR) antagonists also makes BP more sensitive to changes in salt intake despite reducing BP in many hypertensive subjects.[4] Thus, these antihypertensive drugs are generally much more effective when salt intake is normal or reduced than when salt intake in elevated.

Endothelin and Salt Sensitivity

Endothelin-1 (ET-1) is a potent vasoconstrictor but its renal actions, especially in the collecting ducts (CDs), are of special importance in long-term BP regulation and salt sensitivity.[34,35] The CDs produce ET-1 which binds in an autocrine manner to endothelin A/B (ETA/B) receptors, causing inhibition of NaCl reabsorption. Salt/volume loading stimulates CD ET-1 production through local mechanisms that sense salt delivery and shear stress when tubular flow rate increases. Locally released ET-1 then activates ETB receptors and inhibits sodium reabsorption.[34] Moreover, CD-specific deletion of ETB receptors increases BP salt sensitivity.[36] CD-specific deletion of ET-1 production or deletion of ETA/B receptors in CDs produces even greater salt-dependent BP elevation than deficiency of ETB receptors alone.[37,38] Blockade of ET-1 receptors also attenuates or abolishes hypertension in Dahl-salt sensitive rats and DOCA-salt hypertension.[34,35]

Although ET-1 is a potent vasoconstrictor in many tissues, including the kidneys, and may stimulate SNS activity and regulate extravascular sodium storage,[39] whether these extrarenal actions ultimately influence renal-pressure natriuresis, salt sensitivity and chronic BP regulation is uncertain. It is clear, however, that the renal actions of ET-1, especially in the CD, play a major role in protecting against salt-sensitive hypertension.

Genetic Causes of Salt-Sensitive Hypertension

Nearly all monogenic forms of hypertension discovered thus far share the common phenotypes of increased renal NaCl reabsorption and salt-sensitive hypertension (Fig. 5.5). In contrast, those monogenic disorders associated with decreased NaCl reabsorption tend to have salt-sensitive reductions in BP. Although these disorders account for less than 1% of human hypertension, they provide additional examples of salt-sensitive hypertension associated with excessive reabsorption of NaCl in the kidney distal and collecting tubules.

Pseudohypoaldosteronism type 2 (Gordon syndrome) is caused by mutations of genes that encode WNK1 and WNK4, two members of the WNK family of serine-threonine kinases expressed in the distal nephron.[40] Mutations of *WNK1* are large intronic deletions that increase WNK1 expression whereas *WNK4* mutations are missense and cause loss of function. Both mutations increase activity of thiazide-sensitive NaCl transporters in the distal nephron, and patients with these mutations are effectively treated with thiazide diuretics which lower BP chronically by inhibiting NaCl renal reabsorption.[40]

Liddle syndrome is caused by gain of function mutations of the β or γ subunits of the epithelial sodium channel (ENaC) which cause increased sodium reabsorption,

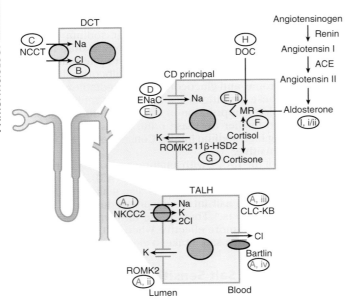

FIG. 5.5 Monogenic forms of hypertension and hypotension in humans affect renal tubular sodium reabsorption directly or through activation of the renin-angiotensin-aldosterone system (RAAS). A diagram of a nephron is shown, with sodium-reabsorbing cells of the thick ascending loop of Henle (TALH), distal convoluted tubule (DCT), and collecting duct (CD) principal cells as well as the RAAS pathway, the major hormonal system for regulating sodium reabsorption. The circled letters indicate: (A, i-iv) types I/II/III/IV Bartter syndrome (loss of function mutation of NKCC2); (B) Gordon syndrome (excess activity of NCCT); (C) Gitelman syndrome (loss of function mutations of NCCT); (D) Liddle syndrome (excess activity of ENaC); (E, i, ii) recessive/dominant pseudohypoaldosteronism type 1 (PHA1, loss of function mutations of ENaC or MR); (F) activating MR exaggerated by pregnancy; (G) syndrome of apparent mineralocorticoid excess because of deficiency of 11β-HSD2; (H) Deoxycorticosterone (DOC) oversecretion because of congenital adrenal hyperplasia, or deficiency of 17α-hydroxylase or 11α-hydroxylase; (I, i, ii) familial hyperaldosteronism I (glucocorticoid-remediable aldosteronism) and II causing excess secretion of aldosterone. *11β-HSD2,* 11β-hydroxysteroid dehydrogenase 2; *ACE,* angiotensin converting enzyme; *CLC-KB,* encodes the basolateral chloride channel in loop of Henle cells; *ENaC,* epithelial sodium channel; *MR,* mineralocorticoid receptor; *NCCT,* sodium-chloride cotransporter; *NKCC2,* sodium-potassium-2chloride cotransporter; *ROMK2,* renal outer medullary potassium channel. *(From Lifton RP, Gharavi AG, Geller DS. Molecular mechanisms of human hypertension.* Cell *2001;104:545-556 and O'Shaughnessy KM, Karet FE. Salt handling and hypertension.* J Clin Invest. *2004;113:1075-1081.)*

hypoaldosteronism and low plasma renin activity.[27,28] This disorder is effectively treated with amiloride or triamterene, which block ENaC and inhibit collecting tubule reabsorption.[27,28] Hypertension also resolved after transplantation of a normal kidney in a patient with Liddle syndrome.[41] The finding that BP remained normal for at least 5 years after kidney transplantation, even though potential extrarenal effects associated with increased ENaC activity were still present, indicates that the kidney dysfunction plays a critical role in the pathogenesis of hypertension.

Apparent mineralocorticoid excess (AME) is a monogenic form of salt-sensitive hypertension caused by deficiency of 11β-HSD2 which causes glucocorticoid activation of MR.[42] Although cortisol binds MR with high affinity, renal epithelial cells are normally "protected" by 11β-HSD2 which locally converts cortisol to cortisone, a steroid that does not avidly bind MR. Therefore, 11β-HSD2 deficiency causes excessive MR stimulation which activates ENaC in aldosterone-sensitive distal nephrons, leading to increased NaCl reabsorption and hypertension with characteristics similar to that caused by primary aldosteronism.[42] After hypertension is established, most indices of kidney function appear normal, except for hypokalemia and impaired renal-pressure natriuresis, and multiple vascular abnormalities begin to appear as a consequence of increased BP. Evidence that kidney dysfunction rather than some extrarenal effect of 11β-HSD2 deficiency mediates this form of salt-sensitive hypertension comes from the finding that transplantation of normal kidneys into patients with AME

caused complete remission of hypertension and electrolyte abnormalities.[43,44]

Glucocorticoid-remediable aldosteronism (GRA), congenital adrenal hyperplasia, familial hyperaldosteronism not remedial by glucocorticoids, and hypertension exacerbated by pregnancy are also monogenic forms of salt-sensitive hypertension associated with excessive activation of the MR.[27] All are effectively treated by drugs that block renal tubular ENaC, MR, or aldosterone secretion. In each case, the primary driving force for salt-sensitive increases in BP is increased distal and collecting tubule NaCl reabsorption.[27]

Kidney Disorders That Cause Salt-Resistant Hypertension

Not all kidney disorders increase salt sensitivity of BP. Generalized increases in preglomerular resistance caused by suprarenal aortic coarctation or constriction of one renal artery and removal of the contralateral kidney (1-kidney, 1-clip Goldblatt hypertension) cause *salt-resistant* hypertension. After constriction of the renal artery or aorta, GFR and sodium excretion initially decrease and renin secretion increases. As BP rises and pressure distal to the stenosis returns toward normal, most measurements of kidney function, including sodium excretion and renin secretion, return to nearly normal if the constriction is not too severe.[45] If renal artery constriction of a sole remaining kidney is severe, malignant hypertension may develop.

A major reason that high salt intake does not usually exacerbate hypertension caused by increased preglomerular resistance is that after BP increases sufficiently to restore renal perfusion pressure and renin secretion to normal, the RAAS is fully capable of appropriate suppression during high salt intake.[3] As discussed previously, the ability to effectively modulate RAAS activity is a key mechanism for preventing salt sensitivity of BP.

Gain-of-function phosphodiesterase 3A (PDE3A) mutations, in contrast to all other forms of monogenic hypertension that have been discovered, cause increased vascular resistance and salt-resistant hypertension.[46,47] This is an autosomal-dominant form of hypertension associated with brachydactyly and is caused by increased activity of PDE3A which catalyzes hydrolysis of intracellular second messengers, cAMP and cGMP. The mutated PDE3A causes vascular smooth muscle cell proliferation and vasoconstriction, leading to increased TPR and presumably increased renal vascular resistance. Sympathetic blockade and hydrochlorothiazide treatment are ineffective in reducing BP whereas nitroprusside caused acute decreases in BP, consistent with an intrinsic vascular abnormality.[47,48] Despite marked vasoconstriction and increased TPR, these patients are not salt-sensitive and have normal renin, aldosterone and norepinephrine.[47]

Thus, generalized vasoconstriction does not appear to increase BP salt sensitivity in the absence of kidney abnormalities that increase tubular reabsorption, decrease glomerular filtration coefficient, and/or reduce responsiveness of the RAAS. Renal preglomerular vasoconstriction can increase BP but the hypertension is usually not salt-sensitive.

Clinical Assessment and Significance of Salt Sensitivity

Although various experimental methods have been used to assess salt sensitivity, none are widely used in clinical practice. Most salt sensitivity protocols involve relatively short-term changes in sodium intake, usually over a few days. For example, salt sensitivity has also been defined as a 10 mm Hg or greater increase in mean BP from the level measured after a 4-hour infusion of 2 L of normal saline compared with the level measured the morning after 1 day of a low-sodium

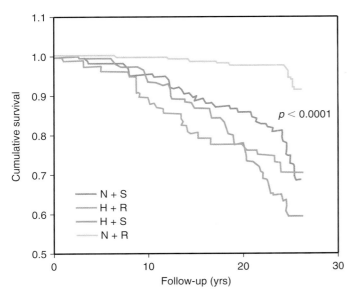

FIG. 5.6 Kaplan-Meier survival curves for normotensive salt-resistant subjects (N+R), normotensive salt-sensitive subjects (N+S), hypertensive salt-resistant subjects (H+R), and hypertensive salt-sensitive subjects (N+S) over the follow-up period. As noted, only the N+R group had an increased survival. *(From Weinberger MH, Fineberg NS, Fineberg SE, et al. Salt sensitivity, pulse pressure, and death in normal and hypertensive humans. Hypertension. 2001;37:429-432.)*

(10 mmol) diet and administration of three doses of furosemide.[49] Using this protocol, Weinberger reported that 51% of hypertensive and 26% of normotensive subjects were salt-sensitive.[49] However, it is unclear whether these short-term protocols reliably predict the long-term effects of changes in salt intake.

In most cases, salt sensitivity is determined empirically by encouraging patients to reduce their salt intake and measuring their BP responses. Some studies suggest that those patients who are salt sensitive may have greatest risk for hypertensive target-organ injury and early death compared with those who are salt-resistant. Weinberger et al followed subjects for more than 20 years and found that normotensive individuals with increased salt sensitivity died almost at the same rate as hypertensive individuals and much faster than salt-resistant individuals who were normotensive[50] (Fig. 5.6). Whether this increased mortality was related to BP effects of salt or to other effects is still unclear. It is also not known whether chronic high salt intake, lasting over many years, may cause a person who is initially "salt-insensitive" to become "salt-sensitive" as a consequence of gradual renal injury.

There is evidence that salt-sensitive forms of hypertension are often associated with glomerular hyperfiltration and increased glomerular hydrostatic pressure that is further amplified by the hypertension[51]; together the hypertension and renal hyperfiltration may promote glomerular injury and may eventually cause loss of nephron function. Clinical studies support this concept and demonstrate that salt-sensitive individuals typically have substantially higher glomerular hydrostatic pressure and albumin excretion when given a salt load compared with salt-resistant individuals.[4,52] Further studies are needed to assess the overall impact of BP salt sensitivity in normotensive and hypertensive subjects and the mechanisms that may link salt sensitivity to target organ injury and premature death.

RENIN-ANGIOTENSIN ALDOSTERONE SYSTEM

The RAAS is one of the body's most powerful systems for regulating sodium balance and BP as evidenced by the effectiveness of RAAS blockers in reducing renal tubular sodium reabsorption and lowering BP in normotensive as well as hypertensive subjects. Although the RAAS has many components its most important effects on sodium excretion and chronic BP regulation are exerted by Ang II and aldosterone. Both Ang II and aldosterone potently increase sodium reabsorption whereas Ang II also has important renal hemodynamic effects that contribute its antinatriuretic actions and long-term BP regulation.[3]

Ang II and Long-Term Blood Pressure Regulation

Ang II has powerful vasoconstrictor effects that help maintain BP during hemorrhage, dehydration, heart failure and other disturbance that cause circulatory depression and/or volume depletion. However, Ang II also plays a key role in chronic BP regulation via its sodium-retaining effects on the kidneys.[3,32] As discussed previously, activation of the RAAS during low salt intake and appropriate suppression during high salt intake permits maintenance of balance with minimal changes in BP over a wide range of sodium intakes.

RAAS antagonists (ACE inhibitors, ARBs, renin inhibitors, MR antagonists) improve the kidneys' ability to excrete sodium and permit sodium balance at lower BP. However, RAAS blockade also makes BP more salt-sensitive because the actions of Ang II and/or aldosterone are already blocked and therefore cannot be effectively suppressed during high salt intake. Conversely, RAAS antagonists are more effective in lowering BP with concomitant diuretic treatment or after reducing salt intake.

Ang II causes salt and water retention by direct actions on the kidneys that increase NaCl reabsorption and by stimulating the adrenal glands to release aldosterone.[32] Ang II also constricts renal efferent arterioles which reduces renal blood flow and peritubular capillary hydrostatic pressure while increasing filtration fraction and peritubular colloid osmotic pressure; together these renal hemodynamics effects enhance peritubular capillary reabsorption and consequently tubular reabsorption of salt and water.[32] In addition, reductions in renal medullary blood flow or direct effects of Ang II on the vasa recta may enhance sodium reabsorption in the loop of Henle and CDs.

Ang II directly stimulates sodium reabsorption through its actions on luminal and basolateral membranes of the renal tubules.[53] Ang II stimulates proximal tubular sodium reabsorption by increasing activities of the Na^+/H^+ exchanger and Na^+/K^+ ATPase. Furthermore, Ang II stimulates $Na^+/K^+/2Cl^-$ transport in the loop of Henle as well as multiple ion transporters in the distal nephron and collecting tubules to increase NaCl reabsorption.[32]

Ang II acts primarily on two receptors. Activation of the AT1 receptor leads to vasoconstriction, increased renal NaCl transport, and release of aldosterone which all ultimately lead to salt and water retention. The AT2 receptor opposes the function of the AT1 receptors and inhibits cell proliferation, promotes cell differentiation, and causes vasodilation and natriuresis.[54] Compared with the AT1 receptor, AT2 receptor expression is relatively low in adult animals, although in some circumstances (eg, wound healing) AT2 receptor expression may increase significantly.

Although the chronic BP effects of Ang II have often been attributed to its effects on the brain, adrenal gland, and non-renal blood vessels, activation of kidney AT1 receptors is required for Ang II to cause chronic hypertension[55,56] (Fig. 5.7). Crowley and colleagues found that Ang II infusion in wild-type (WT) mice increased BP and caused cardiac hypertrophy and fibrosis. In contrast, WT mice that received transplanted kidneys from AT1 receptor knock-out mice (ie, AT1 receptors were present in the peripheral vasculature, brain, heart and other organs, but not in the kidneys), Ang II infusion did not raise BP chronically or cause cardiac hypertrophy/fibrosis. In AT1 receptor knock-out mice that received transplanted

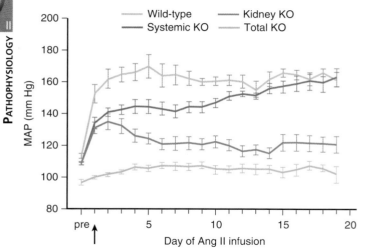

FIG. 5.7 Blood pressures in wild-type mice and in mice with Ang II AT1 receptor deletion after kidney cross-transplantation. Daily, 24-h blood pressures in the experimental groups before ("pre") and during 21 days of Ang II infusion versus wild-type mice with AT1 receptors in the entire body; Systemic knock out (KO) with AT1 receptors present only in the transplanted kidney; Kidney KO with AT1 receptors present everywhere except the kidney; Total KO with AT1 receptors deleted in the entire body. *(From Crowley SD, Gurley SB, Herrera MJ, et al. Angiotensin II causes hypertension and cardiac hypertrophy through its receptors in the kidney. Proc Natl Acad Sci U S A. 2006;103:17985-17990.)*

kidneys from WT mice (ie, AT1 receptors were present only in the kidneys and not in peripheral blood vessels, brain, heart or other organs), Ang II infusion caused chronic increases in BP, albeit more slowly, as well as cardiac hypertrophy/fibrosis that were similar to that found in WT mice. These observations indicate that kidney AT1 receptor activation by Ang II, instead of peripheral vascular or other nonrenal effects, mediate chronic increases in BP and cardiac hypertrophy.

Mechanisms of Ang II-Mediated Target Organ Injury

Ang II has been suggested to cause damage to the kidneys, heart and other organs by both hemodynamic and direct tissue effects. Much of the evidence for nonhemodynamic effects of Ang II in promoting target organ injury comes from *in vitro* studies, often using supraphysiologic doses of Ang II, but also from *in vivo* studies suggesting that RAS blockers (ACE inhibitors and ARBs) reduce target organ damage (ie, chronic kidney disease [CKD] and left ventricular hypertrophy) more than other antihypertensive drugs. However, high Ang II levels in the absence of elevated BP do not appear to cause target organ damage. One example is the two-kidney, one-clip Goldblatt hypertension model where the clipped kidney is exposed to very high Ang II levels but is protected from high BP by the clip.[57] The clipped kidney (as long as the stenosis is not too severe) is protected from renal injury whereas the nonclipped kidney which is exposed to lower Ang II levels but higher BP demonstrates substantial injury. Convincing evidence that the hemodynamic effects of Ang II are essential for target organ injury comes from the experiments by Crowley et al[56] discussed previously. In these studies, cardiac fibrosis and hypertrophy did not occur during chronic Ang II infusion unless BP also increased, and BP did not increase unless AT1 receptors were present in the kidneys.

Aldosterone, Mineralocorticoid Receptor Activation, and Long-Term Blood Pressure Regulation

Aldosterone, a mineralocorticoid synthesized in the zona glomerulosa of the adrenal cortex, is secreted mainly in response to increases in extracellular concentrations of Ang II and potassium, but several other factors associated with changes in body fluid volumes and stress can also influence aldosterone secretion. In humans about 90% of mineralocorticoid activity is normally from aldosterone. Aldosterone stimulates MR in the principal cells of the distal tubules, cortical collecting tubules and the CDs to increase sodium reabsorption and potassium secretion.

Aldosterone exhibits both genomic and nongenomic effects on the cardiovascular and renal systems. Genomic effects are those mediated by gene transcription and require 60 to 90 minutes to occur after the MR is activated. Genomic effects of aldosterone include synthesis and insertion of Na^+/K^+-ATPase pump proteins into the basolateral membrane as well as amiloride-sensitive sodium channels in the luminal membrane of the principal cells, leading to increases in renal sodium reabsorption and potassium secretion.[58] Although the membrane receptor and the cell-signaling mechanisms responsible for nongenomic actions of aldosterone are not well-understood, the effects are rapid. For example, aldosterone may activate the Na^+-H^+ exchanger in vascular smooth muscle in less than 4 minutes.[58,59] Currently, the functional significance of aldosterone's nongenomic effects on BP regulation has not been elucidated.

The effects of aldosterone on renal-pressure natriuresis are similar to those of Ang II. When salt intake is reduced, aldosterone is released to increase renal sodium reabsorption, thereby attenuating sodium loss and preventing large reductions in BP. With high salt intake, aldosterone is suppressed, attenuating sodium retention and increased BP. Excessive aldosterone, by stimulating renal sodium reabsorption, impairs pressure natriuresis and makes BP more salt-sensitive. However, even when aldosterone levels are elevated up to ten-fold, BP may not be elevated if sodium intake is low. Normal or high salt intake also appears to be a requirement for target organ damage associated with increased aldosterone. Thus, high concentrations of aldosterone during low sodium diet are not associated with increased BP or target organ injury.

When occurring concomitantly with normal or high sodium intakes, high levels of aldosterone and MR activation cause excess sodium retention, hypertension and target organ injury. Hyperaldosteronism or failure to adequately suppress aldosterone in response to sodium retention may be more common than previously believed, especially in patients with hypertension resistant to treatment with the usual antihypertensive medications. Some investigators have suggested that the prevalence of primary aldosteronism is as high as 20% of patients referred to specialty clinics for resistant hypertension.[60] Moreover, blockade of MR or amiloride-sensitive sodium channels lowers BP and attenuates cardiovascular and renal injury in many treatment resistant hypertensive subjects even when aldosterone levels are not substantially elevated above normal.[60-62] Convincing evidence for the effectiveness of MR blockade in treatment resistant hypertension not associated with high levels of aldosterone comes from the PATHWAY-2 (The Prevention And Treatment of Hypertension With Algorithm based therapY) study which also provided evidence that sodium retention plays a key role in the hypertension of the patients.[63]

Many treatment-resistant hypertensive patients who respond to MR blockers or amiloride are overweight or obese.[60] As discussed later, obesity may activate MR and increase renal ENaC activity independent of aldosterone. Furthermore, administration of MR antagonists to obese hypertensive patients reduced BP despite concomitant treatment with ACE inhibitors, ARBs, calcium channel blockers or thiazide diuretics suggesting that MR activation in obese humans may occur independently of Ang II-mediated aldosterone secretion.[64]

SYMPATHETIC NERVOUS SYSTEM

The SNS plays a major role in short-term and long-term control of BP. Almost all components of the vasculature and the heart are innervated by sympathetic fibers. SNS activation can increase BP within seconds through its vasoconstrictor effects and by increasing cardiac output (increased chronotropic and inotropic effects). There are multiple levels of the nervous system that can modulate SNS activation including the central nervous system (CNS), ganglionic transmission, release, clearance and reuptake of neurotransmitters, and sensitivity or density of adrenergic receptors.[65]

The renal sympathetic nerves appear to play a major role in long-term control of BP and in the pathogenesis of hypertension. This is evidenced by the effect of renal denervation (RDN) to lower BP in several animal models of experimental hypertension.[66] The renal blood vessels, juxtaglomerular apparatus, and renal tubules are extensively innervated and excessive activation of these nerves promotes sodium retention, increased renin secretion, and impaired renal-pressure natriuresis. Although SNS activation in most forms of hypertension is generally not great enough to reduce renal blood flow and GFR, even mild SNS activation can increase renin release and renal sodium reabsorption in various parts of the nephron including the proximal tubules, loop of Henle, distal tubule, and collecting tubules.[67] The renal nerves therefore provide a mechanism to connect the SNS with control of body fluid volumes and long-term BP regulation.

Multiple studies (eg, SYMPLICITY HTN-1 and HTN-2) suggest that the SNS may contribute to human hypertension via activation of the renal sympathetic nerves. As discussed later in the section on obesity-induced hypertension, renal sympathetic activity is often increased in obese individuals, especially those with increased visceral adiposity.[2] Clinical trials that have ablated the renal nerves using percutaneous procedures to treat resistant hypertensive patients have reported substantial reductions in BP that persisted for as long as 3 years.[68,69] However, the SYMPLICITY HTN-3 trial, which included a sham surgery arm, failed to demonstrate significant reductions in 24-hour ambulatory BP after RDN beyond those observed in the sham control group.[70] The reasons for these differences in BP responses in the SYMPLICITY HTN-1, HTN-2 and HTN-3 trials of RDN in treatment-resistant hypertension are still unclear and have been the subject of much speculation.[71,72]

One obvious explanation for failure of RDN to lower BP in these trials is that the patients were already on at least three antihypertensive medications, including blockers of the RAAS which may mediate at least part of the effect of the renal nerves on BP. Another possible explanation is that the effectiveness of the procedures may have differed in various trials because the extent of RDN was not verified. The usual radiofrequency method causes only 40% to 50% RDN even under optimal procedures.[73,74] Experimental studies indicate that up to 75% ablation of the renal nerves can be achieved if the radiofrequency ablation includes all branches of the main renal artery close to the hilum of kidneys.[75] However, this extensive denervation was not achieved in any of the SYMPLICITY trials. Further studies will be required to determine whether RDN is an effective therapy for patients with resistant hypertension and improved methods are needed to predict which patients will benefit most from RDN. Also, longer follow-up periods will be needed to determine if the renal nerves eventually regrow and reinitiate increases in BP as observed in experimental animal models of RDN.[76]

Excessive sympathetic activation clearly plays a major role in contributing to hypertension in many patients, especially those who have visceral obesity.[2] As discussed previously, obesity accounts for much of the risk for human essential hypertension. In the section on primary hypertension, we discuss some of the mechanisms that may contribute to SNS activation and hypertension in obese subjects. There are, however, many additional factors besides obesity that have been proposed to cause SNS activation in hypertension, as discussed in several excellent reviews.[65,77,78] Two factors that have recently received considerable attention include baroceptor dysfunction and chemoreceptor activation of the SNS.

Arterial Baroreceptors and Long-Term Blood Pressure Regulation

The role of the arterial baroreflex system in moment-to-moment regulation of BP is well known but its importance in long-term BP control remains controversial. Although unloading the baroreceptors by carotid sinus denervation markedly increases BP variability, the average 24-hour mean arterial pressure is not substantially altered after a few days.[21] Also, in chronic hypertension there may be resetting of the arterial baroreceptors to higher BPs, leading to the suggestion that the baroreflex may have little role in long-term BP regulation.[21,77] To the extent that resetting of baroreceptors occurs, their potency as a long-term controller of BP would be diminished. This suggestion is bolstered by the observation that arterial baroreceptor denervation in dogs may increase the rapidity of the rise in BP but not the eventual severity of several forms of chronic hypertension.[21] In contrast, studies in rodents suggest that baroreceptor denervation exacerbates increased BP induced by a chronic high salt diet.[79] Other studies also suggest that baroreceptors may not completely reset in hypertension and therefore buffer increases in BP.[78] Thus, it is still unclear whether baroreceptor dysfunction merely alters the time course for onset of hypertension or plays an important role in long-term BP regulation.

Chronic electric stimulation of the afferent nerves of the carotid sinus baroreceptors produces sustained reductions in SNS activity and BP in normotensive dogs and hypertensive obese dogs.[80] Although baroreflex activation by electric stimulation of carotid sinus nerves also caused transient reductions in BP in dogs infused with Ang II or aldosterone, minimal long-term effects on BP were observed in these models of hypertension.[71] In humans with treatment-resistant hypertension, however, electrical stimulation of baroreceptors caused significant and sustained reductions in BP.[81] These observations indicate that strong chronic activation of the carotid sinus nerves can lower BP in humans with treatment-resistant hypertension and in some, but not all, forms of experimental hypertension.

Electric stimulation of the carotid sinus afferent nerves bypasses the mechanosensors that may contribute to baroreceptor resetting in chronic hypertension. Therefore, the observation that chronic stimulation of baroreceptor afferents lowers BP does not necessarily reveal the physiologic importance of the arterial baroreceptors in long-term BP regulation.

Although the physiologic role of baroreceptor dysfunction in contributing to chronic hypertension is still controversial, there is little doubt that impaired baroreflexes lead to increased BP lability. There is also evidence that large swings in BP associated with impaired baroreflexes eventually cause renal injury that could exacerbate the impact of other hypertensive stimuli. For example, baroreceptor-denervated animals have significant glomerular injury as well as cardiac hypertrophy.[82,83] Therefore, it seems likely that the arterial baroreceptors play a significant role in protecting the heart, blood vessels and kidneys against injury that would otherwise occur with heightened lability of BP.

Peripheral Chemoreceptors and Blood Pressure Regulation

The carotid bodies are chemosensors that initiate reflex increases in ventilation and SNS activity in response to hypoxemia.[84] These chemoreceptors may interact with arterial baroreceptors such that chemoreceptor activation impairs baroreceptor sensitivity whereas carotid body inhibition and/or resection improve baroreflex function. Studies in spontaneous hypertensive rats (SHR) and in patients with primary hypertension suggest that tonic increases in peripheral chemoreceptor activity may contribute to sustained increases in SNS activity, including renal sympathetic nerve activity (RSNA), and hypertension.[85,86] For example, denervation of the carotid body reduced RSNA and attenuated hypertension in SHR.[86] Deactivation of carotid body chemoreceptors by respiration with 100% oxygen reduced muscle SNS activity in hypertensive men but not in control subjects.[87]

Surgical removal of the carotid body for treatment of bronchial asthma or chronic obstructive pulmonary disease has been reported to cause a significant decrease in BP that was sustained for 6 months in hypertensive patients, whereas no reduction in BP was seen in normotensive patients and a rise in BP was found in hypotensive patients.[88] However, there have been no clinical trials to examine the effect of unilateral carotid body resection for hypertension in humans.

Repeated activation of peripheral chemoreceptor in sleep apnea has been suggested to contribute to increased BP as well as metabolic derangements in metabolism in obese subjects.[89] However, establishing cause and effect relationships between chemoreceptor activation and hypertension in obese patients with sleep apnea have been challenging. Even in the absence of obstructive sleep apnea, obesity may activate or sensitize the carotid chemoreceptors. Hypoxemia has been reported in some subjects with obesity,[90,91] although its overall prevalence in obesity is unclear. Lohmeier and colleagues reported that obese dogs fed a high fat diet for only 5 weeks had increases in BP and respiratory rate along with hypoxemia.[92] Moreover, denervation of the carotid sinus region attenuated increases in BP in obese dogs and transiently reduced respiratory rate while exacerbating hypoxemia. These findings suggest that hypoxemia may account for stimulation of peripheral chemoreceptors in obese dogs and that this activation may cause compensatory increases in ventilation and central sympathetic outflow that contributes to neurogenically-mediated increases in BP. However, the role of hypoxemia and peripheral chemoreceptor stimulation in contributing to hypertension in humans is still unclear.

ENDOTHELIN

Endothelial cells can also release vasoconstrictor substances such as endothelin (ET) which only requires nanogram quantities to cause vasoconstriction. Although ET can be expressed as three peptides, ET-1 is the predominant isoform expressed in the cardiovascular system and is the most powerful vasoconstrictor known in humans. Tissue concentrations of ET-1 may be elevated in some forms of hypertension but circulating levels of ET-1 are typically not elevated in patients with essential hypertension or in most models of experimental hypertension unless accompanied by renal failure, endothelial damage, or atherosclerosis.[93-96] However, circulating ET-1 levels do not reflect the local vascular production. ET-1 acts on nearby vascular smooth muscle cells (VSMCs) in a paracrine fashion to cause vasoconstriction.

ET-1 has differential effects depending on which receptor it activates. Activation of ET type A (ET_A) receptors can elicit a hypertensive effect via vasoconstriction and impaired renal-pressure natriuresis as well as exerting a proliferative effect on VSMCs.[97] Chronic ET-1 activation of ET_A receptors in the kidneys may contribute to the development of hypertension and renal injury. ET-1 decreases GFR and renal blood flow by VSMC and mesangial cell contraction. Furthermore, chronic ET-1 may stimulate mesangial cell proliferation, extracellular matrix deposition and VSMC hypertrophy which can increase renal vascular resistance.[98] Augmented ET-1 expression has been noted in animal models of hypertension and renal injury.[99-102] Furthermore, chronic blockade of the ET_A receptor attenuated hypertension and renal injury in these models.[103,104]

Activation of the ET type B (ET_B) receptors can exert an antihypertensive effect by inducing endothelial-dependent vasodilation likely mediated by release of nitric oxide (NO) and prostaglandins.[105,106] ET_B receptors may also play an important role in renal sodium and water handling.[107] ET_B receptor knockout mice develop severe salt-sensitive hypertension and pharmacologic blockade of ET_B receptors causes elevated BP in rats.[108-110] Studies in animals have demonstrated that ET-1modulates renal tubular transport. ET_B receptor deletion in endothelial cells causes endothelial dysfunction without hypertension; however, as mentioned before, total body knockout of ET_B receptors resulted in salt-sensitive hypertension. This discrepancy suggests that inactivation of ET_B receptors in nonendothelial cells can cause hypertension. To this point, genetic deletion of ET_B receptors in the CD causes hypertension suggesting ET_B receptor activation in the CD has a powerful natriuretic effect to reduce BP. The natriuretic and diuretic effects of ET-1 on ET_B receptors in the CD as well as in the thick ascending limb to reduce BP appear to be at least partly mediated by NO.[111,112]

ET-1 may also cause renal cellular proliferation and over-expression of ET-1 causes glomerulosclerosis and interstitial fibrosis.[106,113] ET-1 also appears to play an important role in mediating vascular remodeling, vasoconstriction and cellular proliferation in the lungs and therefore is a target for treating pulmonary arterial hypertension.[114] Although ET-1 receptor antagonists have been beneficial in patients with pulmonary arterial hypertension, their role in treatment of human essential hypertension is unclear. Currently these agents are not used for management of primary hypertension because of their side effects including fluid retention and edema. Initially, the nonselective ET receptor antagonist bosentan was evaluated in patients with primary hypertension and lowered diastolic BP. Darusentan, a more selective ET_A receptor antagonist, was subsequently evaluated in patients with resistant hypertension and found to reduce systolic and diastolic BPs significantly compared with placebo.[115] Despite the BP lowering effects of these drugs, adverse side effects have limited their use in patients with primary hypertension.

Theoretically, selective blockade of ET_A receptors would have advantages for treating hypertension while not antagonizing the antihypertensive effects of ET_B receptors. Although large clinical trials of these agents have not demonstrated acceptable tolerability for treatment of patients with primary hypertension, it is possible that ET receptor antagonists may have beneficial effects in resistant hypertensive patients attributable to certain pathophysiologic states such as pre-eclampsia or cancer patients treated with antiangiogenic agents.[106]

NITRIC OXIDE

NO, a lipophilic gas and potent vasodilator, is released from healthy endothelial cells in response to multiple chemical or physical stimuli. Vascular NO is produced mainly from L-arginine by endothelial NO synthase (eNOS). NO has a short half-life (approximately 6 seconds) and mainly acts locally in the tissues where it is secreted. NO activates soluble guanylate cyclase which catalyzes the conversion of cGTP to cyclic cGMP and activates kinases which mediate vasodilation. cGMP is degraded by phosphodiesterases (PDEs). NO also plays an important role to blunt the vasoconstrictor actions of ET-1 and NOS inhibition amplifies the vasoconstrictor effects of ET-1.[116,117] However, it is not clear if this effect is simply related to NO inhibition of vasoconstriction because of endogenously released ET-1 or whether NO inhibits ET-1 release.[118]

NO plays an important role in chronic regulation of renal blood flow and BP. Intrarenal NO production reduces renal vascular resistance, increases natriuresis, and helps buffer vasoconstrictor-induced reductions in renal medullary blood flow and tissue hypoxia.[119] Long-term inhibition of NOS causes sustained hypertension and impaired renal-pressure natriuresis[120] by several mechanisms, including hemodynamic and tubular effects, each of which may be modulated by processes that are intrinsic or extrinsic to the kidneys.[121-123] Decreased production of NO via reduced L-arginine synthesis and bioinactivation of NO because of increased oxidative stress leads to NO deficiency in chronic kidney disease patients which ultimately contributes to resistant hypertension.[124]

Increased renal NO production, as reflected by increased urinary excretion of NO metabolites or cGMP, the NO second messenger, appears to be essential for maintenance of normotension during dietary salt challenges. Prevention of increased renal NO production resulted in salt-sensitive hypertension. Genetic models of hypertension, such as Dahl salt-sensitive (DS) rat, have impaired pressure natriuresis associated with NO deficiency. Stimulation of NO production with chronic L-arginine supplementation normalizes the blunted pressure natriuretic response in DS rats by improving the kidneys' ability to generate increased renal interstitial hydrostatic pressure during increased renal perfusion pressure.[123]

OXIDATIVE STRESS

Oxidative stress, because of an imbalance of reactive oxygen species (ROS), is a risk factor for cardiovascular disease. Experimental evidence suggests that ROS play an important role in hypertension.[125] Common ROS include superoxide, hydrogen peroxide and peroxynitrite among others. Although these free radicals have important functions to maintain normal cell signaling and homeostasis, when levels exceed the body's antioxidant mechanisms ROS can cause damage to cells and tissues.[126] In some forms of hypertension, increased ROS appear to be derived mainly from nicotinamide adenine dinucleotide phosphate (NADPH) oxidases, which could serve as a trigger for uncoupling endothelial NOS by oxidants. Four members of the NADPH oxidase (Nox) enzyme family have been identified as important sources of ROS in the vasculature: Nox1, Nox2, Nox4, and Nox5.

Experimental studies have demonstrated a role for oxidative stress in the pathophysiology of hypertension. For example, Ang II-mediated hypertension is associated with increased vascular superoxide production and impaired vasodilation.[127] The DS rat has increased vascular and renal superoxide production and increased levels of H_2O_2. Renal expression of superoxide dismutase is decreased in kidneys of DS rats, and long-term administration of tempol, a superoxide dismutase mimetic, significantly decreases BP and attenuates renal damage.[128] Mice deficient in p47(phox), a subunit of the NAPDH oxidase, exhibit lower BP than wild-type mice as well as attenuated hypertensive responses to Ang II and no increased vascular production of superoxide. Administration of tempol to salt-loaded stroke-prone SHR attenuated vascular remodeling, reduced superoxide levels and prevented worsening hypertension compared with controls.[129]

ROS also appear to regulate several vascular transcriptional factors and other vascular signaling pathways that regulate cell growth, migration, and inflammation. In addition, ROS appear to play a role in regulation of vascular smooth muscle cell calcium concentrations and vascular contraction. In SHR, hydrogen peroxide enhances activation of L-type calcium channels and increases calcium influx but superoxide blunts these actions suggesting differential activation of calcium channels by ROS.[130]

Patients with essential hypertension have higher plasma hydrogen peroxide levels than normotensive patients.[131] Although increased ROS production is believed to contribute to human hypertension, clinical studies using chronic antioxidant therapy have failed to confirm this idea. Some, but not all, studies of human primary hypertension have reported an imbalance between total oxidant production and the antioxidant capacity in human primary hypertension. Equivocal findings in human studies are partly caused by the difficulty of assessing oxidative stress. Measurement of ROS in tissues is challenging because of their low levels and short half-lives.[132,133] Most human studies have found that chronic antioxidant therapy with vitamin E and C supplementation has little or no effect on BP.[132,133] However, high concentrations of these vitamins may function as prooxidants, causing cell damage and perhaps explaining some of the negative clinical trial results.[134] Some of the beneficial effects of antihypertensive agents such as RAAS blockers (ACEIs or ARBs) or β blockers may be caused, in part, by reduced generation of ROS because carvedilol and candesartan have been shown to have antioxidant actions.[135,136]

PRIMARY (ESSENTIAL) HYPERTENSION

Primary hypertension (also called "essential" or "idiopathic" hypertension) accounts for at least 90% of human hypertension. In only a small percentage of patients who have "secondary" hypertension is a specific cause of increased BP apparent, based on patient history, clinical features, physical examination, and lab tests. Box 5.1 summarizes some of the most frequently diagnosed causes of secondary hypertension including those caused by drugs that raise BP or exacerbate underlying disorders that contribute to hypertension. Many of these forms of hypertension are associated with renal injury, renal ischemia, or SNS/endocrine disorders that cause kidney dysfunction. A more detailed discussion of the pathogenesis of secondary hypertension is presented in other chapters of this book.

As discussed earlier, many of the long-term BP controllers either directly or indirectly influence renal function. In patients with primary hypertension, sodium balance is maintained at higher BP indicating that pressure natriuresis has been reset. In some hypertensive subjects, this resetting is related to increased renal tubular reabsorption whereas others have renal vasoconstriction and reduced GFR, as a result of intrarenal, neurohormonal, or immune-mediated mechanisms. After hypertension is established, many of these kidney changes are difficult to detect because increased BP often returns many of the indices of renal function (eg, GFR, tubular reabsorption, plasma renin) to nearly normal.

Mild primary hypertension associated with aging, obesity, atherosclerosis, high sodium chloride intake, low potassium intake, or excess alcohol consumption may evolve into secondary hypertension, especially as renal injury occurs. Thus, the distinction between primary and secondary forms of hypertension is not always clear in many patients who have had poorly controlled hypertension for many years.

POSSIBLE ROLE OF GENE VARIANTS, GENE-ENVIRONMENT INTERACTIONS, AND EPIGENETICS IN PRIMARY HYPERTENSION

Considerable effort has been devoted to searching for genetic causes of hypertension. Although several monogenic disorders that increase renal sodium reabsorption and BP have been discovered, together they account for only a tiny percentage (<1%) of human hypertension. Despite limited success, the search for gene variants that contribute to primary

BOX 5.1 Some Secondary Causes of Hypertension

A. Renovascular
- Renal artery stenosis/compression
- Intrarenal vasculitis
- Suprarenal aortic coarctation

B. Renal Parenchymal Disease
- Acute and chronic glomerulonephritis
- Chronic nephritis (eg, pyelonephritis, radiation)
- Polycystic disease
- Diabetic nephropathy
- Hydronephrosis
- Neoplasms

C. Renoprival (Renal Failure, Loss of Kidney Tissue)

D. Endocrine Disorders
- Primary aldosteronism
- Cushing syndrome
- Pheochromocytoma (adrenal or extraadrenal chromaffin tumors)
- Renin-producing tumors
- Pheochromocytoma (adrenal or extraadrenal chromaffin tumors)
- Acromegaly

E. Pregnancy-Induced Hypertension

F. Sleep Apnea

G. Increased Intracranial Pressure (Brain Tumors, Encephalitis)

H. Exogenous Hormones and Drugs (Partial List)
- Excess alcohol use
- Nonsteroidal antiinflammatory drugs
- Drug abuse (eg, amphetamines, cocaine)
- Sympathomimetics
- Glucocorticoids
- Mineralocorticoids
- Tyramine-containing foods and monoamine oxidase inhibitors
- Apparent mineralocorticoid excess (eg, licorice)
- Cyclosporine

hypertension has been spurred by studies of BP patterns in families suggesting that genetic factors may account for as much as 30% to 50% of BP variance.[137,138]

Multiple studies indicate that the closer the genetic relatedness, the greater the similarity of BP.[139,140] For monozygotic twins (with genetic similarity of 100%), the correlation coefficient for systolic BP has ranged from 0.5 to 0.8 (average 0.6), for dizygotic twins it has ranged from 0.19 to 0.46 (average 0.35), and for nontwin siblings (genetic similarity of around 50%) the correlation coefficient has averaged around 0.23. There is also a better correlation of BP values in biologic children than in adopted children.

Although many studies have shown associations of gene polymorphisms and BP, the genetic alterations that contribute to primary hypertension remain elusive. Mixed results have been obtained even for widely studied polymorphisms such as the ACE insertion/deletion and angiotensinogen polymorphisms.[138,141] Polymorphisms and mutations in other genes such as uromodulin, α-adducin, atrial natriuretic factor, the insulin receptor, β2-adrenergic receptor, calcitonin gene-related peptide, angiotensinase C, renin-binding protein, endothelin-1 precursor, G-protein β3-subunit have also been associated with hypertension in some studies[142]; however, all of these polymorphisms show weak associations with BP and many of the early studies have not been confirmed.

Large-scale genome-wide association studies (GWAS) in which hundreds of thousands of common genetic variants were genotyped and analyzed for BP association had limited success in identifying genes that contribute to hypertension.[143,144] The International Consortium for Blood Pressure Genome-Wide Association Studies, which used a multistage design in 200,000 individuals of European descent, identified 16 novel functional genetic variants, associated with high BP.[145] Six of these loci involved genes that were already known to regulate BP whereas the other gene variants suggested novel pathways. However, even with these heroic attempts, the discovered genetic variants collectively account for only a tiny fraction of BP variation and hypertension risk.[146]

Considering the complexity of the multiple neural, hormonal, renal, and vascular mechanisms for short-term and long-term BP regulation it is perhaps not surprising that it has been challenging to find a few variant alleles that account for a major portion of BP variation. The complexity of the problem is compounded by the likelihood that genetic variation of BP is caused not only by single gene variations, but also by polymorphic genetic differences, complex interactions among several genes and interaction among genetic and environmental factors.[138,140]

Hypertension has been suggested to result from additive effects of multiple variant genes acting in concert to elevate BP. Each gene variant is presumed to have a weak impact on BP but when acting together in the presence of the necessary environmental conditions may produce significant hypertension. However, despite the use of sophisticated mathematic models for calculating gene-gene and gene-environment interactions, the likelihood of nonlinear interactions makes it difficult to quantify the precise roles of genes and environment in BP variation.

Further complicating efforts to find genetic contributions to hypertension is the possibility that epigenetic modifications may alter the protein products of genes through mitosis or meiosis without altering the DNA sequence.[147,148] These epigenetic changes can arise throughout life from early embryos to old age, and some studies suggest that epigenetic variants can be transmitted via parental gametes for several generations.[146] However, the contribution of epigenetic modifications to human hypertension is still largely unexplored.

The key role of environmental factors in primary hypertension is supported by the observation that hypertension and age-related increases in BP rarely develop in hunter-gatherers living in nonindustrialized societies. Also, comprehensive familial analyses that include other relatives in addition to twins suggest that the environment contributes at least 30% of BP variance.[140] These observations obviously do not imply that genetic factors are unimportant in hypertension. Genetic variation may be responsible for differences in baseline BP and the normal BP distribution in a population. When hypertension-producing environmental factors (eg, excess weight gain, high sodium intake, low potassium intake) are added to the population baseline BP, the normal frequency distribution is shifted toward higher BP and the curve flattens with increased variability in the overall population BP. Yet, experimental, clinical and population studies suggest that modern sedentary lifestyles associated with excessive weight gain are playing an increasing important role in primary hypertension.

ROLE OF OVERWEIGHT AND OBESITY IN PRIMARY HYPERTENSION

Obesity has rapidly become a major health care challenge. obesity has nearly doubled since 1980 and current estimates indicate that more than 1.4 billion adults are overweight or obese.[149] In the United States alone, approximately 65% of the adults are overweight and 35% are obese.[150,151] Major consequences of being overweight or obese include higher prevalence of hypertension and a cascade of associated

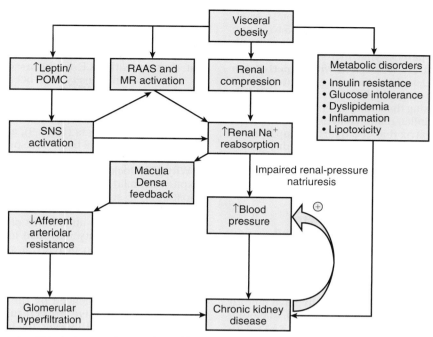

FIG. 5.8 Summary of mechanisms by which obesity causes hypertension and kidney injury. Visceral obesity increases blood pressure by activation of the sympathetic nervous system (SNS) and the renin–angiotensin–aldosterone system (RAAS), and by physical compression of the kidneys from the fat surrounding the kidneys. These effects increase renal sodium reabsorption and impair pressure natriuresis. SNS activation may be caused, in part, by the central nervous system effects of leptin, which acts on proopiomelanocortin (POMC) neurons in the hypothalamus and brainstem. Obesity-induced hypertension and glomerular hyperfiltration may cause kidney injury, especially when combined with dyslipidemia, hyperglycemia and other metabolic disorders. Renal injury then exacerbates the hypertension and makes it more difficult to control. *MR*, Mineralocorticoid receptor.

cardiovascular, renal and metabolic disorders. Studies in diverse populations throughout the world have shown that the relationship between body mass index (BMI) and BP is linear and population studies suggest that 65% to 78% of the risk for hypertension is because of excess weight gain.[1,11,152] Clinical studies also indicate that maintenance of a BMI less than 25 kg/m^2 is effective in preventing hypertension and that weight loss reduces BP in most hypertensive subjects.[153,154]

Although there is impressive evidence that excessive weight gain raises BP, not all obese persons are hypertensive. Some individuals may be more susceptible to the effects of obesity on BP but it is also clear that excess weight gain shifts the BP frequency distribution toward higher levels increasing the probability that a person's BP will register in the hypertensive range. Therefore, even though some obese people have BPs lower than 140/90 mm Hg, the level usually considered as "hypertension," these obese "normotensives" have higher BP than they would at a lower body weight. Moreover, weight loss lowers BP in "normotensive" as well as "hypertensive" obese subjects.[155] The impact of obesity on BP also depends on how long a person has been overweight and how much target organ injury has occurred. When obesity is sustained over many years leading to diabetes, dyslipidemia and kidney injury, hypertension typically worsens and becomes more resistant to treatment.

Another factor that influences the impact of obesity on BP is the distribution of the excess fat. Most population studies of obesity have investigated the relationship between BP and body mass index (BMI) rather than visceral or retroperitoneal fat which appear to be better predictors of increased BP than subcutaneous fat.[156]

Hemodynamic and Renal Changes in Obesity-Induced Hypertension

Obesity is associated with extracellular fluid volume expansion and, in many tissues, higher blood flows which increase venous return and cardiac output.[157,158] Blood flows in tissues such as the kidneys, skeletal muscle, and heart are increased in obese subjects even when normalized for increased tissue weight.[2] Thus, obesity is associated with functional vasodilation that is likely because of increases in metabolic rate and tissue oxygen consumption. Despite higher resting blood flows, however, there is endothelial dysfunction, arterial stiffening and reduced blood flow "reserve" in tissues such as skeletal muscle which limits exercise–induced hyperemia.[2]

The mechanisms responsible for vascular dysfunction in obesity are not fully understood but likely involve interactions of increased BP, inflammation, hyperglycemia, "lipotoxicity" caused by excessive non-β-oxidative metabolism of fatty acids, oxidative stress, and activation of multiple neurohormonal systems. Excess visceral fat is also an important source of cytokines and other factors that lead to oxidative stress, inflammation, endothelial dysfunction, vascular stiffening, and eventually atherosclerosis.[159]

Obesity Increases Renal Sodium Reabsorption and Impairs Pressure Natriuresis

Increased renal sodium reabsorption and impaired renal-pressure natriuresis play a major role in initiating the rise in BP associated with excess weight gain.[160] At least three major factors increase renal sodium reabsorption and BP during rapid, excessive weight gain (Fig. 5.8): (1) Compression of the kidneys by increased visceral, retroperitoneal and renal sinus fat; (2) RAAS activation, including stimulation of MR independent of aldosterone; and (3) SNS activation and increased renal sympathetic nerve activity (RSNA). Also, CKD may, over a much longer time, amplify the BP effects of these mechanisms and, make obesity-associated hypertension more difficult to control and less easily reversed by weight loss.[2,161]

Increases in Visceral, Retroperitoneal and Renal Sinus Fat Compress the Kidneys

Excess fat accumulation in and around the kidneys may cause renal compression and increased BP. In patients with visceral obesity, intraabdominal pressure rises in proportion to sagittal abdominal diameter, reaching levels as high as 35 to 40 mm Hg.[162] These high pressures compress the renal veins, lymph vessels, ureters and renal parenchyma. Increases in retroperitoneal and renal sinus fat are associated with hypertension and increased risk for CKD in obese humans even after adjustment for BMI and visceral adiposity.[163,164]

In addition to compressing the kidneys, retroperitoneal and renal sinus fat may cause inflammation and expansion of renal medullary extracellular matrix that could further impair renal function.[2] Accumulation of fat in and around the kidneys may have additional "lipotoxic" effects on the kidneys because of increased oxidative stress, mitochondrial dysfunction, and endoplasmic reticulum stress.

Renin-Angiotensin-Aldosterone System Activation Contributes to Obesity-Induced Hypertension

The importance of the RAAS in BP regulation was discussed previously in this chapter and its role in obesity hypertension has been extensively reviewed.[155,165,166] Obese subjects, especially those with visceral obesity, generally have mild to moderate increases in plasma renin activity (PRA), angiotensinogen, ACE activity, Ang II, and aldosterone.[167] RAAS activation occurs despite sodium retention and hypertension which normally suppress Ang II formation. Compression of the kidneys and increased SNS activation likely contribute to increased renin secretion.

Some studies also suggest a role for a local RAAS in adipose tissue.[168] Angiotensinogen is produced in adipocytes but the importance of adipose tissue as a source of Ang II formation is still unclear. There have been no studies, to our knowledge, directly demonstrating that adipocyte-specific derived angiotensinogen or Ang II have a major influence on BP regulation in obesity.

Ang II Increases Sodium Reabsorption in Obesity Hypertension

An important role for Ang II in stimulating renal sodium reabsorption in obesity hypertension is supported by studies demonstrating that ARBs or ACE inhibitors attenuate sodium retention, volume expansion, and increased BP in obese rodents and dogs fed a high fat diet.[169,170] In obese Zucker rats there is increased sensitivity to the BP effects of Ang II and ARB lowers BP to a greater extent than in lean rats despite lower PRA.[171]

Although smaller clinical trials have demonstrated that ARBs, renin inhibitors, or ACE inhibitors are effective in lowering BP in obese hypertensive patients,[172-174] there have been no large-scale clinical studies comparing the effectiveness of RAAS blockers in obese and lean hypertensive patients.

Activation of the RAAS contributes to kidney injury in obese subjects by increasing BP and through intrarenal effects. Constriction of efferent arterioles by Ang II exacerbates the rise in glomerular hydrostatic pressure caused by systemic arterial hypertension. ACE inhibitors or ARBs slow progression of CKD in obese type II diabetic patients.[175,176] However, further studies are needed to assess the efficacy of RAAS blockers compared with other antihypertensive agents in treating hypertension and reducing the risk of renal injury in nondiabetic, obese subjects.

Mineralocorticoid Receptor Activation Increases Sodium Reabsorption in Obesity Hypertension

Blockade of MR with spironolactone or eplerenone provides an important therapeutic tool for lowering BP and attenuating target organ injury in obesity hypertension. In obese dogs, for example, MR antagonism markedly attenuated sodium retention, hypertension, and glomerular hyperfiltration. MR

blockade provided antihypertensive benefit in treatment-resistant obese patients, although there was no correlation between plasma aldosterone levels and BP responses[60,64,177]; BP reductions after MR antagonism occurred despite concurrent therapy with ACE inhibitors or ARBs, suggesting that MR activation in obesity can occur independently of Ang II-mediated stimulation of aldosterone secretion.[64] In fact, combined blockade of MR and Ang II receptors may be especially effective in reducing BP and preventing target organ injury in obese subjects (Fig. 5.9), although no large randomized controlled clinical trials have provided definitive support for this therapeutic approach.

Why MR blockade is so effective in lowering BP in obesity despite only mild increases or even slight decreases in plasma aldosterone is still unclear. One explanation is that obesity enhances sensitivity to aldosterone-mediated MR activation because of increased abundance of the α subunit of ENaC in the kidneys.[178] Obesity may also increase renal tubular epithelial cell expression of Rac1, a small GTP-binding protein member of the Rho family of GTPases that activates MR signal transduction.[64] The glucocorticoid cortisol may also contribute to MR activation in obesity. The ability of cortisol to activate MR may be influenced by the intracellular redox state, with increased oxidative stress resulting in increased MR activation by cortisol.[179] However, the importance of these mechanisms is unclear and further studies are needed to determine the mechanisms by which MR blockade lowers BP in obesity hypertension.

Sympathetic Nervous System Activation Contributes to Obesity-Induced Hypertension

Studies in experimental animals and humans indicate that increased SNS activity contributes to obesity hypertension.[11,180] (1) SNS activity, assessed by direct recordings of muscle sympathetic nerve activity (MSNA) or renal norepinephrine spillover, is increased in obese hypertensive subjects; (2) administration of α/β-adrenergic blockers or clonidine, which stimulates central α-2 adrenergic receptors and reduces SNS activity, prevents most of the obesity-induced rise in BP in obese animals and α/β-adrenergic blockade reduces ambulatory BP significantly more in obese than in lean hypertensive patients[155,181,182]; and (3) renal denervation (RDN) markedly attenuates sodium retention and hypertension in obese animals and obese patients with resistant hypertension.[68,73,80]

Several mediators of SNS activation in obesity have been suggested, including: (1) impaired baroreceptor reflexes; (2) activation of chemoreceptor-mediated reflexes associated with sleep apnea and intermittent hypoxia; (3) hyperinsulinemia;

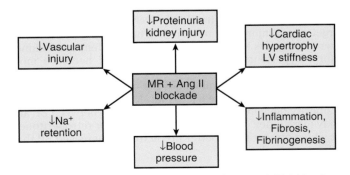

FIG. 5.9 Combined blockade of mineralocorticoid receptor (MR) (with spironolactone or eplerenone) and Ang II (with Ang II receptor blockers or angiotensin-converting enzyme inhibitors) may be especially effective in reducing blood pressure and preventing target organ injury in obese, treatment-resistant subjects. Adverse effects of MR antagonism in some patients include gynecomastia (~6%), hyperkalemia (~ 4%, plasma K+ > 5.5 mmol/L, although diabetic patients may have higher prevalence), and hyponatremia (~1%, plasma Na+ < 130 mmol/L).[205] *LV*, Left ventricle.

(4) Ang II; (5) cytokines released from adipocytes such as leptin, tumor necrosis factor-α (TNF-α) and interleukin-6 (IL-6); and (6) the CNS proopiomelanocortin (POMC) pathway. We discussed earlier in the chapter the potential role of impaired baroreflexes and activation of peripheral chemoreceptors. Although the role of many of these factors is still uncertain, leptin secreted by adipocytes and the CNS POMC pathway appears to mediate at least part of the obesity-induced SNS activation and hypertension.[180,183-185]

Leptin May Link Increased Adiposity With Sympathetic Nervous System Activation

Leptin is a cytokine peptide released from adipocytes in proportion to the degree of adiposity. There is a positive association between plasma leptin concentration and MSNA activity and acute leptin administration in rodents increases SNS activity in various tissues including the kidneys.[180] Acute hyperleptinemia also increases MSNA in humans.[186] Chronic increases in plasma leptin, comparable to those found in severe obesity, causes sustained increases in BP and HR in rodents.[187] Leptin-mediated BP increases occur gradually over several days, consistent with modest increases in SNS activity that are not sufficient to directly cause vasoconstriction but sufficient to increase renal sodium reabsorption. The BP effects of leptin were completely abolished by combined α/β-adrenergic receptor blockade and enhanced by blockade of NO.[181,188] Thus, physiologic levels of leptin can increase BP by SNS activation and these effects are exacerbated when there is NO deficiency, which often occurs in obese subjects with endothelial dysfunction.

A role for endogenous leptin in obesity hypertension is supported by the finding that administration of a leptin receptor antagonist reduced BP and renal SNS activity in obese rabbits fed a high fat diet.[189] Also, obese children with leptin gene mutations have normal BP despite early onset morbid obesity and many other characteristics of the metabolic syndrome, including severe insulin resistance, hyperinsulinemia, and hyperlipidemia.[190] These observations suggest that the functional effects of leptin may be critical in linking obesity with SNS activation and hypertension.

The Central Nervous System Proopiomelanocortin Pathway May Contribute to Sympathetic Nervous System Activation in Obesity

The CNS POMC pathway regulates appetite, energy expenditure and body weight.[191] POMC-expressing neurons in the hypothalamus and brainstem release α-melanocyte stimulating hormone (α-MSH), an agonist for melanocortin 4 receptors (MC4R) (Fig. 5.10). In addition to regulating energy balance, the CNS POMC-MC4R system may contribute to obesity-induced SNS activation and hypertension. Chronic pharmacologic activation of CNS MC4R increases BP while reducing appetite and body weight in rodents and in humans.[192-194] Conversely, blockade of CNS MC4R increases food intake and causes rapid weight gain but reduces rather than increases BP.[195,196] The BP-lowering effects of MC4R antagonism are especially pronounced in SHR, a genetic model of hypertension characterized by increased SNS activity.[195]

Hypertension prevalence is lower in MC4R deficient humans compared with control subjects, despite severe

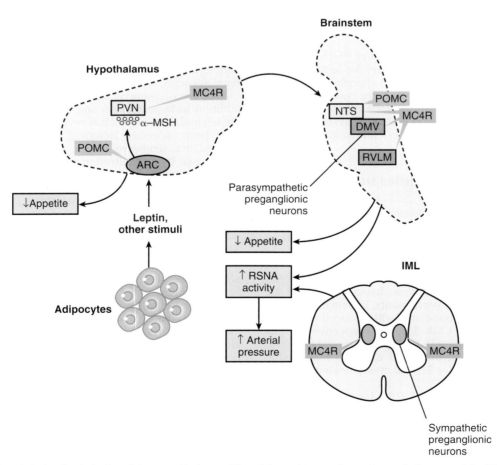

FIG. 5.10 Leptin-melanocortin signaling in the hypothalamus and brainstem differentially regulate appetite, renal sympathetic nerve activity (RSNA) and arterial pressure. Leptin receptor activation in proopiomelanocortin (POMC) neurons causes release α-melanocyte stimulating hormone (α-MSH) which stimulates melanocortin 4 receptors (MC4R) in second-order neurons of the hypothalamus, brainstem, and spinal cord intermediolateral nucleus (IML). *ARC,* Arcuate; *DMV,* dorsal motor nucleus of the vagus; *IML,* intermediolateral cell column; *NTS,* nucleus tractus solitaries; *PVN,* paraventricular; *RVLM,* rostral ventrolateral medulla.

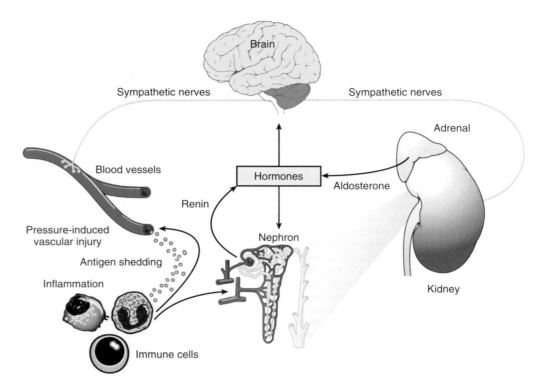

FIG. 5.11 Long-term blood pressure (BP) is regulated by a complex array of intrarenal and extrarenal factors (eg, neural, hormonal, and immune system). Chronic hypertension occurs when one or more of these factors impairs the kidneys' ability to excrete sodium and water and resets pressure natriuresis to a higher BP. This resetting can occur as a result of initial increases in tubular reabsorption or effects on the renal blood vessels that reduce glomerular filtration rate (GFR). After hypertension is established, many of these renal abnormalities may be obscured by increased BP which returns GFR and tubular reabsorption toward normal. Some of these pathways are targets of current antihypertensive therapies but research is uncovering new pathways, including immune and inflammatory mechanisms,[206] that also influence kidney function and control of BP and are discussed in other chapters of this book.

obesity and associated metabolic disorders.[194,197] Moreover, an intact CNS-POMC pathway is necessary for leptin to raise BP. In mice with leptin receptors deleted specifically in POMC neurons, leptin's hypertensive effects were completely abolished.[198] Thus, in humans and rodents, chronic activation of MC4R raises BP and a functional POMC-MC4R system appears to be necessary for obesity and hyperleptinemia to increase SNS activity and BP.

Chronic Kidney Injury Amplifies the Impact of Obesity on Hypertension

The impact of obesity on CKD is clear when one considers that type II diabetes and hypertension, both of which are closely associated with obesity, account for more than 70% of end-stage renal disease (ESRD). Also, the rapid rise in CKD in the past three decades has paralleled increasing obesity and there is evidence that obesity may be an independent risk factor for CKD, beyond its effects to cause hypertension and diabetes.[161] In 6500 nondiabetic participants, increasing BMI and waist circumference were associated with reduced estimated GFR (eGFR) and increased CKD.[199] In a retrospective analysis of 320,252 adults followed for 15 to 35 years, the rate of ESRD increased stepwise as BMI increased and this relationship remained after adjustment for BP, diabetes, smoking, age, and several other variables.[200]

Early in the development of obesity, there is often interstitial fibrosis, microalbuminuria or proteinuria, expansion of mesangial matrix, glomerulomegaly, focal segmental glomerular sclerosis, and podocyte disorder associated with glomerular hyperfiltration.[201-203] As obesity hypertension and metabolic abnormalities are sustained, glomerular hyperfiltration subsides and may be replaced by declining GFR associated with nephron loss.[161] With nephron loss there is increasing salt sensitivity of BP.[4] Obesity also aggravates the

deleterious effects of other primary kidney insults, including unilateral nephrectomy, kidney transplantation, unilateral renal agenesis, and IgA nephropathy.[202]

The mechanisms by which obesity causes renal injury, in addition to hypertension and diabetes, are still unclear and are beyond the scope of this review. However, multiple factors have been proposed including inflammation, mitochondrial dysfunction, oxidative stress, dyslipidemia and "lipotoxicity" caused by fat infiltration into and around the kidneys.[202] Regardless of the mechanisms involved, it is likely that the gradual decline in kidney function contributes to treatment resistant hypertension in overweight or obese subjects.[204]

SUMMARY AND PERSPECTIVES

Although chronic hypertension is a heterogeneous disorder, kidney dysfunction and impaired renal pressure natriuresis have been found in all forms of experimental and human hypertension studied thus far. Kidney dysfunction can be caused by a complex interplay of genetic and environmental factors that influence intrarenal, neurohormonal, immune and inflammatory systems (Fig. 5.11). In many instances abnormal kidney function is obscured by compensatory changes that permit the kidneys to maintain salt and water balance, albeit at higher BPs. Vascular dysfunction may occur concomitantly or secondarily to increased BP, but increases in nonrenal vascular resistance have not been shown to cause chronic hypertension unless renal-pressure natriuresis is also impaired.

Although there are many different causes of secondary hypertension associated with renal injury, renal ischemia, or SNS/endocrine disorders, they are responsible for less than 10% of human hypertension. Current evidence suggests that overweight and obesity may account for as much as 65% to 75% of the risk for increased BP in patients with primary hypertension, although other factors such as high salt intake, sedentary lifestyle, and genetic predisposition may compound the impact of excess weight gain on BP. The mediators of abnormal kidney function and increased BP in obese subjects are complex and include physical compression of the kidneys by fat in and around the kidneys, activation of the RAAS, and increased SNS activity. With prolonged obesity and development of organ injury, especially renal injury, hypertension becomes more difficult to control, often requiring multiple antihypertensive drugs and treatment of other risk factors, including dyslipidemia, insulin resistance and diabetes, and inflammation. Unless effective antiobesity drugs are developed, the impact of obesity on hypertension and related cardiorenal and metabolic disorders is likely to become even more important in the future as the prevalence of obesity continues to increase.

References

1. Garrison RJ, Kannel WB, Stokes J III, et al. Incidence and precursors of hypertension in young adults: the Framingham Offspring Study. *Prev Med*. 1987;16:235-251.
2. Hall JE, do Carmo JM, da Silva AA, et al. Obesity-induced hypertension: interaction of neurohumoral and renal mechanisms. *Circ Res*. 2015;116:991-1006.
3. Hall JE, Granger JP, do Carmo JM, et al. Hypertension: physiology and pathophysiology. *Compr Physiol*. 2012;2:2393-2442.
4. Hall JE. Renal Dysfunction, Rather Than Nonrenal Vascular Dysfunction, Mediates Salt-Induced Hypertension. *Circulation*. 2016;133:894-906.
5. Cowley AW Jr.. The concept of autoregulation of total blood flow and its role in hypertension. *Am J Med*. 1980;68:906-916.
6. Carlstrom M, Wilcox CS, Arendshorst WJ. Renal autoregulation in health and disease. *Physiol Rev*. 2015;95:405-511.
7. Coleman TG, Hall JE. Systemic hemodynamics and regional blood flow regulation. In Izzo JL Jr., Sica DA, Black HC, eds. *Hypertension Primer*. Washington, DC, American Heart Association; 2008:129-132.
8. Linz P, Santoro D, Renz W, et al. Skin sodium measured with ^{23}Na MRI at 7.0 T. *NMR Biomed*. 2015;28:54-62.
9. Kotchen TA, Cowley AW Jr., Frohlich ED. Salt in health and disease—a delicate balance. *N Engl J Med*. 2013;368:1229-1237.
10. Averina VA, Othmer HG, Fink GD, et al. A mathematical model of salt-sensitive hypertension: the neurogenic hypothesis. *J Physiol*. 2015;593:3065-3075.
11. Hall JE. The kidney, hypertension, and obesity. *Hypertension*. 2003;41:625-633.
12. Guyton AC. The surprising kidney-fluid mechanism for pressure control—its infinite gain! *Hypertension*. 1990;16:725-730.
13. Hall JE, Mizelle HL, Hildebrandt DA, et al. Abnormal pressure natriuresis. A cause or a consequence of hypertension? *Hypertension*. 1990;15:547-559.
14. Mizelle HL, Montani JP, Hester RL, et al. Role of pressure natriuresis in long-term control of renal electrolyte excretion. *Hypertension*. 1993;22:102-110.
15. Hall JE, Granger JP, Smith MJ Jr., et al. Role of renal hemodynamics and arterial pressure in aldosterone "escape". *Hypertension*. 1984;6:I183-I192.
16. Hall JE, Granger JP, Hester RL, et al. Mechanisms of escape from sodium retention during angiotensin II hypertension. *Am J Physiol*. 1984;246:F627-F634.
17. Hall JE, Montani JP, Woods LL, et al. Renal escape from vasopressin: role of pressure diuresis. *Am J Physiol*. 1986;250:F907-F916.
18. Hall JE, Mizelle HL, Woods LL, et al. Pressure natriuresis and control of arterial pressure during chronic norepinephrine infusion. *J Hypertens*. 1988;6:723-731.
19. Woods LL, Mizelle HL, Hall JE. Control of sodium excretion in NE-ACTH hypertension: role of pressure natriuresis. *Am J Physiol*. 1988;255:R894-R900.
20. Brands MW, Hall JE. Renal perfusion pressure is an important determinant of sodium and calcium excretion in DOC-salt hypertension. *Am J Hypertens*. 1998;11:1199-1207.
21. Cowley AW Jr.. Long-term control of arterial blood pressure. *Physiol Rev*. 1992;72:231-300.
22. Guyton AC. *Arterial pressure and hypertension: circulatory physiology III*. Philadelphia, WB Saunders; 1980:1-564.
23. Schrier RW, Howard RL. Unifying hypothesis of sodium and water regulation in health and disease. *Hypertension*. 1991;18:III164-III168.
24. Appel LJ, Frohlich ED, Hall JE, et al. The importance of population-wide sodium reduction as a means to prevent cardiovascular disease and stroke: a call to action from the American Heart Association. *Circulation*. 2011;123:1138-1143.
25. Whelton PK, Appel LJ, Sacco RL, et al. Sodium, blood pressure, and cardiovascular disease: further evidence supporting the American Heart Association sodium reduction recommendations. *Circulation*. 2012;126:2880-2889.
26. Kawasaki T, Delea CS, Bartter FC, et al. The effect of high-sodium and low-sodium intakes on blood pressure and other related variables in human subjects with idiopathic hypertension. *Am J Med*. 1978;64:193-198.
27. Rossier BC, Staub O, Hummler E. Genetic dissection of sodium and potassium transport along the aldosterone-sensitive distal nephron: importance in the control of blood pressure and hypertension. *FEBS Lett*. 2013;587:1929-1941.
28. Lifton RP, Gharavi AG, Geller DS. Molecular mechanisms of human hypertension. *Cell*. 2001;104:545-556.
29. Langston JB, Guyton AC, Douglas BH, et al. Effect of changes in salt intake on arterial pressure and renal function in partially nephrectomized dogs. *Circ Res*. 1963;12:508-512.
30. Koomans HA, Roos JC, Boer P, et al. Salt sensitivity of blood pressure in chronic renal failure. Evidence for renal control of body fluid distribution in man. *Hypertension*. 1982;4:190-197.
31. Johnson RJ, Lanaspa MA, Gabriela Sanchez-Lozada L, et al. The discovery of hypertension: evolving views on the role of the kidneys, and current hot topics. *Am J Physiol Renal Physiol*. 2015;308:F167-F178.
32. Hall JE. Control of sodium excretion by angiotensin II: intrarenal mechanisms and blood pressure regulation. *Am J Physiol*. 1986;250:R960-R972.
33. Hall JE, Guyton AC, Smith MJ Jr., et al. Blood pressure and renal function during chronic changes in sodium intake: role of angiotensin. *Am J Physiol*. 1980;239:F271-F280.
34. Kohan DE. Role of collecting duct endothelin in control of renal function and blood pressure. *Am J Physiol Regul Integr Comp Physiol*. 2013;305:R659-R668.
35. Kohan DE, Rossi NF, Inscho EW, et al. Regulation of blood pressure and salt homeostasis by endothelin. *Physiol Rev*. 2011;91:1-77.
36. Ge Y, Bagnall A, Stricklett PK, et al. Collecting duct-specific knockout of the endothelin B receptor causes hypertension and sodium retention. *Am J Physiol Renal Physiol*. 2006;291:F1274-F1280.
37. Ge Y, Bagnall A, Stricklett PK, et al. Combined knockout of collecting duct endothelin A and B receptors causes hypertension and sodium retention. *Am J Physiol Renal Physiol*. 2008;295:F1635-F1640.
38. Ahn D, Ge Y, Stricklett PK, et al. Collecting duct-specific knockout of endothelin-1 causes hypertension and sodium retention. *J Clin Invest*. 2004;114:504-511.
39. Speed JS, Heimlich JB, Hyndman KA, et al. Endothelin-1 as a master regulator of whole-body Na+ homeostasis. *FASEB J*. 2015.
40. Hoorn EJ, Nelson JH, McCormick JA, et al. The WNK kinase network regulating sodium, potassium, and blood pressure. *J Am Soc Nephrol*. 2011;22:605-614.
41. Botero-Velez M, Curtis JJ, Warnock DG. Brief report: liddle's syndrome revisited—a disorder of sodium reabsorption in the distal tubule. *N Engl J Med*. 1994;330:178-181.
42. Chapman K, Holmes M, Seckl J. 11beta-hydroxysteroid dehydrogenases: intracellular gate-keepers of tissue glucocorticoid action. *Physiol Rev*. 2013;93:1139-1206.
43. Palermo M, Cossu M, Shackleton CH. Cure of apparent mineralocorticoid excess by kidney transplantation. *N Engl J Med*. 1998;339:1787-1788.
44. Khattab AM, Shackleton CH, Hughes BA, et al. Remission of hypertension and electrolyte abnormalities following renal transplantation in a patient with apparent mineralocorticoid excess well documented throughout childhood. *J Pediatr Endocrinol Metab*. 2014;27:17-21.
45. Hall JE. Renal function in one-kidney, one-clip hypertension and low renin essential hypertension. *Am J Hypertens*. 1991;4:523S-533S.
46. Toka O, Tank J, Schachterle C, et al. Clinical effects of phosphodiesterase 3A mutations in inherited hypertension with brachydactyly. *Hypertension*. 2015;66:800-808.
47. Schuster H, Toka O, Toka HR, et al. A cross-over medication trial for patients with autosomal-dominant hypertension with brachydactyly. *Kidney Int*. 1998;53:167-172.
48. Jordan J, Toka HR, Heusser K, et al. Severely impaired baroreflex-buffering in patients with monogenic hypertension and neurovascular contact. *Circulation*. 2000;102:2611-2618.
49. Weinberger MH. Salt sensitivity of blood pressure in humans. *Hypertension*. 1996;27:481-490.
50. Weinberger MH, Fineberg NS, Fineberg SE, et al. Salt sensitivity, pulse pressure, and death in normal and hypertensive humans. *Hypertension*. 2001;37:429-432.
51. Hall JE, Guyton AC, Brands MW. Pressure-volume regulation in hypertension. *Kidney Int Suppl*. 1996;55:S35-S41.
52. Campese VM. Salt sensitivity in hypertension. Renal and cardiovascular implications. *Hypertension*. 1994;23:531-550.
53. Hall JE, Brands MW, Henegar JR. Angiotensin II and long-term arterial pressure regulation: the overriding dominance of the kidney. *J Am Soc Nephrol*. 1999;10(Suppl 12):S258-S265.
54. Carey RM, Wang ZQ, Siragy HM. Role of the angiotensin type 2 receptor in the regulation of blood pressure and renal function. *Hypertension*. 2000;35:155-163.
55. Crowley SD, Coffman TM. The inextricable role of the kidney in hypertension. *J Clin Invest*. 2014;124:2341-2347.
56. Crowley SD, Gurley SB, Herrera MJ, et al. Angiotensin II causes hypertension and cardiac hypertrophy through its receptors in the kidney. *Proc Natl Acad Sci U S A*. 2006;103:17985-17990.
57. Eng E, Veniant M, Floege J, et al. Renal proliferative and phenotypic changes in rats with two-kidney, one-clip Goldblatt hypertension. *Am J Hypertens*. 1994;7:177-185.
58. Rossier BC, Baker ME, Studer RA. Epithelial sodium transport and its control by aldosterone: the story of our internal environment revisited. *Physiol Rev*. 2015;95:297-340.
59. Funder JW. The nongenomic actions of aldosterone. *Endocr Rev*. 2005;26:313-321.
60. Calhoun DA. Hyperaldosteronism as a common cause of resistant hypertension. *Annu Rev Med*. 2013;64:233-247.
61. de SF, Muxfeldt E, Fiszman R, et al. Efficacy of spironolactone therapy in patients with true resistant hypertension. *Hypertension*. 2010;55:147-152.
62. Ferrario CM, Schiffrin EL. Role of mineralocorticoid receptor antagonists in cardiovascular disease. *Circ Res*. 2015;116:206-213.
63. Williams B, MacDonald TM, Morant S, et al. Spironolactone versus placebo, bisoprolol, and doxazosin to determine the optimal treatment for drug-resistant hypertension (PATHWAY-2): a randomised, double-blind, crossover trial. *Lancet*. 2015;386:2059-2068.
64. Fujita T. Mechanism of salt-sensitive hypertension: focus on adrenal and sympathetic nervous systems. *J Am Soc Nephrol*. 2014;25:1148-1155.
65. Grassi G, Mark A, Esler M. The sympathetic nervous system alterations in human hypertension. *Circ Res*. 2015;116:976-990.
66. DiBona GF. Sympathetic nervous system and hypertension. *Hypertension*. 2013;61:556-560.
67. DiBona GF. Physiology in perspective: the Wisdom of the Body. Neural control of the kidney. *Am J Physiol Regul Integr Comp Physiol*. 2005;289:R633-R641.
68. Hering D, Marusic P, Walton AS, et al. Sustained sympathetic and blood pressure reduction 1 year after renal denervation in patients with resistant hypertension. *Hypertension*. 2014;64:118-124.
69. Krum H, Schlaich MP, Sobotka PA, et al. Percutaneous renal denervation in patients with treatment-resistant hypertension: final 3-year report of the Symplicity HTN-1 study. *Lancet*. 2014;383:622-629.
70. Bhatt DL, Kandzari DE, O'Neill WW, et al. A controlled trial of renal denervation for resistant hypertension. *N Engl J Med*. 2014;370:1393-1401.
71. Iliescu R, Lohmeier TE, Tudorancea I, et al. Renal denervation for the treatment of resistant hypertension: review and clinical perspective. *Am J Physiol Renal Physiol*. 2015;309:F583-F594.
72. Kandzari DE, Bhatt DL, Brar S, et al. Predictors of blood pressure response in the SYMPLICITY HTN-3 trial. *Eur Heart J*. 2015;36:219-227.
73. Henegar JR, Zhang Y, Rama RD, et al. Catheter-based radiorefrequency renal denervation lowers blood pressure in obese hypertensive dogs. *Am J Hypertens*. 2014;27:1285-1292.
74. Krum H, Schlaich M, Whitbourn R, et al. Catheter-based renal sympathetic denervation for resistant hypertension: a multicentre safety and proof-of-principle cohort study. *Lancet*. 2009;373:1275-1281.
75. Henegar JR, Zhang Y, Hata C, et al. Catheter-Based Radiofrequency Renal Denervation: Location Effects on Renal Norepinephrine. *Am J Hypertens*. 2015;28:909-914.
76. Mulder J, Hokfelt T, Knuepfer MM, et al. Renal sensory and sympathetic nerves reinnervate the kidney in a similar time-dependent fashion after renal denervation in rats. *Am J Physiol Regul Integr Comp Physiol*. 2013;304:R675-R682.
77. Malpas SC. Sympathetic nervous system overactivity and its role in the development of cardiovascular disease. *Physiol Rev*. 2010;90:513-557.
78. Lohmeier TE, Iliescu R. The baroreflex as a long-term controller of arterial pressure. *Physiology (Bethesda)*. 2015;30:148-158.
79. Osborn JW, Provo BJ. Salt-dependent hypertension in the sinoaortic-denervated rat. *Hypertension*. 1992;19:658-662.
80. Lohmeier TE, Iliescu R, Liu B, et al. Systemic and renal-specific sympathoinhibition in obesity hypertension. *Hypertension*. 2012;59:331-338.

81. Wustmann K, Kucera JP, Scheffers I, et al. Effects of chronic baroreceptor stimulation on the autonomic cardiovascular regulation in patients with drug-resistant arterial hypertension. *Hypertension.* 2009;54:530-536.

82. Orfila C, Damase-Michel C, Lepert JC, et al. Renal morphological changes after sinoaortic denervation in dogs. *Hypertension.* 1993;21:758-766.

83. Van Vliet BN, Hu L, Scott T, et al. Cardiac hypertrophy and telemetered blood pressure 6 wk after baroreceptor denervation in normotensive rats. *Am J Physiol.* 1996;271:R1759-R1769.

84. Guyenet PG. Regulation of breathing and autonomic outflows by chemoreceptors. *Compr Physiol.* 2014;4:1511-1562.

85. McBryde FD, Abdala AP, Hendy EB, et al. The carotid body as a putative therapeutic target for the treatment of neurogenic hypertension. *Nat Commun.* 2013;4:2395.

86. Paton JF, Sobotka PA, Fudim M, et al. The carotid body as a therapeutic target for the treatment of sympathetically mediated diseases. *Hypertension.* 2013;61:5-13.

87. Sinski M, Lewandowski J, Przybylski J, et al. Tonic activity of carotid body chemoreceptors contributes to the increased sympathetic drive in essential hypertension. *Hypertens Res.* 2012;35:487-491.

88. Oparil S, Schmieder RE. New approaches in the treatment of hypertension. *Circ Res.* 2015;116:1074-1095.

89. Narkiewicz K, van de Borne PJ, Montano N, et al. Contribution of tonic chemoreflex activation to sympathetic activity and blood pressure in patients with obstructive sleep apnea. *Circulation.* 1998;97:943-945.

90. Verbraecken J, McNicholas WT. Respiratory mechanics and ventilatory control in overlap syndrome and obesity hypoventilation. *Respir Res.* 2013;14:132.

91. Salome CM, King GG, Berend N. Physiology of obesity and effects on lung function. *J Appl Physiol.* (1985) 2010;(108):206-211.

92. Lohmeier TE, Iliescu R, Tudorancea I, et al. Chronic interactions between carotid baroreceptors and chemoreceptors in obesity hypertension. *Hypertension.* 2016;68:227-235.

93. Dhaun N, Goddard J, Kohan DE, et al. Role of endothelin-1 in clinical hypertension: 20 years on. *Hypertension.* 2008;52:452-459.

94. Granger JP, Abram S, Stec D, et al. Endothelin, the kidney, and hypertension. *Curr Hypertens Rep.* 2006;8:298-303.

95. LaMarca BD, Alexander BT, Gilbert JS, et al. Pathophysiology of hypertension in response to placental ischemia during pregnancy: a central role for endothelin? *Gend Med.* 2008;5(Suppl A):S133-S138.

96. Granger JP. Endothelin. *Am J Physiol Regul Integr Comp Physiol.* 2003;285:R298-R301.

97. Ihara M, Noguchi K, Saeki T, et al. Biological profiles of highly potent novel endothelin antagonists selective for the ETA receptor. *Life Sci.* 1992;50:247-255.

98. Davenport AP, Hyndman KA, Dhaun N, et al. Endothelin. *Pharmacol Rev.* 2016;68:357-418.

99. Kassab S, Novak J, Miller T, et al. Role of endothelin in mediating the attenuated renal hemodynamics in Dahl salt-sensitive hypertension. *Hypertension.* 1997;30:682-686.

100. Alexander BT, Cockrell KL, Rinewalt AN, et al. Enhanced renal expression of preproendothelin mRNA during chronic angiotensin II hypertension. *Am J Physiol Regul Integr Comp Physiol.* 2001;280:R1388-R1392.

101. Ballew JR, Fink GD. Role of ET(A) receptors in experimental ANG II-induced hypertension in rats. *Am J Physiol Regul Integr Comp Physiol.* 2001;281:R150-R154.

102. De MC, Pollock DM, Pollock JS. Endothelium-derived ET-1 and the development of renal injury. *Am J Physiol Regul Integr Comp Physiol.* 2015;309:R1071-R1073.

103. Kassab S, Miller MT, Novak J, et al. Endothelin-A receptor antagonism attenuates the hypertension and renal injury in Dahl salt-sensitive rats. *Hypertension.* 1998;31:397-402.

104. d'Uscio LV, Moreau P, Shaw S, et al. Effects of chronic ETA-receptor blockade in angiotensin II-induced hypertension. *Hypertension.* 1997;29:435-441.

105. Lin H, Smith MJ Jr, Young DB. Roles of prostaglandins and nitric oxide in the effect of endothelin-1 on renal hemodynamics. *Hypertension.* 1996;28:372-378.

106. Laffin LJ, Bakris GL. Endothelin antagonism and hypertension: an evolving target. *Semin Nephrol.* 2015;35:168-175.

107. Kohan DE. The renal medullary endothelin system in control of sodium and water excretion and systemic blood pressure. *Curr Opin Nephrol Hypertens.* 2006;15:34-40.

108. Gariepy CE, Cass DT, Yanagisawa M. Null mutation of endothelin receptor type B gene in spotting lethal rats causes aganglionic megacolon and white coat color. *Proc Natl Acad Sci U S A.* 1996;93:867-872.

109. Gariepy CE, Ohuchi T, Williams SC, et al. Salt-sensitive hypertension in endothelin-B receptor-deficient rats. *J Clin Invest.* 2000;105:925-933.

110. Pollock DM, Pollock JS. Evidence for endothelin involvement in the response to high salt. *Am J Physiol Renal Physiol.* 2001;281:F144-F150.

111. Schneider MP, Ge Y, Pollock DM, et al. Collecting duct-derived endothelin regulates arterial pressure and Na excretion via nitric oxide. *Hypertension.* 2008;51:1605-1610.

112. Plato CF, Pollock DM, Garvin JL. Endothelin inhibits thick ascending limb chloride flux via ET(B) receptor-mediated NO release. *Am J Physiol Renal Physiol.* 2000;279:F326-F333.

113. Hocher B, Thone-Reineke C, Rohmeiss P, et al. Endothelin-1 transgenic mice develop glomerulosclerosis, interstitial fibrosis, and renal cysts but not hypertension. *J Clin Invest.* 1997;99:1380-1389.

114. Miyagawa K, Emoto N. Current state of endothelin receptor antagonism in hypertension and pulmonary hypertension. *Ther Adv Cardiovasc Dis.* 2014;8:202-216.

115. Weber MA, Black H, Bakris G, et al. A selective endothelin-receptor antagonist to reduce blood pressure in patients with treatment-resistant hypertension: a randomised, double-blind, placebo-controlled trial. *Lancet.* 2009;374:1423-1431.

116. Ito S, Juncos LA, Nushiro N, et al. Endothelium-derived relaxing factor modulates endothelin action in afferent arterioles. *Hypertension.* 1991;17:1052-1056.

117. Lerman A, Sandok EK, Hildebrand FL Jr, et al. Inhibition of endothelium-derived relaxing factor enhances endothelin-mediated vasoconstriction. *Circulation.* 1992;85:1894-1898.

118. Rapoport RM. Nitric oxide inhibition of endothelin-1 release in the vasculature: in vivo relevance of in vitro findings. *Hypertension.* 2014;64:908-914.

119. Cowley AW Jr., Mori T, Mattson D, et al. Role of renal NO production in the regulation of medullary blood flow. *Am J Physiol Regul Integr Comp Physiol.* 2003;284:R1355-R1369. 2003.

120. Schnackenberg C, Patel AR, Kirchner KA, et al. Nitric oxide, the kidney and hypertension. *Clin Exp Pharmacol Physiol.* 1997;24:600-606.

121. Ortiz PA, Garvin JL. Role of nitric oxide in the regulation of nephron transport. *Am J Physiol Renal Physiol.* 2002;282:F777-F784.

122. Lu Y, Wei J, Stec DE, et al. Macula Densa Nitric Oxide Synthase 1beta Protects against Salt-Sensitive Hypertension. *J Am Soc Nephrol.* 2016;27:2346-2356.

123. Granger JP, Alexander BT. Abnormal pressure-natriuresis in hypertension: role of nitric oxide. *Acta Physiol Scand.* 2000;168:161-168.

124. Brown KE, Dhaun N, Goddard J, et al. Potential therapeutic role of phosphodiesterase type 5 inhibition in hypertension and chronic kidney disease. *Hypertension.* 2014;63:5-11.

125. Sinha N, Dabla PK. Oxidative stress and antioxidants in hypertension—a current review. *Curr Hypertens Rev.* 2015;11:132-142.

126. Hamza SM, Dyck JR. Systemic and renal oxidative stress in the pathogenesis of hypertension: modulation of long-term control of arterial blood pressure by resveratrol. *Front Physiol.* 2014;5:292.

127. Rajagopalan S, Kurz S, Munzel T, et al. Angiotensin II-mediated hypertension in the rat increases vascular superoxide production via membrane NADH/NADPH oxidase activation. Contribution to alterations of vasomotor tone. *J Clin Invest.* 1996;97:1916-1923.

128. Cowley AW Jr., Abe M, Mori T, et al. Reactive oxygen species as important determinants of medullary flow, sodium excretion, and hypertension. *Am J Physiol Renal Physiol.* 2015;308:F179-F197.

129. Park JB, Touyz RM, Chen X, et al. Chronic treatment with a superoxide dismutase mimetic prevents vascular remodeling and progression of hypertension in salt-loaded stroke-prone spontaneously hypertensive rats. *Am J Hypertens.* 2002;15:78-84.

130. Tabet F, Savoia C, Schiffrin EL, et al. Differential calcium regulation by hydrogen peroxide and superoxide in vascular smooth muscle cells from spontaneously hypertensive rats. *J Cardiovasc Pharmacol.* 2004;44:200-208.

131. Lacy F, O'Connor DT, Schmid-Schonbein GW. Plasma hydrogen peroxide production in hypertensives and normotensive subjects at genetic risk of hypertension. *J Hypertens.* 1998;16:291-303.

132. Dikalov S, Griendling KK, Harrison DG. Measurement of reactive oxygen species in cardiovascular studies. *Hypertension.* 2007;49:717-727.

133. Pechanova O, Simko F. Chronic antioxidant therapy fails to ameliorate hypertension: potential mechanisms behind. *J Hypertens Suppl.* 2009;27:S32-S36.

134. Montezano AC, Touyz RM. Molecular mechanisms of hypertension—reactive oxygen species and antioxidants: a basic science update for the clinician. *Can J Cardiol.* 2012;28:288-295.

135. Weseler AR, Bast A. Oxidative stress and vascular function: implications for pharmacologic treatments. *Curr Hypertens Rep.* 2010;12:154-161.

136. Chen S, Ge Y, Si J, et al. Candesartan suppresses chronic renal inflammation by a novel antioxidant action independent of AT1R blockade. *Kidney Int.* 2008;74:1128-1138.

137. Kupper N, Willemsen G, Riese H, et al. Heritability of daytime ambulatory blood pressure in an extended twin design. *Hypertension.* 2005;45:80-85.

138. Padmanabhan S, Caulfield M, Dominiczak AF. Genetic and molecular aspects of hypertension. *Circ Res.* 2015;116:937-959.

139. Longini IM Jr., Higgins MW, Hinton PC, et al. Environmental and genetic sources of familial aggregation of blood pressure in Tecumseh, Michigan. *Am J Epidemiol.* 1984;120:131-144.

140. Cui J, Hopper JL, Harrap SB. Genes and family environment explain correlations between blood pressure and body mass index. *Hypertension.* 2002;40:7-12.

141. Luft FC. Molecular genetics of human hypertension. *J Hypertens.* 1998;16:1871-1878.

142. Luft FC. Geneticism of essential hypertension. *Hypertension.* 2004;43:1155-1159.

143. Levy D, Ehret GB, Rice K, et al. Genome-wide association study of blood pressure and hypertension. *Nat Genet.* 2009;41:677-687.

144. Newton-Cheh C, Johnson T, Gateva V, et al. Genome-wide association study identifies eight loci associated with blood pressure. *Nat Genet.* 2009;41:666-676.

145. Ehret GB, Munroe PB, Rice KM, et al. Genetic variants in novel pathways influence blood pressure and cardiovascular disease risk. *Nature.* 2011;478:103-109.

146. Cowley AW Jr., Nadeau JH, Baccarelli A, et al. Report of the National Heart, Lung, and Blood Institute Working Group on epigenetics and hypertension. *Hypertension.* 2012;59:899-905.

147. Feinberg AP, Fallin MD. Epigenetics at the Crossroads of Genes and the Environment. *JAMA.* 2015;314:1129-1130.

148. Kotchen TA, Cowley AW Jr., Liang M. Ushering Hypertension into a New Era of Precision Medicine. *JAMA.* 2016;315:343-344.

149. World Health Organization. Obesity and Overweight Fact Sheet N°311. http://www.who.int/mediacentre/factsheets/fs311/en/2014.

150. U.S. Department of Health and Human Services—Center for Disease Control and Prevention. Overweight & Obesity Data & Statistics. www.cdc.gov/obesity/data/index.html; 2014.

151. Ogden CL, Carroll MD, Kit BK, et al. Prevalence of childhood and adult obesity in the United States, 2011-2012. *JAMA.* 2014;311:806-814.

152. Jones DW, Kim JS, Andrew ME, et al. Body mass index and blood pressure in Korean men and women: the Korean National Blood Pressure Survey. *J Hypertens.* 1994;12:1433-1437.

153. Jones DW, Miller ME, Wofford MR, et al. The effect of weight loss intervention on antihypertensive medication requirements in the hypertension Optimal Treatment (HOT) study. *Am J Hypertens.* 1999;12:1175-1180.

154. Stevens VJ, Obarzanek E, Cook NR, et al. Long-term weight loss and changes in blood pressure: results of the Trials of Hypertension Prevention, phase II. *Ann Intern Med.* 2001;134:1-11.

155. Hall JE, Crook ED, Jones DW, et al. Mechanisms of obesity-associated cardiovascular and renal disease. *Am J Med Sci.* 2002;324:127-137.

156. Tchernof A, Despres JP. Pathophysiology of human visceral obesity: an update. *Physiol Rev.* 2013;93:359-404.

157. Hall JE, Brands MW, Dixon WN, et al. Obesity-induced hypertension. Renal function and systemic hemodynamics. *Hypertension.* 1993;22:292-299.

158. Messerli FH, Christie B, DeCarvalho JG, et al. Obesity and essential hypertension. Hemodynamics, intravascular volume, sodium excretion, and plasma renin activity. *Arch Intern Med.* 1981;141:81-85.

159. Lyon CJ, Law RE, Hsueh WA. Minireview: adiposity, inflammation, and atherogenesis. *Endocrinology.* 2003;144:2195-2200.

160. Hall JE. Mechanisms of abnormal renal sodium handling in obesity hypertension. *Am J Hypertens.* 1997;10:49S-55S.

161. Hall ME, do Carmo JM, da Silva AA, et al. Obesity, hypertension, and chronic kidney disease. *Int J Nephrol Renovasc Dis.* 2014;7:75-88.

162. Sugerman H, Windsor A, Bessos M, et al. Intra-abdominal pressure, sagittal abdominal diameter and obesity comorbidity. *J Intern Med.* 1997;241:71-79.

163. Chandra A, Neeland IJ, Berry JD, et al. The relationship of body mass and fat distribution with incident hypertension: observations from the Dallas heart study. *J Am Coll Cardiol.* 2014;64:997-1002.

164. Chughtai HL, Morgan TM, Rocco M, et al. Renal sinus fat and poor blood pressure control in middle-aged and elderly individuals at risk for cardiovascular events. *Hypertension.* 2010;56:901-906.

165. DeMarco VG, Aroor AR, Sowers JR. The pathophysiology of hypertension in patients with obesity. *Nat Rev Endocrinol.* 2014;10:364-376.

166. Putnam K, Shoemaker R, Yiannikouris F, et al. The renin-angiotensin system: a target of and contributor to dyslipidemias, altered glucose homeostasis, and hypertension of the metabolic syndrome. *Am J Physiol Heart Circ Physiol.* 2012;302:H1219-H1230.

167. Engeli S, Sharma AM. The renin-angiotensin system and natriuretic peptides in obesity-associated hypertension. *J Mol Med.* 2001;79:21-29.

168. Marcus Y, Shefer G, Stern N. Adipose tissue renin-angiotensin-aldosterone system (RAAS) and progression of insulin resistance. *Mol Cell Endocrinol.* 2013;378:1-14.

169. Boustany CM, Brown DR, Randall DC, et al. AT1-receptor antagonism reverses the blood pressure elevation associated with diet-induced obesity. *Am J Physiol Regul Integr Comp Physiol.* 2005;289:R181-R186.

170. Robles RG, Villa E, Santirso R, et al. Effects of captopril on sympathetic activity, lipid and carbohydrate metabolism in a model of obesity-induced hypertension in dogs. *Am J Hypertens.* 1993;6:1009-1015.

171. Alonso-Galicia M, Brands MW, Zappe DH, et al. Hypertension in obese Zucker rats. Role of angiotensin II and adrenergic activity. *Hypertension.* 1996;28:1047-1054.

172. Dorresteijn JA, Schrover IM, Visseren FL, et al. Differential effects of renin-angiotensin-aldosterone system inhibition, sympathoinhibition and diuretic therapy on endothelial function and blood pressure in obesity-related hypertension: a double-blind, placebo-controlled cross-over trial. *J Hypertens.* 2013;31:393-403.

173. Grassi G, Seravalle G, Dell'Oro R, et al. Comparative effects of candesartan and hydrochlorothiazide on blood pressure, insulin sensitivity, and sympathetic drive in obese hypertensive individuals: results of the CROSS study. *J Hypertens.* 2003;21:1761-1769.

174. Reisin E, Weir MR, Falkner B, et al. Lisinopril versus hydrochlorothiazide in obese hypertensive patients: a multicenter placebo-controlled trial. Treatment in Obese Patients with Hypertension (TROPHY) Study Group. *Hypertension.* 1997;30:140-145.

175. Lewis EJ, Hunsicker LG, Clarke WR, et al. Renoprotective effect of the angiotensin-receptor antagonist irbesartan in patients with nephropathy due to type 2 diabetes. *N Engl J Med.* 2001;345:851-860.

176. Brenner BM, Cooper ME, de ZD, et al. Effects of losartan on renal and cardiovascular outcomes in patients with type 2 diabetes and nephropathy. *N Engl J Med.* 2001;345:861-869.

177. de Paula RB, da Silva AA, Hall JE. Aldosterone antagonism attenuates obesity-induced hypertension and glomerular hyperfiltration. *Hypertension.* 2004;43:41-47.

178. Bickel CA, Verbalis JG, Knepper MA, et al. Increased renal Na-K-ATPase, NCC, and beta-ENaC abundance in obese Zucker rats. *Am J Physiol Renal Physiol.* 2001;281:F639-F648.

179. Funder JW. Reconsidering the roles of the mineralocorticoid receptor. *Hypertension.* 2009;53:286-290.

180. Hall JE, da Silva AA, do Carmo JM, et al. Obesity-induced hypertension: role of sympathetic nervous system, leptin, and melanocortins. *J Biol Chem.* 2010;285:17271-17276.

181. Carlyle M, Jones OB, Kuo JJ, et al. Chronic cardiovascular and renal actions of leptin: role of adrenergic activity. *Hypertension.* 2002;39:496-501.

182. Wofford MR, Anderson DC Jr., Brown CA, et al. Antihypertensive effect of alpha- and beta-adrenergic blockade in obese and lean hypertensive subjects. *Am J Hypertens.* 2001;14:694-698.

183. da Silva AA, do Carmo JM, Wang Z, et al. The brain melanocortin system, sympathetic control, and obesity hypertension. *Physiology (Bethesda).* 2014;29:196-202.

184. do Carmo JM, da Silva AA, Dubinion J, et al. Control of metabolic and cardiovascular function by the leptin-brain melanocortin pathway. *IUBMB Life.* 2013;65:692-698.

185. da Silva AA, do Carmo JM, Hall JE. Role of leptin and central nervous system melanocortins in obesity hypertension. *Curr Opin Nephrol Hypertens.* 2013;22:135-140.

186. Machleidt F, Simon P, Krapalis AF, et al. Experimental hyperleptinemia acutely increases vasoconstrictory sympathetic nerve activity in healthy humans. *J Clin Endocrinol Metab.* 2013;98:E491-E496.

187. Shek EW, Brands MW, Hall JE. Chronic leptin infusion increases arterial pressure. *Hypertension.* 1998;31:409-414.

188. Kuo JJ, Jones OB, Hall JE. Inhibition of NO synthesis enhances chronic cardiovascular and renal actions of leptin. *Hypertension.* 2001;37:670-676.

189. Lim K, Burke SL, Head GA. Obesity-related hypertension and the role of insulin and leptin in high-fat-fed rabbits. *Hypertension.* 2013;61:628-634.

190. Ozata M, Ozdemir IC, Licinio J. Human leptin deficiency caused by a missense mutation: multiple endocrine defects, decreased sympathetic tone, and immune system dysfunction indicate new targets for leptin action, greater central than peripheral resistance to the effects of leptin, and spontaneous correction of leptin-mediated defects. *J Clin Endocrinol Metab.* 1999;84:3686-3695.

191. Cone RD. Studies on the physiological functions of the melanocortin system. *Endocr.* 2006;27:736-749.

192. Kuo JJ, Silva AA, Hall JE. Hypothalamic melanocortin receptors and chronic regulation of arterial pressure and renal function. *Hypertension.* 2003;41:768-774.

193. Kuo JJ, da Silva AA, Tallam LS, et al. Role of adrenergic activity in pressor responses to chronic melanocortin receptor activation. *Hypertension.* 2004;43:370-375.

194. Greenfield JR. Melanocortin signalling and the regulation of blood pressure in human obesity. *J Neuroendocrinol.* 2011;23:186-193.

195. da Silva AA, do Carmo JM, Kanyicska B, et al. Endogenous melanocortin system activity contributes to the elevated arterial pressure in spontaneously hypertensive rats. *Hypertension.* 2008;51:884-890.

196. Tallam LS, da Silva AA, Hall JE. Melanocortin-4 receptor mediates chronic cardiovascular and metabolic actions of leptin. *Hypertension.* 2006;48:58-64.

197. Greenfield JR, Miller JW, Keogh JM, et al. Modulation of blood pressure by central melanocortinergic pathways. *N Engl J Med.* 2009;360:44-52.

198. do Carmo JM, da Silva AA, Cai Z, et al. Control of blood pressure, appetite, and glucose by leptin in mice lacking leptin receptors in proopiomelanocortin neurons. *Hypertension.* 2011;57:918-926.

199. Burton JO, Gray LJ, Webb DR, et al. Association of anthropometric obesity measures with chronic kidney disease risk in a non-diabetic patient population. *Nephrol Dial Transplant.* 2012;27:1860-1866.

200. Hsu CY, McCulloch CE, Iribarren C, et al. Body mass index and risk for end-stage renal disease. *Ann Intern Med.* 2006;144:21-28.

201. Amann K, Benz K. Structural renal changes in obesity and diabetes. *Semin Nephrol.* 2013;33:23-33.

202. Hall JE, Henegar JR, Dwyer TM, et al. Is obesity a major cause of chronic kidney disease? *Adv Ren Replace Ther.* 2004;11:41-54.

203. Henegar JR, Bigler SA, Henegar LK, et al. Functional and structural changes in the kidney in the early stages of obesity. *J Am Soc Nephrol.* 2001;12:1211-1217.

204. Egan BM, Li J. Role of aldosterone blockade in resistant hypertension. *Semin Nephrol.* 2014;34:273-284.

205. Chapman N, Dobson J, Wilson S, et al. Effect of spironolactone on blood pressure in subjects with resistant hypertension. *Hypertension.* 2007;49:839-845.

206. McMaster WG, Kirabo A, Madhur MS, et al. Inflammation, immunity, and hypertensive end-organ damage. *Circ Res.* 2015;116:1022-1033.

6 Genetics of Hypertension

Georg B. Ehret

Hypertension genetics is of interest to different health care professionals: The clinician is often embarrassed by patient questioning on the origins of the blood pressure (BP) elevation in the absence of risk factors and in the clinic, signs indicating the presence of a rare monogenic hypertensive syndrome are important to be recognized. The clinical-trialist can find proof for causality between BP and for example, target organ damage in Mendelian randomization studies.[1] BP is of interest to the scientist in genetic or genomic medicine as it is a classic quantitative trait in the population[2] and monogenic disease in rare families.[3]

Hypertension (HTN) or BP genetics has been proceeding at two separate paces for primary hypertension and the rare familial forms of monogenic hypertension. The former requires genotyping of hundreds of thousands of variants that only became practical with microarrays and the implementation of genome-wide association studies (GWAS).[4] Genes underlying monogenic family traits can be identified with a few hundred genetic markers, and the identification of causal genes was therefore feasible much earlier. Both types of experiments have largely contributed to our understanding of the architecture of BP genetics.

THE CONTRIBUTION OF GENETICS TO THE BLOOD PRESSURE DISTRIBUTION

The contribution of genetics to the BP distribution is of two types: Rare mutations segregating in families drive up BP substantially in many cases and make affected individuals outliers in the BP distribution. This is secondary hypertension caused by single genes and is discussed in more detail in the first part of this chapter. The first such defect was described in 1991[5] and the latest was described in 2015,[6] such monogenic hypertension is a typical example of classic medical genetics.

On the other hand, the distribution of systolic BP (SBP) and diastolic BP (DBP) in the general population has a skewed, but otherwise close to normal distribution, and is a classic quantitative trait.[2] BP in the general population has surprising high heritability at 30% to 50%,[7,8] opening an opportunity to an improved understanding of the interindividual differences in BP levels by understanding the origins of the heritability observed. The nature of the genetic architecture of primary HTN has been the subject of the combative controversy between Robert Platt and George Pickering around 1950, where Dr. Platt advocated a monogenic *dominant disease* and Dr. Pickering multigenic inheritance and a *continuous trait*.[9] Today Dr. Pickering's model of primary hypertension is clearly documented by a large body of data. Because HTN is defined as an arbitrary threshold of BP, causes that explain the interindividual variability of BP values also explain HTN (or primary hypertension when other specific causes of HTN are excluded).[10] BP (continuous phenotype) is preferred over HTN (dichotomous phenotype) in many genetic experiments because the use of a continuous phenotype has greater precision and therefore greater statistical power. The second part of this chapter will describe in more detail the advances made over the last decade to better describe the genetic architecture of primary hypertension.

MONOGENIC (SECONDARY) HYPERTENSION

Monogenic hypertension should be considered secondary hypertension because an underlying genetic defect is clearly identifiable. The genetic defects that are necessary and sufficient for monogenic hypertension have distinctive characteristics that make them different from genetic variants underlying primary hypertension (Table 6.1). Eight different monogenic hypertensive syndromes (MHS) have been described and are summarized in Table 6.2. Three MHS have typically elevated aldosterone levels and are listed above the two MHS with typically low aldosterone. Three additional MHS have special features (occurring in pregnancy, brachydactily, or virilization features). Among the three groups there is considerable overlap.

Even collectively, monogenic familial hypertension is thought to be rare with an incidence of likely below 1/5000 in the general population.[11] But these estimations have been challenged and pathologic mutations might occur more frequently than previously thought,[12] definite proof of significance of these genes for the general population is outstanding. Even though likely rare, the genetic variants underlying MHS are important in two respects:

1. For the occasional patient with hypertension who carries a pathogenic monogenic hypertension variant, the *recognition of the syndrome* is important because in some cases, specific treatment approaches exist that can have spectacular treatment effects and because the recognition of the familiarity makes cascade screening possible. In MHS, untreated hypertension is often very elevated and can be severe with target organ damage occurring early in life, precocious death by stroke is observed in some cases.[13]

2. It is without question that the pathways and mechanisms illuminated by the defects induced by monogenic hypertension have permitted great advances in the understanding of *general BP pathways*. All but one monogenic hypertension gene act either in the kidney or in the steroid metabolism or at the mineralocorticoid receptor (Fig. 6.1). The one exception is the latest identified member of the monogenic hypertension genes, *PDE3A*, a phosphodiesterase that

TABLE 6.1 Key Features of the Genetics of Monogenic Hypertension in Rare Families and Common Primary Hypertension in the General Population

CHARACTERISTIC	MONOGENIC HYPERTENSION	PRIMARY HYPERTENSION
Allele frequency in the population	rare (<1/1000)	~30%
Effect size per genetic variant	Large (likely average ~20 mm Hg)	Small (average ~0.5-1 mm Hg so far)
Total number of known genes (loci) involved	13	~90
Estimated number of all genes (loci) involved	Likely ~15-20	>500

TABLE 6.2 Monogenic Hypertensive Syndromes

SHORT DISEASE NAME	COMPLETE DISEASE NAME	OMIM NUMBER	GENES	RENIN BLOOD LEVEL	ALDOSTERONE BLOOD LEVEL	INHERITANCE
Elevated Aldosterone						
GRA	glucocorticoid remediable aldosteronism = familial hyperaldosteronism type I = glucocorticoid suppressible hyperaldosteronism	#103900	CYP11B2[15]	↓	↑	AD
Gordon syndrome	= pseudohypoaldosteronism type II (PHA2) = Gordon hyperkalemia-hypertension syndrome = familial hyperkalemic hypertension (FHHt)	%145260	WNK1, WNK4[24] KLHL3[25,26] CUL3[25]	↓	↑	AR and AD
FH III	Familial hyperaldosteronism type III	#613677	KCNJ5[28]	↓	↑	AD
Low Aldosterone						
Liddle syndrome	= pseudoaldosteronism	#177200	SCNN1B[31], SCNN1G[30]	↓	↓	AD
AME	cortisol 11-beta-ketoreductase deficiency = syndrome of apparent mineralocorticoid excess	#218030	HSD11B2[37]	↓	↓	AR
Low Aldosterone and Associated Features						
HTNB	hypertension and brachydactyly syndrome = Bilginturan syndrome	#112410	PDE3A[6]	↓	↓	AD
Autosomal dominant hypertension with exacerbation in pregnancy	hypertension, early-onset, autosomal dominant, with exacerbation in pregnancy	#605115	NR3C2[44]	↓	↓	AD
CAH	CAH type IV (congenital adrenal hyperplasia, because of 11-beta-hydroxylase deficiency) and CAH type V (congenital adrenal hyperplasia, because of 17-alpha-hydroxylase deficiency)	#202010 #202110	CYP11B1[5] CYP17A1[46]	↓	↓	AR

Not included in this table are entities that lead indirectly to the elevation of BP (e.g., hereditary pheochromocytoma and monogenic diabetes).
AD, Autosomal dominant; AR, autosomal recessive; OMIM, Online Mendelian inheritance in man database.
(Amberger J, Bocchini C and Hamosh A. A new face and new challenges for Online Mendelian Inheritance in Man (OMIM®). Hum Mutat. 2011;32:564-567.)

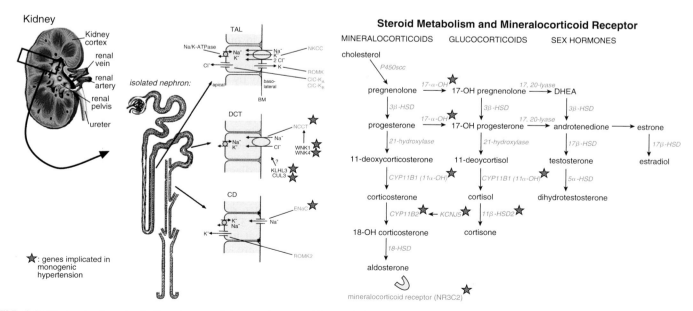

FIG. 6.1 Tissue and pathway localization of monogenic hypertension genes. *Blue stars* indicate the location of monogenic hypertension genes. *(From Ehret GB and Caulfield, MJ. Genes for blood pressure: an opportunity to understand hypertension. Eur Heart J. 2013;34:951-61.)*

likely mediates the hypertensive effect in the vasculature.[6] Many of the 13 genes in which mutations can cause monogenic hypertension have been described by the group of Dr. Richard Lifton[3] and consequently the genes are also referred to as "Lifton genes." Gene mutations found in families leading to low blood pressure have also been described and these are not discussed in more detail here.[14] Note that although classically the renin levels are always low and aldosterone levels high for some entities and low for others, levels are often borderline or normal. Features that should prompt the clinician to suspect a monogenic form of hypertension are summarized in Table 6.3 and the family history is of particular importance. Once a monogenic hypertension syndrome is identified, there are special treatment approaches available for some forms that permit, in general, to obtain large treatment effects. The entities in which specific treatment is possible are summarized in Table 6.4.

Glucocorticoid-Remediable Aldosteronism

Through unequal crossover, a chimeric gene is formed between portions of the *11-beta-hydroxylase* gene and the *aldosterone synthase* gene in such a unique way that adrenocorticotropic hormone (ACTH) stimulates aldosterone synthesis.[15,16] Similar to other monogenic hypertensive disease, the pattern of inheritance is autosomal dominant (see Table 6.2) and therefore the disease is usually readily apparent in families. Hypertension is often observed at a young age, in one study all affected members of a large pedigree were diagnosed with hypertension before the age of 21 and hypokalemia is not usually present.[16] The diagnosis can be made by demonstrating the overproduction of the cortisol C-18 oxidation products in the urine.[17] When defining the disease by criteria based on steroids, it is rare with about 100 cases described worldwide,[18] but affected individuals might have mild hypertension and normal electrolyte levels, making the entity difficult to distinguish from primary hypertension, potentially leading to underdiagnosis.[19] The therapeutic approach is a physiologic dose of an intermediary-acting glucocorticoid (e.g., prednisone) administered at bedtime to suppress the early morning surge of ACTH.[20] An alternative approach is

TABLE 6.3 Clinical Recognition of Monogenic Hypertension

CHARACTERISTIC	TYPICALLY ENCOUNTERED IN MONOGENIC HYPERTENSION
Renin level	Always low
Family history	Usually positive for early-onset hypertension
Patient age	Usually young
Blood pressure elevation	Often important

TABLE 6.4 Monogenic Hypertension Responsive to Special Treatment

MONOGENIC HYPERTENSIVE DISEASE	TREATMENT WITH USUALLY LARGE EFFECT
GRA	Glucocorticoid at physiologic doses or mineralocorticoid receptor antagonist
Gordon syndrome	Low-salt diet or thiazide
Liddle syndrome	Amiloride or triamterene
AME	High doses of mineralocorticoid antagonists, glucocorticoids (long term treatment with important side effects)

treatment with mineralocorticoid receptor antagonists that may be just as effective and avoids the potential disruption of the hypothalamic-pituitary-adrenal axis and risk of iatrogenic side effects.[21]

Gordon Syndrome

Clinical hallmarks of this entity are hypertension, hyperkalemia, and metabolic acidosis. Because of the hyperkalemia, aldosterone levels are classically elevated despite the volume overload. Around 100 individuals with Gordon syndrome have been reported worldwide, the precise prevalence is unknown. In one large French pedigree all affected adults were hypertensive whereas all affected children had normal blood pressure.[22] The mean age of hypertensives with Gordon syndrome was 27 years in another report.[23] The causal mutations for Gordon syndrome have been in part only recently identified: Mutations of the genes encoding the WNK kinases 1 and 4[24] or the *KLHL3* and *CUL3* genes[25,26] result in increased chloride and sodium reabsorption in the kidney with consequent volume expansion. The increased chloride reabsorption leads to potassium retention and hyperkalemia through a reduction in luminal electronegativity.[27] Blood pressure can usually be rapidly corrected by thiazide diuretics or, more slowly, by a low-salt diet.[23]

Familial Hyperaldosteronism Type III

This entity is very rare and is because of loss of function mutations in the potassium channel KCNJ5 (inwardly-rectifying channel, subfamily J, member 5). Pathogenic mutations result in membrane depolarization of the zona glomerulosa in the adrenal cortex, opening of voltage-activated calcium channels triggering inappropriate aldosterone biosynthesis. The pattern of inheritance is dominant. Typically, there is severe hypokalemia with hypertension in childhood and elevated aldosterone blood levels.[28] Enlarged adrenal glands can be observed, in part with massive enlargement. Treatment is either medical, identical to other cases of primary hyperaldosteronism, or surgical.[29]

Liddle Syndrome

This is also a rare entity with close to 100 cases reported in the literature worldwide. The causal defect is a gain-of-function mutation in one of two subunits (SCNN1B, SCNN1G) of the ENaC sodium channel. Pathogenic mutations lead to a large increase in sodium transport and loss of inhibition of channel activity by elevated levels of intracellular sodium.[30,31] Hypertension is usually severe with an onset in young adulthood, but some cases are only diagnosed later.[32] Usually there is prominent hypokalemia, metabolic alkalosis, and associated low plasma renin and aldosterone levels, but some patients do not have all those characteristics and can have near to normal potassium levels.[33] Children usually have normal blood pressure. The diagnosis is suspected based on the typical clinical, blood, and urinary features and a positive family history (dominant inheritance, see Table 6.2), although sporadic cases have been described.[34] Diagnostic confirmation is by genetic testing. Targeted treatment options are amiloride or triamterene that inhibit ENaC activity.[35] Other antihypertensive therapies are largely inefficient. The patients should also follow a low-salt diet.

Syndrome of Apparent Mineralocorticoid Excess

This is one of the rare recessive forms of monogenic hypertension, with less than 100 cases reported worldwide. The causal defects are loss-of-function mutations or deletions of the *HSD11B2* gene, encoding for the kidney isoform of the

11-β-hydroxysteroid dehydrogenase[36] usually responsible for the conversion of cortisol to cortisone, permitting cortisol to activate the mineralocorticoid receptor.[37] Cortisol has an affinity for the mineralocorticoid receptor similar to aldosterone and is therefore converted to cortisone at aldosterone sensitive sites such as the kidney. Clinically the disease is of usually very early onset with severe hypertension, low renin and aldosterone levels, hypokalemia, alkalosis, and often nephrocalcinosis. Strokes in children with apparent mineralocorticoid excess have been observed. But much milder forms also exist that manifest themselves later in life.[38] As treatment approaches spironolactone or other mineralocorticoid antagonists are usually used at high doses,[39] combined with thiazides to prevent nephrocalcinosis. The mineralocorticoid blockers other than spironolactone might be preferable because less elevated doses can be used with fewer side-effects.[40] Exogenous glucocorticoids can be used to decrease the endogenous secretion of cortisol, but a long term treatment has important side effects. Often additional nonspecific antihypertensive medications are required. The syndrome of apparent mineralocorticoid excess can be mimicked by the chronic ingestion of high doses of licorice: glycyrrhetinic acid, contained in licorice, inhibits the 11-β-hydroxysteroid dehydrogenase.

Autosomal Dominant Hypertension With Brachydactyly

Initially described in 1976,[41] the underlying gene for this syndrome has been identified very recently.[6] Activating mutations in the *cGMP-inhibited phosphodiesterase 3A (PDE3A)* gene appear to lead to inhibition of phosphorylation-dependent vasodilation.[42] The typical clinical presentation of severe, age-dependent hypertension is associated with brachydactyly type E (short fingers, predominantly because of malformation of the metacarpal bones). Affected family members are reported to die frequently before the age of 50 of stroke. Neurovascular compression as cause for the hypertension had been postulated, but remains unproven.[43] Currently there is no specific treatment known for this syndrome.

Early-Onset Autosomal Dominant Hypertension With Exacerbation in Pregnancy

This condition is extremely rare with one pedigree identified so far. The defect has been mapped to the mineralocorticoid receptor gene *(NR3C2)*[44] and activating mutations induce spontaneous activity and nonspecific activation of the receptor. Affected individuals present with early-onset hypertension, before 21 years in the initial description, and hypertension is largely exacerbated during pregnancy in women.[44] Although delivery improves hypertension related to the condition in pregnancy, the BP elevation is largely resistant to standard antihypertensive therapy and no clear treatment algorithm could be established so far.[45]

Congenital Adrenal Hyperplasia

There are two forms of the congenital adrenal hyperplasias that lead to hypertension, both because of reduced cortisol production that leads to an ACTH-mediated stimulation of the adrenal gland. The consequent increase of steroid precursors with a mineralocorticoid effect leads to hypertension and hypokalemia while the aldosterone levels are low. One type is attributed to 11-beta-hydroxylase deficiency, the other is because of 17-alpha-hydroxylase deficiency. In the former mutations in the *CYP11B1* gene[5] also induce variable degrees of virilization and often occur during the first years of life, but can also be observed later. In the forms attributed to *CYP17A1*

mutations, hypertension frequently presents together with hypogonadism.[46] These distinctive associated features are associated with steroid metabolism imbalances that can be found in the urine permit usually a diagnosis.

GENOMICS OF PRIMARY HYPERTENSION

The rarity of the monogenic hypertension syndromes implies that they can at most explain very little of primary hypertension with a population prevalence around 30%, quantitatively the most important cardiovascular risk factor of our times.[47,48] As BP in the population is moderately heritable as outlined above, there is a great interest to also understand the genetic basis of primary hypertension.

Linkage and candidate-gene studies performed in large numbers over the past 30 years have only yielded few reproducible genetic results. Building on modern microarray platforms, millions of genetic variants can be genotyped permitting to interrogate close to the entire genome for association with a trait such as BP. The most frequent type of variant is the single nucleotide polymorphism (SNP), but other types exist such as copy number polymorphisms and structural variants, methylation marks, and additional variability. As SNPs constitute, by far, the most common type of variant, it was therefore likely that they influence traits such as BP most significantly.

Key Challenges of Blood Pressure Genome-Wide Association Studies

When association statistics are calculated between many thousands of SNPs and BP traits in GWAS, low p-values are produced by multiple testing and consequently the p-values require to be adjusted for the number of tests. It is generally assumed for common variants that the effective number of tests is 1×10^6, therefore the p-value significance threshold is 5×10^{-8} when applying a multiple-test correction by Bonferroni.

When assessing the frequency of SNPs throughout the genome in GWAS, it becomes rapidly clear that there are many rarer SNPs than frequent SNPs.[49] On the other hand it is also clear from many genetic studies, including the BP variants identified so far, that the effect size of a variant is in general inversely proportional to the frequency of the variant. For blood pressure genes this is exemplified by the rare monogenic familial gene-variants having large effect sizes (beyond 20 mm Hg in many cases), whereas the frequent BP-GWAS variants have low effect sizes (around 1 mm Hg), too little to be of significance individually (Fig. 6.2). This has profound consequences on the design of genetic studies of blood pressure because statistical power depends on both, the effect size and the frequency of the variant.

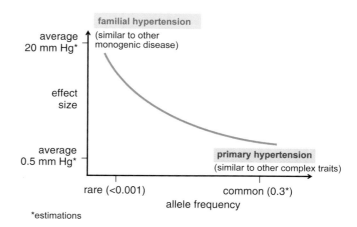

FIG. 6.2 The allele frequency spectrum in hypertension genetics/genomics.

Genome-wide association studies using hundreds of thousands of SNPs have changed the understanding of blood pressure genomics of the general population and demonstrated the presence of clearly reproducible BP loci although they have, by far, not yet explained the majority of blood pressure. The advantage of the method is the unbiased approach that is hypothesis generating. The disadvantage is overall low statistical power because of the multiple testing burden.

Current Findings From Blood Pressure Genome-Wide Association Studies Efforts

A number of BP GWAS studies have been published, starting in 2008, that identify loci and specific variants consistently associated with BP. All currently published BP loci with their sentinel SNPs are listed in Table 6.5. From the GWAS studies on BP so far,[50-63] the following overall conclusions on the origin of primary hypertension and the genomic architecture of BP in the general population can be drawn.

Total Number of Blood Pressure Loci, Their Allele Frequency in the Population, and Blood Pressure Variance Explained

The total number of genetic variants that influence primary hypertension is unknown. Currently 83 independent variants are described (see Table 6.5) and based on predictions[50] and unpublished data, the list will be growing substantially further before a plateau is reached. It appears therefore likely that primary hypertension is as a result of at least hundreds, possibly thousands of independent BP loci (see Table 6.1). Almost all of the BP variants identified so far are frequent in the population (see Fig. 6.2) and have individually low effect sizes, mostly below 1 mm Hg for SBP and below 0.5 mm Hg for DBP per variant, corresponding to close to 0.05 standard deviations of the phenotype distribution. Even taking together collectively all currently known BP loci, only a small fraction of the BP heritability is explained so far (~4-6%). The current studies, even with sample sizes above 100,000 participants, are still underpowered to detect rare variants because of the statistical multiple-testing burden that a genome-wide analysis entails. It will therefore be interesting to see results of larger studies that are underway.

Location of the Blood Pressure Variants Identified by Blood Pressure Genome-Wide Association Studies and Their Multiethnic Nature

The great majority of BP loci discovered so far are not near known hypertension genes. With one or two exceptions the signals are far away from genes described to be causal in familial hypertension (see previous section). Conversely, a similar set of variants appears to act in multiple ethnicities, implying a panethnic action of underlying genes.[50,51] A substantial number of BP loci appear to have multiple independent signals. The demonstration of gene-gene interactions is still outstanding, although large effects of this sort should have been detected with the current studies.

Making Clinical Use of Blood Pressure Genomics

Although the findings of BP loci by GWAS have been very instructive to better understand the genetic architecture of primary hypertension, there is currently no direct clinical application. The variants identified predict BP, but the size of the effect predicted is small and does not currently permit prediction of hypertension in individuals in a clinically meaningful way.

Most applied use of the findings can currently be made by the search of pathways through which multiple genes near BP variants act. There is little evidence for specific pathways so far, but some limited signals for potential involvement of microvascular endothelial cells[64] and the natriuretic peptide pathways.[65]

The most important application yielding clinical evidence are Mendelian randomization studies[1] that help to prove the causal impact of blood pressure on other outcomes. A genetic risk score using multiple BP SNPs will clearly predict BP. If this same risk score also predicts for example, target organ damage (e.g., myocardial infarction or stroke), then this finding is a strong argument for a causal implication of BP in the pathogenesis of myocardial infarction or stroke. Such a relationship could be shown for all commonly recognized types of target organ damage, except for kidney phenotypes (renal failure, clearance, microalbuminuria),[50,54] where no impact of the BP risk score on this type of target organ damage could be shown. This might be an indication that BP is not a causal factor for renal failure or a weak one.[50]

TABLE 6.5 List of Genome-Wide Association Studies Loci Identified. Genomic Positions Are Indicated in hg38 Coordinates

LOCUS NAME	SNP	CHR	POSITION	PHENOTYPE	INITIAL REPORT
CASZ1	rs880315	1	10,736,809	SBP/DBP	66
MTHFR-NPPB	rs17367504	1	11,802,721	SBP/DBP	65
ST7L-CAPZA1-MOV10	rs2932538	1	112,673,921	SBP/DBP	50,55
MDM4	rs2169137	1	204,528,785	DBP	67
AGT	rs2004776	1	230,712,956	SBP/DBP/HTN	68
OSR1	rs1344653	2	19,531,084	PP	54
KCNK3	rs1275988	2	26,691,496	SBP/DBP	52
FER1L5	rs7599598	2	96,686,103	SBP/DBP	52
FIGN-GRB14	rs16849225	2	164,050,310	SBP/DBP	55,62
STK39	rs6749447	2	168,184,876	SBP/DBP	69
PDE1A	rs16823124	2	182,359,400	DBP/MAP	61
HRH1-ATG7	rs347591	3	11,248,436	SBP/DBP	67
SLC4A7	rs13082711	3	27,496,418	SBP	50
ULK4	rs9815354	3	41,871,159	SBP/DBP	56
MAP4	rs319690	3	47,885,994	SBP/DBP	62

TABLE 6.5 List of Genome-Wide Association Studies Loci Identified. Genomic Positions Are Indicated in hg38 Coordinates—cont'd

LOCUS NAME	SNP	CHR	POSITION	PHENOTYPE	INITIAL REPORT
CDC25A	rs6797587	3	48,156,124	MAP	60
MIR1263	rs16833934	3	164,019,462	DBP	60
MECOM	rs419076	3	169,383,098	SBP/DBP	50
CHIC2	rs871606	4	53,933,078	PP	62
CHIC2	rs11725861	4	53,936,138	multi-phen	63
FGF5	rs16998073	4	80,263,187	SBP/DBP	57
ARHGAP24	rs2014912	4	85,794,517	SBP	54
SLC39A8	rs13107325	4	102,267,552	SBP/DBP	50
ENPEP	rs6825911	4	110,460,482	SBP/DBP	55
GUCY1A3-GUCY1B3	rs13139571	4	155,724,361	SBP/DBP	50
NPR3-C5orf23	rs1173771	5	32,814,922	SBP/DBP	50,55
GPR98/ARRDC3	rs10474346	5	91,268,322	DBP	70
PRDM6	rs13359291	5	123,140,763	SBP	54
ABLIM3-SH3TC2	rs9687065	5	149,011,577	DBP	54
EBF1	rs11953630	5	158,418,394	SBP/DBP	50
HFE	rs1799945	6	26,090,951	SBP/DBP	50
BAT2-BAT5	rs805303	6	31,648,589	SBP/DBP	50
TTBK1-ZNF318	rs1563788	6	43,340,625	SBP	54
ZNF318-ABCC10	rs10948071	6	43,312,975	SBP/DBP	52
RSPO3	rs13209747	6	126,794,309	SBP/DBP	51
PLEKHG1	rs17080102	6	150,683,634	SBP/DBP	51
HDAC9	rs2107595	7	19,009,765	PP	54
HOXA-EVX1	rs11564022	7	27,297,427	multi-phen	63
HOXA-EVX1	rs17428471	7	27,298,248	SBP/DBP	51
IGFBP1-IGFBP3	rs11977526	7	45,968,511	multi-phen	63
IGFBP3	rs10260816	7	45,970,501	PP	54
CDK6	rs2282978	7	92,635,096	PP	61
PIK3CG	rs17477177	7	106,771,412	SBP/DBP/PP	62
NOS3	rs3918226	7	150,993,088	DBP	53
PRKAG2	rs10224002	7	151,717,955	SBP	61
BLK-GATA4	rs2898290	8	11,576,400	SBP/DBP	67
CDH17	rs2446849	8	94,091,269	multi-phen	63
NOV	rs2071518	8	119,423,572	PP	62
SMARCA2-VLDLR	rs872256	9	2,496,480	SBP-age spec.	71
CACNB2	rs11014166	10	18,419,869	SBP/DBP	56
C10orf107	rs1530440	10	61,764,833	SBP/DBP	57
VCL	rs4746172	10	74,096,084	DBP, MAP	61
PLCE1	rs932764	10	94,136,183	SBP/DBP	50
CYP17A1-NT5C2	rs1004467	10	102,834,750	SBP/DBP	56,57
ADRB1	rs1801253	10	114,045,297	SBP/DBP/MAP	62,68
LSP1-TNNT3	rs661348	11	1,884,062	SBP/DBP/MAP	53
H19	rs217727	11	1,995,678	SBP	61
ADM	rs7129220	11	10,328,991	SBP/DBP	50
PLEKHA7	rs381815	11	16,880,721	SBP/DBP/MAP	56
NUCB2	rs757081	11	17,330,136	SBP/PP/MAP	61
LRRC10B-SYT7	rs751984	11	61,510,774	MAP	54
RELA	rs3741378	11	65,641,466	SBP/MAP	61
FLJ32810-TMEM133	rs633185	11	100,722,807	SBP/DBP	50
ADAMTS8	rs11222084	11	130,403,335	PP	62
PDE3A	rs12579720	12	20,020,830	DBP	54

Continued

TABLE 6.5 List of Genome-Wide Association Studies Loci Identified. Genomic Positions Are Indicated in hg38 Coordinates—cont'd

LOCUS NAME	SNP	CHR	POSITION	PHENOTYPE	INITIAL REPORT
HOXC4	rs7297416	12	54,049,306	SBP	61
ATP2B1	rs2681492	12	89,619,312	SBP/DBP/HTN	56
SH2B3	rs3184504	12	111,446,804	SBP/DBP	56,57
RPL6-PTPN11-ALDH2	rs11066280	12	112,379,979	SBP/DBP	55
TBX5-TBX3	rs2384550	12	114,914,926	SBP/DBP	55,56
FBN1	rs1036477	15	48,622,729	PP	61
ITGA11	rs1563894	15	68,343,437	SBP-age spec.	71
CYP1A1-ULK3	rs6495122	15	74,833,304	SBP/DBP	56,57
FURIN-FES	rs2521501	15	90,894,158	SBP/DBP	50
UMOD	rs13333226	16	20,354,332	SBP/DBP	58
NFAT5	rs33063	16	69,606,314	PP	61
PLCD3	rs12946454	17	45,130,754	SBP/DBP	57
GOSR2	rs17608766	17	46,935,905	SBP/DBP	50
ZNF652	rs16948048	17	49,363,104	SBP/DBP	57
C17orf82-TBX2	rs2240736	17	61,408,032	MAP	54
AMH-SF3A2	rs740406	19	2,232,222	PP	54
JAG1	rs1327235	20	10,988,382	SBP/DBP	50
GNAS-EDN3	rs6015450	20	59,176,062	SBP/DBP	50

An updated version of this table can be found at www.bloodpressuregenetics.org.

SUMMARY

The genetics of hypertension comes in two types: rare familial monogenic syndromes that should be labeled as secondary hypertension when they are recognized and the genomics of primary hypertension. The elucidation of genetic mechanisms for monogenic familial hypertension has been invaluable for understanding general blood pressure pathways and the entities are important to recognize clinically because specific treatments can be provided in some cases. On the contrary, the genomics of primary hypertension cannot be explained by the rare monogenic hypertension genes. Large number of small-effect size genetic variants have been identified by GWAS over the last decade that begin to be helpful to better understand the pathways that lead to primary hypertension.

References

1. Burgess S, Timpson NJ, Ebrahim S, Davey Smith G. Mendelian randomization: where are we now and where are we going? *Int J Epidemiol.* 2015;44:379-388.
2. McKusick VA. Genetics and the nature of essential hypertension. *Circulation.* 1960;22:857-863.
3. Lifton RP. Genetic dissection of human blood pressure variation: common pathways from rare phenotypes. *Harvey Lect.* 2004;100:71-101.
4. Antonarakis SE, Chakravarti A, Cohen JC, Hardy J. Mendelian disorders and multifactorial traits: the big divide or one for all? *Nat Rev Genet.* 2010;11:380-384.
5. White PC, Dupont J, New MI, Leiberman E, Hochberg Z, Rösler A. A mutation in CYP11B1 (Arg-448—His) associated with steroid 11 beta-hydroxylase deficiency in Jews of Moroccan origin. *J Clin Invest.* 1991;87:1664-1667.
6. Maass PG, et al. PDE3A mutations cause autosomal dominant hypertension with brachydactyly. *Nat Genet.* 2015;47:647-653.
7. Levy D, et al. Framingham Heart Study 100K Project: genome-wide associations for blood pressure and arterial stiffness. *BMC Med Genet.* 2007;8(Suppl 1):S3.
8. Miall WE, Oldham PD. The hereditary factor in arterial blood-pressure. *BMJ.* 1963;1:75-80.
9. Swales JD. *Platt versus Pickering: an episode in recent medical history.* London: Keynes Press (British Medical Association); 1985.
10. Freitag MH, Vasan RS. What is normal blood pressure? *Curr Opin Nephrol. Hypertens.* 2003;12:285-292.
11. Ehret GB, Caulfield MJ. Genes for blood pressure: an opportunity to understand hypertension. *Eur Heart J.* 2013;34:951-961.
12. Ji W, et al. Rare independent mutations in renal salt handling genes contribute to blood pressure variation. *Nat Genet.* 2008;40:592-599.
13. Schuster H, et al. A cross-over medication trial for patients with autosomal-dominant hypertension with brachydactyly. *Kidney Int.* 1998;53:167-172.
14. Simon DB, et al. Bartter's syndrome, hypokalaemic alkalosis with hypercalciuria, is caused by mutations in the Na-K-2Cl cotransporter NKCC2. *Nat Genet.* 1996;13:183-188.
15. Lifton RP, et al. A chimaeric 11 beta-hydroxylase/aldosterone synthase gene causes glucocorticoid-remediable aldosteronism and human hypertension. *Nature.* 1992;355:262-265.
16. Rich GM, et al. Glucocorticoid-remediable aldosteronism in a large kindred: clinical spectrum and diagnosis using a characteristic biochemical phenotype. *Ann Intern Med.* 1992;116:813-820.
17. Ulick S, Chan CK, Wang JZ. Measurement of 4 urinary C-18 oxygenated corticosteroids by stable isotope dilution mass fragmentography. *J Steroid Biochem Mol Biol.* 1991;38:59-66.
18. Ulick S. Two uncommon causes of mineralocorticoid excess. Syndrome of apparent mineralocorticoid excess and glucocorticoid-remediable aldosteronism. *Endocrinol Metab Clin North Am.* 1991;20:269-276.
19. Gates LJ, MacConnachie AA, Lifton RP, Haites NE, Benjamin N. Variation of phenotype in patients with glucocorticoid remediable aldosteronism. *J Med Genet.* 1996;33:25-28.
20. Stowasser M, Bachmann AW, Huggard PR, Rossetti TR, Gordon RD. Treatment of familial hyperaldosteronism type I: only partial suppression of adrenocorticotropin required to correct hypertension. *J Clin Endocrinol Metab.* 2000;85:3313-3318.
21. Young WF. Familial Hyperaldosteronism. In: Post TW, ed. *UpToDate.* Waltham, MA: UpToDate. Accessed May 6, 2016.
22. Achard JM, et al. Familial hyperkalaemic hypertension: phenotypic analysis in a large family with the WNK1 deletion mutation. *Am J Med.* 2003;114:495-498.
23. Gordon RD. Syndrome of hypertension and hyperkalemia with normal glomerular filtration rate. *Hypertension.* 1986;8:93-102.
24. Wilson FH, et al. Human hypertension caused by mutations in WNK kinases. *Science.* 2001;293:1107-1112.
25. Boyden LM, et al. Mutations in kelch-like 3 and cullin 3 cause hypertension and electrolyte abnormalities. *Nature.* 2012;482:98-102.
26. Louis-Dit-Picard H, et al. KLHL3 mutations cause familial hyperkalemic hypertension by impairing ion transport in the distal nephron. *Nat Genet.* 2012;44:456-460. S1-3.
27. Milford DV. Investigation of hypertension and the recognition of monogenic hypertension. *Arch Dis Child.* 1999;81:452-455.
28. Choi M, et al. K+ channel mutations in adrenal aldosterone-producing adenomas and hereditary hypertension. *Science.* 2011;331:768-772.
29. Young WF. Primary aldosteronism: renaissance of a syndrome. *Clin Endocrinol. (Oxf).* 2007;66:607-618.
30. Hansson JH, et al. Hypertension caused by a truncated epithelial sodium channel gamma subunit: genetic heterogeneity of Liddle syndrome. *Nat Genet.* 1995;11:76-82.
31. Shimkets RA, et al. Liddle's syndrome: heritable human hypertension caused by mutations in the beta subunit of the epithelial sodium channel. *Cell.* 1994;79:407-414.
32. Findling JW, Raff H, Hansson JH, Lifton RP. Liddle's syndrome: prospective genetic screening and suppressed aldosterone secretion in an extended kindred. *J Clin Endocrinol Metab.* 1997;82:1071-1074.
33. Botero-Velez M, Curtis JJ, Warnock DG. Brief report: liddle's syndrome revisited—a disorder of sodium reabsorption in the distal tubule. *N Engl J Med.* 1994;330:178-181.
34. Yamashita Y, et al. Two sporadic cases of Liddle's syndrome caused by De novo ENaC mutations. *Am J Kidney Dis.* 2001;37:499-504.
35. Wang C, et al. The effect of triamterene and sodium intake on renin, aldosterone, and erythrocyte sodium transport in Liddle's syndrome. *J Clin Endocrinol Metab.* 1981;52:1027-1032.
36. Funder JW. 11 beta-Hydroxysteroid dehydrogenase: new answers, new questions. *Eur J Endocrinol.* 1996;134:267-268.
37. Mune T, Rogerson FM, Nikkila H, Agarwal AK, White PC. Human hypertension caused by mutations in the kidney isozyme of 11 beta-hydroxysteroid dehydrogenase. *Nat Genet.* 1995;10:394-399.
38. Lavery GG, et al. Late-onset apparent mineralocorticoid excess caused by novel compound heterozygous mutations in the HSD11B2 gene. *Hypertension.* 2003;42:123-129.
39. Speiser PW, Riddick LM, Martin K, New MI. Investigation of the mechanism of hypertension in apparent mineralocorticoid excess. *Metabolism.* 1993;42:843-845.
40. Quinkler M, Stewart PM. Hypertension and the cortisol-cortisone shuttle. *J Clin Endocrinol Metab.* 2003;88:2384-2392.
41. Bilginturan N, Zileli S, Karacadag S, Pirnar T. Hereditary brachydactyly associated with hypertension. *J Med Genet.* 1973;10:253-259.
42. Toka O, et al. Clinical effects of phosphodiesterase 3A mutations in inherited hypertension with brachydactyly. *Hypertension.* 2015;66:800-808.

43. Naraghi R, et al. Neurovascular compression at the ventrolateral medulla in autosomal dominant hypertension and brachydactyly. *Stroke*. 1997;28:1749-1754.

44. Geller DS, et al. Activating mineralocorticoid receptor mutation in hypertension exacerbated by pregnancy. *Science*. 2000;289:119-123.

45. Garovic VD, Hilliard AA, Turner ST. Monogenic forms of low-renin hypertension. *Nat Clin Pract Nephrol*. 2006;2:624-630.

46. Goldsmith O, Solomon DH, Horton R. Hypogonadism and mineralocorticoid excess. The 17-hydroxylase deficiency syndrome. *N Engl J Med*. 1967;277:673-677.

47. James PA, et al. 2014 evidence-based guideline for the management of high blood pressure in adults: report from the panel members appointed to the Eighth Joint National Committee (JNC 8). *JAMA*. 2014;311:507-520.

48. Mancia G, et al. 2013 ESH/ESC guidelines for the management of arterial hypertension: the Task Force for the Management of Arterial Hypertension of the European Society of Hypertension (ESH) and of the European Society of Cardiology (ESC). *Eur Heart J*. 2013;34:2159-2219.

49. The 1000 Genomes Project Consortium. A global reference for human genetic variation. *Nature*. 2015;526:68-74.

50. Ehret GB, et al. Genetic variants in novel pathways influence blood pressure and cardiovascular disease risk. *Nature*. 2011;478:103-109.

51. Franceschini N, et al. Genome-wide association analysis of blood-pressure traits in African-ancestry individuals reveals common associated genes in African and non-African populations. *Am J Hum Genet*. 2013;93:545-554.

52. Ganesh SK, et al. Effects of long-term averaging of quantitative blood pressure traits on the detection of genetic associations. *Am J Hum Genet*. 2014;95:49-65.

53. Johnson T, et al. Blood pressure loci identified with a gene-centric array. *Am J Hum Genet*. 2011;89:688-700.

54. Kato N, et al. Trans-ancestry genome-wide association study identifies 12 genetic loci influencing blood pressure and implicates a role for DNA methylation. *Nat Genet*. 2015;47:1282-1293.

55. Kato N, et al. Meta-analysis of genome-wide association studies identifies common variants associated with blood pressure variation in east Asians. *Nat Genet*. 2011;43:531-538.

56. Levy D, et al. Genome-wide association study of blood pressure and hypertension. *Nat Genet*. 2009;41:677-687.

57. Newton-Cheh C, et al. Genome-wide association study identifies eight loci associated with blood pressure. *Nat Genet*. 2009;41:666-676.

58. Padmanabhan S, et al. Genome-wide association study of blood pressure extremes identifies variant near UMOD associated with hypertension. *PLoS Genet*. 2010;6. e1001177.

59. Salvi E, et al. Genome-wide association study using a high-density single nucleotide polymorphism array and case-control design identifies a novel essential hypertension susceptibility locus in the promoter region of endothelial NO synthase. *Hypertension*. 2012;59:248-255.

60. Simino J, et al. Gene-age interactions in blood pressure regulation: a large-scale investigation with the CHARGE, Global BPgen, and ICBP Consortia. *Am J Hum Genet*. 2014;95:24-38.

61. Tragante V, et al. Gene-centric meta-analysis in 87,736 individuals of European ancestry identifies multiple blood-pressure-related loci. *Am J Hum Genet*. 2014;94:349-360.

62. Wain LV, et al. Genome-wide association study identifies six new loci influencing pulse pressure and mean arterial pressure. *Nat Genet*. 2011;43:1005-1011.

63. Zhu X, et al. Meta-analysis of correlated traits via summary statistics from GWASs with an application in hypertension. *Am J Hum Genet*. 2015;96:21-36.

64. Chasman DI, Giulianini F. Cell-specific enrichment metrics for overlap of signals from GWAS with DNase hypersensitivity sites. In: *American Society of Human Genetics Annual Meeting 2013*. Boston: American Society of Human Genetics; 2013.

65. Newton-Cheh C, et al. Association of common variants in NPPA and NPPB with circulating natriuretic peptides and blood pressure. *Nat Genet*. 2009;41:348-353.

66. Takeuchi F, et al. Blood pressure and hypertension are associated with 7 loci in the Japanese population. *Circulation*. 2010;121:2302-2309.

67. Ganesh SK, et al. Loci influencing blood pressure identified using a cardiovascular gene-centric array. *Hum Mol Genet*. 2013;22:1663-1678.

68. Johnson AD, et al. Association of hypertension drug target genes with blood pressure and hypertension in 86,588 individuals. *Hypertension*. 2011;57:903-910.

69. Wang Y, et al. From the Cover: whole-genome association study identifies STK39 as a hypertension susceptibility gene. *Proc Natl Acad Sci USA*. 2009;106:226-231.

70. Fox ER, et al. Association of genetic variation with systolic and diastolic blood pressure among African Americans: the Candidate Gene Association Resource study. *Hum Mol Genet*. 2011;20:2273-2284.

71. Parmar PG, et al. International GWAS consortium identifies novel loci associated with blood pressure in children and adolescents. *Circ Cardiovasc Genet*. 2016;9:266-278.

7

Inflammation and Immunity in Hypertension

David G. Harrison and Kenneth E. Bernstein

Approximately one-third of the Western population has hypertension, and this disease becomes more frequent with aging. This disease is also a major risk factor for cardiovascular disease, causing stroke, heart failure, renal failure, and cognitive decline. Despite the frequency of hypertension and its profound impact on human health, the precise cause of most cases of human hypertension remains essentially unknown. Rare monogenic causes of hypertension have been identified, but are extremely rare and are not thought to underlie most cases of hypertension. Dysregulation of central neural signaling, renal dysfunction, and alterations of vascular reactivity have all been implicated, but a concise understanding of how these become abnormal and how they interact to produce clinical hypertension has been elusive. Multiple genome-wide association studies (GWAS) have identified genetic loci associated with hypertension, but what might tie these together and actually instigates clinical disease is unknown. In the past several years, it has become apparent that hypertension is often accompanied by an inflammatory process in which immune cells infiltrate and alter function and structure of the kidney and the vasculature. As stressed in this chapter, an emerging paradigm is that this inflammatory reaction promotes not only blood pressure elevation, but also the end-organ damage associated with hypertension.

Inflammation is the biologic response to invading organisms, irritants or injury, and is essential to combat invading organisms, foreign bodies and neoplasia. Unfortunately, inflammation occasionally becomes excessive and persists beyond the initial insult, contributing to numerous chronic degenerative processes. Celsus described the cardinal signs of inflammation as dolor, rubor, calor and tumor (i.e., pain, heat, redness, and swelling). Notably, these are largely vascular phenomena mediated by vasodilatation, increased permeability and in some cases release of pain mediators such as endothelin-1 and substance P from vascular cells. A fundamental aspect of inflammation is infiltration of immune cells through the vessel wall into the interstitium of the affected tissue, governed by endothelial production of adhesion molecules that promote initially sticking of immune cells to the endothelial surface and chemokines that promote diapedesis of these cells through junctions between endothelial cells. This latter event involves molecular interactions between leukocytes and the endothelium and rearrangement and loosening of endothelial cell junctions.[1] A truly miraculous aspect of this process is that there is a concomitant increase on the immune cells of ligands that recognize the adhesion molecules expressed by the activated endothelium, localizing the inflammatory process to sites of infection or injury.

GENERAL CONSIDERATIONS OF THE IMMUNE SYSTEM

The two major arms of the immune system are innate and adaptive immunity. Innate immunity includes chemical and humoral mediators such as nitric oxide, reactive oxygen species (ROS), complement, acute phase proteins, chemokines, and cytokines.[2] Natural immunoglobulin M (IgM) and immunoglobulin G3 (IgG3) antibodies, produced largely by B1 cells, are present in infants and adults before exposure to an antigen and confer innate protection to viruses and bacteria but can also participate in autoimmune diseases like rheumatoid arthritis and systemic lupus erythematosus.[3] Some natural antibodies target lectins, present on the surface of microbes and apoptotic cells. Cellular components of innate immunity include phagocytic cells, including granulocytes, monocytes and macrophages and natural killer (NK) cells. Other cells of the innate immune system include dendritic cells, newly identified innate γ/δ T cells and epithelial cells, which provide a barrier to invading organisms. These features of innate immunity have been reviewed in depth recently.[2]

Several components of the innate immune system will be discussed in greater detail later, however special mention of monocytes and monocyte-derived cells is warranted. Approximately 5% to 10% of circulating leukocytes are monocytes. These survive in the circulation for approximately one to two days, and do not undergo further proliferation, but are capable of enormous phenotypic differentiation.[4] A major impetus for this differentiation is transmigration of these cells through the endothelium which, as mentioned earlier, is triggered by various inflammatory stimuli. Upon entry of monocytes into the interstitial space, monocytes can undergo at least three fates (Fig. 7.1). Most commonly recognized is their conversion to macrophages, which remain in the interstitium and can phagocytose injurious bodies and release potent mediators including reactive oxygen species (ROS), nitric oxide (NO), cytokines, and matrix metalloproteinases. It is now recognized that there is also a population of tissue resident macrophages, not derived from circulating monocytes, which participate in tissue healing. Unlike monocyte-derived macrophages, tissue resident macrophages undergo proliferation and self-renewal.[5] A second fate of monocytes is to differentiate into dendritic cells, powerful antigen-presenting cells for T cell activation, which are discussed more fully later. A final fate of monocytes is to reemerge from the vessel wall without differentiation.[6] It is now recognized that monocytes can enter tissues, acquire antigens and transport these to lymph nodes where they can activate T cells without becoming either dendritic cells or macrophages. These minimally differentiated monocytes are typified by their surface expression of major histocompatibility complex type II and the activation marker Ly-6C and an enhanced ability to activate T cells.

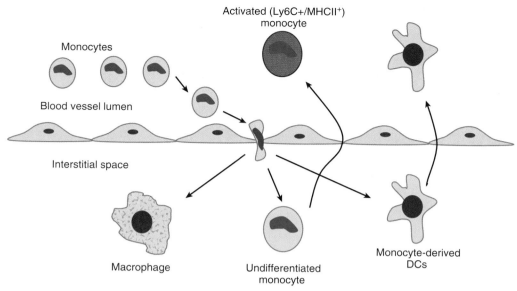

FIG. 7.1 Fates of monocytes. Upon endothelial transmigration, monocytes can become inflammatory macrophages, monocyte derived-dendritic cells or remain monocytes and reemerge in an activated state.

Although the innate immune system is nonspecific and provides immediate protection, it does not have the ability to augment protection upon repeated antigenic challenges. In contrast, adaptive immunity provides powerful and specific defense against previously encountered antigens. Components of the adaptive immune response include T cells, responsible for cellular immunity, and B cells, which upon activation by T cells differentiate into either short or long-lived antibody producing plasma cells.

A critical step in initiation of the adaptive immune response is uptake and processing of antigens by antigen presenting cells (APCs). Although several cells can present antigens, the major APCs are macrophages, B cells, and dendritic cells (DCs). CD4+ T cells are generally activated by peptides that have been derived from extracellular antigens presented in the context of type II major histocompatibility complexes (MHCs), whereas CD8+ T cells are activated by intracellular antigens, such as invading viruses, that are presented by type I MHCs. APCs that have acquired antigen undergo maturation, increasing expression of costimulatory molecules and production of cytokines that can direct T cell polarization. The activated APC migrates to secondary lymphoid organs and seeks a T cell with a T cell receptor that recognizes and binds the MHC/peptide complex. The subsequent immunologic synapse formed by these two cells leads to T cell activation, involving proliferation, an increase in cytokine production and a change in surface receptors that arm the cell to leave the secondary lymphoid organ and migrate to inflamed peripheral tissues. B cells also phagocytose and present antigen, and their formation of an immunologic synapse with T helper cells promoting their proliferation and formation of germinal centers in lymph nodes and tertiary sites.

T cell subsets exhibit division of duty. CD4+ T cells are conditioned or polarized by the cytokines they encounter upon initial stimulation, leading to unique T helper phenotypes. T_H1 cells produce proinflammatory cytokines such as interferon (IFN)-γ, IL-2 and tumor necrosis factor (TNF)α. T_H2 cells produce IL-4, IL-5 and IL-13, cytokines involved in response to allergens and helminth infections. T_H17 cells produce the unique cytokine IL-17, and play critical roles in diseases such as psoriasis, experimental allergic encephalitis and inflammatory bowel disease. T regulatory cells represent another subset of T cells that suppress the immune response. Activated CD8+ T cells have cytolytic activity, manifested principally by their release of isoforms of granzyme and perforin, but they can also release cytokines, and in fact are major sources of IFN-γ. These features of adaptive immunity have been reviewed in depth elsewhere.[7]

HISTORICAL ASPECTS REGARDING INFLAMMATION AND HYPERTENSION

It has been recognized that there is an inflammatory component in human hypertension for more than half of a century, and that immune cells contribute to blood pressure elevation in several experimental models. In 1953, Heptinstall reported that lymphocytic infiltrates were commonly observed in the kidneys of humans undergoing sympathectomy and or adrenalectomy for hypertension.[8] In 1964 White and Olsen showed that cortisone and mercaptopurine could lower blood pressure in a rat model of hypertension caused by renal infarction.[9] Subsequently Okuda and Grollman found that transfer of lymph node cells from these rats could passively raise blood pressure in otherwise normal recipients.[10] In 1970, Olsen showed that chronic angiotensin II infusion in rats lead to a striking periarteriolar infiltrate of lymphocytic and monocytic cells.[11] Soon thereafter, Dr. Olsen demonstrated a striking periarteriolar infiltration of immune cells in humans with hypertension, and pointed out that these appeared to be lymphocytes and monocytes.[12] In 1976, Svendsen demonstrated that athymic nude mice exhibit blunted hypertension in response to deoxycorticosterone acetate (DOCA)-salt challenge but that this phenotype was normalized by grafting of thymus tissue into these animals.[13] Subsequently, Olsen showed that transfer of splenocytes from rats with DOCA-salt hypertension conferred an increase in blood pressure in recipient rats.[14] Antithymocyte serum was shown to reduce hypertension in spontaneously hypertensive rats.[15] These studies among others strongly supported the idea that the immune system contributes to hypertension via mechanisms that were poorly understood at the time.

Recent Evidence Implicating Immune Cells in Hypertension

Advancements in the field of immunology have markedly enhanced our ability to understand the role of immune cells in hypertension. As an example, the development of mice lacking recombination activating gene-1 allowed Guzik et al to show that T cells are essential for the development of hypertension. These mice lack both T and B lymphocytes, and were found to exhibit blunted hypertensive responses to either chronic Ang II infusion or DOCA-salt challenge. Reconstituting T cells completely restored hypertension in these mice. Studies of Dahl salt sensitive rats have confirmed a role of T cells in this salt sensitive model of hypertension. Mechanistic studies in mice lacking T cell costimulatory proteins or various cytokines including IL-17A, IFN-γ and IL-6 have illustrated an important role for these mediators in hypertension. An evolving notion is that CD8+ T cells seem to play an important role, via mechanisms that are incompletely understood. Mice specifically lacking CD8+ T cells are more protected against hypertension than mice lacking CD4+ T cells.[16] Moreover, circulating CD8+ T cells in humans with hypertension display a senescent phenotype and evidence of activation. These cells produce large amounts of IFN-γ, which has been implicated in producing renal injury and promoting local angiotensinogen production in the kidney.

B lymphocytes have also been implicated in hypertension. Chen et al found that Ang II-induced hypertension is associated with a striking increase in serum IgG and in the aortic adventitia and that the hypertensive response to Ang II is attenuated in mice lacking B cells.[17] The precise roles of B cells, their production of antibody and their ability to present antigen to T cells in hypertension remain unclear. In preeclampsia, agonistic antibodies against the angiotensin II type 1 receptor play an important role in blood pressure elevation.[18]

There is also substantial evidence supporting a role of innate immune cells in hypertension. Wenzel et al showed that hypertension increases the accumulation of monocyte/macrophages in the artery wall and deletion of monocyte/macrophages completely prevents Ang II-induced hypertension in mice.[19] The authors provided evidence that these cells contribute to the production of vascular reactive oxygen species and vascular dysfunction. There is also increasing evidence that dendritic cells, and in particular inflammatory dendritic cells derived from monocytes, play a crucial role in T cell activation and contribute to hypertension.[20] Natural killer (NK) cells, which are important sources of IFN-γ, infiltrate the arterial wall in hypertension and seem to contribute to vascular dysfunction and formation of reactive oxygen species.[21]

Recently, myeloid-derived suppressor cells (MDSCs) have been found to have a protective effect in hypertension.[22] These are immature cells that can suppress T cells responses and reduce inflammation, most notably in the setting of neoplasia. MDSCs increase in experimental models of hypertension and depletion of these cells exacerbates blood pressure elevation and kidney injury, whereas adoptive transfer of these cells blunts hypertension.

The previous discussion illustrates that almost all components of the immune system contribute to hypertension. This is typical of many inflammatory conditions, and reflects the interdependence of innate, adaptive, cellular and humoral immunity.

BASIC MECHANISMS BY WHICH INFLAMMATION CONTRIBUTES TO HYPERTENSION

Before discussing how immune cells contribute to hypertension, it is useful to consider currently accepted mechanisms of hypertension to begin to understand how inflammatory cells might affect these processes. As discussed in the introduction, there is substantial debate as to the etiology of most cases of adult hypertension. Indeed, the origins of hypertension are probably diverse. Nonetheless, perturbations of renal function, vascular function, and central neural control are supported by extensive investigation. There is compelling evidence that some degree of renal dysfunction must be present

to sustain hypertension. This is based on the concept of the pressure natriuresis curve in which an elevation of blood pressure leads to a brisk diuresis, restoring blood pressure to its initial set point. In contrast, a lowering of blood pressure leads to a reduction in urine output, leading to volume and sodium retention until blood pressure rises to the set point. Guyton pointed out that all forms of hypertension are therefore associated with a resetting of this set point to a higher level, such that the kidneys no longer respond with diuresis at this higher level of pressure.[23] Although overt renal failure is often associated with hypertension, alterations of the pressure natriuresis curve can involve subtle alterations of renal function not manifested by reduced glomerular filtration rate or elevations of blood urea nitrogen or serum creatinine.[24] In fact, monogenic causes of hypertension, including Liddle syndrome and pseudohyperaldosteronism type II, involve enhanced sodium resorption in the distal nephron with otherwise normal renal function. Autocrine and paracrine factors including Ang II, nitric oxide, reactive oxygen species, endothelin-1 and prostaglandins influence renal sodium transport and their actions on the nephron have been implicated in hypertension. Many extrarenal stimuli, including catecholamines, aldosterone, vasopressin and as discussed later, inflammatory cytokines, can affect the pressure natriuresis curve without causing overt changes in renal function parameters. As discussed later in this chapter, several immune cell released cytokines affect tubular and vascular function and seem to promote sodium and volume retention in hypertension (Fig. 7.2).

Blood pressure is the product of cardiac output and systemic vascular resistance, and thus an increase in blood volume and cardiac output would be expected to increase blood pressure. Vascular resistance, and particularly renal vascular resistance, is elevated in many cases of human essential hypertension, suggesting a vascular etiology.[24] Indeed hypertension is associated with several perturbations of resistance vessel function and structure (Fig. 7.3). Vasodilatation, particularly that mediated by endothelial nitric oxide production, is often compromised in hypertension and vascular remodeling, involving an increase in medial thickness and a decrease in lumen diameter, is common.[25] These effects are in part mediated by cytokine stimulation of reactive oxygen species.[26,27] Vascular fibrosis occurs at both the level of the resistance circulation and as discussed later, in larger vessels. Vascular rarefaction, or disappearance of capillaries and small resistance vessels, is also a common consequence of hypertension.[28] These processes disable proper autoregulation and result in increased systemic vascular resistance.

An emerging vascular mechanism of hypertension relates to stiffening of the central large arteries, and particularly the aorta. Although large vessels have not been considered important in regulating systemic vascular resistance, it has become clear that aortic stiffening is a common harbinger of hypertension.[29] Central arteries expand during systole, accommodating a portion of the ejected blood, and recoil in diastole, propelling blood to the distal tissues. In this way healthy arteries maintain diastolic perfusion. Aortic stiffening is clinically detected as an increase in pulse wave velocity and becomes abnormal in a variety of conditions, including aging, diabetes, obesity, tobacco abuse and hypertension. In large population studies, aortic stiffening precedes the development of hypertension by several years. The precise mechanisms linking aortic stiffening to gradual onset of hypertension remain undefined, but likely involve alterations of pulse wave contour reaching peripheral tissues like the kidney,[30] the microcirculation and the brain, ultimately leading to damage of these tissues. Indeed, aortic stiffening portends conditions such as renal failure, heart failure, atherosclerosis, stroke and dementia.

In addition to renal and vascular causes of hypertension, there is convincing evidence that perturbations of the central

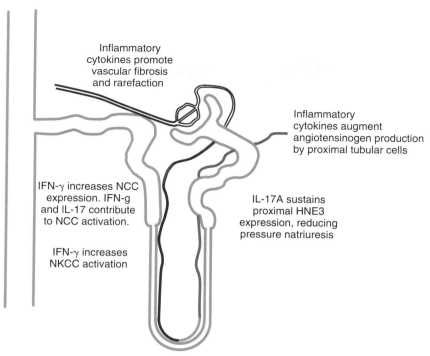

FIG. 7.2 Alterations in renal vascular and tubular function caused by inflammatory cytokines derived from knockout mice studies. IL-17A prevents downregulation of the hydrogen/sodium exchanger-3 (HNE3) in the proximal tubule. IFN-γ increases activation of the sodium/potassium/chloride cotransporter (NKCC) in the thick ascending limb of the loop of Henle. Both IFN-γ and IL-17A increase phosphorylation and activation of the sodium/chloride cotransporter (NCC) and IFN-γ increases protein levels of this transporter in the distal convoluted tubule. Several cytokines have been shown to enhance angiotensinogen production by renal tubular cells, promoting intrarenal Ang II production.

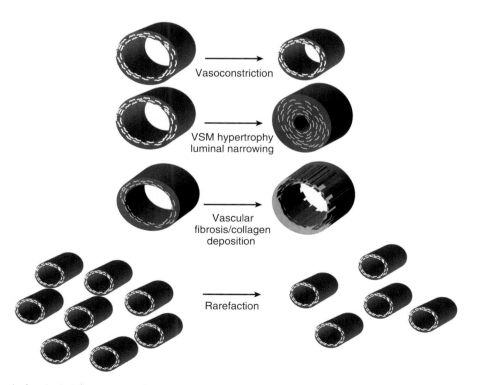

FIG. 7.3 Alterations of vascular function by inflammatory cytokines. Studies using knockout mice and cytokine antagonist indicate that IL-17A and TNFα contribute to reductions of endothelium-dependent vasodilatation, in part by increasing vascular superoxide production. IL-17A and TNFα have likewise been shown to enhance vascular smooth muscle superoxide production. IL-17A stimulates phosphorylation of the endothelial nitric oxide synthase at an inhibitory site (threonine 495), reducing nitric oxide production. Treatment with TNFα antagonists or knockout of IL-17A reduces vascular smooth muscle hypertrophy in response to hypertension. Cytokines including IL-17A and TNFα promote vascular smooth muscle production of reactive oxygen species that in turn alter vasomotion and can enhance vascular smooth muscle hypertrophy. T cell-released cytokines also seem to mediate both vascular fibrosis and rarefaction.

64

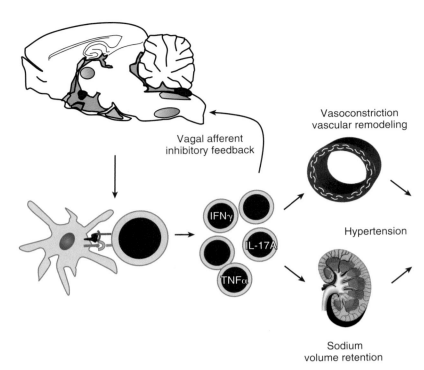

FIG. 7.4 The neuroimmune axis in hypertension integrates renal and vascular dysfunction. Signals from the central nervous system promote T cell activation, in part by stimulating antigen presenting cells. Activated T cells and monocyte/macrophages infiltrate the kidney and vasculature, enhancing vasoconstriction, vascular remodeling and renal sodium retention. Vagal afferents arising from inflamed tissues send inhibitory signals to reduce inflammation. This neuroimmune reflex can be disrupted in hypertension, promoting further inflammation.

nervous system contribute to hypertension. The lamina terminalis of the forebrain is composed of the subfornical organ (SFO), the median preoptic area (MPO) and the organum vasculosum of the lateral terminalis (OVLT). The SFO and OVLT possess poorly developed blood-brain barriers, and are sensitive to circulating mediators such as angiotensin II and salt, which increase neuronal firing in these structures and have input into the hypothalamus, and in particular the paraventricular nucleus. The paraventricular nucleus (PVN) in turn provides input to the rostroventral lateral medulla of the brainstem. This latter structure integrates baroreflex input with signals arising from the higher centers to regulate blood pressure. Hypertension is associated with abnormal neuronal firing, increased angiotensin II signaling and oxidative signaling in all of these structures. Importantly, lesions within these structures and local blockade of the renin angiotensin system have profound effects on blood pressure. As an example, lesions of the anteroventral third ventricle (AV3V) region, which disrupt fibers from the SFO to the OVLT, prevent most forms of experimental hypertension. Likewise, injection of angiotensin receptor blocking agents into the rostral ventrolateral medulla (RVLM) prevents hypertension. An emerging concept is that of the neuroimmune axis, in which sympathetic outflow modulates immune cell activation (Fig. 7.4), whereas afferent signals from the periphery inhibit further sympathetic outflow. There is evidence that this inhibitory loop is disrupted in hypertension.[31]

THE ROLE OF IMMUNITY AND INFLAMMATION AS MEDIATORS OF HYPERTENSION

It has been difficult to understand how the kidney, vasculature, and brain interact to regulate blood pressure. An emerging concept is that immune cells are activated and infiltrate these various organs, and may serve to transmit and intensify alterations of function of the brain, vasculature, and kidney. It should be stressed that inflammation is generally not thought

to cause hypertension on its own, but to intensify dysfunction of the kidney, vasculature, and central nervous system and exacerbate hypertension. Thus, the transformation of mild or prehypertension to clinical hypertension might mark activation of the immune system and inflammation in various end organs. Several general events mediated by inflammatory cells contribute to this process as discussed later.

Cytokine Release

A predominant role of almost all immune cells is to release various cytokines. These are extremely powerful and act locally to affect adjacent cells, including vascular and renal tubular cells. Several T cell, macrophage and dendritic cell-derived cytokines have been implicated in hypertension, including interleukin IL-6, IL-17A, IFN-γ and TNFα. As an example, hypertension in mice lacking IL-17A is blunted and these mice do not exhibit alterations of endothelium-dependent vasodilatation or increases in vascular superoxide production in response to Ang II infusion.[32] Direct application of this cytokine to vascular segments inhibits endothelial NO production and infusion of IL-17A elevates blood pressure via mechanisms involving activation of Rho kinase.[33] IFN-γ has likewise been implicated in causing tissue damage and dysfunction in hypertension. Ang II-induced hypertension increases T cell production of IFN-γ in rats and mice, and this cytokine has been implicated in cardiac and renal injury.[34-36] Mice lacking the transcription factor T box expressed in T cells (Tbet), which is essential for IFN-γ production, are protected against endothelial dysfunction and have reduced vascular expression of several NADPH oxidase subunits.[21] Likewise, mice lacking IL-6 are markedly protected against Ang II-induced hypertension via mechanisms involving the Janus kinase 2/signal transduction and activator of transcription 3 (JAK2/STAT3) pathway.[37]

Although substantial research has focused on the vascular actions of these cytokines, there is also substantial evidence that these mediators alter renal function in ways that could promote hypertension. Interleukin 6 produced by innate cells plays a critical role in skewing T cells to produce IL-17, but also promotes production of angiotensinogen by renal tubular cells, promoting intrarenal production of Ang II. IFN-γ has also been shown to induce angiotensinogen production in these cells. Another major effect of cytokines is to enhance renal tubular sodium retention. We have recently shown that the changes in renal tubular sodium transporter expression and activation caused by Ang II are blunted in mice lacking either IFN-γ or IL-17A. These changes are paralleled by a reduction in the antidiuretic and antinatriuretic effects of Ang II. Thus, immune cells that infiltrate the kidney in hypertension likely produce these cytokines, which in turn affect local Ang II production and enhance sodium retention.

There is increasing evidence that inflammation in the central nervous system contributes to hypertension. Shi et al demonstrated that microglial cells within the paraventricular nucleus (PVN) of the hypothalamus of rats with Ang II-induced hypertension produce increased amounts of IL-1β, IL-6 and TNFα compared to sham-infused rats.[38] Intracerebroventricular (ICV) infusion of the antibiotic minocycline, which suppresses microglial activation, decreased production of these cytokines, lowered systemic norepinephrine levels and reduced both blood pressure and left ventricular hypertrophy in these animals. The authors further demonstrated that adenoviral expression of the antiinflammatory cytokine IL-10 in the paraventricular nucleus also lowered blood pressure and reduced left ventricular hypertrophy whereas ICV infusion of IL-1β induced hypertension. In a related study, these investigators showed that transplant of bone marrow from normal Wistar Kyoto rats to spontaneously hypertensive rats reduced activation of microglial cells and blood pressure in the recipient mice.[39] Pallow et al showed that Ang II-induced hypertension is associated with an increase in infiltration of T cells around the subfornical organ of the brain, and that this is sex-dependent[40] Deletion of an antioxidant enzyme in the paraventricular organs of the brain, which increased sympathetic outflow, raised both blood pressure and activation of T cells.[41] In contrast, deletion of a component of NADPH oxidase, which decreases sympathetic outflow, reduced T cell activation.[42] Recently, we showed that renal denervation markedly reduced activation of dendritic cells and T cells in the kidney and provided evidence that the kidney might be a major site of immune activation.[43] Mice exposed to an emotional stress paradigm develop hypertension and T cell activation whereas mice lacking T cells are protected against stress-induced hypertension.[44]

Oxidative Injury

Many of the effects of these cytokines and immune cells are related to oxidative stress and injury. Phagocytic cells like monocyte/macrophages use the NADPH oxidase to generate large amounts of ROS upon activation and are likely sources of ROS when they accumulate in blood vessels or kidney. Mice lacking various components of this enzyme complex are partially protected against various forms of experimental hypertension.[45-48] Moreover, cytokines like IFN-γ, TNFα, IL-6 and IL-17 enhance expression of NADPH oxidase subunits in various cells increasing vascular superoxide production.[26,49-51] In vessels, ROS inactivate nitric oxide, promote vasoconstriction, enhance vascular smooth muscle hypertrophy and growth, and activate matrix metalloproteinases, which facilitate vascular remodeling. ROS also promote apoptosis, which contributes to vascular rarefaction. In the kidney, in addition to promoting renal vasoconstriction, ROS have been shown to activate sodium transport within the proximal tubule, the medullary thick ascending limb and in the cortical collecting duct. There is also evidence to support a role of ROS in modulating podocyte injury.[52] These effects of ROS in hypertension have previously been reviewed in depth.[53]

Matrix Reorganization

Vascular hypertrophy, luminal narrowing and rarefaction are commonplace in hypertension, and predispose to the increases in systemic vascular resistance encountered in this disease. For cells to proliferate, change size or migrate, there must be degradation of the extracellular matrix that encases cells. Matrix metalloproteinases (MMPs) are major mediators of this process. Although almost all cells can produce these potent enzymes, cells of the innate immune system, including macrophages, monocytes, neutrophils, and mast cells are major sources.[54] These pluripotent enzymes not only degrade matrix, but can activate other enzymes, liberate cell bound mediators, promote tissue calcification and enhance apoptosis, necrosis and cell senescence.[55] Short peptides released by MMPs have been referred to as matrikines that activate other immune cells.[56] An important consequence of MMP activation is the conversion of latent transforming growth factor β (TGFβ) to active TGFβ, which via its signaling through Smad pathways, plays multiple roles in matrix deposition.[57] The Smads act as transcription factors that promote collagen synthesis and also signal formation of myofibroblasts, major sources of extracellular matrix. TGFβ is a product of antigen presenting cells, including macrophages and dendritic cells, and is also an important modulator of T regulatory cell formation.[58] IL-17A, released by activated CD4+ T cells stimulates fibroblasts to produce several isoforms of collagen and fibronectin via p38MAP kinase.[59] An important renal consequence of matrix deposition is nephrosclerosis, a hallmark of hypertensive renal disease, a major cause of renal failure.[60]

It has become increasingly apparent that specialized monocyte-like cells, often termed fibrocytes, play a major role in tissue fibrosis.[61,62] These are bone marrow-derived cells that are recruited to sites of inflammation in a fashion similar to other monocytes, and are characterized by robust production of collagen and fibronectin. We recently found that about 60% of the collagen forming cells in the aorta are bone marrow derived in experimental hypertension.[63] Interestingly, resident fibroblasts seem to represent less than 20% of the collagen-forming cells of the aorta, emphasizing the complexity of this process and the importance of immune cells in tissue fibrosis.

Enhanced Chemotaxis

A recurring observation in hypertension is that products of immune cells in the kidney and blood vessels enhance accumulation of other immune cells. As an example, when hypertension is induced in mice lacking IL-17A, there is a marked decrease in the presence of T cells and monocyte/macrophages in blood vessels. Likewise, the vascular accumulation of all leukocytes caused by chronic Ang II infusion is reduced in mice lacking lymphocytes.[64] This is likely because cytokines such as IL-17A and TNFα promote production of chemokines that attract other immune cells.[65] In addition, these cytokines can promote endothelial activation and expression of adhesion molecules that enhance attraction of other immune cells.[66] This interaction emphasizes the feed forward nature of the inflammatory response that can occur in hypertension and illustrates the importance of local interactions between the innate and adaptive immune cells.

MECHANISMS OF IMMUNE ACTIVATION IN HYPERTENSION: POSSIBLE ROLE OF NEOANTIGENS

The mechanisms underlying T cell activation in hypertension and related cardiovascular disease remain undefined. As discussed earlier, this generally involves presentation of an antigen to a T cell that has a T cell receptor that recognizes the antigenic peptide bound to a major histocompatibility complex protein. In several conditions, including neoplasia, atherosclerosis, type 1 diabetes and autoimmunity, it is thought that self-proteins are altered to become neoantigens. Recently we discovered such a posttranslational modification involving adduction of gamma ketoaldehydes or isoketals to proteins, which seems to yield neoantigens in hypertensive mice.[20,67] Gamma ketoaldehydes are oxidation products of fatty acids, and rapidly ligate to protein lysines. These protein adducts are formed in dendritic cells of hypertensive animals, and are presented in the context of class 1 major histocompatibility complexes (Fig. 7.5). Exposure of murine dendritic cells to gamma ketoaldehyde-adducted proteins primes them to drive proliferation of memory T cells of hypertensive mice, and scavenging gamma ketoaldehydes prevents hypertension and prevents the immunogenicity of dendritic cells. We also observed increased amounts of these adducts in monocytes of humans with hypertension. Thus, alteration of self-proteins in this fashion might serve as a trigger for T cell activation in hypertension and related cardiovascular diseases. This process also illustrates a new mechanism by which oxidative events can contribute to hypertension.

The Relevance of Immune Memory in Hypertension

A cardinal feature of adaptive immunity is memory, or the ability of the immune system to respond to a second antigenic exposure with a response that is more rapid and robust than the response to the first exposure. Upon an initial antigen exposure, naïve T cells proliferate and become activated effector cells. Most of these cells ultimately die; however, a few remain as memory T cells. We found that these memory T cells are major sources of cytokines within

the kidney, and that these cells accumulate in the bone marrow of mice exposed to repeated hypertensive stimuli.[68] Moreover, we observed that these memory cells seem to promote severe hypertension to a second hypertensive stimulus that normally would not raise blood pressure on its own. These findings might have relevance to clinical conditions such as repeated emotional stress, sleep apnea (which causes repeated surges of blood pressure during the apneic episodes), or preeclampsia. Relevant to this last condition, preeclampsia predisposes women to cardiovascular events and hypertension throughout the remainder of their lives.[69,70] It is interesting to speculate that memory T cells, which can survive for decades in humans, might sensitize these individuals to develop hypertension in response to otherwise mild insults that would normally not raise blood pressure. A paradigm of how memory T cells are likely activated in response to repeated hypertensive stimuli is illustrated in Fig.7.6.

CLINICAL IMPLICATIONS REGARDING INFLAMMATION IN HYPERTENSION

Although there are substantial data supporting a role of inflammation in experimental models of hypertension, there is a paucity of such data in humans. Levels of C-reactive protein (CRP) correlate with systolic blood pressure and are associated with an increased risk for the development of hypertension.[71,72] CRP levels also correspond to subsequent end-organ damage in hypertension.[73] Other biomarkers of inflammation have been noted to be elevated in hypertension. As discussed previously, Youn et al found an increase in circulating senescent and activated CD8+ T cells in humans with hypertension.[74] Circulating plasma levels of IL-17A are

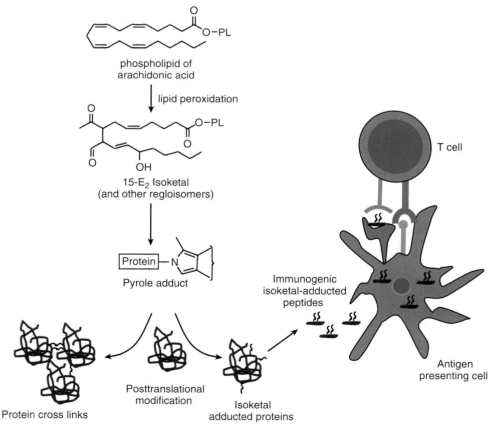

FIG. 7.5 Formation of immunogenic isoketal-adducts promote inflammation in hypertension. Various hypertensive stimuli increase oxidation of lipids, including arachidonic acid, leading to formation of highly reactive gamma-ketoaldehyde, or isoketals. These rapidly form pyrrole adducts with lysine on various proteins. These modified proteins are immunogenic and are processed by antigen-presenting cells and presented in major histocompatibility complexes, leading to T cell activation.

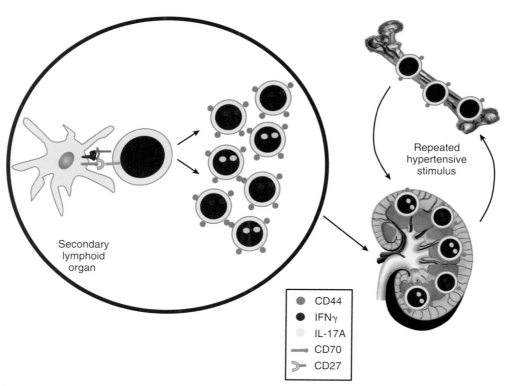

FIG. 7.6 Trafficking of effector memory T cells in hypertension. Effector memory cells formed in secondary lymphoid organs infiltrate the kidney and vasculature in hypertension. These cells are long-lived and can persist in the bone marrow and secondary lymphoid organs, and can be reactivated by mild repeated hypertensive stimuli. *(Adapted from Itani HA, Xiao L, Saleh MA, et al. CD70 Exacerbates Blood Pressure Elevation and Renal Damage in Response to Repeated Hypertensive Stimuli. Circ Res. 2016;118:1233-1243.)*

likewise elevated in patients with diabetes and hypertension as compared with those with diabetes alone.[32] Others have reported higher levels of IL-1β, IL-10, and TNFα in humans with resistant hypertension.[75]

Recent genome wide association studies have identified a single nucleotide polymorphism of *SH2B3* at position 262 (R262W) of LNK (SNP rs3184504) to be associated with many autoimmune and cardiovascular disorders, including type 1 diabetes, celiac disease, hypercholesterolemia, myocardial infarction, and hypertension.[76] LNK is a member of the Src Homology 2B (SH2B) family of adaptor proteins, and seems to integrate multiple cell signaling pathways. LNK is expressed primarily in hematopoietic and endothelial cells, and functions as a negative regulator of hematopoiesis and endothelial cell signaling. A recent study by Saleh et al showed that mice lacking LNK develop profound striking vascular and renal infiltration of T cells and monocyte/macrophages and marked vascular dysfunction hypertension upon infusion of a normally subpressor dose of Ang II (Fig. 7.7A).[77] This was associated with a marked hypertensive response, not observed in normal mice (Fig. 7.7B). Transplant of LNK-deficient bone marrow completely conferred the propensity for hypertension to normal wild-type mice. This study demonstrated key role of *SH2B3* as a potential driver of inflammation in hypertension. In related studies, Huan et al recently used a systems biology approach involving genome wide association data with whole blood messenger RNA expression profiles in 3679 individuals in the Framingham population to discover novel gene modules involved in the genesis of human hypertension.[78] *SH2B3* was identified as a key driver gene in a large protein-protein interaction network (Fig. 7.8). Several of the genes in this network were found to be differentially expressed between normal mice and mice lacking LNK. The function of these genes and their products in hypertension remain undefined, but many are involved in inflammation, immune-mediated cytotoxicity and cellular homeostasis.

There is a paucity of data indicating that antiinflammatory treatment can lower blood pressure, in part because of difficulties of experimental design and a reluctance to use such agents in patients that can be successfully treated using traditional and effective antihypertensive agents. In one small study, Herra et al found that mycophenolate mofetil, a T cell suppressing agent, lowered blood pressure in a small group of patients with autoimmune disease.[79] Recently, Yoshida et al demonstrated that the TNFα antagonist infliximab lowers blood pressure in patients with rheumatoid arthritis.[80] Anti-TNFα therapy has also been shown to improve aortic stiffening in a group of patients with inflammatory arthropathies.[81] Of note, some agents, such as nonsteroidal antiinflammatory drugs (NSAIDs) and cyclosporine, paradoxically raise blood pressure. This likely reflects the fact that there are multiple complex pathways leading to immune activation that are not blocked by NSAIDs and the fact that these agents have off target effects that raise blood pressure. In particular, the T cell suppressing agent cyclosporine is nephrotoxic, increases sympathetic outflow and stimulates renal expression of endothelin-1.[82] It has become increasingly apparent that there is substantial specificity of effect of immune modulating agents. As an example, anti-IL-17 is effective for treatment of psoriasis but not other autoimmune diseases.[83] In depth studies of these pathways, are essential before such interventions can be made in humans. It should be stressed that the major purpose for treating hypertension is to prevent end-organ damage and reduce mortality. As stressed in this chapter, a major cause of end-organ damage in hypertension is the local inflammatory response that leads to cell dysfunction, death, and replacement. Thus, therapeutic interventions to limit inflammation will likely be useful, particularly in population subsets where end-organ damage is poorly controlled by traditional therapy.

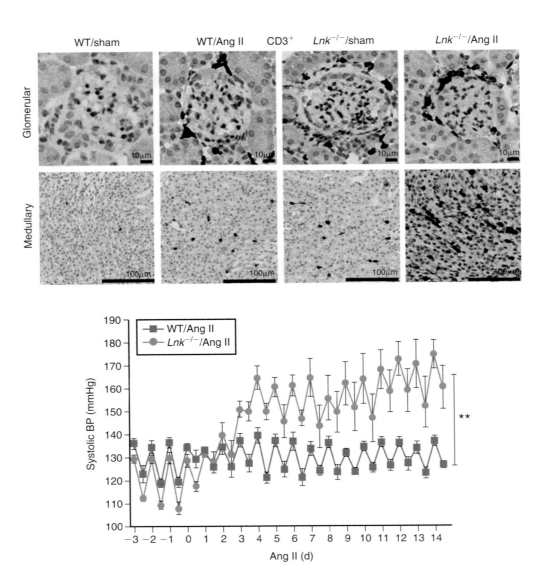

FIG. 7.7 Role of LNK (SH2B3) in hypertension. Renal T cell infiltration is markedly enhanced in mice lacking LNK (panel A) upon Ang II infusion. Panel B illustrates the markedly augmented hypertensive response to a generally suppressor infusion of Ang II. (*Data are from Saleh MA, McMaster WG, Wu J, et al. Lymphocyte adaptor protein LNK deficiency exacerbates hypertension and end-organ inflammation.* J Clin Invest. 2015;125:1189-1202.)

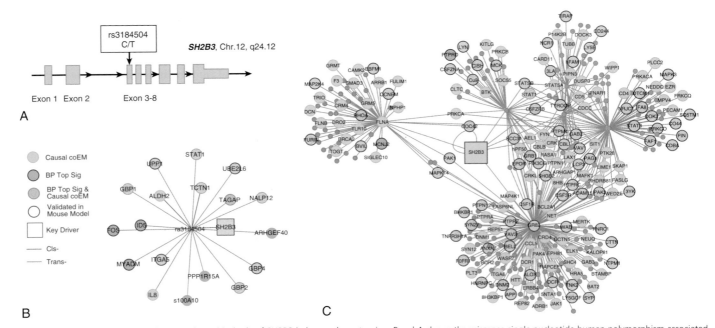

FIG. 7.8 Integrative network analysis reveals a critical role of SH2B3 in human hypertension. Panel A shows the missense single nucleotide human polymorphism associated with hypertension. Panel B shows that SH2B3 is associated either in cis or trans with 19 genes based on analysis of expression quantitative trait loci. Panel C shows the predicted SH2B3 protein–protein interaction (PPI) subnetwork. Green nodes indicate differentially expressed BP genes identified in the Framingham Heart Study data; turquoise nodes represent BP causal coexpression network modules; yellow nodes indicate genes that exist in the BP Top Sig set and the BP causal coexpression network modules. The nodes marked with a red border indicate genes that were also identified as differentially expressed between wild-type mice and mice lacking LNK. (*Data are from Huan T, Meng Q, Saleh MA, et al. Integrative network analysis reveals molecular mechanisms of blood pressure regulation.* Mol Syst Biol. 2015;11:799.)

References

1. Muller WA. The regulation of transendothelial migration: new knowledge and new questions. *Cardiovasc Res.* 2015;107:310-320.
2. Riera Romo M, Perez-Martinez D, Castillo Ferrer C. Innate immunity in vertebrates: an overview. *Immunology.* 2016;148:125-139.
3. Panda S, Ding JL. Natural antibodies bridge innate and adaptive immunity. *J Immunol.* 2015;194:13-20.
4. Ingersoll MA, Platt AM, Potteaux S, et al. Monocyte trafficking in acute and chronic inflammation. *Trends Immunol.* 2011;32:470-477.
5. Hashimoto D, Chow A, Noizat C, et al. Tissue-resident macrophages self-maintain locally throughout adult life with minimal contribution from circulating monocytes. *Immunity.* 2013;38:792-804.
6. Jakubzick C, Gautier EL, Gibbings SL, et al. Minimal differentiation of classical monocytes as they survey steady-state tissues and transport antigen to lymph nodes. *Immunity.* 2013;39:599-610.
7. Abbas A, Lichtman A, Pillai S. *Cellular and Molecular Immunology*. 8th ed. Philadelphia, PA: Elsevier Saunders; 2014.
8. Heptinstall RH. Renal biopsies in hypertension. *Br Heart J.* 1954;16:133-141.
9. White FN, Grollman A. Autoimmune factors associated with infarction of the kidney. *Nephron.* 1964;204:93-102.
10. Okuda T, Grollman A. Passive transfer of autoimmune induced hypertension in the rat by lymph node cells. *Tex Rep Biol Med.* 1967;25:257-264.
11. Olsen F. Type and course of the inflammatory cellular reaction in acute angiotensin-hypertensive vascular disease in rats. *Acta Pathol Microbiol Scand. A.* 1970;78:143-150.
12. Olsen F. Inflammatory cellular reaction in hypertensive vascular disease in man. *Acta Pathol Microbiol Scand. A.* 1972;80:253-256.
13. Svendsen UG. Evidence for an initial, thymus independent and a chronic, thymus dependent phase of DOCA and salt hypertension in mice. *Acta Pathol Microbiol Scand A.* 1976;84:523-528.
14. Olsen F. Transfer of arterial hypertension by splenic cells from DOCA-salt hypertensive and renal hypertensive rats to normotensive recipients. *Acta Pathol Microbiol Scand C.* 1980;88:1-5.
15. Bendich A, Belisle EH, Strausser HR. Immune system modulation and its effect on the blood pressure of the spontaneously hypertensive male and female rat. *Biochem Biophys Res Commun.* 1981;99:600-607.
16. Trott DW, Thabet SR, Kirabo A, et al. Oligoclonal CD8+ T cells play a critical role in the development of hypertension. *Hypertension.* 2014;64:1108-1115.
17. Chan CT, Sobey CG, Lieu M, et al. Obligatory role for B cells in the development of angiotensin II-dependent hypertension. *Hypertension.* 2015;66:1023-1033.
18. LaMarca B, Wallace K, Granger J. Role of angiotensin II type I receptor agonistic autoantibodies (AT1-AA) in preeclampsia. *Curr Opin Pharmacol.* 2011;11:175-179.
19. Wenzel P, Knorr M, Kossmann S, et al. Lysozyme M-positive monocytes mediate angiotensin II-induced arterial hypertension and vascular dysfunction. *Circulation.* 2011;124:1370-1381.
20. Kirabo A, Fontana V, de Faria AP, et al. DC isoketal-modified proteins activate T cells and promote hypertension. *J Clin Invest.* 2014;124:4642-4656.
21. Kossmann S, Schwenk M, Hausding M, et al. Angiotensin II-induced vascular dysfunction depends on interferon-gamma-driven immune cell recruitment and mutual activation of monocytes and NK-cells. *Arterioscler Thromb Vasc Biol.* 2013;33:1313-1319.
22. Shah KH, Shi P, Giani JF, et al. Myeloid Suppressor Cells Accumulate and Regulate Blood Pressure in Hypertension. *Circ Res.* 2015;117:858-869.
23. Guyton AC. Renal function curve—a key to understanding the pathogenesis of hypertension. *Hypertension.* 1987;10:1-6.
24. Derchi LE, Leoncini G, Parodi D, et al. Mild renal dysfunction and renal vascular resistance in primary hypertension. *Am J Hypertens.* 2005;18:966-971.
25. Gkaliagkousi E, Gavriilaki E, Triantafyllou A, et al. Clinical Significance of Endothelial Dysfunction in Essential Hypertension. *Curr Hypertens Rep.* 2015;17:85.
26. De Keulenaer GW, Alexander RW, Ushio-Fukai M, et al. Tumour necrosis factor alpha activates a p22phox-based NADH oxidase in vascular smooth muscle. *Biochem J.* 1998;329(Pt 3):653-657.
27. Miller Jr FJ, Filali M, Huss GJ, et al. Cytokine activation of nuclear factor kappa B in vascular smooth muscle cells requires signaling endosomes containing Nox1 and ClC-3. *Circ Res.* 2007;101:663-671.
28. Bobik A. The structural basis of hypertension: vascular remodeling, rarefaction and angiogenesis/arteriogenesis. *J Hypertens.* 2005;23:1473-1475.
29. Mitchell GF, Hwang SJ, Vasan RS, et al. Arterial stiffness and cardiovascular events: the Framingham Heart Study. *Circulation.* 2010;121:505-511.
30. Cooper LL, Rong J, Benjamin EJ, et al. Components of hemodynamic load and cardiovascular events: the Framingham Heart Study. *Circulation.* 2015;131:354-361. discussion 361.
31. Harwani SC, Chapleau MW, Legge KL, et al. Neurohormonal modulation of the innate immune system is proinflammatory in the prehypertensive spontaneously hypertensive rat, a genetic model of essential hypertension. *Circ Res.* 2012;111:1190-1197.
32. Madhur MS, Lob HE, McCann LA, et al. Interleukin 17 promotes angiotensin II-induced hypertension and vascular dysfunction. *Hypertension.* 2010;55:500-507.
33. Nguyen H, Chiasson VL, Chatterjee P, et al. Interleukin-17 causes Rho-kinase-mediated endothelial dysfunction and hypertension. *Cardiovasc Res.* 2013;97:696-704.
34. Shao J, Nangaku M, Miyata T, et al. Imbalance of T-cell subsets in angiotensin II-infused hypertensive rats with kidney injury. *Hypertension.* 2003;42:31-38.
35. Crowley SD, Song YS, Lin EE, et al. Lymphocyte responses exacerbate angiotensin II-dependent hypertension. *Am J Physiol Regul Integr Comp Physiol.* 2010;298:R1089-R1097.
36. Marko L, Kvakan H, Park JK, et al. Interferon-gamma signaling inhibition ameliorates angiotensin II-induced cardiac damage. *Hypertension.* 2012;60:1430-1436.
37. Brands MW, Banes-Berceli AK, Inscho EW, et al. Interleukin 6 knockout prevents angiotensin II hypertension: role of renal vasoconstriction and janus kinase 2/signal transducer and activator of transcription 3 activation. *Hypertension.* 2010;56:879-884.
38. Shi P, Diez-Freire C, Jun JY, et al. Brain microglial cytokines in neurogenic hypertension. *Hypertension.* 2010;56:297-303.
39. Santisteban MM, Ahmari N, Marulanda Carvajal J, et al. Involvement of bone marrow cells and neuroinflammation in hypertension. *Circ Res.* 2015;113:178-191.
40. Pollow DP, Uhrlaub J, Romero-Aleshire MJ, et al. Sex differences in T-lymphocyte tissue infiltration and development of angiotensin II hypertension. *Hypertension.* 2014;64:384-390.
41. Lob HE, Marvar PJ, Guzik TJ, et al. Induction of hypertension and peripheral inflammation by reduction of extracellular superoxide dismutase in the central nervous system. *Hypertension.* 2010;55:277-283.
42. Lob HE, Schultz D, Marvar PJ, et al. Role of the NADPH oxidases in the subfornical organ in angiotensin II-induced hypertension. *Hypertension.* 2013;61:382-387.
43. Xiao L, Kirabo A, Wu J, et al. Renal Denervation Prevents Immune Cell Activation and Renal Inflammation in Angiotensin II-Induced Hypertension. *Circ Res.* 2015;117:547-557.
44. Marvar PJ, Vinh A, Thabet S, et al. T lymphocytes and vascular inflammation contribute to stress-dependent hypertension. *Biol Psychiatry.* 2012;71:774-782.
45. Jung O, Schreiber JG, Geiger H, et al. gp91phox-containing NADPH oxidase mediates endothelial dysfunction in renovascular hypertension. *Circulation.* 2004;109:1795-1801.
46. Landmesser U, Dikalov S, Price SR, et al. Oxidation of tetrahydrobiopterin leads to uncoupling of endothelial cell nitric oxide synthase in hypertension. *J Clin Invest.* 2003;111:1201-1209.
47. Landmesser U, Cai H, Dikalov S, et al. Role of p47(phox) in vascular oxidative stress and hypertension caused by angiotensin II. *Hypertension.* 2002;40:511-515.
48. Gavazzi G, Banfi B, Deffert C, et al. Decreased blood pressure in NOX1-deficient mice. *FEBS Lett.* 2006;580:497-504.
49. Cassatella MA, Bazzoni F, Flynn RM, et al. Molecular basis of interferon-gamma and lipopolysaccharide enhancement of phagocyte respiratory burst capability. Studies on the gene expression of several NADPH oxidase components. *J Biol Chem.* 1990;265:20241-20246.
50. Manea A, Tanase LI, Raicu M, et al. Jak/STAT signaling pathway regulates nox1 and nox4-based NADPH oxidase in human aortic smooth muscle cells. *Arterioscler Thromb Vasc Biol.* 2010;30:105-112.
51. Pietrowski E, Bender B, Huppert J, et al. Pro-inflammatory effects of interleukin-17A on vascular smooth muscle cells involve NAD(P)H-oxidase derived reactive oxygen species. *J Vasc Res.* 2011;48:52-58.
52. Yan Q, Gao K, Chi Y, et al. NADPH oxidase-mediated upregulation of connexin43 contributes to podocyte injury. *Free Radic Biol Med.* 2012;53:1286-1297.
53. Harrison DG, Gongora MC. Oxidative stress and hypertension. *Med Clin North Am.* 2009;93:621-635.
54. Krstic J, Santibanez JF. Transforming growth factor-beta and matrix metalloproteinases: functional interactions in tumor stroma-infiltrating myeloid cells. *ScientificWorldJournal.* 2014;2014:521754.
55. Wang M, Kim SH, Monticone RE, et al. Matrix metalloproteinases promote arterial remodeling in aging, hypertension, and atherosclerosis. *Hypertension.* 2015;65:698-703.
56. Wells JM, Gaggar A, Blalock JE. MMP generated matrikines. *Matrix Biol.* 2015;44-46:122-129.
57. Meng XM, Tang PM, Li J, et al. TGF-beta/Smad signaling in renal fibrosis. *Front Physiol.* 2015;6:82.
58. Seeger P, Musso T, Sozzani S. The TGF-beta superfamily in dendritic cell biology. *Cytokine Growth Factor Rev.* 2015;26:647-657.
59. Wu J, Thabet SR, Kirabo A, et al. Inflammation and mechanical stretch promote aortic stiffening in hypertension through activation of p38 mitogen-activated protein kinase. *Circ Res.* 2014;114:616-625.
60. Meyrier A. Nephrosclerosis: update on a centenarian. *Nephrol Dial Transplant.* 2015;30:1833-1841.
61. Sakai N, Wada T, Yokoyama H, et al. Secondary lymphoid tissue chemokine (SLC/CCL21)/CCR7 signaling regulates fibrocytes in renal fibrosis. *Proc Natl Acad Sci USA.* 2006;103:14098-14103.
62. Bucala R, Spiegel LA, Chesney J, et al. Circulating fibrocytes define a new leukocyte subpopulation that mediates tissue repair. *Mol Med.* 1994;1:71-81.
63. Wu J, Montaniel KR, Saleh MA, et al. The origin of matrix-producing cells that contribute to aortic fibrosis in hypertension. *Hypertension.* 2016;67:461-468.
64. Guzik TJ, Hoch NE, Brown KA, et al. Role of the T cell in the genesis of angiotensin II induced hypertension and vascular dysfunction. *J Exp Med.* 2007;204:2449-2460.
65. Liu Y, Mei J, Gonzales L, et al. IL-17A and TNF-alpha exert synergistic effects on expression of CXCL5 by alveolar type II cells in vivo and in vitro. *J Immunol.* 2011;186:3197-3205.
66. Yuan S, Zhang S, Zhuang Y, et al. Interleukin-17 Stimulates STAT3-Mediated Endothelial Cell Activation for Neutrophil Recruitment. *Cell Physiol Biochem.* 2015;36:2340-2356.
67. Wu J, Saleh MA, Kirabo A, et al. Immune activation caused by vascular oxidation promotes fibrosis and hypertension. *J Clin Invest.* 2016;126:50-67.
68. Itani HA, Xiao L, Saleh MA, et al. CD70 Exacerbates Blood Pressure Elevation and Renal Damage in Response to Repeated Hypertensive Stimuli. *Circ Res.* 2016;118:1233-1243.
69. Fraser A, Nelson SM, Macdonald-Wallis C, et al. Associations of pregnancy complications with calculated cardiovascular disease risk and cardiovascular risk factors in middle age: the Avon Longitudinal Study of Parents and Children. *Circulation.* 2012;125:1367-1380.
70. Skjaerven R, Wilcox AJ, Klungsoyr K, et al. Cardiovascular mortality after pre-eclampsia in one child mothers: prospective, population based cohort study. *BMJ.* 2012;345:e7677.
71. Emerging Risk Factors Collaboration, Kaptoge S, Di Angelantonio E, et al. C-reactive protein concentration and risk of coronary heart disease, stroke, and mortality: an individual participant meta-analysis. *Lancet.* 2010;375:132-140.
72. Sesso HD, Buring JE, Rifai N, et al. C-reactive protein and the risk of developing hypertension. *JAMA.* 2003;290:2945-2951.
73. Hage FG. C-reactive protein and hypertension. *J Hum Hypertens.* 2014;28:410-415.
74. Youn JC, Yu HT, Lim BJ, et al. Immunosenescent CD8+ T cells and C-X-C chemokine receptor type 3 chemokines are increased in human hypertension. *Hypertension.* 2013;62:126-133.
75. Barbaro NR, Fontana V, Modolo R, et al. Increased arterial stiffness in resistant hypertension is associated with inflammatory biomarkers. *Blood Press.* 2015;24:7-13.
76. Devalliere J, Charreau B. The adaptor Lnk (SH2B3): an emerging regulator in vascular cells and a link between immune and inflammatory signaling. *Biochem Pharmacol.* 2011;82:1391-1402.
77. Saleh MA, McMaster WG, Wu J, et al. Lymphocyte adaptor protein LNK deficiency exacerbates hypertension and end-organ inflammation. *J Clin Invest.* 2015;125:1189-1202.
78. Huan T, Meng Q, Saleh MA, et al. Integrative network analysis reveals molecular mechanisms of blood pressure regulation. *Mol Syst Biol.* 2015;11:799.
79. Herrera J, Ferrebuz A, Macgregor EG, et al. Mycophenolate mofetil treatment improves hypertension in patients with psoriasis and rheumatoid arthritis. *J Am Soc Nephrol.* 2006;17:S218-S225.
80. Yoshida S, Takeuchi T, Kotani T, et al. Infliximab, a TNF-alpha inhibitor, reduces 24-h ambulatory blood pressure in rheumatoid arthritis patients. *J Hum Hypertens.* 2014;28:165-169.
81. Angel K, Provan SA, Gulseth HL, et al. Tumor necrosis factor-alpha antagonists improve aortic stiffness in patients with inflammatory arthropathies: a controlled study. *Hypertension.* 2010;55:333-338.
82. Sander M, Lyson T, Thomas GD, et al. Sympathetic neural mechanisms of cyclosporine-induced hypertension. *Am J Hypertens.* 1996;9:121S-138S.
83. Yang J, Sundrud MS, Skepner J, et al. Targeting Th17 cells in autoimmune diseases. *Trends Pharmacol Sci.* 2014;35:493-500.

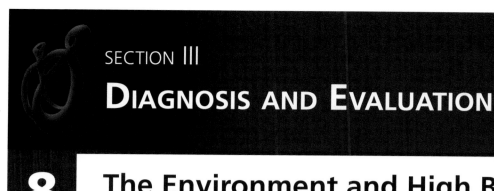

8 The Environment and High Blood Pressure

Robert D. Brook

Hypertension is a polygenetic disorder provoked by remediable (e.g., sodium intake) as well as unmodifiable factors (e.g., aging).[1] It accounts for up to half of cardiovascular events and is the leading risk factor for morbidity and mortality worldwide.[1,2] To combat this public health epidemic, a number of lifestyle interventions (e.g., reduced sodium intake) have been extensively studied and proven over the years to effectively lower blood pressure (BP).[1] As such, a central aspect of hypertension management endorsed by all guidelines is to identify and alleviate these established modifiable risk factors in individual patients.[1] Conversely, little attention has been paid to another important as well as potentially remediable contributor to high BP—*environmental exposures.*[3] Mounting evidence supports that colder ambient temperatures, winter season, higher altitudes, excessive noises, and air pollutants are capable of raising BP.[3] Although the pressor effects are typically modest (5 to 15 mm Hg), billions of people are impacted on a daily basis. Some exposures also tend to overlap in certain settings such as in cities (e.g., noise plus air pollution) and travel destinations (e.g., high altitude plus cold). The full public health burden of environmental exposures remains to be established. However, it is likely to be enormous given their omnipresent nature. This chapter reviews the evidence linking environmental factors with high BP as well as the implications for clinical practice.[3]

ENVIRONMENTAL RISK FACTORS FOR HIGH BLOOD PRESSURE

Colder Ambient Temperature and Winter Season

Colder temperatures increase BP over hours to days[3-10] as well as over more prolonged seasonal periods.[11-13] Studies across a wide range of populations and climates have demonstrated an inverse association between BP and ambient temperature during the same and/or preceding few days.[3-10,14-21] In one of the largest studies (n > 500,000) conducted across China, a colder temperature of 10° C was associated with a 5.7 mm Hg increase in systolic BP.[14] The impact was even more robust among older adults, those with smaller body mass indices; but was obviated by household central heating. Systolic BP was also on average 10 mm Hg higher during winter compared with summer. These results resemble our findings among 2078 cardiac rehabilitation patients in Michigan whereby reductions in outdoor temperatures by 10.4° C during the prior

1 to 7 days promoted a 3.6 mm Hg increase in systolic BP.[21] Moreover, in both studies temperatures below 5° C did not prompt further elevations in BP.[14,21] Similar inverse associations between outdoor temperature and BP have also been reported in other recent studies including patients with cardiovascular disease,[15] individuals living in rural China (e.g., 13% lower hypertension control rate during winter),[16] in a large Dutch population (n = 101,377),[18] and across several locations in Italy.[19,20]

Independent effects of both winter season and cold temperatures on BP have been reported. Cold exposures measured using personal monitors were shown to be associated with higher systolic BP levels during the daytime, even after adjusting for changes in daylight hours (i.e., season).[19] Conversely, nighttime BP was higher during summer (i.e., warmer days) compared with winter months in this[19] as well as in a few other studies.[7,20] We recently demonstrated similar findings using personal monitoring. Warmer nights (independent of season) led to higher BP levels several hours later during the following afternoon.[10] Along with a few prior studies,[7,19,20] these observations support that there is a highly complex interrelationship involving several exposure-related factors (time of day, duration, indoor versus outdoor temperature levels) that determine the true nature of the ensuing BP changes.

Brief exposure to cold induces a rapid thermoregulatory vasoconstriction, thus raising BP.[8] Although the mechanisms responsible for the more persistent pressor responses during winter are likely similar, they may not be entirely identical (Table 8.1).[22-24] Further physiologic adaptations (e.g., lower vitamin D, weight gain, reduced activity, and changes in diet/fluid balance) likely play additional roles. Conversely, changes in other meteorologic factors such as humidity and barometric pressure have not been consistently associated with BP.[3]

The overall evidence supports that both colder ambient temperatures (over a few hours to days) as well as winter seasons (over more prolonged periods) lead to clinically-meaningful elevations in BP. It is possible that this plays a role in the known increase in cardiovascular events during winter.[25,26] From a clinical standpoint, patients with hypertension should be more carefully monitored during colder weather to ensure adequate BP control.[14,16,27] In one study, 38% of patients required added antihypertensive medications during winter.[28] Although some epidemiologic evidence suggests that residential heating might mitigate the prohypertensive effects of cold,[11] further studies are needed before making

TABLE 8.1 Environmental Factors and Blood Pressure

ENVIRONMENTAL FACTOR	EFFECT OF EXPOSURE ON BLOOD PRESSURE	POSSIBLE MECHANISM(S)
Temperature Cold	Overall effect: Inverse association Colder outdoor/indoor ambient temperature associated with higher BP Cold increases BP variability and central aortic pulse pressure	Direct thermoregulation-mediated vasoconstriction HPAA and SNS activation, sodium/volume retention Impaired endothelial-dependent vasodilatation
Heat	Acute heat (e.g., sauna treatment) lowers BP	Reverse of cold mechanisms
Nighttime BP	Warmer daytime associated with higher nocturnal BP	Possibly reduced sleep quality
Nighttime temperature	Warmer nighttime temperature associated with higher next day BP	
Season Winter	Overall effect: Winter season associated with higher BP levels Reduced temperature may be primarily responsible; however, winter may have some additional independent effects	Cold-induced mechanisms plus chronic alterations may play additive roles: lower vitamin D levels, reduced activity, weight gain, shifts in fluid balance (aldosterone increase), and increased arterial stiffness.
Geography Altitude	Overall effect: Higher altitude (>2500 m) raises BP Ascent to higher altitudes raises BP (variable interindividual responses) May be affected by race, acclimatization, rate of climb, or duration of exposure. Long-term population studies are limited in ability to determine effect and show heterogeneous results on chronic BP levels because of many confounding variables.	Altitude-induced hypoxemia activates the chemoreflex along with compensatory responses causing increased SNS and adrenal activity. Long-term acclimatization may lead to differing responsible responses. Other associated factors such as colder temperatures and stress may also play a role. Long-term increases in red blood cell mass may contribute
Loud noises	Overall effect: Exposure to loud noises raises BP Numerous conditions implicated (ambient, traffic, airports)	Acute SNS activation, HPAA activation, endothelial dysfunction Possibly impaired sleep quality because of nocturnal noise
Pollutants Ambient outdoor PM	Overall effect: Exposure to pollutants raises BP Short and long-term PM exposures related to higher BP and hypertension	Acute activation of the SNS via pulmonary autonomic reflexes rapidly raises BP. PM constituents reaching the systemic vasculature and promoting vasoconstriction may also play a role
Indoor PM	Multiple size ranges (fine, coarse, ultrafine) of PM and sources (urban, rural, biomass, and personal-level) of exposures related to higher BP levels	Chronic exposures likely alter vascular tone via endothelial dysfunction or reduced arterial compliance (reduced nitric oxide and higher endothelins) because of PM-mediated systemic inflammation and oxidative stress in the vasculature as well as in the central nervous system
SHS	SHS exposure raises BP	
Others	Lead, cadmium, arsenic, mercury, POP, bisphenol A, strong odors, phthalates	

BP, Blood pressure; *HPAA*, hypothalamic pituitary adrenal axis; *PM*, particulate matter; *POP*, persistent organic pollutants; *SHS*, secondhand smoke; *SNS*, sympathetic nervous system.

definite recommendations in this regard for the sole purposes of preventing winter-induced hypertension. What if any other practical steps (e.g., space heaters, warmer clothes) individuals with hypertension can take to lessen the ill effects of cold exposures on BP require further investigation.

Noise

A diverse array of loud conditions has been implicated in raising BP including traffic, airplanes, and occupational noises.[29-36] Brief exposures can increase BP within minutes.[31,32] Additional studies show that residing at locales chronically impacted by loud noise (e.g., traffic and airplanes) increases the risk for overt hypertension.[29,30,33] Given the variety of conditions implicated and the linear association between decibel intensity and BP elevation, the source appears to be of secondary importance.[33,34] Nevertheless, some studies suggest that nighttime exposures (i.e., aircraft noise) may have a particularly detrimental impact.[32]

Recent reports have furthered our understanding of the adverse effects of noise on promoting hypertension.[35] A metaanalysis of 24 cross-sectional studies demonstrated a 7% increase in the prevalence of hypertension per 10 decibel increase in a 16-hour average traffic noise exposure.[36] Residing within 50 meters of a major roadway has also been independently linked to a 13% higher incidence of hypertension in a large cohort of women (n > 38,000) across the United States.[37] Additional research has attempted to dissociate the ill effects of noise from other coexposures (e.g., traffic noise versus air pollution). Although many studies support that noise is independently linked to higher BP and/or hypertension,[38,39] others have found it difficult to disentangle the individual contributions.[40]

The mechanisms whereby noise triggers an acute increase in BP and promotes chronic hypertension have begun to be elucidated (Table 8.1).[35] The main pathways include an activation of the sympathetic nervous system, the release of stress hormones, and stimulation of the hypothalamic pituitary adrenal axis. Recent experiments show that nocturnal exposures can disrupt sleep quality and impair vascular endothelial function, even when patients are not consciously aware or awoken by the noise.[35,41,42]

More than half of the global population now lives in cities.[37] Roughly 40% of the European population is exposed to excess traffic noise.[35] It has also been estimated that about 150 million people in the United States are exposed to noise levels placing them at excess risk for hypertension.[43] The health importance of the documented BP-raising effect of noise is not entirely clear; however, it may play an important role in the mechanisms linking traffic[44,45] and aircraft[46,47] noise with acute cardiovascular events. Large-scale policies regarding urban planning (e.g., roadway and airport proximities) as well as local ordinances that seek to reduce nuisance noises (e.g., construction) can mitigate exposures.[43,48] It is unclear whether health care providers should recommend patients to take action at work (e.g., wear protective ear muffs), home (e.g., close windows, use noise silencers), or in the health care environment (i.e., hospitalization) to reduce exposures to excessive noise for the sole purposes of lowering BP.

Higher Altitude

During ascent to higher altitudes BP increases over a few days independent of the effect of colder temperatures.[49-54] The magnitude of responses varies within and between individuals and may even differ between races.[49,51] However, the acuity of exposure appears to be an important factor, as those who have acclimatized over weeks tend to exhibit smaller changes.[51] Although the duration of response is not fully elucidated, some studies show that it may persist for weeks to months if remaining at higher altitude.[50,55,56] The overall evidence strongly supports an adverse effect of altitude on BP among individuals undergoing short-term ascents above 2500 meters[49-51]; whereas a few studies suggest that even lower altitudes (1200 m) may also present some risk.[51] Among the various mechanisms responsible, a key factor is hypoxia-induced activation of the chemoreflex and an ensuing augmentation of sympathetic outflow (see Table 8.1).[51,54,55,57,58] Other pathways include increased arterial stiffness, endothelin release and heightened blood viscosity.[51,52] The impact of acclimatization rates, exposure durations, peak altitude, and patient susceptibilities (e.g., black race) require more investigation.[49]

The literature regarding living at higher altitudes and developing chronic hypertension as well as the risk for excess cardiovascular events is more mixed.[53-55,59] This may reflect confounding because of common coexposures (e.g., cold, stress), as well as differences in other ecologic, genetic, and lifestyle variables between populations.[59] However, a recent metaanalysis of eight studies in Tibet (n = 16,913) among individuals living at 3000 to 4300 m above sea level showed a positive relationship between hypertension and higher altitude.[56] Every 100 m increase in altitude was independently associated with a 2% increase in hypertension prevalence. More studies are required given the public health importance of this issue.[59]

Recent studies have also evaluated the effectiveness of pharmacologic interventions to prevent the effects of high altitude on BP.[57,58] Twenty-four hour BP levels were elevated after staying 12 days at Mt. Everest base camp (n = 45).[57] There was a progressive increase in systolic BP (10 to 15 mm Hg) and plasma norepinephrine levels from 3400 m and up to 5400 m that started immediately and persisted throughout prolonged altitude exposure. Moreover, BP normalized upon return to sea level. Angiotensin receptor blockade (ARB) was not capable of mitigating the pressor response to high altitude; whereas it slightly lowered absolute BP levels (4 mm Hg) compared with placebo at 3400 m, but it was ineffective in this regard at the higher altitude (5400 m). This is consistent with the findings that circulating markers of renin-angiotensin activity were suppressed at higher altitudes. Similar results were reported in a study of 89 patients with mild hypertension climbing 3260 m in the Andes.[58] Combined treatment with an ARB plus calcium channel blocker (CCB) did not blunt the magnitude of high altitude-induced increases in BP (10 to 15 mm Hg systolic). However, absolute BP levels remained significantly lower during combination therapy compared with placebo at all altitudes.

From a clinical standpoint, guidelines for managing high BP as well as cardiovascular risk in patients ascending to higher altitudes (typically above 2500 m) have been published.[52,54,60] This issue is of growing public health importance given the roughly 35 million people per year who travel worldwide above this altitude.[55] Recommendations include proper preparation and acclimatization (when warranted) along with careful BP monitoring during time spent at higher altitudes.[54,60] This may even include periods of travel (or seasonal relocation) to relatively lower altitudes (e.g., 1200 m) among at-risk or susceptible patients. A return to lower altitudes may even be justified in some situations, such as for severe or refractory high BP.[57,58] Beta blockers and ARBs do not prevent the pressor response; whereas combination ARB plus CCB therapy has shown some efficacy in controlling absolute BP levels at high altitude.[57,58] The optimal regimen and appropriate clinical scenario when to modify hypertension management (e.g., increase or add medications) to control altitude-induced BP elevations remains to be clarified.[52]

Air Pollution

Air pollution is a leading global risk factor for morbidity and mortality.[2] One of the most important pollutants is fine particulate matter (PM) 2.5 μm, commonly derived from the combustion of fossil fuels (e.g., coal) from a host of modern-day activities (e.g., traffic, power generation, industry).[63] Over the past decade a growing body of studies has demonstrated that exposure to $PM_{2.5}$, along with several different air pollutants, is capable of raising BP.[61-63] As an example, we recently showed among 2078 patients living in southeast Michigan that day-to-day variations of ambient $PM_{2.5}$ levels (8.2 μg/m³) during the prior few days were independently associated with significant increases in BP by 2.1 to 3.5/1.7 to 1.8 mm Hg.[21] This occurred despite the fact that patients were well-treated using contemporary secondary prevention medications (e.g., statins, beta blockers) and the air quality was excellent from a global perspective. In fact, mean $PM_{2.5}$ levels (12.6 μg/m³) were well within daily United States National Ambient Air Quality Standards (<35 μg/m³).[63] At the other end of the dose spectrum, more extreme $PM_{2.5}$ levels (from 50 to >550 μg/m³) in cities such as Beijing are also linked to short-term as well as more chronic elevations in BP.[64,65] A recent metaanalysis of up to 25 studies from across the world concluded that an increase in $PM_{2.5}$ by 10 μg/m³ during the prior few days is associated with an elevation in BP of 1.4/0.9 mm Hg.[66] Chronic exposures over the prior year resulted in even more robust responses (7.3/9.5 mm Hg).[66] In support of these findings, several randomized double-blind controlled trials of exposures to fine, coarse (2.5 to 10 μm) and diesel exhaust (10 to 100 nm) have shown that the acute inhalation of PM across a wide range of size fractions and derived from a variety of sources are capable of rapidly raising BP (2 to 10 mm Hg) over a few hours.[62,63]

Beyond the acute pressor response, exposure to $PM_{2.5}$ on a chronic basis is linked to development of overt hypertension.[62] In a cohort of 33,303 adults living a clean environment (Ontario, Canada), a long-term increase of $PM_{2.5}$ levels of 10 μg/m³ was associated with a 13% higher incidence of hypertension.[67] Similarly, a 14% increase in the onset of hypertension was found in association with chronic exposure to traffic-related pollutants in black women living in Los Angeles.[68] There is even evidence that living in regions across the United States with higher ambient $PM_{2.5}$ levels increases hypertension-related mortality.[69]

A wide array biologic mechanisms have been shown to be involved in air pollution-mediated BP elevations.[62,63] $PM_{2.5}$ inhalation activates the sympathetic nervous system via autonomic reflexes following stimulation of a variety of receptors (e.g., transient receptor potential channels) throughout the pulmonary tree. Another important pathway is the genesis of systemic inflammation resulting from the "spill-over" of numerous circulating factors (cytokines, activated immune cells, oxidized lipoproteins) from the lungs. Thereafter, this can adversely impact the entire cardiovascular system by triggering vasoconstriction and endothelial dysfunction. Finally, there is accruing evidence that some prooxidative constituents of inhaled particles (e.g., nanoparticles, metals, organic compounds) may be capable of reaching the systemic circulation and thereby directly impact the cardiovascular system.

Beyond regional (e.g., industry) and point-sources (e.g., traffic) of widespread ambient air pollution, a more localized source, secondhand smoke (SHS) from cigarettes, can also raise BP.[70-75] SHS increases the risk of elevated home BP values as well as the prevalence of masked hypertension.[72-74] We have shown by controlled exposures[70] as well as personal monitoring[71] that short-term SHS inhalation causes elevations in BP over a few hours-to-days. Perhaps even more important, a number of studies have also began to show that long-term exposures are capable of promoting the development of chronic hypertension.[76,77]

The negative influence of air pollution on BP is of clinical relevance. Emergency department visits for hypertension have been shown to be increased following more air polluted days in several countries including Canada (low levels) and China (extremely high levels).[62,78] Hypertension-related mortality has also been linked to chronic $PM_{2.5}$ exposures.[69] Reductions in citywide and national ambient air pollution levels because of governmental regulations provide substantial improvements in cardiovascular health as well as reductions in all-cause mortality.[79] From a clinical practice standpoint, some studies have shown that several personal-level interventions can be effective in reducing harmful exposures and thereby blunt or mitigate the prohypertensive responses. These include wearing high efficiency filter (HEPA) facemasks while outdoors and/or closing outside windows while in heavily polluted cities, as well as using household and automobile cabin HEPA filtration systems.[79] Decreased exposure to SHS also results in substantial reductions (10% to 20%) in cardiovascular events within a few months of instituting smoking ordinances.[80] Clinical recommendations regarding practical methods to assess and reduce the cardiovascular risks related to air pollution have been outlined in detail.[63]

Other Environmental Factors

Several additional environmental factors common to modern societies have proven capable of increasing BP including exposures to persistent organic pollutants, strong odors (e.g., nearby farm animals), certain metals (i.e., lead, cadmium, mercury, arsenic), and several endocrine-disrupting chemicals used in plastics such as beverage bottles (e.g., bisphenol A) and food wraps (e.g., phthalates).[3,81-89] Facial immersion in cold water also acutely raises BP (i.e., diving reflex).[3] There is additional evidence that living at more extreme northern or southern latitudes is associated with higher BP (possibly related to lower vitamin D).[81,82] Finally, extraordinarily rare exposures shown in a few case reports to significantly alter BP include the inhalation of moon dust by astronauts (elevates BP)[3] and zero gravity space flight (lowers BP because of vasodilatation despite increased cardiac output).[87-89]

Summary of Evidence

The main findings in the published literature and the biologic mechanisms linking environmental exposures to BP changes are summarized in Table 8.1. The majority of studies report average systolic BP elevations between 5 and 15 mm Hg following relevant exposures either commonly or plausibly encountered in real-world scenarios. Note that some patients may experience even larger responses and extreme exposures may produce even greater pressor responses than typically reported.

CLINICAL PRACTICE IMPLICATIONS

Fig. 8.1 outlines a suggested approach for health care providers on when to suspect and evaluate for the potential effects of environmental exposures on BP. Practical recommendations include providing education and counseling to patients regarding the potential risks during relocation (e.g., travel, residential or occupational moves) to settings where increased exposures are expected (e.g., high altitude, colder/polluted location). The precautionary principal also dictates that some high risk patients (e.g., severe or uncontrolled hypertension; patients with unstable cardiovascular conditions) should make serious attempt to avoid unnecessary exposures if possible (e.g., voluntary travel). Completely avoiding exposures may require impractical life changes (e.g., moving) that should only be considered in very rare circumstances among extremely impacted or highly-vulnerable patients. On

When To Consider Environmental Factors May Be Affecting BP
- Increase in BP or worsening of hypertension control (without other ostensible causes)
- "Masked" hypertension (exposures in the daily environment outside of the clinic setting)
- Recognizable or obvious exposure(s) reported by the patient (e.g., loud noises)
- Relocation or travel to settings of higher exposure (high altitude, cold, air pollution)

Other plausible scenarios
- Paucity of traditional risk factors to explain high BP or hypertension
- Potential trigger of a hypertensive urgency/emergency (e.g., air pollution)

Evaluate For Potential Environmental Exposures
- Occupational (PM or noise exposure)
- Residential (especially by roadway or colder/higher altitude region)
- Commutes (especially involving heavy traffic-related PM or noise)
- Travel (especially to cold/high altitude climate or high PM region)
- Ask for common recognizable exposure(s) to:
  - **Noise:** roadway, occupational, air traffic, local nuisance noise (e.g., construction)
  - **PM:** near-roadway, local point sources (factories); moved to polluted region, occupational
  - **SHS:** home. workplace. social exposures
  - **Altitude:** travel, moves, seasonal relocations to higher altitude locations
  - **Season changes:** increase in BP during winter months
  - **Cold:** winter hypertension, recent move to colder local; lack of appropriate residential heating

Consider Prudent Mitigating Actions On a Case-by-case Basis

FIG. 8.1 Clinical algorithm addressing the effects of environmental exposures on blood pressure. *BP*, Blood pressure; *PM*, particulate matter.

the other hand, there is some evidence to support a number of more realistic actions (e.g., air filters, home heating) that patients can implement on a case-by-case basis (outlined in prior sections).

References

1. Mancia G, Fagard R, Narkiewicz K, et al. 2013 ESH/ESC Guidelines for the management of arterial hypertension: the Task Force for the management of arterial hypertension of the European Society of Hypertension (ESH) and of the European Society of Cardiology (ESC). *J Hypertens.* 2013;31:1281-1357.
2. GBD 2013 Risk Factors Collaborators. Global, regional, and national comparative risk assessment of 79 behavioral, environmental and occupational, and metabolic risks or clusters of risks in 188 countries, 1990-2013: a systematic analysis for the Global Burden of Disease Study 2013. *Lancet.* 2015;386:2287-2323.
3. Brook RD, Weder AB, Rajagopalan S. "Environmental hypertensionology" the effects of environmental factors on blood pressure in clinical practice and research. *J Clin Hypertens. (Greenwich).* 2011;13:836-842.
4. Alpérovitch A, Lacombe J-M, Hanon O, et al. Relationship between blood pressure and outdoor temperature in a large sample of elderly individuals. The Three-City Study. *Arch Intern Med.* 2009;169:75-80.
5. Barnett AG, Sans S, Salomaa V, et al. The effect of temperature on systolic blood pressure. *Blood Press Monit.* 2007;12:195-203.
6. Halonen JI, Zanobetti A, Sparrow D, et al. Relationship between outdoor temperature and blood pressure. *Occup Environ Med.* 2011;68:296-301.
7. Modesti PA, Borabito M, Bertolozzi I, et al. Weather-related changes in 24-hour blood pressure profile. Effects of age and implications for hypertension management. *Hypertension.* 2006;47:1-7.
8. Sun Z. Cardiovascular responses to cold exposure. *Front Biosci.* 2010;2:495-503.
9. Luurila AJ, Kohvakka A, Sundberg S. Comparison of blood pressure response to heat stress in sauna in young hypertensive patients treated with atenolol and diltiazem. *Am J Cardiol.* 1989;64:97-99.
10. Brook RD, Shin HH, Bard RL, et al. Can personal exposures to higher nighttime and early morning temperatures increase blood pressure? *J Clin Hypertens.* 2011;13:881-888.

11. Nafstad MC. Associations between environmental exposure and blood pressure among participants in the Oslo Health Study (HUBRO). *Eur J Epidemiol*. 2006;21:485-491.
12. Woodhouse PR, Khaw K-T, Plummer M. Seasonal variation of blood pressure and its relationship to ambient temperature in an elderly population. *J Hypertens*. 1993;11:1267-1274.
13. Al-Tamre YY, Al-Hayali JMT, Al-Ramadhan EAH. Seasonality of hypertension. *J Clin Hypert*. 2008;10:125-129.
14. Lewington S, Li L, Sherliker P, et al. Seasonal variation in blood pressure and its relationship with outdoor temperature in 10 diverse regions of China: the China Kadoorie Biobank. *J Hypertens*. 2012;30:1383-1391.
15. Yang L, Li L, Lewington S, et al. Outdoor temperature, blood pressure, and cardiovascular disease mortality among 23 000 individuals with diagnosed cardiovascular diseases from China. *Eur Heart J*. 2015;36:1178-1185.
16. Su D, Du H, Zhang X, et al. Season and outdoor temperature in relation to detection and control of hypertension in a large rural Chinese population. *Int J Epidemiol*. 2014;43:1835-1845.
17. Chen Q, Wang J, Tian J, et al. Association between ambient temperature and blood pressure and blood pressure regulators: 1831 hypertensive patients followed up for three years. *PLoS One*. 2013;8:e84522.
18. van den Hurk K, de Kort WL, Deinum J, Atsma F. Higher outdoor temperatures are progressively associated with lower blood pressure: a longitudinal study in 100,000 healthy individuals. *J Am Soc Hypertens*. 2015;9:536-543.
19. Modesti PA, Morabito M, Massetti L, et al. Seasonal blood pressure changes: an independent relationship with temperature and daylight hours. *Hypertension*. 2013;61:908-914.
20. Fedecostante M, Barbatelli P, Guerra F, Espinosa E, Dessì-Fulgheri P, Sarzani R. Summer does not always mean lower: seasonality of 24 h, daytime, and night-time blood pressure. *J Hypertens*. 2012;30:1392-1398.
21. Giorgini P, Rubenfire M, Das R, et al. Particulate matter air pollution and ambient temperature: opposing effects on blood pressure in high-risk cardiac patients. *J Hypertens*. 2015;33:2032-2038.
22. Fares A. Winter Hypertension: Potential mechanisms. *Int J Health Sci (Qassim)*. 2013;7:210-219.
23. Cuspidi C, Ochoa JE, Parati G. Seasonal variations in blood pressure: a complex phenomenon. *J Hypertens*. 2012;30:1315-1320.
24. Cui J, Muller MD, Blaha C, Kunselman AR, Sinoway LI. Seasonal variation in muscle sympathetic nerve activity. *Physiol Rep*. 2015;3:e12492.
25. Ye X, Wolff R, Yu W, Vaneckova P, Pan X, Tong S. Ambient temperature and morbidity: a review of epidemiological evidence. *Environ Health Perspect*. 2012;120:19-28.
26. Bhaskaran K, Hajat S, Haines A, Herrett E, Wilkinson P, Smeeth L. Short term effects of temperature on risk of myocardial infarction in England and Wales: time series regression analysis of the Myocardial Ischaemia National Audit Project (MINAP) registry. *BMJ*. 2010;341:c3823.
27. Handler J. Seasonal variability of blood pressure in California. *J Clin Hypertens. (Greenwich)*. 2011;13:856-860.
28. Charach G, Rabinovich PD, Weintraub M. Seasonal changes in blood pressure and frequency of related complications in elderly Israeli patients with essential hypertension. *Gerontology*. 2004;50:315-321.
29. Jarup L, Babisch W, Houthuijs D, et al. Hypertension and exposure to noise near airports: the HYENA study. *Environ Health Perspect*. 2008;116:329-333.
30. Barregard L, Bonde E, Öhrström E. Risk of hypertension from exposure to road traffic noise in a population-based sample. *Occup Environ Med*. 2009;66:410-415.
31. Chang T-Y, Lai Y-A, Hsieh H-H, et al. Effects of environmental noise exposure on ambulatory blood pressure in young adults. *Environ Res*. 2009;109:900-905.
32. Haraladbidis AS, Dimakopoulou K, Vigna-Taglianti F, et al. Acute effects of night-time noise exposure on blood pressure in populations living near airports. *Eur Heart J*. 2008;29:658-664.
33. Davies HW, Vlaanderen JJ, Henderson SB, et al. Correlation between co-exposures to noise and air pollution from traffic sources. *Occup Environ Med*. 2009;66:347-350.
34. Barregard L. Traffic noise and hypertension. *Environ Res*. 2011;111:186-187.
35. Münzel T, Gori T, Babisch W, Basner M. Cardiovascular effects of environmental noise exposure. *Eur Heart J*. 2014;35:829-836.
36. van Kempen E, Babisch W. The quantitative relationship between road traffic noise and hypertension: a meta-analysis. *J Hypertens*. 2012;30:1075-1086.
37. Kingsley SL, Eliot MN, Whitsel EA, et al. Residential proximity to major roadways and incident hypertension in post-menopausal women. *Environ Res*. 2015;142:522-528.
38. Foraster M, Künzli N, Aguilera I, et al. High blood pressure and long-term exposure to indoor noise and air pollution from road traffic. *Environ Health Perspect*. 2014;122:1193-1200.
39. Stansfeld SA. Noise effects on health in the context of air pollution exposure. *Int J Environ Res Public Health*. 2015;12:12735-12760.
40. Babisch W, Wolf K, Petz M, Heinrich J, Cyrys J, Peters A. Associations between traffic noise, particulate air pollution, hypertension, and isolated systolic hypertension in adults: the KORA study. *Environ Health Perspect*. 2014;122:492-498.
41. Akinseye OA, Williams SK, Seixas A, et al. Sleep as a mediator in the pathway linking environmental factors to hypertension: a review of the literature. *Int J Hypertens*. 2015;2015:926414.
42. Schmidt F, Kolle K, Kreuder K, et al. Nighttime aircraft noise impairs endothelial function and increases blood pressure in patients with or at high risk for coronary artery disease. *Clin Res Cardiol*. 2015;104:23-30.
43. Hammer MS, Swinburn TK, Neitzel RL. Environmental noise pollution in the United States: developing an effective public health response. *Environ Health Perspect*. 2014;122:115-119.
44. Babisch W. Updated exposure-response relationship between road traffic noise and coronary heart diseases: a meta-analysis. *Noise Health*. 2014;16:1-9.
45. Halonen JI, Hansell AL, Gulliver J, et al. Road traffic noise is associated with increased cardiovascular morbidity and mortality and all-cause mortality in London. *Eur Heart J*. 2015;36:2653-2661.
46. Floud S, Blangiardo M, Clark C, et al. Exposure to aircraft and road traffic noise and associations with heart disease and stroke in six European countries: a cross-sectional study. *Environ Health*. 2013;12:89.
47. Correia AW, Peters JL, Levy JI, Melly S, Dominici F. Residential exposure to aircraft noise and hospital admissions for cardiovascular diseases: multi-airport retrospective study. *BMJ*. 2013;347:f5561.
48. Babisch W, Swart W, Houthuijs D, et al. Exposure modifiers of the relationships of transportation noise with high blood pressure and noise annoyance. *J Acoust Soc Am*. 2012;132:3788-3808.
49. Hasler E, Suter PM. Vetter. Race specific altitude effects on blood pressure. *J Hum Hypertens*. 1997;11:435-438.
50. Sizlan A, Ogur R, Ozer M, et al. Blood pressure changes in young male subjects exposed to a median altitude. *Clin Auton Res*. 2008;18:84-89.
51. Handler J. Altitude-related hypertension. *J Clin Hypertens*. 2009;11:161-165.
52. Luks AM. Should travelers with hypertension adjust their medications when traveling to high altitude? *High Altitude Med Biol*. 2009;10:11-14.
53. Faeh D, Gutzwiller F, Bopp M, et al. Lower mortality from coronary heart disease and stroke at higher altitudes in Switzerland. *Circulation*. 2009;120:495-501.
54. Rimoldi SF, Sartori C, Seiler C, et al. High-altitude exposure in patients with cardiovascular disease: risk assessment and practical recommendations. *Prog Cardiovasc Dis*. 2010;52:512-524.
55. Dhar P, Sharma VK, Hota KB, et al. Autonomic cardiovascular responses in acclimatized lowlanders on prolonged stay at high altitude: a longitudinal follow up study. *PLoS One*. 2014;9:e84274.
56. Mingji C, Onakpoya IJ, Perera R, Ward AM, Heneghan CJ. Relationship between altitude and the prevalence of hypertension in Tibet: a systematic review. *Heart*. 2015;101:1054-1060.
57. Parati G, Bilo G, Faini A, et al. Changes in 24 h ambulatory blood pressure and effects of angiotensin II receptor blockade during acute and prolonged high-altitude exposure: a randomized clinical trial. *Eur Heart J*. 2014;35:3113-3122.
58. Bilo G, Villafuerte FC, Faini A, et al. Ambulatory blood pressure in untreated and treated hypertensive patients at high altitude: the High Altitude Cardiovascular Research-Andes study. *Hypertension*. 2015;65:1266-1272.
59. Burtscher M. Effects of living at higher altitudes on mortality: a narrative review. *Aging Dis*. 2013;5:274-280.
60. Bärtsch P, Swenson ER. Clinical practice: acute high-altitude illnesses. *N Engl J Med*. 2013;368:2294-2302.
61. Brook RD, Rajagopalan S. Particulate matter air pollution and blood pressure. *J Am Soc Hypertens*. 2009;3:332-350.
62. Giorgini P, Di Giosia P, Grassi D, Rubenfire M, Brook RD, Ferri C. Air pollution exposure and blood pressure: an updated review of the literature. *Curr Pharm Des*. 2015;22:28-51.
63. Brook RD, Rajagopalan S, Pope 3rd CA, et al. Particulate matter air pollution and cardiovascular disease: an update to the scientific statement from the American Heart Association. *Circulation*. 2010;121:2331-2378.
64. Brook RD, Sun Z, Brook JR, et al. Extreme air pollution conditions adversely affect blood pressure and insulin resistance: the air pollution and cardiometabolic disease study. *Hypertension*. 2016;67:77-85.
65. Rich DQ, Kipen HM, Huang W, et al. Association between changes in air pollution levels during the Beijing Olympics and biomarkers of inflammation and thrombosis in healthy young adults. *JAMA*. 2012;307:2068-2078.
66. Liang R, Zhang B, Zhao X, Ruan Y, Lian H, Fan Z. Effect of exposure to PM2.5 on blood pressure: a systematic review and meta-analysis. *J Hypertens*. 2014;32:2130-2140.
67. Chen H, Burnett RT, Kwong JC, et al. Spatial association between ambient fine particulate matter and incident hypertension. *Circulation*. 2014;129:562-569.
68. Coogan PF, White LF, Jerrett M, et al. Air pollution and incidence of hypertension and diabetes mellitus in black women living in Los Angeles. *Circulation*. 2012;125:767-772.
69. Pope 3rd CA, Turner MC, Burnett RT, et al. Relationships between fine particulate air pollution, cardiometabolic disorders, and cardiovascular mortality. *Circ Res*. 2015;116:108-115.
70. Bard RL, Dvonch JT, Kaciroti N, et al. Is acute high-dose secondhand smoke exposure always harmful to microvascular function in healthy adults? *Prevent Cardiol*. 2010;13:175-179.
71. Brook RD, Bard RL, Burnett RT, et al. Differences in blood pressure and vascular responses associated with ambient fine particulate matter exposures measured at the personal versus community level. *Occup Environ Med*. 2011;68:224-230.
72. Makrisk TK, Thomapoulous C, Papadopoulous DP, et al. Association of passive smoking with masked hypertension in clinically normotensive nonsmokers. *Am J Hypertens*. 2009;22:853-859.
73. Yarlioglues M, Kaya MG, Ardic I, et al. Acute effects of passive smoking on blood pressure and heart rate in healthy females. *Blood Press Monit*. 2010;15:251-256.
74. Seki M, Inoue R, Ohkubo T, et al. Association of environmental tobacco smoke exposure with elevated home blood pressure in Japanese women: the Ohasma study. *J Hypertens*. 2010;28:1814-1820.
75. Heiss C, Amabile N, Lee AC, et al. Brief secondhand smoke exposure depresses endothelial progenitor cell activity and endothelial function. *J Am Coll Cardiol*. 2008;51:1760-1771.
76. Alshaarawy O, Xiao J, Shankar A. Association of serum cotinine levels and hypertension in never smokers. *Hypertension*. 2013;61:304-308.
77. Li N, Li Z, Chen S, Yang N, Ren A, Ye R. Effects of passive smoking on hypertension in rural Chinese nonsmoking women. *J Hypertens*. 2015;33:2210-2214.
78. Brook RD, Kousha T. Air pollution and emergency department visits for hypertension in Edmonton and Calgary, Canada: a case-crossover study. *Am J Hypertens*. 2015;28:1121-1126.
79. Morishita M, Thompson KC, Brook RD. Understanding air pollution and cardiovascular diseases: is it preventable? *Curr Cardiovasc Risk Rep*. 2015;9:30.
80. Jones MR, Barnoya J, Stranges S, Losonczy L, Navas-Acien A. Cardiovascular events following smoke-free legislations: an updated systematic review and meta-analysis. *Curr Environ Health Rep*. 2014;1:239-249.
81. Jh Young, Chang Y-PC, Kim JD-O, et al. Differential susceptibility to hypertension is due to selection during the out-of-Africa expansion. *PLOS Genetics*. 2005;1:e82.
82. Rostand SG. Ultraviolet light may contribute to geographic and racial pressure differences. *Hypertension*. 1997;30:150-156.
83. Rancière F, Lyons JG, Loh VH, et al. Bisphenol A and the risk of cardiometabolic disorders: a systematic review with meta-analysis of the epidemiological evidence. *Environ Health*. 2015;14:46.
84. Trasande L, Attina TM. Association of exposure to di-2-ethylhexylphthalate replacements with increased blood pressure in children and adolescents. *Hypertension*. 2015;66:301-308.
85. Lind L, Lind PM. Can persistent organic pollutants and plastic-associated chemicals cause cardiovascular disease? *J Intern Med*. 2012;271:537-553.
86. Wing S, Horton RA, Rose KM. Air pollution from industrial swine operations and blood pressure of neighboring residents. *Environ Health Perspect*. 2013;121:92-96.
87. Hallgren E, Migeotte PF, Kornilova L, et al. Dysfunctional vestibular system causes a blood pressure drop in astronauts returning from space. *Sci Rep*. 2015;5:17627.
88. Mandsager KT, Robertson D, Diedrich A. The function of the autonomic nervous system during spaceflight. *Clin Auton Res*. 2015;25:141-151.
89. Norsk P, Asmar A, Damgaard M, Christensen NJ. Fluid shifts, vasodilatation and ambulatory blood pressure reduction during long duration spaceflight. *J Physiol*. 2015;593:573-584.

Office Blood Pressure Measurement

Clarence E. Grim and Carlene M. Grim

Because patients whose blood pressure (BP) rises to unhealthy levels usually have no symptoms to suggest the presence of this condition the only way to detect the "silent killer" is to measure the BP accurately. Thus, the major reason for measuring BP in the office is to detect the evolution of an unhealthy BP so treatment to lower the BP to healthy levels can be incorporated into the patient's treatment plan. As with any screening test, it is key to minimize false positive and false negative results. This can only be accomplished by strict adherence to guidelines. Unfortunately, these guidelines are almost never adhered to in current medical practice. The goal of this chapter is to assure that BP is measured accurately during every visit as well as during the screening process. It is hoped that standards for "screening" will be followed every time BP is measured to guide therapy in the clinic. The United States Preventive Task Force has studied this critical health care issue and the recommended screening guidelines are in Table 9.1.[1]

Table 9.1 summarizes their recommendations. Note they do not recommend that BP be done every visit (will save time and money), but only at specified intervals depending on the patients' age. Our preference is that BP must be done with a specific protocol at what could be called "Screening or Diagnostic BP" measurements. When this BP is done it should be exactly per the American Heart Association (AHA) protocol by auscultation; rest 5 minutes, 3 readings and average used. At other visits BP should not even be measured unless there are good reasons to do so. They do not incorporate the SPRINT (Systolic Blood Pressure Intervention Trial)[2] data which would suggest that if systolic in greater than 120 mm Hg in high risk subjects should be screened each year and our interpretation of SPRINT is that this should be done with the Omron 907 only.

They recommend screening BPs be done every 3 to 5 years in some and yearly in the rest (Table 9.1).

WHY SHOULD I READ THIS CHAPTER IN GREAT DETAIL?

"The most important skill you will learn in your medical career is to measure blood pressure. Do it correctly and you will help more patients to better health than with any other skill you learn. Do it wrong and you will harm more patients than with any other medical errors you make over your career." CE Grim MD 1991: UCLA Preventive Medicine Curriculum, Blood Pressure Measurement Training and Certification Program, First year.

The goal of this chapter is to update your BP skills so you always obtain or are given the most accurate blood pressure. In our 40 years' experience in assessing and updating practicing physician's (and their staff's) skills in BP measurement, it is very likely that you did not receive the detailed training and guided practice needed to master this skill nor has your ability to measure BP accurately been assessed since your initial training. The delegation of this measurement skill to others is acceptable and perhaps preferred but you must have mastered the knowledge and skills to assure that those doing BP for you are doing it correctly. The continual assessment and updating of your and their skills is critical to the delivery of the highest quality cardiovascular care.

We recommend that you do this quick self-assessment because it will provide a guide to areas of knowledge and practice that you need to update. All of these issues will then be covered in detail.

1. The 2015 SPRINT study[2] tested the hypothesis that lowering systolic BP to less than 120 mm Hg was better than to a goal of 120 to less than 140 mm Hg. The study was stopped early because the lower group had markedly lower rates of death, stroke and congestive heart failure. What was unique about the BP measurement protocol used to diagnose and treat these patients? (BP was measured by the Omron 907 device after resting for 5 minutes with no one else in the room. Three measurements were taken and averaged).

2. You measure the BP with your patient seated on the edge of the examining table. How much and in which direction will this change the BP reading compared with measuring the BP with the patient properly seated in a chair?

3. On the average, what percent of patients who have BP measured by an AAMI (Association for the Advancement of Medical Instrumentation)-approved automatic BP device will the BP recorded be off by more than 5 mm Hg?[3] That is in your patients with a true diastolic pressure of 90 mm Hg, in how many will the automated reading the device records off by more than 5 mm Hg? 5%, 12%, 25% 50%?

4. The recommended gold standard for office blood pressure measurement by the latest AHA is: (1) The auscultatory method using a mercury manometer? (2) Any electronic device that has been validated as accurate by the AAMI?[3]

5. Why should BP be measured in both arms at the first visit?

TABLE 9.1 Recommend Blood Pressure Screenings

EVERY 3-5 YEARS	EVERY YEAR
Age 18-39. If office BP has always been <130/85 mm Hg and no other risk factors.	Age ≥ 40 or BMI > 30 (obese) African Americans BPs 130-39/85-89 mm Hg

(Data from Newsroom. U.S. Preventive Services Task Force. June 2016. http://www.uspreventiveservicestaskforce.org/Page/Name/newsroom.)
BMI, Body mass index; BP, blood pressure.

6. Which head of your stethoscope has been shown to be most accurate in detecting the BP sounds?
7. How accurately do you want your staff to measure your patient's BP? Within 2, 4, 6, 8 or 10 mm Hg?
8. How accurate do you want the device used by your staff to measure BP? Within 2, 4, 6, 8 or 10 mm Hg?
9. Once an office BP above 140/90 mm Hg is recorded in a previously normotensive patient what is the next step recommended to confirm the diagnosis before starting treatment? More office readings, home self BP readings, 24-hour ambulatory BP readings.
10. If your staff positions the center of the BP cuff on your patient's arm correctly at heart level but this is two inches lower than used by your referring doctor's office staff, will the BP measured in your office (all other things being equal) be higher or lower? By about how much?
11. How does your staff validate that the automatic BP device used in your office or by your patient is "accurate enough" for your guidelines on each patient?

The role of a physician measured BP has diminished with the introduction of automated devices and time crunches on physician time. Yet most practitioners do not realize that the auscultatory method is still the gold standard because no automatic device has been shown to be as accurate and reliable. Nor do they understand that all automatic devices must be validated as accurate in each patient using the gold standard auscultatory method. This can only be done by auscultation. Either you or someone on your team must be designated as the gold standard to assure that your patients receive the best of cardiovascular care. This chapter will enable you to update your knowledge and skills in BP measurement as well as to assure that your staff is up to date.

Blood pressure (BP) ranks third (after age and tobacco use) as predictors of mortality and percent of life spent suffering from the cardiovascular complication of an unhealthy BP (duration of suffering from cardiovascular disease [CVD]).[4,5] The reason to measure a patient's blood pressure is to identify if it is unhealthy (which we call hypertension or HTN) as proven by studies showing lowering that level of BP decreases the risk of the CVD because of HTN and increases length of life and decreases disability because of HTN complications. An accurate measurement of BP is essential to assure your patients are not denied the proven benefits of detecting and treating HTN. Unfortunately, BP measurement is almost never performed according to recognized guidelines, published by the AHA periodically since 1938.[6] The World Hypertension League[7] recently issued guidelines for manufacturers to develop an accurate and reliable BP-measuring device for use in low resource settings, because high BP is now the leading cause of death and disability in every country in the world. We argue that such a device currently exists: a trained health care worker using an accurate manometer and a stethoscope. These recommendations stress that every clinic must have a trained BP observer who can validate accuracy of all automatic devices as well as anyone who does auscultatory measurements.

A BRIEF HISTORY OF MORE THAN A CENTURY OF BLOOD PRESSURE MEASUREMENT

In the early 1900s, with the advent of standardized methods for measuring BP, it became apparent that elevated BP was an important predictor of premature death and disability in patients who reported feeling ill. In 1904, Theodore C. Janeway, the first full time professor of Medicine at Hopkins, published the first clinical text[8] on how to measure BP by simply palpating the radial artery using an inflatable cuff and a mercury manometer. The point at which the pulse disappeared on inflation and reappeared on deflation was the "palpated systolic pressure." He then reported eight years later on his observations of morbidity and mortality of 7872 symptomatic patients that he and his father had followed. The 870 hypertensive "well-to-do" patients all had a BP greater than 160 and were followed for nine years.[9] From this analysis, he suggested the term "hypertensive cardiovascular disease." He noted that 53% of men and 32% of women with symptomatic hypertension died in this 9-year period, and 50% of those who died had done so in the first 5 years after being seen. Cardiac insufficiency and stroke accounted for 50%, and uremia for 30%, of the deaths. Thus even a systolic BP determined only by palpation was a remarkable way to predict further cardiovascular death. By 1914, the life insurance industry had learned that even in asymptomatic men, the measurement of BP was the best way (after age) to predict premature death and disability. The goal of the life insurance industry is to insure people who are going to live the longest and not insure those who are at risk in dying prematurely. BP quickly emerged as the best way to do this. Soon all insurance examiners were required to measure BP before a person could obtain a life insurance policy. In 1913, the Chief Medical Officer of the Northwest Mutual Life Insurance Company stated, "No practitioner of medicine should be without a sphygmomanometer. This is a most valuable aid in diagnosis."[10] In 1918, the Medical Director of the Metropolitan Life Insurance Company ordered 1000 Baumanometers from the WA Baum Company for their medical examiners to use for screening applicants to assure that they were only insuring those at the lowest risks at standard rates.[11]

Population-based studies to investigate the role of the factors that predict those who will develop CVD began in 1948 with the Framingham Heart Study. A single BP was measured at the first visit by auscultation with a mercury manometer by a trained physician. Within 6 years it was clear that this single BP was the key predictor of future CVD and the risk increased continuously from the lowest to the highest levels of systolic BP. All of the predictive information was contained in the systolic BP. Furthermore, when BPs were averaged over more visits (examinations were every two years) the better the systolic BP predicted outcomes. At least 91% of those who developed heart failure (HF) had high BP before they developed overt HF.[12] A recent report from Minnesota suggests that the 10-year trajectory of BP may be an even better predictor of years of life lost from CVD.[13] The impact of BP is even more devastating in African Americans in Evans County, Georgia, where 40% of all deaths in African American women were attributed to high BP.[14] Before the advent of effective BP medications, only severe sodium restriction had been demonstrated as an effective way to reduce BP to normal levels and rapidly reverse advanced CHF.[15] However the discovery of drugs in the 1950s that lowered BP, led to the implementation of large-scale trials in the 1960s to determine the level of BP at which the risks of lowering it outweighed the risks of not lowering it. These early trials attempting to modify the natural history of hypertension (see Chapter 18) required design and implementation of mechanisms to ensure that all personnel at the many study centers would measure BP with the highest accuracy and reliability over 5 years. Methods of

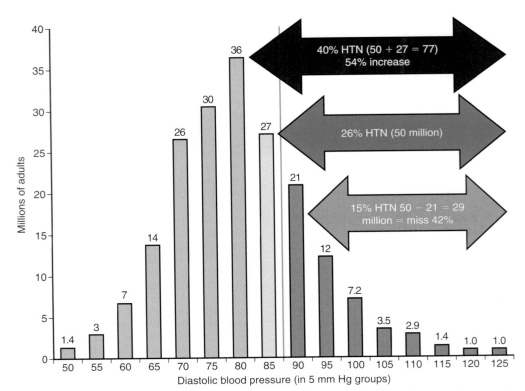

FIG. 9.1 The effect of small errors on blood pressure (BP) measurement in the percentage of the population with and without high BP. See text for further discussion. *(Data from Daugherty SA. Hypertension detection and follow-up program. Description of the enumerated and screened population. Hypertension. 1983;5[6 Pt 2]:IV1-43.)*

training developed for these and other trials, as well as for the population-based National Health And Nutrition Examination Surveys (NHANES), evolved into a standardized training, certification, and quality assurance program.[16] The lessons learned from these training programs have yet to be transferred to the basic training of those who take BP in the practice of medicine today. A video and CD–based training and certification program has been based on their experiences.[17] Implementation of these training and certification programs for personnel working in NHANES has improved the quality of BP measurements in this important program.[18] The States of Michigan[19] and Arkansas[20] have adapted the program to an online venue, to improve the quality of BP measurement in clinical practice (see www.michigan.gov/hbpu for more details; the program is also available online at http://shared care.trainingcampus.net). In Arkansas public health nurses' knowledge and ability to read auscultatory BP was markedly improved by this 1-hour online program. One nurse noted that she had been measuring BP incorrectly for over 30 years!

In most large-scale hypertension trials, the difference in BP between the treated and untreated groups over 5 years has been less than 10/5 mm Hg. Thus errors of this magnitude, if falsely low, will deny the proven benefits of treatment to millions of people who truly have high BP but who will be incorrectly told that their BPs are not high enough to warrant treatment. See Fig. 9.1 and later discussion.

Automated indirect BP by the oscillometric method (see Chapter 10) was first described in 1979 by Ramsey[21] in which the pulse wave oscillations transmitted from the artery under the cuff were converted into estimates of systolic and diastolic BP. Unfortunately the algorithm used by automated devices differs by manufacture and different devices often do not get the same reading on the same person[22] and are often inaccurate in practice.[23] To assure that such devices were "accurate enough" for clinical use the AAMI established that devices that pass their validation be unlikely to read off by more than 10 mm Hg too high or too low. The gold standard

used by AAMI and recommended by the AHA continues to be auscultatory technique.

THE IMPORTANCE OF CAREFUL BLOOD PRESSURE MEASUREMENT FOR THE HEALTH CARE SYSTEM

Fig. 9.1 illustrates the effect of a "small" (5 mm Hg) systematic BP measurement error on the prevalence of hypertension in the largest nationwide screening program for hypertension ever performed,[24] which is still reflective of the U.S. health care system. The horizontal axis is diastolic blood pressure (DBP) in 5 mm Hg intervals. The vertical axis is the percentage of the U.S. population (in 1983) who had a DBP in each 5 mm Hg interval. The vertical yellow line at 90 mm Hg divides the population into those with a DBP 90 mm Hg or higher, who are diagnosed as hypertensive. In this sample, 25% of adults (~50 million persons) had a DBP of 90 mm Hg or higher. If the BP was measured "only" 5 mm Hg too high, then those with a DBP of 85 to 90 mm Hg would have been told they had hypertension. This would have increased the number of Americans diagnosed with HTN by 54% (~27 million) who should have their BP lowered. In other words, the American hypertensive population would have been (erroneously) increased by 54%. This would add a tremendous burden (in time, cost, and effort) to the health care system. If the error was such that DBP was measured systematically "only" 5 mm Hg too low, then those with a DBP from 90 to 95 mm Hg would have been labeled as being not hypertensive, and 42% of all truly hypertensive people would be denied the proven benefits of BP lowering. Because a trained human using a mercury manometer is still the gold standard for BP measurement, and the overwhelming majority of our clinical trial database has been based on this method, true disciples of evidence-based medicine should insist on using this technique to measure BP, rather than accept other methods of BP measurement. The recent SPRINT trial[2] may have changed this as only an automated device was used to enroll and adjust medications during the trial.

ENVIRONMENTAL CONCERNS ABOUT ELEMENTAL MERCURY IN THE MEDICAL WORKPLACE

Since the early 1990s, regulatory authorities (including the U.S. Occupational Health and Safety Administration) have urged reduction/removal of mercury and other known toxic substances from all workplaces.[25-28] In some jurisdictions (e.g., Sweden, Minnesota) and health care systems (e.g., U.S. Department of Veterans Affairs Medical Centers), mercury sphygmomanometers have been prohibited and are being replaced. The contribution of mercury manometers to the global mercury burden must be extremely small, and much smaller than the contribution of the widely recommended mercury-containing, low-energy light bulbs. Nevertheless, the state of Washington forbids the purchase of a new mercury manometer unless it is replacing one already in service. On the other hand, Michigan permits every physician's office to have one mercury device for calibration. This presents both challenges and opportunities.

The obvious benefit of removal of the known toxin, elemental mercury, is that health care workers will no longer be exposed to even low levels of mercury vapor. Chronic inhalation of mercury vapor has been linked to decreased mental acuity, renal impairment, peripheral neuropathy, and death.[29] Problems have not been reported with mercury exposure from BP devices, except among individuals who repaired them many years ago in unventilated facilities. The clear concern is that the mercury sphygmomanometer will be difficult to replace.[30] This traditional, very accurate, highly reproducible, and simple method of measuring BP has been the standard technique for measurement of office BP for more than 100 years. In fact, the design of the mercury sphygmomanometer is essentially unchanged today from what was used 100 years ago, except that today's instruments are less likely to discharge liquid mercury, particularly if dropped. Because of the constant density of mercury at all altitudes and inhabitable environments, and its universal function as "the standard" in all pressure measurements in every branch of science, there is little difference in accuracy across brands, which is certainly not the case with other types of sphygmomanometers. Despite the simplicity of the mercury sphygmomanometer, it must be properly maintained and cleaned occasionally. A survey of mercury sphygmomanometers in Brazilian hospitals found 21% of the devices with technical problems that could reduce their accuracy,[31] a similar study in England found more than 50% of mercury columns that were defective.[32] However the majority of the problems with these devices were related to the bladders, cuffs, and valves, and not the mercury manometers themselves. Thus even when mercury devices are replaced, the office/health system must implement quality control measures for all parts of BP devices that most commonly malfunction.

Unfortunately, there is currently no generally accepted replacement for mercury manometers, and the most recent set of guidelines from both Europe and the AHA continue to recommend the use of mercury, if available.[6,33] Although the most recent report of the Joint National Committee on Prevention, Detection, Evaluation and Treatment of High Blood Pressure (JNC 7) has not fully endorsed the use of alternatives to the mercury sphygmomanometer,[34] newer BP measurement devices (that do not contain mercury) are being adopted in many centers. Unfortunately, very few "professional" BP measurement devices have been thoroughly tested[35] or proved as reliable, accurate, and long-lived as the mercury column. Few automated sphygmomanometers have been validated as accurate in children using Korotkoff phase IV or phase 4 (muffling), as required by the newest AAMI standards. Most of the inexpensive devices currently on the market are meant for home use, where they may be activated perhaps once daily. These are probably neither accurate nor durable enough to be recommended for a busy health care facility, at which BP is measured hundreds of times a day. Nevertheless, such home devices are widely used in offices, especially in geriatric facilities. Because there is no gold standard home electronic device, seven different home BP devices have been tested on a single subject over several weeks, to determine if the average home BPs measured by the devices were similar.[22] Unfortunately, the average 2-week home BP estimated by these devices varied by 31 mm Hg for systolic bool pressure (SBP) and 19 mm Hg for diastolic blood pressure (DBP). Thus the practitioner must validate, in each patient, every automatic device used to make medical judgments. One electronic device that looks like a large aneroid manometer has been validated.[36] The long-term accuracy, durability, drift, and hysteresis problems have not been reported in this or any other electronic BP monitor. Inexpensive aneroid sphygmomanometers are susceptible to damage (particularly after being dropped to the floor), resulting in inaccurate measurements that are not easily recognized.[37] These devices are most commonly used by home health care professionals, such as visiting nurses. Rubber guards and regular calibration have been recommended for these devices. Even validated oscillometric devices will make large errors (>10 mm Hg) in many individual patients. The term Unreliable Oscillometric Blood Pressure Measurement (UOBPM) was coined by Sterigou in 2006[38] when they made the observation that one of the most widely used devices, the BPTru, made errors in which the average of three readings made by the device (compared with the gold standard simultaneous auscultated BP) exceeded 10 mm Hg in at least 40% of subjects. In a detailed analysis of the AAMI validation protocol[39] it was pointed out that up to 50% of readings can be expected to be off by at least 5 mm Hg. It is thus necessary to assess the accuracy of any automatic device on every patient to be certain it is accurate enough to be used to diagnose and treat BP in them. The new revisions of both the European Society of Hypertension (ESH) and the AAMI protocols will increase the number of home devices that will not be able to pass standards. An analysis of the new ESH protocol standard increased the failure rate of published devices on the market from 17% to 42%.[40] The major reason for failure was the requirement that, when tested on 33 subjects, only three could have all three readings by the device that differ by more than 5 mm Hg from sequential human readings that bracket each device reading. The new and more stringent AAMI validation protocol tests the probability (at the 15% level) that a device will have an error greater than 10 mm Hg.[3] The statistical testing protocol is based on the historical definition of a "clinically significant" error in BP measurement of more than 10 mm Hg when AAMI first set their standards. This should now probably be lowered to a minimum of a 5 mm Hg tolerable error, to minimize the likelihood that automatic devices will not overestimate or underestimate BP by more than 5 mm Hg in most patients. Current recommendations from both the AHA and European Expert Committees recommend that whenever a sphygmomanometer that does not contain mercury is to be used, it should be checked regularly against a standard mercury column to ensure accuracy. Even electronic calibrators must be regularly calibrated against mercury to assess and correct for electronic drift over time. There is currently no recommended standard to use in the clinic to calibrate a manometer other than a mercury device.

HOW CAN THE MEASUREMENT OF BLOOD PRESSURE BE IMPROVED IN CLINICAL PRACTICE?

The most recent AHA guidelines include these important conclusions[6]:

In view of the consequences of inaccurate measurement, including both the over-treatment and under-treatment, it is the opinion of this committee that regulatory agencies should establish standards to ensure the use of validated devices, routine calibration of equipment, and the training and retraining of manual observers. Because the use of automated devices does not eliminate all major sources of human error, the training of observers should be required even when automated devices are used.

Although BP measurement is taught in all schools for health care professionals, from office assistant to medical school, correct measurement techniques, according to the AHA's Guidelines,[6] are almost never taught and therefore never practiced. This may be the result of failure to initially master the knowledge, skills, and techniques needed to obtain an accurate BP measurement, and the lack of periodic retraining and reevaluation thereafter, which the AHA recommends on a semi-annual basis.[6] Neither beginning medical students who claim to have learned proper BP measurement technique,[41] nor practicing nurses in Australia[42] or Taiwan,[43] nor physicians in India,[44] nor general practitioners in Newfoundland,[45] nor practicing public health nurses in Arkansas[20] had sufficient knowledge to pass a standardized test regarding correct technique in BP measurement. Instruction in BP measurement should be provided in a standardized fashion, in compliance with current AHA guidelines.

The importance of retraining and retesting was illustrated in the British Regional Heart Study, in which simultaneous BP readings were taken by trained nurses and a triple-headed stethoscope during training.[46] Immediately after the initial training, the interindividual variability in the field (Fig. 9.2) was very small, but it increased progressively during the next 6 months. After the preplanned retraining session at 6 months (see Fig. 9.2), interindividual variability decreased again, nearly to baseline levels. However, because the nurses considered the training tedious and unnecessary, the second retraining session, scheduled for 12 months, was not held. At 14 months into the study, however, the SBPs recorded by observer 1 and 2 differed by an average of 21 mm Hg. After retraining at 18 months, the interindividual variability returned to 0 mm Hg. The authors suggested that retraining and retesting should be done every few months for research studies, but this might not be feasible in routine medical practice. We disagree because their data was used only for epidemiologic research whereas the office and home BP is used to diagnose and guide treatment in the most common chronic disease in the office. This led to the

development, testing, and publication of a video-tutored program that teaches the AHA guidelines and tests mastery of the knowledge, skills, and techniques required to obtain accurate and reliable BP readings.[17] The program requires 6 to 8 hours of contact time, but few curricula in medical, nursing, or health aide professions devote sufficient time to practice and then test a student's mastery of this critical skill. Once trained, few if any curricula retest this skill before graduation, and few health care systems require any retesting or update in knowledge once entering the health care delivery system. Periodic equipment maintenance and observer quality assurance programs should both be part of the curriculum.

BLOOD PRESSURE MEASUREMENT: PROPER TECHNIQUE FOR QUALITY ASSURANCE AND IMPROVEMENT

This section summarizes our published curriculum that reviews, reinforces, and tests the knowledge, skills, and technique needed to obtain an accurate BP.[17] It is based on the AHA recommendations for BP measurement and many years of experience teaching these skills and certifying practitioners around the world in practice or for research studies funded by the National Institutes of Health, the pharmaceutical industry, and public and private health care delivery systems.

Many assume that using an automatic BP measurement device eliminates human error. However, except for those principles and skills needed to perform the auscultatory BP measurement, all of the steps required to get an accurate BP by auscultation must also be followed when an automated device is used. Indeed, unless the guidelines are followed, using an automatic device will give unreliable data as well.

CRITICAL SKILLS FOR ANY BLOOD PRESSURE OBSERVER

Any person who measures BP or interprets the readings made by others must possess the skills, knowledge, and mastery of techniques summarized in Fig. 9.3. Proper measurement of BP involves coordination of hands, eyes, ears, and mind, and deficits in any one of these areas can lead to imprecise and erroneous measurements. In testing of "experienced" observers, some persons were identified who could not hear well enough to recognize Korotkoff sounds. Other individuals could not remember the SBP without writing it down during cuff deflation. Staff in every practice setting can be screened initially

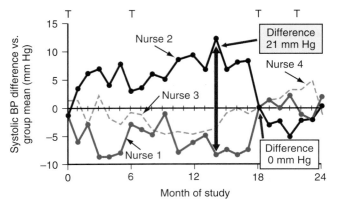

FIG. 9.2 Training decreases between-observer measurement differences in blood pressure. In this 24-month British Regional Heart Study, three nurses measured blood pressure during a population survey, and their interindividual variation is plotted on the y-axis over time. After training sessions (designated by "T" along the top), the interindividual variations decreased markedly. When the training session scheduled at 12 months was omitted, the variation hit a peak, but dropped back to very little after the next training session at 14 months. *(Modified from Bruce NG, Shaper AG, Walker M, Wannamethee G. Observer bias in blood pressure studies. J Hypertens. 1988;6:375-380.)*

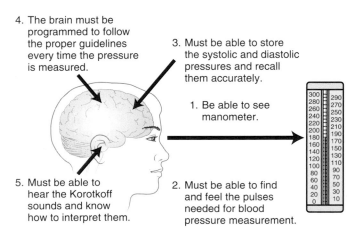

4. The brain must be programmed to follow the proper guidelines every time the pressure is measured.

3. Must be able to store the systolic and diastolic pressures and recall them accurately.

1. Be able to see manometer.

5. Must be able to hear the Korotkoff sounds and know how to interpret them.

2. Must be able to find and feel the pulses needed for blood pressure measurement.

6. Must be able to recall and write down correctly and legibly the sounds heard.

FIG. 9.3 The skills needed to obtain an accurate blood pressure. The observer must master a high-level integration of eye, hand, ear, and brain coordination.

and annually for these problems by testing with standard videotapes and multiearpiece stethoscope BP measurements (described later) and direct observation of the individual's technique. An online update is also available.[20]

MANOMETERS AND THEIR CALIBRATION

A mercury manometer, two aneroid gauges (one intact and one with the face removed), and an electronic BP measuring device are shown in Figs. 9.4 and 9.5. The mercury manometer is the primary (reference) standard for all pressure measurements in science, industry, and medicine. The pressure is read at the top of the liquid mercury meniscus to the nearest 2 mm Hg. Practitioners who measure BP with nonmercury devices should have at least one reference mercury device available to check other devices regularly, or have an electronic calibration device that can be traceable directly to the mercury standard. The tube containing the mercury should be large enough to allow rapid increases and decreases in pressure. The 2-mm graduated markings should be on the tube itself. The standard glass tube, which can break, should be replaced with either a Mylar-wrapped glass tube or a plastic tube. The inside view of the aneroid

device (see Fig. 9.4) shows a delicate system of gears and bellows that can easily be damaged by rough handling. Such devices also develop metal fatigue with time, which leads to inaccuracy. In a recent survey in German hospitals, 60% of aneroid devices were out of calibration and the error was almost always reading too low.[37] To detect an inaccurate aneroid device, inspect the face for cracks and be sure the needle is at zero. If it is cracked or does not read zero, it will nearly always be inaccurate and should be recalibrated before reuse. Once an aneroid device is out of calibration, it is difficult to detect the direction of the variance without calibrating it against a mercury or other reference standard. This process is uncommon in both the United States and Europe. It has been alleged that, "clinicians using equipment which has not been maintained and calibrated may be medically negligent,"[47] but this has not been legally tested.

Calibrating the Manometer

If a mercury device is at zero and the column is clean and rises and falls rapidly with inflation-deflation, the manometer is, by definition, accurate. Other manometers for calibration should be connected in parallel by Y tubes (e.g., see Fig. 9.5). Mercury or aneroid devices should be checked for leaks by wrapping the BP cuff around a cylinder (e.g., a tin can) and inflating the cuff to 200 mm Hg. If the pressure after 1 minute is lower than 170 mm Hg, there is a leak that must be found. If pinching the tubing just before the inflation bulb stops the leak, the leak is in the valve, which can be taken apart and cleaned or replaced. If the leak continues when the tubing is pinched just before the manometer, the leak is in the manometer. If this is the case: (1) note whether the mercury column rises and falls smoothly; (2) locate and correct any leaks by replacing the appropriate part (although a leak of <2 mm/sec can be tolerated because this is the correct deflation rate); and (3) date the device to indicate when it was last inspected/repaired. Now reinflate to 200 mm Hg. Deflate the pressure in the system slowly, and check the aneroid manometer against the mercury column at the critical decision points for BP: 180, 160, 140, 130, 120, 110, 100, 90, 80, and 70 mm Hg. The standard for reading both mercury and aneroid manometers is as follows: (1) if the Korotkoff sound occurs when the column of Hg or the tip of the aneroid needle is at or above the middle of the 2-mm mark, one should round up the reading to the nearest 2 mm Hg; (2) if the reading is below the mid 2-mm mark, the reading is rounded down to the nearest 2 mm; (3) with the Y-tube connecting the aneroid and mercury manometers, if the average of readings from the nonmercury device differs from that of the mercury column by more than 4 mm Hg, the nonmercury device should be recalibrated by trained personnel or discarded.

To calibrate an electronic device, connect the electronic instrument and the mercury column using the Y-tube. If the device has a calibration setting, check the pressures registered on the electronic manometer, as described earlier. If there is no calibration setting, the inflation mechanism of the electronic device must be activated, and the pressure on the digital display compared with the mercury column. Because many automated devices (especially those used in the home) do not have an easy way to calibrate them, it is necessary to rhythmically squeeze the rolled-up cuff to simulate a pulsating arm, to avoid an error signal and automatic deflation of the electronic monitor.

Three steps can be recommended to validate any automatic device for an individual patient:

1. Test the pressure measuring system itself. All electronic pressure systems have unavoidable drift and fatigue. This is tested as described earlier.
2. Test the rough accuracy of the automatic device by performing a palpated SBP as the device inflates and deflates

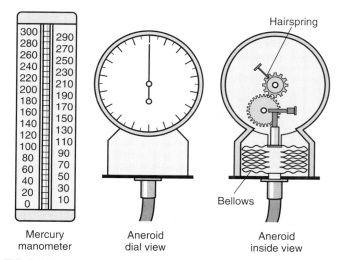

FIG. 9.4 Three manometers commonly used in blood pressure measurement. The mercury column (on the left) has been the traditional gold standard for pressure measurement in science, industry, and medicine; the aneroid manometer (with dial in the center) and with dial removed (at the right) are shown.

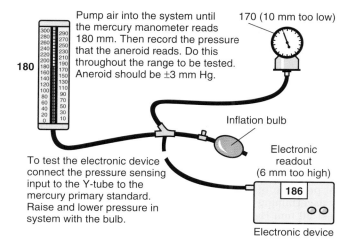

FIG. 9.5 Diagrammatic set-up for calibrating manometers against the mercury column. The Y-tube connects the devices being calibrated with the reference mercury manometer for simultaneous static comparisons of pressure readings in the devices being calibrated. It is recommended that this be done every six months.

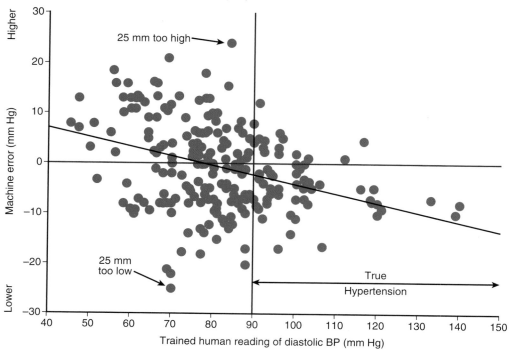

Range of BP Differences Between an Automated Device and Readings by a Trained Human Observer

FIG. 9.6 Bland-Altman plot generated from testing the 85 subjects required for an Advancement of Medical Instrumentation validation protocol. Blood pressure was taken in alternating sequence by two observers using a double stethoscope (four readings) and the device (three readings). The x-axis is the diastolic pressure taken by auscultation, and the y-axis is the difference between the device's reading and the auscultatory human readings. The horizontal line of zero difference (on the y-axis) between the human and device readings is shown. The vertical black line at diastolic blood pressure 90 mm Hg or higher indicates the threshold defining hypertension. There are many subjects for whom this device would have produced both false-positive and false-negative diagnoses of hypertension.

on the patient's arm. Record the palpated SBP; it should be within 15 mm Hg of the device's recorded SBP in most patients.

3. If possible, test the accuracy of the SBPs and DBPs recorded by the machine, by doing an auscultatory BP at the same time the device takes the BP, using the display on the device to estimate the SBP and DBP. These should be within 5 mm Hg for both SBP and DBP. Automatic devices that deflate faster than 3 mm Hg per second are more difficult to validate using the auscultatory method; they may need to be sent back to the manufacturer for calibration.

Fig. 9.6 illustrates the errors seen with one device that passed both AAMI and ESH validation protocols. The horizontal axis shows the average reading taken by two observers with a mercury manometer. The vertical axis plots the machine error for each human reading. On the vertical axis the zero-error line is drawn to the left. A machine reading greater that the human reading will fall above this line, and a machine reading lower than the human reading will fall below the "0" error line. The machine errors have a wide scatter between patients: in one person the machine reads 25 mm Hg too high, and in another subject, it reads 25 mm Hg too low. The AAMI protocol averages these, and the device is graded as having "zero error." The black vertical line at 90 mm Hg DBP (on the x-axis) defines "true hypertension" (DBP ≥90 mm Hg by trained human measurements). This device would produce a large number of both false-positive and false-negative diagnoses of hypertension if used in clinical practice.

Is This Electronic Device Accurate When Used for an Individual Patient?

Now that the electronic manometer has been properly calibrated, the question arises whether this device records an accurate BP in a specific patient. Unfortunately, there is no

standard method for this. The best guide therefore seems to be to follow the new AAMI or ESH guidelines used in validating automatic devices.[3,48] The following is useful if the device deflates at a rate of 2 to 3 mm Hg/second (presuming the reference device provides digital readout during deflation):

(1) Connect the electronic and mercury manometers in parallel with a Y-tube. (2) Cover the digital readout with a piece of paper (to avoid bias). (3) Trigger the automatic device and measure BP in the traditional fashion, watching the mercury manometer and detecting Korotkoff sounds with the stethoscope (see later for more details). (4) Immediately write down the BP reading, then uncover the digital readout and record the electronic device's reading. If another observer is simultaneously measuring BP, both observers should use a double-headed stethoscope. (5) Take at least three readings, and compare the observed average with that of the electronic device (see Table 9.2 for an example). (6) To test a device using the AAMI protocol, two validated human readers using a double stethoscope are blinded to others' readings, and 85 subjects must be tested. A total of seven readings are taken, alternating between the human and device reading in each subject. To meet the current criteria for electronic monitors from the AAMI, the average difference in 85 subjects with three readings each (255 readings) must be less than 5 mm Hg (both SBP and DBP), and the standard deviation of the difference between methods must be 8 mm Hg or less.[3]

It is important to check that the device inflates to an initial pressure of 30 mm Hg or more above SBP; this is done by ascertaining that the device's initial (peak) pressure is at least 30 mm Hg above that which causes the palpated brachial or radial arterial pulse to disappear. Many devices have a switch that patients use to limit the discomfort associated with very high initial pressures; this leads to inaccurate readings if they often have high SBP readings. If the device has no digital readout, deflates faster than 2 mm Hg per second,

TABLE 9.2 Data From a Test of an Automatic Device in an Individual Patient

Reading	SYSTOLIC BLOOD PRESSURE (mm Hg)			DIASTOLIC BLOOD PRESSURE (mm Hg)		
	Human	Device	Error[a]	Human	Device	Error[a]
1	140	144	4	80	88	**8**
2	136	140	4	76	84	**8**
3	132	138	6	74	78	**4**
Average[b]	136.0	140.7	4.7	77	83	**6.7**
SD[c]	4.0	3.1	1.2	3.1	5.0	**2.3**
p for	t test[d]	0.02			0.04	

Enter systolic and diastolic by human and device.
[a]The error is calculated for both systolic and diastolic blood pressure (BP) by subtracting the human reading from the device reading.
[b]The average of each is calculated.
[c]These are typical spreadsheet functions.
[d]The two-tailed paired t-test is calculated.
SD, Standard deviation of each is calculated.
In this example the systolic and diastolic readings by the device are significantly higher for both systolic and diastolic readings. The physician must make a decision if this is a tolerable error for this patient. If the error is too large, another device should be recommended and tested in this patient.

TABLE 9.3 Recommended Cuff Sizes Based on Arm Circumference and Bladder Dimensions From American Heart Association Guidelines

Cuff Name	MOST RECENT GUIDELINES[8]					PREVIOUS GUIDELINES[7]				
	AC Range	W	L	40% W	80% L	AC Range[a]	W	L	40% W	80% L
Newborn	8-10	4	8	10	10	<6	3	6	7.5	7.5
Infant	12-15	6	12	15	15	6-15[b]	5	15	12.5	18.8
Older child	18-22.5	9	18	22.5	22.5	16-21[b]	8	21	20.0	26.3
Small adult	22-27.5	12	22	30	27.5	22-26	10	24	25.0	30.0
Adult	30-37.5	16	30	40	37.5	27-34	13	30	32.5	37.5
Large adult	38-47.5	16	38	40	47.5	35-44	16	38	40.0	47.5
Adult thigh	42-52.5	16	42	40	52.5	45-52	20	42	50.0	52.5

Adapted from each set of guidelines. All measurements are given in cm.
[a]There is some overlap of the recommended range for arm circumferences to limit the number of cuffs; it is recommended that the larger cuff be used when available.
[b]To approximate the bladder width: arm circumference ratio of 0.40 more closely in infants and children, additional cuffs are available.
AC, Arm circumferences; L, length; W, width.

takes readings during inflation, or measures BP at the wrist, alternate sequential readings must be taken. The AAMI guidelines recommend seven readings (four human alternating with three device readings).[3] An error greater than 5 mm Hg or a standard deviation greater than 8 mm Hg is generally considered unacceptable.

In 2002, an expert panel from the ESH proposed a simpler set of validation criteria that requires only four simultaneous readings, and recommended use of the device if both SBP and DBP readings are within 5 mm Hg of the standard in at least two of the four readings.[49] The British Hypertension Society recommends only devices listed on their website that have been validated using the ESH testing protocol. Every 90 days, the dabl Educational Trust (www.dableducational.com/) updates their website that lists available BP monitors by type and validation status. As noted above, many of the devices on the current site would not be acceptable according to the recently updated guidelines. Devices marketed in the U.S. should have also passed the AAMI validation protocol.

STETHOSCOPES

The bell, or low-frequency head, of the stethoscope is designed to more accurately transmit low-frequency (e.g., Korotkoff or K) sounds and can be placed more precisely over the brachial artery pulse than the diaphragm. The origin of the K sounds has recently been reviewed.[50] Electronic stethoscopes are generally not recommended, because it is difficult to adjust the amplification so that the person using it

hears what a standard observer hears with the bell. The tubing connecting the bell to the earpieces should be thick and 12 to 15 inches (30.5 to 38.0 cm) in length. For sound transmission, earpieces should be worn tilted in the direction of the ear canal (i.e., toward the nose). There are a number of types of ear tips available and each observer should determine which type works best for sound transmission into that person's ears. One way to determine this is "the touch test": lightly touch the patient's skin next to the bell placed over the brachial artery. If no sound is heard, ensure that the stethoscope head is rotated to select the bell, ensure that there is an air-tight seal by the bell over the skin, the stethoscope earpieces face forward, and finally, that the earpieces fit well within the ear canals.

SELECTION AND APPLICATION OF THE PROPER BLOOD PRESSURE CUFF

Choosing an incorrectly sized BP cuff has been the most common error in BP measurement for more than 30 years.[51] In a 1983 study of British hypertensives, 83% of the mistakes of this type were choosing a cuff too small for larger arms.[52] These problems can be avoided if the patient's arm circumference at the mid-biceps (measured at the initial visit, and then yearly) can be matched to the appropriately sized cuff (Table 9.3). Unfortunately, there are no standards for BP cuff sizes, and different manufacturers make different sized bladders, sold by the same name. Furthermore, the cuff range marked on many cuffs often does not agree with the AHA recommendations based on the bladder's length and width. The newest

AHA guidelines have radically changed the cuff size recommendations[6] but large inconsistencies exist across manufacturers regarding bladder size (which seldom corresponds exactly to either the new or older guidelines or cuff name.

All guidelines agree that the width of the cuff bladder should be at least 40% of the arm circumference[53] and the length of the bladder must encircle at least 80% of the arm. Because of increasing obesity in the population, a cuff with a width that is at least 40% of the arm circumference would exceed the distance between the axilla and antecubital fossa in many people.[54] Some manufacturers provide markings on the BP cuff that denote the smallest and largest arms for which the cuff has the appropriate size; making such marks on cuffs can be useful (Fig. 9.7). There are two dimensions of the bladder that require proper placement to get an accurate BP reading. The center of the bladder LENGTH must go over the brachial artery, typically just above and medial to the antecubital fossa, just under the medial bicipital groove. The center of the WIDTH of the bladder should be halfway up the length of the upper arm, and this center of the bladder width point must be placed at heart level (fourth intercostal space). See Fig. 9.8.

PREPARING FOR AN ACCURATE READING

In the United States, seated BP measurements are traditional; in most of Europe, supine measurements are routine. DBP is usually higher (by about 5 mm Hg) when seated than when supine, but the differences in SBP are smaller.[55,56] The purpose of preparation (Fig. 9.8) is to inquire about, note, and control factors that can cause BP variability, including pain, recent tobacco use, distended bowel or bladder, food or caffeine ingestion, over-the-counter medications (including cold preparations and nonsteroidal antiinflammatory drugs), or strenuous exercise during the last 30 minutes. The setting should be quiet and relaxed, because talking raises SBP about 10 mm Hg, and listening about half as much. Feet should be relaxed and flat on the floor (if seated), because crossing the legs raises SBP about 5 mm Hg.[57] The arm wearing the BP cuff should be supported, usually at the elbow, by an armrest or nearby table (if seated; see Fig. 9.8), by an adjustable-height table, or by the observer (if standing). Measuring BP with the patient seated on the examination table without back support increases the SBP about 5 mm Hg.[58] The manometer should be placed so the scale is visible at the observer's eye level. The observer is more comfortable when seated, supporting both arms, and focusing efforts on fine movements of the fingers, while coordinating vision, hearing, and bulb deflation.

Where Should the Center of the Cuff Width on the Arm Be Positioned to Get the Most Accurate Pressure?

If the patient is wearing a long-sleeved or tight garment around the arm, provide a gown or remove the arm from the sleeve, and suggest wearing a loose, short-sleeved top at future visits, because gowning involves muscular work of the arms and increases BP. The center of the bladder width on the patient's arm should be at "heart level" (fourth intercostal space). Each inch above this level decreases BP by 2 mm Hg or more, and vice versa[59,60]; the effect is larger in hypertensives (23/10 mm Hg, seated) than in normotensives (8/7 mm Hg). Arm position is especially important when standing, because BP increased by 13/8 mm Hg if the arm was allowed to dangle at the side, rather than having the center of the cuff properly positioned at heart level by placing the forearm on an adjustable Mayo stand. When supine BP is measured, a small pillow is often needed to support the elbow and upper arm in barrel-chested or obese patients.[61] The center of the cuff on the arm would otherwise be 5 to 8 cm below the right atrium, falsely increasing BP.

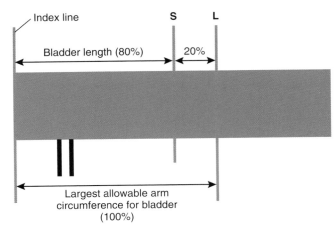

FIG. 9.7 Schematic diagram for marking the blood pressure cuff to designate the lower limit of arm circumference that should be used (same as the bladder length, marked "S"), and the upper limit of arm circumference that should be used (20% longer than the bladder length, marked "L").

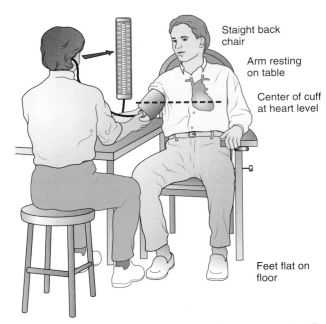

FIG. 9.8 Standardized positioning of the observer, the manometer, the cuff, and the patient for a seated blood pressure measurement. Important features of the positioning include the subject being comfortably seated with his back against the chair, feet flat on the floor, arm bent at the elbow, but supported by the table, with the cuff positioned at the level of the heart (fourth intercostal space) and centered at the midpoint of the humerus. The observer is comfortably seated, with the manometer at eye level, silent, and not touching the cuff with the bell of the stethoscope (the last detail is difficult to appreciate, given the resolution of this figure).

MEASURING THE BLOOD PRESSURE

After a brief explanation of the need for silence, apply the appropriately sized BP cuff; adjust posture, arm, and foot support; and then leave the patient alone (and silent) for 5 minutes. Then take multiple readings (typically three) in short sequence, typically 60 seconds between readings. If the variation between the three readings is greater than 12/8 mm Hg the sequence should be repeated.

Which Arm Should Be Used?

At the first visit, BP should be recorded in both arms. This is the only way to avoid missing a significant difference between the two arms (up to 100 mm Hg), which changes the differential diagnosis. After the first visit, the arm with the higher BP is traditionally used. The most common cause of a between-arm difference in older people is a hemodynamically significant atherosclerotic stenosis of the left subclavian artery. Such a stenosis is 10 times more likely on the left than the right side. Although most coarctations of the aorta result in lower BPs in the lower extremities, those that result in BP differences between the arms also result in lower BP in the left arm. In the screening situation in which BP is to be measured in only one arm, unless the subject knows that one arm is higher, the right arm is traditionally chosen. This recommendation was recently validated in 854 normotensive and 2395 hypertensive subjects, because the right arm BP was significantly higher (by 3/5 mm Hg) than the left in all six sequential BP measurements.[62]

How High Should the Cuff Be Inflated to Avoid Missing an Auscultatory Gap?

An auscultatory gap is the name given to a situation when Korotkoff sounds temporary disappear between phases 1 and 4, only to reappear at a lower BP. Depending on where one begins or ceases to listen during this gap can cause overreading of the DBP or underreading of the SBP. It is more common in older people with wide pulse pressures and target organ damage.[63] To avoid missing this gap, inflate the BP cuff to the maximum inflation level (MIL; 30 mm Hg higher than the palpated SBP, determined by obliteration during inflation and then reappearance during deflation of the palpable radial pulse).

Where Do I Listen to Hear the Best Blood Pressure Sounds?

Korotkoff sounds are louder when the bell is placed directly over the brachial artery, which can be palpated just medial to and usually under the biceps tendon in the antecubital fossa. Extending the forearm with the palm up will make it easier to detect Korotkoff sounds. The edges of the bell must contact the skin to form a seal or external room sounds will be heard and Korotkoff sounds will be softer leading to falsely low systolic and high diastolic pressures. Using too much pressure on the head of the stethoscope can compress the artery beneath and lead to bruitlike sounds even when there is no pressure in the cuff. This will lead to falsely low diastolic readings. In the rare situation in which neither brachial pulse is palpable, the cuff may be placed on the forearm and the radial artery auscultated at the wrist, although this overestimates SBP.[64]

What Are the Steps for Properly Taking and Recording the Pressure?

To take the reading, (1) inflate the cuff quickly to the MIL; (2) immediately begin to deflate at 2 mm Hg per second; (3) determine the SBP at the point where the first of at least two regular or repetitive Korotkoff phase 1 sounds are heard; (4) repeat this number silently at each auscultated sound until Korotkoff phase 5 (i.e., the last regular sound) is detected; this is the DBP, so write down the reading immediately; (5) if Korotkoff sounds are heard to zero, repeat the reading and note the phase 4 Korotkoff (at phase 4 the tapping [Korotkoff] sounds become lower in pitch and muffling occurs; muffling is the point at which the sounds become soft and blowing) and record all three sounds (e.g., 142/66/0 mm Hg); (6) record the arm, position, cuff size used, and the SBP and DBP. Repeat the process two more times. Many experts recommend discarding the first reading and averaging the last two, because this has been the protocol followed for many epidemiologic and intervention studies. The National Committee on Quality Assurance currently accepts the lowest SBP and DBP measurement in any position (and not from the same reading) as

the "BP for that visit," which is why most managed care organizations require every reading to be charted.[65]

How Can the Korotkoff Sounds Be Made Louder?

One or both of two methods can be chosen. The first uses exercise to increase postischemic blood flow. To perform this maneuver, inflate the cuff to the MIL and ask the patient to vigorously open and close the fist 10 times. Then the hand is relaxed and BP measured in the standard fashion. The second technique drains venous blood from the arm by holding the arm straight up over the head for 30 to 60 seconds, and then the cuff is inflated to 30 mm Hg above the MIL, the arm is lowered, and Korotkoff sounds are recorded. Dysrhythmias make BP measurement difficult and less precise, as is widely recognized for many automated devices. The average of several BP readings obtained at one sitting are recommended for routine clinical care, because of the beat-to-beat variability of cardiac output in atrial fibrillation and other cardiac dysrhythmias. In extreme cases, it may be necessary to do an intraarterial BP measurement, particularly if the patient has a positive "Osler maneuver."

STANDARDIZED MONITORING FOR ACCURACY, REPRODUCIBILITY, AND OBSERVER BIAS

The assessment of observer accuracy of BP measurement can be done with a standardized video test and/or a stethoscope with two or more sets of earpieces. Both methods can be recommended, because Korotkoff sounds in real people are frequently more difficult to interpret than carefully selected recorded sounds. Fig. 9.9 shows the test form used to evaluate observer accuracy under two circumstances. In one, observers record 12 BPs, based on video clips (a falling mercury column, an aneroid manometer with falling needle, or the Greenlight with lights replacing the needle) and an audio track with corresponding Korotkoff sounds. The correct answers are then provided and the differences calculated. This same form can be used with a double stethoscope, in which the instructor/supervisor listens to live Korotkoff sounds simultaneously with the observer to be tested; the results are graded in the same fashion. The form can also be used to assess terminal digit preference over 12 random BPs taken by an observer in different patients. Ideally, the terminal digits (0, 2, 4, 6, or 8) should be evenly distributed among the 24 (SBP/DBP) entries.

All staff who measure BP should, on at least an annual basis, be (1) observed while taking seated/standing BPs, and have their technique critiqued and corrected, if needed; (2) tested with a double stethoscope for the ability to hear, interpret, and record BPs accurately; and (3) assessed with a standardized video test for accuracy, reliability, terminal digit bias, and direction bias. Those who make these errors should be counseled and retested every month until there is no bias. Individuals who cannot be certified as accurate and reliable after several training sessions should be directed to other duties and not be permitted to measure BPs.

INSPECT EQUIPMENT FOR QUALITY ASSURANCE

In every health care setting, at least one staff member should undergo training and assume responsibility for performing regular calibration and quality control regarding BP, so that all patients' BPs are measured accurately and reliably. This process involves several steps:
1. Test the mercury manometer. At least once a year, the responsible staff member should inspect each BP-measuring device, document the results, and initiate maintenance if needed.

BP Measurement

GRADING BP ACCURACY AND RELIABILITY

Name _____ Date _____

View the videotape and record your answers in the spaces below.

Example number		Your answer		T	Correct answer	Difference (record sign [±] of diff.)
Example	Sys	1	2	8	126	+2
1	Dias		5	8	62	−4
Example	Sys	2	2	0	220	0
2	Dias	1	1	0	118	−8
Video	Sys					
1	Dias					
Video	Sys					
2	Dias					
Video	Sys					
3	Dias					
Video	Sys					
4	Dias					
Video	Sys					
5	Dias					
Video	Sys					
6	Dias					
Video	Sys					
7	Dias					
Video	Sys					
8	Dias					
Video	Sys					
9	Dias					
Video	Sys					
10	Dias					
Video	Sys					
11	Dias					
Video	Sys					
12	Dias					

BP Measurement — Quality Assessment

GRADING BP ACCURACY AND RELIABILITY ACCURACY:

Subtract the correct answer from your answer and place this difference (with sign) in the "Difference" column. Count and record the differences you have from the correct answers in the table below.

Accuracy table

Range	0	±2	±4	±6	≥±8
Count					

To be graded as accurate you should have at least 22 answers that are ±2 and only 2 can be ±4 mm Hg.

ARE YOU ACCURATE?   YES   NO

If you have answers that are ±8 or greater it is likely that you misread the manometer by about 10 mm Hg.

RELIABILITY:

Each of the examples you saw in the standardized video-test was repeated in the sequence. You should be ±2 mm Hg in all of the repeat pairs. Complete the table below to assess your reliability.

Pair	1 and 11	2 and 8	3 and 10	4 and 7	5 and 9	6 and 12
±2?						

ARE YOU RELIABLE?   YES   NO

If you are not reliable it is likely you need to read the manometer more carefully or you have a memory problem.

DIRECTION BIAS:

If you read above or below the correct answer, you have direction bias. Record the number of times your answers are above the correct answer (number of +'s) and the number of times you were below the correct answer (number of −'s) in the table below.

+'s =	Least freq. sign =	1	2	3	4	5	6	7
−'s =	Sum of +'s, −'s =	8–10	11–12	13–15	16–17	18–20	21–22	23–24

You should have about 50% +'s and −'s. Enter the sum of +'s and −'s here = _____ . If this is ≤7, you do not have direction bias. If ≥8, match your sum of +'s and −'s with the cell in the bottom row of the table above. If your least frequent sign is ≤ the value of the cell above it (in the top row) you have direction bias ($P < 0.05$). If you tend to read the systolic too low and the diastolic too high you may have a hearing problem.

TERMINAL DIGIT BIAS:

The last digit of a BP reading should end in an even number if you follow AHA guidelines. Count the number of times your answers ended in 0 and enter it into the "n" row in the table below under the 0's column. Repeat for 2's, 4's, 6's, and 8's. Any answer ending in an odd number is wrong.

End digit =	0's	2's	4's	6's	8's	odd#?
n =						
n^2 =						

Now square each "n" and enter it in the n^2 = row. Now add the n^2 in this row and enter here Σn^2 = _____ . If $\Sigma n^2 \geq 161$ you have terminal digit bias ($P<0.05$). You need to be more careful.

DO YOU HAVE TERMINAL DIGIT BIAS?   YES   NO

BETWEEN OBSERVER BIAS can be assessed by comparing your answers with others who watched the same video.

FIG. 9.9 Form for testing accuracy, reproducibility, direction bias, and terminal digit bias of 12 blood pressure measurements shown on the authors' standardized videos. *(From Grim CM, Grim CE. A curriculum for the training and certification of blood pressure measurement for health care providers. Can J Cardiol. 1995,11 [Suppl. H]:38H-42H.)*

2. Test all aneroid/electronic manometers. Each should be calibrated against a mercury manometer, using a Y-tube (see Fig. 9.5). At least twice a year, the responsible staff member should inspect each BP-measuring device, document the results, and initiate maintenance if needed.
3. Test all stethoscopes and cuffs. Each stethoscope and BP cuff should be checked periodically for wear, damage, and leaks.

ASSESS KNOWLEDGE ABOUT BLOOD PRESSURE MEASUREMENT

All staff involved in BP measurement should be retrained and retested on hiring, and every 6 months thereafter so that BP measurement can be standardized. A series of questions is often useful in quickly determining which staff members should undergo more frequent retraining about BP measurement. Each question is followed by its indicated answer.

1. Which part of the stethoscope is better for hearing low-pitched Korotkoff sounds? The bell.
2. How does one demonstrate that a person's hearing is good enough to accurately identify Korotkoff sounds? Double stethoscope and video BP testing.
3. How can the accuracy of a BP-measurement device in daily use be demonstrated? Calibrate it against a mercury column.
4. What is the effect of having patients sit on the examination table when their BP is measured? Increases both SBPs and DBPs.
5. Some patients can have an arm difference in BP of 20 mm Hg. Which arm should be used for BP measurements? The one with the higher reading.
6. How is the correct size of BP cuff selected for patients? Measure the mid-arm circumference and match it to the appropriately sized cuff for that patient at that visit.
7. When placing the BP cuff on an arm, where does one place the center of the length of the bladder? On the medial aspect of the arm, centered over the palpated brachial artery.
8. When the patient is seated in a straight-backed chair or stands for a BP measurement, how should the arm be placed, to avoid erroneous measurements resulting from hydrostatic pressure? The center of the cuff should be at heart level (fourth intercostal space) and the flexed forearm supported with the palm facing up.
9. Where should the bell of the stethoscope be placed to get the best Korotkoff sounds? Over the palpated brachial artery, usually over the medial aspect of the antecubital fossa.
10. How high should the pressure be inflated, before starting to listen for Korotkoff sounds? 30 mm Hg above the palpated SBP.
11. How fast (in mm Hg per second) should the manometer be deflated? 2 to 3 mm Hg per second.
12. Which Korotkoff sound defines the SBP reading? Phase 1 or K1
13. Which Korotkoff sound defines the DBP reading? Phase 5 or K5
14. A 75-year-old patient with chronic kidney disease has left ventricular hypertrophy (LVH) by electrocardiogram (ECG), chest radiograph, and echocardiogram. A radial and brachial pulse can be palpated, and no Korotkoff sounds can be heard. Inflating the BP cuff to 300 mm Hg reduces the pulsation at the wrist, but the radial artery can still be palpated. What is the problem? Calcified brachial artery (Mönckeburg sclerosis).
15. An 84-year-old man with angina and claudication has a blood pressure of 122/74 mm Hg in the right arm, and 86/50 mm Hg in the left, but has striking LVH on ECG and echocardiogram and Grade II hypertensive retinopathy. At cardiac catheterization, the aortic BP is 240/140 mm Hg. What is the most likely diagnosis? Bilateral stenosis between the aorta and brachial arteries.
16. What are the likely problems with each of the recorded BP readings in Table 9.4? Answers are provided in the right column of Table 9.4.
17. What is the recommended frequency for demonstration of knowledge, skills, and technique for quality improvement of BP accuracy? AHA recommends every 6 months.

ASSESS PERFORMANCE REGARDING BLOOD PRESSURE MEASUREMENTS

Electronic medical records provide data for analysis to assess and improve quality. The simplest clue is "terminal digit preference." A simple chi-square test can assess whether one

TABLE 9.4 Diagnosing Blood Pressure Measurement Errors: What Is the Problem With These Readings Taken by Auscultation?

READING(S) RECORDED (mm Hg)	PROBLEMS WITH THIS READING
122/74	Only one reading. AHA, JNC 7, and NCQA guidelines recommend recording 2-3 individual BP readings at each visit.
170/75, 165/75, 160/65	These BP readings end in an odd number (5). AHA guidelines recommend that BP should be rounded to the nearest 2 mm Hg.
140/80, 150/90, 140/80	Terminal digit bias for 0. Likely deflating too fast, or rounding to the nearest 10 mm Hg instead of the nearest 2 mm Hg.
146/84, 146/84, 146/84	Failure to take a second and third BP, and instead just rerecording the first reading for the last two.
188/166, 180/164, 182/162	Failure to recognize an auscultatory gap, leading to a falsely high diastolic pressure.

AHA, American Heart Association; *BP,* blood pressure; *JNC 7,* Joint National Committee on Prevention, Detection, Evaluation and Treatment of High Blood Pressure; *NCQA,* National Committee for Quality Assurance.

terminal digit (typically "0" or "8") is recorded significantly more commonly than the 20% expected by chance. If serial readings are taken at the same visit by different staff members, interobserver variation can be assessed (as in the British Regional Heart Study)[47] and the person who should benefit from retraining can be identified.

Incorrect or uncertain answers to any of criterion based questions above, or troublesome performance measures, should motivate health care professionals to update the rationale and techniques required to obtain an accurate BP measurement.

SUMMARY

With continuous quality control of measurements your patients will continue to benefit from one of the most important of all Cardiology skills: the use of the stethoscope to detect the Korotkoff sounds to measure BP.

References

1. Siu AL, Bibbins-Domingo K, Grossman D, et al. Screening for high blood pressure in adults: US preventive services task force recommendation statement. *Ann Intern Med.* 2015;163(10):778-786.
2. Wright JT Jr, Williamson JD, Whelton PK. A Randomized Trial of Intensive versus Standard Blood-Pressure Control. *N Engl J Med.* 2015;373:2103-2116.
3. Association for the Advancement of Medical Instrumentation. Non-invasive sphygmomanometers. Part 2. Clinical validation of automated measurement. *ANSI/AAMI/ISO.* 2009:81060-81062.
4. Prospective Studies Collaborative. Age-specific relevance of usual blood pressure to vascular mortality. A meta-analysis of individual data for one million adults in 61 prospective studies. *Lancet.* 2002;360:1903-1913.
5. Franco OH, Peeters A, Bonneux L, et al. Blood pressure in adulthood and life expectancy with cardiovascular disease in men and women: life course analysis. *Hypertension.* 2005;46:280-286.
6. Pickering TG, John E, Hall JE, et al. Recommendations for blood pressure measurement in humans and experimental animals. Part 1. Blood pressure measurement in humans: a statement for professionals from the Subcommittee of Professional and Public Education of the American Heart Association Council on High Blood Pressure Research. *Hypertension.* 2005;45:142-161.
7. Campbell NR, Berbari AE, Cloutier L, et al. Policy statement of the world hypertension league on noninvasive blood pressure measurement devices and blood pressure measurement in the clinical or community setting. *J Clin Hypertens.* 2014;16:320-322.
8. Janeway TC. *The clinical study of blood-pressure a guide to the use of the sphygmomanometer in medical, surgical, and obstetrical practice, with a summary of the experimental and clinical facts relating to the blood-pressure in health and in disease.* New York and London D; Appleton and Company: 1904.
9. Janeway TC. A clinical study of hypertensive cardiovascular disease. *Arch Intern Med.* 1913;12:752-786.
10. Fisher JW. The diagnostic value of the sphygmomanometer in examinations for life insurance. *JAMA.* 1914;63:1752-1754.
11. Personal communication from the WA Baum Company.
12. Levy D, Larson MG, Vasan RS, et al. The progression from hypertension to congestive heart failure. *JAMA.* 1996;275:1557-1562.
13. Tielemans SMAJ, Geleijnse JM, Menotti A. Ten year blood pressure trajectories, cardiovascular mortality, and life years lost in 2 extinction cohorts: the Minnesota Business and Professional Men Study and the Zutphen Study. *J Am Heart Assoc.* 2015;4:e001378.

14. Deubner DC, Tyroler HA, Cassel JC, et al. Attributable risk, population risk and population attributable risk fraction of death associated with hypertension in a biracial community. *Circulation.* 1975;52:901-908.
15. Kempner W. Some effects of the rice diet treatment of kidney disease and hypertension. *Bull N Y Acad Med.* 1946;22:358-370.
16. Curb JD, Labarthe DR, Cooper SP, et al. Training and certification of blood pressure observers. *Hypertension.* 1983;5:610-614.
17. Grim CM, Grim CE. A curriculum for the training and certification of blood pressure measurement for health care providers. *Can J Cardiol.* 1995;11(Suppl. H):38H-42H.
18. Ostchega Y, Prineas RJ, Paulose-Ram R, et al. National Health and Nutrition Examination Survey 1999-2000: effect of observer training and protocol standardization on reducing blood pressure measurement error. *J Clin Epidemiol.* 2003;56:768-774.
19. www.michigan.gov/hbpu. For more details; the program itself is available online at http://sharedcare.trainingcampus.net.
20. Grim CE, Grim CM, Zahoori N, Faulkner L. An online update of knowledge and skills required to get an accurate blood pressure for public health personnel who measure blood pressure. *Abstracts. J Am Soc Hypertens.* 2014;8(4S):e46. Course available at http://sharedcare.trainingcampus.net.
21. Ramsey M III. Non-invasive automatic determination of mean arterial pressure. *Med Biol Eng Comput.* 1979;17:11-18.
22. Grim CE. Some home blood pressure devices get remarkably different blood pressures on the same person [abstract]. *J Clinical Hypertens (Greenwich).* 2008;10(Suppl):A70-A71.
23. Akpolat TI, Aydogdu T, Erdem E, Karatas A. Inaccuracy of home sphygmomanometers: a perspective from clinical practice. *Blood Press Monit.* 2011;16:168-171.
24. Daugherty SA. Hypertension detection and follow-up program. Description of the enumerated and screened population. *Hypertension.* 1983;5(6 Pt 2):IV1-43.
25. O'Brien E. Has conventional sphygmomanometry ended with the banning of mercury? *Blood Press Monit.* 2002;7:37-40.
26. Aylett M. Pressure for change: unresolved issues in blood pressure measurement. *Br J Gen Pract.* 1999;49:136-139.
27. O'Brien E. Replacing the mercury sphygmomanometer requires clinicians to demand better automated devices. *BMJ.* 2000;320:815-816.
28. Padfield PL. The demise of the mercury sphygmomanometer. *Scot Med J.* 1998;43:87-88.
29. Clarkson TW, Magos L, Myers GJ. The toxicology of mercury: current exposures and clinical manifestations. *N Engl J Med.* 2003;349:1731-1737.
30. Jones DW, Frohlich ED, Grim CM, et al. Mercury sphygmomanometers should not be abandoned: an advisory statement from the Council on High Blood Pressure Research, American Heart Association. Professional Education Committee, Council for High Blood Pressure Research. *Hypertension.* 2001;37:185-186.
31. Mion D, Pierin AM. How accurate are sphygmomanometers? *J Hum Hypertens.* 1998;12:245-248.
32. Markandu ND, Whitcher F, Arnold A, Carney C. The mercury sphygmomanometer should be abandoned before it is proscribed. *J Hum Hypertens.* 2000;14:31-36.
33. O'Brien E, Asmar R, Beilin L, et al. Practice guidelines of the European Society of Hypertension for clinic, ambulatory and self blood pressure measurement. *J Hypertens.* 2005;23:697-701.
34. Chobanian AV, Bakris GL, Black HR, et al. Seventh Report of the Joint National Committee on Prevention, Detection, Evaluation and Treatment of High Blood Pressure. National High Blood Pressure Education Program Coordinating Committee. *Hypertension.* 2003;42:1206-1252.
35. White WB, Anwar YA. Evaluation of the overall efficacy of the Omron office digital blood pressure HEM-907 monitor in adults. *Blood Press Monit.* 2001;6:107-110.
36. Graves JW, Tibor M, Murtagh B, et al. The Accuson Greenlight 300, the first non-automated mercury-free blood pressure measurement device to pass the International Protocol for Blood Pressure Measuring Devices in Adults. *Blood Press Monit.* 2004;9:13-17.
37. Cozanitis DA, Jones CJ. The extent of inaccurate aneroid sphygmomanometers in a hospital setting. *Wien Med Wochenschr.* 2010;160:356-361.
38. Stergiou GS, Lourida P, Tzamouranis D, Baibas NM. Unreliable oscillometric blood pressure measurement: prevalence, repeatability and characteristics of the phenomenon. *J Hum Hypertens.* 2009;23:794-800.
39. Gerin W, Schwartz AR, Schwartz JE, et al. Limitations of current validation protocols for home blood pressure monitors for individual patients. *Blood Press Monit.* 2002;7:313-318.
40. Stergiou GS, Karpettas N, Atkins N, O'Brien E. Impact of applying the more stringent validation criteria of the revised European Society of Hypertension International Protocol 2010 on earlier validation studies. *Blood Press Monit.* 2011;16:67-73.
41. Grim CE, Grim CM, Li J. Entering medical students who say they have been trained to take blood pressure do not follow American Heart Association guidelines [abstract]. *Am J Hypertens.* 1999;12:122A.
42. Armstrong RS. Nurses' knowledge of error in blood pressure measurement technique. *Internat J Nursing Pract.* 2003;8:118-126.
43. Chen HL, Liu PF, Liu PW, Tsai PS. Awareness of hypertension guidelines in Taiwanese nurses: a questionnaire survey. *J Cardiovasc Nurs.* 2011;26:129-136.
44. Mohan B, Aslam N, Ralhan U, et al. Office blood pressure measurement practices among community health providers (medical and paramedical) in northern district of India. *Indian Heart J.* 2014;66:401-407.
45. McKay DW, Campbell NR, Parab A, et al. Clinical assessment of blood pressure. *J Hum Hypertens.* 1990;4:639-645.
46. Bruce NG, Shaper AG, Walker M, Wannamethee G. Observer bias in blood pressure studies. *J Hypertens.* 1988;6:375-380.
47. Rouse A, Marshall T. The extent and implications of sphygmomanometer calibration error in primary care. *J Hum Hypertens.* 2001;15:587-591.
48. O'Brien E, Atkins N, Stergiou G, et al. European Society of Hypertension International Protocol: revision 2010 for the validation of blood pressure measuring devices in adults. Working Group on Blood Pressure Monitoring of the European Society of Hypertension. *Blood Press Monit.* 2010;15:23-38.
49. O'Brien E, Pickering T, Asmar R for the Working Group on Blood Pressure Monitoring of the European Society of Hypertension, et al. International protocol for validation of blood pressure measuring devices in adults. *Blood Press Monit.* 2002;7:3-17.
50. Babbs CF. The origin of Korotkoff sounds and the accuracy of auscultatory blood pressure measurements. *J Am Soc Hypertens.* 2015;9:935-950.
51. Maxwell MH, Waks AU, Schroth PC, et al. Error in blood-pressure measurement due to incorrect cuff size in obese patients. *Lancet.* 1982;ii:33-36.
52. Manning DM, Kuchirka C, Kaminski J. Miscuffing: inappropriate blood pressure cuff application. *Circulation.* 1983;68:763-766.
53. Marks LA, Groch A. Optimizing cuff width for noninvasive measurement of blood pressure. *Blood Press Monit.* 2005;5:153-158.
54. Graves JW, Darby CH, Bailey K, Sheps SG. The changing prevalence of arm circumference in NHANES III and NHANES 2000 and its impact on the utility of the "standard adult" blood pressure cuff. *Blood Press Monit.* 2003;8:223-227.
55. Netea RT, Lenders JW, Smits P, Thien T. Influence of body and arm position on blood pressure readings: an overview. *J Hypertens.* 2003;21:237-241.
56. Minor DS, Butler KR Jr, Artman KL, et al. Evaluation of blood pressure measurement and agreement in an academic health sciences center. *J Clin Hypertens.* 2012;14:222-227.
57. Peters GL, Binder SK, Campbell NR. The effect of crossing legs on blood pressure: a randomized single-blind cross-over study. *Blood Press Monit.* 1999;4:97-101.
58. Cushman WC, Cooper KM, Horne RA, Meydrech EF. Effect of back support and stethoscope head on seated blood pressure. *Am J Hypertens.* 1990;3:240-241.
59. Mitchell PL, Parlin RW, Blackburn H. Effect of vertical displacement of the arm on indirect blood pressure measurement. *N Engl J Med.* 1964;271:72-74.
60. Mourad A, Carney S, Gillies A, et al. Arm position and blood pressure: a risk factor for hypertension? *J Hum Hypertens.* 2003;17:389-395.
61. Ljungvall P, Thorvinger B, Thulin T. The influence of a heart level pillow on the result of blood pressure measurement *J Hum Hypertens.* 1989;6:471-474.
62. Arnett DK, Tang W, Province MA, et al. Interarm differences in seated systolic and diastolic blood pressure: the Hypertension Genetic Epidemiology Network study. *J Hypertens.* 2005;23:1141-1147.
63. Cavallini MC, Roman MJ, Blank SG, et al. Association of the auscultatory gap with vascular disease in hypertensive patients. *Ann Intern Med.* 1996;124:877-883.
64. Leblanc MÉ, Croteau S, Ferland A, et al. Blood pressure assessment in severe obesity: validation of a forearm approach. *Obesity.* 2013;12:E533-41.
65. National Committee for Quality Assurance (NCQA). Healthplan Employee Data Information Set (HEDIS®) 2007. Washington, DC: NCQA; 2007, www.ncqa.org. Accessed July 19, 2011.

10 Home Monitoring of Blood Pressure

George S. Stergiou and Anastasios Kollias

Despite the fact that conventional measurement of blood pressure (BP) in the office (OBP) has been the cornerstone for hypertension diagnosis and management for decades, it is recognized that this method might often be misleading, mainly because of the white-coat and masked hypertension phenomena, which are common among both untreated and treated subjects.[1-5] Furthermore, the small number of BP readings, the usually unstandardized setting and conditions, and the observer bias and error, further weaken the reliability of OBP in the diagnosis and management of hypertension.[1-5]

In the last decades, self-monitoring of BP by patients at home (HBPM) and 24-hour ambulatory BP monitoring (ABPM) have both gained ground compared with OBP for hypertension management, aiming to overcome the abovementioned drawbacks. These methods have major similarities, because they both provide multiple measurements taken in the individual's usual environment. However, they have also important differences, as HBPM is performed only at home and in the sitting posture, whereas ABPM is performed in ambulatory conditions, at work, at home and during sleep.[1-6] Therefore, it is still debated whether their role in the clinical management of hypertension is interchangeable or complementary.

The clinical value of ABPM is strongly supported by evidence from short-term and longitudinal trials, whereas HBPM has been less well investigated. However, evidence has recently accumulated from studies investigating the diagnostic value of HBPM and its association with target organ damage and cardiovascular risk, aiming to support the utility of this method as an indispensable tool for the initial evaluation of elevated BP, for treatment initiation and adjustment, as well as for long-term follow-up of treated hypertension.[1-5]

ADVANTAGES AND LIMITATIONS

Table 10.1 presents the main advantages and limitations of HBPM. HBPM is widely available and well accepted by patients for long-term use, it has superior reproducibility to OBP and similar to ABPM, identifies the white-coat and the masked hypertension phenomena allowing accurate diagnosis of hypertension, and improves long-term compliance with treatment and thereby hypertension control rates.[1-5,7,8] On the other hand, HBPM requires patient education and training, as well as the use of validated devices. In addition, patients often misreport their self-taken BP readings, which is the "Achilles' heel" of HBPM and might lead in overtreatment or undertreatment, especially in high risk hypertensives or those with high BP variability.[9] It should be mentioned that even if HBPM is performed under ideal circumstances, it only provides BP readings at home and in the sitting posture under fully standardized conditions and thus not representing the dynamic behavior of BP during usual daily activities.[1-5]

CLINICAL INDICATIONS

The main clinical indications for HBPM include the detection of white-coat and masked hypertension, identification of white-coat reaction and masked hypertension effect in treated hypertensives, overcoming considerable variability of OBP over the same or different visit(s), identification of true and false resistant hypertension.[2,3]

Several previous cross-sectional studies have investigated the diagnostic performance of HBPM by taking ABPM as reference. Most of these studies have looked at selected diagnostic phenotypes of hypertension (sustained, white-coat, masked, or resistant) and included populations with different characteristics (untreated subjects, treated hypertensives, patients with type 2 diabetes, chronic kidney disease). Overall, these data suggest considerable diagnostic agreement between the two methods ranging from about 70% to 90%, with consistently high specificity and negative predictive value (>80%) and lower sensitivity and positive predictive value (60% to 70%).[10] One of these studies examined the diagnostic accuracy of HBPM separately in 613 untreated and treated subjects and reported that the sensitivity for hypertension diagnosis varied between 48% and 100% in untreated subjects and 52% and 97% in treated subjects and specificity between 44% and 93% and 63% and 84% respectively.[11] Another study in resistant hypertension also showed that HBPM was a reliable alternative diagnostic method to ABPM.[12] These findings should be interpreted with caution because they are based on the assumption that ABPM, which was used as reference method, is perfectly reproducible and reliable, which certainly is not the case. Moreover, the diagnostic disagreement between the two methods is mostly present in subjects whose BP levels are very close to the diagnostic thresholds, and is probably attributed, to a great extent, to the imperfect reproducibility of all BP measurement methods.

As mentioned previously, the usefulness of HBPM is manifested through the identification of white-coat and masked hypertension phenomena, which remain undiagnosed and inadequately treated when considering exclusively OBP measurements.[2,3] White-coat hypertension is defined by normal HBPM (<135/85 mm Hg) but elevated OBP values (≥140/90 mm Hg), thus not truly reflecting the "true" BP of an individual. These individuals should not be considered as normotensives because they present an intermediate cardiovascular risk between normotensives and hypertensives and are more likely to develop sustained hypertension within the next years.[13-15] On the other hand, masked hypertensives have elevated HBPM (≥135/85 mm Hg) but normal OBP levels (<140/90 mm Hg), and present higher prevalence of preclinical target organ damage and increased cardiovascular risk, similar to that of the sustained hypertensives.[15-17] The masked hypertension phenomenon is also frequent in treated hypertensives (masked uncontrolled hypertension). In these patients OBP

TABLE 10.1 Advantages and Limitations of Home Blood Pressure Monitoring

ADVANTAGES	LIMITATIONS
• Large sample of BP readings • Absence of placebo effect • Absence of observer error and bias (automated devices with memory or PC link) • Good reproducibility • Detection of white-coat and masked hypertension phenomena • Association with preclinical organ damage • Prediction of cardiovascular events • Wide availability • Need of minimal training (with automated devices) • Good acceptance by users • Improvement of patients' compliance with drug therapy • Improvement of hypertension control rates • Cost-effectiveness	• Devices often not properly validated • Misreporting (over- or under-) of readings by patients • Need of user training (minimal with automated devices) and medical supervision • May induce anxiety in some patients • Some patients may self-modify their drug treatment on the basis of casual BP readings • Measurements do not reflect usual daily activities • Inability to monitor nocturnal BP (possible with some novel home monitors) • Questionable accuracy of oscillometric devices in the presence of arrhythmias

BP, Blood pressure, *PC*, personal computer.

measurements often reflect the peak effect of morning antihypertensive drug treatment on BP, whereas morning and evening HBPM readings can reveal trough or plateau effect respectively. When the diagnosis of these phenomena is confirmed by repeat OBP and HBPM or ABPM, treatment adjustment should be considered, particularly in subjects with high cardiovascular risk.[2]

PROGNOSTIC VALUE

Association With Target-Organ Damage

Preclinical organ damage is recognized as an intermediate stage in the continuum of the cardiovascular disease and its presence indicates increased cardiovascular risk while assessing asymptomatic hypertensive subjects.[2] Several cross-sectional studies have evaluated the association of HBPM with indices of preclinical target-organ damage including the heart, large arteries, and kidneys. Two recent metaanalyses included studies that evaluated the association of HBPM with preclinical target-organ damage.[18,19] The first one examined the association of HBPM versus OBP and ABPM with indices of organ damage. Most of the available data regarded echocardiographic left ventricular mass index and analysis of 10 studies revealed stronger correlation coefficients for HBPM versus OBP (systolic/diastolic, pooled r = 0.46/0.28 versus 0.23/0.19 respectively).[18] Data from nine studies indicated similar coefficients for HBPM and ABPM.[18] Less evidence was available for carotid intima-media thickness, pulse wave velocity and urine protein excretion, with a consistent trend towards stronger coefficients for HBPM than OBP, with the latter not reaching statistical significance.[18] The second metaanalysis included more data and demonstrated that HBPM is a stronger determinant of proteinuria than OBP.[19]

Prediction of Cardiovascular Events

The superiority of HBPM over OBP in determining target-organ damage confirms the hypothesis that HBPM better reflects the true BP status; yet this superiority refers to intermediate (surrogate) endpoints and, by itself, does not imply superiority in terms of cardiovascular risk stratification or prediction of

outcome (cardiovascular events or deaths). Indeed, the ultimate criterion to identify a useful method for the assessment of a cardiovascular risk factor in clinical practice is its actual ability to predict future cardiovascular events. Two metaanalyses have investigated the evidence sourced from outcome trials in the general population, in primary care and in hypertensive patients and assessed the prognostic ability of HBPM compared with OBP measurements.[20,21] Both were based on data from eight prospective studies and 17,688 patients followed for 3.2 to 10.9 years, which resulted in the availability of information based on almost 100,000 person/years of follow-up, and showed HPBM to be superior to OBP measurements, with this difference being beyond chance for systolic BP.[20,21] Moreover, in the metaanalysis by Ward et al, HBPM remained a significant predictor of cardiovascular mortality and cardiovascular events even after adjusting for OBP, suggesting its independent prognostic value over and beyond that of OBP.[21] However, one major limitation of the abovementioned metaanalyses was that these were based on aggregate data.

In 2012, the International Database of HOme blood pressure in relation to Cardiovascular Outcome (IDHOCO) was constructed using individual participants' data of published population studies (n = 6753, mean follow-up 9.2 years) that evaluated the prognostic value of HBPM.[22] One of the major findings of this analysis was that HBPM substantially refined risk stratification at OBP levels assumed to carry no or only mildly increased risk, in particular in the presence of masked hypertension.[23] More specifically, in participants with optimal or normal OBP, hazard ratios for a composite cardiovascular endpoint associated with a 10-mm Hg higher systolic home BP were 1.28 (95% CI 1.01 to 1.62) and 1.22 (1.00 to 1.49), respectively.[23] At high-normal OBP and in mild hypertension, the hazard ratios were at about 1.20 for all cardiovascular events and 1.30 for stroke.[23] A further analysis of the same dataset was performed separately in untreated and treated subjects.[15] Among untreated subjects, cardiovascular risk was higher in those with white-coat hypertension (adjusted hazard ratio 1.42), masked hypertension (1.55) and sustained hypertension (2.13) compared with normotensive subjects.[15] Among treated patients, the cardiovascular risk did not differ between those with high office and low home BP (white-coat) and treated controlled subjects (low office and home BP).[15] However, treated subjects with masked hypertension (low office and high home BP) and uncontrolled hypertension (high office and home BP) had higher cardiovascular risk than treated controlled patients.[15]

In conclusion, HBPM has independent prognostic value and allows more accurate risk stratification than OBP, particularly in cases with masked hypertension.

HOME BLOOD PRESSURE MONITORING AND MANAGEMENT OF HYPERTENSION

Treatment Adjustment

As mentioned earlier, the diagnostic accuracy of HBPM in identifying the hypertension phenotypes, as well as the prognostic significance of these phenotypes detected by HBPM in untreated and treated subjects, have rendered this method very important for treatment initiation and titration.

The association between treatment-induced changes in home, ambulatory, and office BP and treatment-induced changes in indices of preclinical organ damage has been investigated in two studies. In the Study on Ambulatory Monitoring of Blood Pressure and Lisinopril Evaluation (SAMPLE) in 206 hypertensives followed for 12 months, the treatment-induced regression in left ventricular hypertrophy was more closely associated with treatment-induced changes in ambulatory than in office or home BP.[24] However, only two HBPM readings were obtained in this study, in contrast to the recommended minimum 3-day schedule and therefore the potential of HBPM was not exhausted.[3] Another study in 116 hypertensives with 13.4 months follow-up, showed that treatment-induced changes in both 24-hour ABPM and 7-day HBPM were more closely related than OBP measurements with treatment-induced changes in organ damage (left ventricular mass index, pulse wave velocity, albuminuria).[25] Interestingly, there were differences between HBPM and ABPM in their associations with the changes in different indices of organ damage, which implies that these methods are complementary rather than interchangeable in monitoring the effects of antihypertensive treatment on target-organ damage.[25]

Nine randomized studies assessed treatment adjustment based on HBPM compared with OBP (seven studies)[26-32] or ABPM (two studies).[33,34] It should be noted that there are important differences among these studies regarding the inclusion criteria, population characteristics, BP measurement methodology, BP goals, and duration of follow-up. Three of the studies used the same threshold for OBP and HBPM,[27,28,30] which is not in line with current guidelines[2] and led to inferior BP control with HBPM. Four other studies showed larger BP decline with treatment adjustment based on HBPM rather than OBP measurements.[26,29,31,32] Two studies compared HBPM versus ABPM for treatment adjustment. The first in 98 subjects followed for 6 months found no difference in BP control when using HBPM or ABPM.[33] The second one randomized 116 subjects to treatment initiation and titration based either on HBPM alone or on combined use of OBP and ABPM.[34] After an average follow-up of 13.4 months there was no difference between the two arms in BP decline and hypertension control assessed by HBPM or ABPM and, more important, there was no difference in treatment induced changes in several indices of preclinical target-organ damage.[34]

Long-Term Follow-Up

HBPM has the unique advantage to enable patients to take multiple measurements not only through a period of days, but weeks, months and even years, and at minimal cost. Moreover, this method motivates the patients by increasing their awareness and rendering them active in their follow-up. The long-term use of HBPM by patients treated for hypertension is recommended by current guidelines, as it enhances their compliance to therapy, and prevents them from adhering to therapy only before an office visit, a phenomenon known as "white-coat adherence," which is associated with increased cardiovascular risk.[2,3] However, comparative data regarding the effects of long-term monitoring of treated hypertensives based on HBPM or ABPM are lacking.

Improvement of Patients' Adherence and Blood Pressure Control

Several randomized controlled trials have shown that treated hypertensives who perform HBPM have improved long-term adherence to drug therapy, and thereby higher hypertension control rates.[35,36] A systematic review of 72 randomized controlled trials that evaluated the effectiveness of several interventions aiming to improve BP control (HBPM, educational interventions, pharmacist- or nurse-led care, organizational interventions, appointment reminder systems) showed HBPM to be the most efficient method.[37] The MONITOR study in treated uncontrolled hypertensives showed that a two-month HBPM protocol without medication titration led to superior ABPM control than the usual care control group.[38] Another study in 1350 hypertensive patients attending a BP clinic showed that those using HBPM had higher BP control rates.[39]

Nocturnal Home Blood Pressure Monitoring

Accumulating evidence suggests that nighttime BP evaluated by ABPM carries superior prognostic value in terms of cardiovascular risk.[6,40] Novel HBPM monitors allow automated BP monitoring during nighttime sleep. A few studies have provided comparative data between nighttime HBPM and ABPM regarding their differences as well as their association with indices of preclinical target-organ damage.[41-44] Four studies, mainly including hypertensives, reported similar values for nighttime systolic/diastolic HBPM and ABPM.[41-44] Moreover, three studies reported correlation coefficients between systolic/diastolic BP derived from nighttime HBPM and ABPM ranging from 0.6 to 0.8.[42-44] The agreement between nighttime HBPM and ABPM in detecting nondippers was examined in two studies and was at 74% to 79%.[42,43] Two studies reported correlation coefficients of similar range for nighttime HBPM versus ABPM in terms of association with indices of target-organ damage (left ventricular mass index, common carotid intima-media thickness, urinary albumin excretion); however, in multivariate analyses, nighttime HBPM appeared to be a better determinant of urinary albumin excretion.[43,44]

In conclusion, preliminary data suggest that nighttime HBPM appears to provide similar values with nighttime ABPM and most importantly seems to be at least as reliable in determining preclinical target-organ damage. However, these data are cross-sectional and outcome studies are needed to confirm the value of nighttime HBPM in predicting cardiovascular morbidity and mortality.

HOME BLOOD PRESSURE MONITORING IN SPECIAL POPULATIONS

Children

As in the adults, in children and adolescents, OBP might lead to incorrect diagnosis because of the white-coat and masked hypertension phenomena. Therefore, out-of-office BP measurements are often needed and several studies have demonstrated the indispensable value of ABPM in the management of pediatric hypertension.[45,46] The data regarding HBPM in children are fewer, but increasing evidence suggests that HBPM is feasible, can provide reliable readings, and appears to have similar diagnostic value as in the adults regarding the detection of the hypertension phenotypes when ABPM is taken as reference.[47,48] One study in children and adolescents showed HBPM to be comparable to ABPM and superior to OBP in terms of relationship with indices of preclinical target-organ damage, but further data are lacking.[46,49] A school-based study in 778 children and adolescents provided the first home BP normalcy data and it appears that home BP in children and adolescents is lower than daytime ambulatory BP, whereas no such difference exists in the adults.[47,50,51] Three-day HBPM with duplicate morning and evening measurements seems to be the minimum schedule required, yet 6- to 7-day monitoring is recommended.[47]

Elderly

Out of office BP monitoring in the elderly is highly important for the accurate assessment of the hypertension because of the higher prevalence of the white-coat hypertension, the increased BP variability and the potential hazards of an excessive BP reduction.[3,4] Despite the limited data regarding HBPM in the elderly, the recommended thresholds for hypertension diagnosis and management are the same as in other adults.[3] One of the limitations of HBPM in the elderly is the inability to assess orthostatic hypotension which is identified by ABPM. However, HBPM readings might be taken with the subject both sitting and standing.

Pregnancy

BP presents a dynamic pattern during pregnancy with an initial fall and a subsequent increase. Thus, frequent and accurate measurement of BP during pregnancy is of paramount importance in terms of prompt recognition of preeclampsia which can develop abruptly and is associated with maternal and fetal mortality.[3,4] HBPM is theoretically ideal for monitoring changes in BP during pregnancy, because it can provide multiple readings over prolonged periods of time and can reduce the number of antenatal office visits without increasing anxiety.[3,4] It should be mentioned however that there are no established thresholds or algorithms for the management of hypertension during pregnancy with HBPM. Another concern is that the altered hemodynamics during pregnancy requires special validation studies of the oscillometric devices in pregnant women with and without preeclampsia.[3] Only a few devices have been validated in pregnancy by methodologically acceptable studies and can be recommended. As recommended for OBP, HBPM should also be performed with the woman seated or lying on her side at a 45 degree angle, with her arm at the level of the heart.[3]

Obesity

The measurement of BP in obese subjects can be problematic. First, obesity is associated with a higher prevalence of both white-coat and masked hypertension phenomena.[3] Second, inappropriate cuff size may lead to inaccurate BP readings and more specifically provide overestimated values.[3] In addition, not only the cuff size, but also its shape may be equally important. A conical shaped arm, which is the case in obese subjects, can make it difficult to fit the cuff and moreover can predispose to inconvenience with pain during inflation and inaccurate measurement.[3] Thus, special validation studies of BP monitors with different cuffs in obese individuals are necessary. The use of wrist devices could be an alternative choice by avoiding some of these difficulties, however further investigation, technological improvement and special validation studies are required.[3]

Atrial Fibrillation

Hypertension and atrial fibrillation often coexist particularly in the elderly and are strong risk factors for stroke. Current guidelines for BP measurement in atrial fibrillation recommend repeated measurements using the auscultatory method, whereas the accuracy of the automated devices is regarded as questionable.[2] Studies evaluating the use of automated BP monitors in atrial fibrillation are limited and have significant heterogeneity in methodology and protocols.[52,53] Overall, the oscillometric method is feasible and appears to be more accurate for systolic than diastolic BP measurement.[52] Given that systolic hypertension is particularly common and important in the elderly, the automated BP measurement method may be acceptable for HBPM as long as repeated (duplicate or triplicate) measurements are performed.[53] An embedded algorithm for the automated detection of asymptomatic atrial fibrillation during routine HBPM has been developed and appears to have high diagnostic accuracy and therefore to be a useful screening tool in the elderly hypertensives.[53,54]

Diabetes

The usefulness of HBPM in diabetic patients is related to the detection of masked hypertension which appears to be higher in this population and carries an adverse prognosis if uncontrolled.[3,55] In patients with type 2 diabetes, HBPM is superior to OBP measurements, and allows more accurate detection of hypertension.[56]

Chronic Kidney Disease

Hypertension is highly prevalent in patients with chronic kidney disease and associated with poor outcome.[3,4] In such patients, HBPM presents better prognostic value compared with OBP in terms of cardiovascular events, end-stage renal disease and all-cause mortality.[3,57] HBPM can also provide useful information in the dialysis population, where BP is very variable and cannot be assessed in the office in a representative way.[3,4] Although these patients have increased arterial stiffness, the oscillometric method may still be accurate, but special validation studies in this population are required.[3,4]

COST-EFFECTIVENESS

The cost-effectiveness of HBPM has not been thoroughly investigated. HBPM has the potential for significant cost savings made through the prevention of unnecessary treatment in untreated or treated subjects with white-coat phenomenon, the lesser need for office visits, and the optimal treatment of masked hypertensives that is expected to reduce the incidence of cardiovascular complications.[4,10] On the other hand, there are several costs such as that of the HBPM devices, the cost related to the implementation and use of HBPM, and those related to the necessary validation of devices, the training of users, the review of HBPM data and advice to patients regarding changes in treatment.[4,10] An old review showed that the estimated annualized resource cost of HBPM was less than half of that of ABPM.[58] A decision tree model based on data from the Ohasama home BP outcome study applied on a Japanese national database concluded that the introduction of HBPM for the diagnosis and treatment of hypertension would be very effective to save costs.[59,60] This was mainly attributed to avoidance of treatment of white-coat hypertensives and improvement of prognosis because of better control of hypertension.[59,60] A recent study in 116 untreated hypertensive subjects who were randomized to use HBPM or OBP/ABPM for antihypertensive treatment initiation and titration showed that the cost related to health resources used within 12-months follow-up was lower in the HBPM arm.[61] Interestingly, this difference in favor of HBPM became more evident in a 5-year projection.[61] Another study performed a cost-benefit analysis from the perspective of the insurer by using a decision-analytic model that simulated the transitions among health states from initial physician visit to hypertension diagnosis, to treatment, to hypertension-related cardiovascular diseases, and patient death or resignation from the plan.[62] This study concluded that reimbursement of HBPM is cost beneficial from an insurer's perspective for diagnosing and treating hypertension.[62]

HOME BLOOD PRESSURE TELEMONITORING

Tele-HBPM is based on registration of BP data obtained by the patient at home and their transmission to a remote computer through telephone or internet connection. Accumulating evidence suggests that tele-HBPM allows more accurate evaluation and is associated with higher BP control rates and increased patient satisfaction.[63-66] As technology is being improved and the cost is reduced, tele-HBPM might become more cost-effective, particularly in high-risk patients or when combined with monitoring of other vital signs or cardiovascular risk factors (i.e., diabetes).[65] More research is needed to provide direct comparison against usual HBPM and with long-term endpoints including BP reduction, hypertension control, quality of life, and cost-effectiveness.[67]

HOME BLOOD PRESSURE MONITORING IN RESEARCH

HBPM has great potential in several research fields, such as outcome trials, and those evaluating drug effects or BP variability.

As mentioned previously, large longitudinal prospective studies conducted in Europe and Japan, have confirmed the superior prognostic value of HBPM compared with OBP.[20] The IDHOCO database of outcome HBPM studies allowed powered analyses of individual subject data and provided important information for outcome-based HBPM thresholds, the predictive value of white-coat and masked hypertension detected by HBPM in treated and untreated subjects, and more.[15,22,23,68,69]

Regarding the assessment of drug effects, a metaanalysis of 30 studies in 6794 subjects showed that antihypertensive treatment reduced home BP by about 20% less than OBP, which was attributed to difference in baseline BP levels.[70] Regression to the mean, as well as other factors, such as the white-coat effect and the placebo effect, may have resulted in larger OBP decline. Thus, HBPM appears to be more accurate than OBP in the assessment of drug-induced BP changes. Furthermore, studies have shown that the morning/evening home BP ratio provides similar information about the duration of action of antihypertensive drugs, as the trough/peak ratio assessed by ABPM.[71,72]

Preliminary data from heterogeneous studies suggest an important and independent role of day-by-day home BP variability in the progression of target-organ damage as well as in cardiovascular morbidity and mortality.[73] However, fundamental questions remain unanswered, including the optimal variability index, the optimal HBPM schedule required, the threshold for increased home BP variability and the impact of treatment-induced variability change on organ damage and cardiovascular events.

HOME VERSUS AMBULATORY BLOOD PRESSURE MONITORING

Although both HBPM and ABPM provide multiple measurements in the usual environment of each individual, there are several methodologic differences because home BP is always measured after a few minutes' rest in the sitting posture at home, whereas ABPM is performed in fully ambulatory conditions and posture (walking, standing, sitting, lying), without a period of rest before each measurement, at home, work, or during sleep. Despite these differences, average HBPM and daytime ABPM appear to have similar normalcy thresholds, similar reproducibility, similar diagnostic accuracy for white-coat and masked hypertension and prediction of target-organ damage and cardiovascular events, with all these features being superior to those of the conventional OBP measurements.[10] However, the abovementioned features do not render these methods interchangeable. This was clearly demonstrated in two populations outcome studies (PAMELA, Ohasama) where subjects with elevated ambulatory but low home BP or the reverse were at increased cardiovascular risk compared with normotensives (low home and ambulatory BP), implying independent prognostic information provided by each method.[74,75] Thus, these methods should be regarded as complementary rather than competitive in the assessment of hypertensive patients. In an ideal setting, one would like to have both methods to obtain a complete picture of the BP profile during the 24-hour period and on multiple days. When deciding which method to use, equipment availability and patients' preference should also be taken into account, both of which usually favor HBPM, particularly for repeated application. HBPM is widely available in many countries, and is relatively inexpensive and well-accepted by patients, whereas ABP is not widely available and is rather expensive because of device costs and physician time required for device initialization, download, and interpretation. This difference is expected to decrease as the cost of ambulatory monitors is being reduced and the technique is becoming accessible even in pharmacies.[6]

TABLE 10.2 Practical Recommendations for Optimal Application of Home Blood Pressure Monitoring.

Device	Automated upper-arm device validated according to an established protocol.
Cuff	Bladder size according to individual arm circumference.
Conditions	Relaxed, after 5 min. sitting rest.
Monitoring schedule	7-day monitoring before each office visit with duplicate morning (before drug intake) and evening measurements. Not fewer than 3 days (12 readings).
Evaluation	Calculation of average BP of all readings after discarding the first day. Casual readings have little clinical relevance.
Diagnostic thresholds	Normal home BP: <130/80 mm Hg; hypertension: ≥135/85 mm Hg; intermediate levels are considered borderline.
Long-term follow-up	1-2 duplicate measurements per week. Too frequent monitoring and self-modification of treatment on the basis of casual measurements to be avoided.

HOME BLOOD PRESSURE MONITORING RECOMMENDATIONS (TABLE 10.2)

Devices

Validated automated electronic devices, especially those using an oscillometric algorithm and having an upper-arm cuff are currently recommended for HBPM because they are relatively accurate, devoid of the observer bias, and require little training.[3] Aneroid or hybrid auscultatory devices can also be used, but require skills, training, and more regular calibration, which often are not feasible in general practice. Auscultatory devices might be preferred only in case of arrhythmias, or preeclampsia, yet these indications are also debatable. Some automated wrist devices have passed the internationally accepted validation protocols, however these are regarded as less accurate than upper-arm devices, mainly because of anatomic differentiations of the wrist and of difficulty in following the correct wrist position (at heart level and relaxed).[3] Finger devices are not accurate and have been withdrawn from the market.[3]

The accuracy of electronic BP monitors should be tested against conventional mercury sphygmomanometry according to established validation protocols.[76-79] However, many of the electronic devices for HBPM available on the market have not been subjected to independent validation or have failed. Updated lists of devices which have passed at least one of the aforementioned validation protocols are available at the British Hypertension Society website (www.bhsoc.org) and the Medaval website for the evaluation of BP monitors (www.medaval.org). It should be mentioned that even validated devices may present significant measurement errors in some cases for reasons that remain rather unclear and might be related to the individual's arterial wall properties.

The use of a cuff with appropriate inflatable bladder size for the arm circumference of each individual is of equal importance as the accuracy of the device.[3] The length of the inflatable bladder should cover 80% to 100% of the arm circumference and the width should be about half of the length.[3] Cuffs which are too small for the arm circumference tend to overestimate BP (common in obese subjects), whereas cuffs which are too large (in children or lean women) tend to underestimate BP. It is recommended that subjects with arm circumference larger than 32 cm should use a cuff larger than the standard size, whereas those with arm circumference smaller than 24 cm a smaller cuff than the standard.[3]

Monitoring Conditions and Procedure

The conditions of HBPM should be similar to those recommended for OBP.[3] The patient should be relaxed in the sitting posture, with the back supported, without crossing legs, in a quiet room at a comfortable temperature and at least 5 minutes of rest should precede the measurement.[3] Talking during the measurement and coffee or smoking for at least 30 minutes before the measurement should be discouraged.[3] The cuff should be placed at heart level with the center of the bladder over the brachial artery.[3] BP on both arms should be measured by the doctor in the first office visit to exclude occlusive arterial disease. In individuals without a consistent between-arm difference (e.g., >10 mm Hg systolic and/or >5 mm Hg diastolic) on repeated measurements, HBPM should be performed sequentially on the same, usually the nondominant, arm.[3]

Monitoring Schedule

Current HBPM guidelines[3,4] recommend a standard HBPM schedule for the initial evaluation of BP levels (untreated subjects) and before each visit to the physician (for treated hypertensives), which includes duplicate measurements (with one minute interval) in the morning (before drug intake if treated), and the evening, for 7 routine work days (not less than 3 days), with weekends preferably excluded as the corresponding BP values are usually lower than in workdays.[3] For decision making, a total of 24 home BP readings (7 days and exclusion of the first one) should be routinely obtained and 12 readings seem to be the minimum acceptable sample.[1,3] Home BP readings of the first monitoring day should be better discarded, as they are typically higher and more variable than of the next days.[1,3] For the long-term follow-up of treated hypertensives, HBPM once or twice per week might seem to be appropriate to ensure maintenance of adequate BP control.

Reporting of Home Blood Pressure Values

Accurate reporting of all systolic/diastolic BP readings and heart rate must be ensured, as it has been shown that HBPM reported by patients frequently differs from the actually measured values.[3,9] The use of monitors with automated memory and averaging, or PC download is recommended. In addition, patients should be encouraged to report all HBPM readings in a form according to the recommended schedule.

Diagnostic Threshold and Interpretation

Based on evidence derived from metaanalyses, cross-sectional and also long-term observational studies, the current guidelines recommend a hypertension threshold for average home BP at 135/85 mm Hg, which is the same as recommended for awake ABPM.[3,4] Levels exceeding this threshold are considered elevated. Home BP levels ranging between 130 to 135 mm Hg for systolic and 80 to 85 mm Hg for diastolic BP are regarded as borderline (prehypertension range), and those less than 130/80 mm Hg as normal.[3]

SUMMARY

Increasing and considerable evidence on HBPM has accumulated during the last two decades and current guidelines recommend its wide application in clinical practice. Its primary role in hypertension management is supported from data regarding its prognostic ability, its contribution in accurate diagnosis, and its usefulness in treatment adjustment and in long-term follow-up leading to improved hypertension control, combined with wide availability, low cost, and good acceptance by patients.

References

1. Stergiou GS, Kollias A, Zeniodi M, et al. Home blood pressure monitoring: primary role in hypertension management. Curr Hypertens Rep. 2014;16:462.
2. Mancia G, Fagard R, Narkiewicz K, et al. ESH/ESC Guidelines for the management of arterial hypertension: the Task Force for the management of arterial hypertension of the European Society of Hypertension (ESH) and of the European Society of Cardiology (ESC). J Hypertens. 2013;31:1281-1357.
3. Parati G, Stergiou GS, Asmar R, et al. European Society of Hypertension guidelines for blood pressure monitoring at home: a summary report of the Second International Consensus Conference on Home Blood Pressure Monitoring. J Hypertens. 2008;26:1505-1526.
4. Pickering TG, Miller NH, Ogedegbe G, et al. Call to action on use and reimbursement for home blood pressure monitoring: a joint scientific statement from the American Heart Association, American Society Of Hypertension, and Preventive Cardiovascular Nurses Association. Hypertension. 2008;52:10-29.
5. McManus RJ, Glasziou P, Hayen A, et al. Blood pressure self-monitoring: questions and answers from a national committee. BMJ. 2008;337:a2732.
6. O'Brien E, Parati G, Stergiou G, et al. European Society of Hypertension position paper on ambulatory blood pressure monitoring. J Hypertens. 2013;31:1731-1768.
7. Stergiou GS, Baibas NM, Gantzarou AP, et al. Reproducibility of home, ambulatory, and clinic blood pressure: implications for the design of trials for the assessment of antihypertensive drug efficacy. Am J Hypertens. 2002;15:101-104.
8. Cappuccio FP, Kerry SM, Forbes L, et al. Blood pressure control by home monitoring: meta-analysis of randomised trials. BMJ. 2004;329:145.
9. Myers MG, Stergiou GS. Reporting bias: Achilles' heel of home blood pressure monitoring. J Am Soc Hypertens. 2014;8:350-357.
10. Stergiou GS, Bliziotis IA. Home blood pressure monitoring in the diagnosis and treatment of hypertension: a systematic review. Am J Hypertens. 2011;24:123-134.
11. Nasothimiou EG, Tzamouranis D, Rarra V, et al. Diagnostic accuracy of home vs. ambulatory blood pressure monitoring in untreated and treated hypertension. Hypertens Res. 2012;35:750-755.
12. Nasothimiou EG, Tzamouranis D, Roussias LG, et al. Home versus ambulatory blood pressure monitoring in the diagnosis of clinic resistant and true resistant hypertension. J Hum Hypertens. 2012;26:696-700.
13. Kollias A, Ntineri A, Stergiou GS. Is white-coat hypertension a harbinger of increased risk? Hypertens Res. 2014;37:791-795.
14. Briasoulis A, Androulakis E, Palla M, et al. White-coat hypertension and cardiovascular events: a meta-analysis. J Hypertens. 2016;34:593-599.
15. Stergiou GS, Asayama K, Thijs L, et al. Prognosis of white-coat and masked hypertension: International Database of HOme blood pressure in relation to Cardiovascular Outcome. Hypertension. 2014;63:675-682.
16. Cuspidi C, Sala C, Tadic M, et al. Untreated masked hypertension and subclinical cardiac damage: a systematic review and meta-analysis. Am J Hypertens. 2015;28:806-813.
17. Bobrie G, Chatellier G, Genes N, et al. Cardiovascular prognosis of "masked hypertension" detected by blood pressure self-measurement in elderly treated hypertensive patients. JAMA. 2004;291:1342-1349.
18. Bliziotis IA, Destounis A. Stergiou GS. Home versus ambulatory and office blood pressure in predicting target organ damage in hypertension: a systematic review and meta-analysis. J Hypertens. 2012;30:1289-1299.
19. Fuchs SC, Mello RG, Fuchs FC. Home blood pressure monitoring is better predictor of cardiovascular disease and target organ damage than office blood pressure: a systematic review and meta-analysis. Curr Cardiol Rep. 2013;15:413.
20. Stergiou GS, Siontis KC, Ioannidis JP. Home blood pressure as a cardiovascular outcome predictor: it's time to take this method seriously. Hypertension. 2010;55:1301-1303.
21. Ward AM, Takahashi O, Stevens R, et al. Home measurement of blood pressure and cardiovascular disease: systematic review and meta-analysis of prospective studies. J Hypertens. 2012;30:449-456.
22. Niiranen TJ, Thijs L, Asayama K, et al. IDHOCO Investigators. The International Database of HOme blood pressure in relation to Cardiovascular Outcome (IDHOCO): moving from baseline characteristics to research perspectives. Hypertens Res. 2012;35:1072-1079.
23. Asayama K, Thijs L, Brguljan-Hitij J, et al. International Database of Home Blood Pressure in Relation to Cardiovascular Outcome (IDHOCO) investigators. Risk stratification by self-measured home blood pressure across categories of conventional blood pressure: a participant-level meta-analysis. PLoS Med. 2014;11:e1001591.
24. Mancia G1, Zanchetti A, Agabiti-Rosei E, et al. Ambulatory blood pressure is superior to clinic blood pressure in predicting treatment-induced regression of left ventricular hypertrophy. SAMPLE Study Group. Study on Ambulatory Monitoring of Blood Pressure and Lisinopril Evaluation. Circulation. 1997;95:1464-1470.
25. Karpettas N, Destounis A, Kollias A, et al. Prediction of treatment-induced changes in target-organ damage using changes in clinic, home and ambulatory blood pressure. Hypertens Res. 2014;37:543-547.
26. Zarnke KB, Feagan BG, Mahon JL, et al. A randomized study comparing a patient-directed hypertension management strategy with usual office-based care. Am J Hypertens. 1997;10:58-67.
27. Broege PA, James GD, Pickering TG. Management of hypertension in the elderly using home blood pressures. Blood Press Monit. 2001;6:139-144.
28. Staessen JA, Den Hond E, Celis H, et al. Treatment of Hypertension Based on Home or Office Blood Pressure (THOP) Trial Investigators. Antihypertensive treatment based on blood pressure measurement at home or in the physician's office: a randomized controlled trial. JAMA. 2004;291:955-964.
29. Halme L, Vesalainen R, Kaaja M, et al. Home MEasuRement of blood pressure study group. Self-monitoring of blood pressure promotes achievement of blood pressure target in primary health care. Am J Hypertens. 2005;18:1415-1420.
30. Verberk WJ, Kroon AA, Lenders JW, et al. Home versus office measurement, reduction of unnecessary treatment study investigators. Self-measurement of blood pressure at home reduces the need for antihypertensive drugs: a randomized, controlled trial. Hypertension. 2007;50:1019-1025.
31. Tobe SW, Hunter K, Geerts R, et al. Canadian Hypertension Society. IMPPACT: Investigation of Medical Professionals and Patients Achieving Control Together. Can J Cardiol. 2008;24:205-208.
32. McManus RJ, Mant J, Bray EP, et al. Telemonitoring and self-management in the control of hypertension (TASMINH2): a randomized controlled trial. Lancet. 2010;376:163-172.
33. Niiranen TJ, Kantola IM, Vesalainen R, et al. A comparison of home measurement and ambulatory monitoring of blood pressure in the adjustment of antihypertensive treatment. Am J Hypertens. 2006;19:468-474.
34. Stergiou GS, Karpettas N, Destounis A, et al. Home blood pressure monitoring alone vs. combined clinic and ambulatory measurements in following treatment-induced changes in blood pressure and organ damage. Am J Hypertens. 2014;27:184-192.
35. Ogedegbe G, Schoenthaler A. A systematic review of the effects of home blood pressure monitoring on medication adherence. J Clin Hypertens. (Greenwich) 2006;8:174-180.

36. Agarwal R, Bills JE, Hecht TJ, et al. Role of home blood pressure monitoring in overcoming therapeutic inertia and improving hypertension control: a systematic review and meta-analysis. *Hypertension.* 2011;57:29-38.

37. Glynn LG, Murphy AW, Smith SM, et al. Self-monitoring and other non-pharmacological interventions to improve the management of hypertension in primary care: a systematic review. *Br J Gen Pract.* 2010;60:e476-e488.

38. Fuchs SC, Ferreira-da-Silva AL, Moreira LB, et al. Efficacy of isolated home blood pressure monitoring for blood pressure control: randomized controlled trial with ambulatory blood pressure monitoring—MONITOR study. *J Hypertens.* 2012;30:75-80.

39. Cuspidi C, Meani S, Fusi V, et al. Home blood pressure measurement and its relationship with blood pressure control in a large selected hypertensive population. *J Hum Hypertens.* 2004;18:725-731.

40. Hansen TW, Li Y, Boggia J, et al. Predictive role of the nighttime blood pressure. *Hypertension.* 2011;57:3-10.

41. Ushio H, Ishigami T, Araki N, et al. Utility and feasibility of a new programmable home blood pressure monitoring device for the assessment of nighttime blood pressure. *Clin Exp Nephrol.* 2009;13:480-485.

42. Stergiou GS, Nasothimiou EG, Destounis A, et al. Assessment of the diurnal blood pressure profile and detection of non-dippers based on home or ambulatory monitoring. *Am J Hypertens.* 2012;25:974-978.

43. Andreadis EA, Agaliotis G, Kollias A, et al. Night-time home versus ambulatory blood pressure in determining target organ damage. *J Hypertens.* 2016;34:438-444.

44. Ishikawa J, Hoshide S, Eguchi K, et al. Nighttime home blood pressure and the risk of hypertensive target organ damage. *Hypertension.* 2012;60:921-928.

45. Flynn JT, Daniels SR, Hayman LL, et al. American Heart Association Atherosclerosis, Hypertension and Obesity in Youth Committee of the Council on Cardiovascular Disease in the Young. Update: ambulatory blood pressure monitoring in children and adolescents: a scientific statement from the American Heart Association. *Hypertension.* 2014;63:1116-1135.

46. Kollias A, Dafni M, Poulidakis E, et al. Out-of-office blood pressure and target organ damage in children and adolescents: a systematic review and meta-analysis. *J Hypertens.* 2014;32:2315-2331.

47. Stergiou GS, Karpettas N, Kapoyiannis A, et al. Home blood pressure monitoring in children and adolescents: a systematic review. *J Hypertens.* 2009;27:1941-1947.

48. Stergiou GS, Nasothimiou E, Giovas P, et al. Diagnosis of hypertension in children and adolescents based on home versus ambulatory blood pressure monitoring. *J Hypertens.* 2008;26:1556-1562.

49. Stergiou GS, Giovas PP, Kollias A, et al. Relationship of home blood pressure with target-organ damage in children and adolescents. *Hypertens Res.* 2011;34:640-644.

50. Stergiou GS, Yiannes NG, Rarra VC, et al. Home blood pressure normalcy in children and adolescents: the Arsakeion School study. *J Hypertens.* 2007;25:1375-1379.

51. Stergiou GS, Karpettas N, Panagiotakos DB, et al. Comparison of office, ambulatory and home blood pressure in children and adolescents on the basis of normalcy tables. *J Hum Hypertens.* 2011;25:218-223.

52. Stergiou GS, Kollias A, Destounis A, et al. Automated blood pressure measurement in atrial fibrillation: a systematic review and meta-analysis. *J Hypertens.* 2012;30:2074-2082.

53. Kollias A, Stergiou GS. Automated measurement of office, home and ambulatory blood pressure in atrial fibrillation. *Clin Exp Pharmacol Physiol.* 2014;41:9-15.

54. Verberk WJ, Omboni S, Kollias A, et al. Screening for atrial fibrillation with automated blood pressure measurement: Research evidence and practice recommendations. *Int J Cardiol.* 2016;203:465-473.

55. Eguchi K, Ishikawa J, Hoshide S, et al. Masked hypertension in diabetes mellitus: a potential risk. *J Clin Hypertens.* (Greenwich) 2007;9:601-607.

56. Masding MG, Jones JR, Bartley E, et al. Assessment of blood pressure in patients with Type 2 diabetes: comparison between home blood pressure monitoring, clinic blood pressure measurement and 24-h ambulatory blood pressure monitoring. *Diabet Med.* 2001;18:431-437.

57. Agarwal R, Andersen MJ. Prognostic importance of clinic and home blood pressure recordings in patients with chronic kidney disease. *Kidney Int.* 2006;69:406-411.

58. Appel LJ, Stason WB. Ambulatory blood pressure monitoring and blood pressure self-measurement in the diagnosis and management of hypertension. *Ann Intern Med.* 1993;118:867-882.

59. Funahashi J, Ohkubo T, Fukunaga H, et al. The economic impact of the introduction of home blood pressure measurement for the diagnosis and treatment of hypertension. *Blood Press Monit.* 2006;11:257-267.

60. Fukunaga H, Ohkubo T, Kobayashi M, et al. Cost-effectiveness of the introduction of home blood pressure measurement in patients with office hypertension. *J Hypertens.* 2008;26:685-690.

61. Boubouchairopoulou N, Karpettas N, Athanasakis K. Cost estimation of hypertension management based on home blood pressure monitoring alone or combined office and ambulatory blood pressure measurements. *J Am Soc Hypertens.* 2014;8:732-738.

62. Arrieta A, Woods JR, Qiao N, et al. Cost-benefit analysis of home blood pressure monitoring in hypertension diagnosis and treatment: an insurer perspective. *Hypertension.* 2014;64:891-896.

63. AbuDagga A, Resnick HE, Alwan M. Impact of blood pressure telemonitoring on hypertension outcomes: a literature review. *Telemed J E Health.* 2010;16:830-838.

64. Zullig LL, Melnyk SD, Goldstein K, et al. The role of home blood pressure telemonitoring in managing hypertensive populations. *Curr Hypertens Rep.* 2013;15:346-355.

65. Omboni S, Gazzola T, Carabelli G, et al. Clinical usefulness and cost effectiveness of home blood pressure telemonitoring: meta-analysis of randomized controlled studies. *J Hypertens.* 2013;31:455-467.

66. Margolis KL, Asche SE, Bergdall AR, et al. Effect of home blood pressure telemonitoring and pharmacist management on blood pressure control: a cluster randomized clinical trial. *JAMA.* 2013;310:46-56.

67. Stergiou GS, Nasothimiou EG. Hypertension: Does home telemonitoring improve hypertension management? *Nat Rev Nephrol.* 2011;7:493-495.

68. Aparicio LS, Thijs L, Boggia J, et al. International Database on Home Blood Pressure in Relation to Cardiovascular Outcome (IDHOCO) Investigators. Defining thresholds for home blood pressure monitoring in octogenarians. *Hypertension.* 2015;66:865-873.

69. Niiranen TJ, Asayama K, Thijs L, et al. IDHOCO Investigators. Optimal number of days for home blood pressure measurement. *Am J Hypertens.* 2015;28:595-603.

70. Ishikawa J, Carroll DJ, Kuruvilla S, et al. Changes in home versus clinic blood pressure with antihypertensive treatments: a meta-analysis. *Hypertension.* 2008;52:856-864.

71. Ménard J, Chatellier G, Day M, et al. Self-measurement of blood pressure at home to evaluate drug effects by the trough:peak ratio. *J Hypertens Suppl.* 1994;12:S21-S25.

72. Stergiou GS, Efstathiou SP, Skeva II, et al. Comparison of the smoothness index, the trough:peak ratio and the morning:evening ratio in assessing the features of the antihypertensive drug effect. *J Hypertens.* 2003;21:913-920.

73. Stergiou GS, Ntineri A, Kollias A, et al. Blood pressure variability assessed by home measurements: a systematic review. *Hypertens Res.* 2014;37:565-572.

74. Mancia G, Facchetti R, Bombelli M, et al. Long-term risk of mortality associated with selective and combined elevation in office, home, and ambulatory blood pressure. *Hypertension.* 2006;47:846-853.

75. Satoh M, Asayama K, Kikuya M, et al. Long-term stroke risk due to partial white-coat or masked hypertension based on home and ambulatory blood pressure measurements: The Ohasama Study. *Hypertension.* 2016;67:48-55.

76. Association for the Advancement of Medical Instrumentation. American National Standard. Electronic or automated sphygmomanometers. ANSI/AAMI; 1987; SP10-1987. 3330.

77. O'Brien E, Petrie J, Littler W, et al. The British Hypertension Society Protocol for the evaluation of automated and semi-automated blood pressure measuring devices with special reference to ambulatory systems. *J Hypertens.* 1990;8:607-619.

78. O'Brien E, Pickering T, Asmar R, et al. Working Group on Blood Pressure Monitoring of the European Society of Hypertension International Protocol for validation of blood pressure measuring devices in adults. *Blood Press Monit.* 2002;7:3-17.

79. O'Brien E, Atkins N, Stergiou G, et al. European Society of Hypertension International Protocol revision 2010 for the validation of blood pressure measuring devices in adults. *Blood Press Monit.* 2010;15:23-38.

11 Ambulatory Blood Pressure Monitoring in Clinical Hypertension Management

William B. White and Line Malha

Before the early 1970s, intraarterial recordings provided the only means of following changes in blood pressure (BP) during the typical activities of daily living over a period of time. The development and commercial availability of lightweight, quiet, easy-to-wear automated noninvasive BP recorders has facilitated the collection of large volumes of data (~100 measurements in 24 hours) while a subject pursues his or her everyday activities. Data derived from ambulatory BP monitoring (ABPM) have made important contributions to our understanding of the pathophysiology of hypertension and its complications, the definition of daytime and nighttime normotension, the prognostic value of ambulatory BP, and the evaluation of therapies.

CIRCADIAN VARIATION OF BLOOD PRESSURE

The circadian variation in BP and its association with cardiovascular events, including both myocardial infarction and stroke, are well-established.[1-5] Blood pressure follows a highly reproducible pattern characterized by: (1) a low period during sleep; (2) an early morning, postawakening rise, coinciding with the transition from sleep to wakefulness; and (3) a higher, sustained and more variable period thereafter. Evidence for the circadian periodicity of BP being synchronized with the sleep–wake cycle also comes from observations in shift workers.[6,7] For example, a complete and immediate reversal of the circadian BP rhythm occurs on the first occasion of a session of night shifts.[6] As a result of the shift in work schedules (and sleep times), the peak systolic blood pressure (SBP) in night workers is recorded at about 11 PM and the diastolic blood pressure (DBP) peaks at about 10 PM.[7] Night shift work is also associated with a conversion from a dipping to nondipping pattern in BP which is reversed when the nocturnal work is stopped.[8,9] Night shift and rotating patterns in shifts have been associated with an increased incidence of metabolic syndrome,[10,11] inflammatory markers[12] and dyslipidemia.[13]

Clinical Importance of Nighttime Decline ("Dipping") in Blood Pressure

A dipping pattern is characterized by nighttime BP reductions of 10% to 30% relative to the "awake" period and is consistently found in the majority of normotensive and hypertensive people. However, about 25% to 35% of hypertensive patients (and probably a smaller proportion of normotensive people) do not display this decline in nocturnal BP.[14] Instead, this population expresses a blunted or total absence in decline in nocturnal BP. The absence of a nocturnal decline in BP varies according to the patient population and is more prevalent in the older persons,[15] African Americans,[16] and postmenopausal women (especially African-American women).[17] The term "nondippers" was coined by O'Brien[18] to describe those individuals in whom the decline in nighttime BP is less than 10% of the daytime value; such people were found to be at increased risk for

stroke. There is strong evidence that a persistent nondipping pattern is associated with more pronounced cardiac involvement, particularly left ventricular hypertrophy (LVH).[19] It has been proposed that the nondipping pattern may be associated with atherosclerosis,[20] cardiovascular and kidney disease.[21] Of particular relevance is a large cohort study of 8711 patients demonstrating that even in normotensive people, isolated nocturnal hypertension predicts cardiovascular outcomes.[22] However, patients with blunted nocturnal dipping patterns frequently belong to high-risk categories that confound outcomes; they are often older, obese, diabetic, or have overt cardiovascular or renal disease.[23,24] Nondipping also confounds the higher cardiovascular risk observed in African Americans.[25-27] Even among patients with treated hypertension, half do not adequately drop their nocturnal BPs.[28] After adjusting for age, sex and diabetes, a mean 5 mm Hg reduction in systolic nocturnal BP is associated with a 17% drop in cardiovascular risk.[29]

Despite the clinical findings associated with the lack of decline in BP during sleep, the validity of an arbitrary proportional threshold to define dipping status has been questioned.[30] The reproducibility of the fall in nighttime BP compared with daytime values has been poor in some studies,[31,32] because sleep quality and depth of sleep may influence the degree of dipping. Rather than a proportional reduction in BP, an absolute BP value may be more appropriate to define nocturnal hypertension.[21,30,33,34] Many years ago, a consensus panel of the American Society of Hypertension originally proposed a definition of nocturnal hypertension as being a mean nighttime BP of greater than 125/80 mm Hg,[35] based on epidemiologic and cross-sectional studies of target organ disease at that time. A committee, later organized by the American Heart Association, suggested using a value of 125/75 mm Hg.[36] This threshold was further lowered by the European Society of Hypertension (ESH) updated practice guidelines that considered a nighttime BP of greater than 120/70 mm Hg to be abnormal.[37,38]

In the past decade, the examination of ambulatory BP data has established the reproducibility of an absolute definition of nocturnal hypertension compared with proportional decreases.[30] Data were extracted from high-quality 24-hour recordings obtained during the placebo run-in phase of a series of clinical trials conducted in hypertensive patients diagnosed according to the standard office BP. Patients with nocturnal hypertension were identified using three different criteria: those with a less than 5% decrease in nighttime BP compared with daytime; those with a less than 10% decrease in nighttime compared with daytime; and those with a mean nocturnal BP of greater than 125/80 mm Hg. The analyses confirmed that a mean nighttime BP of greater than 125/80 mm Hg is more reproducible than the other two criteria. About half of the patients identified as nondippers on the first ABPM assessment were considered nondippers on the second assessment performed after 4 to 8 weeks.[30] The dipper status was more

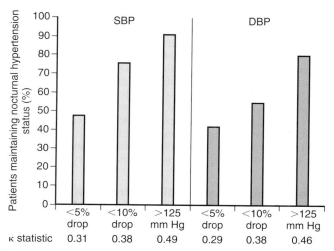

FIG. 11.1 Proportion of patients maintaining nocturnal hypertension status (defined as <5% drop, <10% drop, or an absolute value of >125/80 mm Hg) after two 24-hour ambulatory blood pressure monitoring sessions 4 to 8 weeks apart. κ, The agreement between the sets of data; *DBP,* diastolic blood pressure; *SBP,* systolic blood pressure. *(Data from White WB, Larocca GM. Improving the utility of the nocturnal hypertension definition by using absolute sleep blood pressure rather than the "dipping" proportion. Am J Cardiol. 2003;92:1439-1441.)*

reproducible using absolute criteria for SBP rather than similar criteria for DBP (Fig. 11.1). These findings suggested that the absolute nocturnal BP may have provided a more appropriate approach than proportional declines in BP for evaluating the efficacy of antihypertensive agents.

Clinical Importance of the Early-Morning Blood Pressure Surge

In most individuals who sleep at night, a rapid rise in both BP and heart rate occurs in the morning upon awakening. During this period of the "early morning BP surge," there is also an increase in the incidence of cardiovascular events, including myocardial infarction and stroke. Many non-hemodynamic factors, including plaque vulnerability and increased coagulability, contribute to the early morning prothrombotic state.[39] Studies have consistently shown that acute myocardial infarction is more prevalent between 6 AM and noon than at other times of the day or night.[40] In addition, the incidence of subarachnoid hemorrhage,[41] ischemic stroke,[42] hemorrhagic stroke,[42,43] and transient ischemic attacks[44] is highest in the morning period after awakening.

The primary evidence for a link between a steep increase in BP and morbidities associated with hypertension comes from a study conducted in elderly Japanese hypertensive patients.[45] Using ABPM, the early morning BP surge was defined as the difference between the SBP during the 2 hours after awakening minus the lowest sleep SBP. The 519 patients studied were divided into two groups, according to the extent of the surge. In the group of 53 patients who had a surge of 55 mm Hg or more (average 69 mm Hg) at baseline, there was a 57% incidence of silent cerebral infarcts, as opposed to only 33% in the remaining patients whose average increase in SBP was a more modest 29 mm Hg. During the follow-up period that averaged 41 months, 19% of patients with a large early-morning BP surge suffered a stroke, compared with 7.3% of those with a relatively small surge. The control of the early-morning BP surge was regarded as being an important stratagem to prevent vascular disease in hypertensive patients. The authors concluded that, in the future, large randomized trials should investigate the ability of antihypertensive agents to suppress the morning BP surge.[45] Later, larger studies in more diverse populations exposed an increased risk for renal disease[46]

and even death[47] associated with a morning blood pressure rise. However, a relationship between morning BP surge and cardiovascular outcomes has been controversial.[48,49] A diminished surge in morning BP has been associated with a blunting in dipping pattern and with worse cardiovascular outcomes.[49] Importantly, there are no data showing that inhibiting this surge pharmacologically is of specific benefit to patients. The logical approach to treatment would be to prescribe an antihypertensive medication that is effective for 24 hours or longer, to provide target organ protection throughout the dosing interval. Controlling morning BP is a reasonable therapeutic target, if assisted by the use of ABPM and home BP, as well as appropriate timing of medications that mirror the circadian variation of both the renin-angiotensin and the sympathetic nervous systems.

PROGNOSTIC VALUE OF AMBULATORY BLOOD PRESSURE

Data from both prospective clinical and population-based studies show that ambulatory BP predicts the risk for a cardiovascular event, after adjustment for conventional (office) BP. A now-historic prospective study by Perloff and associates[50] established that cardiovascular risk was greater in patients with higher daytime ambulatory BP than in those with lower daytime value, independent of the office BP values. Subsequent outcomes-based studies have shown that ambulatory BP is superior to conventional clinic BP measurements in predicting adverse cardiovascular clinical events.[4,5,29,50-57] Of these, two considered the prognostic value of ambulatory BP in the general population.[51,52] In both studies, after adjustment for gender, age, smoking status, baseline clinic BP, and antihypertensive treatment, ambulatory BP proved to be a superior predictor of cardiovascular death compared with clinic BP. In addition, the BP at night and the ambulatory SBPs were the best predictors of cardiovascular death. Similar results were also observed in the Dublin outcome study that followed over 5000 patients for 5 years.[57]

In most studies, ambulatory BP data used to predict cardiovascular endpoints were recorded in untreated subjects participating in clinical trials while receiving placebo during the run-in phase. The absence of data on the prognostic value of ambulatory BP in patients with treated hypertension was addressed in the Office versus Ambulatory Blood Pressure Study.[55] This study followed 1963 patients for a median of 5 years, during which 157 patients had documented new cardiovascular events. After adjustment for age, sex, body mass index, use of lipid-lowering drugs, and a history of cardiovascular events, higher 24-hour mean ambulatory SBPs and DBPs were independent risk factors for new cardiovascular events. Even after adjusting for clinic BP, 24-hour and daytime SBP and DBP predicted outcomes. Patients with a 24-hour mean ambulatory SBP of less than 135 mm Hg had higher cardiovascular risk than those with a mean value of 135 mm Hg or higher. This was true especially when the patients were classified according to their clinic BPs.

USE OF AMBULATORY BLOOD PRESSURE MONITORING IN THE MANAGEMENT OF HYPERTENSION

Diagnosis of hypertension and the decision to initiate drug treatment are traditionally based on office BP measurements. Prospective cohort studies clearly show that the prognostic capabilities of office BP, however, are inferior to ambulatory BP.[58-60] Most notably, clinic BP measurements correlate poorly with 24-hour mean ambulatory BP, especially in men both before and during antihypertensive treatment.[59] The

Spanish ABPM Registry, which has incorporated 190,000 clinical records of people with hypertension, shows that the use of ABPM in clinical practice may double the rates of hypertension control.[61] The findings of both the Office versus Ambulatory Blood Pressure Study[55] and the Spanish registry[61] support more extensive utilization of ABPM in clinical practice.[61] ABPM has potential advantages, but its use needs to be considered in relation to the cost of the equipment and data evaluation, poor insurance coverage in most countries, information gained, additional consultations required, and possible inconvenience to the patient. A developed algorithm for the use of self-monitoring of BP and ABPM may help to minimize the excessive use of ABPM while identifying patients who would benefit from antihypertensive therapy (Fig. 11.2).[62]

Self-monitoring of BP may restrict the use of ABPM to those patients in whom there is a large disparity between clinic measurements and out-of-clinic values. Ideally, patients should measure their BP twice daily at home and/or while at work over a minimum of a 1-week period. In 2015, for the first time, the U.S. Preventive Services Task Force recommended the use of ABPM to confirm the diagnosis of hypertension in people with an elevated office BP.[60] The National Clinical Guideline Centre in the United Kingdom had already issued a similar recommendation in 2011 to use ABPM to diagnose hypertension in any person with an elevated office blood pressure and also to consider its use for therapeutic monitoring.[63] Other societies, including, the World Health Organization,[64] British Hypertension Society,[65] American Heart Association,[36] American Society of Hypertension,[66] and European Society of Hypertension,[67] have not recommended the use of ABPM to diagnose hypertension in all patients but in many instances

these groups do not have recent updates to their guidelines. In most guidelines the indications for ABPM had been limited to: ruling out white-coat hypertension, ascertaining resistant hypertension, evaluating episodic hypotension or hypertension and assessing dipping patterns. The major impediments to recommending ABPM for all patients with an elevated BP have been costs, coverage and practical concerns of device acquisition and maintenance. The recent U.S. Preventive Services Task Force recommendations[60] now clearly encourage practitioners to look beyond these logistic difficulties and develop programs and protocols for ABPM to be disseminated more into the hypertension and cardiovascular communities.

Impact of Ambulatory Blood Pressure Monitoring on Advances in Treatment

In addition to its use in everyday clinical practice for the identification of patients at risk, ABPM has become the gold standard for the evaluation of drug therapy in clinical trials. ABPM reveals important differences between antihypertensive agents, most notably regarding duration of action; many commonly used once-daily antihypertensive drugs were determined to provide suboptimal control toward the end of the dosing interval.[59] With once-daily dosing and drug administration in the morning on arising to encourage patient adherence to therapy, incomplete BP control at the end of the dosing interval could actually coincide with the time of the greatest risk of an acute cardiovascular event.

To illustrate the utility of ABPM to differentiate antihypertensive therapies, we evaluated two angiotensin receptor blockers (ARB): valsartan, an ARB with a half-life of about 7 hours, versus telmisartan, an ARB with a half-life of 24 hours. The study proved that telmisartan provided better BP control at the end of the once-daily dosing interval.[68] A clear benefit of ABPM in clinical trials is its enhanced reproducibility compared with office BP measurements; this leads to improved precision in evaluating drug effects, and a smaller number of subjects, especially when comparisons are made between two drugs.

Analyses of Ambulatory Blood Pressure Data in Antihypertensive Drug Trials

Data from ambulatory BP studies in hypertension trials may be analyzed in a number of ways. Despite numerous attempts by different committees across the globe, a consensus regarding a single superior method of analysis for ABPM data has never been reached. The use of 24-hour means, daytime and nighttime means (or preferably awake and sleep values), BP loads (the proportion of values above a cutoff value during wakefulness [typically >140/90 mm Hg] or sleep [typically >120/80 mm Hg] divided by the total number of BP readings), area under the 24-hour BP curve, and smoothing techniques designed to remove some of the variability from the raw BP data analysis are among the most popularly used methods of analysis.[69,70]

Features of any method of analysis for ambulatory BP data should include the statistical ease of calculation, clinical relevance of the measure, and relationship of the parameter to the hypertensive disease process. Many of these analytic methods meet all of these criteria. For example, the 24-hour mean BP remains an important parameter for evaluation in antihypertensive drug trials because it appears to be a strong predictor of hypertensive target organ disease, is easy to calculate, uses all of the ambulatory BP data, and, as previously mentioned, is remarkably reproducible in both short-term and long-term studies.[71-73]

The BP load has been used as a simple method of analysis in evaluating the effects of antihypertensive drugs. BP load has been defined in our laboratory as the percentage of BPs

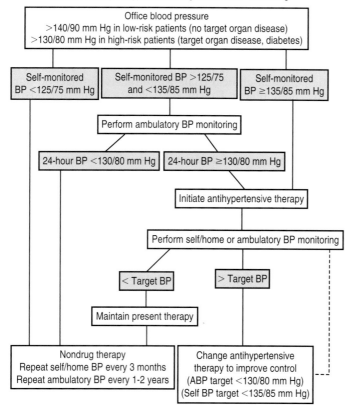

American Society of Hypertension Algorithm for BP Monitering

Office blood pressure
>140/90 mm Hg in low-risk patients (no target organ disease)
>130/80 mm Hg in high-risk patients (target organ disease, diabetes)

- Self-monitored BP <125/75 mm Hg
- Self-monitored BP >125/75 and <135/85 mm Hg
- Self-monitored BP ≥135/85 mm Hg

Perform ambulatory BP monitoring

- 24-hour BP <130/80 mm Hg
- 24-hour BP ≥130/80 mm Hg

Initiate antihypertensive therapy

Perform self/home or ambulatory BP monitoring

- < Target BP → Maintain present therapy
- > Target BP

Nondrug therapy
Repeat self/home BP every 3 months
Repeat ambulatory BP every 1-2 years

Change antihypertensive therapy to improve control
(ABP target <130/80 mm Hg)
(Self BP target <135/85 mm Hg)

FIG. 11.2 Role of ambulatory and home blood pressure monitoring in clinical practice. *ABP,* Ambulatory blood pressure; *BP,* blood pressure. (*Adapted from Pickering TG, White WB. ASH Position Paper: When and how to use self (home) and ambulatory blood pressure monitoring. J Clin Hypertens [Greenwich]. 2008;10:850-856.*)

exceeding 140/90 mm Hg while the patient is awake, plus the percentage of BPs exceeding 120/80 mm Hg during sleep.[74] A number of years ago, we evaluated the relationship between this BP load and cardiac target organ indices in previously untreated hypertensives. At a 40% DBP load, the prevalence of LVH was nearly 80%, but below a 40% DBP load, it was only about 8%. In contrast, the office BP and even the 24-hour average BP were not as discriminating in predicting LVH in this group of previously untreated patients. Thus, in most stage 1 hypertensive patients, one would desire a low BP load (conservatively, <30%), during treatment with antihypertensive drug therapy.

In studies in which the patient population has a greater range in BP, the proportional (or percentage) BP load becomes unhelpful. Because the upper limit of the BP load is 100%, this value may represent a substantial number of individuals with broad ranges of high stage 2 hypertension. To overcome this problem, we devised a method to integrate the area under the ambulatory BP curve and relate its values to predicting hemodynamic indices in untreated essential hypertensives.[75] Areas under the BP curve (AUC) were computed separately for periods of wakefulness and sleep, and combined to form the 24-hour area under the BP curve. Threshold values were used to calculate AUC such as 135 or 140 mm Hg systolic while awake and 85 or 90 mm Hg diastolic while awake. Values during sleep were reduced to 115 and 120 mm Hg systolic and 75 and 80 mm Hg diastolic. This method allowed simplification of the data processing and improved the diagnostic performance of the ABPM.

Smoothing of ambulatory BP data may be used to aid in the identification of the peak and trough effects of an antihypertensive drug.[69] The extent of variability in an individual's BP curve may be large because of both mental and physical activity; thus evaluating the peak antihypertensive effect of a short- or intermediate-acting drug may be difficult. Other than the benefits associated with examining pharmacodynamic effects of new antihypertensive drugs, data and curve smoothing for 24-hour BP monitoring appear to have little clinical relevance. Furthermore, editing protocols are not uniform in the literature and missing data may alter the balance of mean values for shorter periods of time. To avoid excessive data reduction in a clinical trial, one statistical expert suggested that data smoothing should be performed on individual BP profiles rather than on group means.[76]

USEFUL SITUATIONS FOR AMBULATORY BLOOD PRESSURE MONITORING IN ANTIHYPERTENSIVE DRUG TRIALS

Utility of Ambulatory Blood Pressure Monitoring in Dose-Finding Studies

Since the early 1990s, numerous studies have been performed with ABPM to fully assess the efficacy of a wide range of doses of new antihypertensive agents. The advantage of ABPM in dose-finding studies is related in part to the improved statistical power to show differences among the treatment groups compared with clinic pressures. Examples are shown in the following section.

Eprosartan

To determine the dose responsiveness of the then-new angiotensin II receptor antagonist eprosartan during phase II of development, the drug was studied at doses of 100, 200, 300, and 400 mg daily (in twice-daily divided doses) using ABPM.[77] Compared with placebo, only the 400-mg daily dose showed consistently significant reductions in ambulatory systolic and diastolic BP. These findings led to the use of

higher doses in the phase III clinical development program and a larger trial using 600 and 1200 mg once daily versus placebo.[77] The trough BP (last 4 hours of the dosing period) changes from baseline were significantly greater than placebo for both doses of the drug, with a trend for greater reductions at 1200 mg versus 600 mg once daily. When assessing the changes from baseline using clinic BPs, the differences for 1200 mg versus 600 mg once daily against placebo were not significant.

Eplerenone

The efficacy of a novel selective aldosterone receptor antagonist, eplerenone, was studied in 417 patients with essential hypertension using a multicenter, randomized, placebo-controlled design.[78] In this trial, the drug was assessed using either a once daily dosing regimen of 50, 100, or 400 mg or a twice-daily dosing regimen of 25, 50, or 200 mg. Clinic and ambulatory BPs were compared with both baseline values and with the effects of placebo. As shown in Fig. 11.3, there was a dose-related reduction in SBP at trough for both clinic and ambulatory BP (similar results were seen for the changes in DBP). Twice daily dosing of eplerenone led to greater reductions in BP compared with the once-daily dosing regimen, but these differences were not statistically significant.

Utility of Ambulatory Blood Pressure Monitoring in Clinical Comparator Trials

ABPM has been very helpful in comparing antihypertensive drugs, especially when assessing their duration of action. There are numerous examples in the literature that now illustrate this benefit, including the superiority of ambulatory BP over clinic BP in assessing the trough to peak ratio of various agents.[69]

Comparisons within the Same Class

In a now-classic multicenter study, Neutel and associates[70] compared the beta-blockers bisoprolol and atenolol in 606 patients using both clinic and ambulatory BPs. Following therapy, trough BP in the clinic was reduced 12/12 mm Hg by bisoprolol and 11/12 mm Hg by atenolol. Although these changes were significantly different from baseline, they were not significantly different between drugs. In contrast, daytime systolic and diastolic BPs (6 AM to 10 PM) and the last 4 hours of the dosing interval (6 AM to 10 PM) were lowered to a significantly greater extent by bisoprolol than by atenolol. This

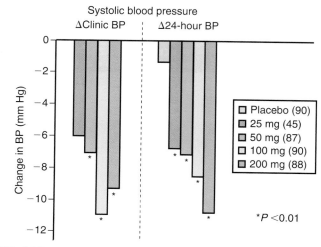

FIG. 11.3 Changes from baseline in the clinic and ambulatory BP with eplerenone. *(Data from White WB, Carr AA, Krause S, et al. Assessment of the novel selective aldosterone blocker eplerenone using ambulatory and clinical blood pressure in patients with systemic hypertension. Am J Cardiol. 2003;92:38-42.)*

finding was present whether the assessment was made by examination of the overall means, area under the curve, or BP loads. These data demonstrated that despite no difference in office BPs, bisoprolol had significant differences in efficacy and duration of action compared with atenolol when assessed by 24-hour BP monitoring.

More recently, the antihypertensive efficacy of the selective angiotensin II receptor antagonists azilsartan medoxomil, valsartan, and olmesartan medoxomil were compared with placebo in randomized, parallel group, double-blind trial of 1291 patients with stages I and II hypertension.[71] After 2 to 3 weeks of single-blind placebo treatment, patients were randomized to receive azilsartan medoxomil at either 40 or 80 mg, valsartan 320 mg, olmesartan 40 mg, or placebo once daily. Based on ambulatory SBP measurements, the reductions in BP were significantly greater with azilsartan 80 mg daily compared with both other angiotensin receptor blockers (Table 11.1). The ability of ABPM to reveal small but statistically significant changes between treatment groups is most likely related to the lower variance that occurs with repeated ambulatory BP studies compared with repeated clinic BPs.[27,32,69]

Comparisons of Drugs Across Different Classes

In a study performed by Lacourcière and coworkers[72] in Canada, the angiotensin II receptor blocker telmisartan (doses of 40 to 120 mg once daily) was compared with the long-acting calcium antagonist amlodipine (5 to 10 mg once daily) in a clinical trial that used 24-hour ABPM at baseline and following 12 weeks of double-blind treatment. Although these agents have similar plasma half-lives (>24 hours), they have entirely different mechanisms of action. This bears relevance because it is known that as BP and heart rate fall during sleep, plasma renin activity gradually increases. In the morning upon awakening, the sympathetic nervous system is activated, which enhances renin secretion from the juxtaglomerular apparatus in the kidney. Thus the renin-angiotensin-aldosterone system is further activated in the early morning upon awakening, increasing the contribution of angiotensin to the postawakening surge in BP.[79]

Both amlodipine and telmisartan lowered clinic BP to similar extents at the end of the dosing period.[72] However, reductions in ambulatory diastolic BP with telmisartan were greater than those with amlodipine during the nighttime, as well as during the last 4 hours of the dosing interval. In addition, the ambulatory BP control rates (24-hour diastolic BP <85 mm Hg) were higher following telmisartan treatment (71%) than following amlodipine (55%). Thus these findings serve

as additional data that demonstrate the improved ability of ABPM to discern pharmacodynamic changes between two drugs with relatively similar pharmacokinetic profiles.

Use of Ambulatory Blood Pressure Monitoring to Assess the Effects of Chronotherapeutic Agents

In general, chronotherapeutics attempt to match the effects of a drug to the timing of the disease being treated or prevented.[77,78,80] In the case of hypertension and coronary heart disease, this is clinically relevant because BP and heart rate have distinct, reproducible circadian rhythms. In most people, the BP and heart rate are lowest during sleep and highest during the day, particularly in the early morning hours after awakening. Most cardiovascular diseases, including myocardial infarction, angina, myocardial ischemia, stroke, cardiovascular death, and atrial fibrillation have circadian patterns that are all characterized by the highest incidences in the early morning hours.[40,80]

Timing of Drug Administration

The approach for the chronotherapeutic treatment of hypertension and angina pectoris differs from conventional "homeostatic" treatments that deliver medication to achieve a constant effect, regardless of the circadian rhythm of BP. Several authors have made attempts to alter the effects of conventional drugs by dosing them before sleep versus upon arising.[81-89] In one of these studies[86] ABPM and actigraphy were used to prospectively evaluate the effect of time of dosing of antihypertensives in more than 2000 patients. Subjects administered medication at bedtime showed significantly lower mean sleep-time BPs, a reduced prevalence of nondipping (34% versus 62%; $p < 0.001$), and a higher prevalence of controlled ambulatory BPs (62% versus 53%; $p < 0.001$). After a median follow-up of 5.6 years, subjects on one or more antihypertensive medication(s) at bedtime exhibited a significantly lower relative risk of total cardiovascular events than those on an antihypertensive drug dosed in the morning (odds ratio, 0.39; 95% confidence interval [CI], 0.29-0.51) because of a smaller number of events (187 versus 68; $p < 0.001$). These data suggest that nocturnal delivery of BP-lowering medications, compared with conventional morning antihypertensive therapy, may reduce cardiovascular morbidity. Another large study in Spain, the MAPEC (Monitorización Ambulatoria para Predicción de Eventos Cardiovasculares) study, randomized 2156 subjects to either taking all of their antihypertensive medications upon awakening or, to taking at least one of

TABLE 11.1 Changes From Baseline in 24-Hour Mean Ambulatory Systolic Blood Pressure on Angiotensin Receptor Blockers Dosed Once Daily

	PLACEBO n = 134	AZILSARTAN 40 MG n = 237	AZILSARTAN 80 MG n = 229	VALSARTAN 320 MG n = 234	OLMESARTAN 40 MG N = 254
Baseline SBP, mmHg (SEM)	144.3 (0.9)	144.4 (0.6)	144.6 (0.7)	146.3 (0.7)	144.4 (0.6)
Change from baseline, mmHg (SEM)	−0.3 (0.9)	−13.4 (0.7)	−14.5 (0.7)	−10.2 (0.7)	−12.0 (0.7)
Mean difference vs. placebo (95% CI)		−13.2 (−15.5, −10.9)	−14.3 (−16.5, −12.0)	−10.0 (−12.2, −7.7)	−11.7 (−14.0, −9.5)
p value vs. placebo		<0.001[a]	<0.001[a]	<0.001[a]	<0.001[a]
Mean difference vs. olmesartan (95% CI)		−1.4 (−3.3, 0.5)	−2.5 (−4.4, −0.6)		
p value vs. olmesartan		0.14	0.009[a]		
Mean difference vs. valsartan (95% CI)		−3.5 (−5.1, −1.3)	−4.3 (−6.3, −2.4)		
p value vs. valsartan		<0.001[a]	<0.001[a]		

[a]Indicates significant difference at $p < 0.05$ level; values are expressed as least-squares mean from baseline and standard error of the mean (SEM).
CI, Confidence interval; SBP, systolic blood pressure.
(Data from White WB, Weber MA, Sica D, et al. Effects of the angiotensin receptor blocker azilsartan medoxomil versus olmesartan and valsartan on ambulatory and clinic blood pressure in patients with stages 1 and 2 hypertension. Hypertension. 2011;57:413-420.)

them at bedtime.[86] The group taking at least one medication at bedtime was found to have improvement in ambulatory BP control, dipping pattern and cardiovascular risk profile at a median follow-up of 5.6 years.

Use of Ambulatory Blood Pressure Monitoring in Device Therapy Studies

Over the past decade, renal sympathetic denervation devices have been developed to treat severe, difficult to control, drug-resistant hypertension. Multiple devices and technical procedures have been designed to ablate the sympathetic nerves supplying the renal arteries using radiofrequency catheters thereby decreasing catecholamine mediated elevation in BP.[90,91] Early on, unblinded and nonrandomized clinical trials showed remarkable reductions in office systolic BP associated with this therapy and created great enthusiasm for the field. However, ambulatory BP changes following renal denervation were less than one-third of those seen using clinic BP measurements at 3 and 6 months probably because of the removal of observer bias.[90,91] The SYMPLICITY

HTN-3[92] trial was the first randomized, sham-controlled, and blinded clinical trial using a renal nerve ablation catheter. The study evaluated the effects of renal denervation in 535 severely hypertensive patients on a mean of five antihypertensive drugs using ambulatory systolic BP at a time point of 6 months. The results of the study did not demonstrate a statistically significant difference in ambulatory[92] or nocturnal[93] systolic BPs between the denervation and sham groups. The discrepancy between open label and randomized blinded trials are complex and may have been caused by study design, the catheter itself, and changes in patient behavior during the trial. In addition, results for ambulatory BP were quite consistent with the findings for the clinic BP measurements in SYMPLICITY HTN-3.[90]

In a metaanalysis of 346 subjects who underwent renal denervation from German registry studies,[90] it was found that renal denervation significantly decreased ambulatory BP in patients with true resistant hypertension, but not in those with pseudo-resistant hypertension (24-hour mean systolic BP was <130 mm Hg). As depicted in Fig. 11.4, this difference in response between these two groups could not be detected

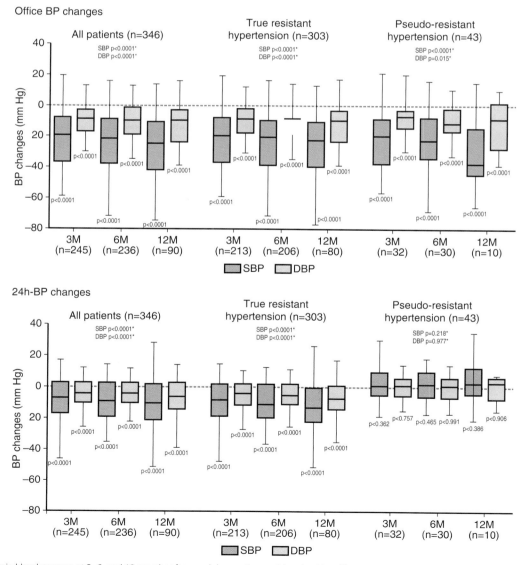

FIG. 11.4 Changes in blood pressure at 3, 6, and 12 months after renal denervation as determined by office measurements and 24h ambulatory monitoring. *DBP*, Diastolic blood pressure; *SBP*, systolic blood pressure. Whiskers span from 5th to 95th percentile. *p-value computed using linear mixed-effects models comparing the specified time point to baseline values (*Data from Mahfoud F, Ukena C, Schmieder RE, et al. Ambulatory blood pressure changes after renal sympathetic denervation in patients with resistant hypertension.* Circulation. 2013;128:132-140).

based solely on office BP. These findings highlight the importance of thorough characterization of study participants before randomization in clinical trials.

CONCLUSIONS

Data generated by ABPM have established that, even after adjustment for well-known cardiac risk factors, there is a progressive increase in the risk of cardiovascular morbidity and mortality with elevated 24-hour, daytime, and nighttime BPs. Studies from the International Database of Ambulatory Monitoring and Cardiovascular Outcomes (IDACO) have shown the importance of the early morning BP surge on hypertensive target organ involvement as well as cardiovascular events. The technique of ambulatory BP measurements has become widely adopted to identify effective therapeutic options that provide BP control throughout the dosing interval.

In the primary care setting, the contribution of ABPM to the management of patients with hypertension is increasingly being acknowledged. Although this technology was considered "experimental" for a very long time between the 1980s and 2000s, this has changed in the United States with improved insurance coverage for performing ABPM in specific patients and support for its use in certain subgroups of hypertensive patients by a number of consensus groups, including the Joint National Committee on Prevention, Detection, Evaluation, and Treatment of High Blood Pressure; the Council on High Blood Pressure Research of the American Heart Association; and the American Society of Hypertension. Ambulatory BP monitoring is now the recognized gold standard for the evaluation of elevated office BP by the U.S. Preventive Services Task Force[60] and the National Clinical Guideline Centre in the United Kingdom.[63]

References

1. White WB. Circadian variation of blood pressure: clinical relevance and implications for cardiovascular chronotherapeutics. *Blood Press Monitor.* 1997;2:47-51.
2. Perloff D, Sokolow M, Cowan RM, Juster RP. Prognostic value of ambulatory blood pressure measurements: further analyses. *J Hypertens. Suppl.* 1989;7:S3-S10.
3. Verdecchia P, Angeli F, Cavallini C. Ambulatory blood pressure for cardiovascular risk stratification. *Circulation.* 2007;115:2091-2093.
4. Verdecchia P, Porcellati C, Schillaci G, et al. Ambulatory blood pressure. An independent predictor of prognosis in essential hypertension. *Hypertension.* 1994;24:793-801.
5. Staessen JA, Thijs L, Fagard R, et al. Predicting cardiovascular risk using conventional vs ambulatory blood pressure in older patients with systolic hypertension. Systolic Hypertension in Europe Trial Investigators. *JAMA.* 1999;282:539-546.
6. Sundberg S, Kohvakka A, Gordin A. Rapid reversal of circadian blood pressure rhythm in shift workers. *J Hypertens.* 1988;6:393-396.
7. Sternberg H, Rosenthal T, Shamiss A, Green M. Altered circadian rhythm of blood pressure in shift workers. *J Hum Hypertens.* 1995;9:349-953.
8. Kitamura T, Onishi K, Dohi K, et al. Circadian rhythm of blood pressure is transformed from a dipper to a non-dipper pattern in shift workers with hypertension. *J Hum Hypertens.* 2002;16:193-197.
9. Lo SH, Liau CS, Hwang JS, Wang JD. Dynamic blood pressure changes and recovery under different work shifts in young women. *Am J Hypertens.* 2008;21:759-764.
10. Lajoie P, Aronson KJ, Day A, Tranmer J. A cross-sectional study of shift work, sleep quality and cardiometabolic risk in female hospital employees. *BMJ open.* 2015;5:e007327.
11. De Bacquer D, Van Risseghem M, Clays E, Kittel F, De Backer G, Braeckman L. Rotating shift work and the metabolic syndrome: a prospective study. *Int J Epidemiol.* 2009;38:848-854.
12. Sookoian S, Gemma C, Fernandez Gianotti T, et al. Effects of rotating shift work on biomarkers of metabolic syndrome and inflammation. *J Intern Med.* 2007;261:285-292.
13. Karlsson B, Knutsson A, Lindahl B. Is there an association between shift work and having a metabolic syndrome? Results from a population based study of 27,485 people. *Occup Environ Med.* 2001;58:747-752.
14. White WB, Mansoor GA, Tendler BE, Anwar YA. Nocturnal blood pressure epidemiology, determinants, and effects of antihypertensive therapy. *Blood Press Monitor.* 1998;3:43-51.
15. Di Iorio A, Marini E, Lupinetti M, Zito M, Abate G. Blood pressure rhythm and prevalence of vascular events in hypertensive subjects. *Age Ageing.* 1999;28:23-28.
16. Muntner P, Lewis CE, Diaz KM, et al. Racial differences in abnormal ambulatory blood pressure monitoring measures: Results from the Coronary Artery Risk Development in Young Adults (CARDIA) study. *Am J Hypertens.* 2015;28:640-648.
17. Sherwood A, Thurston R, Steffen P, Blumenthal JA, Waugh RA, Hinderliter AL. Blunted nighttime blood pressure dipping in postmenopausal women. *Am J Hypertens.* 2001;14:749-754.
18. O'Brien E, Sheridan J, O'Malley K. Dippers and non-dippers. *Lancet.* 1988;2:397.
19. Cuspidi C, Giudici V, Negri F, Sala C. Nocturnal nondipping and left ventricular hypertrophy in hypertension: an updated review. *Expert Rev Cardiovasc Ther.* 2010;8:781-792.
20. Vasunta RL, Kesaniemi YA, Ylitalo A, Ukkola O. Nondipping pattern and carotid atherosclerosis in a middle-aged population: OPERA Study. *Am J Hypertens.* 2012;25:60-66.
21. de la Sierra A, Gorostidi M, Banegas JR, Segura J, de la Cruz JJ, Ruilope LM. Nocturnal hypertension or nondipping: which is better associated with the cardiovascular risk profile? *Am J Hypertens.* 2014;27:680-687.
22. Fan HQ, Li Y, Thijs L, et al. Prognostic value of isolated nocturnal hypertension on ambulatory measurement in 8711 individuals from 10 populations. *J Hypertens.* 2010;28:2036-2045.
23. Gorostidi M, Sobrino J, Segura J, et al. Ambulatory blood pressure monitoring in hypertensive patients with high cardiovascular risk: a cross-sectional analysis of a 20,000-patient database in Spain. *J Hypertens.* 2007;25:977-984.
24. de la Sierra A, Segura J, Gorostidi M, Banegas JR, de la Cruz JJ, Ruilope LM. Diurnal blood pressure variation, risk categories and antihypertensive treatment. *Hypertens Res.* 2010;33:767-771.
25. Pickering TG, Shimbo D, Haas D. Ambulatory blood-pressure monitoring. *New Engl J Med.* 2006;354:2368-2374.
26. Cuspidi C, Macca G, Sampieri L, et al. Target organ damage and non-dipping pattern defined by two sessions of ambulatory blood pressure monitoring in recently diagnosed essential hypertensive patients. *J Hypertens.* 2001;19:1539-1545.
27. Verdecchia P. Prognostic value of ambulatory blood pressure: current evidence and clinical implications. *Hypertension.* 2000;35:844-851.
28. de la Sierra A, Redon J, Banegas JR, et al. Prevalence and factors associated with circadian blood pressure patterns in hypertensive patients. *Hypertension.* 2009;53:466-472.
29. Hermida RC, Ayala DE, Mojon A, Fernandez JR. Decreasing sleep-time blood pressure determined by ambulatory monitoring reduces cardiovascular risk. *J Am Coll Cardiol.* 2011;58:1165-1173.
30. White WB, Larocca GM. Improving the utility of the nocturnal hypertension definition by using absolute sleep blood pressure rather than the "dipping" proportion. *Am J Cardiol.* 2003;92:1439-1441.
31. Mochizuki Y, Okutani M, Donfeng Y, et al. Limited reproducibility of circadian variation in blood pressure dippers and nondippers. *Am J Hypertens.* 1998;11:403-409.
32. Omboni S, Parati G, Palatini P, et al. Reproducibility and clinical value of nocturnal hypotension: prospective evidence from the SAMPLE study. Study on Ambulatory Monitoring of Pressure and Lisinopril Evaluation. *J Hypertens.* 1998;16:733-738.
33. Androulakis E, Papageorgiou N, Chatzistamatiou E, Kallikazaros I, Stefanadis C, Tousoulis D. Improving the detection of preclinical organ damage in newly diagnosed hypertension: nocturnal hypertension versus non-dipping pattern. *J Hum Hypertens.* 2015;29:689-695.
34. Perez-Lloret S, Toblli JE, Cardinali DP, Malateste JC, Milei J. Nocturnal hypertension defined by fixed cut-off limits is a better predictor of left ventricular hypertrophy than non-dipping. *Int J Cardiol.* 2008;127:387-389.
35. Pickering T. Recommendations for the use of home (self) and ambulatory blood pressure monitoring. American Society of Hypertension Ad Hoc Panel. *Am J Hypertens.* 1996;9:1-11.
36. Pickering TG, Hall JE, Appel LJ, et al. Recommendations for blood pressure measurement in humans and experimental animals: part 1: blood pressure measurement in humans: a statement for professionals from the Subcommittee of Professional and Public Education of the American Heart Association Council on High Blood Pressure Research. *Circulation.* 2005;111:697-716.
37. O'Brien E, Parati G, Stergiou G, et al. European Society of Hypertension position paper on ambulatory blood pressure monitoring. *J Hypertens.* 2013;31:1731-1768.
38. Parati G, Stergiou G, O'Brien E, et al. European Society of Hypertension practice guidelines for ambulatory blood pressure monitoring. *J Hypertens.* 2014;32:1359-1366.
39. Kario K, White WB. Early morning hypertension: what does it contribute to overall cardiovascular risk assessment? *JASH.* 2008;2:397-402.
40. White WB. Cardiovascular risk and therapeutic intervention for the early morning surge in blood pressure and heart rate. *Blood Press Monitor.* 2001;6:63-72.
41. Wroe SJ, Sandercock P, Bamford J, Dennis M, Slattery J, Warlow C. Diurnal variation in incidence of stroke: Oxfordshire community stroke project. *BMJ.* 1992;304:155-157.
42. Elliott WJ. Circadian variation in the timing of stroke onset: a meta-analysis. *Stroke.* 1998;29:992-996.
43. Casetta I, Granieri E, Portaluppi F, Manfredini R. Circadian variability in hemorrhagic stroke. *JAMA.* 2002;287:1266-1267.
44. Gallerani M, Manfredini R, Ricci L, et al. Chronobiological aspects of acute cerebrovascular diseases. *Acta Neurol Scand.* 1993;87:482-487.
45. Kario K, Pickering TG, Umeda Y, et al. Morning surge in blood pressure as a predictor of silent and clinical cerebrovascular disease in elderly hypertensives: a prospective study. *Circulation.* 2003;107:1401-1406.
46. Turak O, Afsar B, Siriopol D, et al. Morning blood pressure surge as a predictor of development of chronic kidney disease. *J Clin Hypertens (Greenwich, Conn).* 2016;18:444-448.
47. Amodeo C, Guimaraes GG, Picotti JC, et al. Morning blood pressure surge is associated with death in hypertensive patients. *Blood Press Monitor.* 2014;19:199-202.
48. Bombelli M, Fodri D, Toso E, et al. Relationship among morning blood pressure surge, 24-hour blood pressure variability, and cardiovascular outcomes in a white population. *Hypertension.* 2014;64:943-950.
49. Verdecchia P, Angeli F, Mazzotta G, et al. Day-night dip and early-morning surge in blood pressure in hypertension: prognostic implications. *Hypertension.* 2012;60:34-42.
50. Perloff D, Sokolow M, Cowan R. The prognostic value of ambulatory blood pressures. *JAMA.* 1983;249:2792.
51. Fagard RH, Staessen JA, Thijs L, et al. Response to antihypertensive therapy in older patients with sustained and nonsustained systolic hypertension. Systolic Hypertension in Europe (Syst-Eur) Trial Investigators. *Circulation.* 2000;102:1139-1144.
52. Imai Y, Ohkubo T, Sakuma M, et al. Predictive power of screening blood pressure, ambulatory blood pressure and blood pressure measured at home for overall and cardiovascular mortality: a prospective observation in a cohort from Ohasama, northern Japan. *Blood Press Monitor.* 1996;1:251-254.
53. Khattar RS, Swales JD, Banfield A, Dore C, Senior R, Lahiri A. Prediction of coronary and cerebrovascular morbidity and mortality by direct continuous ambulatory blood pressure monitoring in essential hypertension. *Circulation.* 1999;100:1071-1076.
54. Redon J, Campos C, Narciso ML, Rodicio JL, Pascual JM, Ruilope LM. Prognostic value of ambulatory blood pressure monitoring in refractory hypertension: a prospective study. *Hypertension.* 1998;31:712-718.
55. Clement DL, De Buyzere ML, De Bacquer DA, et al. Prognostic value of ambulatory blood-pressure recordings in patients with treated hypertension. *New Engl J Med.* 2003;348:2407-2415.
56. Sega R, Facchetti R, Bombelli M, et al. Prognostic value of ambulatory and home blood pressures compared with office blood pressure in the general population: follow-up results from the Pressioni Arteriose Monitorate e Loro Associazioni (PAMELA) study. *Circulation.* 2005;111:1777-1783.
57. Dolan E, Stanton A, Thijs L, et al. Superiority of ambulatory over clinic blood pressure measurement in predicting mortality: the Dublin outcome study. *Hypertension.* 2005;46:156-161.
58. White WB. Ambulatory blood-pressure monitoring in clinical practice. *New Engl J Med.* 2003;348:2377-2378.
59. Neutel JM. The importance of 24-h blood pressure control. *Blood Press Monitor.* 2001;6:9-16.

60. Piper MA, Evans CV, Burda BU, Margolis KL, O'Connor E, Whitlock EP. Diagnostic and predictive accuracy of blood pressure screening methods with consideration of rescreening intervals: a systematic review for the U.S. Preventive Services Task Force. *Ann Intern Med.* 2015;162:192-204.

61. Gorostidi M, Banegas JR, de la Sierra A, Vinyoles E, Segura J, Ruilope LM. Ambulatory blood pressure monitoring in daily clinical practice—the Spanish ABPM Registry experience. *Eur J Clin Invest.* 2016;46:92-98.

62. Pickering TG, White WB. ASH Position Paper: home and ambulatory blood pressure monitoring. When and how to use self (home) and ambulatory blood pressure monitoring. *J Clin Hypertens (Greenwich, Conn).* 2008;10:850-855.

63. Hypertension: The Clinical Management of Primary Hypertension in Adults: Update of Clinical Guidelines 18 and 34. London: National Clinical Guideline Centre; 2011.

64. 1999 World Health Organization-International Society of Hypertension Guidelines for the Management of Hypertension. Guidelines Subcommittee. *J Hypertens.* 1999;17:151-183.

65. Williams B, Poulter NR, Brown MJ, et al. Guidelines for management of hypertension: report of the fourth working party of the British Hypertension Society, 2004-BHS IV. *J Hum Hypertens.* 2004;18:139-185.

66. Pickering TG, White WB, Giles TD, et al. When and how to use self (home) and ambulatory blood pressure monitoring. *J Clin Hypertens (Greenwich, Conn).* 2008;10:850-855.

67. Mancia G, Fagard R, Narkiewicz K, et al. 2013 ESH/ESC Guidelines for the management of arterial hypertension: the Task Force for the management of arterial hypertension of the European Society of Hypertension (ESH) and of the European Society of Cardiology (ESC). *J Hypertens.* 2013;31:1281-1357.

68. Bakris G. Comparison of telmisartan vs. valsartan in the treatment of mild to moderate hypertension using ambulatory blood pressure monitoring. *J Clin Hypertens (Greenwich, Conn).* 2002;4:26-31.

69. White WB, Malha L. Ambulatory blood pressure monitoring in clinical trials of drugs and devices. In: W.B. White, ed. *Blood Pressure Monitoring in Cardiovascular Medicine and Therapeutics.* 3rd ed. Totowa, NJ: Humana Press; 2016:371-394.

70. Neutel JM, Smith DH, Ram CV, et al. Application of ambulatory blood pressure monitoring in differentiating between antihypertensive agents. *Am J Med.* 1993;94:181-187.

71. White WB, Weber MA, Sica D, et al. Effects of the angiotensin receptor blocker azilsartan medoxomil versus olmesartan and valsartan on ambulatory and clinic blood pressure in patients with stages 1 and 2 hypertension. *Hypertension.* 2011;57:413-420.

72. Lacourciere Y, Lenis J, Orchard R, et al. A comparison of the efficacies and duration of action of the angiotensin II receptor blockers telmisartan and amlodipine. *Blood Press Monitor.* 1998;3:295-302.

73. White WB. A chronotherapeutic approach to the management of hypertension. *Am J Hypertens.* 1996;9:29s-33s.

74. White WB. Blood pressure load and target organ effects in patients with essential hypertension. *J Hypertens Suppl.* 1991;9:S39-41.

75. White WB, Lund-Johansen P, Weiss S, Omvik P, Indurkhya N. The relationships between casual and ambulatory blood pressure measurements and central hemodynamics in essential human hypertension. *J Hypertens.* 1994;12:1075-1081.

76. Dickson D, Hasford J. 24-hour blood pressure measurement in antihypertensive drug trials: data requirements and methods of analysis. *Stat Med.* 1992;11:2147-2158.

77. White WB, Anwar YA, Mansoor GA, Sica DA. Evaluation of the 24-hour blood pressure effects of eprosartan in patients with systemic hypertension. *Am J Hypertens.* 2001;14:1248-1255.

78. White WB, Carr AA, Krause S, Jordan R, Roniker B, Oigman W. Assessment of the novel selective aldosterone blocker eplerenone using ambulatory and clinical blood pressure in patients with systemic hypertension. *Am J Cardiol.* 2003;92:38-42.

79. Larochelle P. Circadian variation in blood pressure: dipper or nondipper. *J Clin Hypertens (Greenwich, Conn).* 2002;4:3-8.

80. Deedwania PC, Nelson JR. Pathophysiology of silent myocardial ischemia during daily life. Hemodynamic evaluation by simultaneous electrocardiographic and blood pressure monitoring. *Circulation.* 1990;82:1296-1304.

81. Palatini P, Racioppa A, Raule G, Zaninotto M, Penzo M, Pessina AC. Effect of timing of administration on the plasma ACE inhibitory activity and the antihypertensive effect of quinapril. *Clin Pharmacol Ther.* 1992;52:378-383.

82. Mengden T, Binswanger B, Gruene S. Dynamics of drug compliance and 24 hour blood pressure control of once daily morning vs evening amlodipine. *J Hypertens.* 1992;10:S136-S142.

83. Lemmer B. Differential effects of antihypertensive drugs on circadian rhythm in blood pressure from the chronobiological point of view. *Blood Press Monitor.* 1996;1:161-169.

84. White WB, Mansoor GA, Pickering TG, et al. Differential effects of morning and evening dosing of nisoldipine ER on circadian blood pressure and heart rate. *Am J Hypertens.* 1999;12:806-814.

85. Hermida RC, Ayala DE, Mojon A, et al. Comparison of the effects on ambulatory blood pressure of awakening versus bedtime administration of torasemide in essential hypertension. *Chronobiol Int.* 2008;25:950-970.

86. Hermida RC, Ayala DE, Mojon A, Fernandez JR. Influence of circadian time of hypertension treatment on cardiovascular risk: results of the MAPEC study. *Chronobiol Int.* 2010;27:1629-1651.

87. Hermida RC, Ayala DE, Mojon A, Fontao MJ, Fernandez JR. Chronotherapy with valsartan/hydrochlorothiazide combination in essential hypertension: improved sleep-time blood pressure control with bedtime dosing. *Chronobiol Int.* 2011;28:601-610.

88. Hermida RC, Rios MT, Crespo JJ, et al. Treatment-time regimen of hypertension medications significantly affects ambulatory blood pressure and clinical characteristics of patients with resistant hypertension. *Chronobiol Int.* 2013;30:192-206.

89. Moya A, Crespo JJ, Ayala DE, et al. Effects of time-of-day of hypertension treatment on ambulatory blood pressure and clinical characteristics of patients with type 2 diabetes. *Chronobiol Int.* 2013;30:116-131.

90. Mahfoud F, Ukena C, Schmieder RE, et al. Ambulatory blood pressure changes after renal sympathetic denervation in patients with resistant hypertension. *Circulation.* 2013;128:132-140.

91. Krum H, Schlaich M, Whitbourn R, et al. Catheter-based renal sympathetic denervation for resistant hypertension: a multicentre safety and proof-of-principle cohort study. *Lancet.* 2009;373:1275-1281.

92. Kandzari DE, Bhatt DL, Sobotka PA, et al. Catheter-based renal denervation for resistant hypertension: rationale and design of the SYMPLICITY HTN-3 trial. *Clin Cardiol.* 2012;35:528-535.

93. Bakris GL, Townsend RR, Liu M, et al. Impact of renal denervation on 24-hour ambulatory blood pressure: results from SYMPLICITY HTN-3. *J Am Coll Cardiol.* 2014;64:1071-1078.

White-Coat and Masked Hypertension

Gianfranco Parati and Juan Eugenio Ochoa

Traditionally, identification and management of hypertension has been based on office blood pressure (BP) measurements. However, after the introduction of methods to assess BP values under everyday life conditions, through either 24-hour ambulatory BP monitoring (ABPM) or home BP monitoring (HBPM), there has been growing awareness about the substantial discrepancies between information on BP provided by these "out-of-office BP" methodologies and conventional office BP (OBP) measurements. This has led to identification of four specific hypertension phenotypes, characterized by variable agreement or disagreement between OBP and out-of-office BP: (1) "true" or "sustained" normotension (SN) when both office and out-of-office BP are within currently defined normal limits; (2) "sustained" hypertension (SH), when both office and out-of-office BP are above normal limits; (3) "white-coat" hypertension (WCH), also defined as "isolated office hypertension," when office BP is elevated but out-of-office BP levels are within normal limits; and (4) "masked" hypertension (MH), when office is normal, but out-of-office BP levels are elevated. WCH and MH have for years been matter of debate, regarding their actual clinical significance. However, recent observational studies and metaanalyses[1,2] have indicated that both these BP phenotypes, compared with true or sustained normotension, are associated with some negative impact on cardiovascular prognosis, which in the case of MH may indeed be very similar to that of SH. However, in clinical practice these conditions have been often treated rather simplistically, ignoring important problems associated with their identification and management.

In its first part, this chapter will address the clinical significance and the initial diagnostic and therapeutic approach to white-coat and masked hypertension in untreated subjects. Because these discrepancies between office and out-of-office BP may continue to be present even after initiation of antihypertensive treatment, the second part of this chapter will address the persistence of an elevated OBP combined with normal out-of-office BP during treatment (so called "white-coat resistant" hypertension), as well as the condition characterized by the persistence of elevated out-of-office BP combined with normal OBP (defined as "masked uncontrolled" hypertension) in treated hypertensive patients.

WHITE-COAT HYPERTENSION AND MASKED HYPERTENSION IN UNTREATED INDIVIDUALS

Definition

White-Coat Hypertension

The BP rise associated with the alerting reaction during the medical visit, the so called "white-coat effect" (WCE)[3,4] represents a major problem associated with conventional BP measurement because it may lead to overestimation of initial BP levels. As a consequence of this, there will be a significant number of subjects with elevated BP values in the office but with persistently normal out-of-office BP levels (a condition defined as "white-coat" hypertension, WCH, or "isolated office" hypertension).[3,5,6] Traditionally, WCH has been defined as BP levels measured in the office persistently equal to or higher than 140 mm Hg for systolic and/or 90 mm Hg for diastolic, associated with persistently

normal out-of-office BP values either on ambulatory or on home BP monitoring.[7] Because BP levels are different during the day and night, and BP may be elevated during either of these periods or throughout the 24-hours, definition of normality in out-of-office BP levels must take into consideration the whole BP recording period. In recognition of this, as well as of the prevailing prognostic relevance of nighttime blood pressure levels over other components of ABPM, current European Society of Hypertension/European Society of Cardiology (ESH/ESC) hypertension guidelines[8] and ABPM guidelines have expanded the definition of WCH, requiring normality in ambulatory BP values during either daytime (i.e., <135/85 mm Hg); 24-hours (i.e., <130/80 mm Hg) and nighttime (i.e., <120/70 mm Hg) and also normality in average home BP levels (i.e., <135/85 mm Hg) when this methodology is used[9-11] (Fig. 12.1 and Table 12.1).

Masked Hypertension

The condition characterized by normal in-office but elevated out-of-office BP levels has been defined as masked hypertension. For its diagnosis, conventional BP in the office is considered to be normal if it is less than 140/90 mm Hg. However, when defining elevation in out-of-office BP, according to recent guidelines,[10,11] it is now considered inappropriate to exclude nocturnal BP and to focus on daytime BP levels only, as done in the past. Indeed, masked hypertension might be attributed not only to elevated daytime BP levels, but also to isolated nocturnal hypertension, which characterizes 7% of hypertensive individuals and can at present only be diagnosed with 24h ABPM. The definition of masked hypertension, has thus been extended to include elevation in ambulatory BP levels during either daytime (i.e., ≥135/85 mm Hg), and/or 24-hours (i.e., ≥130/80 mm Hg) and/or nighttime (i.e., ≥120/70 mm Hg); and/or elevation in average home BP levels (i.e., 135/85 mm Hg) (see Fig. 12.1 and Table 12.1).

Although, ABPM is currently considered the standard method for estimating out-of-office BP,[12] and for assessing daily life BP control in treated hypertensive patients,[8,10,13] it is not easily available everywhere and requires trained clinic staff and specialized equipment and software for its analysis.[9] Conversely, HBPM could be easily used on a routine basis, as recommended by recent ESH guidelines.[9] Indeed, when performed on a regular basis and following standardized protocols,[9] repeated BP measures obtained by patients at home offer the possibility to accurately and frequently assess out-of-office BP not only during a single day, but also over several days, weeks, or months in a usual life setting, thus providing a reliable assessment not only of the degree but also of the consistency of BP control over time.[9]

Besides, recent studies have indicated that HBPM is almost as reliable as ABPM in identifying WCH and MH[14-16] although it provides complementary rather than superimposable information on out-of-office BP as compared with ABPM. Based on its undeniable advantages, as well as on the predictive value of HBP values over and above the information provided by OBP, current hypertension guidelines recommend the extensive use of HBPM not only for the initial diagnostic approach to hypertension, but also and more specifically, for the long-term follow-up of treated hypertensive patients[8,9,17] as well as an additional useful method for

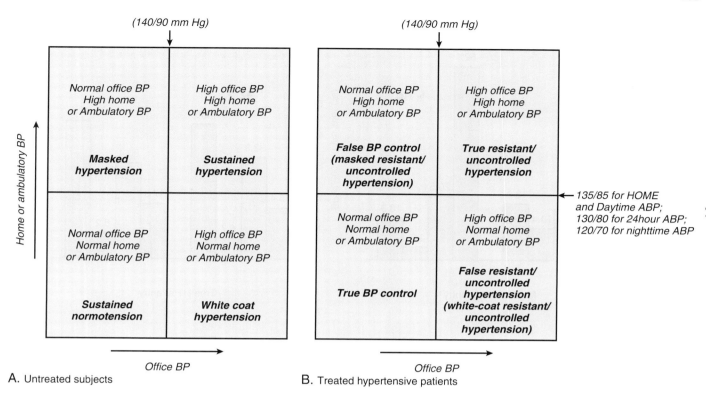

(140/90 mm Hg)   *(140/90 mm Hg)*

A. Untreated subjects   **B.** Treated hypertensive patients

FIG. 12.1 Classification of patients based on the comparison of conventional office and home ambulatory blood pressure (ABP) levels, separately in untreated individuals (A) and in treated hypertensive patients (B). Reference threshold values for ABP levels during daytime (i.e., 135/85 mm Hg); 24 hours (i.e., 130/80 mm Hg) and nighttime (i.e., 120/70 mm Hg) and for average threshold home BP levels (i.e., 135/85 mm Hg) are provided according to recent guidelines in O'Brien E, Parati G, Stergiou G, et al. European society of hypertension position paper on ambulatory blood pressure monitoring. *J Hypertens.* 2013;31:1731-1768 and Parati G, Stergiou G, O'Brien E, Asmar R, Beilin L, Bilo G, et al. European Society of Hypertension practice guidelines for ambulatory blood pressure monitoring. *J Hypertens.* 2014;32:1359-1366.

TABLE 12.1 Defining Criteria for White-Coat and Masked Hypertension

White-coat (or isolated office) hypertension	Untreated patients with elevated office blood pressure ≥140/90 mm Hg[a] and 24-hour ambulatory blood pressure measurement <130/80 mm Hg and awake ambulatory blood pressure measurement <135/85 mm Hg and sleep measurement <120/70 mm Hg or home blood pressure <135/85 mm Hg
Masked hypertension	Untreated individuals with office BP <140/90 mm Hg and 24-hour ABP ≥130/80 mm Hg and/or awake ABP ≥135/85 mm Hg and/or sleep ABP ≥120/70 mm Hg[b] or home BP ≥135/85 mm Hg
Masked uncontrolled hypertension	Treated individuals with office BP <140/90 mm Hg and 24-hour ABP ≥130/80 mm Hg and/or awake ABP ≥135/85 mm Hg and/or sleep ABP ≥120/70 mm Hg[b] or home BP ≥135/85 mm Hg

Diagnoses require confirmation by repeating ambulatory blood pressure monitoring or home blood pressure monitoring within 3-6 months, depending on the individual's total cardiovascular risk.
[a]Ambulatory blood pressure values obtained in the clinic during the first or last hour of a 24-h recording may also partly reflect the white-coat effect.
[b]Patients with office BP<140/90 mm Hg, 24-h BP<130/80 mm Hg, awake BP <135/85 mm Hg but sleep BP ≥120/70 mm Hg should be defined as having 'Isolated Nocturnal Hypertension,' to be considered as a form of masked hypertension.
(Adapted from O'Brien E, Parati G, Stergiou G, et al. European society of hypertension position paper on ambulatory blood pressure monitoring. J Hypertens. *2013;31:1731-1768.)*
ABP, Ambulatory blood pressure; BP, blood pressure.

assessment of WCH and MH. The currently proposed threshold values for definition of WCH and MH based on this methodology, are shown in Table 12.1.[8,10] Of note, the cutoff BP values of 135/85 mm Hg or higher for diagnosing hypertension pertain to both daytime ABPM and to average self measured BP values obtained through HBPM.

In particular, a report of the Pressioni Arteriose Monitorate e Loro Associazioni study, (PAMELA study) in which the initial diagnosis of WCH (identified as office BP ≥140/90 mm Hg with 24-hour BP mean <125/79 mm Hg or home BP <132/82 associated mm Hg) was reassessed 10 years later, showed similar results in the ability of HBPM and ABPM to identify WCH, sustained hypertension, true normotension and masked hypertension, even if a substantial percentage of subjects, changed from one category to another, including progression from normotension, WCH or MH to sustained hypertension (true hypertension) (Fig. 12.2).

However, as mentioned previously, although HBPM shares many of the advantages of ABPM, resulting more cost-effective for the diagnosis of WCH and MH, it cannot be considered as a substitute but rather a complement to ABPM, as these methods are likely to pick up different moments of BP behavior in a subject's daily life.[8,10]

Prevalence

White-Coat Hypertension

WCH or isolated office hypertension (IOH) has been shown to be a rather common phenomenon, reasonably reproducible when properly studied with OBP measurements along with real-life ABPM or HBPM.[18] The prevalence reported in literature for WCH is quite variable across different studies, ranging from less than 10%[19] to more than 60%[20] with several intermediate values.[10,21,22] After the evidence from several population studies and their metaanalyses[19,23-25] supporting a threshold value equal or higher than 135/85 mm Hg to define hypertension with average daytime ambulatory BP, the frequency of WCH has been reported to range from 9% to 16% in the general population (average 13%) and from 25% to 46% (average about 32%) among hypertensive subjects defined only based

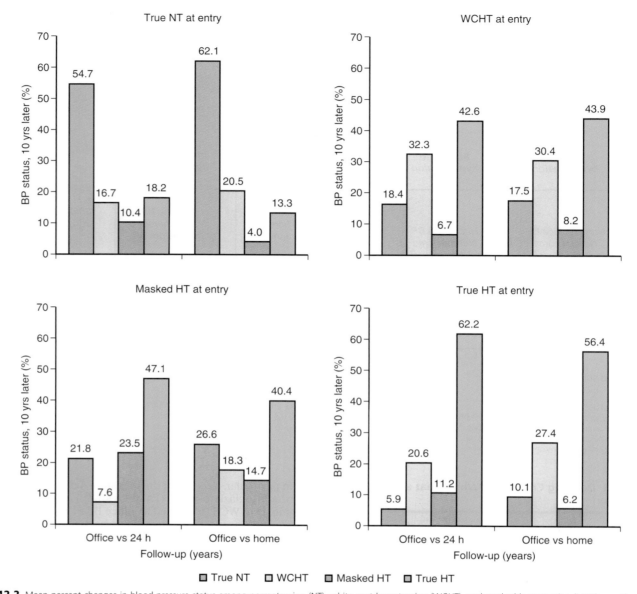

FIG. 12.2 Mean percent changes in blood pressure status among normotension (NT), white-coat hypertension (WCHT), and masked hypertension (MHT) over the 10-year period of the study. Data referring to true hypertension (true HT) are shown for comparison. *(From Mancia G, Bombelli M, Facchetti R, et al. Long-term risk of sustained hypertension in white-coat or masked hypertension.* Hypertension. *2009;54:226-232.)*

on OBP.[2,10,19,21,22] The frequency of WCH has been shown to increase in the presence of certain clinical characteristics, such as office systolic (S)BP in the range of 140 to 159 mmHg or diastolic (D)BP in the range of 90 to 99 mm Hg[6,26-29]; female sex; increasing age[30]; nonsmoking status; hypertension of recent diagnosis; limited number of BP measurements in the doctor's office; and normal left ventricular mass at echocardiography.[3,22,31] It should be emphasized that despite having home and ambulatory BP within "normal" limits, subjects with WCH have nevertheless slightly higher out-of-office BP levels than normotensive controls[32] (Fig. 12.3).

Masked Hypertension

Overall, the prevalence of masked hypertension in the general population ranges from 8.5% to 16.6%, and may increase up to 30.4% in populations with high normal clinic BP. The variability in prevalence estimates is attributed to the heterogeneous definition of masked hypertension, and to differences in the characteristics of the populations being investigated across studies. In the International Database on Ambulatory Blood Pressure in Relation to Cardiovascular Outcomes (IDACO)

study, the prevalence of MH was 44.5% among middle-aged and elderly patients (mean age, 64 years).[33] A subsequent report of the IDACO showed a prevalence for MH of 18.8% among subjects from a nondiabetic population, and of 29.3% among normotensive diabetic patients.[34] Masked hypertension is more likely to occur in elderly male patients with increased BP variability,[35] in whom a marked reduction in OBP immediately after a large meal may contribute to a diagnosis of MH[36]; in subjects who experience mental stress at work or at home (i.e., BP rise to hypertensive levels during working hours with normal BP at the time of conventional office measurements)[37,38]; in smokers,[39] further supporting a previous observation from our group that smoking one cigarette may increase ambulatory BP over 15 minutes[40]; in case of excessive alcohol consumption[41]; in sedentary obese individuals who are characterized by poor exercise tolerance throughout the daytime activities, whereas they often display normal BP values while at rest in the physician's office[42,43]; the presence of metabolic risk factors[44] or diabetes mellitus[34]; in chronic kidney disease[45]; in association with shortened sleep time, or obstructive sleep apnea[46] and with other conditions

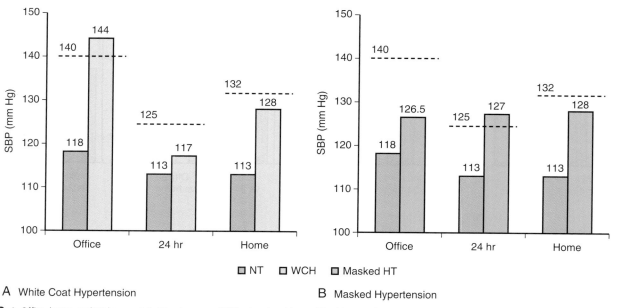

FIG. 12.3 A, Office, home, and 24-hour systolic blood pressure (SBP) values in subjects with white-coat hypertension (WCH) versus normotensive (NT) subjects or B, in patients with masked hypertension (masked HT) versus NT subjects. Data are shown as means. Dashed lines indicate reference normal blood pressure (BP) levels for each technique of BP measurement. Although having normal home and ambulatory BP, subjects with WCH have nevertheless slightly higher out-of-office BP levels than normotensive controls. *(Modified from Mancia G, Facchetti R, Bombelli M, Grassi G, Sega R. Long-term risk of mortality associated with selective and combined elevation in office, home, and ambulatory blood pressure.* Hypertension. *2006;47:846-853.)*

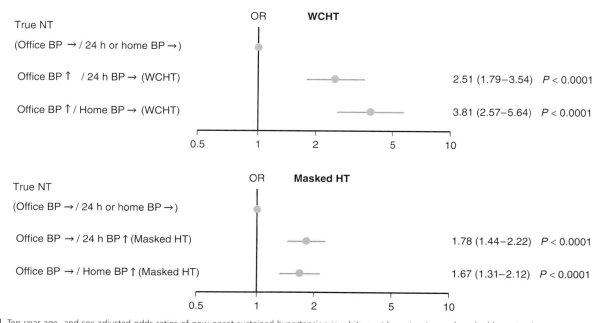

FIG. 12.4 Ten-year age- and sex-adjusted odds ratios of new-onset sustained hypertension in white-coat hypertension and masked hypertension versus true normotension at entry. *(From Mancia G, Bombelli M, Facchetti R, et al. Long-term risk of sustained hypertension in white-coat or masked hypertension.* Hypertension. *2009;54:226-232.)*

characterized by isolated nocturnal hypertension, nondipping or rising nocturnal BP patterns whenever these patterns are associated with normal conventional office BP values.[47,48]

Clinical Significance

White-Coat Hypertension

Population studies have indicated that compared with true normotension, WCH may increase the risk of developing sustained hypertension[15,49] leading to consider this condition as a prehypertensive state[50] (Fig. 12.4).

Moreover, compared with sustained normotension, patients with WCH have been shown to exhibit a greater prevalence/severity of alterations in glucose and lipid metabolism

(blood glucose, serum cholesterol, impaired fasting glucose or diabetes mellitus, etc.), albeit less than in patients with true hypertension that make the overall cardiovascular risk profile of this condition unfavorable when compared with the true normotensive fraction of the population[32] (Fig. 12.5).

Evidence has also been provided that compared with sustained normotension, WCH is associated with an increased risk of development and progression of renal, cerebral, vascular and cardiac organ damage (i.e., increased left ventricular [LV] mass index and carotid intima-media thickness).[51-53] Besides, most population studies (although not all)[33] and their meta-analyses have also indicated that WCH is associated with an increased risk of cardiovascular morbidity and mortality compared with true normotension, although such a risk remains

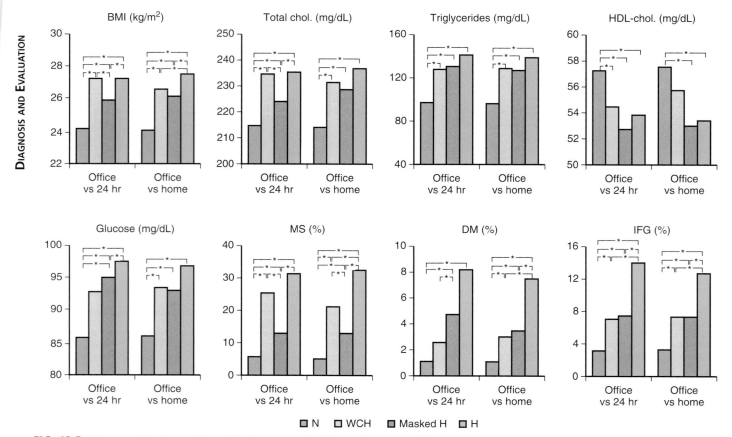

FIG. 12.5 Anthropometric and metabolic variables in normotensive subjects and in patients with white-coat and masked hypertension. Groups are classified according to office versus 24 hour and office versus home blood pressure (BP) differences. *Asterisks* refer to the statistical significance to between-group differences (*, $p < 0.05$). *H*, Hypertension; *Masked HT*, masked hypertension; *WCH*, white-coat hypertension. *(Modified from Mancia G, Facchetti R, Bombelli M, Grassi G, Sega R. Long-term risk of mortality associated with selective and combined elevation in office, home, and ambulatory blood pressure. Hypertension. 2006;47:846-853.)*

lower than that of MH and sustained hypertension[1,2,32,54-63] (Fig. 12.6). Thus, on the background of the evidence summarized above, the idea that WCH is a clinically innocent condition that should be regarded as not being substantially different from true normotension, cannot be supported.

Masked Hypertension

Evidence from large cohort studies has demonstrated that MH is associated with an increased risk of new-onset sustained hypertension[15] (see Fig. 12.4, lower panel) and with an increased prevalence of metabolic alterations and cardiovascular risk factors (see Fig. 12.5).[32] Consistent evidence from large population studies and their metaanalyses have also indicated that compared with their true normotensive counterparts, subjects with MH have a higher risk of development and progression of cardiac (i.e., LV structural alterations)[64] and vascular subclinical organ damage (i.e., early carotid atherosclerosis)[65] and an increased incidence of cardiovascular events and mortality.[60,61,66] Although in some reports only sustained hypertension and not MH was significantly associated with cardiovascular outcomes,[67] the metaanalyses of available studies including subjects from the general population and from primary care and specialty clinics have provided more consistent evidence in this regard.[1,2] In one of such metaanalyses, after a mean follow-up of 8 years, compared with sustained normotension, the adjusted hazard ratios for cardiovascular disease events were 1.12 (95% confidence interval [CI] 0.84 to 1.50) for white-coat hypertension, 2.00 (95% CI 1.58 to 2.52) for masked hypertension, and 2.28 (95% CI 1.87 to 2.78) for sustained hypertension. The results did not differ significantly across the studies ($p = 0.89$).[2] Of note, other metaanalyses have found an increased risk of cardiovascular

events for subjects with masked hypertension (HR 1.62, 95% CI 1.35 to 1.96) which not only was higher than that of WCH (hazard ratio [HR] 1.22, 95% CI 0.96 to 1.53) but was also not significantly different from that of sustained hypertension (HR 1.80, 95% CI 1.59 to 2.03)[1] (Fig. 12.7).

Management

White-Coat Hypertension

In recognition of the prognostic relevance and frequent occurrence of this condition in clinical practice, current hypertension guidelines have included suspicion of WCH in untreated individuals among the compelling clinical indications for out-of-office BP monitoring.[8,10,11] They recommend confirming the diagnosis of WCH within 3 to 6 months, along with follow-up visits at yearly intervals accompanied by out-of-office BP measurements (i.e., ABPM, or home BP monitoring), so as to detect whether and when sustained hypertension may develop.[8,10,11] There is still uncertainty regarding the question on whether patients with WCH should or should not be given antihypertensive treatment, with some experts suggesting that because it does not differ from normotension, WCH needs no therapeutic intervention. Along this line of thinking, identification of WCH would thus avoid administering "unnecessary" treatment to subjects who have otherwise normal BP levels in daily life conditions, thus preserving them from the possible adverse effects associated with inappropriate long-term drug administration, improving their quality of life, and reducing the health care costs. This could be particularly true in elderly subjects or in presence of severe atherosclerotic disease, where unnecessary BP lowering treatment, might compromise renal and/or cardiac perfusion leading to

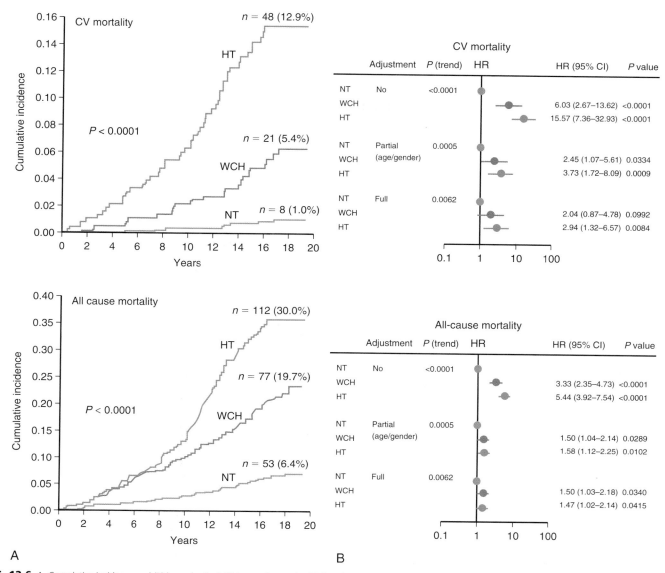

FIG. 12.6 A, Cumulative incidence and (B) hazard ratio (HR) for cardiovascular (CV) and all-cause mortality in normotensives (NT), white-coat hypertensives (WCH), and true hypertensives (HT) of PAMELA study over a long observation period (average 16 years). NT and true HT were defined by office, home, and ambulatory blood pressure normality and elevation, respectively. WCH was defined by elevation of office blood pressure accompanied by ambulatory or home blood pressure normality. Full adjustment refers to adjustment for age, sex, smoking, blood glucose, serum total cholesterol, body mass index, antihypertensive treatment, and history of cardiovascular events. *(Adapted from Mancia G, Bombelli M, Brambilla G, et al. Long-term prognostic value of white-coat hypertension: an insight from diagnostic use of both ambulatory and home blood pressure measurements. Hypertension. 2013;62:168-174.)*

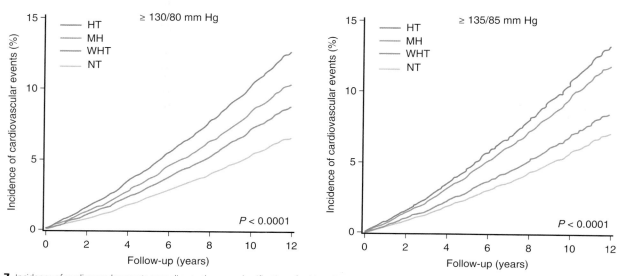

FIG. 12.7 Incidence of cardiovascular events according to the cross classification of subjects by conventional and daytime ambulatory blood pressure. *NT*, Normotension; *WHT*, white-coat hypertension (WCH); *MH*, masked hypertension; *HT*, sustained hypertension. The analyses were based on (a) lower (≥130/80 mm Hg) or (b) higher (≥135/85 mm Hg) cut-off limits for daytime ambulatory hypertension. Incidence was standardized to the sex distribution and mean age in the whole study population. The p-values are for trend across the blood pressure groups. *(Adapted from Hansen TW, Kikuya M, Thijs L, et al. Prognostic superiority of daytime ambulatory over conventional blood pressure in four populations: a meta-analysis of 7,030 individuals. J Hypertens. 2007;25:1554-1564.)*

episodes of acute kidney injury or coronary ischemia.[68,69] On the other hand, on the background of the more recent evidence that patients with WCH are at greater risk of developing sustained hypertension, metabolic alterations and cardiovascular complications compared with truly normotensive individuals (although still remaining at a lower risk than in true hypertension), it has been suggested that WCH subjects could benefit from an active therapeutic intervention.[49] Because no evidence is yet available that antihypertensive drugs are beneficial in WCH, this intervention has in most cases to be limited, however, to close follow-up and lifestyle changes, aimed at improving the adverse risk profile of these subjects. In line with the 2013 ESH/ESC Guidelines on hypertension management, drug treatment could be considered in presence of organ damage and with a history of cardiovascular disease.[8]

Masked Hypertension

Although the evidence on the adverse cardiovascular consequences associated with MH strongly suggests a potential benefit from BP lowering, no clinical trial up to date has specifically addressed whether or not treatment of MH may translate into improved cardiovascular prognosis. Despite this lack of evidence, the 2013 ESH/ESC guidelines have suggested that in patients with MH, drug treatment could also be considered because in these subjects the risk of hypertensive subclinical organ damage and adverse cardiovascular outcomes is very close to that of subjects with sustained hypertension.[8,10] A first step in the management of patients with MH should thus include a careful diagnostic work up to assess the presence of additional risk factors including a deranged metabolic profile and search for the presence of target organ involvement. Initially, nonpharmacologic strategies such as lifestyle changes should be implemented to decrease out-of-office BP levels and to ameliorate metabolic alterations. If nonpharmacologic measures are insufficient to normalize BP levels, pharmacologic treatment could be initiated, although evidence from randomized control trials is still lacking in this regard. The ongoing MASTER trial (MASked-unconTrolled hypERtension management based on office BP or on out-of-office [ambulatory] BP measurement [NCT028047074]), a research project of the European Society of Hypertension and the ARTEMIS Consortium, is aimed at filling this gap in the next few years.

When ambulatory blood pressure is measured, pharmacologic treatment may be modulated according to whether blood pressure is elevated either during daytime or during nighttime hours.

WHITE-COAT RESISTANT AND MASKED UNCONTROLLED HYPERTENSION IN TREATED HYPERTENSIVE SUBJECTS

Definition

White-Coat Resistant Hypertension

The BP rise associated with the alerting reaction during the medical visit, the so-called "white-coat effect" (WCE), is also present in subjects receiving antihypertensive treatment and represents a major problem with conventional BP measurement as it may lead to falsely underestimate the effect of antihypertensive drugs in treated subjects. As a consequence of this, there will be a significant number of treated subjects with apparent resistant hypertension in the office, despite achieving adequate out-of-office BP control with antihypertensive drugs, a condition defined as white-coat resistant hypertension (WCRH), or false resistant hypertension. Indeed, when combining office BP readings with either ambulatory or home BP monitoring to assess BP control in treated patients, and when considering the threshold values to assess BP control recommended by current guidelines for these different BP measuring techniques (office BP <140/90 mm Hg; ambulatory

BP levels during daytime <135/85 mm Hg, during 24 hours <130/80 mm Hg and during nighttime <120/70 mm Hg; average of 3 to 6 days home BP levels <135/85 mm Hg),[9-11] a treated hypertensive patient may fall into one of four categories: (1) true BP control (normal office and out-of-office BP levels); (2) true resistant hypertension (elevated office and out-of-office BP levels); (3) false resistant/uncontrolled hypertension (elevated office but normal out-of-office BP levels) also known as white-coat resistant/uncontrolled hypertension (WCRH); and (4) false BP control (normal office but elevated out-of-office BP levels) also known as masked resistant/uncontrolled hypertension (MRH) (see Fig. 12.1B).

Masked Uncontrolled Hypertension

Concerning the question as to whether or not the definition of masked hypertension should also be applied to individuals on BP lowering medication and not only to untreated individuals, it is agreed that the term should not be applied to individuals on treatment, because by definition in treated individuals, hypertension has been already diagnosed, and thus it cannot be "masked." Therefore, "masked uncontrolled hypertension" has been proposed as a more appropriate term for treated individuals.

Although ABPM is considered the reference standard to characterize different subtypes of hypertension and resistant hypertension, HBPM has proved to be similarly effective in discriminating between false and true hypertension/resistant hypertension, and between true and false normotension/BP control, thus reducing misclassification also of treated hypertensive subjects.[70] Because there are individuals in whom an elevated clinic BP is associated with a normal home BP, but an elevated ambulatory BP, or vice versa, for a precise identification of white-coat resistant hypertension either office, ambulatory, or home BP monitoring should ideally be implemented.[32]

Prevalence

White-Coat Resistant Hypertension

Analyses of large databases of observational and interventional studies in hypertension implementing ABPM and HBPM in addition to OBP have overwhelmingly shown that a substantial and sometimes larger than expected number of treated subjects initially diagnosed with resistant hypertension actually correspond to false resistant hypertension (white-coat resistant hypertension, WCRH). Overall, about 10% to 30% of subjects within the hypertensive population may be resistant to antihypertensive treatment.[71-74] However, this prevalence may falsely increase not only as a result of inadequate doses of antihypertensive therapy, improper use of diuretics and poor adherence to medical treatment after increases in dosing or in number of drugs, but also because of the persistency of a "white-coat" effect.[74,75] Indeed, analyses of observational studies and clinical trials in hypertension have indicated that in a significant proportion of subjects with resistant hypertension, the persistent elevation in OBP actually corresponds to WCRH (false resistance hypertension).[73,74,76] In a recent report of the Spanish Ambulatory Blood Pressure Monitoring Registry on about 68,000 hypertensive patients who had OBP and 24-hour ABPM performed,[73] the prevalence of resistant hypertension when considering OBP only (i.e., OBP ≥140/90 mm Hg while taking three antihypertensive drugs) was 12% (n = 8295 subjects). Remarkably, about 37.5% of these subjects had relatively normal 24-hour ABP (24-hour systolic/diastolic ambulatory BP <130/80 mm Hg) so that their elevated OBP could be explained by a "white-coat" effect. This high prevalence of false resistant hypertension exceeds previously reported estimates (18% to 33%) of this phenomenon in the general hypertensive population.[77] In the frame of the J-HOME Study in which cut-off values of 140/90 mm Hg for office and 135/85 mm Hg for home BP, were used, the prevalence of WCRH (false resistant hypertension) among patients with apparently resistant hypertension based on office BP readings amounted to 27.4%.[76]

Masked Uncontrolled Hypertension

The prevalence of masked uncontrolled hypertension (MUCH) has been found to be variable among studies. In the Spanish Registry, MUCH (defined as OBP <140/90 and 24-hour ambulatory SBP >130 and/or DBP >80 mm Hg) was found to be present in 31% of treated hypertensive patients apparently controlled based on OBP measures[78] whereas in the J-HOME STUDY, the prevalence was even higher amounting to 43.1%.[76] Of note, the prevalence of masked hypertension was found to be higher in treated hypertensives than in untreated individuals[34] likely as a consequence of the differential effect of antihypertensive treatment on office and out-of-office BP (i.e., reductions in ABP values may correspond to only 60% of the reduction of conventional in-office BP).[79] The reductions in OBP levels induced by antihypertensive treatment have been shown to be even higher than in ambulatory BP,[79] in particular among patients with higher pretreatment SBP levels.[80] In contrast to masked hypertension, the white-coat effect has been shown to decrease on average by 10/5 mm Hg in SBP/DBP respectively, after beginning antihypertensive treatment, thus further contributing to the reduction of office BP but not of ABP values.[81] Finally, measuring OBP levels in the morning, that is, often at the peak of plasma levels of antihypertensive drugs most commonly administered in the morning hours, may not necessarily reflect the trough BP levels achieved later in the day and night (i.e., when plasma levels of medications commonly taken in the morning are lower). If these discrepancies are substantial, then the prevalence of MUCH may further increase.

Clinical Significance

White-Coat Resistant Hypertension

Although a number of studies have supported the prognostic relevance of WCH for cardiovascular morbidity and mortality in nontreated subjects, the evidence is less regarding WCRH in treated patients. A study by Ben-Dov et al, aimed at determining the prognostic implications of the white-coat phenomenon in treated patients, found that compared with MRH and sustained hypertension, WCRH is a rather benign condition.[82] A study by Pierdomenico et al comparatively evaluated the occurrence of fatal and nonfatal cardiovascular events in patients with true BP control (OBP <140/90 mm Hg and daytime BP <135/85 mm Hg), masked uncontrolled hypertension (clinic BP <140/90 mm Hg and daytime BP >135 or 85 mm Hg), white-coat resistant hypertension (clinic BP ≥140 and/or 90 mm Hg and daytime BP <135/85 mm Hg), and true resistant hypertension (clinic BP ≥140 and/or 90 mm Hg and daytime BP >135 or 85 mm Hg). After almost 5-year follow-up, the cardiovascular risk in patients with WCRH was lower compared with subjects with masked and true resistant hypertension, and it was not different from that of subjects with true BP control.[62] More recently, a longitudinal, event-based cohort study with follow-up time of 10.6 years[33] found incidence rate of cardiovascular events in 334 participants with untreated white-coat hypertension to be no greater than in the untreated normotensive control population (relative risk [RR] 1.17 95% CI 0.87 to 1.57).[33] Moreover, 162 subjects with a diagnosis of white-coat hypertension who had been prescribed antihypertensive drugs had similar cardiovascular risk as compared with treated normotensives. In contrast, subjects with treated white-coat hypertension had about twice as high the cardiovascular risk when compared with untreated normotensives (RR 1.98, 95% CI 1.49 to 2.62).[33]

Masked Uncontrolled Hypertension

Available evidence indicates that MUCH is associated with an increased cardiovascular risk. A study by Pierdomenico et al showed a significantly higher risk of fatal and nonfatal cardiovascular events among treated subjects with MUCH (hazard ratio [HR] 2.28, 95% CI 1.1 to 4.7) and true resistant hypertension (RR 2.94, 95% CI 1.02 to 8.41) compared with those who achieved true BP control.[62] Another report in 2285 treated hypertensives found a significantly higher risk for all-cause mortality in subjects with MUCH (HR 1.88, 95% CI 1.08 to 3.27) and sustained uncontrolled hypertension (HR 2.02 95% CI 1.30 to 3.13) when compared with those with WCRH.[82] More recently, evidence has indicated that antihypertensive treatment (often prescribed at suboptimal doses in relation to out-of-office BP control), not only increases the prevalence of masked uncontrolled hypertension, but might be associated with an increased cardiovascular risk in these subjects. In a recent report of the IDACO study in nondiabetic individuals addressing the effects of antihypertensive treatment versus no treatment on the cardiovascular risk of sustained hypertension, there was an increased cardiovascular risk among treated subjects who achieved a condition of MUCH and of sustained normotension, compared with untreated subjects with masked hypertension and sustained normotension[34] (Fig. 12.8). Such an increased risk is likely to occur when subjects initially identified as having sustained hypertension are converted into masked hypertension, by suboptimal antihypertensive treatment which is enough to achieve OBP control, but not to normalize out-of-office BP levels. In due course, suboptimal BP lowering not only is not effective in eliminating the lifetime burden associated with previous elevated 24-hour BP (risk, in part, being dependent on the duration of hypertension), but may not further effectively prevent development and progression of subclinical organ damage and cardiovascular events. In contrast, optimal treatment of masked hypertension, using out-of-office BP monitoring to monitor the BP-lowering effects of antihypertensive treatment will promote conversion to sustained normotension of a larger number of subjects, thus reducing the prevalence of MUCH. However, the study by Franklin et al suggests that even sustained normotension achieved by treatment is not completely deprived by a residual increase in cardiovascular risk, albeit lower than in MUCH, as compared with spontaneously normotensive never

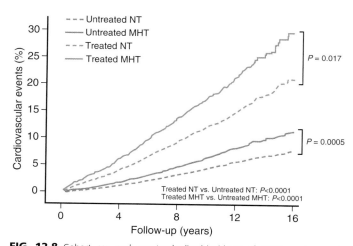

FIG. 12.8 Cohort, sex, and age-standardized incidence of cardiovascular events in untreated and treated normotensive (NT) and in untreated masked hypertensive (MHT) and in treated masked uncontrolled hypertensive (MUCH) nondiabetic subjects, as derived from an IDACO (International Database on Ambulatory Blood Pressure in Relation to Cardiovascular Outcomes) metaanalysis. Fully adjusted hazard ratios (HRs) for treated versus untreated masked hypertensives were as follows: HR, 2.27 (95% confidence interval, 1.6-3.2; *p* < 0.0001). (*Adapted from Franklin SS, Thijs L, Li Y, et al. Masked hypertension in diabetes mellitus: treatment implications for clinical practice. Hypertension. 2013;61:964-971.*)

treated individuals (see Fig. 12.8). Further insights into these complex clinical issues are likely to be provided by the above mentioned ongoing MASTER study (NCT028047074).

Management

White-Coat Resistant Hypertension

As mentioned earlier, up to one-third of treated hypertensives may be mistakenly classified as having resistant hypertension, whereas on the contrary they are only affected by WCRH (white-coat resistant hypertension, that is, false resistant hypertension because of a persisting white-coat effect).[73] In view of the limitations characterizing OBP measurements, it becomes clearer and clearer that an adequate assessment of BP control cannot be based on isolated OBP readings only, the identification of a WCRH requiring its combination with out-of-office BP monitoring. In consideration of this, current hypertension guidelines have included WCRH as a compelling clinical indication to perform ABPM.[10,11] Identification of WCRH (false resistant hypertension) on one hand, would prevent performing unnecessary and costly diagnostic tests for identification of secondary causes of hypertension; on the other hand, it would avoid introducing unnecessary modifications of antihypertensive treatment, that is, a nonrequired increase in dosing or number of antihypertensive drugs, thus reducing the chance of adverse effects associated with improperly prescribed multidrug therapy that often interferes with patients' quality of life, leading in the end to poor compliance with treatment. On the other hand, it would reduce the costs associated with unnecessary additional pharmacologic treatment and/or interventional device-based strategies (i.e., carotid baroreceptor activation[83] and renal denervation[84]) which have recently been introduced for the management of resistant hypertension. Indeed, given the elevated costs and invasive character of these approaches, as well as their potential adverse effects when not properly indicated, discarding WCRH based on out-of-office BP measures is currently considered among the eligibility criteria before proceeding with interventional treatment of resistant hypertension.[85] Fig. 12.9 presents the initial diagnostic approach for identifying white-coat resistant hypertension in treated hypertensives through the combined use of OBP and/or ABPM/HBPM.

Masked Resistant Hypertension

Analyses of large databases have shown that up to 30% of treated subjects may be mistakenly classified as having BP controlled based on OBP only, whereas their out-of-office BP levels actually remain elevated (masked resistant hypertension or false BP control).[76,78] On the background of the prognostic implications of MUCH, current hypertension guidelines advise performing ABPM whenever possible in already treated hypertensive individuals, to assess effective BP control with

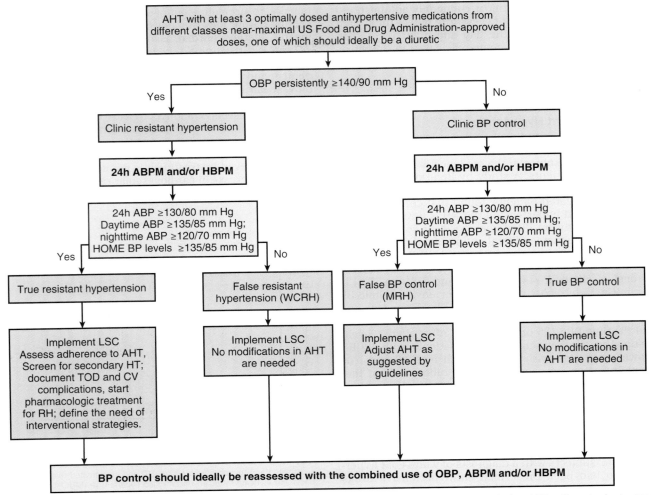

FIG.12.9 Initial diagnostic approach to the patient with clinic resistant hypertension. *ABPM,* Ambulatory blood pressure monitoring; *AHT,* antihypertensive treatment; *BP,* blood pressure; *CKD,* chronic kidney disease; *CV,* cardiovascular; *DM,* diabetes mellitus; *HBPM,* home blood pressure monitoring; *HT,* hypertension; *MRH,* masked resistant hypertension; *OBP,* office blood pressure; *RH,* resistant hypertension; *WCRH,* "white-coat" resistant hypertension. *(Modified from Parati G, Ochoa JE, Bilo G. False versus true resistant hypertension. In: Mancia G, ed. Resistant Hypertension: Epidemiology, Pathophysiology, Diagnosis and Treatment, 1st ed. Springer Milan Heidelberg New York Dordrecht London: Springer-Verlag Italia Srl; 2013: 277.)*

treatment not only for office BP but also for ambulatory BP levels during daytime, nighttime and 24 hours[10] thus preventing the cardiovascular consequences of uncontrolled out-of-office hypertension.[10,11] In particular, guaranteeing optimal nighttime BP control is of upmost importance in treated hypertensive subjects.[86] A recent report of the Spanish ABPM registry showed that, after a 4-year follow-up for cardiovascular events, nighttime but not daytime SBP predicted cardiovascular outcome, being the single, most important predictor of cardiovascular risk.[86] A recent report from a large population (n = 14,840) of treated hypertensive subjects with apparent BP control based on conventional BP,[87] identified 31% of patients who had MUCH when applying 24-hour ABPM, in whom poorer control of nocturnal BP was twice as frequent as poor daytime ABPM control. Indeed, many patients with resistant MUCH had persistent failure to control elevated nighttime BP, which was indeed the exclusive abnormality in 24% of them.[87] Identification and management of MUCH in treated hypertensives would thus require combined use of OBP and/or ABPM/HBPM.

The results provided by the few available studies on this issue strongly emphasize the need of additional evidence on the importance of identifying and properly managing patients with either WCRH or MUCH, which should come from properly designed, longitudinal, randomized intervention outcome trials.

SUMMARY

The important discrepancies between office and out-of-office BP levels lead to significant overestimation/underestimation and misclassification of BP levels in a substantial number of subjects (whether or not hypertensive and whether or not receiving antihypertensive treatment).

Based on the evidence provided by several studies on the clinical value of ABPM either for selecting patients for treatment or for assessing the effects of antihypertensive drug therapy, ABPM is currently considered the standard method for identifying WCH and MH in clinical practice.[10,11] Of remark, in recognition of the prevailing prognostic value of nighttime BP levels over other components of the 24-hour ABPM, current guidelines for hypertension management,[8,10,11] have expanded the definition of WCH and MH accounting for nighttime and 24-hour ambulatory BP levels. In the future, studies are required to determine the prevalence of WCH and MH according to this new definitions, as well as for better defining outcome-driven thresholds for out-of-the-office BP measurement, and the time intervals (24 hours versus daytime versus nighttime) to be considered to diagnose WCH and MH.

Additional studies are also needed to clarify the role of HBPM in this regard, aimed at defining when and how ABPM and HBPM should be used, and whether they could be used alternatively in specific clinical conditions, or should always be combined. In particular, HBPM appears to be of specific importance in the long-term follow-up of treated hypertensive patients although a number of practical issues still remain to be adequately defined, such as the number and timing of self-measurements required when using home BP monitoring.[9-11] From a treatment perspective, evidence from recent studies indicates that WCH may have potential, long-term implications, by carrying a higher risk for developing sustained hypertension, metabolic alterations and cardiovascular outcomes. This suggests that subjects with this condition could benefit from active follow-up and lifestyle counselling, whereas the possible need of drug treatment requires further investigation. Despite the recognized adverse cardiovascular prognosis associated with MH which may be similar to that of sustained hypertension, whether or not treating this condition may translate into improved cardiovascular protection needs documentation from prospective studies having

a proper control group, and focusing on outcomes of undisputable prognostic significance as endpoints. In particular, studies focusing on masked (untreated) hypertensive patients and/or on masked uncontrolled (on treatment) hypertensive patients are needed to assess the actual role of out-of-office BP measurements as a tool to guide the management of hypertension, and whether antihypertensive treatment guided by out-of-office BP measurements could be superior to a treatment strategy guided by office BP in terms of morbidity, mortality, intermediate endpoints and costs reduction.

References

1. Hansen TW, Kikuya M, Thijs L, et al. Prognostic superiority of daytime ambulatory over conventional blood pressure in four populations: a meta-analysis of 7,030 individuals. J Hypertens. 2007;25:1554-1564.
2. Fagard RH, Cornelissen VA. Incidence of cardiovascular events in white-coat, masked and sustained hypertension versus true normotension: a meta-analysis. J Hypertens. 2007;25:2193-2198.
3. Pickering TG, James GD, Boddie C, Harshfield GA, Blank S, Laragh JH. How common is white coat hypertension? JAMA. 1988;259:225-228.
4. Mancia G, Bertinieri G, Grassi G, et al. Effects of blood-pressure measurement by the doctor on patient's blood pressure and heart rate. Lancet. 1983;2:695-698.
5. Julius S, Mejia A, Jones K, et al. "White coat" versus "sustained" borderline hypertension in Tecumseh. Michigan. Hypertension. 1990;16:617-623.
6. Verdecchia P, Schillaci G, Borgioni C, et al. White coat hypertension and white coat effect. Similarities and differences. Am J Hypertens. 1995;8:790-798.
7. Pickering T. Recommendations for the use of home (self) and ambulatory blood pressure monitoring. American Society of Hypertension Ad Hoc Panel. Am J Hypertens. 1996;9:1-11.
8. Mancia G, Fagard R, Narkiewicz K, et al. 2013 ESH/ESC Guidelines for the management of arterial hypertension: the Task Force for the management of arterial hypertension of the European Society of Hypertension (ESH) and of the European Society of Cardiology (ESC). J Hypertens. 2013;31:1281-1357.
9. Parati G, Stergiou GS, Asmar R, et al. European Society of Hypertension guidelines for blood pressure monitoring at home: a summary report of the Second International Consensus Conference on Home Blood Pressure Monitoring. J Hypertens. 2008;26:1505-1526.
10. O'Brien E, Parati G, Stergiou G, et al. European society of hypertension position paper on ambulatory blood pressure monitoring. J Hypertens. 2013;31:1731-1768.
11. Parati G, Stergiou G, O'Brien E, et al. European Society of Hypertension practice guidelines for ambulatory blood pressure monitoring. J Hypertens. 2014;32:1359-1366.
12. Pickering TG, Miller NH, Ogedegbe G, Krakoff LR, Artinian NT, Goff D. Call to action on use and reimbursement for home blood pressure monitoring: a joint scientific statement from the American Heart Association, American Society of Hypertension, and Preventive Cardiovascular Nurses Association. Hypertension. 2008;52:10-29.
13. Ritchie LD, Campbell NC, Murchie P. New NICE guidelines for hypertension. BMJ. 2011;343:d5644.
14. Hara A, Ohkubo T, Kikuya M, et al. Detection of carotid atherosclerosis in individuals with masked hypertension and white-coat hypertension by self-measured blood pressure at home: the Ohasama study. J Hypertens. 2007;25:321-327.
15. Mancia G, Bombelli M, Facchetti R, et al. Long-term risk of sustained hypertension in white-coat or masked hypertension. Hypertension. 2009;54:226-232.
16. Stergiou GS, Salgami EV, Tzamouranis DG, Roussias LG. Masked hypertension assessed by ambulatory blood pressure versus home blood pressure monitoring: is it the same phenomenon? Am J Hypertens. 2005;18:772-778.
17. Chobanian AV, Bakris GL, Black HR, et al. Seventh report of the Joint National Committee on Prevention, Detection, Evaluation, and Treatment of High Blood Pressure. Hypertension. 2003;42:1206-1252.
18. Ben-Dov IZ, Ben-Arie L, Mekler J, Bursztyn M. Reproducibility of white-coat and masked hypertension in ambulatory BP monitoring. Int J Cardiol. 2007;117:355-359.
19. Mancia G, Sega R, Bravi C, et al. Ambulatory blood pressure normality: results from the PAMELA study. J Hypertens. 1995;13(12 Pt 1):1377-1390.
20. Spence JD, Bass M, Robinson HC, et al. Prospective study of ambulatory monitoring and echocardiography in borderline hypertension. Clinical and Investigative Medicine Medecine Clinique et Experimentale. 1991;14:241-250.
21. Pickering TG, Hall JE, Appel LJ, et al. Recommendations for blood pressure measurement in humans and experimental animals: Part 1: blood pressure measurement in humans: a statement for professionals from the Subcommittee of Professional and Public Education of the American Heart Association Council on High Blood Pressure Research. Hypertension. 2005;45:142-161.
22. Dolan E, Stanton A, Atkins N, et al. Determinants of white-coat hypertension. Blood Press Monitor. 2004;9:307-309.
23. Staessen JA, Bieniaszewski L, O'Brien ET, Imai Y, Fagard R. An epidemiological approach to ambulatory blood pressure monitoring: the Belgian Population Study. Blood Press Monitor. 1996;1:13-26.
24. Imai Y, Nagai K, Sakuma M, et al. Ambulatory blood pressure of adults in Ohasama. Japan. Hypertension. 1993;22:900-912.
25. Staessen JA, Fagard RH, Lijnen PJ, Thijs L, Van Hoof R, Amery AK. Mean and range of the ambulatory pressure in normotensive subjects from a meta-analysis of 23 studies. Am J Cardiol. 1991;67:723-727.
26. Hoegholm A, Kristensen KS, Madsen NH, Svendsen TL. White coat hypertension diagnosed by 24-h ambulatory monitoring. Examination of 159 newly diagnosed hypertensive patients. Am J Hypertens. 1992;5:64-70.
27. Martinez MA, Garcia-Puig J, Martin JC, et al. Frequency and determinants of white coat hypertension in mild to moderate hypertension: a primary care-based study. Monitorizacion Ambulatoria de la Presion Arterial (MAPA)-Area 5 Working Group. Am J Hypertens. 1999;12:251-259.
28. Hoegholm A, Kristensen KS, Bang LE, Nielsen JW. White coat hypertension and target organ involvement: the impact of different cut-off levels on albuminuria and left ventricular mass and geometry. J Hum Hypertens. 1998;12:433-439.
29. Staessen JA, O'Brien ET, Amery AK, et al. Ambulatory blood pressure in normotensive and hypertensive subjects: results from an international database. J Hypertens Suppl. 1994;12:S1-S12.
30. Sega R, Cesana G, Milesi C, Grassi G, Zanchetti A, Mancia G. Ambulatory and home blood pressure normality in the elderly: data from the PAMELA population. Hypertension. 1997;30(1 Pt 1):1-6.

31. Verdecchia P, Palatini P, Schillaci G, Mormino P, Porcellati C, Pessina AC. Independent predictors of isolated clinic ('white-coat') hypertension. *J Hypertens*. 2001;19:1015-1020.

32. Mancia G, Facchetti R, Bombelli M, Grassi G, Sega R. Long-term risk of mortality associated with selective and combined elevation in office, home, and ambulatory blood pressure. *Hypertension*. 2006;47:846-853.

33. Franklin SS, Thijs L, Hansen TW, et al. Significance of white-coat hypertension in older persons with isolated systolic hypertension: a meta-analysis using the International Database on Ambulatory Blood Pressure Monitoring in Relation to Cardiovascular Outcomes population. *Hypertension*. 2012;59:564-571.

34. Franklin SS, Thijs L, Li Y, Hansen TW, Boggia J, Liu Y, et al. Masked hypertension in diabetes mellitus: treatment implications for clinical practice. *Hypertension*. 2013;61:964-971.

35. Cacciolati C, Tzourio C, Hanon O. Blood pressure variability in elderly persons with white-coat and masked hypertension compared to those with normotension and sustained hypertension. *Am J Hypertens*. 2013;26:367-372.

36. Tabara Y, Okada Y, Uetani E, et al. Postprandial hypotension as a risk marker for asymptomatic lacunar infarction. *J Hypertens*. 2014;32:1084-1090. discussion 90.

37. Trudel X, Brisson C, Milot A. Job strain and masked hypertension. *Psychosom Med*. 2010;72:786-793.

38. Landsbergis PA, Dobson M, Koutsouras G, Schnall P. Job strain and ambulatory blood pressure: a meta-analysis and systematic review. *Am J Public Health*. 2013;103:e61-e71.

39. Seki M, Inoue R, Ohkubo T, et al. Association of environmental tobacco smoke exposure with elevated home blood pressure in Japanese women: the Ohasama study. *J Hypertens*. 2010;28:1814-1820.

40. Groppelli A, Giorgi DM, Omboni S, Parati G, Mancia G. Persistent blood pressure increase induced by heavy smoking. *J Hypertens*. 1992;10:495-499.

41. Ohira T, Tanigawa T, Tabata M, et al. Effects of habitual alcohol intake on ambulatory blood pressure, heart rate, and its variability among Japanese men. *Hypertension*. 2009;53:13-19.

42. Schultz MG, Hare JL, Marwick TH, Stowasser M, Sharman JE. Masked hypertension is "unmasked" by low-intensity exercise blood pressure. *Blood Press*. 2011;20:284-289.

43. Sharman JE, Hare JL, Thomas S, et al. Association of masked hypertension and left ventricular remodeling with the hypertensive response to exercise. *Am J Hypertens*. 2011;24:898-903.

44. Hanninen MR, Niiranen TJ, Puukka PJ, Jula AM. Metabolic risk factors and masked hypertension in the general population: the Finn-Home study. *J Hypertens*. 2014;28:421-426.

45. Bangash F, Agarwal R. Masked hypertension and white-coat hypertension in chronic kidney disease: a meta-analysis. *CJASN*. 2009;4(3):656-664.

46. Hermida RC, Ayala DE, Mojon A, Fernandez JR. Sleep-time blood pressure and the prognostic value of isolated-office and masked hypertension. *Am J Hypertens*. 2012;25:297-305.

47. Fan HQ, Li Y, Thijs L, et al. Prognostic value of isolated nocturnal hypertension on ambulatory measurement in 8711 individuals from 10 populations. *J Hypertens*. 2010;28:2036-2045.

48. de la Sierra A, Gorostidi M, Banegas JR, Segura J, de la Cruz JJ, Ruilope LM. Nocturnal hypertension or nondipping: which is better associated with the cardiovascular risk profile? *Am J Hypertens*. 2014;27:680-687.

49. Siven SS, Niiranen TJ, Kantola IM, Jula AM. White-coat and masked hypertension as risk factors for progression to sustained hypertension: the Finn-Home study. *J Hypertens*. 2016;34:54-60.

50. Bidlingmeyer I, Burnier M, Bidlingmeyer M, Waeber B, Brunner HR. Isolated office hypertension: a prehypertensive state? *J Hypertens*. 1996;14:327-332.

51. Sega R, Trocino G, Lanzarotti A, et al. Alterations of cardiac structure in patients with isolated office, ambulatory, or home hypertension: data from the general population (Pressione Arteriose Monitorate E Loro Associazioni [PAMELA] Study). *Circulation*. 2001;104:1385-1392.

52. Fukuhara M, Arima H, Ninomiya T, et al. White-coat and masked hypertension are associated with carotid atherosclerosis in a general population: the Hisayama study. *Stroke*. 2013;44:1512-1517.

53. Verdecchia P, Schillaci G, Borgioni C, et al. Identification of subjects with white-coat hypertension and persistently normal ambulatory blood pressure. *Blood Press Monitor*. 1996;1:217-222.

54. Verdecchia P, Reboldi GP, Angeli F, et al. Short- and long-term incidence of stroke in white-coat hypertension. *Hypertension*. 2005;45:203-208.

55. Strandberg TE, Salomaa V. White coat effect, blood pressure and mortality in men: prospective cohort study. *Eur Heart J*. 2000;21:1714-1718.

56. Dawes MG, Bartlett G, Coats AJ, Juszczak E. Comparing the effects of white coat hypertension and sustained hypertension on mortality in a UK primary care setting. *Ann Fam Med*. 2008;6:390-396.

57. Khattar RS, Senior R, Lahiri A. Cardiovascular outcome in white-coat versus sustained mild hypertension: a 10-year follow-up study. *Circulation*. 1998;98:1892-1897.

58. Verdecchia P, Porcellati C, Schillaci G, et al. Ambulatory blood pressure. An independent predictor of prognosis in essential hypertension. *Hypertension*. 1994;24:793-801.

59. Kario K, Shimada K, Schwartz JE, Matsuo T, Hoshide S, Pickering TG. [Silent and clinically overt stroke in older Japanese subjects with white-coat and sustained hypertension]. *J Cardiol*. 2002;39:52-54.

60. Ohkubo T, Kikuya M, Metoki H, Asayama K, Obara T, Hashimoto J, et al. Prognosis of "masked" hypertension and "white-coat" hypertension detected by 24-h ambulatory blood pressure monitoring 10-year follow-up from the Ohasama study. *J Am Coll Cardiol*. 2005;46:508-515.

61. Bobrie G, Chatellier G, Genes N, Clerson P, Vaur L, Vaisse B, et al. Cardiovascular prognosis of "masked hypertension" detected by blood pressure self-measurement in elderly treated hypertensive patients. *JAMA*. 2004;291:1342-1349.

62. Pierdomenico SD, Lapenna D, Bucci A, et al. Cardiovascular outcome in treated hypertensive patients with responder, masked, false resistant, and true resistant hypertension. *Am J Hypertens*. 2005;18:1422-1428.

63. Mancia G, Bombelli M, Brambilla G, et al. Long-term prognostic value of white coat hypertension: an insight from diagnostic use of both ambulatory and home blood pressure measurements. *Hypertension*. 2013;62:168-174.

64. Cuspidi C, Sala C, Tadic M, Rescaldani M, Grassi G, Mancia G. Untreated masked hypertension and subclinical cardiac damage: a systematic review and meta-analysis. *AM J Hypertens*. 2015;28:806-813.

65. Cuspidi C, Sala C, Tadic M, et al. Untreated masked hypertension and carotid atherosclerosis: a meta-analysis. *Blood Press*. 2015;24:65-71.

66. Bjorklund K, Lind L, Zethelius B, Andren B, Lithell H. Isolated ambulatory hypertension predicts cardiovascular morbidity in elderly men. *Circulation*. 2003;107:1297-1302.

67. Hansen TW, Jeppesen J, Rasmussen S, Ibsen H, Torp-Pedersen C. Ambulatory blood pressure monitoring and risk of cardiovascular disease: a population based study. *Am J Hypertens*. 2006;19:243-250.

68. Tomlinson LA, Holt SG, Leslie AR, Rajkumar C. Prevalence of ambulatory hypotension in elderly patients with CKD stages 3 and 4. *Nephrol Dial Transplant*. 2009;24:3751-3755.

69. Messerli FH, Mancia G, Conti CR, et al. Dogma disputed: can aggressively lowering blood pressure in hypertensive patients with coronary artery disease be dangerous? *Ann Intern Med*. 2006;144:884-893.

70. Nasothimiou EG, Tzamouranis D, Roussias LG, Stergiou GS. Home versus ambulatory blood pressure monitoring in the diagnosis of clinic resistant and true resistant hypertension. *J Hum Hypertens*. 2011;26:696-700.

71. Cushman WC, Ford CE, Cutler JA, et al. Success and predictors of blood pressure control in diverse North American settings: the antihypertensive and lipid-lowering treatment to prevent heart attack trial (ALLHAT). *J Clin Hypertens. (Greenwich)*. 2002;4:393-404.

72. Hajjar I, Kotchen TA. Trends in prevalence, awareness, treatment, and control of hypertension in the United States, 1988-2000. *JAMA*. 2003;290:199-206.

73. de la Sierra A, Segura J, Banegas JR, et al. Clinical features of 8295 patients with resistant hypertension classified on the basis of ambulatory blood pressure monitoring. *Hypertension*. 2011;57:898-902.

74. Persell SD. Prevalence of resistant hypertension in the United States, 2003-2008. *Hypertension*. 2011;57:1076-1080.

75. Ahmed MI, Calhoun DA. Resistant hypertension: bad and getting worse. *Hypertension*. 2011;57:1045-1046.

76. Oikawa T, Obara T, Ohkubo T, et al. Characteristics of resistant hypertension determined by self-measured blood pressure at home and office blood pressure measurements: the J-HOME study. *J Hypertens*. 2006;24:1737-1743.

77. Elliott WJ. High prevalence of white-coat hypertension in Spanish resistant hypertensive patients. *Hypertension*. 2011;57:889-890.

78. de la Sierra A, Banegas JR, Oliveras A, Gorostidi M, Segura J, de la Cruz JJ, et al. Clinical differences between resistant hypertensives and patients treated and controlled with three or less drugs. *J Hypertens*. 2012;30:1211-1216.

79. Mancia G, Parati G. Office compared with ambulatory blood pressure in assessing response to antihypertensive treatment: a meta-analysis. *J Hypertens*. 2004;22:435-445.

80. Schmieder RE, Schmidt ST, Riemer T, et al. Disproportional decrease in office blood pressure compared with 24-hour ambulatory blood pressure with antihypertensive treatment: dependency on pretreatment blood pressure levels. *Hypertension*. 2014;64:1067-1072.

81. Parati G, Ulian L, Sampieri L, et al. Attenuation of the "white-coat effect" by antihypertensive treatment and regression of target organ damage. *Hypertension*. 2000;35:614-620.

82. Ben-Dov IZ, Kark JD, Mekler J, Shaked E, Bursztyn M. The white coat phenomenon is benign in referred treated patients: a 14-year ambulatory blood pressure mortality study. *J Hypertens*. 2008;26:699-705.

83. Papademetriou V, Doumas M, Faselis C, et al. Carotid baroreceptor stimulation for the treatment of resistant hypertension. *Int J Hypertens*. 2011;2011:964394.

84. Doumas M, Faselis C, Papademetriou V. Renal sympathetic denervation in hypertension. *Curr Opin Nephrol Hypertens*. 2011;20:647-653.

85. Schmieder RE, Redon J, Grassi G, et al. ESH position paper: renal denervation—an interventional therapy of resistant hypertension. *J Hypertens*. 2012;30:837-841.

86. de la Sierra A, Banegas JR, Segura J, Gorostidi M, Ruilope LM. Ambulatory blood pressure monitoring and development of cardiovascular events in high-risk patients included in the Spanish ABPM registry: the CARDIORISC Event study. *J Hypertens*. 2012;30:713-719.

87. Banegas JR, Ruilope LM, de la Sierra A, de la Cruz JJ, Gorostidi M, Segura J, et al. High prevalence of masked uncontrolled hypertension in people with treated hypertension. *Eur Heart J*. 2014;35:3304-3312.

13 Renovascular Hypertension and Ischemic Nephropathy

Stephen C. Textor

ADVANCES AND MAJOR POINTS OF EMPHASIS

1. Definition of the spectrum of progressive clinical manifestations attributable to renovascular disease
2. Recognition that moderate reductions in renal blood flow do not induce tissue hypoxia or damage, thereby allowing ongoing medical therapy of renovascular hypertension.
3. Integration of limited prospective trial results into clinical practice in favor of optimized medical therapy using agents that block the renin-angiotensin system.
4. Identification of high-risk subsets that have mortality benefits associated with renal revascularization
5. Establishing the limits of kidney adaptation to reduced blood, beyond which tissue hypoxia and activation of inflammatory pathways ensue

More than 80 years have passed since the original observations indicating that constriction of the renal arteries produces a rise in systemic arterial pressures. These studies established the primal role of the kidney in regulating the circulation and blood pressure. Since then, occlusive renovascular lesions have been recognized as a major form of "secondary hypertension" and have been a widely applied model for understanding the role of the renin-angiotensin-aldosterone system (RAAS). In clinical terms, this has produced an odyssey of surgical and endovascular attempts to restore the kidney circulation, and eventually led to pharmacologic blockade of the RAAS. The range of clinical manifestations particularly associated with atherosclerotic renovascular disease (RVD) is highly variable and continues to challenge clinicians. Despite the intuitive benefits of restoring kidney blood flow, results of several prospective, randomized clinical trials attempting to clarify the modern role of adding renal revascularization to optimized medical therapy have been ambiguous. Enrollment for these studies has been hampered by the history of major clinical benefits after successful revascularization for cases of severe disease that limited physicians' willingness to randomize patients. As a result, the clinical decision regarding when to move forward with renal revascularization most commonly falls to experienced clinicians after failure of medical therapy. It behooves those caring for complex vascular and renal disease to be familiar with the pathophysiology and management of these disorders.

DISEASE DEFINITION

Renovascular hypertension (RVH) and ischemic nephropathy both refer to clinical conditions related to occlusive renovascular disease. RVH identifies a variety of disorders in which a rise in arterial pressure is induced by reduction in renal perfusion pressure. Experiments in the 1930s linked reduced renal perfusion to a rise in systemic pressure.[1] It should be emphasized that this can occur at levels of renal pressure above those that impair kidney function, although further reduction in renal

blood flow ultimately leads to additional sequelae, including impaired volume control, circulatory congestion, and ultimately irreversible kidney injury. Hence, occlusive renovascular disease (RVD) comprises a spectrum of clinical disorders ranging from incidental, minor disease to incipient occlusion with tissue ischemia as illustrated in Fig. 13.1 for atherosclerotic disease. Ischemic nephropathy refers to advanced hemodynamic impairment of glomerular filtration that ultimately threatens kidney survival. Recognizing this spectrum and its specific manifestations within an individual patient is an important responsibility of the cardiovascular clinician or nephrologist.

EPIDEMIOLOGY

Within western countries the dominant (at least 85%) cause of RVD is atherosclerotic renal artery stenosis (ARAS). This develops invariably as part of systemic atherosclerotic disease affecting various vascular beds, including coronary, cerebral, and peripheral vascular territories. Risk factors for ARAS include advancing age, smoking, dyslipidemia, preexisting essential hypertension, and diabetes. Community-based studies suggest that up to 6.8% of individuals older than 65 have ARAS producing more than 60% occlusion.[2] Screening studies indicate rising prevalence of detectable ARAS in hypertensive subjects from 3% (ages 50 to 59 years) to 25% (above age 70 years) with older ages.[3] Imaging studies of patients with symptomatic coronary or peripheral vascular disease indicate that more than 50% lumen occlusion of the renal arteries may be detected in 14% to 33% of such individuals.[4] It must be emphasized that many such cases are incidental in nature and have minimal hemodynamic or clinical importance. Clinically significant atherosclerotic RVD most often appears as worsening or accelerating blood pressure elevation in older individuals with preexisting hypertension. Establishing the clinical significance of incidentally detected atherosclerotic RVD remains challenging but should be considered carefully before embarking on vascular interventional procedures.

Alternative causes of RVH derive from other flow-limiting lesions affecting the renal circulation. These can arise from various fibromuscular dysplasias (FMD), such as medial fibroplasia that typically presents an appearance of "string-of-beads" (Fig. 13.2). Some form of FMD may be detected incidentally in up to 3% of normotensive men or women presenting as potential kidney donors.[5] Those that progress to develop renovascular hypertension are predominantly females, some of whom are smokers. This gender predominance suggests that hormonal factors modulate the progression of this disorder and its clinical phenotype. Other disorders that produce RVH include renal trauma, arterial occlusion from dissection or thrombosis, and embolic occlusion of the renal artery (Table 13.1). Particularly in Southeast Asia, inflammatory vascular disorders such as Takayasu arteritis commonly impinge

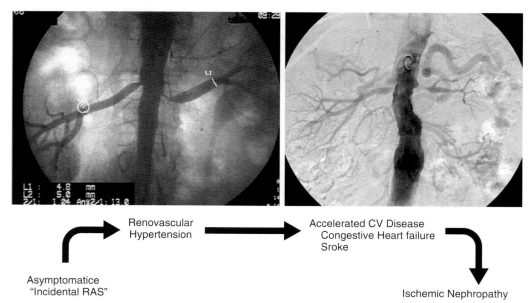

Asymptomatice
"Incidental RAS"

Renovascular
Hypertension

Accelerated CV Disease
Congestive Heart failure
Sroke

Ischemic Nephropathy

FIG. 13.1 Schematic view of progressively more severe clinical manifestations associated with occlusive renovascular disease (RVD). Minor degrees of lumen obstruction are manifest as "incidental" lesions of minimal hemodynamic importance. As obstruction leads to reduced pressures and flow beyond the lesion, renovascular hypertension and acceleration of cardiovascular events ensue, particularly when bilateral disease is associated with impaired sodium excretion. Ultimately, severe and longstanding RVD activates injury pathways within the kidney parenchyma that may no longer depend primarily upon hemodynamic effects of stenosis and respond only partially to restoring vessel patency.

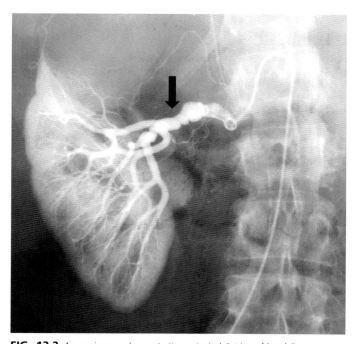

FIG. 13.2 An angiogram demonstrating a typical "string-of-beads" appearance as an example of fibromuscular dysplasia. Indentation of the vessel wall represents a series of internal webs that reduce distal perfusion and trigger renovascular hypertension. Such lesions can respond to percutaneous transluminal renal angioplasty (PTRA) with reduced arterial pressure (see text).

TABLE 13.1 Examples of Vascular Lesions Producing Renal Hypoperfusion and the Syndrome of Renovascular Hypertension

Unilateral Disease (Analogous to 1-Clip-2-Kidney Hypertension)	• Unilateral atherosclerotic renal artery stenosis
	 • Unilateral fibromuscular dysplasia (FMD)
	   • Medial fibroplasia
	   • Perimedial fibroplasia
	   • Intimal fibroplasia
	   • Medial hyperplasia
	 • Renal artery aneurysm
	 • Arterial embolus
	 • Arteriovenous fistula (congenital/traumatic)
	 • Segmental arterial occlusion (posttraumatic) or segmental arteriomediolysis (SAM)
	 • Extrinsic compression of renal artery, e.g., pheochromocytoma
	 • Renal compression, e.g., metastatic tumor

Bilateral Disease or Solitary Functioning Kidney (Analogous to 1-Clip-1-Kidney Model)	• Stenosis to a solitary functioning kidney • Bilateral renal arterial stenosis • Aortic coarctation • Systemic vasculitis (e.g., Takayasu, Polyarteritis) • Atheroembolic disease • Vascular occlusion because of endovascular aortic stent graft

(Modified from Textor SC. Renovascular Hypertension and Ischemic Nephropathy. In: Skorecki K, Taal MW, Chertow GM, Yu ASL, Marsden PA, ed. Brenner and Rector's The Kidney. Philadelphia: Elsevier; 2016: 1567-609.)

upon the renal circulation. An emerging iatrogenic form of RVD includes occlusion of the renal arteries from endovascular aortic stent grafts, for which landing zones may migrate or be deliberately placed across the origins of the renal arteries.[6] Loss of renal function from vascular compromise limits the clinical success of endovascular aortic repair.

PATHOPHYSIOLOGY

RVH is triggered initially by activation of release of pressor hormones, primarily renin from the juxtaglomerular

apparatus within the kidney. Circulating renin acts upon its substrate, angiotensinogen, to release angiotensin I, which is converted to angiotensin II (Ang II) in many sites, particularly the lung. Studies over several decades have identified numerous actions of Ang II, including direct vasoconstriction, stimulation of adrenal release of aldosterone, and induction of sodium retention. Ang II also mobilizes additional pressor mechanisms, such as sympathetic adrenergic pathways,

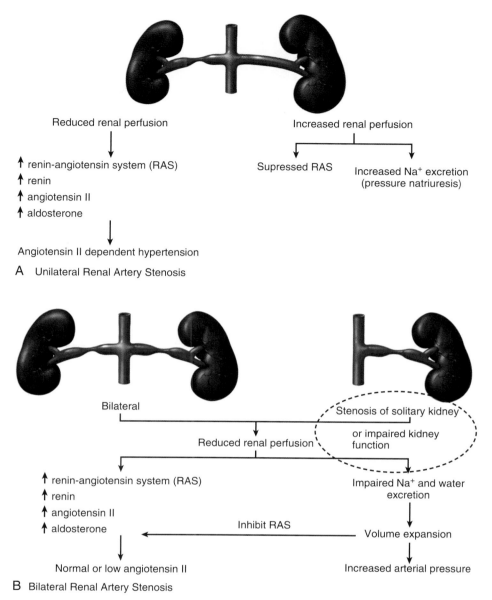

Reduced renal perfusion

Increased renal perfusion

↑ renin-angiotensin system (RAS)
↑ renin
↑ angiotensin II
↑ aldosterone

Supressed RAS

Increased Na⁺ excretion
(pressure natriuresis)

Angiotensin II dependent hypertension

A Unilateral Renal Artery Stenosis

Bilateral

Stenosis of solitary kidney
or impaired kidney
function

Reduced renal perfusion

↑ renin-angiotensin system (RAS)
↑ renin
↑ angiotensin II
↑ aldosterone

Impaired Na⁺ and water
excretion

Inhibit RAS

Volume expansion

Normal or low angiotensin II

Increased arterial pressure

B Bilateral Renal Artery Stenosis

FIG. 13.3 A, Depiction of initial hormonal responses to reducing renal perfusion pressures to one kidney in the presence of a normal "contralateral" kidney (designated 2-kidney-1-clip renovascular hypertension [RVH]). The rise in systemic pressure suppresses renin release from the contralateral kidney and promotes pressure-natriuresis from the contralateral side. B, Summary of hormonal responses when both kidneys are stenosed or in the presence of a solitary functioning kidney (designated 1-kidney-1-clip RVH). In this instance, initial rise in renin release triggers a rise in pressure and eventual sodium retention which suppresses circulating levels of plasma renin activity. Both of these are triggered initially by reduced renal perfusion and can respond with lower arterial pressures after restoring renal blood flow with revascularization. In practice, the contralateral kidney often fails to function normally, making clinical measurement of plasma renin activity of limited diagnostic value.

vascular remodeling, and modification of prostaglandin dependent vasodilation.[7] Experimental studies demonstrate that blockade of the renin-angiotensin system or genetic knockout of AT-1 receptors prevents the development of RVH.[8] Ang II is recognized to induce T-cell activation leading to accelerating hypertension and end-organ inflammatory injury.[9] After initial activation of the RAAS, the secondary vasoconstrictor pathways can become dominant with the result that pharmacologic RAAS blockade and/or renal revascularization may no longer completely reverse RVH.

Two classic models of RVH have been proposed, depending upon the functional role of the remaining kidney (the nonstenotic or "contralateral" kidney)[10] (Fig. 13.3A and B). When the contralateral kidney is normal, it responds to rising systemic pressure with suppression of its own renin release and enhanced sodium excretion, termed *pressure natriuresis*. This 2-kidney-1-clip condition is characterized by unilateral release of renin into the renal veins, elevated levels of plasma renin

activity and arterial pressure demonstrably dependent upon the pressor effects of Ang II. These features have been used as diagnostic tests to establish the diagnosis of RVH and the likely response of arterial hypertension to revascularization of the stenotic kidney. Such testing was undertaken routinely in the era of surgical renal revascularization aimed specifically for the treatment of renovascular hypertension. The second model has been designated 1-kidney-1-clip RVD in which no functional contralateral kidney is present or capable of ongoing pressure natriuresis (see Fig. 13.3B). This occurs typically in the setting of a solitary functioning kidney or severe RVD affecting both kidneys. As a result, the rise in systemic pressure no longer is offset by increased sodium excretion, leading to volume expansion and secondary reduction in renin release from the stenotic kidney. These events lead to lower values for circulating plasma renin activity, loss of renal vein renin lateralization, and loss of detectable angiotensin dependence of systemic hypertension, unless or until diuresis and

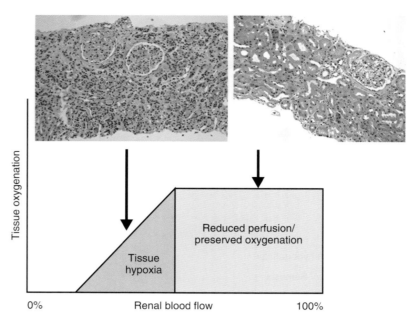

FIG. 13.4 Schematic view of the relationship between reduced renal blood flow and tissue oxygenation in the poststenotic kidney. Moderate reductions in blood flow do not induce overt hypoxia, in part because of overabundant baseline blood flow and in part because of reduced filtration and reabsorptive energy consumption (see text). Such moderate reductions do not necessarily damage kidney parenchyma, as illustrated by the biopsy of the poststenotic kidney on the right. With more severe and prolonged vascular occlusion, however, ischemic nephropathy with hypoxia and inflammatory injury develops as illustrated in the left biopsy. These inflammatory changes with destruction of renal tubules may not reverse after restoring vascular patency. The clinical outcome of renal revascularization therefore depends heavily upon the condition of the poststenotic kidney.

volume contraction are accomplished. In reality, the contralateral kidney in 2-kidney-1-clip renovascular hypertension is rarely entirely normal,[11] possibly as a result of tissue injury from direct effects of angiotensin II and/or other pathways. As a result, impaired contralateral kidney function commonly impairs sodium excretion and renal function in many patients with longstanding RVH. Hence, clinical laboratory manifestations in human subjects vary widely between the extremes predicted by 1-kidney and 2-kidney experimental models.

"Ischemic nephropathy" is used to designate parenchymal kidney injury that develops beyond vascular occlusive lesions. Remarkably, clinical studies using blood oxygen level dependent (BOLD) magnetic resonance (MR) indicate that substantial reductions in blood flow (up to 35% to 40%) can occur without demonstrable tissue hypoxia or evident long-term kidney fibrosis[12] (Fig. 13.4). This is partly because of the abundant perfusion of the kidney cortex as part of its filtration function, reflected by the fact that less than 10% of oxygen is required for fulfilling the energy requirements of the kidney.[13] The medulla, by contrast, is supplied by postglomerular arterioles with lower blood flow and has greater oxygen extraction because of energy-dependent active solute transport.[14] Thus, the kidney normally has a large cortical-medullary oxygen gradient with areas of reduced oxygen tension in deep medullary areas.[15] Moderate reductions in blood flow therefore exert only minor effects on oxygen delivery to the cortex and the reductions in glomerular filtration that result also reduce net solute transport and thereby reduce oxygen requirements in medullary regions. Taken together, the kidney normally adapts to heterogeneous blood flows and regional hypoxia. An important corollary of these observations is that medical therapy of renovascular hypertension (albeit necessarily reducing perfusion pressure and blood flow to the poststenotic kidney) can be tolerated, sometimes for many years, without necessarily inducing parenchymal kidney damage.

Renal tolerance to reduced blood flow has limits, of course. More severe and prolonged reductions in blood flow eventually threaten both tissue oxygenation and viability of the poststenotic kidney.[16] Studies of both experimental and human RVD indicate that cortical hypoxia eventually is associated with activation of inflammatory pathways.[17] These are characterized by abundant renal vein levels of proinflammatory cytokines, such as tumor necrosis factor-alpha (TNF-α, monocyte chemoattractant protein 1 [MCP-1]), biomarkers of injury (e.g., neutrophil gelatinase-associated lipocalin (NGAL) in addition to the appearance of t-lymphocytes and macrophages within the tissue parenchyma[18,19] (see Fig. 13.4). Inflammatory changes associated with severe ischemia lead to obliteration of tubules with failure to regenerate intratubular epithelial cells with resulting atubular glomeruli.[20] At some point, these processes become refractory to restoring vessel patency with revascularization, despite partial restoration of renal blood flow and reversal of tissue hypoxia.[21]

DIAGNOSIS

Clinical Manifestations

RVH and ischemic nephropathy are diagnosed primarily by recognition of a clinical syndrome consistent with these disorders, particularly progressive or secondary hypertension with or without unexplained chronic kidney disease (CKD). Occlusive RVD is expressed across a range of manifestations generally related to the severity and/or duration of vascular occlusion, as illustrated in Fig. 13.1. Many incidental lesions are now identified during imaging procedures for other indications, including computed tomography (CT) and/or MR angiography. It should be emphasized that hemodynamic effects of lumen occlusion such as changes in either translesional pressure or flow are barely detectable until lumen occlusion reaches a "critical level" in the vicinity of 70% to 80% lumen occlusion.[22] Studies in humans subjected to stepwise partial balloon obstruction of the renal artery indicate that gradients of at least 10% to 20% reductions in postobstruction pressures are required to detect measurable renin release.[23] An important corollary is that failure to identify a pressure gradient across such a vascular lesion makes it unlikely that renal revascularization will have detectable hemodynamic benefits.

Clinical characteristics of atherosclerotic RVH include rapid changes in arterial pressure, often in subjects with preexisting hypertension (Table 13.2). The average age of recent interventional reports for RVH is above 70 years. Arterial pressure rises

TABLE 13.2 Syndromes Associated With Renovascular Hypertension

1. Early or late onset hypertension (<30 years >50 years)
2. Acceleration of treated essential hypertension
3. Deterioration of renal function in treated essential hypertension
4. Acute renal failure during treatment of hypertension
5. "Flash" pulmonary edema
6. Progressive renal failure
7. Refractory congestive cardiac failure

The above "syndromes" should alert the clinician to the possible contribution of renovascular disease in a given patient. The bottom three are most common in patients with bilateral disease, many of whom are treated as "essential hypertension" until these characteristics appear (see text).

TABLE 13.3 Clinical Features Favoring Renovascular Hypertension

- Duration less than 1 year
- Onset over age 50 years
- Grade 3-4 optic fundi
- Abdominal bruit/other vascular disease

with age in Western societies, so the majority of these individuals will have previously identified hypertension. Recognizing recent progression and rising antihypertensive drug requirements should raise the question of a superimposed secondary process such as atherosclerotic RVH. As compared with essential hypertension, patients with RVH have more evident activation of the renin-angiotensin system and increased sympathetic nerve activation, sometimes associated with wide pressure fluctuations and variability. Clinical findings suggestive of RVH as opposed to essential hypertension are listed in Table 13.3. Target organ manifestations including vascular injury, left ventricular hypertrophy, and renal dysfunction are more common with RVH as compared with age-matched subjects with essential hypertension of similar levels.[24]

Based on clinical features alone, some authors indicate that a scoring system based on age, gender, smoking history, recent onset of hypertension, and elevated serum creatinine allows excellent estimates of pretest probability of identifying renovascular lesions.[25]

The presence of occlusive RVD and RVH can accelerate manifestations of other vascular disease. Impaired volume control related to RVD worsens circulatory congestion associated with left-ventricular dysfunction. When RVD triggers additional rises in arterial pressure, the resulting left-ventricular outflow resistance can precipitate congestive heart failure, sometimes designated "flash" pulmonary edema.[26,27] This is a recognizable clinical syndrome and is often associated with rapid worsening of renal function as arterial pressure is lowered and/or diuresis is achieved. Observational series report higher rates of mortality and rehospitalization for patients with combined congestive heart failure and RVD.[28,29]

Ultimately, progressive atherosclerotic RVD leads to loss of kidney function in the affected kidney(s). Prospective trials including ASTRAL (Angioplasty and Stenting for Renal Artery Lesions) and CORAL (Cardiovascular Outcomes in Renal Atherosclerotic Lesions) indicate that 15% to 22% of subjects with RVD progress to a renal "endpoint" over a follow-up period between 3 and 4 years.[30] As a practical matter, establishing whether this progression poses a clinical problem in a specific individual is often the central element in management of atherosclerotic RVD.

Physical Examination

Detailed review of blood pressure measurement is beyond the scope of this chapter (for more information, see American Heart Association recommendations).[31] Ambulatory blood pressure monitoring with RVH commonly identifies disturbed day-night circadian rhythms with loss of the normal nocturnal fall.[32] Retinal examination may reveal vascular changes of long-term hypertension, although grading these is notoriously variable between physicians. Peripheral pulses may be diminished and/or asymmetric as a result of vascular occlusive disease in other vascular beds. Audible bruits are sometimes heard over the abdomen and/or other vascular sites, such as carotid or aortic regions, but are nonspecific and relatively insensitive. Other evidence of peripheral arterial occlusive disease, including claudication, temperature differences, loss of limb perfusion with elevation, hair loss over the extremities, and peripheral atheroembolic lesions may provide clues to underlying peripheral arterial disease.

Laboratory Studies

General values for hematologic and electrolyte levels are normal or consistent with the degree of glomerular filtration rate (GFR) reduction (stage of CKD). Unexplained elevations of serum creatinine merit further evaluation with at least ultrasound duplex imaging. Urinalyses are typically "bland" with few cellular elements or proteinuria. The presence of significant albuminuria (or elevation of urinary albumin/creatinine ratio) should raise consideration of other parenchymal renal disorders, including diabetic nephropathy.

Measurement of circulating plasma renin activity warrants consideration. As noted previously, elevated levels are consistent with RVH, although sodium retention, drug effects, and transitions to alternative pressor pathways sometimes leave these levels normal or low. Examination of the aldosterone/renin ratio typically is consistent with secondary aldosterone excess, and may account for hypokalemia observed either spontaneously or during diuretic therapy. These hormonal and electrolyte levels are affected by many other factors, making their diagnostic value limited. They are most useful when positive and identify distinctly abnormal patterns.

Measurement of renal vein renin levels was commonly performed during planning for surgical renal artery procedures when this was the primary therapy for RVH. Identification of overt lateralization to the poststenotic kidney along with suppression of renin release from the contralateral kidney has been associated with substantial pressure reduction in more than 90% of subjects.[33] Once again, the utility of this procedure is limited by variable conditions under which the measurements are made, which are often associated with saline administration during the imaging procedure that suppresses renin. Hence, failure to identify lateralization was associated with improved blood pressure in at least 50% of cases, rendering it of limited sensitivity and specificity. Repeated measurement after sodium depletion has been shown to "unmask" renal vein lateralization and identify RVH.[34] As a clinical measure, identifying a specific kidney as a "pressor kidney" with unilateral renin release is most useful when contemplating therapeutic nephrectomy for blood pressure control.

Imaging Studies

Establishing the diagnosis of occlusive RVD intrinsically requires demonstrating renal arterial obstruction. Hence, imaging studies are a sine qua non for this diagnosis. Before embarking on detailed imaging procedures, some of which are expensive and potentially hazardous, clinicians would do well to establish exactly what goals of the imaging study should be. Is the purpose simply to identify if one or both arteries have evident occlusive disease? Is it to establish the viability and functional characteristics of the poststenotic kidney? Is it to identify the specific location and severity of RVD for revascularization? Is it to identify translesional gradient information and/or response to revascularization? Perhaps most importantly, to what degree do the clinical conditions of the specific patient warrant acting on the imaging data, specifically regarding either renal revascularization or nephrectomy? As a result, the choice and pace of diagnostic imaging depend partly on the response to medical therapy and the clinical status of the specific patient.

Duplex Ultrasonography

Duplex Doppler renal ultrasonography is an excellent initial imaging tool and provides both some degree of functional and structural assessment. Because it is relatively inexpensive, ultrasound can be used to follow patients serially and to evaluate vascular patency after revascularization. The peak systolic velocity (PSV) has the highest performance characteristics and reaches a sensitivity of 85% and a specificity of 92% for the diagnosis of atherosclerotic RVD in experienced laboratories.[35] An example of extremely high PSV is illustrated in Fig. 13.5. The limitations of this technique hinge upon its dependence upon operator skills and patient body habitus, leading to reported accuracy estimates that range from 60% to more than 90%. The resistive index (RI) is determined from segmental arterial flow characteristics. The RI is defined as height of the peak systolic velocity minus height of the end-diastolic velocity (EDV) divided by the peak systolic velocity (RI= (PSV − EDV) ÷ PSV) and thus reflects the status of the flow characteristics in the renal microcirculation beyond the main renal arteries. An elevated RI indicates limited diastolic flow and may reflect intrinsic parenchymal or small vessel disease. In conjunction with clinical findings, RI has been promoted as a useful parameter to predict benefit after revascularization.

Initial reports indicate that patients with RI below 0.8 before angioplasty have better outcomes regarding both blood pressure and renal function as compared with those with RI above 0.8,[36] as we have reviewed. Other authors find less consistent separation based on segmental artery resistance, although the general condition of the poststenotic kidney and likely recovery after revascularization are better with a low RI.[33] Hence, reliance upon RI as a predictive parameter for ARAS management remains ambiguous. Our interpretation of these studies is that lower RI is likely associated with more preserved renal flow characteristics and better kidney function overall, but should not be the final determinant regarding the decision for revascularization.

Computed Tomography and Magnetic Resonance Angiography

Advances in imaging technology favor expanded use of spiral multidetector CT angiography (CTA) and magnetic resonance angiography (MRA) as valid methods to visualize ARAS. Compared with catheter-based renal angiography, these modalities are less invasive, allow multiplanar imaging of the arteries and soft tissue, and are suitable for complex reconstruction analysis.[37] CTA and MRA are of comparable accuracy, reaching sensitivity and specificity above 90% in a number of single center studies compared with catheter angiography. Use of breath-hold contrast enhanced MRA in 96 renovascular patients without fibromuscular dysplasia demonstrated MRA to have a sensitivity of 97% and negative predictive value of 98% for the detection of renal artery stenoses of at least 60%. An example of MR angiography is shown

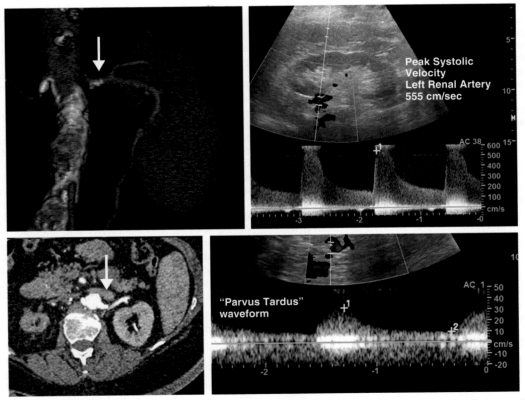

FIG. 13.5 Determining both the hemodynamic effects of vascular occlusive disease and the condition of the poststenotic kidney may benefit from combined imaging modalities. The upper left panel depicts a reconstructed computed tomography angiogram from a 72-year-old woman with a solitary functioning kidney. Duplex ultrasound (upper right panel) identifies peak systolic velocities of 555 cm/sec that reflect a severe degree of vascular occlusion, although the nephrogram appears well-preserved. The delayed upstroke illustrated as a parvus tardus segmental arterial waveform confirms the sluggish arterial flow (lower right panel) produced by an arterial plaque extending from the aortic orifice (lower left). This individual had developed serum creatinine values above 4.5 mg/dL during antihypertensive drug therapy with an angiotensin receptor blocker (ARB). Withdrawal of the ARB was associated with reduction in serum creatinine, but severe hypertension and episodes of flash pulmonary edema. Renal revascularization was associated with elimination of episodes of congestive heart failure, reinstitution of ARB therapy, and stable kidney function with serum creatinine 1.7 mg/dL. This individual would not have been a candidate for prospective, randomized trials such as CORAL. (Modified from Textor SC, McKusick MM. Renal artery stenosis: if and when to intervene. Curr Opin Nephrol Hypertens. 2016;25:144-151.)

in Fig. 13.6A. Even though CTA currently offers better spatial resolution, MRA has the advantage of avoiding radiation. The main limitations of these imaging studies include the risk of contrast nephropathy with CTA and concerns regarding the potential for nephrogenic systemic fibrosis in MRA patients receiving gadolinium contrast with significant renal insufficiency (GFR < 30 mL/min/1.73m^2).

Blood Oxygen Level Dependent Magnetic Resonance

Blood Oxygen Level Dependent (BOLD) MR imaging has been applied to examine tissue oxygenation within kidneys beyond a vascular occlusive lesion.[38,39] This technique relies upon the paramagnetic properties of deoxyhemoglobin, requires no contrast, and allows real-time estimation of oxygen delivery and consumption. Experimental and clinical studies identify a major oxygen gradient between cortical and deep medullary areas of the kidney that is magnified in severe vascular occlusive disease.[40] Optimizing its analysis remains difficult and BOLD imaging remains primarily a research tool, although it can identify both whole kidney and cortical hypoxia associated with vascular disease.[41]

Radionuclide Studies: Captopril Renography

Radionuclide studies using captopril have been used to evaluate RVD. Diethylenetriaminepentaacetic acid (DTPA) and mercapto-acetyltriglycine (MAG 3) are the most commonly used agents with the latter being more reliable in renal insufficiency. Criteria for RVD include (1) a decrease in the percentage of uptake of the isotope by the affected kidney to less than 40% of the total, (2) delayed time to peak uptake of the isotope to greater than 10 to 11 min, well above the normal value of 6 min, and (3) delayed excretion of the isotope with retention at 25 min or greater than 20%. The addition of captopril and comparison with a baseline (noncaptopril) renogram allow estimation of the functional role of angiotensin in maintaining glomerular filtration. However, this test does not distinguish reliably unilateral and bilateral ARAS. Among patients with bilateral disease, asymmetry was identified in the more severely affected kidney, but the presence or absence of stenosis in the contralateral kidney could not be assured. Importantly, renogram sensitivity and specificity decrease with decline of renal function, especially for patients who have serum creatinine levels greater than 2 mg/dL. As a result,

isotope renography is less commonly used in the current era and has value primarily to evaluate the relative function of each kidney before considering therapeutic nephrectomy of a "pressor" kidney.[42]

Intraarterial Angiography

Intraarterial angiography currently remains the gold standard for definition of vascular anatomy and stenotic lesions in the kidney. Often it is completed at the time of a planned intervention, such as endovascular angioplasty and/or stenting (Fig. 13.7). Screening or drive-by angiography is less commonly performed because the publication of prospective randomized trials suggesting limited benefit from renal revascularization for stable patients with atherosclerotic renovascular disease (see later). Hence, endovascular procedures for RVD lesions normally should be confined to individuals with strong indications for renal revascularization.

Contrast toxicity remains an issue with conventional iodinated agents. Intravascular ultrasound procedures have been undertaken using papaverine to evaluate flow reserve beyond stenotic lesions. Previous studies of pressure gradients measured across stenotic lesions failed to predict the clinical response to renal revascularization. Measurements using currently available low-profile wire probes do, however, indicate a relationship between pressure gradients and activation of the renin-angiotensin system.[23] Outcomes of patients with translesional pressure gradients measured after vasodilation suggest that measurement of hyperemic systolic gradient above 21 mm Hg most accurately predicts high-grade stenosis (average 78% by intravascular ultrasonography) and a beneficial response of blood pressure after stenting.[43]

Differential Diagnosis

RVH remains one of the most common contributors to resistant hypertension. The differential diagnosis for resistant hypertension comprises other secondary causes, including obstructive sleep apnea, primary renal diseases, inappropriate aldosterone production/activity, and others.[44] Most commonly, the question arises as to whether renal dysfunction represents parenchymal renal injury from hypertension itself (hypertensive nephrosclerosis). The latter is largely a diagnosis of exclusion, and it has been questioned whether or not

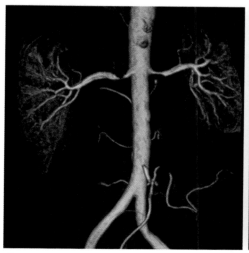

A MR Angiography

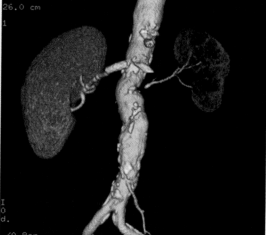

B CT Angiography

FIG. 13.6 A, Magnetic resonance angiogram (MRA) with gadolinium identifying bilateral renal arterial stenosis in an individual treated with "mantle" radiation more than twenty years earlier. MRA offers excellent imaging of the main renal vessels, although gadolinium has been associated with nephrogenic systemic fibrosis in subjects with reduced glomerular filtration rate (less than 30 mL/min/1.73 m^2). B, Computed tomography angiogram with iodinated contrast can provide excellent vascular imaging and delineation of perfusion nephrogram. This individual has well-preserved parenchyma beyond a vascular stent to the right renal artery, but major occlusive disease and reduction in tissue perfusion to the left kidney.

nonmalignant forms of hypertension actually lead to renal failure.[45] Recent studies indicate that other factors, including specific genetic predisposition in African Americans, may determine the risk for renal dysfunction in such individuals. Some individuals have small vessel disease with or without thrombotic phenomena that mimics large vessel RVD, for which little can be done at present. Exclusion of RVD is an important diagnostic step in the evaluation of otherwise unexplained renal dysfunction with or without hypertension.

TREATMENT OF RENOVASCULAR HYPERTENSION AND ISCHEMIC NEPHROPATHY

Few conditions have undergone more radical paradigm shifts in nephrology than the management of RVH. It remains a prototype for reversible causes of secondary hypertension, insofar as restoring vessel patency (see Fig. 13.7) and perfusion pressures sometimes can lower blood pressure to normal. This is particularly applicable to younger individuals, such as women with renovascular hypertension from fibromuscular disease, whose hypertension sometimes regresses completely with technically successful renal artery angioplasty.[46] By contrast, older individuals with widespread atherosclerotic vascular disease and preexisting hypertension will likely require ongoing medical antihypertensive therapy regardless of the success of revascularization. Before the advent of agents capable of blocking the renin-angiotensin system, drug therapy effectively controlled RVH approximately 40% to 50% of the time. After introduction of these agents, medical therapy has achieved goal blood pressures more than 80% of the time, although multiple agents may be required.[47] Selecting the optimal approach to these individuals over the long term remains a major challenge to clinicians.

Management of RVH begins with optimizing medical therapy, which necessarily includes withholding tobacco use, introduction of statins, glucose control, and effective antihypertensive drug treatment, most often including either an angiotensin converting enzyme (ACE) inhibitor or angiotensin receptor blocker (ARB)[48] (Fig. 13.8). Evaluation of subjects enrolled in the CORAL trial indicates that only 50% of patients with atherosclerotic RAS were treated with ACE/ARB before randomization,[49] despite multiple registry reports of a survival benefit.[48,50] Such reports suggest that ACE/ARB therapy is underused in patients with RVH, particularly in the United States and for patients with reduced GFR. If this medical approach achieves excellent blood pressure levels with stable renal function, no further action may be required, other than surveillance for disease progression.

Atherosclerosis is intrinsically progressive, albeit at variable rates between individuals. Poststenotic perfusion pressures are lower than those in the aorta or prestenosis levels, thereby subjecting the kidney to reduced renal perfusion. As noted earlier, the kidney can tolerate moderate reductions in pressure without developing tissue hypoxia or structural renal injury,[51] sometimes for many years. At some point, however, overt hypoxia does develop, along with inflammatory injury. Glomerular filtration at reduced renal perfusion pressure eventually depends upon the postglomerular efferent arteriolar effects of angiotensin II. Hence blockade of the RAAS is particularly capable of reducing filtration pressure at critical levels of kidney perfusion. Progressive loss of GFR in such patients can sometimes recover substantially by withholding these ACE inhibitors and/or ARBs, as some have advocated routinely.[52] Such a critical dependence signals near critical levels of occlusive disease that may benefit from renal revascularization.

Renal Revascularization

Restoration of blood flow to the kidney beyond a stenotic lesion is an obvious approach to improving renovascular hypertension and halting progressive vascular occlusive injury. A major shift from surgical reconstruction ensued in the 1990s in favor of endovascular stent procedures. Although some patients benefit enormously, revascularization procedures have both benefits and risks. With older patients developing renal artery stenosis in the context of preexisting hypertension, the likelihood of a cure for hypertension is small, particularly in atherosclerotic disease. Although complications are not common, they can be catastrophic, including atheroembolic disease and aortic dissection. Knowing when the benefits of revascularization outweigh the risks is central to the dilemma of managing renovascular disease.

Angioplasty for Fibromuscular Disease

Most lesions of medial fibroplasia are located at a distance away from the renal artery ostium. Many of these have multiple webs within the vessel, which can be successfully traversed and opened by balloon angioplasty. Experience in the 1980s indicated more than 94% technical success rates. Some of these lesions (approximately 10% to 15%) develop restenosis

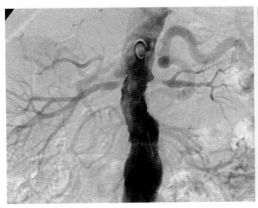

Bilateral atherosclerotic renal artery stenosis
(pre-stent)

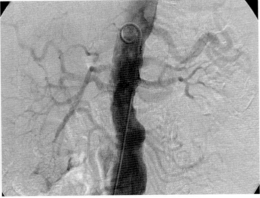

Post-stent(s)

FIG. 13.7 Angiograms of high-grade atherosclerotic renovascular disease before (left panel) and after (right panel) technically successful endovascular renal artery stenting. The ability to restore vessel patency using endovascular techniques allows treatment of many individuals previously not suited to surgical repair. Using low-profile guidewires and careful techniques, serious complication rates in experienced centers have fallen, for example, to less than 3% in CORAL (Cardiovascular Outcomes in Renal Atherosclerotic Lesions).[7]

for which repeat procedures have been used. Clinical benefit regarding blood pressure control has been reported in observational outcome studies in 65% to 75% of patients, although the rates of cure are less secure.[53] Cure of hypertension, defined as sustained blood pressure levels less than 140/90 mm Hg with no antihypertensive medications, may be obtained in 35% to 50% of patients. Predictors of cure (normal arterial pressures without medication beyond 6 months after angioplasty) include lower systolic blood pressures, younger age, and shorter duration of hypertension. A majority of patients with FMD are female and generally have less aortic disease and are at lower risk for major complications of angioplasty. Most clinicians favor early intervention for hypertensive patients with FMD with the hope of reduced antihypertensive medication requirements after successful angioplasty.

Angioplasty and Stenting for Atherosclerotic Renal Artery Stenosis

Angioplasty alone commonly fails to maintain patency for proximal or ostial atherosclerotic lesions, in part because of extensive recoil of the plaque extending into the main portion of the aorta. These lesions develop restenosis rapidly even after early success. Introduction of endovascular stents provide an indisputable advantage. An example of successful renal artery stenting is shown in Fig. 13.7. As technical success continues to improve, many reports suggest nearly 100% technical success in early vessel patency, although rates of in-stent restenosis continue to reach 14% to 25%.[54]

Several observational studies suggest that progression of renal failure attributed to ischemic nephropathy may be reduced by endovascular procedures. Harden and associates presented reciprocal creatinine plots in 23 (of 32) patients suggesting that the slope of loss of GFR could be favorably changed after renal artery stenting.[55] It should be emphasized that 69% of patients improved or stabilized, indicating that 31% worsened, consistent with results from other series. Perhaps the

most convincing group data in this regard derives from serial renal functional measurement in 33 patients with high-grade (>70%) stenosis to the entire affected renal mass (bilateral disease or stenosis to a solitary functioning kidney) with creatinine levels between 1.5 and 4.0 mg/dL. Follow-up over a mean of 20 months indicates that the slope of GFR loss converted from negative (–0.0079 dL/mg per month) to positive (0.0043 dL/mg per month).[56] These studies agree with other observations that long-term survival is reduced in bilateral disease and that the potential for renal dysfunction and accelerated cardiovascular disease risk is highest in such patients.[29,57]

Treatment Trials

Over the past two decades, several prospective RCTs have attempted to quantify the role for renal revascularization when added to medical therapy. Three early trials in renovascular hypertension from the 1990s addressed the added value of endovascular repair using PTRA without stenting as compared with medical therapy for atherosclerotic RVH. Crossover rates for failure of medical therapy ranged from 22% to 44%, suggesting a role for PTRA in refractory hypertension, although the overall intention-to-treat analyses were negative.[58] There was greater blood pressure benefit after PTRA in those with bilateral renal artery stenosis.

Recent prospective trials include STAR (Stent Placement and Blood Pressure and Lipid-Lowering for the Prevention of Progression of Renal Dysfunction Caused by Atherosclerotic Ostial Stenosis of the Renal Artery), ASTRAL and CORAL as summarized in Table 13.4. In some cases, revascularization achieved slightly improved blood pressure levels and/ or reduced drug requirements, but the differences have been minor. No definitive benefits regarding recovery of renal function, blood pressure control, or reduction of serious comorbid vascular events have been identified in any of these trials lasting 3 to 5 years.[59,60] These negative results have dampened the argument for early intervention in atherosclerotic RVD. As

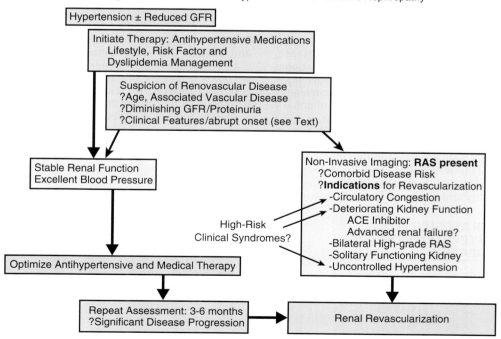

Management of Renovascular Hypertension and Ischemic Nephropathy

FIG. 13.8 Schematic algorithm for the management of renovascular hypertension and ischemic nephropathy. The overriding goal is lower morbidity associated with hypertension by reaching goal blood pressure with preserved kidney function. Should that not be achievable by medical therapy or should renovascular disease progress to produce "high-risk clinical syndromes" as shown, renal revascularization should be considered, either by endovascular or surgical intervention (see text). *(Modified from Textor SC. Renovascular Hypertension and Ischemic Nephropathy. In: Skorecki K, Taal MW, Chertow GM. Yu ASL, Marsden PA, ed. Brenner and Rector's The Kidney. Philadelphia: Elsevier; 2016: 1567-1609.)*

TABLE 13.4 Randomized Clinical Trials: Percutaneous Transluminal Renal Angioplasty With Stenting Versus Medical Therapy Alone for Renal Function and/or Cardiovascular Outcomes With Atherosclerotic Renovascular Disease

TRIALS	N	POPULATION	INCLUSION CRITERIA	EXCLUSION CRITERIA	OUTCOMES
STAR (2009) 10 centers f/up 2 years	Med Tx:76 PTRA: 64	Patients with impaired renal function, ostial ARVD detected by various imaging studies and stable blood pressure on statin and aspirin	ARVD >50% Creatinine clearance <80 mL/min/1.73 m² Controlled blood pressure one month before inclusion	Kidney <8 cm and, renal artery diameter <4 mm, eCrCl < 15 mL/min per 1.73 m2, DM with proteinuria (>3 g/d), malignant hypertension	No difference in GFR decline (primary endpoint ≥20% change in clearance), but many did not undergo PTRA due ARVD <50% on angiography Serious complication in the PTRA group Study was underpowered
ASTRAL (2009) 57 centers f/up 5 years	Med Tx:403 PTRA: 403	Patients with uncontrolled or refractory hypertension or unexplained renal dysfunction with unilateral or bilateral ARVD on statin and aspirin	ARVD substantial disease suitable for endovascular intervention and patient's doctor uncertainty of clinical benefit from revascularization	High likelihood of PTRA in <6 months Without ARVD, previous ARVD PTRA FMD	No difference in BP, renal function, mortality, CV events (primary endpoint: 20% reduction of the mean slope of the reciprocal of the serum creatinine level) Substantial risk in the PTRA group
CORAL (2014) 109 centers f/up 5 years	Med Tx:480 PTRA:467	Hypertension 2 or more antihypertensives or CKD stage ≥3 with ARVD with unilateral or bilateral disease on statin	SBP >155 mm Hg, at least two drugs ARVD >60% Subsequent changes included that the SBP >155 mm Hg for defining systolic hypertension was no longer specified as long as patient had CKD stage 3	FMD Creatinine >4.0 mg/dL kidney length <7 cm and use of >1 stent	No difference of death from CV or renal causes. Modest improvement of SBP in the stented group Total 26 complications (5.5%)

(Summarized from Herrmann SM, Saad A, Textor SC. Management of atherosclerotic renovascular disease after Cardiovascular Outcomes in Renal Atherosclerotic Lesions (CORAL). Nephrol Dial Transplant. 2015;30:366-375.)
ARVD, Acute viral respiratory disease; *ASTRAL,* Angioplasty and Stenting for Renal Artery Lesions; *CKD,* chronic kidney disease; *CORAL,* Cardiovascular Outcomes in Renal Atherosclerotic Lesions; *CV,* cardiovascular; *DM,* diabetes mellitus; *eCRCL,* estimates of creatinine clearance; *FMD,* fibromuscular dysplasia; *f/up,* follow-up; *GFR,* glomerular filtration rate; *N,* number of patients; *PTRA,* percutaneous transluminal renal angioplasty; *SBP,* systolic blood pressure; *STAR,* Stent Placement and Blood Pressure and Lipid-Lowering for the Prevention of Progression of Renal Dysfunction Caused by Atherosclerotic Ostial Stenosis of the Renal Artery; *Tx,* therapy.

a result, rates of endovascular stent procedures have fallen in recent years.

The limitations of these trials have been substantial, however, particularly as many severe cases of rapidly progressive renal insufficiency, intractable hypertension, and/or episodic pulmonary edema have not been enrolled.[30,61] Hence, these trials suffer from underrepresentation of high-risk disease, as has been emphasized from registry[29,57] and observational reports.[62] These additional reports and series identify high-risk subsets of patients with rapidly advancing disease and/or clinical problems related to fluid retention (pulmonary edema), acute kidney injury (AKI) during initiation of ACE/ARB therapy, or rapidly developing renal failure that benefit enormously from revascularization. Such a case developing progressive stenosis to a solitary functioning kidney associated with episodes of acute renal failure and circulatory congestion is illustrated in Fig. 13.5. It remains an important role for the clinician to identify and intervene for such individuals.

MANAGEMENT STRATEGIES FOR RENOVASCULAR HYPERTENSION AND ISCHEMIC NEPHROPATHY

A clinical algorithm for managing RVH and ischemic nephropathy is presented in Fig. 13.8. In most cases, RVH surfaces as progressive (or de novo) hypertension with some decrement in kidney function. Reduction of cardiovascular risk is paramount and includes antihypertensive drug therapy to goal levels, along with removal of tobacco use, likely initiation of statins and aspirin, particularly with atherosclerotic disease. Duplex imaging will evaluate basic kidney structure, size, and whether occlusive disease is present, unilateral or bilateral. In most cases, drug therapy will be sufficient to achieve BP goals. If kidney function and BP are stable on therapy, results of prospective, randomized trials suggest that little further is to be gained immediately from revascularization, at least in follow-up intervals between 3 to 5 years. However, rates of progression and stability vary widely between individual patients. Important considerations include whether kidney function deteriorates in the presence of RAAS blockade and/or if a high-risk syndrome develops, including circulatory congestion (pulmonary edema) and/or rapidly progressive renal insufficiency with failure to achieve BP targets. Several professional societies have proposed a consensus statement (Table 13.5) to acknowledge the appropriate application of renal revascularization for such individuals.[63] In such cases, clinicians must carefully weigh the potential benefits and risks of restoring vessel patency and blood flow to the affected kidney at a point when renal function can be salvaged.

TABLE 13.5 Clinical Scenarios in Which Revascularization of Significant Renal Artery Stenosis May Be Considered

Appropriate Care	• Cardiac disturbance syndromes (flash pulmonary edema or acute coronary syndrome[ACS]) with severe hypertension • Resistant hypertension (HTN) (Uncontrolled HTN with failure of maximally tolerated doses of at least three antihypertensive agents, one of which is a diuretic, or intolerance to medications • Ischemic nephropathy with chronic kidney disease (CKD) with estimate glomerular filtration rate (eGFR) <45 mL/min and global renal ischemia (unilateral significant renal artery stenosis [RAS] with a solitary kidney or bilateral significant RAS) without other explanation
May Be Appropriate Care	• Unilateral RAS with CKD (eGFR <45 mL/min) • Unilateral RAS with prior episodes of congestive heart failure (stage C) • Anatomically challenging or high risk lesion (early bifurcation, small vessel, severe concentric calcification, and severe aortic atheroma or mural thrombus)
Rarely Appropriate Care	• Unilateral, solitary, or bilateral RAS with • controlled blood pressure and normal renal function • Unilateral, solitary, or bilateral RAS with kidney size <7 cm in pole-to-pole length • Unilateral, solitary, or bilateral RAS with chronic endstage renal disease on hemodialysis >3 months • Unilateral, solitary, or bilateral renal artery chronic total occlusion

Significant renal artery stenosis is an angiographically moderate lesion (50%-70%) with physiologic confirmation of severity or greater than 70% stenosis.
(Modified from Parikh SA, Shishehbor MH, Gray BH, et al. SCAI expert consensus statement for renal artery stenting appropriate use. Catheter Cardiovasc. *2014;84:1163-1171.)*

References

1. Basso N, Terragno NA. History about the discovery of the renin-angiotensin system. *Hypertension*. 2001;38:1246-1249.
2. Hansen KJ, Edwards MS, Craven TE, et al. Prevalence of renovascular disease in the elderly: a population based study. *J Vasc Surg*. 2002;36:443-451.
3. Coen G, Manni M, Giannoni MF, et al. Ischemic nephropathy in an elderly nephrologic and hypertensive population. *Am J Nephrol*. 1998;18:221-227.
4. de Mast Q, Beutler JJ. The prevalence of atherosclerotic renal artery stenosis in risk groups: a systematic literature review. *J Hypertens*. 2009;27:1333-1340.
5. Lorenz EC, Vrtiska TJ, Lieske JC, et al. Prevalence of renal artery and kidney abnormalities by computed tomography among healthy adults. *Clin J Am Soc Nephrol*. 2010;5:431-438.
6. Textor SC, Misra S, Oderich G. Percutaneous revascularization for ischemic nephropathy: the past, present and future. *Kidney Int*. 2013;83:28-40.
7. Lerman LO, Nath KA, Rodriguez-Porcel M, et al. Increased oxidative stress in experimental renovascular hypertension. *Hypertension*. 2001;37(2 Pt 2):541-546.
8. Cervenka L, Horacek V, Vaneckova I, et al. Essential role of AT1-A receptor in the development of 2K1C hypertension. *Hypertension*. 2002;40:735-741.
9. Harrison DG, Guzik TJ, Lob HE, et al. Inflammation, immunity and hypertension. *Hypertension*. 2010;57:132-140.
10. Brunner HR, Kirshmann JD, Sealey JE, Laragh JH. Hypertension of renal origin: Evidence for two different mechanisms. *Science*. 1971;174:1344-1346.
11. Herrmann SM, Saad A, Eirin A, et al. Differences in GFR and Tissue Oxygenation, and Interactions between Stenotic and Contralateral Kidneys in Unilateral Atherosclerotic Renovascular Disease. *Clin J Am Soc Nephrol*. 2016;11:458-469.
12. Gloviczki ML, Glockner JF, Lerman LO, et al. Preserved oxygenation despite reduced blood flow in poststenotic kidneys in human atherosclerotic renal artery stenosis. *Hypertension*. 2010;55:961-966.
13. Epstein FH. Oxygen and renal metabolism. *Kidney Int*. 1997;51:381-385.
14. Evans RG, Gardiner BS, Smith DW, O'Connor PM. Intrarenal oxygenation: unique challenges and the biophysical basis of homeostasis. *Am J Physiol Renal Physiol*. 2008;295:F1259-F1270.
15. Epstein FH, Prasad P. Effects of furosemide on medullary oxygenation in younger and older subjects. *Kidney Int*. 2000;57:2080-2083.
16. Lerman LO, Chade AR. Angiogenesis in the kidney: a new therapeutic target? *Curr Opin Nephrol Hyper*. 2009;18:160-165.
17. Lerman LO, Textor SC. Gained in translation: protective paradigms for the poststenotic kidney. *Hypertension*. 2015;65:976-982.
18. Gloviczki ML, Glockner JF, Crane JA, et al. BOLD magnetic resonance imaging identifies cortical hypoxia in severe renovascular disease. *Hypertension*. 2011;58:1066-1072.
19. Gloviczki ML, Keddis MT, Garovic VD, et al. TGF expression and macrophage accumulation in atherosclerotic renal artery stenosis. *Clin J Am Soc Nephrol*. 2013;8:546-553.
20. Lech M, Grobmayr R, Ryu M, et al. Macrophage phenotype controls long-term AKI outcomes—kidney regeneration versus atrophy. *J Am Soc Nephrol*. 2014;25:292-304.
21. Saad A, Herrmann SMS, Crane J, et al. Stent revascularization restores cortical blood flow and reverses tissue hypoxia in atherosclerotic renal artery stenosis but fails to reverse inflammatory pathways or glomerular filtration rate. *Circ Cardiovasc Interv*. 2013;6:428-435.
22. Romero JC, Lerman LO. Novel noninvasive techniques for studying renal function in man. *Sem Nephrol*. 2000;20:456-462.
23. De Bruyne B, Manoharan G, Pijls NHJ, et al. Assessment of renal artery stenosis severity by pressure gradient measurements. *J Am Coll Cardiol*. 2006;48:1851-1855.
24. Losito A, Fagugli RM, Zampi I, et al. Comparison of target organ damage in renovascular and essential hypertension. *Am J Hypertens*. 1996;9:1062-1067.
25. Krijnen P, van Jaarsveld BC, Steyerberg EW, et al. A clinical prediction rule for renal artery stenosis. *Ann Int Med*. 1998;129:705-711.
26. Messerli FH, Bangalore S, Makani H, et al. Flash pulmonary oedema and bilateral renal artery stenosis: the Pickering Syndrome. *Eur Heart J*. 2011;32:2231-2237.
27. Gandhi SK, Powers JC, Nomeir AM, et al. The pathogenesis of acute pulmonary edema associated with hypertension. *N Engl J Med*. 2001;344:17-22.
28. Kane GC, Xu N, Mistrik E, et al. Renal artery revascularization improves heart failure control in patients with atherosclerotic renal artery stenosis. *Nephrol Dial Transplant*. 2010;25:813-820.
29. Ritchie J, Green D, Chrysochou C, et al. High-risk clinical presentations in atherosclerotic renovascular disease: prognosis and response to renal artery revascularization. *Am J Kidney Dis*. 2014;63:186-197.
30. Herrmann SM, Saad A, Textor SC. Management of atherosclerotic renovascular disease after Cardiovascular Outcomes in Renal Atherosclerotic Lesions (CORAL). *Nephrol Dial Transplant*. 2015;30:366-375.
31. Pickering TG, Hall JE, Appel LJ, et al. Recommendations for blood pressure measurement in humans and experimental animals. Part 1: Blood pressure measurement in humans. A statement for professionals from the subcommittee of professional and public education of the American Heart Association Council on High Blood Pressure Research. *Hypertension*. 2005;45:142-161.
32. Iantorno M, Pola R, Schinzari F, et al. Association between altered circadian blood pressure profile and cardiac end-organ damage in patients with renovascular hypertension. *Cardiology*. 2003;100:114-119.
33. Herrmann SMS, Textor SC. Diagnostic criteria for renovascular disease: where are we now? *Nephrol Dial Transplant*. 2012;27:2657-2663.
34. Strong CG, Hunt JC, Sheps SG, et al. Renal venous renin activity: enhancement of sensitivity of lateralization by sodium depletion. *Am J Cardiol*. 1971;27:602-611.
35. Weinberg I, Jaff MR. Renal artery duplex ultrasonography. In: Lerman LO, Textor SC, editors. *Renal Vascular Disease*. 1st ed. London: Springer; 2014:211-230.
36. Radermacher J, Chavan A, Bleck J, et al. Use of Doppler ultrasonography to predict the outcome of therapy for renal-artery stenosis. *N Engl J Med*. 2001;344:410-417.
37. Glockner JF, Vrtiska TJ. Renal MR and CT angiography: current concepts. *Abdom Imaging*. 2007;32:407-420.
38. Juillard L, Lerman LO, Kruger DG, et al. Blood oxygen level-dependent measurement of acute intra-renal ischemia. *Kidney Int*. 2004;65:944-950.
39. Textor SC, Glockner JF, Lerman LO, et al. The use of magnetic resonance to evaluate tissue oxygenation in renal artery stenosis. *J Am Soc Nephrol*. 2008;19:780-788.
40. Saad A, Crane J, Glockner JF, et al. Human renovascular disease: estimating fractional tissue hypoxia to analyze blood oxygen level dependent (BOLD) MR in human renovascular disease. *Radiology*. 2013;268:770-778.
41. Chrysochou C, Mendichovszky IA, Buckley DL, et al. BOLD imaging: a potential predictive biomarker of renal functional outcome following revascularization in atheromatous renovascular disease. *Nephrol Dial Transplant*. 2012;27:1013-1019.
42. Elliott WJ. Renovascular hypertension: an update. *J Clin Hypertens*. 2008;10:522-533.
43. Mangiacapra F, Trana C, Sarno G, et al. Translesional pressure gradients to predict blood pressure response after renal artery stenting in patients with renovascular hypertension. *Circ Cardiovasc Interven*. 2010;3:537-542.
44. Calhoun DA, Jones D, Textor S, et al. Resistant hypertension: diagnosis, evaluation, and treatment: a scientific statement from the American Heart Association Professional Education Committee of the Council for High Blood Pressure Research. *Circulation*. 2008;117:e510-526.
45. Freedman BI, Sedor JR. Hypertension-associated kidney disease—perhaps no more. *J Am Soc Nephrol*. 2008;19:2047-2051.
46. Olin JW, Sealove BA. Diagnosis, management, and future developments of fibromuscular dysplasia. *J Vasc Surg Cases*. 2011;53:826-836.
47. Canzanello VJ. Medical management of renovascular disease. In: Lerman LO, Textor SC, editors. *Renal Vascular Disease*. 1st ed. London: Springer; 2014:305-316.
48. Chrysochou C, Foley RN, Young JF, et al. Dispelling the myth: the use of renin-angiotensin blockade in atheromatous renovascular disease. *Nephrol Dial Transplant*. 2012;27:1403-1409.
49. Evans KL, Tuttle KR, Folt DA, et al. Use of renin-angiotensin inhibitors in people with renal artery stenosis. *Clin J Am Soc Nephrol*. 2014;9:1199-1206.
50. Hackam DG, Duong-Hua ML, Mamdani M, et al. Angiotensin inhibition in renovascular disease: a population-based cohort study. *Am Heart J*. 2008;156:549-555.
51. Textor SC, Lerman LO. Paradigm Shifts in atherosclerotic renovascular disease: where are we now? *J Am Soc Nephrol*. 2015;26:2074-2080.
52. Onuigbo MAC. Is renoprotection with RAAS blockade a failed paradigm? Have we learnt any lessions so far? *Int J Clin Pract*. 2010;64:1341-1346.
53. Slovut DP, Olin JW. Current concepts: Fibromuscular dysplasia. *N Engl J Med*. 2004;350:1862-18671.
54. Boateng FK, Greco BA. Renal Artery Stenosis: prevalence of, risk factors for and management of in-stent stenosis. *Am J Kidney Dis*. 2013;61:147-160.
55. Harden PN, Macleod MJ, Rodger RS, et al. Effect of renal-artery stenting on progression of renovacular renal failure. *Lancet*. 1997;349:1133-1136.
56. Watson PS, Hadjipetrou P, Cox SV, et al. Effect of renal artery stenting on renal function and size in patients with atherosclerotic renovascular disease. *Circulation*. 2001;102:1671-1677.
57. Kalra PA, Chrysochou C, Green D, et al. The benefit of renal artery stenting in patients with atheromatous renovascular disease and advanced chronic kidney disease. *Catheter Cardiovasc Interven*. 2010;75:1-10.
58. Balk E, Raman G, Chung M, et al. Effectiveness of management strategies for renal artery stenosis: a systematic review. *Ann Int Med*. 2006;145:901-912.
59. Cooper CJ, Murphy TP, Cutlip DE, et al. Stenting and medical therapy for atherosclerotic renal-artery stenosis. *N Engl J Med*. 2014;370:13-22.
60. The AI. Revascularization versus medical therapy for renal-artery stenosis. *N Engl J Med*. 2009;361:1953-1962.
61. Textor SC, Lerman L, McKusick M. The uncertain value of renal artery interventions: where are we now? *JAAC Cardiovasc Intervent*. 2009;2:175-182.
62. Textor SC. Attending rounds: a patient with accelerated hypertension and an atrophic kidney. *Clin J Am Soc Nephrol*. 2014;9:1117-1123.
63. Parikh SA, Shishehbor MH, Gray BH, et al. SCAI expert consensus statement for renal artery stenting appropriate use. *Catheter Cardiovasc Intervent*. 2014;84:1163-1171.

14 Secondary Hypertension: Primary Hyperaldosteronism and Mineralocorticoid Excess States

William F. Young, Jr.

Hypertension resulting from mineralocorticoid excess can be categorized based on levels of renin and aldosterone (Box 14.1). Aldosterone, deoxycorticosterone, and cortisol are the three major mineralocorticoid receptor ligands. This chapter reviews the clinical presentation, diagnostic evaluation, and treatment of these three types of renin-independent mineralocorticoid excess states.

PRIMARY ALDOSTERONISM

Hypertension, suppressed plasma renin activity (PRA), and increased aldosterone excretion characterize the syndrome of primary aldosteronism, first described in 1955.[1] Aldosterone-producing adenoma (APA) and bilateral idiopathic hyperaldosteronism (IHA) are the most common subtypes of primary aldosteronism (see Box 14.1). Somatic mutations account for about half of APAs and include mutations in genes encoding components of: the Kir 3.4 (GIRK4) potassium channel (KCNJ5); the sodium/potassium and calcium ATPases (ATP1A1 and ATP2B3); and a voltage-dependent C-type calcium channel (CACNA1D).[2] A much less common form, unilateral hyperplasia or primary adrenal hyperplasia (PAH), is caused by micronodular or macronodular hyperplasia of the zona glomerulosa of predominantly one adrenal gland. Familial hyperaldosteronism (FH) is also rare, and three types have been described (see later).[2]

In the past, clinicians would not consider the diagnosis of primary aldosteronism unless the patient presented with spontaneous hypokalemia, and then the diagnostic evaluation would require discontinuation of antihypertensive medications for at least 2 weeks. This diagnostic approach resulted in predicted prevalence rates of less than 0.5% of hypertensive patients.[3-9] However, it is now recognized that most patients with primary aldosteronism are not hypokalemic[10-12] and that screening can be completed while the patient is taking antihypertensive drugs with a simple blood test that yields the ratio of plasma aldosterone concentration (PAC) to PRA.[12] Use of the PAC/PRA ratio as a case-detection test, followed by aldosterone suppression for confirmatory testing, has resulted in much higher prevalence estimates for primary aldosteronism; 5% to 10% of all patients with hypertension.[11-14]

CLINICAL PRESENTATION

The diagnosis of primary aldosteronism is usually made in patients who are in the third to sixth decade of life. Few symptoms are specific to the syndrome. Patients with marked hypokalemia may have muscle weakness and cramping, headaches, palpitations, polydipsia, polyuria, nocturia, or a combination of these.[10] Periodic paralysis is a very rare presentation in Caucasians, but it is not an infrequent presentation in patients of Asian descent.[15] For example, in a series of 50 patients with APA reported from Hong Kong, 21 (42%)

presented with periodic paralysis.[15] Another rare presentation is tetany associated with the decrease in ionized calcium with marked hypokalemic alkalosis. The polyuria and nocturia are a result of hypokalemia-induced renal concentrating defect, and the presentation is frequently mistaken for prostatism in men. There are no specific physical findings. Edema is not a common finding because of the phenomenon of mineralocorticoid escape, described earlier. The degree of hypertension is typically moderate to severe and may be resistant to usual pharmacologic treatments.[10,16] In the first 262 cases of primary aldosteronism diagnosed at Mayo Clinic (1957 to 1986), the highest blood pressure was 260/155 mm Hg; the mean (± standard deviation [SD]) was 184/112 ± 28/16 mm Hg.[16] Patients with APA tend to have higher blood pressures than those with IHA.

Hypokalemia is frequently absent, so all patients with hypertension are candidates for this disorder. In other patients, the hypokalemia becomes evident only with the addition of a potassium-wasting diuretic (e.g., hydrochlorothiazide, furosemide). Deep-seated renal cysts are found in up to 60% of patients with chronic hypokalemia.[17] Because of a reset osmostat, the serum sodium concentration tends to be high-normal or slightly above the upper limit of normal. This clinical clue is very useful in the initial assessment for potential primary aldosteronism.

Several studies have shown that patients with primary aldosteronism are at higher risk than other patients with hypertension for target-organ damage of the heart and kidney.[18,19] Chronic kidney disease is common in patients with long standing primary aldosteronism.[20] When matched for age, blood pressure, and duration of hypertension, patients with primary aldosteronism have greater left ventricular mass measurements than patients with other types of hypertension (e.g., pheochromocytoma, Cushing syndrome, essential hypertension).[21] In patients with APA, the left ventricular wall thickness and mass were markedly decreased 1 year after adrenalectomy.[22] A case-control study of 124 patients with primary aldosteronism and 465 patients with essential hypertension (matched for age, sex, and systolic and diastolic blood pressure) found that patients presenting with either APA or IHA had a significantly higher rate of cardiovascular events (e.g., stroke, atrial fibrillation, myocardial infarction) than the matched patients with essential hypertension.[19] A negative effect of circulating aldosterone on cardiac function was found in young nonhypertensive subjects with GRA who had increased left ventricular wall thickness and reduced diastolic function compared with age- and sex-matched controls.[18]

DIAGNOSTIC INVESTIGATION

The diagnostic approach to primary aldosteronism can be considered in three phases: case-detection tests, confirmatory tests, and subtype evaluation tests.

BOX 14.1 Mineralocorticoid Excess States

Low Renin and High Aldosterone
Primary Aldosteronism
Aldosterone-producing adenoma (APA)—35% of cases
Bilateral idiopathic hyperplasia (IHA)—60% of cases
Primary (unilateral) adrenal hyperplasia—2% of cases
Aldosterone-producing adrenocortical carcinoma—<1% of cases
Familial hyperaldosteronism (FH)
    Glucocorticoid-remediable aldosteronism (FH type I)—<1% of cases
    FH type II (APA or IHA)—<2% of cases
    FH type III (associated with the germline mutation in the KCNJ5 potassium channel)—<1% of cases
Ectopic aldosterone-producing adenoma or carcinoma—<0.1% of cases

Low Renin and Low Aldosterone
Hyperdeoxycorticosteronism
Congenital adrenal hyperplasia
    11β-Hydroxylase deficiency
    17α-Hydroxylase deficiency
Deoxycorticosterone-producing tumor
Primary cortisol resistance
Apparent Mineralocorticoid Excess (AME)/11β-Hydroxysteroid Dehydrogenase Deficiency

Genetic
Acquired
    Licorice or carbenoxolone ingestion
    Cushing syndrome

Cushing Syndrome
Exogenous glucocorticoid administration—most common cause
Endogenous
    ACTH-dependent—85% of cases
        Pituitary
        Ectopic
    ACTH-independent—15% of cases
        Unilateral adrenal disease
        Bilateral adrenal disease
            Bilateral macronodular adrenal hyperplasia (rare)
            Primary pigmented nodular adrenal disease (rare)

High Renin and High Aldosterone
Renovascular hypertension
Diuretic use
Renin-secreting tumor
Malignant-phase hypertension
Coarctation of the aorta

ACTH, Adrenocorticotropin hormone, *AME*, apparent mineralocorticoid excess; *APA*, aldosterone-producing adenoma; *FH*, familial hyperaldosteronism; *IHA*, idiopathic hyperaldosteronism.

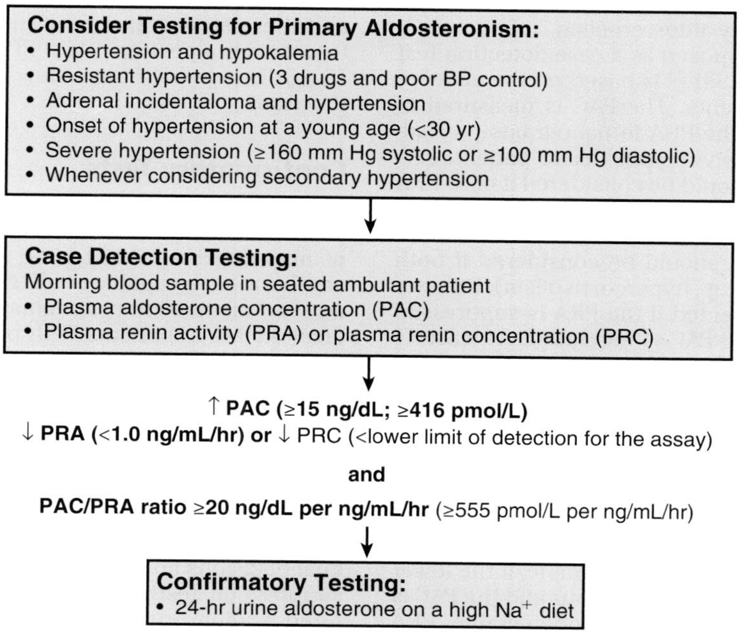

Consider Testing for Primary Aldosteronism:
• Hypertension and hypokalemia
• Resistant hypertension (3 drugs and poor BP control)
• Adrenal incidentaloma and hypertension
• Onset of hypertension at a young age (<30 yr)
• Severe hypertension (≥160 mm Hg systolic or ≥100 mm Hg diastolic)
• Whenever considering secondary hypertension

↓

Case Detection Testing:
Morning blood sample in seated ambulant patient
• Plasma aldosterone concentration (PAC)
• Plasma renin activity (PRA) or plasma renin concentration (PRC)

↓

↑ **PAC (≥15 ng/dL; ≥416 pmol/L)**
↓ **PRA (<1.0 ng/mL/hr) or** ↓ PRC (<lower limit of detection for the assay)

and

PAC/PRA ratio ≥20 ng/dL per ng/mL/hr (≥555 pmol/L per ng/mL/hr)

↓

Confirmatory Testing:
• 24-hr urine aldosterone on a high Na⁺ diet

FIG. 14.1 When to consider testing for primary aldosteronism and use of the plasma aldosterone concentration–to–plasma renin activity ratio as a case-detection tool. *PAC*, Plasma aldosterone concentration, *PRA*, plasma renin activity, *PRC*, plasma renin concentration.

Case-Detection Tests

Spontaneous hypokalemia is uncommon in patients with uncomplicated hypertension; when present, it strongly suggests associated mineralocorticoid excess. However, several studies have shown that most patients with primary aldosteronism have baseline serum levels of potassium in the normal range.[12,13] Therefore, hypokalemia should not be the major criterion used to trigger case detection testing for primary aldosteronism. Patients with hypertension and hypokalemia (regardless of presumed cause), treatment-resistant hypertension (poor control on three antihypertensive drugs), severe hypertension (≥160 mm Hg systolic or ≥100 mm Hg diastolic), hypertension, and an incidental adrenal mass, or onset of hypertension at a young age should undergo screening for primary aldosteronism (Fig. 14.1).[10,12]

In patients with suspected primary aldosteronism, screening can be accomplished (see Fig. 14.1) by paired measurements of PAC and PRA in a random morning ambulatory blood sample (preferably obtained between 8.00 and 10.00 AM). This test may be performed while the patient is taking antihypertensive medications (with some exceptions, discussed later) and without posture stimulation.[10] Marked hypokalemia reduces the secretion of aldosterone, and it is optimal to restore the serum level of potassium to normal before performing diagnostic studies.

It may be difficult to interpret data obtained from patients treated with a mineralocorticoid receptor antagonist (spironolactone and eplerenone). These drugs prevent aldosterone from activating the receptor, resulting sequentially in sodium loss, a decrease in plasma volume, and an elevation in PRA, which will reduce the utility of the PAC/PRA ratio. For this reason, spironolactone and eplerenone should not be initiated until the evaluation is completed and the final decisions about treatment are made. However, there are rare exceptions to this rule. For example, if the patient is hypokalemic despite treatment with spironolactone or eplerenone, then the mineralocorticoid receptors are not fully blocked and PRA or PRC should be suppressed in such a patient with primary aldosteronism. In this unique circumstance, the evaluation for primary aldosteronism can proceed despite treatment with mineralocorticoid receptor antagonists. However, in most patients already receiving spironolactone, therapy should be discontinued for at least six weeks. Other potassium-sparing diuretics, such as amiloride and triamterene, usually do not interfere with testing unless the patient is on high doses.

Angiotensin-converting-enzyme (ACE) inhibitors and angiotensin receptor blockers (ARBs) have the potential to falsely elevate the PRA. Therefore, the finding of a detectable PRA level or a low PAC/PRA ratio in a patient taking one of these drugs does not exclude the diagnosis of primary aldosteronism. However, an undetectably low PRA level in a patient taking an ACE inhibitor or ARB makes primary aldosteronism likely, and the PRA is suppressed (<1.0 ng/mL per hour) in almost all patients with primary aldosteronism.

The PAC/PRA ratio, first proposed as a case-detection test for primary aldosteronism in 1981,[23] is based on the concept of paired hormone measurements. The PAC is measured in nanograms per deciliter, and the PRA in nanograms per milliliter per hour. In a hypertensive hypokalemic patient, secondary hyperaldosteronism should be considered if both PRA and PAC are increased and the PAC/PRA ratio is less than 10 (e.g., renovascular disease). An alternative source of mineralocorticoid receptor agonism should be considered if both PRA and PAC are suppressed (e.g., hypercortisolism). Primary aldosteronism should be suspected if the PRA is suppressed (<1.0 ng/mL per hour) and the PAC is increased. At least 14 prospective studies have been published on the use of the PAC/PRA ratio in detecting primary aldosteronism.[24] Although there is some uncertainty about test characteristics and lack of standardization (see later discussion), the PAC/PRA ratio is widely accepted as the case-detection test of choice for primary aldosteronism.[12]

It is important to understand that the lower limit of detection varies among different PRA assays and can have a dramatic effect on the PAC/PRA ratio. As an example, if the lower limit of detection for PRA is 0.6 ng/mL per hour and the PAC is 16 ng/dL, then the PAC/PRA ratio with an "undetectable" PRA would be 27; however, if the lower limit of detection for PRA is 0.1 ng/mL per hour, the same PAC level would yield a PAC/PRA ratio of 160. Thus, the cutoff for a "high" PAC/PRA ratio is laboratory dependent and, more specifically, PRA assay dependent. In a retrospective study, the combination of a PAC/PRA ratio greater than 30 and a PAC level greater than 20 ng/dL had a sensitivity of 90% and a specificity of 91% for APA.[25] At Mayo Clinic, the combination of a PAC/PRA ratio of 20 or higher, and a PAC level of at least 15 ng/dL is found in more than 90% of patients with surgically confirmed APA. In patients without primary aldosteronism, most of the variation occurs within the normal range.[26] A high PAC/PRA ratio is a positive screening test result, a finding that warrants further testing.[12]

It is critical for the clinician to recognize that the PAC/PRA ratio is only a case-detection tool, and all positive results should be followed by a confirmatory aldosterone suppression test to verify autonomous aldosterone production before treatment is initiated.[12] In a systematic review of 16 studies with 3136 participants, the PAC/PRA cutoff levels used varied between 7.2 and 100.[24] The sensitivity for APA varied between 64% and 100%, and the specificity between 87% and 100%. However, the description of the reference standard and the attribution of diagnosis at the end of the studies were incomplete, and there was a lack of standardization concerning the origin of the study cohort, ongoing antihypertensive medications, use of high-salt versus low-salt diet, and circumstances during blood sampling. The authors concluded that none of the studies provided any valid estimates of test characteristics (sensitivity, specificity, and likelihood ratio at various cutoff levels).[24] In a study of 118 subjects with essential hypertension, neither antihypertensive medications nor acute variation of dietary sodium affected the accuracy of the PAC/PRA ratio adversely; the sensitivities on and off therapy were 73% and 87%, respectively, and the specificities were 74% and 75%, respectively.[27] In a study of African American and Caucasian subjects with resistant hypertension, the PAC/PRA ratio was elevated (>20) in 45 of 58 subjects with primary aldosteronism and in 35 of 207 patients without primary aldosteronism (sensitivity, 78%; specificity, 83%).[28]

The measurement of PRA is time-consuming, shows high interlaboratory variability, and requires special preanalytic prerequisites. To overcome these disadvantages, a monoclonal antibody against active renin is being used by several reference laboratories to measure the plasma renin concentration (PRC) instead of PRA. However, few studies have compared the different methods of testing for primary aldosteronism, and these studies lack confirmatory testing. It is reasonable to consider a positive PAC/PRC test if the PAC is greater than 15 ng/dL and the PRC is below the lower limit of detection for the assay.

Confirmatory Tests

An increased PAC/PRA ratio is not diagnostic by itself, and primary aldosteronism must be confirmed by demonstration of inappropriate aldosterone secretion.[11] The list of drugs and hormones capable of affecting the RAA axis is extensive, and a "medication-contaminated" evaluation is frequently unavoidable in patients with poorly controlled hypertension despite a three-drug program. Calcium channel blockers and α1-adrenergic receptor blockers do not affect the diagnostic accuracy in most cases.[12] It is impossible to interpret data obtained from patients receiving treatment with mineralocorticoid receptor antagonists (e.g., spironolactone, eplerenone) when the PRA is not suppressed (see earlier). Therefore, treatment with a mineralocorticoid receptor antagonist should not be initiated until the evaluation has been completed and the final decisions about treatment have been made. Aldosterone suppression testing can be performed with orally administered sodium chloride and measurement of urinary aldosterone or with intravenous sodium chloride loading and measurement of PAC.[10,12]

Oral Sodium Loading Test

After hypertension and hypokalemia have been controlled, patients should receive a high-sodium diet (supplemented with sodium chloride tablets if needed) for 3 days, with a goal sodium intake of 5000 mg (equivalent to 218 mEq of sodium or 12.8 g sodium chloride).[16] The risk of increasing dietary sodium in patients with severe hypertension must be assessed in each case.[29] Because the high-salt diet can increase kaliuresis and hypokalemia, vigorous replacement of potassium chloride may be needed, and the serum level of potassium should be monitored daily. On the third day of the high-sodium diet, a 24-hour urine specimen is collected for measurement of aldosterone, sodium, and creatinine. To

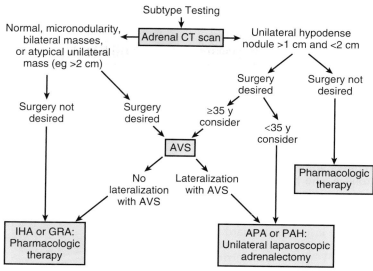

FIG. 14.2 Subtype evaluation of primary aldosteronism. For patients who want to pursue a surgical treatment for their hypertension, adrenal venous sampling is frequently a key diagnostic step. See text for details. *APA*, Aldosterone-producing adenoma; *AVS*, adrenal venous sampling; *CT*, computed tomography; *IHA*, idiopathic hyperaldosteronism; *PAH*, primary adrenal hyperplasia. *(Modified from Young WF, Jr., Hogan MJ. Renin-Independent hypermineralocorticoidism. Trends Endocrinol Metab. 1994;5:97-106.)*

document adequate sodium repletion, the 24-hour urinary sodium excretion should exceed 200 mEq. Urinary aldosterone excretion of more than 12 μg/24 hours in this setting is consistent with autonomous aldosterone secretion.[16] The sensitivity and specificity of the oral sodium loading test are 96% and 93%, respectively.[30]

Intravenous Saline Infusion Test

The intravenous saline infusion test has also been used widely for the diagnosis of primary aldosteronism.[11,31] Normal subjects show suppression of PAC after volume expansion with isotonic saline; subjects with primary aldosteronism do not show this suppression. The test is done after an overnight fast. Two liters of 0.9% sodium chloride solution is infused intravenously with an infusion pump over 4 hours with the patient recumbent. Blood pressure and heart rate are monitored during the infusion. At the completion of the infusion, blood is drawn for measurement of PAC. PAC levels in normal subjects decrease to less than 5 ng/dL, whereas most patients with primary aldosteronism do not suppress to less than 10 ng/dL. Postinfusion PAC values between 5 and 10 ng/dL are indeterminate and may be seen in patients with IHA. Historically, the saline infusion test has been performed in the supine position and the false-negative rate has been excessive; preliminary data suggest that if the saline infusion test is performed in the seated position the accuracy is improved.[32]

Fludrocortisone Suppression Test

In the fludrocortisone suppression test, fludrocortisone acetate is administered for 4 days (0.1 mg every 6 hours) in combination with sodium chloride tablets (2 g three times daily with food). Blood pressure and serum potassium levels must be monitored daily. In the setting of low PRA, failure to suppress the upright 10 AM PAC to less than 6 ng/dL on day 4 is diagnostic of primary aldosteronism.[33] Increased QT dispersion and deterioration of left ventricular function have been reported during fludrocortisone suppression tests.[29] Most centers no longer use this test.

Subtype Studies

After case-detection and confirmatory testing, the third management issue guides the therapeutic approach by distinguishing APA and PAH from IHA and GRA. Unilateral adrenalectomy in patients with APA or PAH results in normalization

of hypokalemia in all cases; hypertension is improved in all cases and is cured in 30% to 60% of patients.[34-36] In IHA and GRA, unilateral or bilateral adrenalectomy seldom corrects the hypertension.[16] IHA and GRA should be treated medically. APA is found in approximately 35% of cases and bilateral IHA in approximately 60% (see Box 14.1). APAs are usually small hypodense adrenal nodules (<2 cm in diameter) on computed tomography (CT) and are golden yellow in color when resected. IHA adrenal glands may be normal on CT or may show nodular changes. Aldosterone-producing adrenal carcinomas are almost always larger than 4 cm in diameter and have an inhomogeneous phenotype on CT.[37,38]

Adrenal Computed Tomography

Primary aldosteronism subtype evaluation may require one or more tests, the first of which is imaging of the adrenal glands with CT. If a solitary unilateral hypodense (HU < 10) macroadenoma (>1 cm) and normal contralateral adrenal morphology are found on CT in a young patient (<35 years) with severe primary aldosteronism, unilateral adrenalectomy is a reasonable therapeutic option (Fig. 14.2).[39] However, in many cases, CT shows normal-appearing adrenals, minimal unilateral adrenal limb thickening, unilateral microadenomas (≤1 cm), or bilateral macroadenomas. In these cases, additional testing is required to determine the source of excess aldosterone secretion.

Small APAs may be labeled incorrectly as IHA on the basis of CT findings of bilateral nodularity or normal-appearing adrenals. Also, apparent adrenal microadenomas may actually represent areas of hyperplasia, and unilateral adrenalectomy would be inappropriate. In addition, nonfunctioning unilateral adrenal macroadenomas are not uncommon, especially in older patients (>40 years).[40] Unilateral PAH may be visible on CT, or the PAH adrenal may appear normal on CT. In general, patients with APAs have more severe hypertension, more frequent hypokalemia, and higher levels of plasma aldosterone (>25 ng/dL) and urinary aldosterone (>30 μg/24 hours), and are younger (<50 years), compared with those who have IHA.[16] Patients fitting these descriptors are considered to have a "high probability of APA" regardless of the CT findings, and 41% of patients with a "high probability of APA" and a normal adrenal CT scan prove to have unilateral aldosterone hypersecretion.[41]

Adrenal CT is not accurate in distinguishing between APA and IHA.[39,41,42] In one study of 203 patients with primary aldosteronism who were evaluated with both CT and adrenal venous sampling, CT was accurate in only 53% of patients; based on the CT findings, 42 patients (22%) would have been incorrectly excluded as candidates for adrenalectomy, and 48 (25%) might have had unnecessary or inappropriate surgery.[41] In a systematic review of 38 studies involving 950 patients with primary aldosteronism, adrenal CT/magnetic resonance imaging (MRI) results did not agree with the findings from adrenal venous sampling in 359 patients (38%); based on CT/MRI, 19% of the 950 patients would have undergone noncurative surgery, and 19% would have been offered medical therapy instead of curative adrenalectomy.[42] Therefore, adrenal venous sampling is essential to direct appropriate therapy in patients with primary aldosteronism who have a high probability of APA and are seeking a potential surgical cure.

Adrenal Venous Sampling

Adrenal venous sampling (AVS) is the criterion standard test to distinguish between unilateral and bilateral disease in patients with primary aldosteronism.[31,39,42] AVS is an intricate procedure because the right adrenal vein is small and may be difficult to locate and cannulate; the success rate depends on the proficiency of the angiographer.[43] A review of 47 reports found that the success rate for cannulation of the right adrenal vein in 384 patients was 74%.[16] With experience and focusing the expertise to one or two radiologists at a referral center, the AVS success rate can be as high as 96%.[41,44,45]

The five keys to a successful AVS program are: (1) appropriate patient selection, (2) careful patient preparation, (3) focused technical expertise, (4) defined protocol, and (5) accurate data interpretation.[43] A center-specific, written protocol is mandatory. The protocol should be developed by an interested group of endocrinologists, hypertension specialists, internists, radiologists, and laboratory personnel. Safeguards should be in place to prevent mislabeling of the blood tubes in the radiology suite and to prevent sample mix-up in the laboratory.[43]

At Mayo Clinic, we use continuous cosyntropin infusion during AVS (50 μg/hour starting 30 minutes before sampling and continuing throughout the procedure) for the following reasons: (1) to minimize stress-induced fluctuations in aldosterone secretion during nonsimultaneous AVS; (2) to maximize the gradient in cortisol from adrenal vein to inferior vena cava (IVC) and thus confirm successful sampling of the adrenal veins; and (3) to maximize the secretion of aldosterone from an APA.[41,43] The adrenal veins are catheterized through the percutaneous femoral vein approach, and the position of the catheter tip is verified by gentle injection of a small amount of nonionic contrast medium and radiographic documentation. Blood is obtained from both adrenal veins and from the IVC below the renal veins and assayed for aldosterone and cortisol concentrations. To be sure that there is no cross-contamination, the IVC sample should be obtained from the external iliac vein. The venous sample from the left side typically is obtained from the common phrenic vein immediately adjacent to the entrance of the adrenal vein. The cortisol concentrations from the adrenal veins and IVC are used to confirm successful catheterization; the adrenal vein/IVC cortisol ratio is typically greater than 10:1.

Dividing the right and left adrenal vein PAC values by their respective cortisol concentrations corrects for the dilutional effect of the inferior phrenic vein flow into the left adrenal vein; these are termed *cortisol-corrected ratios* (Figs. 14.3A and 14.3B). In patients with APA, the mean cortisol-corrected aldosterone ratio (i.e., the ratio of PAC/cortisol from the APA side to that from the normal side) is 18:1.[41] A cutoff point of 4:1 for this ratio is used to indicate unilateral aldosterone excess. In patients with IHA, the mean cortisol-corrected aldosterone ratio is 1.8:1 (high side to low side), and a ratio of less than 3.0:1 suggests bilateral aldosterone hypersecretion.[41]

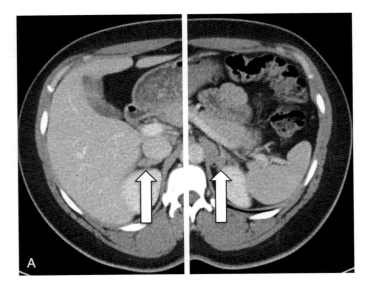

Results of Bilateral Adrenal Venous Sampling[a]

Vein	Aldosterone (A), ng/dL	Cortisol (C), μg/dL	A/C ratio	Aldosterone ratio[b]
R adrenal vein	250	647	0.4	
L adrenal vein	4,267	495	8.6	21.5
Inferior vena cava	98	22	4.5	

[a]Performed with continuous cosyntropin infusion, 50 μg/hr.
[b]Dominant adrenal vein A/C ratio divided by non-dominant adrenal vein A/C ratio.

B

FIG. 14.3 A 39-year-old woman had an 8-year history of hypertension and hypokalemia. The case detection test for primary aldosteronism was positive, with a plasma aldosterone concentration (PAC) of 41 ng/dL and low plasma renin activity (PRA) at less than 0.6 ng/mL per hour (PAC/PRA ratio >68). The confirmatory test for primary aldosteronism was also positive, with 24-hour urinary excretion of aldosterone of 28 μg on a high sodium diet (urinary sodium, >200 mEq/24 hours). A, Adrenal computed tomography with a 9-mm nodule (*arrow*, left panel) in the right adrenal and an 8-mm nodule (*arrow*, right panel) within the left adrenal gland. B, Adrenal venous sampling lateralized aldosterone secretion to the left adrenal gland, and two small cortical adenomas were found at laparoscopic left adrenalectomy. The postoperative plasma aldosterone concentration was less than 1.0 ng/dL. Hypokalemia was cured and blood pressure was normal without the aid of antihypertensive medications.

Therefore, most patients with a unilateral source of aldosterone have cortisol-corrected aldosterone lateralization ratios greater than 4.0, and ratios greater than 3.0 but less than 4.0 represent a zone of overlap. Ratios no higher than 3.0 are consistent with bilateral aldosterone secretion. The test characteristics of adrenal vein sampling for detection of unilateral aldosterone hypersecretion (APA or PAH) are 95% sensitivity and 100% specificity.[41] At centers with experience with AVS, the complication rate is 2.5% or less.[41,44] Complications can include symptomatic groin hematoma, adrenal hemorrhage, and dissection of an adrenal vein. However, adrenocortical function remains intact in most patients who experience AVS-related adrenal hemorrhage.[46]

Some centers and clinical practice guidelines recommend that AVS should be performed in all patients who have the diagnosis of primary aldosteronism.[31] The use of AVS should be based on patient preference, patient age, clinical comorbidities, and the clinical probability of finding an APA. A more practical approach is the selective use of AVS (see Fig. 14.2).[12,47]

As more aldosterone-specific imaging agents are developed, it is hoped that an accurate and widely available noninvasive subtype test will be available.[48]

Familial Hyperaldosteronism

Glucocorticoid-Remediable Aldosteronism: Familial Hyperaldosteronism Type 1

GRA (FH type 1) was first described in a single family in 1966.[49] Twenty-six years later the causative CYP11B1/CYP11B2 chimeric gene was discovered.[50] GRA is a form of hyperaldosteronism in which the hypersecretion of aldosterone can be reversed with physiologic doses of glucocorticoid.[51] It is rare, as illustrated by a study of 300 consecutive patients with primary aldosteronism; only two patients were diagnosed with GRA (prevalence = 0.66%) (see Box 14.1).[52] GRA is characterized by early-onset hypertension that is usually severe and refractory to conventional antihypertensive therapies, aldosterone excess, suppressed PRA, and excess production of 18-hydroxycortisol and 18-oxycortisol. Mineralocorticoid production is regulated by adrenocorticotropin hormone (ACTH) instead of by the normal secretagogue, angiotensin II. Therefore, aldosterone secretion can be suppressed by glucocorticoid therapy. In the absence of glucocorticoid therapy, this mutation results in overproduction of aldosterone and the hybrid steroids 18-hydroxycortisol and 18-oxycortisol, which can be measured in the urine to make the diagnosis.

Genetic testing is a sensitive and specific means of diagnosing GRA and obviates the need to measure the urinary levels of 18-oxycortisol and 18-hydroxycortisol or to perform dexamethasone suppression testing. Genetic testing for GRA should be considered for patients with primary aldosteronism who have a family history of primary aldosteronism, onset of primary aldosteronism at a young age (<20 years), or a family history of strokes at a young age.

Familial Hyperaldosteronism Type 2

FH-2 is autosomal dominant and may be monogenic.[2,53,54] The hyperaldosteronism in FH-2 does not suppress with dexamethasone, and GRA mutation testing is negative. FH-2 is more common than FH-1, but it still accounts for fewer than 6% of all patients with primary aldosteronism.[52] The molecular basis for FH-2 is unclear, although a recent linkage analysis study showed an association with chromosomal region 7p22.[53,54]

Familial Hyperaldosteronism Type 3

FH-3 was first described in a single family in 2008.[55] This initial report included a father and two daughters who all presented with refractory hypertension before seven years of age and all three were treated with bilateral adrenalectomy. The adrenal glands showed massive hyperplasia. Three years later the causative germline mutation in this family was discovered: a point mutation in and near the selectivity filter of the potassium channel KCNJ5.[56] This KCNJ5 mutation produces increased sodium conductance and cell depolarization, triggering calcium entry into glomerulosa cells, the signal for aldosterone production and cell proliferation. Other families with early onset hyperaldosteronism have also been identified to have germline point mutations in the KCNJ5 gene.[57,58] In families in Europe with FH (GRA excluded), a new germline G151E KCNJ5 mutation was found in two patients with primary aldosteronism from Italy and they presented a remarkably milder clinical and biochemical phenotype.[59] In four families with early onset primary aldosteronism, germline G151R KCNJ5 mutations were found in two with severe hyperplasia requiring surgery; two kindreds had G151E mutations and mild primary aldosteronism.[60]

Somatic Mutations in KCNJ5, ATP1A1, ATP2B3, and CACNA1D Genes

Somatic mutations in KCNJ5, ATP1A1, ATP2B3, and CACNA1D are found in approximately 50% of resected aldosterone-producing adenomas.[61] In a study of 474 unselected patients with aldosterone-producing adenomas, somatic heterozygous KCNJ5 mutations were present in 38%, CACNA1D mutations in 9.3%, ATP1A1 mutations in 5.3%, and ATP2B3 mutations in 1.7%. A metaanalysis that included 1636 patients with primary aldosteronism who had somatic KCNJ5 mutations showed that more pronounced hyperaldosteronism, young age, female gender, and larger tumors are the phenotypic features of APA patients with KCNJ5 mutations.[62] In addition, patients with KCNJ5 mutations were more frequently female and diagnosed younger, compared with CACNA1D mutation carriers or noncarriers.[61] However, the presence of one of these somatic mutations does not affect diagnosis or treatment.

Additional somatic APA mutations have been identified in three other genes: ATP1A1 and ATP2B3, encoding Na+/K+-ATPase 1 and Ca++-ATPase 3, respectively; and, CACNA1D, encoding a voltage-gated calcium channel.[63,64] In a subsequent study, somatic APA mutations in ATP1A1, ATP2B3, and KCNJ5 were present in 6.3%, 0.9%, and 39.3% of 112 APAs, respectively.[65] In addition, germline mutations in CACNA1D have now been reported in two children with primary aldosteronism.[66]

TREATMENT

The treatment goal is to prevent the morbidity and mortality associated with hypertension, hypokalemia, and cardiovascular damage. Knowing the cause of the primary aldosteronism helps to determine the appropriate treatment. Normalization of blood pressure should not be the only goal. In addition to the kidney and colon, mineralocorticoid receptors are present in the heart, brain, and blood vessels. Excessive secretion of aldosterone is associated with increased risk of cardiovascular disease and morbidity. Therefore, normalization of circulating aldosterone or mineralocorticoid receptor blockade should be part of the management plan for all patients with primary aldosteronism. However, clinicians must understand that most patients with long-standing primary aldosteronism have some degree of renal insufficiency that is masked by the glomerular hyperfiltration associated with aldosterone excess.[67,68] The true degree of renal insufficiency may become evident only after effective pharmacologic or surgical therapy.[67,68]

Unilateral Adrenalectomy

Unilateral laparoscopic adrenalectomy is an excellent treatment option for patients with APA or unilateral hyperplasia.[69,70] Although blood pressure control improves in almost 100% of patients postoperatively, average long-term cure rates of hypertension after unilateral adrenalectomy for APA range from 30% to 60%.[34,39] Persistent hypertension after adrenalectomy is correlated directly with having more than one first-degree relative with hypertension, use of more than two antihypertensive agents preoperatively, older age, increased serum creatinine level, and duration of hypertension and is most likely caused by coexistent primary hypertension.[34,71,72]

Laparoscopic adrenalectomy is the preferred surgical approach and is associated with shorter hospital stays and less long-term morbidity than the open approach. Because APAs are small and may be multiple, the entire adrenal gland should be removed.[73] To decrease the surgical risk, hypokalemia should be corrected with potassium supplements or a mineralocorticoid receptor antagonist, or both, preoperatively. These medications should be discontinued postoperatively. PAC should be measured 1 to 2 days after the operation to confirm a biochemical cure.[39] Serum potassium levels should be monitored weekly for 4 weeks after surgery, and a generous sodium diet should be followed to avoid the hyperkalemia of hypoaldosteronism that may occur because of the chronic suppression of the RAA axis.[74,75] Clinically significant hyperkalemia develops after surgery in approximately 5% of APA patients, and short-term fludrocortisone supplementation may be required. Typically, the hypertension that was associated with aldosterone excess resolves in 1 to 3 months after the surgery. It has been found that adrenalectomy for APA is significantly less expensive than long-term medical therapy.[76]

Pharmacologic Treatment

IHA and GRA should be treated medically. In addition, APA may be treated medically if the medical treatment includes mineralocorticoid receptor blockade.[77,78] A sodium-restricted diet (<100 mEq of sodium per day), maintenance of ideal body weight, tobacco avoidance, and regular aerobic exercise contribute significantly to the success of pharmacologic treatment. No placebo-controlled, randomized trials have evaluated the relative efficacy of drugs in the treatment of primary aldosteronism.[79]

Spironolactone has been the drug of choice to treat primary aldosteronism for more than four decades. It is available as 25-mg, 50-mg, and 100-mg tablets. The dosage is 12.5 to 25 mg per day initially and can be increased to 400 mg per day if necessary to achieve a high-normal serum potassium concentration without the aid of oral potassium chloride supplementation. Hypokalemia responds promptly, but hypertension can take as long as 4 to 8 weeks to be corrected. After several months of therapy, the dosage of spironolactone often can be decreased to as little as 25 to 50 mg per day; dosage titration is based on a goal serum potassium level in the high-normal range. Serum potassium and creatinine should be monitored frequently during the first 4 to 6 weeks of therapy (especially in patients with renal insufficiency or diabetes mellitus). Spironolactone increases the half-life of digoxin, and the digoxin dosage may need to be adjusted when treatment with spironolactone is started. Concomitant therapy with salicylates should be avoided because they interfere with the tubular secretion of an active metabolite and decrease the effectiveness of spironolactone. However, spironolactone is not selective for the mineralocorticoid receptor. For example, antagonism at the testosterone receptor may result in painful gynecomastia, erectile dysfunction, and decreased libido in men, and agonist activity at the progesterone receptor results in menstrual irregularity in women.[80]

Eplerenone is a steroid-based antimineralocorticoid that acts as a competitive and selective mineralocorticoid receptor antagonist and was approved by the United States Food and Drug Administration (FDA) for the treatment of uncomplicated essential hypertension in 2003. The 9,11-epoxide group in eplerenone results in a marked reduction of the molecule's progestational and antiandrogenic actions; compared with spironolactone, eplerenone has 0.1% of the binding affinity to androgen receptors and less than 1% of the binding affinity to progesterone receptors. In a randomized, double-blinded trial comparing the efficacy, safety, and tolerability of eplerenone with that of spironolactone (100 to 300 versus 75 to 225 mg, respectively) in patients with primary aldosteronism found spironolactone to be superior in terms of blood pressure lowering, but to be associated with higher rates of male gynecomastia (21% versus 5% for eplerenone) and female mastodynia (21% versus 0%).[81] Eplerenone is available as 25-mg and 50-mg tablets. For primary aldosteronism, it is reasonable to start with a dose of 25 mg twice daily (twice daily because of the shorter half-life of eplerenone compared with spironolactone) and titrated upward; the target is a high-normal serum potassium concentration without the aid of potassium supplements. The maximum dose approved by the FDA for hypertension is 100 mg per day. Potency studies with eplerenone show 25% to 50% less milligram-per-milligram potency compared with spironolactone. As with spironolactone, it is important to monitor blood pressure, serum potassium, and serum creatinine levels closely. Side effects include dizziness, headache, fatigue, diarrhea, hypertriglyceridemia, and elevated liver enzymes.

Patients with IHA frequently require a second antihypertensive agent to achieve good blood pressure control. Hypervolemia is a major reason for resistance to drug therapy, and low doses of a thiazide (e.g., 12.5 to 50 mg of hydrochlorothiazide daily) or a related sulfonamide diuretic are effective in combination with the mineralocorticoid receptor antagonist. Because these agents often lead to further hypokalemia, serum potassium levels should be monitored.

Before treatment for GRA is initiated, the diagnosis of GRA should be confirmed with genetic testing. In the GRA patient, chronic treatment with physiologic doses of a glucocorticoid normalizes blood pressure and corrects hypokalemia. The clinician should be cautious about iatrogenic Cushing syndrome with excessive doses of glucocorticoids, especially when dexamethasone is used in children. Shorter-acting agents such as prednisone or hydrocortisone should be prescribed, using the smallest effective dose in relation to body surface area (e.g., hydrocortisone, 10 to 12 mg/m^2 per day). Target blood pressure in children should be guided by age-specific blood pressure percentiles. Children should be monitored by pediatricians with expertise in glucocorticoid therapy, with careful attention paid to preventing retardation of linear growth as a result of overtreatment. Treatment with mineralocorticoid receptor antagonists in these patients may be just as effective as glucocorticoids and avoids the potential disruption of the hypothalamic-pituitary-adrenal axis and risk of iatrogenic side effects. In addition, glucocorticoid therapy or mineralocorticoid receptor blockade may even have a role in normotensive GRA patients.[18]

Pregnancy

Primary aldosteronism is uncommon in pregnancy with fewer than 40 patients reported in the medical literature and most patients have had APAs.[82-85] Primary aldosteronism can lead to intrauterine growth retardation, preterm delivery, intrauterine fetal demise, and placental abruption.[86] Case detection testing for primary aldosteronism in the pregnant woman is the same as for nonpregnant patients: morning blood sample for the measurement of aldosterone and plasma renin activity or renin mass measurement. Suppressed renin and an aldosterone level greater than 15 ng/dL is a positive case detection test for primary aldosteronism. If spontaneous hypokalemia is present in the woman with high aldosterone and suppressed renin, confirmatory testing is not needed. In the normokalemic woman with a positive case detection test, confirmatory testing should be pursued. However, the captopril stimulation test is contraindicated in pregnancy and the saline infusion test may not be well tolerated. One option is measurement of sodium and aldosterone in a 24-hour urine collection on an ambient sodium diet.

Subtype testing with abdominal MRI without gadolinium is the test of choice. Adrenal imaging with CT, iodocholesterol scintigraphy, and adrenal venous sampling should be avoided in pregnancy. As highlighted in the revised Endocrine Society guidelines on primary aldosteronism,[12] adrenal venous sampling may not be needed in patients with vigorous primary aldosteronism who are less than 35 years old and have a clear-cut unilateral adrenal adenoma on cross-sectional imaging.[12,39]

Primary aldosteronism in pregnancy is fascinating in that the degree of disease may be improved or aggravated by pregnancy. In some women with primary aldosteronism, the high blood levels of pregnancy-related progesterone are antagonistic at the mineralocorticoid receptor and partially block the action of aldosterone; these patients have an improvement in the manifestations of primary aldosteronism during pregnancy.[87,88] In other pregnant women, increased expression of luteinizing hormone choriogonadotropin receptor (LHCGR) and gonadotropin-releasing hormone receptor (GnRHR) have been documented in APAs and the degree of hyperaldosteronism is aggravated by the increased pregnancy-related blood levels of human chorionic gonadotropin.[89,90]

The type of treatment for primary aldosteronism in pregnancy depends on how difficult it is to manage the hypertension and hypokalemia. If the patient is in the subset of patients who have a remission in the degree of primary aldosteronism, then surgery or treatment with a mineralocorticoid antagonist can be avoided until after delivery. However, if hypertension and hypokalemia are marked, then surgical and/or medical intervention is indicated. Unilateral laparoscopic adrenalectomy during the second trimester can be considered in those women with confirmed primary aldosteronism and a clear-cut unilateral adrenal macroadenoma (>10 mm).

Spironolactone crosses the placenta and is an FDA pregnancy category C drug because feminization of newborn male rats has been documented. However, there is only one human case in the medical literature where treatment with spironolactone in pregnancy led to ambiguous genitalia in a male infant; this occurred in a woman treated with spironolactone for polycystic ovarian disease prepregnancy and through the fifth week of gestation.[91] Eplerenone is an FDA pregnancy category B drug. Therefore, for those pregnant women who will be managed medically, the hypertension should be treated with standard antihypertensive drugs approved for use during pregnancy. Hypokalemia, if present, should be treated with oral potassium supplements. For those patients with refractory hypertension and/or hypokalemia, the addition of eplerenone may be cautiously considered.[92,93]

OTHER FORMS OF MINERALOCORTICOID EXCESS OR EFFECT

The medical disorders associated with excess mineralocorticoid effect from 11-deoxycorticosterone (DOC) and cortisol are listed in Box 14.1. These diagnoses should be considered if PAC and PRA are low in a patient with hypertension and hypokalemia.

Hyperdeoxycorticosteronism

Congenital Adrenal Hyperplasia

Congenital adrenal hyperplasia (CAH) is a group of autosomal recessive disorders caused by enzymatic defects in adrenal steroidogenesis that result in deficient secretion of cortisol.[94,95] Approximately 90% of CAH cases are caused by 21-hydroxylase deficiency, which does not result in hypertension.[96] Deficiencies of 11β-hydroxylase (CYP11B1, P450c11) or 17α-hydroxylase (CYP17, P450c17) cause hypertension and hypokalemia because of hypersecretion of the mineralocorticoid DOC. The mineralocorticoid effect of increased circulating levels of DOC also decreases renin and aldosterone secretion. These mutations are autosomal recessive in inheritance and are typically diagnosed in childhood. However, partial enzymatic defects have been shown to cause hypertension in adults.

11β-Hydroxylase Deficiency

Approximately 5% of all cases of CAH are caused by 11β-hydroxylase deficiency; the prevalence in Caucasians is 1 in 100,000.[97] More than 40 mutations have been described in CYP11B1, the gene encoding 11β-hydroxylase.[98] There is an increased prevalence among Sephardic Jews from Morocco, suggestive of a founder effect. The impaired conversion of DOC to corticosterone results in high levels of DOC and 11-deoxycortisol; the substrate mass effect results in increased levels of adrenal androgens. Girls present in infancy or childhood with hypertension, hypokalemia, acne, hirsutism, and virilization. Boys with CAH as a result of 11β-hydroxylase deficiency present with hypertension, hypokalemia, and pseudoprecocious puberty. Approximately two-thirds of patients have mild

to moderate hypertension. The initial screening tests include measurement of blood levels of DOC, 11-deoxycortisol, androstenedione, testosterone, and DHEA-S; all of which should be increased above the upper limit of the respective reference ranges. Confirmatory testing includes germline mutation testing (www.genetests.org).

17α-Hydroxylase Deficiency

17α-Hydroxylase deficiency is a very rare cause of CAH and good prevalence data are not available, but likely less than 1 in 1,000,000 live births.[99] 17α-Hydroxylase is essential for the synthesis of cortisol and gonadal hormones, and deficiency results in decreased production of cortisol and sex steroids. Genetic 46,XY males present with either pseudohermaphroditism or as phenotypic females, and 46,XX females present with primary amenorrhea. Therefore, a person with this form of CAH may not come to medical attention until puberty. Children, adolescents, and young adults who present with hypertension and spontaneous hypokalemia and low levels of aldosterone and renin should be screened for CAH. Although very rare, there is an increased prevalence of 17α-hydroxylase deficiency among Dutch Mennonites. The initial screening tests include measurement of blood levels of androstenedione, testosterone, DHEA-S, 17-hydroxyprogesterone, aldosterone, and cortisol; all of which should be either low or at the lower quartile of the respective references ranges. The plasma concentrations of DOC and corticosterone should be above the upper limit of the respective reference ranges. Confirmatory testing includes germline mutation testing (www.genetests.org).

Deoxycorticosterone-Producing Tumor

Pure DOC-producing adrenal tumors are very rare and usually large and malignant.[100] Some patients have been documented to have benign DOC-producing adrenocortical adenomas.[101] Some of these adrenal neoplasms cosecrete androgens and estrogens in addition to DOC, which may cause virilization in women or feminization in men. The typical clinical presentation would be that of relatively rapid onset of marked hypertension associated with hypokalemia and low blood levels of aldosterone and renin. A high level of plasma DOC or urinary tetrahydrodeoxycorticosterone and a large adrenal tumor seen on CT confirm the diagnosis. Aldosterone secretion in these patients is typically suppressed.

Primary Cortisol Resistance

Increased cortisol secretion and plasma cortisol concentrations without evidence of Cushing syndrome are found in patients with primary cortisol resistance (or glucocorticoid resistance), a rare familial syndrome.[102,103] Primary cortisol resistance is caused by genetic defects in the glucocorticoid receptor and the steroid-receptor complex. The syndrome is characterized by hypokalemic alkalosis, hypertension, increased plasma concentrations of DOC, and increased adrenal androgen secretion. The hypertension and hypokalemia result from the combined effects of excess DOC and increased cortisol access to the mineralocorticoid receptor, resulting in high rates of cortisol production that overwhelm 11β-hydroxysteroid dehydrogenase type 2 (HSD11B2) activity. Most affected individuals present in childhood with hypertension and spontaneous hypokalemia and low levels of aldosterone and renin. The initial screening tests include measurement of blood levels of cortisol, DOC, 11-deoxycortisol, androstenedione, testosterone, and DHEA-S; all of which should be increased above the upper limit of the respective reference ranges. In addition, 24-hour urinary cortisol excretion is above the upper limit of the reference range and serum ACTH is not suppressed. Confirmatory testing includes germline mutation testing (www.genetests.org).

DIAGNOSIS AND EVALUATION

Apparent Mineralocorticoid Excess Syndrome

Apparent mineralocorticoid excess is the result of impaired activity of the microsomal enzyme HSD11B2, which normally inactivates cortisol in the kidney by converting it to the inactive 11-keto compound, cortisone.[104] Cortisol can be a potent mineralocorticoid, and when HSD11B2 is genetically deficient or its activity blocked, high levels of cortisol accumulate in the kidney. Decreased HSD11B2 activity may be hereditary, or it may be secondary to pharmacologic inhibition of enzyme activity by glycyrrhizic acid, the active principle of licorice root (Glycyrrhiza glabra).[105] The congenital forms are rare autosomal recessive disorders; fewer than 50 patients have been identified worldwide.[106] Congenital apparent mineralocorticoid excess typically presents in childhood with hypertension, hypokalemia, low birth weight, failure to thrive, hypertension, polyuria and polydipsia, and poor growth.[98] Acquired apparent mineralocorticoid excess attributed to licorice root ingestion presents with hypertension and hypokalemia; the cause becomes evident when a good medical history is obtained. In addition, when HSD11B2 is overwhelmed by massive cortisol hypersecretion associated with Cushing syndrome because of ectopic ACTH syndrome, hypokalemic hypertension may be one of the outcomes.[107] The clinical phenotype of patients with apparent mineralocorticoid excess attributed to congenital deficiency of or inhibition of HSD11B2 includes hypertension, hypokalemia, metabolic alkalosis, low renin, low aldosterone, and normal plasma cortisol levels. The diagnosis of apparent mineralocorticoid excess is confirmed by demonstration of an abnormal (high) ratio of cortisol to cortisone in a 24-hour urine collection. The characteristic abnormal urinary cortisol-cortisone metabolite profile reflects decreased HSD11B2 activity; the ratio of cortisol to cortisone is typically increased tenfold above the normal value.[104] DOC levels may also be increased in severe ACTH-dependent Cushing syndrome and contribute to the hypertension and hypokalemia in this disorder.

Liddle Syndrome: Abnormal Renal Tubular Ionic Transport

In 1963, Grant Liddle described an autosomal dominant renal disorder with a presentation similar to primary aldosteronism with hypertension, hypokalemia, and inappropriate kaliuresis.[108] However, blood levels of aldosterone and renin were very low so the disorder was termed pseudoaldosteronism. Liddle syndrome is caused by autosomal dominant mutations in the β or γ subunit of the amiloride-sensitive epithelial sodium channel.[98] It is extremely rare, with less than 30 families reported worldwide.[109] This mutation results in enhanced activity of the epithelial sodium channel and patients present with increased renal sodium reabsorption, potassium wasting, hypertension, and hypokalemia. However, as mentioned above, blood levels of aldosterone and renin are low. Affected individuals usually present as children or young adults with hypertension and spontaneous hypokalemia and low levels of aldosterone and renin. A family history of hypertension associated with hypokalemia makes Liddle syndrome more likely. The finding of low aldosterone and renin levels in the hypokalemic hypertensive patient should raise the possibility of Liddle syndrome. When the other causes of this presentation have been excluded, then a treatment trial with amiloride or triamterene should be considered. Liddle syndrome can easily be distinguished from apparent mineralocorticoid excess based on the good clinical response to amiloride or triamterene combined with a sodium-restricted diet, lack of efficacy of spironolactone and dexamethasone, and normal 24-hour urine cortisone/cortisol ratio. Clinical genetic testing is available (see www.genetests.org).

References

1. Conn JW. Presidential address. I. Painting background. II. Primary aldosteronism, a new clinical syndrome. J Lab Clin Med. 1955;45:3-17.
2. Funder JW. Genetics of primary aldosteronism. Front Horm Res. 2014;43:70-78.
3. Fishman LM, Kuchel O, Liddle GW, Michelakis AM, Gordon RD, Chick WT. Incidence of primary aldosteronism uncomplicated "essential" hypertension. A prospective study with elevated aldosterone secretion and suppressed plasma renin activity used as diagnostic criteria. JAMA. 1968;205:497-502.
4. Kaplan NM. Hypokalemia in the hypertensive patient, with observations on the incidence of primary aldosteronism. Ann Intern Med. 1967;66:1079-1090.
5. Andersen GS, Toftdahl DB, Lund JO, Strandgaard S, Nielsen PE. The incidence rate of phaeochromocytoma and Conn's syndrome in Denmark, 1977-1981. J Hum Hypertens. 1988;2:187-189.
6. Berglund G, Andersson O, Wilhelmsen L. Prevalence of primary and secondary hypertension: studies in a random population sample. Br Med J. 1976;2:554-556.
7. Streeten DH, Tomycz N, Anderson GH. Reliability of screening methods for the diagnosis of primary aldosteronism. Am J Med. 1979;67:403-413.
8. Tucker RM, Labarthe DR. Frequency of surgical treatment for hypertension in adults at the Mayo Clinic from 1973 through 1975. Mayo Clin Proc. 1977;52:549-545.
9. Sinclair AM, Isles CG, Brown I, Cameron H, Murray GD, Robertson JW. Secondary hypertension in a blood pressure clinic. Arch Intern Med. 1987;147:1289-1293.
10. Young WF. Primary aldosteronism: renaissance of a syndrome. Clin Endocrinol. (Oxf). 2007;66:607-618.
11. Stowasser M. Update in primary aldosteronism. J Clin Endocrinol Metab. 2015;100:1-10.
12. Funder JW, Carey RM, Mantero F, et al. The management of primary aldosteronism: case detection, diagnosis, and treatment: An Endocrine Society Clinical Practice guideline. J Clin Endocrinol Metab. 2016:jc20154061.
13. Mulatero P, Stowasser M, Loh KC, et al. Increased diagnosis of primary aldosteronism, including surgically correctable forms, in centers from five continents. J Clin Endocrinol Metab. 2004;89:1045-1050.
14. Piaditis G, Markou A, Papanastasiou L, Androulakis I, Kaltsas G. Progress in primary aldosteronism: a review of the prevalence of primary aldosteronism in pre-hypertension and hypertension. Eur J Endocrinol. 2015;172:191-203.
15. Ma JT, Wang C, Lam KS, et al. Fifty cases of primary hyperaldosteronism in Hong Kong Chinese with a high frequency of periodic paralysis. Evaluation of techniques for tumour localisation. Q J Med. 1986;61:1021-1037.
16. Young WF, Jr., Klee GG. Primary aldosteronism. Diagnostic evaluation. Endocrinol Metab Clin North Am. 1988;17:367-395.
17. Torres VE, Young WF, Jr., Offord KP, Hattery RR. Association of hypokalemia, aldosteronism, and renal cysts. N Engl J Med. 1990;322:345-351.
18. Stowasser M, Sharman J, Leano R, et al. Evidence for abnormal left ventricular structure and function in normotensive individuals with familial hyperaldosteronism type I. J Clin Endocrinol Metab. 2005;90:5070-5076.
19. Milliez P, Girerd X, Plouin PF, Blacher J, Safar ME, Mourad JJ. Evidence for an increased rate of cardiovascular events in patients with primary aldosteronism. J Am Coll Cardiol. 2005;45:1243-1248.
20. Iwakura Y, Morimoto R, Kudo M, et al. Predictors of decreasing glomerular filtration rate and prevalence of chronic kidney disease after treatment of primary aldosteronism: renal outcome of 213 cases. J Clin Endocrinol Metab. 2014;99:1593-1598.
21. Tanabe A, Naruse M, Naruse K, et al. Left ventricular hypertrophy is more prominent in patients with primary aldosteronism than in patients with other types of secondary hypertension. Hypertens Res. 1997;20:85-90.
22. Rossi GP, Sacchetto A, Visentin P, et al. Changes in left ventricular anatomy and function in hypertension and primary aldosteronism. Hypertension. 1996;27:1039-1045.
23. Hiramatsu K, Yamada T, Yukimura Y, et al. A screening test to identify aldosterone-producing adenoma by measuring plasma renin activity. Results in hypertensive patients. Arch Intern Med. 1981;141:1589-1593.
24. Montori VM, Young WF, Jr. Use of plasma aldosterone concentration-to-plasma renin activity ratio as a screening test for primary aldosteronism. A systematic review of the literature. Endocrinol Metab Clin North Am. 2002;31:619-632, xi.
25. Weinberger MH, Fineberg NS. The diagnosis of primary aldosteronism and separation of two major subtypes. Arch Intern Med. 1993;153:2125-2129.
26. Young WF, Jr. Primary aldosteronism: diagnosis. In: Mansoor GA, ed. Secondary Hypertension: Clinical Presentation, Diagnosis, and Treatment. Totowa, New Jersey: Humana Press; 2004:119-37.
27. Schwartz GL, Turner ST. Screening for primary aldosteronism in essential hypertension: diagnostic accuracy of the ratio of plasma aldosterone concentration to plasma renin activity. Clin Chem. 2005;51:386-394.
28. Nishizaka MK, Pratt-Ubunama M, Zaman MA, Cofield S, Calhoun DA. Validity of plasma aldosterone-to-renin activity ratio in African American and white subjects with resistant hypertension. Am J Hypertens. 2005;18:805-812.
29. Lim PO, Farquharson CA, Shiels P, Jung RT, Struthers AD, MacDonald TM. Adverse cardiac effects of salt with fludrocortisone in hypertension. Hypertension. 2001;37:856-861.
30. Bravo EL, Tarazi RC, Dustan HP, et al. The changing clinical spectrum of primary aldosteronism. Am J Med. 1983;74:641-651.
31. Funder JW, Carey RM, Fardella C, et al. Case detection, diagnosis, and treatment of patients with primary aldosteronism: an endocrine society clinical practice guideline. J Clin Endocrinol Metab. 2008;93:3266-3281.
32. Ahmed AH, Cowley D, Wolley M, et al. Seated saline suppression testing for the diagnosis of primary aldosteronism: a preliminary study. J Clin Endocrinol Metab. 2014;99:2745-2753.
33. Stowasser M, Gordon RD. Primary aldosteronism—careful investigation is essential and rewarding. Mol Cell Endocrinol. 2004;217:33-39.
34. Sawka AM, Young WF, Thompson GB, et al. Primary aldosteronism: factors associated with normalization of blood pressure after surgery. Ann Intern Med. 2001;135:258-261.
35. Citton M, Viel G, Rossi GP, Mantero F, Nitti D, Iacobone M. Outcome of surgical treatment of primary aldosteronism. Langenbecks Arch Surg. 2015;400:325-331.
36. Wachtel H, Cerullo I, Bartlett EK, et al. Long-term blood pressure control in patients undergoing adrenalectomy for primary hyperaldosteronism. Surgery. 2014;156:1394-1403.
37. Hussain S, Panteliou E, Berney DM, et al. Pure aldosterone-secreting adrenocortical carcinoma in a patient with refractory primary hyperaldosteronism. Endocrinol Diabetes Metab Case Rep. 2015;2015:150064.
38. Kendrick ML, Curlee K, Lloyd R, et al. Aldosterone-secreting adrenocortical carcinomas are associated with unique operative risks and outcomes. Surgery. 2002;132:1008-1011; discussion 12.
39. Lim V, Guo Q, Grant CS, et al. Accuracy of adrenal imaging and adrenal venous sampling in predicting surgical cure of primary aldosteronism. J Clin Endocrinol Metab. 2014;99:2712-2719.
40. Kloos RT, Gross MD, Francis IR, Korobkin M, Shapiro B. Incidentally discovered adrenal masses. Endocr Rev. 1995;16:460-484.

41. Young WF, Stanson AW, Thompson GB, Grant CS, Farley DR, van Heerden JA. Role for adrenal venous sampling in primary aldosteronism. *Surgery*. 2004;136:1227-1235.
42. Kempers MJ, Lenders JW, van Outheusden L, et al. Systematic review: diagnostic procedures to differentiate unilateral from bilateral adrenal abnormality in primary aldosteronism. *Ann Intern Med*. 2009;151:329-337.
43. Young WF, Stanson AW. What are the keys to successful adrenal venous sampling (AVS) in patients with primary aldosteronism? *Clin Endocrinol. (Oxf)*. 2009;70:14-17.
44. Daunt N. Adrenal vein sampling: how to make it quick, easy, and successful. *Radiographics*. 2005;25(Suppl 1):S143-S158.
45. Rossi GP, Auchus RJ, Brown M, et al. An expert consensus statement on use of adrenal vein sampling for the subtyping of primary aldosteronism. *Hypertension*. 2014;63:151-160.
46. Monticone S, Satoh F, Dietz AS, et al. Clinical Management and Outcomes of Adrenal Hemorrhage Following Adrenal Vein Sampling in Primary Aldosteronism. *Hypertension*. 2016;67:146-152.
47. Young WF, Jr., Hogan MJ. Renin-Independent hypermineralocorticoidism. *Trends Endocrinol Metab*. 1994;5:97-106.
48. Abe T, Naruse M, Young WF, Jr., et al. A Novel CYP11B2-Specific Imaging Agent for Detection of Unilateral Subtypes of Primary Aldosteronism. *J Clin Endocrinol Metab*. 2016;101:1008-1015.
49. Sutherland DJ, Ruse JL, Laidlaw JC. Hypertension, increased aldosterone secretion and low plasma renin activity relieved by dexamethasone. *Can Med Assoc J*. 1966;95:1109-1119.
50. Lifton RP, Dluhy RG, Powers M, et al. A chimaeric 11 beta-hydroxylase/aldosterone synthase gene causes glucocorticoid-remediable aldosteronism and human hypertension. *Nature*. 1992;355:262-265.
51. Rich GM, Ulick S, Cook S, Wang JZ, Lifton RP, Dluhy RG. Glucocorticoid-remediable aldosteronism in a large kindred: clinical spectrum and diagnosis using a characteristic biochemical phenotype. *Ann Intern Med*. 1992;116:813-820.
52. Mulatero P, Tizzani D, Viola A, et al. Prevalence and characteristics of familial hyperaldosteronism: the PATOGEN study (Primary Aldosteronism in TOrino-GENetic forms). *Hypertension*. 2011;58:797-803.
53. Sukor N, Mulatero P, Gordon RD, et al. Further evidence for linkage of familial hyperaldosteronism type II at chromosome 7p22 in Italian as well as Australian and South American families. *J Hypertens*. 2008;26:1577-1582.
54. Carss KJ, Stowasser M, Gordon RD, O'Shaughnessy KM. Further study of chromosome 7p22 to identify the molecular basis of familial hyperaldosteronism type II. *J Hum Hypertens*. 2011;25:560-564.
55. Geller DS, Zhang J, Wisgerhof MV, Shackleton C, Kashgarian M, Lifton RP. A novel form of human mendelian hypertension featuring nonglucocorticoid-remediable aldosteronism. *J Clin Endocrinol Metab*. 2008;93:3117-3123.
56. Choi M, Scholl UI, Yue P, et al. K+ channel mutations in adrenal aldosterone-producing adenomas and hereditary hypertension. *Science*. 2011;331:768-772.
57. Mussa A, Camilla R, Monticone S, et al. Polyuric-polydipsic syndrome in a pediatric case of non-glucocorticoid remediable familial hyperaldosteronism. *Endocr J*. 2012;59:497-502.
58. Charmandari E, Sertedaki A, Kino T, et al. A novel point mutation in the KCNJ5 gene causing primary hyperaldosteronism and early-onset autosomal dominant hypertension. *J Clin Endocrinol Metab*. 2012;97:E1532-E1539.
59. Mulatero P, Tauber P, Zennaro MC, et al. KCNJ5 mutations in European families with nonglucocorticoid remediable familial hyperaldosteronism. *Hypertension*. 2012;59:235-240.
60. Scholl UI, Nelson-Williams C, Yue P, et al. Hypertension with or without adrenal hyperplasia due to different inherited mutations in the potassium channel KCNJ5. *Proc Natl Acad Sci USA*. 2012;109:2533-2538.
61. Fernandes-Rosa FL, Williams TA, Riester A, et al. Genetic spectrum and clinical correlates of somatic mutations in aldosterone-producing adenoma. *Hypertension*. 2014;64:354-361.
62. Lenzini L, Rossitto G, Maiolino G, Letizia C, Funder JW, Rossi GP. A Meta-analysis of somatic KCNJ5 K(+) channel mutations in 1636 patients with an aldosterone-producing adenoma. *J Clin Endocrinol Metab*. 2015;100:E1089-E1095.
63. Beuschlein F, Boulkroun S, Osswald A, et al. Somatic mutations in ATP1A1 and ATP2B3 lead to aldosterone-producing adenomas and secondary hypertension. *Nat Genet*. 2013;45:440-444, 4e1-2.
64. Azizan EA, Poulsen H, Tuluc P, et al. Somatic mutations in ATP1A1 and CACNA1D underlie a common subtype of adrenal hypertension. *Nat Genet*. 2013;45:1055-1060.
65. Williams TA, Monticone S, Schack VR, et al. Somatic ATP1A1, ATP2B3, and KCNJ5 mutations in aldosterone-producing adenomas. *Hypertension*. 2014;63:188-195.
66. Scholl UI, Goh G, Stolting G, et al. Somatic and germline CACNA1D calcium channel mutations in aldosterone-producing adenomas and primary aldosteronism. *Nat Genet*. 2013;45:1050-1054.
67. Sechi LA, Di Fabio A, Bazzocchi M, Uzzau A, Catena C. Intrarenal hemodynamics in primary aldosteronism before and after treatment. *J Clin Endocrinol Metab*. 2009;94:1191-1197.
68. Reincke M, Rump LC, Quinkler M, et al. Risk factors associated with a low glomerular filtration rate in primary aldosteronism. *J Clin Endocrinol Metab*. 2009;94:869-875.
69. Assalia A, Gagner M. Laparoscopic adrenalectomy. *Br J Surg*. 2004;91:1259-1274.
70. Muth A, Ragnarsson O, Johannsson G, Wangberg B. Systematic review of surgery and outcomes in patients with primary aldosteronism. *Br J Surg*. 2015;102:307-317.
71. Celen O, O'Brien MJ, Melby JC, Beazley RM. Factors influencing outcome of surgery for primary aldosteronism. *Arch Surg*. 1996;131:646-650.
72. Worth PJ, Kunio NR, Siegfried I, Sheppard BC, Gilbert EW. Characteristics predicting clinical improvement and cure following laparoscopic adrenalectomy for primary aldosteronism in a large cohort. *Am J Surg*. 2015;210:702-709.
73. Ishidoya S, Ito A, Sakai K, et al. Laparoscopic partial versus total adrenalectomy for aldosterone producing adenoma. *J Urol*. 2005;174:40-43.
74. Chiang WF, Cheng CJ, Wu ST, et al. Incidence and factors of post-adrenalectomy hyperkalemia in patients with aldosterone producing adenoma. *Clin Chim Acta*. 2013;424:114-118.
75. Yorke E, Stafford S, Holmes D, Sheth S, Melck A. Aldosterone deficiency after unilateral adrenalectomy for Conn's syndrome: a case report and literature review. *Int J Surg Case Rep*. 2015;7C:141-144.
76. Sywak M, Pasieka JL. Long-term follow-up and cost benefit of adrenalectomy in patients with primary hyperaldosteronism. *Br J Surg*. 2002;89:1587-1593.
77. Ghose RP, Hall PM, Bravo EL. Medical management of aldosterone-producing adenomas. *Ann Intern Med*. 1999;131:105-108.
78. Sechi LA, Colussi GL, Novello M, Uzzau A, Catena C. Mineralocorticoid receptor antagonists and clinical outcomes in primary aldosteronism: as good as surgery? *Horm Metab Res*. 2015;47:1000-1006.
79. Lim PO, Young WF, MacDonald TM. A review of the medical treatment of primary aldosteronism. *J Hypertens*. 2001;19:353-361.
80. Jeunemaitre X, Chatellier G, Kreft-Jais C, et al. Efficacy and tolerance of spironolactone in essential hypertension. *Am J Cardiol*. 1987;60:820-825.
81. Parthasarathy HK, Menard J, White WB, et al. A double-blind, randomized study comparing the antihypertensive effect of eplerenone and spironolactone in patients with hypertension and evidence of primary aldosteronism. *J Hypertens*. 2011;29:980-990.
82. Eschler DC, Kogekar N, Pessah-Pollack R. Management of adrenal tumors in pregnancy. *Endocrinol Metab Clin North Am*. 2015;44:381-397.
83. Monticone S, Auchus RJ, Rainey WE. Adrenal disorders in pregnancy. *Nat Rev Endocrinol*. 2012;8:668-678.
84. Riester A, Reincke M. Progress in primary aldosteronism: mineralocorticoid receptor antagonists and management of primary aldosteronism in pregnancy. *Eur J Endocrinol*. 2015;172:R23-R30.
85. Krysiak R, Samborek M, Stojko R. Primary aldosteronism in pregnancy. *Acta Clin Belg*. 2012;67:130-134.
86. Eguchi K, Hoshide S, Nagashima S, Maekawa T, Sasano H, Kario K. An adverse pregnancy-associated outcome due to overlooked primary aldosteronism. *Intern Med*. 2014;53:2499-2504.
87. Campino C, Trejo P, Carvajal CA, et al. Pregnancy normalized familial hyperaldosteronism type I: a novel role for progesterone? *J Hum Hypertens*. 2015;29:138-139.
88. Ronconi V, Turchi F, Zennaro MC, Boscaro M, Giacchetti G. Progesterone increase counteracts aldosterone action in a pregnant woman with primary aldosteronism. *Clin Endocrinol*. (Oxf) 2011;74:278-279.
89. Albiger NM, Sartorato P, Mariniello B, et al. A case of primary aldosteronism in pregnancy: do LH and GNRH receptors have a potential role in regulating aldosterone secretion? *Eur J Endocrinol*. 2011;164:405-412.
90. Teo AE, Garg S, Shaikh LH, et al. Pregnancy, Primary Aldosteronism, and Adrenal CTNNB1 Mutations. *N Engl J Med*. 2015;373:1429-1436.
91. Shah A. Ambiguous genitalia in a newborn with spironolactone exposure. 93rd Annual Meeting of the Endocrine Society 2011;4:227.
92. Cabassi A, Rocco R, Berretta R, Regolisti G, Bacchi-Modena A. Eplerenone use in primary aldosteronism during pregnancy. *Hypertension*. 2012;59:e18-e19.
93. Gunganah K, Carpenter R, Drake WM. Eplerenone use in primary aldosteronism during pregnancy. *Clin Case Rep*. 2016;4:81-82.
94. Speiser PW, Azziz R, Baskin LS, et al. Congenital adrenal hyperplasia due to steroid 21-hydroxylase deficiency: an Endocrine Society clinical practice guideline. *J Clin Endocrinol Metab*. 2010;95:4133-4160.
95. Krone N, Arlt W. Genetics of congenital adrenal hyperplasia. *Best Pract Res Clin Endocrinol Metab*. 2009;23:181-192.
96. White PC, Dupont J, New MI, Leiberman E, Hochberg Z, Rosler A. A mutation in CYP11B1 (Arg-448—His) associated with steroid 11 beta-hydroxylase deficiency in Jews of Moroccan origin. *J Clin Invest*. 1991;87:1664-1667.
97. Merke DP, Bornstein SR. Congenital adrenal hyperplasia. *Lancet*. 2005;365:2125-2136.
98. New MI, Geller DS, Fallo F, Wilson RC. Monogenic low renin hypertension. *Trends Endocrinol Metab*. 2005;16:92-97.
99. Kim YM, Kang M, Choi JH, et al. A review of the literature on common CYP17A1 mutations in adults with 17-hydroxylase/17,20-lyase deficiency, a case series of such mutations among Koreans and functional characteristics of a novel mutation. *Metabolism*. 2014;63:42-49.
100. Mussig K, Wehrmann M, Horger M, Maser-Gluth C, Haring HU, Overkamp D. Adrenocortical carcinoma producing 11-deoxycorticosterone: a rare cause of mineralocorticoid hypertension. *J Endocrinol Invest*. 2005;28:61-65.
101. Ishikawa SE, Saito T, Kaneko K, Okada K, Fukuda S, Kuzuya T. Hypermineralocorticism without elevation of plasma aldosterone: deoxycorticosterone-producing adrenal adenoma and hyperplasia. *Clin Endocrinol*. (Oxf) 1988;29:367-375.
102. Nicolaides NC, Roberts ML, Kino T, et al. A novel point mutation of the human glucocorticoid receptor gene causes primary generalized glucocorticoid resistance through impaired interaction with the LXXLL motif of the p160 coactivators: dissociation of the transactivating and transreppressive activities. *J Clin Endocrinol Metab*. 2014;99:E902-E907.
103. Charmandari E, Kino T, Chrousos GP. Primary generalized familial and sporadic glucocorticoid resistance (Chrousos syndrome) and hypersensitivity. *Endocr Dev*. 2013;24:67-85.
104. Chapman K, Holmes M, Seckl J. 11beta-hydroxysteroid dehydrogenases: intracellular gate-keepers of tissue glucocorticoid action. *Physiol Rev*. 2013;93:1139-1206.
105. Robles BJ, Sandoval AR, Dardon JD, Blas CA. Lethal liquorice lollies (liquorice abuse causing pseudohyperaldosteronism). *BMJ Case Rep*. 2013;2013.
106. Stewart PM, Krozowski ZS, Gupta A, et al. Hypertension in the syndrome of apparent mineralocorticoid excess due to mutation of the 11 beta-hydroxysteroid dehydrogenase type 2 gene. *Lancet*. 1996;347:88-91.
107. Nieman LK, Biller BM, Findling JW, et al. The diagnosis of Cushing's syndrome: an Endocrine Society Clinical Practice Guideline. *J Clin Endocrinol Metab*. 2008;93:1526-1540.
108. Liddle GW. A familial renal disorder simulating primary aldosteronism but with negligible aldosterone secretion. *Trans Assoc Am Physicians*. 1963;76:199-213.
109. Rossier BC, Schild L. Epithelial sodium channel: mendelian versus essential hypertension. *Hypertension*. 2008;52:595-600.

15 Secondary Hypertension: Pheochromocytoma and Paraganglioma

Debbie L. Cohen and Lauren Fishbein

Endocrine disorders account for about 5% to 10% of secondary hypertension.[1] Pheochromocytoma and paraganglioma tumors are a well-established, albeit rare, cause of secondary hypertension. Pheochromocytomas and paragangliomas are tumors of the autonomic nervous system that arise from chromaffin tissue in the adrenal medulla and extraadrenal ganglia, respectively. Pheochromocytomas and most paragangliomas are derived from sympathetic nervous system tissue which secretes catecholamines and metanephrines. Some paragangliomas, however, are derived from parasympathetic ganglia, especially those in the head and neck, and most are nonsecretory.

Pheochromocytomas and paragangliomas occur in only 2 to 8 per million people and are rare cause of hypertension (0.2% to 0.6% of all patients with hypertension)[2]; however, pheochromocytomas make up 4% to 7% of adrenal incidentalomas.[3] When left undiagnosed, these tumors are associated with high morbidity and mortality secondary to the uncontrolled catecholamine levels leading to hypertension, heart disease, stroke, and even death. Interestingly, pheochromocytomas and paragangliomas are the tumors most commonly associated with inherited genetic mutations.[4] Although most tumors are benign, up to 25% can be malignant and are associated with a poor prognosis.[5] Making the diagnosis in this disease is key; and once diagnosed, appropriate medical management is necessary to decrease morbidity of the tumor and of the associated surgical risks. Pheochromocytomas used to be thought of as the "tumor of tens," with 10% of tumors being bilateral, 10% being extraadrenal, 10% being malignant, and 10% being asymptomatic. This is no longer true. In this chapter, we will discuss the unique features of pheochromocytomas and paragangliomas, diagnosis and management of these tumors, and the associated genetic disorders.

SCREENING AND DIAGNOSIS

Secondary causes for hypertension, including pheochromocytoma and paraganglioma, should be sought in young adults with hypertension and in patients of any age with new onset difficult to control hypertension.[1] Screening for pheochromocytomas is also part of the adrenal incidentaloma evaluation for both hypertensive and normotensive patients.[6] In addition, screening should be done when patients have symptoms suggestive of pheochromocytoma and paraganglioma, including the classic triad of headaches, palpitations, and diaphoresis, as well as anxiety, tremors, new onset or worsening of previously established diabetes mellitus, syncope, or presyncope. Patients may also be asymptomatic at a rate higher than previously appreciated.[7] Often times, patients, especially those with episodic events, are dismissed for having anxiety or panic attacks. The differential diagnosis is long (Table 15.1), and clinicians must suspect pheochromocytoma and paraganglioma to make the diagnosis.

Laboratory Testing

Once suspected, screening can be done in two ways, testing for plasma free metanephrines or 24-hour urine fractionated metanephrines. Both plasma and urine tests have over 90% sensitivity for pheochromocytoma and paraganglioma. Plasma metanephrines are favored because this test is easier to collect and has a higher specificity compared with the 24-hour urine tests (ranging from 79% to 98% versus 69% to 95%, respectively).[8] Catecholamine and metanephrine measurements are susceptible to false-positive elevations for many reasons. An upright position or recent exercise can increase levels. Therefore, guidelines recommend the plasma tests be performed with the patient resting for 20 minutes in the supine position[8] although this is not usually practical in the clinical setting. Plasma catecholamines are particularly sensitive to this, and therefore, are not recommended as a first line screening test because of increased likelihood of false-positive results. Most laboratories have different reference ranges for plasma tests drawn in the supine and upright positions which must be used when interpreting the results. The catecholamine and metanephrine levels for both plasma and urine tests can also be falsely elevated because of interfering medications[9] (Table 15.2).

Imaging

Once elevated levels of catecholamines and/or metanephrines are confirmed, imaging studies should be done to localize the tumor. Cross-sectional imaging with computed tomography (CT) or magnetic resonance imaging (MRI) of the abdomen/pelvis is the first recommended imaging test because the vast majority of tumors will be in the adrenal glands or in the abdomen or pelvis. For patients with known susceptibility gene mutations, imaging other locations may be necessary based on the associated phenotype (see Genetic Syndromes section). Paragangliomas derived from the parasympathetic chain, such as those in the head and neck for example, are often nonsecretory. Therefore, if a parasympathetic paraganglioma is suspected, imaging should be performed regardless of biochemical testing results. Furthermore, because parasympathetic paragangliomas are usually nonsecretory, if patients with a known parasympathetic tumor have elevated metanephrines, abdominal/pelvic imaging studies must be performed to evaluate for an additional sympathetic-derived primary pheochromocytoma or paraganglioma.

Imaging with ^{123}I-metaiodobenzylguanidine (MIBG) is not useful as first line study because normal adrenal glands can have increased symmetric or asymmetric physiologic uptake leading to false-positive results.[10] Instead, ^{123}I-MIBG imaging is usually reserved for the patient in whom cross-sectional imaging did not reveal a tumor despite highly elevated biochemical testing or for the patient with metastatic disease to assess if the lesions are MIBG avid in preparation for possible treatment with ^{131}I-MIBG.[8] Guidelines recommend fluorodeoxyglucose positron emission tomography

TABLE 15.1 Differential Diagnoses for Pheochromocytoma/Paraganglioma by System

SYSTEM	DIFFERENTIAL
Cardiovascular Differential	Angina
	Deconditioning
	Labile essential hypertension
	Orthostatic hypotension
	Paroxysmal cardiac arrhythmia and torsade de pointes
	Renovascular disease
	Syncope or presyncope
Endocrine Differential	Carbohydrate intolerance
	Carcinoid syndrome
	Hyperthyroidism
	Hypoglycemia
	Insulinoma
	Medullary thyroid carcinoma
	Menopause or primary ovarian/testicular failure
	Pheochromocytoma/paraganglioma
Neurologic Differential	Autonomic neuropathy
	Cerebrovascular insufficiency
	Diencephalic epilepsy (autonomic seizures)
	Hyperadrenergic spells
	Migraine headache
	Postural orthostatic tachycardia syndrome
	Stroke
Psychologic Differential	Factitious
	Generalized anxiety disorder
	Hyperventilation
	Panic attacks
	Somatization disorder
Pharmacologic Differential	Illegal drug ingestion
	Sympathomimetic ingestion
	Vancomycin ("red man" syndrome)
	Withdrawal of adrenergic inhibitor
	Withdrawal of psychotropic medications
Other	Mastocytosis
	Recurrent idiopathic anaphylaxis

TABLE 15.2 Medications That Interfere With Screening Tests for Pheochromocytomas and Paragangliomas

Acetaminophen
Levodopa
Monoamine oxidase inhibitors
Selective serotonin reuptake inhibitors
Sympathomimetics
Tricyclic antidepressants
Some beta-blockers (especially nonselective)
Some alpha-blockers (ie, phenoxybenzamine)

(^{18}F-FDG PET)/CT scanning over ^{123}I-MIBG imaging to diagnosis metastatic disease, especially in patients with germline *Succinate Dehydrogenase Subunit B (SDHB)* gene mutations for whom the sensitivity of positron emission tomography (PET) imaging is 74% to 100%.[8]

TREATMENT

Surgery

Surgical resection is the treatment of choice for pheochromocytoma and paraganglioma. Surgical resection was previously associated with a high perioperative morbidity and mortality because of the hypersecretion of catecholamines, but with the introduction of perioperative blockade, surgery is now relatively safe with morbidity and mortality rates as low as

0% to 2%.[11] Improved outcomes have also been associated with laparoscopic surgery for pheochromocytoma and paraganglioma as opposed to open adrenalectomy procedures.[12] In fact, laparoscopic adrenalectomy is the treatment of choice for adrenal pheochromocytoma and is often curative for small adrenal pheochromocytomas. Open adrenalectomy is usually reserved for very large tumors, greater than 8 cm, and extraadrenal paragangliomas. Usually the entire adrenal gland is removed; however, cortical sparing surgery should be attempted in patients with bilateral adrenal pheochromocytomas and in patients with a genetic predisposition to bilateral pheochromocytomas (such as Multiple Endocrine Neoplasia type 2 [MEN2] and von Hippel Lindau [vHL]). If a sufficient part of the cortex can be spared, these patients can avoid lifetime glucocorticoid and mineralocorticoid replacement. There is a higher risk of recurrence with cortical sparing surgery. During adrenalectomy, it is important not to violate the tumor capsule and not to rupture a cystic pheochromocytoma as cells that are spilled during surgery can seed the abdominal cavity resulting in recurrent growth in the adrenal bed or peritoneum. It is essential to have an experienced surgical team with an experienced anesthesiologist.

In preparation for surgery, patients should receive preoperative alpha-blockade for 10 to 14 days before surgery and should be instructed to take these medications on the morning of surgery. Certain induction agents and narcotics should be avoided during surgery (such as fentanyl, ketamine, and morphine) because they can potentially stimulate catecholamine release. Atropine, a parasympathetic nervous system blocking agent, should also be avoided as this causes tachycardia. Preferred induction agents include propofol, etomidate, barbiturates, and synthetic opioids. Most anesthetic gases can be used, but halothane and desflurane should be avoided. It is essential to provide close continuous hemodynamic and cardiovascular monitoring during surgery and in the perioperative period.

During surgery, patients will require either intraoperative intravenous phentolamine or nicardipine. During intubation, surgical excision, and tumor manipulation, it is common to see an increase in blood pressure; and once the tumor is removed, blood pressure can drop precipitously as a result of the large decrease in catecholamine levels. Risk factors for hemodynamic instability include tumors greater than 3 to 4 cm, higher catecholamine levels, uncontrolled blood pressure, or orthostatic hypotension preoperatively.[11] After surgery, patients may require blood pressure support with fluids, colloids, and sometimes alpha-adrenergic agonists for 24 to 48 hours and may need monitoring in an intensive care unit setting. Postoperative hypotension is less common in patients who have received adequate preoperative alpha-blockade. Blood pressure usually returns to normal within a few days of surgery, but patients may remain hypertensive particularly if they have chronic underlying hypertension or widespread metastatic disease.

Perioperative Blockade

Perioperative blockade is important to lower morbidity and mortality associated with tumor resection. Blockade is also required before other surgical procedures and biopsies and should also be considered when undertaking treatment for metastatic disease such as chemotherapy, radiation, and high dose ^{131}I-MIBG therapy, particularly when catecholamine levels are very elevated. There are no standardized guidelines for the perioperative blockade regimen, and the data that exist are sparse with no randomized controlled trials. Preoperative alpha-blockade is usually started as soon as the diagnosis is made, and surgery is usually scheduled within 2 to 3 weeks of the diagnosis. There are many different medical regimens used to control the effects of catecholamine hypersecretion,

TABLE 15.3 Common Medications for Perioperative Blockade of Patients With Pheochromocytoma and Paraganglioma

DRUG	ACTION	CHARACTERISTICS	COMMON DOSING	COMMON SIDE EFFECTS[a]
Phenoxybenzamine	Nonselective alpha-1 and alpha-2 blocker	Noncompetitive antagonist	10 mg 2-3 daily (maximum 60 mg per day)	Orthostasis, nasal congestion
Doxazosin	Selective alpha-1 blocker	Competitive antagonist	2-4 mg 2-3 × daily	Orthostasis, dizziness
Prazosin	Selective alpha-1 blocker	Competitive antagonist	1-2 mg twice daily	Orthostasis, dizziness
Terazosin	Selective alpha-1 blocker	Competitive antagonist	1-4 mg once daily	Orthostasis, dizziness
Nicardipine	Calcium channel blocker	Dihydropyridine long acting	30 mg twice daily	Headache, edema, vasodilatation
Amlodipine	Calcium channel blocker	Dihydropyridine long acting	5-10 mg daily	Headache, edema, palpitations
Metyrosine	Tyrosine hydroxylase inhibitor	Decreases catecholamine production	250-500 mg 4 × daily (dose escalated every 2 days)	Severe lethargy, extrapyramidal neurologic side effects and gastrointestinal upset
Metoprolol	Selective beta-1 blocker	Used to treat reflex tachycardia only after full alpha blockade achieved	25-50 mg 1-2 × daily	Fatigue, dizziness

[a]Many common side effects are expected and are suggestive of complete perioperative blockade. If possible and when appropriate, these side effects should be managed without dose reduction.
(From Fishbein L, Orlowski R, Cohen D. Pheochromocytoma/Paraganglioma: Review of perioperative management of blood pressure and update on genetic mutations associated with pheochromocytoma. J Clin Hypertens (Greenwich). *2013;15:428-434.)*

and these include the use of alpha-blockers, calcium channel blockers and tyrosine hydroxylase inhibition. The typical drugs and dosing regimens are shown in Table 15.3.

Medications

Alpha-Blockers

Alpha-blockers are most commonly used in the perioperative management in patients with pheochromocytoma and paraganglioma. These tumors cause alpha-receptor activation in response to excess catecholamine secretion leading to severe vasoconstriction which can cause hypertension, arrhythmias, and myocardial ischemia. Both competitive and noncompetitive alpha-blockers can be used in perioperative management. The most commonly used alpha-blocker for perioperative management is phenoxybenzamine, which is a noncompetitive inhibitor that covalently binds to alpha-1 and alpha-2 receptors. This noncompetitive inhibition of both alpha receptors by phenoxybenzamine is difficult to displace during the excess release of catecholamines during surgery and tumor manipulation, and therefore, provides more complete blockade of alpha receptors. The irreversible binding significantly lowers the risk of an intraoperative hypertensive crisis; however, this can also result in hypotension after the tumor is resected. Vasopressor support and intravenous fluids may be required for 24 to 48 hours postoperatively to maintain blood pressure.

Selective alpha-1 receptor blockers include doxazosin, terazosin, and prazosin. These competitive inhibitors have a relatively short duration of action; and therefore, the receptor inhibition can be overcome by the excess catecholamine release intraoperatively and can potentially lead to a hypertensive crisis intraoperatively. The shorter half-life, however, results in less hypotension after the tumor is removed. We usually reserve use of selective alpha-blockers for chronic use of alpha-blockade in patients with symptomatic metastatic disease or for use when a lower dose alpha-blockade is required, for example in preparation for a dental extraction in patients with elevated catecholamine levels because of metastatic disease. These agents provide incomplete alpha-blockade but cost significantly less and are better tolerated than phenoxybenzamine.

Calcium Channel Blockers

Calcium channel blockers inhibit norepinephrine mediated transmembrane calcium influx into smooth muscle. Nicardipine is the most commonly used calcium channel blocker and can be given orally preoperatively and intravenously intraoperatively. There are no prospective studies directly comparing alpha blockade and calcium channel blockers for preoperative blockade, but some physicians prefer the use of calcium channel blockers given the cardiac and renal protective effects.

Beta-Blockers

Beta-blockers should never be used before alpha-blockade in patients with pheochromocytoma or paraganglioma because this can result in unopposed alpha-adrenergic stimulation, which can cause severe vasoconstriction and a hypertensive crisis. Selective beta-1 blockers like metoprolol are usually added after the patient has achieved full alpha-blockade and develops reflex tachycardia. This tachyarrhythmia is a desired side effect indicating complete alpha-blockade has been achieved. Metoprolol tartrate is usually added at a dose of 25 mg twice daily and can be titrated up to achieve a heart rate of 60 to 80 beats per minute. Labetalol, which has both alpha-blocking and beta-blocking properties, is not recommended because it has been reported to cause a paradoxical hypertensive response presumably as a result of incomplete alpha-adrenergic blockade. Labetalol may however be effective for management of blood pressure in patients with metastatic disease and chronic elevation of catecholamines.

Metyrosine

Alpha-methyl-tyrosine or metyrosine is a tyrosine hydroxylase inhibitor which blocks conversion of tyrosine to dopamine and thereby inhibits catecholamine biosynthesis. This medication can offer significant hemodynamic stability to patients because the lack of excessive catecholamine production will help prevent the potential intraoperative hypertension and hypotension experienced before and after tumor resection.[13,14] Metyrosine can cause some significant side effects including severe lethargy, gastrointestinal upset, and extrapyramidal neurological symptoms. Nevertheless, metyrosine is used in some centers in combination with phenoxybenzamine, and it is usually started 8 to 10 days before surgery in titrating doses from 250 mg once a day increasing by 250 mg every 1 to 2 days to result in a dose of 250 mg or 500 mg four times daily by the day of surgery. Metyrosine in combination with phenoxybenzamine may offer a cardiovascular advantage and has been shown in a retrospective study to decrease cardiovascular morbidity perioperatively.[15] This agent could be considered for use in patients at high cardiovascular risk or who have very high preoperative catecholamine levels. It also has a role in metastatic disease in patients with a very high catecholamine burden who are symptomatic.

There are several retrospective studies assessing the effects of different perioperative blockade protocols in pheochromocytoma and paraganglioma. The largest retrospective series compared the perioperative management protocol used at the Mayo Clinic versus the one used at the Cleveland Clinic.[16] The Mayo Clinic protocol used phenoxybenzamine for 1 to 4 weeks before surgery, and patients were dosed until they had orthostatic hypotension to ensure full alpha-blockade. Beta-blockers were added if the patient's heart rate was above 80 beats per minute, and a calcium channel blocker was added if the patient was still hypertensive. In addition, metyrosine was added if the tumor was very large. The Cleveland Clinic protocol involved treating with doxazosin as first line therapy often adding a calcium channel blocker to the regimen. Beta-blockade was added if needed to treat tachycardia. The retrospective analysis showed that there was a trend towards a shorter duration of severe intraoperative hypertension with phenoxybenzamine but more postoperative hypotension with 56% of phenoxybenzamine treated patients requiring phenylephrine pressor support versus 27% of doxazosin treated patients.[16] Nevertheless, there were no differences between treatment regimens with regard to postoperative surgical outcomes or length of hospital stay. This study has significant limitations including that it was retrospective and compared nonstandardized protocols from two institutions with different patient populations, surgeons, and intraoperative care. Other small retrospective single center studies each with 39 patients or less also have found no difference in outcomes when comparing phenoxybenzamine with selective alpha-blockers perioperative blockades regimens.[17,18]

In our experience, we recommend using noncompetitive alpha-blockade with phenoxybenzamine for surgical procedures. Phenoxybenzamine is usually dosed at 10 mg twice daily and this is titrated up usually to the maximum dose of 20 mg three times a day. Common side effects include orthostatic hypotension and nasal congestion. The goal is to maintain blood pressure in the high normal range with systolic blood pressure 120 to 140 mm Hg and diastolic blood pressure 70 to 90 mm Hg. We expect to see a reflex tachycardia when full alpha-blockade is achieved. We add a beta-blocker if the heart rate is consistently above 100 beats per minute. If patients have very large tumors or very high catecholamine levels, we will add metyrosine for 8 to 14 days before surgery to decrease catecholamine production. We often see some postoperative hypotension which rarely lasts more than 24 hours and can be an indication of complete and appropriate preoperative blockade. To treat postoperative hypotension, we recommend administering intravenous fluids and, if needed, vasopressor support with alpha-agonists such as levophed.

Historically, our treatment regimen consisted of metyrosine and phenoxybenzamine for all patients with pheochromocytoma and paraganglioma; however, there was a metyrosine shortage requiring that phenoxybenzamine be used alone. Therefore, we conducted a retrospective cohort study to determine the impact of preoperative phenoxybenzamine and metyrosine versus phenoxybenzamine alone.[15] Of 174 patients, 142 (81.6%) were in the combined therapy group versus 32 in the phenoxybenzamine only group. Both groups of patients had comparable intraoperative use of antihypertensives (83.9 versus 78.1%; p = 0.443), vasopressors (74.6 versus 87.5%; p = 0.120), and fluid resuscitation (mean, 24.4 versus 24.8 mL per min; p = 0.761). Although the perioperative complication rate did not differ significantly between the two groups, the phenoxybenzamine only patients had a 15.8% higher rate of cardiovascular complications after controlling for confounders (p = 0.034). Compared with the combined therapy group, the phenoxybenzamine only patients had

significantly more hemodynamic instability intraoperatively, with a greater range in heart rate (7.4 beats per minute; p = 0.034) and systolic blood pressure (14.8 mm Hg; p = 0.020). This study demonstrated that preoperative metyrosine improved intraoperative hemodynamic stability and decreased cardiovascular complication rates in patients undergoing surgery for pheochromocytoma/paraganglioma resection.

Acute Hypertensive Crisis

Acute hypertensive crisis can be the presenting symptom in patients with an undiagnosed pheochromocytoma or paraganglioma and can occur in patients with a known tumor. In the setting of a hypertensive emergency, we recommend controlling blood pressure with an intravenous alpha-blockade with phentolamine. If needed, other intravenous vasodilators can be used such as sodium nitroprusside or nicardipine.

PHEOCHROMOCYTOMA AND PARAGANGLIOMA IN PREGNANCY

Pheochromocytoma and paraganglioma in pregnancy can be dangerous and even fatal for both the mother and the fetus. Perioperative blockade is the same as for nonpregnant patients; however, timing of surgery is often tricky. It is usually recommended to proceed with surgical resection around 18 to 22 weeks of pregnancy. If diagnosis is only made in the third trimester, it is recommended to perform a cesarean section and surgical resection of the pheochromocytoma/paraganglioma at the same surgery. Spontaneous labor and delivery should be avoided. In patients with genetic predisposition to pheochromocytoma, such as patients with vHL and MEN2, it is recommended to screen the patient with plasma metanephrine levels for early detection of pheochromocytoma when contemplating conception and/or when pregnancy is confirmed to avoid late detection and pregnancy related morbidity because of an undetected pheochromocytoma. If patients develop a hypertensive crisis during pregnancy, treatment is the same as for nonpregnant patients except nitroprusside should not be used because of the risk of cyanide toxicity in the fetus.

FOLLOW-UP

All patients should have catecholamine biochemistries (preferably plasma metanephrines) checked about 4 to 6 weeks after surgery to ensure levels have returned to normal. If levels remain elevated, this may indicate residual or metastatic disease. If the patient has had bilateral adrenalectomies, they will need lifelong mineralocorticoid and glucocorticoid replacement therapy. Pheochromocytomas and paragangliomas do tend to recur, and we have seen recurrences up to 25 years later. Patients also can develop additional primary tumors. Therefore, all patients should have annual plasma metanephrines levels checked for life. In addition, all patients should be referred for genetic testing because of the high rate of germline mutation detection in this tumor type.[8] There is no need for follow-up cross-sectional imaging in most patients with complete adrenal pheochromocytoma resection. There is, however, a need for follow-up imaging in patients with known germline susceptibility gene mutations which, depending on the gene, are associated with an increased risk of recurrence or additional primary tumors, and, in the case of *SDHB* mutations, high rates of malignant or metastatic disease (see Genetic Syndromes section for recommendations). ^{123}I-MIBG scanning should also be considered if catecholamines remain elevated or if metastatic disease is suspected. Guidelines suggest ^{18}F-FDG PET/CT scanning over ^{123}I-MIBG imaging to diagnosis metastatic disease, especially in patients with germline *SDHB* mutations for whom the sensitivity of PET imaging is significantly higher.[8]

MALIGNANCY

It is not possible to diagnose malignancy based on the histologic findings of a pheochromocytoma or paraganglioma. Malignancy is defined by the World Health Organization as involvement of metastatic disease in nonchromaffin tissue remote from the primary tumor site.[2] Common metastatic sites for pheochromocytoma and paraganglioma include lymph nodes, liver, bones including the skull, lung, and peritoneal metastases. Local vascular invasion is common in pheochromocytoma and is not considered malignancy without distant metastatic disease. Unfortunately, there are no reliable markers to predict malignant pheochromocytoma. The Pheochromocytoma of the Adrenal Gland Scaled Score (PASS) is a histologic scoring system developed in 2002 to predict malignant potential.[19] Histologic features are scored from 0 to 20, and in the initial study, a score of less than 4 was associated with benign tumors, whereas scores of 4 or greater carried an increased risk of malignant potential. The PASS score is prone to great interobserver and intraobserver variability[20] and should be used with caution; however, it may be especially useful to predict benign disease and determine which patients do not need close follow-up. Another pathologic score was developed called the Grading system for Adrenal Pheochromocytoma and Paraganglioma (GAPP), and includes histopathologic features, biochemical secretion, and Ki67 proliferation index.[21] This scoring system classifies tumors as well-differentiated, moderately differentiated, and poorly differentiated. The GAPP has not yet been used clinically but may be more useful than the PASS to predict malignancy if future validation studies can support the initial findings. Adrenal tumors are less likely to be malignant than extraadrenal tumors with metastatic disease arising from approximately 10% of adrenal primary tumors and approximately 20% of extraadrenal tumors.[5] Metastatic disease is more likely to occur in large tumors, extraadrenal paragangliomas and in patients with *SDHB* mutations.[5] Metastases can be present at diagnosis of the primary tumor or can occur even 20 to 25 years later. Patients with metastatic pheochromocytomas have an overall five-year survival rate of 50%.[5]

Treatment Options

All treatments for metastatic disease can slow disease progression but none are curative. Surgical debulking is still the best option as an initial treatment for malignant disease. If the tumor is MIBG avid, this presents a good treatment option for patients with metastatic disease. There are protocols to use both low and high dose ^{131}I-MIBG therapy, with the higher doses being associated with more bone marrow toxicity. A systematic review and meta-analysis was done to examine the effect of ^{131}I-MIBG treatment on tumor volume in patients with metastatic disease.[22] A total of 243 patients in seven studies were analyzed. The patients may or may not have had prior treatments and received various doses and regimens of ^{131}I-MIBG. The results showed a complete or partial tumor response in 3% and 27% of patients, respectively, and a complete or partial hormonal response in 11% and 40% of patients, respectively.[22] There is also a new formulation of MIBG (Azedra [Ultratrace iobenguane I-131]), which is currently being evaluated in trials. This compound has more specificity for tumor cells that secrete catecholamines.

External beam radiation therapy and proton therapy is often used for bone metastases and control of unresectable head and neck paragangliomas. Radiation therapy has also been shown to be effective for metastatic disease which is limited to a few index bulky or symptomatic lesions when used alone[23,24] or in combination with ^{131}I-MIBG therapy[23] because these therapies have nonoverlapping toxicities.

Chemotherapeutic regimens have not been very successful in the treatment of metastatic disease. The most commonly used regimen consists of cyclophosphamide, vincristine, and dacarbazine (CVD). No prospective clinical trials exist; but a systematic review and meta-analysis was done to evaluate the effects of CVD chemotherapy in patients with metastatic pheochromocytoma and paraganglioma.[25] This analysis included a total of 50 patients across four studies. Results showed a complete or partial tumor response rate in 4% and 37% of patients, respectively, and a complete or partial biochemical response rate of 14% and 40% of patients, respectively.[25] Responses occurred after 2 to 4 cycles of CVD therapy, and the median duration of response was 20 and 40 months in the two studies which included these data.

Temozolomide, a DNA alkylating agent, was used in a very small study of 15 patients with metastatic pheochromocytoma and paraganglioma (10 patients had *SDHB* mutations).[26] The investigators hypothesized that because *SDHB*-associated pheochromocytoma and paraganglioma have global hypermethylation, these tumors may respond better to treatment with temozolomide because they may have epigenetically silenced the enzyme needed for DNA repair response to temozolomide. This study found that the median progression-free survival was longer in *SDHB* mutation carriers (19.7 months) compared with nonmutation carriers (2.9 months) ($p = 0.007$).[26]

Some newer agents are being used to treat metastatic pheochromocytoma including targeted therapies with tyrosine kinase inhibitors such as sunitinib and pazopanib, which are multi-targeted agents with antiangiogenic and antitumor activity. Clinical trials are ongoing, but some initial results with sunitinib have been disappointing with a median progression-free survival of 4.1 months with grade 4 hypertension being common and a limiting factor.[27] Some patients with metastatic disease may have positive uptake on an octreotide scan indicating upregulation of somatostatin receptors, and if present, octreotide or the longer acting lanreotide may also be considered as another therapeutic option.[28,29] Solitary hepatic metastases can be treated with resection, and if multiple liver metastases are present, chemoembolization of liver is also a treatment option.

Hypertensive Effects of Medical Treatment for Malignant Pheochromocytoma

Treatment of malignant pheochromocytoma may increase catecholamine secretion and induce a hypertensive crisis. In addition, some of the therapies themselves may induce a hypertensive crisis. CVD treatment requires careful monitoring after therapy because there can be large releases of catecholamines from tumor cell lysis causing hemodynamic instability. High dose ^{131}I-MIBG therapy has been shown in trials to be associated with significant grade 3 hypertension in about 15% of patients usually within 30 minutes after injection.[30] The mechanism of action of the worsening hypertension is not clear. Hypertension is a common side effect of tyrosine kinase inhibitor (TKI) use in other cancer types and is particularly a problem in patients with metastatic pheochromocytoma and paraganglioma because they already have severe hypertension. The mechanism of action for TKIs to induce or worsen hypertension is not known, but it is postulated that by blocking vascular endothelial growth factor (VEGF) action, nitric oxide synthetase production is decreased, preventing generation of nitric oxide with unopposed action of endothelin resulting in hypertension.[31] Another hypothesis is that decreased VEGF function leads to remodeling of the capillary beds and to endothelial dysfunction.[31] Alternatively, TKIs may cause tumor cell apoptosis leading to release of stored catecholamines and metanephrines.[27] We suggest that patients with malignant pheochromocytoma and paraganglioma receiving any systemic therapy should be evaluated for pre-treatment with alpha-blockers or calcium channel blockers, similar to the perioperative blockade, to prevent exacerbation of hypertension. In addition, as tumors respond to systemic therapy and catecholamine secretion decreases, these patients require close monitoring for hypotension while on antihypertensive medications.

GENETIC SYNDROMES

Up to 40% of patients with pheochromocytomas and para-gangliomas will have a germline mutation in one of over 14 genes known to increase risk of this tumor type[4] (Table 15.4). Because pheochromocytomas and paragangliomas are the tumors with the highest rate of hereditary mutations, guidelines recommend that all patients with these tumors be referred for clinical genetic testing.[8] Knowing the presence of a germline mutation has screening and surveillance implications for the patient and the family members. The first syndromes noted to increase risk of pheochromocytomas were the classic tumor suppressor syndromes of Neurofibromatosis type 1 (NF1), MEN2, and vHL. Over time, several other syndromes and susceptibility genes have been identified.

Neurofibromatosis Type 1

NF1 occurs in 1 in 3000 people and is an autosomal dominant syndrome caused by inactivating germline mutations in the *NF1* tumor suppressor gene.[32] The *NF1* gene product, neuro-fibromin, negatively regulates the MAPK (mitogen-activated protein kinases) pathway for cell proliferation. NF1 is diagnosed based on clinical criteria[33] which includes patients having two or more of the following: six or more café au lait spots of certain size based on pubertal status, Lisch nodules which are benign iris hamartomas, two or more cutaneous neurofibromas, one or more plexiform neurofibroma, axillary or inguinal freckling, optic glioma, sphenoid dysplasia or thinning of the long bones, and a first degree relative with NF1. These criteria do not include pheochromocytomas or paragangliomas, but patients with NF1 are at increased risk of developing adrenal pheochromocytomas compared with the general population. Still, pheochromocytomas in patients with NF1 are rare, but once present, the risk of malignancy is up to 12%.[34] Screening with biochemical testing for

pheochromocytoma in patients with NF1 is recommended for any patient who is hypertensive.

Multiple Endocrine Neoplasia Type 2

MEN2 is an autosomal dominant syndrome occurring in 1 in 30,000 people and caused by activating germline mutations in the *RET* protooncogene. The RET protein is a membrane tyrosine kinase receptor, which activates PI3K signaling pathways in the cell. MEN2 has two subtypes: MEN2A and MEN2B. Over 90% of patients with MEN2 have the MEN2A subtype. These patients are at risk for medullary thyroid carcinoma, pheochromocytomas, and hyperparathyroidism from parathyroid adenomas or hyperplasia. This subtype can also include patients who develop Hirshsprung's disease and those who develop only medullary thyroid carcinoma. The minority of patients with MEN2 have MEN2B and develop medullary thyroid carcinoma, pheochromocytomas, and have additional features of mucosal neuromas, gastrointestinal ganglioneuromas, and a marfanoid habitus. The risk of developing pheochromocytomas with MEN2 varies depending on the specific *RET* gene mutation[35]; overall, 50% of patients with MEN2 developed pheochromocytomas and approximately 50% of those have bilateral disease. Paragangliomas are rare in this syndrome but can occur.[36] The 2015 revised guidelines suggest annual screening with biochemical testing for pheochromocytomas and paragangliomas in patients with MEN2 should begin by age 11 for those with high-risk mutations (including those in codons 634 and 918) and by age 16 for those with moderate-risk mutations.[35] The mean age of diagnosis of pheochromocytoma in patients with MEN2 is between ages 30 and 40 years, and the risk of malignancy is less than 5%.[37]

von Hippel Lindau Disease

vHL occurs in 1 in 36,000 and is an autosomal dominant syndrome caused by inactivating germline mutations in the *VHL* gene.[38] In response to oxygen levels in the cell, the VHL protein regulates hypoxia inducible factor alpha (HIFalpha) function in controlling transcription of genes involved in angiogenesis. vHL disease is characterized by multiple different tumors and cysts including pheochromocytomas, hemangioblastomas of the nervous system, renal cysts, and clear cell renal cell carcinoma, pancreatic cysts, and pancreatic neuroendocrine tumors, endolymphatic sac tumors, and epididymal cysts.[38] Approximately 10% to 20% of patients with vHL develop

TABLE 15.4 Pheochromocytoma and Paraganglioma Susceptibility Genes

GENE	SYNDROME	PRIMARY PHEOCHROMOCYTOMA OR PARAGANGLIOMA LOCATION
NF1	Neurofibromatosis type 1	Adrenal pheochromocytomas
VHL	von Hippel Lindau	Adrenal pheochromocytomas
RET	Multiple Endocrine Neoplasia type 2	Adrenal pheochromocytomas
SDHA	Hereditary paraganglioma syndrome	Any location
SDHB	Hereditary paraganglioma syndrome	Extraadrenal paraganglioma (any location)
SDHC	Hereditary paraganglioma syndrome	Head and neck paragangliomas (thoracic paragangliomas)
SDHD	Hereditary paraganglioma syndrome	Head and neck paragangliomas (any location)
SDHAF2	Hereditary paraganglioma syndrome	Head and neck paragangliomas
TMEM127	Familial pheochromocytoma/paraganglioma syndrome	Adrenal pheochromocytoma (any location)
MAX	Familial pheochromocytoma/paraganglioma syndrome	Adrenal pheochromocytomas
FH	Hereditary leiomyomatosis and renal cell cancer syndrome	Any location
MDH2	Familial pheochromocytoma/paraganglioma syndrome	Any location
EPAS1	Polycythemia paraganglioma syndrome	Any location

unilateral or bilateral pheochromocytomas with paragangliomas occurring extremely rarely.[36] Screening with biochemical testing for pheochromocytoma in vHL patients should begin at age 5 years for families with high-risk mutations. The mean age at diagnosis of pheochromocytoma in patients with vHL is 30 years,[39] and around 5% develop metastatic disease.[38]

Hereditary Paraganglioma Syndromes

The next group of syndromes associated with pheochromocytomas and paragangliomas are called the hereditary paraganglioma syndromes. The hereditary paraganglioma syndromes are caused by germline mutations in the succinate dehydrogenase (SDH) complex, which is complex II of the mitochondrial respiratory chain and also coverts succinate to fumarate in the Krebs cycle. The complex is made up of four genes, SDHA, SDHB, SDHC, SDHC, and a cofactor, SDHAF2. Mutations in any of those genes increase risk for pheochromocytomas and paragangliomas. There are some genotype/phenotype correlations. SDHB mutations are the most common in the complex and are often associated with extraadrenal paragangliomas, but patients can develop adrenal pheochromocytomas and head and neck paragangliomas as well.[40] Patients who carry germline SDHB mutations have the highest risk (23%) of developing metastatic disease[41] compared with any other SDH gene mutations (less than 5%). SDHD mutations are the next most common mutations in the complex and are associated most often with head and neck paraganglioma, but patients can also develop adrenal or extraadrenal tumors as well.[40] SDHD mutations are paternally expressed, meaning tumors only develop if the mutation was inherited from the proband's father with extremely rare exception.[42,43] Mutations in the remaining subunits occur much more rarely. SDHC germline mutations are most commonly associated with head and neck paragangliomas (over 80%), but patients have an increased risk of thoracic paraganglioma as well as abdominal paraganglioma and adrenal pheochromocytoma.[44] Rare patients with pheochromocytomas and paragangliomas have germline mutations in SDHA or SDHAF2.[45,46] SDHAF2 mutations have a parent-of-origin effect with paternal transmission of disease, and affected patients appear to develop multiple head and neck paraganglioma only.[46]

SDHx mutation carriers are at risk for developing multiple primary pheochromocytomas and paragangliomas as well as other tumors including clear cell renal cell carcinoma, gastrointestinal stromal tumors, and pituitary adenomas.[40,47-49] Because of this, SDHx mutation carriers require life-long screening. However, there are no formal guidelines regarding how to screen unaffected SDHx mutation carriers. Long-term surveillance studies of mutation carrier families are needed to determine the true rates of malignancy and penetrance of disease. Until these data are available, most experts recommend screening starting between ages 5 and 10 years with annual biochemistries and full body imaging every two years.[50] Most centers use MRI imaging to screen these patients to avoid the radiation exposure from life-long CT scanning.

Other Hereditary Causes

Several other susceptibility genes have been identified in a small percentage of patients with pheochromocytomas and paragangliomas. Transmembrane protein 127 (TMEM127) and Myc-associated protein X (MAX) germline mutations are usually associated with adrenal pheochromocytomas, but patients may have extraadrenal paragangliomas as well.[51,52] TMEM127 is thought to have a role in the mTOR pathway and MAX is a transcription factor which heterodimerizes with MYC. Patients with mutations in Fumarate hydratase (FH) develop hereditary leiomyomatosis and renal cell cancer syndrome, and recently a few families been found to have pheochromocytomas/

paragangliomas with mutations in this gene.[53,54] FH is involved in the Krebs cycle. Another gene playing a role in the Kreb cycle, Malate dehydrogenase 2 (MDH2), has also been found to be mutated in the germline of a few families with pheochromocytomas and paragangliomas.[55] Mutations in EPAS1, the gene encoding the transcription factor hypoxia inducible factor 2-alpha, have been found in some patients with pheochromocytomas with or without polycythemia and/or somatostatinomas.[56-58] Because so little is known about the penetrance of these mutations for pheochromocytoma and paraganglioma, most experts recommend annual biochemical testing and cross-sectional imaging every two years for patients who carry one of these rare susceptibility gene mutations.[4,50]

Somatic Genetics

Despite the high rate of germline mutations in this disease, still more than half of pheochromocytomas and paragangliomas are not believed to be hereditary. In these sporadic tumors, somatic mutations in the classic susceptibility genes NF1, VHL, and RET occur at low rates, but interestingly, somatic mutations are rarely if ever seen in the SDHx genes.[59,60] Up to 10% of sporadic tumors have somatic mutations in HRAS.[61] Approximately 13% of paragangliomas/pheochromocytomas were found to have somatic mutations in ATRX, and these mutations are associated with clinically aggressive disease.[62] ATRX is a chromatin remodeling gene which is mutated in other neuroendocrine tumors as well, such as neuroblastomas and well-differentiated pancreatic neuroendocrine tumors. The role of ATRX in tumorigenesis is not clearly understood. The Cancer Genome Atlas (TCGA) consortium through the National Institutes of Health is completing a study on the integrative genomics of pheochromocytomas and paragangliomas which may provide further insight in the biology of these tumors, identify markers for aggressive disease and offer novel targets for therapy.

CONCLUSION

Pheochromocytomas and paragangliomas are rare but important causes of secondary hypertension. Unrecognized tumors are associated with high cardiovascular morbidity and mortality. Surgery is the mainstay of treatment, and patients require appropriate perioperative alpha-blockade. Up to 40% of patients have germline mutations in known susceptibility genes. Knowing if a germline mutation is present has implications for treatment, screening, and surveillance of patients and their family members; consequently, all patients with pheochromocytomas and paragangliomas should be referred for clinical genetic testing.

References

1. Velasco A, Vongpatanasin W. The evaluation and treatment of endocrine forms of hypertension. Curr Cardiol Rep. 2014;16:528.
2. DeLellis RA, Lloyd RV, Heitz PU, Eng C, eds. World Health Organization Classification of Tumours. Pathology and Genetics of Tumours of Endocrine Organs. Lyon, France: IARC Press; 2004.
3. Nieman LK. Approach to the patient with an adrenal incidentaloma. J Clin Endocrinol Metab. 2010;95:4106-4113.
4. Favier J, Amar L, Gimenez-Roqueplo AP. Paraganglioma and phaeochromocytoma: from genetics to personalized medicine. Nat Rev Endocrinol. 2015;11:101-111.
5. Ayala-Ramirez M, Feng L, Johnson MM, et al. Clinical risk factors for malignancy and overall survival in patients with pheochromocytomas and sympathetic paragangliomas: primary tumor size and primary tumor location as prognostic indicators. J Clin Endocrinol Metab. 2011;96:717-725.
6. Zeiger MA, Thompson GB, Duh QY, et al. The American Association of Clinical Endocrinologists and American Association of Endocrine Surgeons medical guidelines for the management of adrenal incidentalomas. Endocr Pract. 2009;15:1-20.
7. Cohen DL, Fraker D, Townsend RR. Lack of symptoms in patients with histologic evidence of pheochromocytoma: a diagnostic challenge. Ann N Y Acad Sci. 2006;1073:47-51.
8. Lenders JW, Duh QY, Eisenhofer G, et al. Pheochromocytoma and paraganglioma: an endocrine society clinical practice guideline. J Clin Endocrinol Metab. 2014;99:1915-1942.
9. Neary NM, King KS, Pacak K. Drugs and pheochromocytoma—don't be fooled by every elevated metanephrine. N Engl J Med. 2011;364:2268-2270.
10. Mozley PD, Kim CK, Mohsin J, Jatlow A, Gosfield E, 3rd, Alavi A. The efficacy of iodine-123-MIBG as a screening test for pheochromocytoma. J Nucl Med. 1994;35:1138-1144.
11. Bruynzeel H, Feelders RA, Groenland TH, et al. Risk factors for hemodynamic instability during surgery for pheochromocytoma. J Clin Endocrinol Metab. 2010;95:678-685.

12. Dickson PV, Alex GC, Grubbs EG, et al. Posterior retroperitoneoscopic adrenalectomy is a safe and effective alternative to transabdominal laparoscopic adrenalectomy for pheochromocytoma. *Surgery*. 2011;150:452-458.
13. Steinsapir J, Carr AA, Prisant LM, Bransome ED, Jr. Metyrosine and pheochromocytoma. *Arch Intern Med*. 1997;157:901-906.
14. Perry RR, Keiser HR, Norton JA, et al. Surgical management of pheochromocytoma with the use of metyrosine. *Ann Surg*. 1990;212:621-628.
15. Wachtel H, Kennedy EH, Zaheer S, et al. Preoperative metyrosine improves cardiovascular outcomes for patients undergoing surgery for pheochromocytoma and paraganglioma. *Ann Surg Oncol*. 2015;22(Suppl 3):646-654.
16. Weingarten TN, Cata JP, O'Hara JF, et al. Comparison of two preoperative medical management strategies for laparoscopic resection of pheochromocytoma. *Urology*. 2010;76:508:e6-e11.
17. Kocak S, Aydintug S, Canakci N. Alpha blockade in preoperative preparation of patients with pheochromocytomas. *Int Surg*. 2002;87:191-194.
18. Prys-Roberts C, Farndon JR. Efficacy and safety of doxazosin for perioperative management of patients with pheochromocytoma. *World J Surg*. 2002;26:1037-1042.
19. Thompson LD. Pheochromocytoma of the Adrenal gland Scaled Score (PASS) to separate benign from malignant neoplasms: a clinicopathologic and immunophenotypic study of 100 cases. *Am J Surg Pathol*. 2002;26:551-566.
20. Wu D, Tischler AS, Lloyd RV, et al. Observer variation in the application of the Pheochromocytoma of the Adrenal Gland Scaled Score. *Am J Surg Pathol*. 2009;33:599-608.
21. Kimura N, Takayanagi R, Takizawa N, et al. Pathological grading for predicting metastasis in phaeochromocytoma and paraganglioma. *Endocr Relat Cancer*. 2014;21:405-414.
22. van Hulsteijn LT, Niemeijer ND, Dekkers OM, Corssmit EP. (131)I-MIBG therapy for malignant paraganglioma and phaeochromocytoma: systematic review and meta-analysis. *Clin Endocrinol. (Oxf)*. 2014;80:487-501.
23. Fishbein L, Bonner L, Torigian DA, et al. External beam radiation therapy (EBRT) for patients with malignant pheochromocytoma and non-head and -neck paraganglioma: combination with 131I-MIBG. *Horm Metab Res*. 2012;44:405-410.
24. Vogel J, Atanacio AS, Prodanov T, et al. External beam radiation therapy in treatment of malignant pheochromocytoma and paraganglioma. *Front Oncol*. 2014;4:166.
25. Niemeijer ND, Alblas G, van Hulsteijn LT, Dekkers OM, Corssmit EP. Chemotherapy with cyclophosphamide, vincristine and dacarbazine for malignant paraganglioma and pheochromocytoma: systematic review and meta-analysis. *Clin Endocrinol. (Oxf)*. 2014;81:642-651.
26. Hadoux J, Favier J, Scoazec JY, et al. SDHB mutations are associated with response to temozolomide in patients with metastatic pheochromocytoma or paraganglioma. *Int J Cancer*. 2014;135:2711-2720.
27. Ayala-Ramirez M, Chougnet CN, Habra MA, et al. Treatment with sunitinib for patients with progressive metastatic pheochromocytomas and sympathetic paragangliomas. *J Clin Endocrinol Metab*. 2012;97:4040-4050.
28. Elshafie O, Al Badaai Y, Alwahaibi K, et al. Catecholamine-secreting carotid body paraganglioma: successful preoperative control of hypertension and clinical symptoms using high-dose long-acting octreotide. *Endocrinol Diabetes Metab Case Rep*. 2014;2014:140051.
29. Duet M, Guichard JP, Rizzo N, Boudiaf M, Herman P. Tran Ba Huy P. Are somatostatin analogs therapeutic alternatives in the management of head and neck paragangliomas? *Laryngoscope*. 2005;115:1381-1384.
30. Gonias S, Goldsby R, Matthay KK, et al. Phase II study of high-dose [131I]metaiodobenzylguanidine therapy for patients with metastatic pheochromocytoma and paraganglioma. *J Clin Oncol*. 2009;27:4162-4168.
31. Aparicio-Gallego G, Afonso-Afonso FJ, Leon-Mateos L, et al. Molecular basis of hypertension side effects induced by sunitinib. *Anticancer Drugs*. 2011;22:1-8.
32. Williams VC, Lucas J, Babcock MA, Gutmann DH, Korf B, Maria BL. Neurofibromatosis type 1 revisited. *Pediatrics*. 2009;123:124-133.
33. Ferner RE, Huson SM, Thomas N, et al. Guidelines for the diagnosis and management of individuals with neurofibromatosis 1. *J Med Genet*. 2007;44:81-88.
34. Bausch B, Borozdin W, Neumann HP. Clinical and genetic characteristics of patients with neurofibromatosis type 1 and pheochromocytoma. *N Engl J Med*. 2006;354:2729-2731.
35. Wells A, Jr., Asa SL, Dralle H, et al. Revised American Thyroid Association guidelines for the management of medullary thyroid carcinoma. *Thyroid*. 2015;25:567-610.
36. Boedeker CC, Erlic Z, Richard S, et al. Head and neck paragangliomas in von Hippel-Lindau disease and multiple endocrine neoplasia type 2. *J Clin Endocrinol Metab*. 2009;94:1938-1944.
37. Modigliani E, Vasen HM, Raue K, et al. Pheochromocytoma in multiple endocrine neoplasia type 2: European study. The Euromen Study Group. *J Intern Med*. 1995;238:363-367.
38. Maher ER, Neumann HP, Richard S. von Hippel-Lindau disease: a clinical and scientific review. *Eur J Hum Genet*. 2011;19:617-623.
39. Delman KA, Shapiro SE, Jonasch EW, et al. Abdominal visceral lesions in von Hippel-Lindau disease: incidence and clinical behavior of pancreatic and adrenal lesions at a single center. *World J Surg*. 2006;30:665-669.
40. Ricketts CJ, Forman JR, Rattenberry E, et al. Tumor risks and genotype-phenotype-proteotype analysis in 358 patients with germline mutations in SDHB and SDHD. *Hum Mutat*. 2010;31:41-51.
41. van Hulsteijn LT, Dekkers OM, Hes FJ, Smit JW, Corssmit EP. Risk of malignant paraganglioma in SDHB-mutation and SDHD-mutation carriers: a systematic review and meta-analysis. *J Med Genet*. 2012;49:768-776.
42. Bayley JP, Oldenburg RA, Nuk J, et al. Paraganglioma and pheochromocytoma upon maternal transmission of SDHD mutations. *BMC Med Genet*. 2014;15:111.
43. Yeap PM, Tobias ES, Mavraki E, et al. Molecular analysis of pheochromocytoma after maternal transmission of SDHD mutation elucidates mechanism of parent-of-origin effect. *J Clin Endocrinol Metab*. 2011;96:E2009-2013.
44. Else T, Marvin ML, Everett JN, et al. The clinical phenotype of SDHC-associated hereditary paraganglioma syndrome (PGL3). *J Clin Endocrinol Metab*. 2014;99:E1482-1486.
45. Burnichon N, Briere JJ, Libe R, et al. SDHA is a tumor suppressor gene causing paraganglioma. *Hum Mol Genet*. 2010;19:3011-3020.
46. Kunst HP, Rutten MH, de Monnink JP, et al. SDHAF2 (PGL2-SDH5) and hereditary head and neck paraganglioma. *Clin Cancer Res*. 2011;17:247-254.
47. Evenepoel L, Papathomas TG, Krol N, et al. Toward an improved definition of the genetic and tumor spectrum associated with SDH germ-line mutations. *Genet Med*. 2014;17:610-620.
48. Pasini B, Stratakis CA. SDH mutations in tumorigenesis and inherited endocrine tumours: lesson from the phaeochromocytoma-paraganglioma syndromes. *J Intern Med*. 2009;266:19-42.
49. Xekouki P, Szarek E, Bullova P, et al. Pituitary adenoma with paraganglioma/pheochromocytoma (3PAs) and succinate dehydrogenase defects in humans and mice. *J Clin Endocrinol Metab*. 2015;100:E710-719.
50. Fishbein L, Nathanson KL. Pheochromocytoma and paraganglioma: understanding the complexities of the genetic background. *Cancer Genet*. 2012;205:1-11.
51. Comino-Mendez I, Gracia-Aznarez FJ, Schiavi F, et al. Exome sequencing identifies MAX mutations as a cause of hereditary pheochromocytoma. *Nat Genet*. 2011;43:663-667.
52. Jiang S, Dahia PL. Minireview: the busy road to pheochromocytomas and paragangliomas has a new member, TMEM127. *Endocrinology*. 2011;152:2133-2140.
53. Castro-Vega LJ, Buffet A, De Cubas AA, et al. Germline mutations in FH confer predisposition to malignant pheochromocytomas and paragangliomas. *Hum Mol Genet*. 2014;23:2440-2446.
54. Clark GR, Sciacovelli M, Gaude E, et al. Germline FH mutations presenting with pheochromocytoma. *J Clin Endocrinol Metab*. 2014;99:E2046-2050.
55. Cascon A, Comino-Mendez I, Curras-Freixes M, et al. Whole-exome sequencing identifies MDH2 as a new familial paraganglioma gene. *J Natl Cancer Inst*. 2015;107.
56. Buffet A, Smati S, Mansuy L, et al. Mosaicism in HIF2A-related polycythemia-paraganglioma syndrome. *J Clin Endocrinol Metab*. 2014;99:E369-673.
57. Comino-Mendez I, de Cubas AA, Bernal C, et al. Tumoral EPAS1 (HIF2A) mutations explain sporadic pheochromocytoma and paraganglioma in the absence of erythrocytosis. *Hum Mol Genet*. 2013;22:2169-2176.
58. Zhuang Z, Yang C, Lorenzo F, et al. Somatic HIF2A gain-of-function mutations in paraganglioma with polycythemia. *N Engl J Med*. 2012;367:922-930.
59. Burnichon N, Vescovo L, Amar L, et al. Integrative genomic analysis reveals somatic mutations in pheochromocytoma and paraganglioma. *Hum Mol Genet*. 2011;20:3974-3985.
60. Welander J, Larsson C, Backdahl M, et al. Integrative genomics reveals frequent somatic NF1 mutations in sporadic pheochromocytomas. *Hum Mol Genet*. 2012;21:5406-5416.
61. Oudijk L, de Krijger RR, Rapa I, et al. H-RAS mutations are restricted to sporadic pheochromocytomas lacking specific clinical or pathological features: data from a multi-institutional series. *J Clin Endocrinol Metab*. 2014;99:E1376-1380.
62. Fishbein L, Khare S, Wubbenhorst B, et al. Whole-exome sequencing identifies somatic ATRX mutations in pheochromocytomas and paragangliomas. *Nat Commun*. 2015;6:6140.

16 Secondary Hypertension: Sleep Disturbances Including Sleep Apnea

Ailia W. Ali and Patrick J. Strollo, Jr.

OBSTRUCTIVE SLEEP APNEA AND HYPERTENSION

Obstructive sleep apnea (OSA) and hypertension are common medical conditions which often coexist. Is there is a causal relationship between these two conditions? This question has been repeatedly raised in literature and has remained an area of interest for many years. The association between OSA and hypertension was initially reported by Tilkian et al[1] in 1976 who demonstrated a substantial cyclical elevation in blood pressure with each apneic episode. Systemic hypertension was also noted in one-third of the patients with OSA.[1]

In this chapter we will review the epidemiology of OSA and hypertension; mechanisms by which OSA leads to development and/or progression of hypertension; and the effect of treating OSA on hypertension.

DEFINITION OF OBSTRUCTIVE SLEEP APNEA

OSA is defined by the occurrence of daytime sleepiness, loud snoring, witnessed breathing interruptions, or awakenings as a result of gasping or choking in the presence of at least five obstructive respiratory events (apneas, hypopneas, or respiratory effort–related arousals) per hour of sleep. The presence of 15 or more obstructive respiratory events per hour of sleep in the absence of sleep-related symptoms is also sufficient for the diagnosis of OSA because of a greater association of this severity of obstruction with important consequences such as increased cardiovascular disease risk.

Obstructive apneas or hypopneas occur when the upper airway dilator muscles fail to maintain the patency of the upper airway and airflow during sleep. Various factors that can increase the risk for developing OSA include altered facial structure, small upper airway lumen, poor upper airway muscle function, respiratory control instability, increased arousal response, small lung volumes, fluid retention, male sex, obesity, advancing age, genetic factors, menopause, and smoking.[2]

PREVALENCE OF OBSTRUCTIVE SLEEP APNEA AND HYPERTENSION

Sleep apnea occurs in 3% to 7% of adult males and 2% to 5% of adult females in the general population.[3] Peppard et al[4] recently reported the prevalence of OSA of 26% among patients between 30 to 70 years of age. A population-based, age-stratified case control study done in Sweden assessed the prevalence of OSA in men. This study reported that the prevalence of OSA in primary hypertension was 35%.[5] In the Wisconsin Sleep Cohort, the odds ratios for the presence of hypertension at 4-year follow-up was 2.89 with an apnea-hypopnea index (AHI) of 15 or more events per hour compared with those with an AHI of 0.[6] This study demonstrated

a dose-response relationship between the severity of OSA and presence of hypertension, independent of the confounding factors. The Sleep Heart Health Study showed similar findings with an increase in prevalence of hypertension with increasing AHI.[7]

Rapid eye movement (REM) sleep is generally associated with a greater propensity for upper airway closure because of inhibition of muscle tone during this stage of sleep. As a result, the likelihood of OSA or worsening of OSA in REM sleep is increased. In addition, REM sleep is also associated with increased sympathetic activity which can contribute to a rise in blood pressure. The Wisconsin Sleep cohort reported a significant dose-relationships between REM AHI and prevalent hypertension. The higher relative odds of prevalent hypertension were most evident with REM AHI 15 or more. In individuals with a non-REM AHI 5 or less, a two-fold increase in REM AHI was associated with 24% higher odds ratio of hypertension. Longitudinal analysis also revealed a significant association between higher REM AHI and the development of hypertension (p trend = 0.017).[8]

A recent report with a 5-year follow-up from the Sleep Heart Health Study concluded that the association between hypertension and AHI was not significant after adjusting for body mass index (BMI).[9] Similarly, the Vitoria Sleep Cohort also found no association between OSA and incidence of hypertension after adjustment for confounders.[10] It is unclear why there are variations in the results of these studies but these could be accounted by differences in the populations sampled and techniques used to diagnose sleep apnea or AHI cutoff points may account for the variation related to the impact of OSA on prevalent and incident hypertension.

There is a striking association between drug-resistant hypertension and OSA. Prevalence of OSA in patients with drug-resistant hypertension has been reported to be approximately 64% to 83%.[11,12] Pedrosa et al[12] identified OSA as the most common secondary cause of hypertension in patients with drug-resistant hypertension (Fig. 16.1).

Treatment of OSA with continuous positive airway pressure (CPAP) has been shown to lower blood pressure (BP) in this patient cohort.[13] Similar impact of CPAP on BP was observed in a recent study including patients with resistant and nonresistant hypertension and OSA.[14] These findings support the role of OSA in the pathogenesis of hypertension in these patients (Fig. 16.2).

MECHANISM OF OBSTRUCTIVE SLEEP APNEA

Anatomically, the upper airway has a limited bony support. There are multiple anatomic and physiologic factors which promote the collapse of this portion of the airway. These influences are offset by the factors which dilate the airway to maintain airway patency.

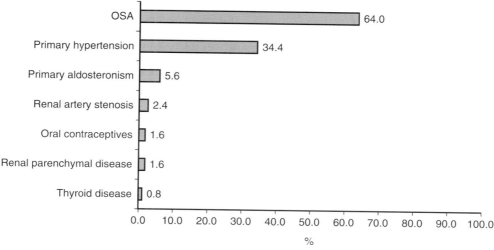

FIG. 16.1 Prevalence of secondary causes of hypertension associated with resistant hypertension. *OSA,* Obstructive sleep apnea. *(Reused with permission from Pedrosa RP, Drager LF, Gonzaga CC, et al. Obstructive sleep apnea: the most common secondary cause of hypertension associated with resistant hypertension. Hypertension. 2011;58:811-817.)*

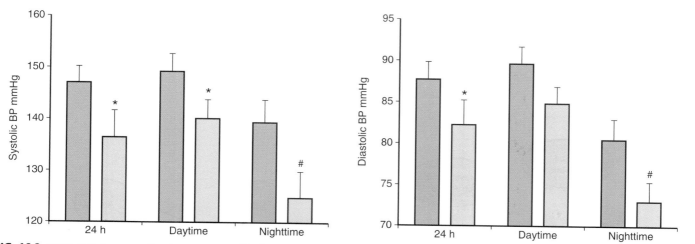

FIG. 16.2 Impact of continuous positive airway pressure on blood pressure. *(Reused with permission from Logan AG, Tkacova R, Perlikowski SM, et al. Refractory hypertension and sleep apnea: effect of CPAP on blood pressure and baroreflex. Eur Respir J. 2003;21:241-247.)*

The two primary forces promoting airway collapse are intraluminal negative pressure generated by the diaphragm during inspiration and the extraluminal tissue pressure produced by tissues surrounding the airway. These influences are overcome by the action of pharyngeal dilator muscles, specifically genioglossus muscle along with the impact of tracheal traction on the airway from lung inflation.[15-17] In addition, low lung volumes during nonrapid eye movement (NREM) sleep lead to less tension on the airway wall and are associated with increased airflow resistance and collapsibility.[18]

OSA results from complete or partial collapse of the upper airway lumen during sleep. During state of wakefulness, upper airway patency is maintained by the activity of pharyngeal dilator muscles. This muscle activity tends to be reduced during sleep along with the decrease in lung volumes, increasing the likelihood of airway closure during sleep.[19] Factors that affect the functioning of pharyngeal dilator muscles include fatigue, and neuropathic and myopathic injury also contribute to airway obstruction.[20,21] Most patients with obstructive apnea have an anatomically small upper airway, either because of increased soft tissue surrounding the airway or a small bony structure surrounding the airway.[22,23]

Stability of the respiratory control system may fluctuate during sleep leading to variation in activity of the upper airway dilator muscles. Low central respiratory drive leads to low upper airway dilator muscle activity, high airway resistance, and propensity to airway collapse.[24]

Any disease state contributing to fluid retention and mobilization of fluid overnight from the legs to the neck may lead to narrowing of the airway lumen and increase the propensity to airway closure. This can be an important factor for OSA in conditions such as heart failure and end-stage renal disease (Fig. 16.3).[25,26]

Obesity and male gender are risk factors for OSA. Obesity promotes airway collapsibility by increasing extraluminal tissue pressure as a result of fat deposition.[27] Men have greater total neck soft tissue volume and longer length of airway, independent of height, that may account for higher airway collapsibility.[28,29]

Aging is a risk factor for OSA because of multiple reasons. Older individuals have an increased collapsibility of the airway caused by a loss of collagen and an increased deposition of parapharyngeal fat,[30] an impairment of pharyngeal dilator muscles response to negative intraluminal pressure, a loss of elastic recoil of the lung leading to reduction in lung volumes, and a less tethering effect on the upper airways.[17]

The ability to arouse from sleep can also be involved in pathogenesis of OSA. In general, after arousal, people hyperventilate for a short duration which may lead to drop in CO_2

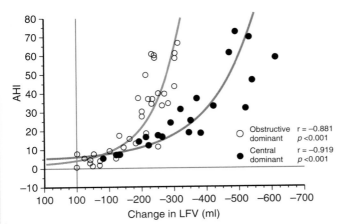

FIG. 16.3 Changes in AHI relative to leg fluid volume (LFV). Relationship between change in LFV and AHI in the obstructive- and central-dominant groups. The open circles and solid line represent the relationship between the AHI and the change in LFV in the obstructive-dominant group [$y = 2.4 \times e^{(-0.011 \times x)}$]. The closed circles and dashed line represent the relationship between the AHI and the change in LFV in the central-dominant group [$y = 5.18 \, e^{(-0.004 \times x)}$]. The slopes of these curves differed significantly ($p < 0.001$). (*Reused with permission from Yumino D, Redolfi S, Ruttanaumpawan P, Su MC, et al. Nocturnal rostral fluid shift: a unifying concept for the pathogenesis of obstructive and central sleep apnea in men with heart failure.* Circulation. *2010;121:1598-1605.*)

concentration. If this drop is below the apnea threshold, central apnea occurs. As the upper airway dilator muscles receive respiratory input, hypocapnia reduces the activity of the upper airway dilator muscles and leads to collapse of the airway.[2]

Other risk factors for OSA include genetic causes and ethnicity which affects craniofacial anatomy and may predispose to obesity. Menopause has also been identified as a risk factor for OSA because of central redistribution of body fat. Smoking has been associated with OSA and is likely as a result of increased upper airway inflammation and nasal stuffiness (Fig. 16.4).[2]

CARDIOVASCULAR EFFECTS OF OBSTRUCTIVE SLEEP APNEA

Airway closure leads to a decrement or cessation of ventilation and development of hypoxia and hypercapnia. These changes lead to an arousal from sleep and increase in respiratory drive until the upper airway opens and blood gas abnormalities are reversed. Each episode of airway occlusion initiates a sequence of hemodynamic, autonomic, and chemical changes (Fig. 16.5).[31]

Each episode of OSA leads to a generation of negative intrathoracic pressure as an effort is made to breathe against a closed glottis. This leads to an increase in left ventricular (LV) transmural pressure, which in turn increases the LV afterload.

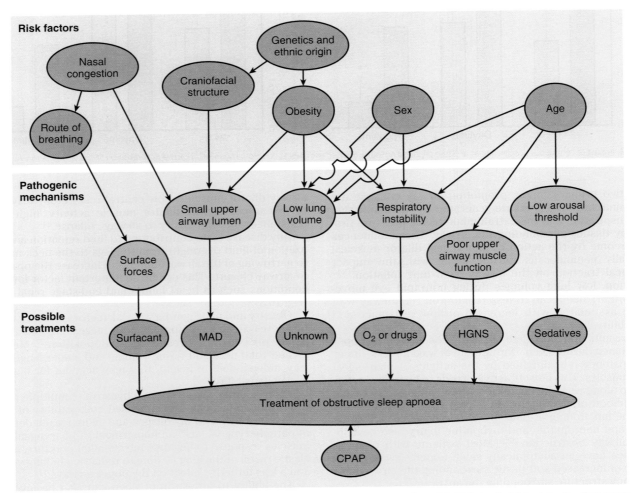

FIG. 16.4 Risk Factors Impacting obstructive sleep apnea. (*Reused with permission from Jordan AS, McSharry DG, Malhotra A. Adult obstructive sleep apnoea.* Lancet. *2014;383:736-747.*)

It also increases venous return which increases right ventricular (RV) preload. RV afterload also increases simultaneously as a result of hypoxic pulmonary vasoconstriction. These changes lead to RV distention and leftward displacement of the interventricular septum which impairs LV filling. The combination of increased LV afterload and diminished LV preload during obstructive apneas lead to a reduction in stroke volume and cardiac output.[32,33] This increase in cardiac afterload raises the myocardial oxygen demand whereas OSA related hypoxia has reduced the oxygen supply. These changes can potentially precipitate myocardial ischemia in those with preexisting coronary artery disease, impair cardiac contractility, and diastolic relaxation.[34] These repetitive episodes over time can induce LV hypertrophy (Fig. 16.6).[35,36]

Each episode of apnea leads to hypoxia and hypercapnia which are potent stimuli to chemoreceptors and lead to sympathetic stimulation. Apnea also induces sympathetic stimulation via elimination of inhibitory effects of pulmonary stretch receptors. Reductions in stroke volume during obstructive apneas reduce sympathetic inhibitory input from carotid sinus, in turn augmenting sympathetic outflow. Arousal from sleep at the end of apnea causes further adrenergic surge which leads to a rise in blood pressure and heart rate.[37] Once the sleep ensues, the same cycle repeats itself (Fig. 16.7).

The episodes of hypoxia followed by reoxygenation lead to generation of free radicals and induces inflammation. Induction of inflammation leads to vascular endothelial injury and atherogenesis.[38] Patients with OSA have a reduction in nitric oxide levels, which in turn impairs endothelially mediated vasodilation and can lead to hypertension.[39] Treating OSA with CPAP has been shown to reduce oxidative stress and improve nitrate levels (Fig. 16.8).[40]

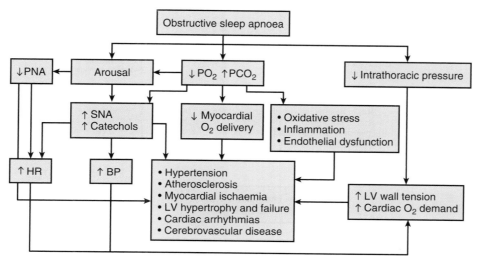

FIG. 16.5 Pathophysiologic effects of obstructive sleep apnea on the cardiovascular system. *BP*, Blood pressure; *HR*, heart rate; *LV*, left ventricular; *PCO2*, partial pressure of carbon dioxide; *PNA*, parasympathetic nervous system activity; *PO2*, partial pressure of oxygen; *SNA*, sympathetic nervous system activity. *(Reused with permission Floras JS. Hypertension and Sleep Apnea. Can J Cardiol. 2015;31:889-897.)*

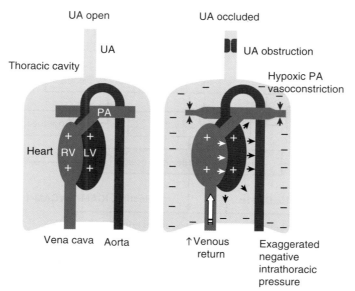

FIG. 16.6 Effects of obstructive sleep apnea (OSA) on the right and left ventricle. During OSA, negative intrathoracic pressure generated against the occluded upper airway (UA) increases left ventricular (LV) transmural pressure (intracardiac minus intrathoracic pressure) and LV afterload. It also increases venous return, augmenting right ventricular (RV) preload, whereas OSA-induced hypoxia causes pulmonary artery vasoconstriction and pulmonary hypertension. These cause RV distension and leftward displacement of the interventricular septum during diastole, which impairs LV filling and diminishes LV preload and stroke volume. +, Positive intracardiac pressure; −, negative intrathoracic pressure. *(Reused with permission from Kasai T, Bradley TD. Obstructive sleep apnea and heart failure: pathophysiologic and therapeutic implications. J Am Coll Cardiol. 2011 Jan 11;57(2):119-127.)*

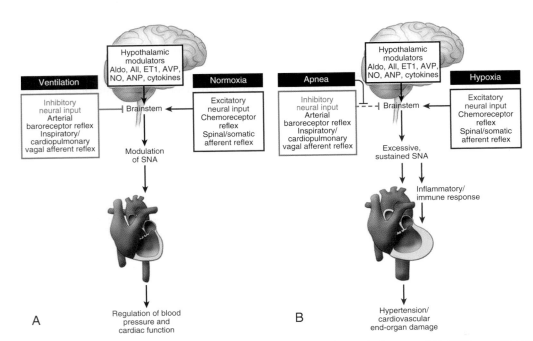

FIG. 16.7 Obstructive sleep apnea and mechanisms of sympathetic overactivity. Enhancement of sympathetic nerve activity (SNA) promotes cardiovascular disease. A, Under normal conditions, hypothalamic modulators, including aldosterone (Aldo), angiotensin II (AII), endothelin 1 (ET1), arginine vasopressin (AVP), nitric oxide, atrial natriuretic peptide (ANP), and cytokines, influence SNA. In healthy individuals, SNA is promoted by excitatory neural input *(red)* in response to peripheral stress. Simultaneously, peripheral responses *(green)*, such as the arterial baroreceptor reflex and the cardiopulmonary and other vagal afferent reflexes, buffer the increase in SNA and maintain homeostasis. B, Patients with obstructive sleep apnea exhibit sustained excessive SNA, because of a pathologic increase of excitatory neural input *(red)* and prevention and/or decrease of the protective inhibitory signals *(green)*. Sustained SNA promotes proinflammatory immune responses and, ultimately, cardiovascular disease–associated end-organ damage. *(From Abboud F, Kumar R. Obstructive sleep apnea and insight into mechanisms of sympathetic overactivity. J Clin Invest. 2014 Apr;124(4):1454-1457.)*

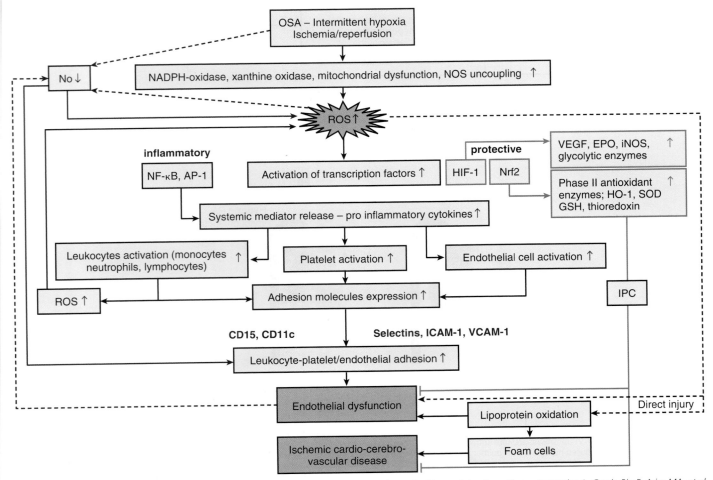

FIG. 16.8 Molecular pathways related to intermittent hypoxia in obstructive sleep apnea. *(Reused with permission from Alonso-Fernandez A, Garcia-Rio F, Arias MA, et al. Effects of CPAP on oxidative stress and nitrate efficiency in sleep apnoea: a randomised trial. Thorax. 2009;64:581-586.)*

Secondary Hypertension: Sleep Disturbances Including Sleep Apnea

A randomized trial has also reported a reduction in carotid intima-media thickness, pulse-wave velocity, C-reactive protein, and catecholamine levels in patients treated with CPAP.[41]

MECHANISM OF OBSTRUCTIVE SLEEP APNEA IN A SELECTED POPULATION

Hypertension

OSA is associated with surges in sympathetic outflow which in turn raises the blood pressure and heart rate. Somers et al[42] reported that patients with OSA have high sympathetic activity when awake with further increases in blood pressure and sympathetic activity during sleep, especially stage II and REM sleep. Peak sympathetic activity was noted at the end of each episode of apnea and was followed by a surge in blood pressures (Fig. 16.9). Interestingly, peak mean blood

pressures remained higher than wakefulness during all stages of sleep (116 ± 5 mm Hg during stage II and 127 ± 7 mm Hg during REM both ($p < 0.0001$). This study also showed that treatment with CPAP attenuates sympathetic activity and blood pressure during sleep ($p < 0.03$).

A similar observation was made by Spaak et al[43] who showed a sustained augmented effect of OSA on muscle sympathetic nerve activity during wakefulness in patients with systolic heart failure compared with systolic heart failure control subjects without OSA. This finding further strengthens the hypothesis that OSA increases the central sympathetic outflow. Sin et al[44] also reported a significant relationship between AHI and systolic blood pressure after adjusting for confounding variables.

All these studies point towards the role of OSA in the pathogenesis of hypertension. Multiple clinical trials have shown an association of OSA with nondipping blood pressure (BP) profile. The most recent observation supporting this finding came from the study which included participants of Heart BEAT trial. It showed an increase in the prevalence of nondipping systolic blood pressure (SBP) with increasing levels of AHI and Oxygen Desaturation Index (ODI) (4% increase in the odds of nondipping systolic blood pressure per 1 unit increase in both AHI and ODI) in participants with moderate-to-severe untreated OSA and with cardiovascular risk factors or established cardiovascular disease recruited from cardiology practices who had well controlled resting BP profiles (Fig. 16.10).[45] The most noteworthy observation from this trial is the fact that despite expert medical management by cardiology service and well-controlled resting BP indices, there is a relationship between increasing OSA severity and nondipping SBP. This finding emphasizes the role of OSA in the pathophysiology of nondipping BP profiles.

Another mechanism implicated in the pathogenesis of hypertension attributed to OSA is the renal sympathetic nerve stimulation. Renal sympathetic nerve has three major effects in the kidney. Increased renal sympathetic nerve activity (RSNA) leads to an increased renin secretion via stimulation of beta-1 adrenoceptors on juxtaglomerular granular cells, an increased renal tubular sodium reabsorption via stimulation of alpha-1B adrenoceptors on renal tubular epithelial cells, and decreased renal blood flow via stimulation of alpha-1A adrenoceptors on the renal artery. Kidneys regulate blood pressure by regulating total body fluid volume via altering

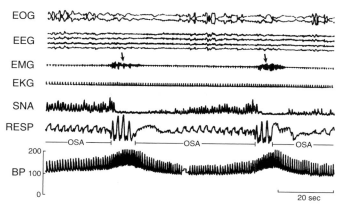

FIG. 16.9 Sympathetic neural mechanisms during rapid eye movement (REM) sleep. Superimposed records of the electrooculogram (EOG), electroencephalogram (EEG), electromyogram (EMG), electrocardiogram (EKG), sympathetic nerve activity, respiration (RESP), and blood pressure (BP) during REM sleep in a patient with obstructive sleep apnea. BP during REM, even during the lowest phases (~160/105 mm Hg), was higher than in the awake state (130/75 mm Hg). BP surges at the end of the apneic periods reached levels as high as 220/130 mm Hg. EOG shows the sharp eye movements characteristic of REM sleep. Increase in muscle tone (EMG) and cessation of rapid eye movements toward the end of the apneic period indicates arousal from REM sleep (arrows). (From Somers VK, Dyken ME, Clary MP, Abboud FM. Sympathetic neural mechanisms in obstructive sleep apnea. J Clin Invest. 1995;96:1897-904.)

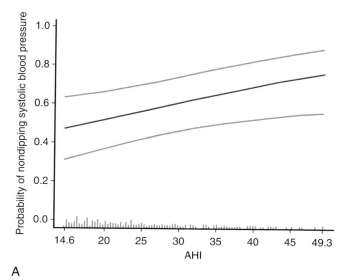

A

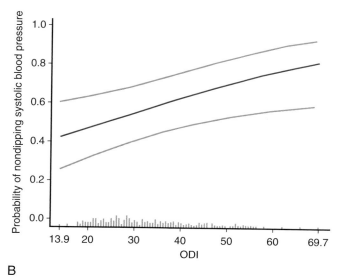

B

FIG. 16.10 Impact of apnea hypopnea index (AHI) and oxygen desaturation index (ODI) on nondipping blood pressure (BP). Solid line represents the model-based probability of nondipping systolic BP for white men at Case Medical Center with an AHI between 14.6 and 49.3 (A) or an ODI between 13.9 and 69.7 (B) who are 63.2-years-old with a body mass index of 33.3 kg/m², 6.4 smoking pack years with hypertension, dyslipidemia, and cardiovascular disease and without diabetes mellitus. Dotted lines represent the associated 95% confidence intervals (CIs). (Reused with permission from Seif F, Patel SR, Walia HK, et al. Obstructive sleep apnea and diurnal nondipping hemodynamic indices in patients at increased cardiovascular risk. J Hypertens. 2014;32:267-275.)

the excretion of sodium in the face of varying sodium intake. Increased RSNA can result in enhanced renal tubular sodium reabsorption, decreased urinary sodium excretion, and renal sodium retention, ultimately leading to development of hypertension.[46] Given the evidence of augmented sympathetic outflow in the setting of OSA, improvement in 6-month office systolic BP noted in subjects with OSA (-17.0 ± 22.4 versus -6.3 ± 26.1 mm Hg, $p = 0.01$) who were treated with renal denervation therapy point towards the role of increased RSNA in the pathogenesis of hypertension in individuals with OSA.[47]

OSA is associated with an impairment in endothelium dependent vasodilation which could lead to hypertension.[39] A similar observation was made by Jelic et al[48] who demonstrated a significantly lower expression of endothelial nitric oxide (NO) synthase and lower flow-mediated dilation of brachial artery in patients with OSA whereas the expression of nitrotyrosine, marker of oxidative stress was significantly greater in OSA group, independent of obesity. Synthesis of NO from L-arginine is an oxygen dependent process and hypoxia induced by OSA could potentially influence NO formation in vascular beds leading to the aforementioned effects.

DRUG-RESISTANT HYPERTENSION

OSA has been identified as the most common secondary cause of drug-resistant hypertension and has been reported in 64% of patient with drug-resistant hypertension.[12] The etiology of drug-resistant hypertension in patients with OSA is likely multifactorial. As mentioned earlier in the discussion of mechanisms of hypertension in OSA, increased sympathetic outflow,[42] increased RSNA,[47] and impairment in NO-mediated vasodilation[39,48] play a significant role in the pathogenesis. Drug-resistant hypertensive patients are in a state of volume overload and have been shown to have a greater overnight rostral fluid shift from legs which strongly relates to the severity of their AHI, compared with controlled hypertensive patients.[49] There has been a significant correlation between plasma aldosterone concentration and the severity of OSA in patients with drug-resistant hypertension compared with normotensive or controlled hypertensive individuals which points towards the role of aldosterone-mediated fluid retention in the pathogenesis of drug-resistant hypertension.[50] This observation is further supported by a significant reduction in AHI (39.8 ± 19.5 versus 22.0 ± 6.8 events/hour; $p < 0.05$), hypoxic index (13.6 ± 10.8 versus 6.7 ± 6.6 events/hour; $p < 0.05$), weight, clinic,

and ambulatory BP in patients with drug-resistant hypertension with the addition of aldosterone receptor antagonist for 8 weeks.[51]

TREATMENT

One of the primary reasons for treating OSA is excessive daytime sleepiness. However, there is no correlation between self-reported daytime sleepiness measured via Epworth Sleepiness Score and severity of sleep apnea.[52] Results of 18-year follow-up of Wisconsin Sleep Cohort showed that sleep disordered breathing is associated with increased mortality, irrespective of symptoms of sleepiness. There is a strikingly high all-cause mortality and cardiovascular mortality of patient with untreated severe sleep disordered breathing (AHI more than 30) which suggests that treatment decision should not be contingent on symptoms of daytime sleepiness.[53]

Historically, treatment options for OSA have included positive airway pressure, oral appliance, upper airway surgery, positional therapy, and conservative measures including weight loss. Emerging therapeutic modalities include upper airway stimulation and renal denervation.

How these various therapeutic options for OSA impact BP control will be reviewed later.

CPAP was first reported as an effective treatment option for OSA in 1981.[54] It works by preventing collapse of pharyngeal airway wall through a positive pharyngeal transmural pressure. Multiple clinical trials assessing the impact of CPAP on BP in patients with OSA have yielded mixed results. These variable findings are likely as a result of variation in characteristics of patient population studied. Some of these trials have included normotensive or well-controlled hypertensive patients which may have underestimated the role of CPAP in improving BP in patients with OSA. In addition, the BP endpoint measured in each of these clinical trials has also differed. As mentioned previously, peak sympathetic activity and elevation in BP occur at the end of apneic events during sleep.[42] This nocturnal cyclical hypertension seems to be a reasonable endpoint to monitor the impact of CPAP on BP but has not been used in most of the clinical trials.

Somers et al[42] demonstrated reduction in average and peak sympathetic nerve activity during sleep with the application of CPAP in four subjects with moderate to severe OSA. Average and peak BP increases were also attenuated in these subjects with the CPAP (Fig. 16.11).

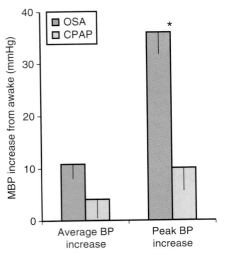
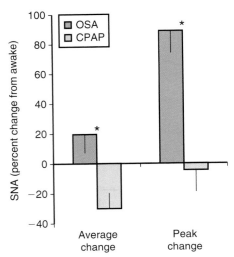

FIG. 16.11 Impact of continuous positive airway pressure (CPAP) on blood pressure (BP) and sympathetic activity. Bar graphs comparing changes in average and peak BP and sympathetic activity in four participants with OSA during sleep (with correction for sleep stage) as compared to measurements when awake. *Blue bars* indicate untreated OSA (control condition) and *gold bars* indicate CPAP (treatment condition). *(Reused with permission from Somers VK, Dyken ME, Clary MP, Abboud FM. Sympathetic neural mechanisms in obstructive sleep apnea. J Clin Invest. 1995;96:1897-904.)*

The randomized trials assessing the effect of CPAP on BP parameters in nonsleepy hypertensive patients with OSA have shown minimal, if any improvement BP with CPAP therapy. Robinson et al[55] found no significant change in mean 24-hour BP with 4 weeks of CPAP treatment whereas the results of Spanish Sleep and Breathing group showed minimal but statistically significant decrement in daytime office BP after 1 year of CPAP use. (systolic blood pressure by 1.89 mm Hg, $p = 0.0654$, diastolic blood pressure by 2.19 mm Hg, $p = 0.0008$)[56] The Spanish Sleep and Breathing group also found no statistically significant reduction in the incidence of hypertension or cardiovascular events with 4 years of CPAP treatment in nonsleepy patient with OSA. The hypertension or cardiovascular event incidence density rate was 9.20 per 100 person-years (95% confidence interval [CI], 7.36 to 11.04) in the CPAP group and 11.02 per 100 person-years (95% CI, 8.96 to 13.08) in the control group.[57]

CPAP therapy in moderate to severe OSA patient has been associated with significant reduction in BP. Becker et al[58] showed mean arterial blood pressure reduction of 10 mm Hg whereas Spanish Sleep and Breathing group showed small but statistically significant reduction in mean 24-hour ambulatory blood pressure by 1.5 mm Hg (95% CI: 0.4 to 2.7 $p = 0.01$) in CPAP group.[59]

CPAP therapy in drug-resistant hypertensive patient with moderate to severe OSA has resulted in a reduction of 24-hour BP after 3 months of CPAP compared with medical treatment alone.[60]

A recently published study comparing the impact of CPAP on BP in resistant and nonresistant hypertensive patients with OSA showed comparable improvement in systolic BP, diastolic BP, and mean arterial pressure following CPAP initiation in both the groups.[14]

Based on these findings, it can be concluded that treatment of moderate to severe OSA by CPAP can lower BP in hypertensive patients. The current body of literature suggests that the magnitude of improvement of BP specifically in nonsleepy hypertensive OSA patient is at best, minimal.

Although intermittent hypoxemia attributed to OSA has been considered an important factor in the pathogenesis of cardiovascular complications, the use of oxygen for treating OSA has continued to be an area of controversy. Heart BEAT trial[61] evaluated the effects of nocturnal supplemental oxygen and CPAP on markers of cardiovascular risk. In patients with cardiovascular disease or multiple cardiovascular risk factors, the treatment of obstructive sleep apnea with CPAP, but not nocturnal supplemental oxygen, resulted in a significant reduction in blood pressure.

Because obesity is implicated in the pathogenesis of both OSA[2] and hypertension,[62] weight loss can be an attractive therapeutic option for treating hypertension. This was shown in a randomized clinical trial comparing the effects of CPAP, weight loss, or both in adults with obesity (BMI ≥ 30), moderate-to-severe obstructive sleep apnea (AHI ≥ 15), and serum level of C-reactive protein (CRP) greater than 1.0 mg per liter. Adherence to a regimen of weight loss and CPAP resulted in incremental reductions in blood pressure as compared with either intervention alone (reduction in systolic blood pressure at 24 weeks in the combined-intervention group of 14.1 mm Hg versus the weight-loss group of 6.8 mm Hg versus the CPAP group of 3.0 mm Hg).[63]

Although CPAP is the most widely used treatment for OSA, it is often cumbersome for patients which makes the compliance suboptimal.[64] This makes oral appliance (OA) therapy an attractive alternative treatment option. How the treatment of OSA with OA impacts cardiovascular outcomes, including hypertension, is an important consideration. There is paucity of well-designed randomized clinical trials assessing the impact of OA on hypertension. The majority of the data comes from nonrandomized, small observational studies.

A prospective observational study from Canada including 11 patients with OSA who received OA had significant reductions in diastolic blood pressure (DBP) and mean arterial pressure (MAP) for the 20-hour periods, and systolic blood pressure (SBP), DBP, and MAP while asleep. It is notable that these results were seen after posttitration Respiratory Disturbance Index (RDI) had significantly decreased from a mean of 24.7 to 6.1.[65] In an another observational study by Andren et al[66] OA led to significant reductions BP from baseline to 3 months ($p < 0.001$). These BP changes were sustained at the 3-year follow-up in both systolic BP of −15.4 ± 18.7 mm Hg and diastolic BP of −10.3 ± 10.0 mm Hg.

A randomized clinical trial of 72 patients with OSA and hypertension assigned to intervention with either an OA with mandibular advancement (active group) or an OA without advancement (control group), showed a modest trend toward effect on reducing BP. A stronger trend toward a treatment effect was seen after excluding patients with normal baseline ambulatory BP. The additional exclusion of patients with baseline AHI 15 or lower showed a significant treatment effect.[67] A recently published study to assess the effect of OA therapy on BP reduction in Japanese patients with mild to moderate OSA showed reduction in systolic and diastolic BP in all patients treated with OA for 8 to 12 weeks. Interestingly, the antihypertensive effect was greater in OSA patients whose BP was higher before receiving OA therapy.[68]

Based on the results of these trials, it can be concluded that OA does lead to significant, albeit modest, BP reduction in hypertensive OSA patients.

Upper airway surgery can be considered in a highly selected group of patients with OSA. To our knowledge, there are no data available regarding the impact of upper airway surgery, other than tracheostomy, on hypertension in patients with OSA.

Given the concern for increased renal sympathetic nerve activity leading to development of hypertension, renal denervation may to be a potential therapeutic option. The SYMPLICITY HTN-3 trial was a large prospective, randomized, blinded, sham-controlled trial of renal denervation for treatment of uncontrolled, treatment-resistant hypertension. In a posthoc analysis, effects of renal denervation versus sham control on office and ambulatory systolic BP in patients with and without OSA was analyzed. Compared with sham control, renal denervation reduced the 6-month office systolic BP in subjects with OSA (−17.0 ± 22.4 versus −6.3 ± 26.1 mm Hg, $p = 0.01$) but not in subjects without OSA (−14.7 ± 24.5 versus −13.4 ± 26.4 mm Hg, $p = 0.64$). In those with OSA, renal denervation was also associated with a reduction in maximum (−4.8 ± 21.8 versus 4.5 ± 24.6 mm Hg, $p = 0.03$) and average peak (−5.6 ± 20.4 versus 3.2 ± 22.4 mm Hg, $p = 0.02$) nighttime systolic BP.[47]

SUMMARY

OSA is present in approximately one-third of individuals with hypertension. The prevalence of OSA is more than 60% in patients with drug-resistant hypertension. Various physiologic changes are brought on by the episodes of apnea which promote the development or progression of hypertension. Each episode of apnea leads to hypoxia and hypercapnia which triggers the sympathetic system, in turn leading to an increase in peripheral vascular tone and heart rate. Renal sympathetic nerve stimulation leads to sodium and water retention. Hypoxia also impairs NO-dependent vasodilation leading to hypertension. Nocturnal rostral shift of fluid from lower extremities to the upper airway leads to airway narrowing with an increased chance of airway closure during sleep. Clinical trials have shown variable improvement in BP with the initiation of CPAP for OSA. This variability could be related to differences in patient population studied with confounding factors. Another possible explanation is that we are not using sensitive-enough tools to detect the impact of change. Most of the trials show some degree of improvement in the cohort with moderate to severe sleep apnea. Oral appliance is an alternative therapeutic option for OSA but methodologically robust clinical trials are lacking to assess the impact of oral appliance on hypertension. Modest reductions in BP are seen with the use of OA in hypertensive individuals with OSA. Upper airway surgery is not a commonly used therapeutic choice for OSA and there are no clinical trials to assess its impact on hypertension other than tracheostomy. Renal denervation appears to be a promising therapeutic option in a highly selected group of uncontrolled treatment-resistant hypertensive patients with OSA.

FUTURE DIRECTIONS

There is significant variability in treatment response among patients with OSA. Currently, there are no tools available to identify patients who will respond to a specific therapeutic option. Identifying a specific biomarker that may reliably predict a favorable therapeutic response would be an exciting and long awaited evolution in the field of sleep medicine.

Microribonucleic acids (miRNAs) are identified as a class of noncoding RNAs that regulate gene expression and may play an important role in achieving a biologic response in selected OSA endotypes.

Sanchez-de-la-Torre et al[69] identified a cluster of three plasma miRNAs functionally associated with the cardiovascular system, that predicted a favorable blood pressure response to CPAP treatment in patients with drug-resistant hypertension and OSA. This study also demonstrated that adherent CPAP treatment is associated with changes in circulating cardiovascular system related miRNAs that may alter the risk for developing cardiovascular disease in these patients.

Further studies are needed in this area to identify additional miRNA profiles and assessing other outcomes of interest with the treatment of OSA. It would also be interesting to examine changes in these biomarker profiles with the concurrent use of CPAP and specific antihypertensive classes of drugs.

In addition to symptomatic response, improvement in BP indices have been the primary focus when treating individuals with OSA and hypertension. Does altering the BP levels in these patients translate into a favorable long-term cardiovascular disease risk? This is yet to be answered.

References

1. Tilkian AG, Guilleminault C, Schroeder JS, Lehrman KL, Simmons FB, Dement WC. Hemodynamics in sleep-induced apnea. Studies during wakefulness and sleep. *Ann Intern Med.* 1976;85:714-719.
2. Jordan AS, McSharry DG, Malhotra A. Adult obstructive sleep apnoea. *Lancet.* 2014;383:736-747.
3. Punjabi NM. The epidemiology of adult obstructive sleep apnea. *Proc Am Thorac Soc.* 2008;5:136-143.
4. Peppard PE, Young T, Barnet JH, Palta M, Hagen EW, Hla KM. Increased prevalence of sleep-disordered breathing in adults. *Am J Epidemiol.* 2013;177:1006-1014.
5. Sjostrom C, Lindberg E, Elmasry A, Hagg A, Svardsudd K, Janson C. Prevalence of sleep apnoea and snoring in hypertensive men: a population based study. *Thorax.* 2002;57:602-607.
6. Peppard PE, Young T, Palta M, Skatrud J. Prospective study of the association between sleep-disordered breathing and hypertension. *N Engl J Med.* 2000;342:1378-1384.
7. Nieto FJ, Young TB, Lind BK, et al. Association of sleep-disordered breathing, sleep apnea, and hypertension in a large community-based study. Sleep Heart Health Study. *JAMA.* 2000;283:1829-1836.
8. Mokhlesi B, Finn LA, Hagen EW, et al. Obstructive sleep apnea during REM sleep and hypertension. results of the Wisconsin Sleep Cohort. *Am J Respir Crit Care Med.* 2014;190:1158-1167.
9. O'Connor GT, Caffo B, Newman AB, et al. Prospective study of sleep-disordered breathing and hypertension: the Sleep Heart Health Study. *Am J Respir Crit Care Med.* 2009;179:1159-1164.
10. Cano-Pumarega I, Duran-Cantolla J, Aizpuru F, et al. Obstructive sleep apnea and systemic hypertension: longitudinal study in the general population: the Vitoria Sleep Cohort. *Am J Respir Crit Care Med.* 2011;184:1299-1304.
11. Logan AG, Perlikowski SM, Mente A, et al. High prevalence of unrecognized sleep apnoea in drug-resistant hypertension. *J Hypertens.* 2001;19:2271-2277.
12. Pedrosa RP, Drager LF, Gonzaga CC, et al. Obstructive sleep apnea: the most common secondary cause of hypertension associated with resistant hypertension. *Hypertension.* 2011;58:811-817.
13. Logan AG, Tkacova R, Perlikowski SM, et al. Refractory hypertension and sleep apnoea: effect of CPAP on blood pressure and baroreflex. *Eur Respir J.* 2003;21:241-247.
14. Walia HK, Griffith SD, Foldvary-Schaefer N, et al. Longitudinal effect of CPAP on BP in resistant and nonresistant hypertension in a large clinic-based cohort. *Chest.* 2016;149:747-755.
15. Kobayashi I, Perry A, Rhymer J, et al. Inspiratory coactivation of the genioglossus enlarges retroglossal space in laryngectomized humans. *J Appl Physiol.* (1985) 1996;80:1595-1604.
16. Remmers JE, deGroot WJ, Sauerland EK, Anch AM. Pathogenesis of upper airway occlusion during sleep. *J Appl Physiol Respir Environ Exerc Physiol.* 1978;44:931-938.
17. Van de Graaff WB. Thoracic traction on the trachea: mechanisms and magnitude. *J Appl Physiol.* (1985) 1991;70:1328-1336.
18. Stanchina ML, Malhotra A, Fogel RB, et al. The influence of lung volume on pharyngeal mechanics, collapsibility, and genioglossus muscle activation during sleep. *Sleep.* 2003;26:851-856.
19. Horner RL, Innes JA, Morrell MJ, Shea SA, Guz A. The effect of sleep on reflex genioglossus muscle activation by stimuli of negative airway pressure in humans. *J Physiol.* 1994;476:141-151.
20. Friberg D, Ansved T, Borg K, Carlsson-Nordlander B, Larsson H, Svanborg E. Histological indications of a progressive snorers disease in an upper airway muscle. *Am J Respir Crit Care Med.* 1998;157:586-593.
21. McSharry D, O'Connor C, McNicholas T, et al. Genioglossus fatigue in obstructive sleep apnea. *Respir Physiol Neurobiol.* 2012;183:59-66.
22. Schwab RJ, Gupta KB, Gefter WB, Metzger LJ, Hoffman EA, Pack AI. Upper airway and soft tissue anatomy in normal subjects and patients with sleep-disordered breathing. Significance of the lateral pharyngeal walls. *Am J Respir Crit Care Med.* 1995;152:1673-1689.
23. Haponik EF, Smith PL, Bohlman ME, Allen RP, Goldman SM, Bleecker ER. Computerized tomography in obstructive sleep apnea. Correlation of airway size with physiology during sleep and wakefulness. *Am Rev Respir Dis.* 1983;127:221-226.
24. Wellman A, Jordan AS, Malhotra A, et al. Ventilatory control and airway anatomy in obstructive sleep apnea. *Am J Respir Crit Care Med.* 2004;170:1225-1232.
25. Hanly PJ, Pierratos A. Improvement of sleep apnea in patients with chronic renal failure who undergo nocturnal hemodialysis. *N Engl J Med.* 2001;344:102-107.
26. Yumino D, Redolfi S, Ruttanaumpawan P, et al. Nocturnal rostral fluid shift: a unifying concept for the pathogenesis of obstructive and central sleep apnea in men with heart failure. *Circulation.* 2010;121:1598-1605.
27. Schwab RJ, Pasirstein M, Pierson R, et al. Identification of upper airway anatomic risk factors for obstructive sleep apnea with volumetric magnetic resonance imaging. *Am J Respir Crit Care Med.* 2003;168:522-530.
28. Malhotra A, Huang Y, Fogel RB, et al. The male predisposition to pharyngeal collapse: importance of airway length. *Am J Respir Crit Care Med.* 2002;166:1388-1395.
29. Whittle AT, Marshall I, Mortimore IL, Wraith PK, Sellar RJ, Douglas NJ. Neck soft tissue and fat distribution: comparison between normal men and women by magnetic resonance imaging. *Thorax.* 1999;54:323-328.
30. Malhotra A, Huang Y, Fogel R, et al. Aging influences on pharyngeal anatomy and physiology: the predisposition to pharyngeal collapse. *Am J Med.* 2006;119:72:e9-e14.
31. Floras JS. Hypertension and Sleep Apnea. *Can J Cardiol.* 2015;31:889-897.
32. Kasai T, Bradley TD. Obstructive sleep apnea and heart failure: pathophysiologic and therapeutic implications. *J Am Coll Cardiol.* 2011;57:119-127.
33. Yumino D, Kasai T, Kimmerly D, Amirthalingam V, Floras JS, Bradley TD. Differing effects of obstructive and central sleep apneas on stroke volume in patients with heart failure. *Am J Respir Crit Care Med.* 2013;187:433-438.
34. Arias MA, Garcia-Rio F, Alonso-Fernandez A, Mediano O, Martinez I, Villamor J. Obstructive sleep apnea syndrome affects left ventricular diastolic function: effects of nasal continuous positive airway pressure in men. *Circulation.* 2005;112:375-383.
35. Chami HA, Devereux RB, Gottdiener JS, et al. Left ventricular morphology and systolic function in sleep-disordered breathing: the Sleep Heart Health Study. *Circulation.* 2008;117:2599-2607.
36. Usui K, Parker JD, Newton GE, Floras JS, Ryan CM, Bradley TD. Left ventricular structural adaptations to obstructive sleep apnea in dilated cardiomyopathy. *Am J Respir Crit Care Med.* 2006;173:1170-1175.
37. Abboud F, Kumar R. Obstructive sleep apnea and insight into mechanisms of sympathetic overactivity. *J Clin Invest.* 2014;124:1454-1457.
38. Savransky V, Nanayakkara A, Li J, et al. Chronic intermittent hypoxia induces atherosclerosis. *Am J Respir Crit Care Med.* 2007;175:1290-1297.
39. Carlson JT, Rangemark C, Hedner JA. Attenuated endothelium-dependent vascular relaxation in patients with sleep apnoea. *J Hypertens.* 1996;14:577-584.
40. Alonso-Fernandez A, Garcia-Rio F, Arias MA, et al. Effects of CPAP on oxidative stress and nitrate efficiency in sleep apnoea: a randomised trial. *Thorax.* 2009;64:581-586.
41. Drager LF, Bortolotto LA, Figueiredo AC, Krieger EM, Lorenzi GF. Effects of continuous positive airway pressure on early signs of atherosclerosis in obstructive sleep apnea. *Am J Respir Crit Care Med.* 2007;176:706-712.
42. Somers VK, Dyken ME, Clary MP, Abboud FM. Sympathetic neural mechanisms in obstructive sleep apnea. *J Clin Invest.* 1995;96:1897-1904.
43. Spaak J, Egri ZJ, Kubo T, et al. Muscle sympathetic nerve activity during wakefulness in heart failure patients with and without sleep apnea. *Hypertension.* 2005;46:1327-1332.
44. Sin DD, Fitzgerald F, Parker JD, et al. Relationship of systolic BP to obstructive sleep apnea in patients with heart failure. *Chest.* 2003;123:1536-1543.
45. Seif F, Patel SR, Walia HK, et al. Obstructive sleep apnea and diurnal nondipping hemodynamic indices in patients at increased cardiovascular risk. *J Hypertens.* 2014;32:267-275.
46. DiBona GF. Physiology in perspective: The wisdom of the body. Neural control of the kidney. *Am J Physiol Regul Integr Comp Physiol.* 2005;289:R633-R641.
47. Kario K, Bhatt DL, Kandzari DE, et al. Impact of renal denervation on patients with obstructive sleep apnea and resistant hypertension—insights from the SYMPLICITY HTN-3 Trial. *Circ J.* 2016;80:1404-1412.
48. Jelic S, Lederer DJ, Adams T, et al. Vascular inflammation in obesity and sleep apnea. *Circulation.* 2010;121:1014-1021.
49. Friedman O, Bradley TD, Chan CT, Parkes R, Logan AG. Relationship between overnight rostral fluid shift and obstructive sleep apnea in drug-resistant hypertension. *Hypertension.* 2010;56:1077-1082.
50. Pratt-Ubunama MN, Nishizaka MK, Boedefeld RL, Cofield SS, Harding SM, Calhoun DA. Plasma aldosterone is related to severity of obstructive sleep apnea in subjects with resistant hypertension. *Chest.* 2007;131:453-459.
51. Gaddam K, Pimenta E, Thomas SJ, et al. Spironolactone reduces severity of obstructive sleep apnoea in patients with resistant hypertension: a preliminary report. *J Hum Hypertens.* 2010;24:532-537.

52. Luyster FS, Buysse DJ, Strollo PJ, Jr. Comorbid insomnia and obstructive sleep apnea: challenges for clinical practice and research. *J Clin Sleep Med.* 2010;6:196-204.

53. Young T, Finn L, Peppard PE, et al. Sleep disordered breathing and mortality: eighteen-year follow-up of the Wisconsin sleep cohort. *Sleep.* 2008;31:1071-1078.

54. Sullivan CE, Issa FG, Berthon-Jones M, Eves L. Reversal of obstructive sleep apnoea by continuous positive airway pressure applied through the nares. *Lancet.* 1981;1:862-865.

55. Robinson GV, Smith DM, Langford BA, Davies RJ, Stradling JR. Continuous positive airway pressure does not reduce blood pressure in nonsleepy hypertensive OSA patients. *Eur Respir J.* 2006;27:1229-1235.

56. Barbe F, Duran-Cantolla J, Capote F, et al. Long-term effect of continuous positive airway pressure in hypertensive patients with sleep apnea. *Am J Respir Crit Care Med.* 2010;181:718-726.

57. Barbe F, Duran-Cantolla J, Sanchez-de-la-Torre M, et al. Effect of continuous positive airway pressure on the incidence of hypertension and cardiovascular events in non-sleepy patients with obstructive sleep apnea: a randomized controlled trial. *JAMA.* 2012;307:2161-2168.

58. Becker HF, Jerrentrup A, Ploch T, et al. Effect of nasal continuous positive airway pressure treatment on blood pressure in patients with obstructive sleep apnea. *Circulation.* 2003;107:68-73.

59. Duran-Cantolla J, Aizpuru F, Montserrat JM, et al. Continuous positive airway pressure as treatment for systemic hypertension in people with obstructive sleep apnoea: randomised controlled trial. *BMJ.* 2010;341:c5991.

60. Lozano L, Tovar JL, Sampol G, et al. Continuous positive airway pressure treatment in sleep apnea patients with resistant hypertension: a randomized, controlled trial. *J Hypertens.* 2010;28:2161-2168.

61. Gottlieb DJ, Punjabi NM, Mehra R, et al. CPAP versus oxygen in obstructive sleep apnea. *N Engl J Med.* 2014;370:2276-2285.

62. Fox CS, Massaro JM, Hoffmann U, et al. Abdominal visceral and subcutaneous adipose tissue compartments: association with metabolic risk factors in the Framingham Heart Study. *Circulation.* 2007;116:39-48.

63. Chirinos JA, Gurubhagavatula I, Teff K, et al. CPAP, weight loss, or both for obstructive sleep apnea. *N Engl J Med.* 2014;370:2265-2275.

64. Meurice JC, Dore P, Paquereau J, et al. Predictive factors of long-term compliance with nasal continuous positive airway pressure treatment in sleep apnea syndrome. *Chest.* 1994;105:429-433.

65. Otsuka R, Ribeiro de Almeida F, Lowe AA, Linden W, Ryan F. The effect of oral appliance therapy on blood pressure in patients with obstructive sleep apnea. *Sleep Breath.* 2006;10:29-36.

66. Andren A, Sjoquist M, Tegelberg A. Effects on blood pressure after treatment of obstructive sleep apnoea with a mandibular advancement appliance—a three-year follow-up. *J Oral Rehabil.* 2009;36:719-725.

67. Andren A, Hedberg P, Walker-Engstrom ML, Wahlen P, Tegelberg A. Effects of treatment with oral appliance on 24-h blood pressure in patients with obstructive sleep apnea and hypertension: a randomized clinical trial. *Sleep Breath.* 2013;17:705-712.

68. Sekizuka H, Osada N, Akashi YJ. Effect of oral appliance therapy on blood pressure in Japanese patients with obstructive sleep apnea. *Clin Exp Hypertens.* 2016;38:404-408.

69. Sanchez-de-la-Torre M, Khalyfa A, Sanchez-de-la-Torre A, et al. Precision medicine in patients with resistant hypertension and obstructive sleep apnea: blood pressure response to continuous positive airway pressure treatment. *J Am Coll Cardiol.* 2015;66:1023-1032.

17 Hypertension in Children: Diagnosis and Treatment

Coral D. Hanevold and Joseph T. Flynn

Over the past decade, there has been increasing interest in childhood hypertension and greater recognition that adult cardiovascular disease has its origins in childhood. Fueling this interest has been the childhood obesity epidemic, which has led to an increase in the prevalence of hypertension and its consequences in the young. This chapter will discuss some of the recent trends in pediatric hypertension, with a focus on the importance of correctly identifying and treating hypertensive children and adolescents. Important differences in clinical practice guidelines for hypertension in adults and children will be highlighted when appropriate. Selected special topics in childhood hypertension, including hypertension in children with chronic kidney disease and management of acute severe hypertension will be briefly reviewed.

EPIDEMIOLOGY OF HYPERTENSION IN CHILDREN AND ADOLESCENTS

Recent screening studies and population-based surveys have provided updated information of the prevalence of elevated blood pressure (BP) in the young. When Fourth Report[1] BP cut-points are used and data from three screening visits included, there is a consistent prevalence of approximately 3% to 4% for hypertension and 7% to 15% for prehypertension (see following section for definitions).[2-4]

Data from national surveys such as the National Health and Examination Survey in the United States have demonstrated an increase in the prevalence of both prehypertension and hypertension over recent years in the pediatric age group.[5] Although there is some disagreement in the literature, most experts attribute this increase to the significantly higher prevalence of childhood obesity that has developed over the past several decades.[5,6] Indeed a recent examination of BP and lipid levels in United States children clearly showed that the prevalence of elevated BP was greater in overweight and obese children than in the population as a whole.[7] This has also been shown in school-based screening studies conducted in both the United States and abroad.[8-9] Potential mechanisms for this phenomenon are beyond the scope of this chapter but have recently been reviewed.[6] As the prevalence of childhood obesity appears to have leveled off in the most recent data from the Centers for Disease Control and Prevention, there is hope that the prevalence of childhood hypertension may stabilize, at least in the United States.

DEFINITION OF HYPERTENSION IN CHILDHOOD

Defining hypertension in children is challenging because there are no outcome data to support a particular level, such as the widely used 140/90 for adults (Table 17.1).[10] Additionally, BP increases with age and linear growth and thus the absolute value that defines an elevated BP will differ greatly as an infant grows into a young adult. As a result, the definition is based on the statistical analysis of normative data obtained from readings on more than 60,000 U.S. children and adolescents.[1] From this analysis tables have been generated that display the 50th, 90th, 95th, and 99th percentiles based on age, gender, and height percentile (see Tables 17.2 and 17.3). Prehypertension and hypertension are defined as noted in Table 17.1. The diagnosis of hypertension is made when the average BP is greater than or equal to the 95th percentile on 3 or more occasions.[1] Use of height percentiles may be problematic for some providers; therefore simplified tables that define the BP percentiles based on absolute height rather than height percentile have been created and are available through the International Pediatric Hypertension Association (http://d706084.u55.profitability.net/wp-core/wp-content/uploads/BPLimitsChart0112.pdf). Categorization of elevated BPs into stages 1 and 2 is explained in Table 17.1, which compares the pediatric definitions to the corresponding definitions for stages of hypertension in adults.

The National High Blood Pressure Education Program Working Group and the European Society of Hypertension both recommend documentation of elevated pressures at three visits before making the diagnosis of hypertension in children and adolescents.[1,11] The value of obtaining readings on three occasions before classifying a child as hypertensive was first noted in the 1970s and has been confirmed in more recent studies.[12,13] For example, in a school-based screening using the 2004 National High Blood Pressure Education Working Group guidelines, McNiece et al found that the prevalence of elevated BPs fell from 9.4% to 3.2% by the third visit.[12] Also, the importance of obtaining multiple readings at each encounter has been verified by previous investigators.[14,15] BP may drop with subsequent measurement between the vital sign station and the examination room.[14] The pressure improves as a result of reduction in anxiety with repeated readings and regression to the mean.[1,14,15] Certainly in symptomatic children or those with marked BP elevation the above mentioned delay in initiating an evaluation and treatment pending verification at multiple visits would not be appropriate. This is recognized in the Fourth Report,[1] which allows for more immediate diagnosis and treatment in those with symptomatic or severely elevated BP.

MEASURING THE BLOOD PRESSURE

Casual Blood Pressure Measurement

Accurate measurement of the BP is critical and can be challenging. Important points to consider include: type of device, appropriate cuffing, and environmental/positional factors. Mercury manometers have been removed from widespread clinical practice but accurate readings can be obtained with properly maintained aneroid devices. Casual manual readings may be compromised by improper technique, tendency to round off

TABLE 17.1 Classification of Childhood Blood Pressure Compared With Adult Classification

BLOOD PRESSURE CLASSIFICATION	CHILDREN AND ADOLESCENTS UNDER 18 YEARS OF AGE[a]	ADULTS 18 YEARS OF AGE OR OLDER[b]
Normal	SBP and DBP <90th percentile	SBP <120 mm Hg and DBP <80 mm Hg
Prehypertension	SBP or DBP 90-95th percentile; or if BP is >120/80 even if <90th percentile	SBP 120-139 mm Hg or DBP 80-89 mm Hg
Stage 1 hypertension	SBP or DBP ≥95th to 99th percentile plus 5 mm Hg	SBP 140-159 mm Hg or DBP 90-99 mm Hg
Stage 2 hypertension	SBP or DBP >99th percentile plus 5 mm Hg	SBP ≥160 mm Hg or DBP ≥100 mm Hg

[a]Adapted from National High Blood Pressure Education Program Working Group on High Blood Pressure in Children and Adolescents. The fourth report on the diagnosis, evaluation, and treatment of high blood pressure in children and adolescents. National Heart, Lung, and Blood Institute, Bethesda, MD 2005;*National Institute of Health publication* 05:5267.
[b]Adapted from Chobanian AV, Bakris GL, Black HR, et al. The seventh report of the Joint National Committee on Prevention, Detection, Evaluation, and Treatment of High Blood Pressure: the JNC 7 report. *JAMA.* 2003;289:2560-2572.
BP, Blood pressure; *DBP,* diastolic blood pressure; *SBP,* systolic blood pressure; *SNP,* systolic blood pressure.

readings, failure to allow adequate rest before measurement, and background noise. As in adults, K5 is used to determine the diastolic reading in children.[1] The reader is directed to an excellent review of the technique of ausculatory measurement for more details.[16] Oscillometric devices offer convenience, objectivity, and are particularly helpful in infants. However, the monitors rapidly inflate to high levels, which may lead to discomfort and be counterproductive by upsetting young children. The first reading is almost always higher than subsequent readings. Measurement may be difficult or impossible in moving or uncooperative children or in those with arrhythmias. Lastly, oscillometric BP monitors detect the oscillations of the artery during inflation of the cuff with maximum oscillations occurring at the mean arterial pressure. Systolic and diastolic values are then back-calculated based on proprietary formulas that vary between machines.[17] Validation of these devices in pediatric populations is not universal and should be confirmed before use, particularly in younger children.[18]

The American Society of Hypertension and the International Society of Hypertension recently indicated that automated readings are preferred over manual readings because of concerns over the inaccuracy of ausculated readings.[19] However, the measurements used to generate the pediatric BP tables were obtained by auscultation.[1] Several studies in children have demonstrated that oscillometric measurements tend to be higher and do not correlate well with ausculated readings.[15,20-22] Thus for consistency, continued use of carefully obtained ausculated readings in the pediatric population for confirmation of hypertension is recommended.

Cuff size is very important and cannot be judged based on the manufacturer's labeling. The width of the bladder should cover at least 40% of the circumference of the arm measured midway between the olecranon and the acromion. The length of the bladder should cover 80% to 100% of the circumference of the upper arm, resulting in a bladder width to length ratio of 1:2.[1] Arm size designations on the cuff can be misleading and cuff size should be selected based on the arm circumference. Finding an appropriate cuff can be difficult in infants and in obese adolescents. Use of wrist and forearm cuffs is not recommended because pediatric thresholds are based on readings obtained in the upper arm. Inappropriately sized cuffs can lead to erroneous readings, with the greatest issue being obtaining falsely high readings if the cuff is too small.

Lastly, BPs should be taken in a quiet environment after allowing the patient to rest for at least 5 minutes. The patient should be seated with the back supported, feet on the floor, and the arm positioned such that the brachial artery is at heart level. Two to three readings should be taken about one minute apart. Readings should be obtained in both arms. Pressures in the right arm may be higher than the left in those with coarctation of the aorta. If the readings are similar the right arm should be used subsequently for consistency. Leg pressures are obtained at least once in children to exclude coarctation of

the aorta or midaortic syndrome. The measurements should be obtained after the patient has been lying down for 5 minutes and are compared with supine arm readings. Measurements in one leg and the right arm are sufficient. Leg pressures typically exceed arm pressures by 10 mm Hg or more and if lower than arm pressures, abnormalities of the aorta should be considered. Standing BPs are not typically considered part of the evaluation unless orthostatic symptoms are reported.

Ambulatory Blood Pressure Monitoring

Ambulatory BP monitoring (ABPM) is increasingly recognized as a valid and valuable procedure in the evaluation of elevated casual office BP readings in children. In the United Kingdom and Canada ABPM is recommended in all adults to confirm the diagnosis of hypertension.[23] Such a universal recommendation has not been made for the pediatric population to date. However, several studies have demonstrated the benefits and cost savings of this procedure as a means of detecting white coat hypertension, thus obviating the need for an extensive diagnostic evaluation.[24,25] White coat hypertension is reported in up to 46% of children and adolescents investigated for hypertension.[24,26,27] Although home BP measurement may be helpful in excluding white coat hypertension, ABPM offers a more complete assessment of the BP pattern over the course of the day because it obtains readings during day-to-day activities and while asleep.[18,28,29] Additional issues with home BP measurement include the scarcity of data on normal values in children and the lack of consistent validation of devices in the pediatric population.[18] As with casual readings, thresholds defining hypertension on ABPM are not limited to one threshold for awake and asleep periods as in adults. Guidelines on performance and interpretation of ABPM in the pediatric population were recently updated and include height and gender-specific 95th percentiles along with recommendations for interpretation.[30] Recordings are classified based on mean systolic/diastolic readings and the BP load (percent of readings above the threshold). An ABPM study is classified as demonstrating sustained hypertension if the mean systolic and/or diastolic pressures are above threshold. If BP loads are above 50% the ABPM is further classified as showing severe ambulatory hypertension. An ABPM study is classified as indicating prehypertension if the mean systolic and/or diastolic pressures are below threshold but the pressure loads are above 25%.[30] As mentioned above in regard to home monitors, there are many ABPM devices on the market but few are actually validated in the pediatric population; it is important to investigate this issue when planning provision of this service. Although ABPM has been used in very young children, we generally reserve this procedure for children ages 7 and up. As shown in Fig. 17.1, at Seattle Children's Hospital we use ABPM as the first step in our evaluation of elevated BPs for children 7 years or older. Only those with

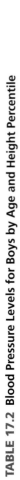

TABLE 17.2 Blood Pressure Levels for Boys by Age and Height Percentile

Age (Years)	BP Percentile	Systolic BP (mm Hg) — Percentile of Height →							Diastolic BP (mm Hg) ← Percentile of Height						
		5	10	25	50	75	90	95	5	10	25	50	75	90	95
1	50	80	81	83	85	87	88	89	34	35	36	37	38	39	39
	90	94	95	97	99	100	102	103	49	50	51	52	53	53	54
	95	98	99	101	103	104	106	106	54	54	55	56	57	58	58
	99	105	106	108	110	112	113	114	61	62	63	64	65	66	66
2	50	84	85	87	88	90	92	92	39	40	41	42	43	44	44
	90	97	99	100	102	104	105	106	54	55	56	57	58	58	59
	95	101	102	104	106	108	109	110	59	59	60	61	62	63	63
	99	109	110	111	113	115	117	117	66	67	68	69	70	71	71
3	50	86	87	89	91	93	94	95	44	44	45	46	47	48	48
	90	100	101	103	105	107	108	109	59	59	60	61	62	63	63
	95	104	105	107	109	110	112	113	63	63	64	65	66	67	67
	99	111	112	114	116	118	119	120	71	71	72	73	74	75	75
4	50	88	89	91	93	95	96	97	47	48	49	50	51	51	52
	90	102	103	105	107	109	110	111	62	63	64	65	66	66	67
	95	106	107	109	111	112	114	115	66	67	68	69	70	71	71
	99	113	114	116	118	120	121	122	74	75	76	77	78	78	79
5	50	90	91	93	95	96	98	98	50	51	52	53	54	55	55
	90	104	105	106	108	110	111	112	65	66	67	68	69	69	70
	95	108	109	110	112	114	115	116	69	70	71	72	73	74	74
	99	115	116	118	120	121	123	123	77	78	79	80	81	81	82
6	50	91	92	94	96	98	99	100	53	53	54	55	56	57	57
	90	105	106	108	110	111	113	113	68	68	69	70	71	72	72
	95	109	110	112	114	115	117	117	72	72	73	74	75	76	76
	99	116	117	119	121	123	124	125	80	80	81	82	83	84	84
7	50	92	94	95	97	99	100	101	55	55	56	57	58	59	59
	90	106	107	109	111	113	114	115	70	70	71	72	73	74	74
	95	110	111	113	115	117	118	119	74	74	75	76	77	78	78
	99	117	118	120	122	124	125	126	82	82	83	84	85	86	86
8	50	94	95	97	99	100	102	102	56	57	58	59	60	60	61
	90	107	109	110	112	114	115	116	71	72	72	73	74	75	76
	95	111	112	114	116	118	119	120	75	76	77	78	79	79	80
	99	119	120	122	123	125	127	127	83	84	85	86	87	87	88
9	50	95	96	98	100	102	103	104	57	58	59	60	61	61	62
	90	109	110	112	114	115	117	118	72	73	74	75	76	76	77

Age	BP %ile	SBP							DBP						
(9)	95	113	114	116	118	119	121	121	76	77	78	79	80	81	81
	99	120	121	123	125	127	128	129	84	85	86	87	88	88	89
10	50	97	98	100	102	103	105	106	58	59	60	61	61	62	63
	90	111	112	114	115	117	119	119	73	73	74	75	76	77	78
	95	115	116	117	119	121	122	123	77	78	79	80	81	81	82
	99	122	123	125	127	128	130	130	85	86	86	88	88	89	90
11	50	99	100	102	104	105	107	107	59	59	60	61	62	63	63
	90	113	114	115	117	119	120	121	74	74	75	76	77	78	78
	95	117	118	119	121	123	124	125	78	78	79	80	81	82	82
	99	124	125	127	129	130	132	132	86	86	87	88	89	90	90
12	50	101	102	104	106	108	109	110	59	60	61	62	63	63	64
	90	115	116	118	120	121	123	123	74	75	75	76	77	78	79
	95	119	120	122	123	125	127	127	78	79	80	81	82	82	83
	99	126	127	129	131	133	134	135	86	87	88	89	90	90	91
13	50	104	105	106	108	110	111	112	60	60	61	62	63	64	64
	90	117	118	120	122	124	125	126	75	75	76	77	78	79	79
	95	121	122	124	126	128	129	130	79	79	80	81	82	83	83
	99	128	130	131	133	135	136	137	87	87	88	89	90	91	91
14	50	106	107	109	111	113	114	115	60	61	62	63	64	65	65
	90	120	121	123	125	126	128	128	75	76	77	78	79	79	80
	95	124	125	127	128	130	132	132	80	80	81	82	83	84	84
	99	131	132	134	136	138	139	140	87	88	89	90	91	92	92
15	50	109	110	112	113	115	117	117	61	62	63	64	65	66	66
	90	122	124	125	127	129	130	131	76	77	78	79	80	80	81
	95	126	127	129	131	133	134	135	81	81	82	83	84	85	85
	99	134	135	136	138	140	142	142	88	89	90	91	92	93	93
16	50	111	112	114	116	118	119	120	63	63	64	65	66	67	67
	90	125	126	128	130	131	133	134	78	78	79	80	81	82	82
	95	129	130	132	134	135	137	137	82	83	83	84	85	86	87
	99	136	137	139	141	143	144	145	90	90	91	92	93	94	94
17	50	114	115	116	118	120	121	122	65	66	66	67	68	69	70
	90	127	128	130	132	134	135	136	80	80	81	82	83	84	84
	95	131	132	134	136	138	139	140	84	85	86	87	87	88	89
	99	139	140	141	143	145	146	147	92	93	93	94	95	96	97

To use the table, first plot the child's height on a standard growth curve (www.cdc.gov/growthcharts). The child's measured systolic blood pressure (SBP) and diastolic blood pressure (DBP) are compared with the numbers provided in the table according to the child's age and height percentile.
(Adapted from National High Blood Pressure Education Program Working Group on High Blood Pressure in Children and Adolescents. The fourth report on the diagnosis, evaluation, and treatment of high blood pressure in children and adolescents. National Heart, Lung, and Blood Institute, Bethesda, MD 2005;National Institute of Health publication 05:5267).

TABLE 17.3 Blood Pressure Levels for Girls by Age and Height Percentile

Age (Years)	BP Percentile	Systolic Blood Pressure (mm Hg) — Percentile of Height							Diastolic Blood Pressure (mm Hg) — Percentile of Height						
		5	10	25	50	75	90	95	5	10	25	50	75	90	95
1	50	83	84	85	86	88	89	90	38	39	39	40	41	41	42
	90	97	97	98	100	101	102	103	52	53	53	54	55	55	56
	95	100	101	102	104	105	106	107	56	57	57	58	59	59	60
	99	108	108	109	111	112	113	114	64	64	65	65	66	67	67
2	50	85	85	87	88	89	91	91	43	44	44	45	46	46	47
	90	98	99	100	101	103	104	105	57	58	58	59	60	61	61
	95	102	103	104	105	107	108	109	61	62	62	63	64	65	65
	99	109	110	111	112	114	115	116	69	69	70	70	71	72	72
3	50	86	87	88	89	91	92	93	47	48	48	49	50	50	51
	90	100	100	102	103	104	106	106	61	62	62	63	64	64	65
	95	104	104	105	107	108	109	110	65	66	66	67	68	68	69
	99	111	111	113	114	115	116	117	73	73	74	74	75	76	76
4	50	88	88	90	91	92	94	94	50	50	51	52	52	53	54
	90	101	102	103	104	106	107	108	64	64	65	66	67	67	68
	95	105	106	107	108	110	111	112	68	68	69	70	71	71	72
	99	112	113	114	115	117	118	119	76	76	76	77	78	79	79
5	50	89	90	91	93	94	95	96	52	53	53	54	55	55	56
	90	103	103	105	106	107	109	109	66	67	67	68	69	69	70
	95	107	107	108	110	111	112	113	70	71	71	72	73	73	74
	99	114	114	116	117	118	120	120	78	78	79	79	80	81	81
6	50	91	92	93	94	96	97	98	54	54	55	56	56	57	58
	90	104	105	106	108	109	110	111	68	68	69	70	70	71	72
	95	108	109	110	111	113	114	115	72	72	73	74	74	75	76
	99	115	116	117	119	120	121	122	80	80	80	81	82	83	83
7	50	93	93	95	96	97	99	99	55	56	56	57	58	58	59
	90	106	107	108	109	111	112	113	69	70	70	71	72	72	73
	95	110	111	112	113	115	116	116	73	74	74	75	76	76	77
	99	117	118	119	120	122	123	124	81	81	82	82	83	84	84
8	50	95	95	96	98	99	100	101	57	57	57	58	59	60	60
	90	108	109	110	111	113	114	114	71	71	71	72	73	74	74
	95	112	112	114	115	116	118	118	75	75	75	76	77	78	78
	99	119	120	121	122	123	125	125	82	82	83	83	84	85	86
9	50	96	97	98	100	101	102	103	58	58	58	59	60	61	61
	90	110	110	112	113	114	116	116	72	72	72	73	74	75	75

Age (year)	BP Percentile	BP	Height %ile 1	2	3	4	5	6	7
(9, cont.)	95th	SBP	114	114	115	117	118	119	120
		DBP	76	76	76	76	77	78	79
	99th	SBP	121	121	123	124	125	127	127
		DBP	83	84	84	85	85	86	87
10	50th	SBP	98	99	100	102	103	104	105
		DBP	59	59	59	60	61	61	62
	90th	SBP	112	112	114	115	116	118	118
		DBP	73	73	73	74	75	76	76
	95th	SBP	116	116	117	119	120	121	122
		DBP	77	77	77	78	79	80	80
	99th	SBP	123	123	125	126	127	129	129
		DBP	84	85	86	86	87	88	88
11	50th	SBP	100	101	102	103	105	106	107
		DBP	60	60	60	61	62	63	63
	90th	SBP	114	114	116	117	118	119	120
		DBP	74	74	74	75	76	77	77
	95th	SBP	118	118	119	121	122	123	124
		DBP	78	78	78	79	80	81	81
	99th	SBP	125	125	126	128	129	130	131
		DBP	85	85	86	87	87	88	89
12	50th	SBP	102	103	104	105	107	108	109
		DBP	61	61	61	62	63	64	64
	90th	SBP	116	116	117	119	120	121	122
		DBP	75	75	75	76	77	78	78
	95th	SBP	119	120	121	123	124	125	126
		DBP	79	79	79	80	81	82	82
	99th	SBP	127	127	128	130	131	132	133
		DBP	86	86	86	87	88	89	90
13	50th	SBP	104	104	106	107	109	110	110
		DBP	62	62	62	63	64	65	65
	90th	SBP	117	117	119	121	122	123	124
		DBP	76	76	76	77	78	79	79
	95th	SBP	121	121	123	124	126	127	128
		DBP	80	80	80	81	82	83	83
	99th	SBP	128	128	130	132	133	134	135
		DBP	87	87	87	88	89	90	91
14	50th	SBP	106	106	107	109	110	111	112
		DBP	63	63	63	64	65	66	66
	90th	SBP	119	120	121	122	124	125	125
		DBP	77	77	77	78	79	80	80
	95th	SBP	123	123	125	126	127	129	129
		DBP	81	81	81	82	83	84	84
	99th	SBP	130	131	132	133	135	136	136
		DBP	88	88	88	89	90	91	92
15	50th	SBP	107	108	109	110	111	113	113
		DBP	64	64	64	65	66	67	67
	90th	SBP	120	121	122	123	125	126	127
		DBP	78	78	78	79	80	81	81
	95th	SBP	124	125	126	127	129	130	131
		DBP	82	82	82	83	84	85	85
	99th	SBP	131	132	133	134	136	137	138
		DBP	89	89	89	90	91	92	93
16	50th	SBP	108	108	110	111	112	114	114
		DBP	64	64	65	66	66	67	68
	90th	SBP	121	122	123	124	126	127	128
		DBP	78	78	79	80	81	81	82
	95th	SBP	125	126	127	128	130	131	132
		DBP	82	82	83	84	85	85	86
	99th	SBP	132	133	134	135	137	138	139
		DBP	90	90	90	91	92	93	93
17	50th	SBP	108	109	110	111	113	114	115
		DBP	64	65	65	66	67	67	68
	90th	SBP	122	122	123	125	126	127	128
		DBP	78	79	79	80	81	81	82
	95th	SBP	125	126	127	129	130	131	132
		DBP	82	83	83	84	85	85	86
	99th	SBP	133	133	134	136	137	138	139
		DBP	90	91	91	92	93	93	93

To use the table, first plot the child's height on a standard growth curve (www.cdc.gov/growthcharts). The child's measured systolic blood pressure (SBP) and diastolic blood pressure (DBP) are compared with the numbers provided in the table according to the child's age and height percentile.

(From National High Blood Pressure Education Program Working Group on High Blood Pressure in Children and Adolescents. The fourth report on the diagnosis, evaluation, and treatment of high blood pressure in children and adolescents. National Heart, Lung, and Blood Institute, Bethesda, MD 2005; National Institute of Health publication 05-5267.)

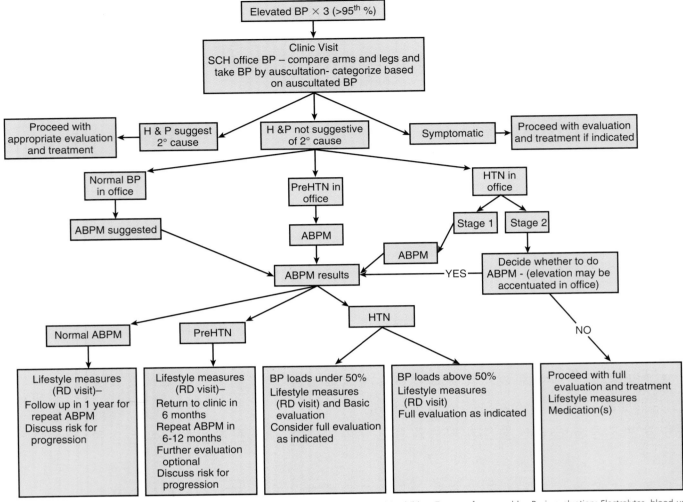

FIG. 17.1 Suggested algorithm for outpatient clinic evaluation of elevated blood pressure (BP) in children 7 years of age or older. Basic evaluation: Electrolytes, blood urea nitrogen, creatinine, calcium, lipid panel, urinalysis, echocardiogram, renal ultrasound. If overweight or obese add fasting glucose. Consider sleep study if obese and concerns for obstructive sleep apnea. Full evaluation: If strong suspicion of secondary hypertension or BP very high, complete basic evaluation and consider other tests listed in Table 17.6 as indicated.

sustained hypertension on ABPM or confirmed stage 2 hypertension in the office undergo a full evaluation, as discussed later. For those with white coat hypertension or prehypertension, lifestyle modifications and repeat ABPM in one year are recommended.

CAUSES OF HYPERTENSION IN THE YOUNG

Traditionally, most hypertension in the pediatric age group has been felt to be secondary to an underlying disorder. This is certainly the case for infants, toddlers, and younger school-aged children. In hypertensive children in these age groups, renal disease, renovascular disease, and cardiac disease will often be found after an appropriate diagnostic evaluation (see Table 17.4). This was recently demonstrated in an analysis of subjects enrolled in two antihypertensive drug studies: 80% of enrolled children younger than 6 years of age had secondary causes of hypertension.[31] Primary hypertension in young children is therefore usually considered a diagnosis of exclusion, and such children do warrant a more extensive diagnostic evaluation (see below).

In adolescents, however, hypertension is most likely to be primary in origin. This was clearly demonstrated 2 decades ago in a study of over 1000 hypertensive children evaluated at a Polish children's hospital.[32] In this series, the vast majority of adolescents with persistent BP elevation had no identifiable underlying cause found. Even many children aged

TABLE 17.4 Differential Diagnosis of Childhood Hypertension by Age

AGE GROUP	CAUSES[a]
Newborn infants	Umbilical catheter-related thromboembolism Bronchopulmonary dysplasia Congenital renal disease/malformations Renal venous thrombosis Aortic coarctation Medications
Infants and toddlers	Renal parenchymal disease Congenital renal disease/malformations Renal artery stenosis Aortic coarctation Endocrine causes
Preadolescent children	Renal parenchymal disease Renal artery stenosis Primary hypertension Aortic coarctation Endocrine causes
Adolescents	Primary hypertension Renal parenchymal disease Renal artery stenosis Substance-induced Aortic coarctation Endocrine causes

[a]Listed roughly in descending order of frequency

between 6 and 12 with mild hypertension are likely to have primary hypertension.[31] Other clinical and demographic features that support the diagnosis of primary hypertension in children and adolescents include obesity, lack of symptoms of hypertension, unremarkable past medical history, and a family history of hypertension.[33,34] Hypertensive youth with these characteristics may not need as extensive an evaluation as younger children.

On the other hand, hypertension in neonates should always be considered secondary in origin (Table 17.4). The most common causes of neonatal hypertension include renovascular disease (most commonly umbilical artery catheterization–related aortic or renal thromboembolism), renal parenchymal disease, bronchopulmonary dysplasia/chronic lung disease, and coarctation of the thoracic aorta. Other potential causes to consider include endocrinopathies, genetic disorders, and the complications of other therapies such as extracorporeal membrane oxygenation.[35,36] Thus, when hypertension is detected in a neonate (or older infant <1 year old), it is appropriate to pursue an extensive diagnostic work up. For a more comprehensive discussion of neonatal/infant hypertension, the reader is encouraged to consult other references.[37]

EVALUATION OF HYPERTENSION IN CHILDREN AND ADOLESCENTS

The extent of the evaluation of hypertension should be guided by multiple factors, including severity of elevation, age, as well as findings on history and physical. An old but valid pearl is that the younger the child and the higher the BP, the more likely it is that a secondary cause will be identified. Additionally, one can add that in young children it is incumbent upon the provider to exclude a secondary cause or at least methodically consider possible etiologies. In contrast, in an older child or adolescent with mild hypertension, the evaluation may be limited.

Medical History

Clues from the history can direct the initial evaluation. A complete history should be obtained regardless of age at presentation. Questioning about the past medical history should include the neonatal period with attention to premature birth, need for umbilical artery catheter, birth weight, neonatal asphyxia, episodes of acute kidney injury, and bronchopulmonary dysplasia. Low birth weight, particularly if coupled with prematurity, has been associated with reduced nephron numbers and potentially an increased risk for the development of hypertension in later life.[38-40] Beyond infancy, a history of voiding irregularities, recurrent urinary tract infections, unexplained fevers, edema, arthralgias, hematuria, rash or other systemic symptoms could suggest renal parenchymal disease or vasculitis. A history of renal trauma, including from motor vehicle accidents or from noncontact sports, should be considered pertinent even if remote, as posttraumatic hypertension occurs more frequently in the adolescent and young adult age group as compared with the general population.[41] Endocrine causes of hypertension are uncommon but might be considered in a child with headaches, tremulousness, palpitations, sweating at rest, episodic pallor or flushing, unexpected weight loss, or weakness. Pheochromocytomas and other neuroendocrine tumors are unusual in childhood but often present with sustained rather than paroxysmal hypertension. Medication history should always be considered, particularly in children under treatment for attention deficit disorder or behavioral/psychiatric issues because some of the medications employed for these indications may cause mild elevation of the BP or rapid weight gain.[42,43] Specific questioning about medication use is recommended as patients may fail to mention the use of birth control pills and over the counter

TABLE 17.5 History and Physical Examination Findings Suggestive of Secondary Causes Of Hypertension

Present in History	Suggests
Known UTI/UTI symptoms	Reflux nephropathy
Joint pains, rash, fever	Vasculitis, SLE
Acute onset of gross hematuria	Glomerulonephritis, renal thrombosis
Renal trauma	Renal infarct, RAS
Abdominal radiation	Radiation nephritis, RAS
Renal transplant	Transplant RAS
Precocious puberty	Adrenal disorder
Muscle cramping, constipation	Hyperaldosteronism
Excessive sweating, headache, pallor and/or flushing	Pheochromocytoma
Known illicit drug use	Drug-induced hypertension
Present on Examination	**Suggests**
BP >140/100 mm Hg at any age	Secondary hypertension
Leg BP < arm BP	Aortic coarctation
Poor growth, pallor	Chronic renal disease
Turner syndrome	Aortic coarctation
Café au lait spots	Renal artery stenosis
Delayed leg pulses	Aortic coarctation
Precocious puberty	Adrenal disorder
Bruits over upper abdomen	Renal artery stenosis
Edema	Renal disease
Excessive sweating	Pheochromocytoma
Excessive pigmentation	Adrenal disorder
Striae in a male	Drug-induced HTN

BP, Blood pressure; *HTN,* hypertension; *RAS,* renal artery stenosis; *SLE,* systemic lupus erythematosus; *UTI,* urinary tract infection.

medications such as decongestants and nonsteroidal antiinflammatory drugs.[44]

Turning to family history, a strong history of early onset hypertension may raise suspicion for monogenic, low renin forms of hypertension such as glucocorticoid remediable aldosteronism. Other pertinent family history could include (among others), a history of collagen vascular disease, hyperlipidemia, obesity, cystic kidney disease, and neurocutaneous disorders. Lifestyle history should also be elicited, including exercise and dietary habits, tobacco or illicit drug and alcohol use, caffeine intake, school performance, or other stress factors. Inquiry into sleep habits is suggested to assess sleep duration and quality. Symptoms of obstructive sleep apnea such as daytime sleepiness, frequent awakenings, or apnea should be noted, as obstructive sleep apnea has been associated with nocturnal hypertension in children.[45,46] Clues from the history to potential secondary causes of hypertension are summarized in Table 17.5.

Physical Examination

Findings on physical examination may also aid in focusing the evaluation. Height, weight, and body mass index should be plotted on growth curves and compared with past data points if available. Leg pulses and BPs should be checked in all children at least once to screen for coarctation of the thoracic aorta and midaortic syndrome. Differences in the quality of pulses in the upper and lower extremity, delay between the brachial and femoral pulses, and reduced leg pressures are suggestive of aortic pathology. Although coarctation of

III

DIAGNOSIS AND EVALUATION

the aorta is generally identified in infants, diagnosis even in teenagers is not uncommon, making this part of the physical examination mandatory in the initial evaluation of all hypertensive children and adolescents.

On general physical exam, the finding of short stature, pallor, edema, or evidence of rickets might suggest chronic kidney disease. Abdominal or pelvic masses, hepatosplenomegaly, or costovertebral angle tenderness may suggest autosomal dominant or recessive polycystic kidney disease, Wilms tumor, hydronephrosis, or pyelonephritis. Abdominal bruits if found, could be a nonspecific finding in a thin child but would certainly prompt evaluation for renovascular disease. Striae and acanthosis nigricans are frequently seen in adolescents with obesity-related hypertension, whereas true Cushing syndrome is quite unusual in childhood outside of iatrogenic exposure to glucocorticoid steroids. Other dermatologic findings such as malar rash, vasculitic lesions, or impetigo may suggest glomerulonephritis. Stigmata of syndromes associated with hypertension such as Turner syndrome, neurofibromatosis, tuberous sclerosis, and Williams syndrome would raise concerns about renal structural abnormalities or renal artery stenosis. Funduscopic examination to assess for hypertensive retinopathy should be conducted in cooperative patients with stage 2 hypertension. Arteriolar narrowing may be appreciated but more severe abnormalities are not typically seen in children.[46] Clues from the physical examination to potential secondary causes of hypertension are summarized in Table 17.5.

Diagnostic Tests

A basic screening evaluation should be undertaken in all children and adolescents with confirmed hypertension. Urinalysis, blood urea nitrogen (BUN), and serum creatinine will screen for renal disease, the most common cause of secondary hypertension in childhood. Many providers will also check a complete blood count to screen for anemia related to chronic kidney disease. Electrolytes are generally included as part of a routine chemistry panel but are most useful as a screen for low renin disorders as will be discussed later. A renal ultrasound will assess for renal anomalies, cysts, and discrepancy in the size of the kidneys. Additional basic testing should include fasting lipids and glucose in older children and adolescents to screen for metabolic disturbances that would increase their risk for future cardiovascular morbidity. An echocardiogram is recommended in all children diagnosed with hypertension to evaluate for left ventricular hypertrophy and rule out coarctation of the thoracic aorta.[1] The calculated left ventricular mass should be indexed to height in meters$^{2.7}$ with readings above the 95th percentile for age and gender indicative of left ventricular hypertrophy (LVH).[47] Multicenter studies have demonstrated that 30% to 40% of newly diagnosed children and adolescents with hypertension have LVH.[48,49]

In an older child or an adolescent with stage 1 hypertension, further evaluation may not be required if the basic screening does not suggest a secondary etiology. In younger children and in those with stage 2 hypertension, additional investigation for an underlying cause is recommended as suggested in Table 17.6. This list is not exhaustive and the evaluation should be expanded to address specific concerns that come up in individual patients. Generally once parenchymal renal disease is excluded, the next step is to evaluate for renovascular disease. Screening for renal artery stenosis with Duplex Doppler ultrasound is challenging because many of the children will be young and unable to cooperate with testing, or may be too obese to obtain an accurate study. The sensitivity of Doppler ultrasound for renovascular disease in children is at best a disappointing 73% to 85%, with a specificity of 71% to 92%.[50] Random plasma renin activity is not a reliable marker and is primarily useful in the evaluation for low-renin

TABLE 17.6 Diagnostic Evaluation of Hypertension in Children and Adolescents

Basic Screening Tests Indicated in All Children With Sustained Blood Pressure Greater Than the 95th Percentile	
Study(ies)	*Purpose*
Electrolytes	Evaluate for hyperaldosteronism
BUN, creatinine, CBC, UA	Evaluate for renal disease
Fasting lipids, glucose	Identify other cardiovascular risk factors
Renal ultrasound	Evaluate size and structure of kidneys
Echocardiogram	Assess for left ventricular hypertrophy, aortic coarctation

Additional Testing Based on Presentation, Age and/or Severity of Blood Pressure Elevation	
Study(ies)	*Purpose*
Drug screen	Identify drugs of abuse that may elevate BP
Renin and aldosterone	Identify low-renin hypertension
Plasma and/or urine metanephrines	Evaluate for catecholamine-secreting tumor
Polysomnography	Evaluate for obstructive sleep apnea
Plasma and urine steroid measurements	Evaluate for steroid-induced hypertension
Renovascular imaging (see text)	Evaluate for renovascular disease

BP, Blood pressure; *BUN,* blood urea nitrogen; *CBC,* complete blood count; *UA,* urinalysis.

hypertension. Computed tomography (CT) angiography and magnetic resonance angiography can be helpful but are still not definitive studies, with false-negative and positive results noted with both modalities. In children with severe hypertension, conditions associated with renovascular disease (such as Williams syndrome), requirement for more than two antihypertensive medications, past history of umbilical catheterization, or an elevated plasma renin level, arteriography should be considered even if preliminary noninvasive imaging is normal.[50] These services are usually best provided at a referral center that can offer the services of experienced pediatric interventional radiologists.

Low renin hypertension is uncommon but should be considered in children with severe hypertension. Family history is usually strong, although sporadic cases do occur so a negative family history does not preclude investigation. Although hypokalemia in association with metabolic alkalosis is the typical picture, normal serum potassium does not exclude these disorders. Further testing with random plasma renin activity in combination with aldosterone is useful as all of these disorders ultimately lead to excessive sodium reabsorption in the distal tubule and suppression of renin. For a detailed discussion, the reader should consult other sources.[51] Lastly, pheochromocytomas and neuroendocrine tumors are uncommon but should be considered if hypertension is severe. Pheochromocytomas may be associated with several genetic syndromes such as von Hippel-Lindau, among others. Evaluation with plasma metanephrines is suggested for initial screening and should be interpreted based on age-specific normal reference ranges.[52] Further testing with abdominal CT and MIBG (metaiodobenzylguanidine) should be performed when indicated. Other endocrine etiologies related to dysfunction of the adrenal cortex with overproduction of cortisol or other steroids, such as Cushing syndrome, congenital adrenal hyperplasia among others, are unusual, but should be considered if indicated based on history, physical exam, and initial screening.

MANAGEMENT OF HYPERTENSION IN CHILDREN AND ADOLESCENTS

Treatment of hypertension in children and adolescents is still largely empiric, because no long-term studies of either non-pharmacologic interventions or drug therapy have been conducted. Although significantly more pediatric data are now available on the antihypertensive efficacy of drug therapy than in the past,[53] the decision as to whether or not a specific child or adolescent should receive medication must be individualized.

Nonpharmacologic Measures

Weight loss, exercise, and dietary modifications have all been shown to reduce BP in children and adolescents, and are therefore considered primary treatment, especially in those with obesity-related hypertension.[1] Studies in obese children have demonstrated that modest weight loss will not only reduce BP, but can also improve other cardiovascular risk factors such as dyslipidemia and insulin resistance.[54,55] Unfortunately, weight loss is difficult and frequently unsuccessful. Additionally, in many families, other family members may also be obese. However, identifying a medical complication of obesity in a child such as hypertension can sometimes provide the necessary motivation for families to make the appropriate lifestyle changes. In this context, family-based interventions should be encouraged, because they have been shown to be reasonably successful long-term.[56]

Aerobic forms of exercise are generally preferred in the management of hypertension. Many children and adolescents may already be participating in one or more appropriate activities and may only need to increase the frequency and/or intensity of these to see a beneficial effect on their BP. Increased physical activity has clear benefit in contributing to weight control and can also lead to improvements in insulin resistance, endothelial function, and other cardiovascular risk factors.[57] Exercise has been shown to lower systolic and diastolic BP in a recent meta-analysis of nine randomized controlled trials including over 400 obese children.[58] The combination of increased physical activity and improved fitness along with decreases in body fat may also prevent or delay the development of type 2 diabetes in at risk individuals. At the very least, the amount of time spent in sedentary activities such as video game playing ("screen time") should be limited to less than 2 hours per day.

Dietary modification in the management of hypertension in children and adolescents usually begins with sodium restriction. Justification for this can be found in national surveys, which repeatedly show that most adults and children eat far more sodium than is recommended by consensus organizations.[59] A high salt intake increases thirst and high dietary sodium intakes of children have been linked to the obesity epidemic through increased consumption of sweetened drinks.[60] Although individual studies of reduced sodium intake in children have not demonstrated consistent effects on BP, a meta-analysis of 10 studies found that a 54% reduction in sodium intake was associated with a 2.47 mm Hg reduction in systolic BP.[61] These findings indicate that limitation of dietary sodium intake could have an additional beneficial effect in the treatment of obese adolescents with hypertension.

Other nutrients that have been examined in patients with hypertension include potassium and calcium, both of which have been shown to have antihypertensive effects. A 2-year trial of potassium and calcium supplementation in hypertensive, salt-sensitive Chinese children demonstrated that this combination significantly reduced systolic BP.[62] Therefore, a low-sodium diet that is also enriched in potassium and calcium content may be more effective in treatment of hypertension

than a diet that restricts sodium intake only. An example of such a diet is the DASH (dietary approaches to stop hypertension) diet, which is high in fruits, vegetables, and low-fat dairy foods, and has been shown to lower BP in adults with hypertension, even in those receiving antihypertensive medication.[63] Couch et al have demonstrated that the DASH eating plan can also reduce BP in children and adolescents with modestly elevated BP.[64]

Nonpharmacologic measures need to be implemented in a systematic manner, with a great deal of family involvement and long-term support, to be most effective. The DASH diet plan was effective in adolescents but successful implementation required the support of trained dietitians.[64] Exercise regimens can be effective as noted above, but as in adults, BP will return to baseline levels once the child or adolescent ceases the additional activity. They should be instituted even if there is an established indication for initiation of antihypertensive medications, as successful lifestyle intervention will complement the efficacy of pharmacologic treatment.

Use of Antihypertensive Medications

Given the intensive nature of nonpharmacologic approaches, and because some hypertensive youth may have hypertensive target-organ damage that could be reversed with effective treatment, antihypertensive medications may be needed. As has already been noted, the long-term consequences of untreated hypertension in an asymptomatic, otherwise healthy child or adolescent remain unknown. Additionally, there are few data available on the long-term effects of antihypertensive medications on the growth and development of children. Therefore, it is recommended to limit use of pharmacologic therapy to children and adolescents with one of the following indications[1]:

- Symptomatic hypertension
- Secondary hypertension
- Hypertensive target-organ damage
- Diabetes (types 1 & 2)
- Persistent hypertension despite nonpharmacologic measures
- Stage 2 hypertension

The historical lack of pediatric drug trials has been largely rectified by passage of the Food and Drug Administration Modernization Act (FDAMA) in the United States in 1997. This legislation contained a provision that granted 6 additional months of patent protection to drug manufacturers if they conducted pediatric trials. Subsequent legislation (Best Pharmaceuticals for Children Act, Pediatric Research Equity Act, FDA Amendments Act of 2007) has extended this provision and also has led to other initiatives, including public posting of internal FDA pharmacology and efficacy reviews on the Internet, and mechanisms to promote studies of medications with lapsed patent protection. These initiatives have led to a significant number of pediatric clinical trials of antihypertensive medications and have also increased the number of such medications with specific pediatric labeling, thereby significantly increasing the amount of clinically useful information for practitioners.[53]

Unlike in adults, large-scale comparative trials of different classes of antihypertensive agents have not been conducted in children. Therefore, the choice of initial antihypertensive agent for use in children still remains up to the preference of the individual practitioner. Diuretics and beta-adrenergic blockers, which were recommended as initial therapy in the First and Second Task Force Reports, have a long track record of safety and efficacy in hypertensive children and are still appropriate for pediatric use, although they are now mostly used as second-line agents. Newer classes of agents, including angiotensin converting enzyme inhibitors (ACEIs), calcium channel blockers, and angiotensin receptor blockers (ARBs),

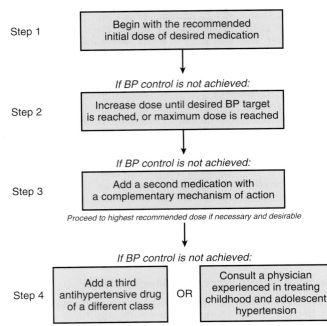

FIG. 17.2 Stepped-care approach to use of antihypertensive medications in children and adolescents. See text for explanation.

have now been shown to be safe and well tolerated in hypertensive children in recent industry-sponsored trials, and may be prescribed if indicated.[1] As a matter of fact, these newer agents, particularly calcium channel blockers and ACE inhibitors, have become the most widely used initial agents in the pediatric age group.

It is reasonable to try to base the choice of agent upon the assumed pathophysiology of the child's hypertension. Additionally, consideration should be given to using specific classes of antihypertensive medications in certain hypertensive children and adolescents with specific underlying or concurrent medical conditions. The best example of this would be the use of ACEIs or ARBs in children with diabetes or proteinuric renal diseases, in whom such agents may have a beneficial effect in slowing progression.[65] An additional example would be a teenager with hypertension who is receiving stimulant medications for attention deficit hyperactivity disorder; such patients are commonly tachycardic and could benefit from treatment with a beta-blocker.

Antihypertensive drugs in children and adolescents are generally prescribed in a stepped-care manner (Fig. 17.2).[1] The patient is started on the lowest recommended dose of the initial agent and the dose is increased until the highest recommended dose is reached, or until the child experiences adverse effects from the medication. At this point a second drug from a different class should be added, until the desired goal BP is reached. Because many antihypertensive drugs now have specific FDA-approved pediatric labeling, the generalist should restrict their choices to those agents. Recommended doses for selected antihypertensive agents for use in hypertensive children and adolescents are given in Table 17.7.

The value of prescribing antihypertensive medications in the young has recently been questioned. In an analysis conducted for the United States Preventative Service Task Force, Thompson et al found that although recent studies have demonstrated that antihypertensive medications do lower BP in children and adolescents, the trials were of short duration and no long-term benefits of such treatment were seen.[66] Similar concerns were raised in an even more recent systematic review; although modest BP reductions were seen, there were limited data available for most

agents, particularly with respect to safety.[67] Thus, until new information regarding risks and benefits of using antihypertensive medications in children and adolescents becomes available, it is important to follow the conservative guidelines discussed above.

Hypertension in Children With Chronic Kidney Disease

As has been discussed, underlying kidney disease is the most common secondary cause of hypertension in children and adolescents. BP reduction in this population is important as it may help slow progression of the underlying renal disease. Both the National High Blood Pressure Education Program Working Group and the European Society of Hypertension have recommended a lower BP target in children with chronic kidney disease than for those with uncomplicated primary hypertension.[1,11] The evidence supporting a lower BP target, as well as the various clinical practice recommendations for BP management in this population have recently been reviewed.[65] Therapy should generally begin with either an ACE inhibitor or an ARB, with additional agents added on as necessary until the target BP is reached. Close follow up and use of repeated ABPM is important to help assure that the BP goal has been attained.

Acute Severe Hypertension

The pathophysiology, management, and outcome of severe hypertension in children and adolescents have been reviewed in detail elsewhere.[68,69] Many aspects are similar to hypertensive emergencies and urgencies in adults as reviewed in elsewhere in this text. However, a few unique aspects warrant consideration.

Medication nonadherence in patients with established hypertension, the most common cause of acute severe hypertension in adults,[70] occurs rarely in pediatric patients, except perhaps in those with established renal disease. Children or adolescents with acute severe hypertension almost always have an underlying condition such as acute or chronic renal disease, solid organ transplantation, or renovascular hypertension.[68]

Hypertensive encephalopathy is the most frequent life-threatening manifestation of severe hypertension in children and adolescents, emphasizing the need for slow, controlled reduction in BP to prevent complications arising through loss of normal auto-regulatory processes.[69] Less severe symptoms may include nausea, vomiting, or unusual irritability; because these may be somewhat nonspecific, especially in younger children, a high degree of clinical suspicion must be maintained.

Although evidence-based recommendations are lacking, the usual goal in the treatment of a hypertensive emergency is to reduce the BP by no more than 25% over the first 8 hours, with a gradual return to normal/goal BP over 24 to 48 hours.[68] Treatment of hypertensive emergencies in children is usually initiated with a continuous infusion of an intravenous antihypertensive, with nicardipine and labetalol being the agents most commonly used. Other intravenous agents that have found use in children with severe hypertension include sodium nitroprusside, esmolol, hydralazine, and fenoldopam.[69] Oral antihypertensive agents can be used in pediatric patients with acute severe hypertension who do not have life-threatening symptoms.[71] The choice of oral antihypertensives for use in management of severe hypertension in pediatric patients is fairly limited. As in adults, short-acting nifedipine is no longer recommended.[68] Recommended doses of both oral and intravenous drugs useful in the treatment of acute severe hypertension in children and adolescents can be found in Table 17.8.

TABLE 17.7 Antihypertensive Medications and Dosing in Children and Adolescents

CLASS	DRUG	STARTING DOSE	INTERVAL	MAXIMUM DOSE[a]
ARAs	Eplerenone	25 mg/day	QD-BID	100 mg/day
	Spironolactone[b]	1 mg/kg/day	QD-BID	3.3 mg/kg/day up to 100 mg/day
ARBs	Candesartan[b]	1-6 years: 0.2 mg/kg/day; 6-17 years: <50 kg 4-8 mg QD >50 kg 8-16 mg QD	QD	1-6 years: 0.4 mg/kg/day; 6-17 years: <50 kg 16 mg daily >50 kg 32 mg daily
	Losartan[b]	0.75 mg/kg/day (up to 50 mg QD)	QD	1.4 mg/kg/day (max 100 mg QD)
	Olmesartan[b]	20-35 kg: 10 mg QD ≥35 kg: 20 mg QD	QD	20-35 kg: 20 mg QD ≥35 kg: 40 mg QD
	Valsartan[b]	<6 years: 5-10 mg/day 6-17 years: 1.3 mg/kg/day (up to 40 mg QD)	QD	<6 years: 80 mg QD 6-17 years: 2.7 mg/kg/day (up to 160 mg QD)
ACE inhibitors	Benazepril[b]	0.2 mg/kg/day (up to 10 mg/day)	QD	0.6 mg/kg/day (up to 40 mg/day)
	Captopril[b]	0.3-0.5 mg/kg/dose	BID-TID	0.6 mg/kg/day (up to 450 mg/day)
	Enalapril[c]	0.08 mg/kg/day	QD-BID	0.6 mg/kg/day (up to 40 mg/day)
	Fosinopril	0.1 mg/kg/day (up to 10 mg/day)	QD	0.6 mg/kg/day (up to 40 mg/day)
	Lisinopril[b]	0.07 mg/kg/day (up to 5 mg/day)	QD	0.6 mg/kg/day (up to 40 mg/day)
	Quinapril	5-10 mg/day	QD	80 mg/day
α- and β-adrenergic antagonists	Carvedilol[b]	0.1 mg/kg/dose (up to 6.25 mg BID)	BID	0.5 mg/kg/dose up to 25 mg BID
	Labetalol[b]	2-3 mg/kg/day	BID	10-12 mg/kg/day (up to 1.2g/day)
β-adrenergic antagonists	Atenolol[b]	0.5-1 mg/kg/day	QD	2 mg/kg/day up to 100 mg day
	Bisoprolol/HCTZ	2.5/6.25 mg daily	QD	10/6.25 mg daily
	Metoprolol	1-2 mg/kg/day	BID	6 mg/kg/day (up to 200 mg/day)
	Propranolol[c]	1 mg/kg/day	BID-QID	8 mg/kg/day (up to 640 mg/day)
CCBs	Amlodipine[b]	0.06 mg/kg/day	QD	0.3 mg/kg/day (up to 10 mg/day)
	Felodipine	2.5 mg/day	QD	10 mg/day
	Isradipine[b]	0.05-0.15 mg/kg/dose	TID-QID	0.8 mg/kg/day up to 20 mg/day
	Extended-release nifedipine	0.25-0.5 mg/kg/day	QD-BID	3 mg/kg/day (up to 120 mg/day)
Central a-agonist	Clonidine[b]	5-20 mcg/kg/day	QD-BID	25 mcg/kg/day (up to 0.9 mg/day)
Diuretics	Amiloride	5-10 mg/day	QD	20 mg/day
	Chlorthalidone	0.3 mg/kg/day	QD	2 mg/kg/day (up to 50 mg/day)
	Furosemide[c]	0.5-2 mg/kg/dose	QD-BID	6 mg/kg/day
	HCTZ	0.5-1 mg/kg/day	QD	3 mg/kg/day (up to 50 mg/day)
Vasodilators	Hydralazine	0.25 mg/kg/dose	TID-QID	7.5 mg/kg/day (up to 200 mg/day)
	Minoxidil	0.1-0.2 mg/kg/day	BID-TID	1 mg/kg/day (up to 50 mg/day)

[a]The maximum recommended adult dose should not be exceeded
[b]Information on preparation of a stable extemporaneous suspension is available for these agents
[c]Available as a United States Food and Drug Administration approved commercially supplied oral solution
ARA, Aldosterone receptor antagonist; ACE, angiotensin converting enzyme; ARB, angiotensin receptor blocker; BID, twice daily; CCB, calcium channel blocker; HCTZ, hydrochlorothiazide; QD, once daily; QID, four times daily; TID, three times daily.

TABLE 17.8 Antihypertensive Agents for Acute Severe Hypertension in Children and Adolescents

Useful for Severely Hypertensive Patients With Life-Threatening Symptoms				
Drug	Class	Dose	Route	Comments
Esmolol	β-adrenergic blocker	100-500 mcg/kg/min	IV infusion	Very short-acting—constant infusion preferred. May cause profound bradycardia.
Hydralazine	Direct vasodilator	0.1-0.2 mg/kg/dose up to 0.6 mg/kg/dose	IV, IM	Should be given q4 hours when given IV bolus.
Labetalol	α- and β-adrenergic blocker	Bolus: 0.20-1.0 mg/kg/dose, up to 40 mg/dose infusion: 0.25-3.0 mg/kg/hour	IV bolus or infusion	Asthma and overt heart failure are relative contraindications.
Nicardipine	Calcium channel blocker	Bolus: 30 mcg/kg up to 2 mg/dose infusion: 0.5-4 mcg/kg/min	IV bolus or infusion	May cause reflex tachycardia. Increases cyclosporine and tacrolimus levels.
Sodium Nitroprusside	Direct vasodilator	Starting: 0.3-0.5 mcg/kg/min Maximum: 10 mcg/kg/min	IV infusion	Monitor cyanide levels with prolonged (>72 hours) use or in renal failure; or coadminister with sodium thiosulfate.

Continued

TABLE 17.8 Antihypertensive Agents for Acute Severe Hypertension in Children and Adolescents—cont'd

Useful for Severely Hypertensive Patients With Less Significant Symptoms

Drug	Class	Dose	Route	Comments
Clonidine	Central α-agonist	2-5 mcg/kg/dose, up to 10 mcg/kg/dose given q6-8 hours	PO	Side effects include dry mouth and drowsiness.
Fenoldopam	Dopamine receptor agonist	0.2-0.5 mcg/kg/min up to 0.8 mcg/kg/min	IV infusion	Higher doses worsen tachycardia without further reducing BP.
Hydralazine	Direct vasodilator	0.2 mg/kg/dose up to 25 mg/dose given q6-8 hours	PO	Half-life varies with genetically determined acetylation rates.
Isradipine	Calcium channel blocker	0.05-0.1 mg/kg/dose up to 5 mg/dose given q6-8 hours	PO	Exaggerated fall in BP can be seen in patients receiving azole antifungals.
Minoxidil	Direct vasodilator	0.1-0.2 mg/kg/dose up to 10 mg/dose given q8-12 hours	PO	Most potent oral vasodilator; long-acting.

ACE, Angiotensin-converting enzyme; *BP,* blood pressure; *IM,* intramuscular; *IV,* intravenous; *kg,* kilogram; *mcg,* microgram; *mg,* milligram; *PO,* per os (oral); *q,* quaque (every).

References

1. National High Blood Pressure Education Program Working Group on High Blood Pressure in Children and Adolescents. The fourth report on the diagnosis, evaluation, and treatment of high blood pressure in children and adolescents. National Heart, Lung, and Blood Institute, Bethesda, MD 2005; *National Institute of Health publication* 05:5267.
2. McNiece KL, Poffenbarger TS, Turner JL, et al. Prevalence of hypertension and pre-hypertension among adolescents. *J Pediatr.* 2007;150:640-644.
3. Steinthorsdottir SD, Eliasdottir SB, Indridason OS, et al. Prevalence of hypertension in 9- to 10-year-old Icelandic school children. *J Clin Hypertens (Greenwich).* 2011;13:774-779.
4. Cao Z-Q, Zhu L, Zhang T, et al. Blood pressure and obesity among adolescents: a school-based population study in China. *Am J Hypertens.* 2012;25:576-582.
5. Din-Dzietham R, Liu Y, Bielo MV, Shamsa F. High blood pressure trends in children and adolescents in national surveys, 1963 to 2002. *Circulation.* 2007;116:1488-1496.
6. Flynn JT. The changing face of pediatric hypertension in the era of the childhood obesity epidemic. *Pediatr Nephrol.* 2013;28:1059-1066.
7. Kit BK, Kuklina E, Carroll MD, et al. Prevalence of and trends in dyslipidemia and blood pressure among US children and adolescents, 1999-2012. *JAMA Pediatr.* 2012;169:272-279.
8. Sorof JM, Lai D, Turner J, et al. Overweight, ethnicity, and the prevalence of hypertension in school-aged children. *Pediatrics.* 2004;113:475-482.
9. Lu X, Shi P, Luo CY, et al. Prevalence of hypertension in overweight and obese children from a large school-based population in Shanghai, China. *BMC Public Health.* 2013;13:24.
10. Chobanian AV, Bakris GL, Black HR, et al. The seventh report of the Joint National Committee on Prevention, Detection, Evaluation, and Treatment of High Blood Pressure: the JNC 7 report. *JAMA.* 2003;289:2560-2572.
11. Lurbe E, Cifkova R, Cruickshank JK, et al. Management of high blood pressure in children and adolescents: recommendations of the European society of hypertension. *J Hypertens.* 2009;27:1719-1742.
12. McNiece KL, Poffenbarger TS, Turner JL, et al. Prevalence of hypertension and pre-hypertension among adolescents. *J Pediatr.* 2007;150:640-644, 644.e1.
13. Chiolero A, Cachat F, Burnier M, et al. Prevalence of hypertension in schoolchildren based on repeated measurements and association with overweight. *J Hypertens.* 2007;25:2209-2217.
14. Podoll A, Grenier M, Croix B, Feig D. Inaccuracy in pediatric outpatient blood pressure measurement. *Pediatrics.* 2007;119, e538-e543.
15. Eliasdottir SB, Steinthorsdottir SD, Indridason OS, et al. Comparsion of aneroid and oscillometric blood pressure measurements in children. *J Clin Hypertens (Greenwich).* 2013;15:776-783.
16. Beevers G, Lip GYH, O'Brien E. ABC of hypertension. Blood pressure measurement. Part II—conventional sphygmomanometry: technique of auscultatory blood pressure measurement. *BMJ.* 2001;322:1043-1047.
17. Alpert BS, Quinn D, Gallick D. Oscillometric blood pressure: a review for clinicians. *J Am Soc Hypertens.* 2014;8:930-938.
18. Karpettas N, Nasothimiou e, Kollias A, et al. Ambulatory and home blood pressure monitoring in children and adolescents: diagnosis of hypertension and assessment of target-organ damage. *Hypertens Res.* 2013;36:285-292.
19. Weber MA, Schiffrin EL, White WB, et al. Clinical practice guidelines for the management of hypertension in the community. A statement by the American Society of Hypertension and the International Society of Hypertension. *J Clin Hypertens.* 2014;16:14-26.
20. Park MK, Menard SW, Yuan C. Comparison of auscultatory and oscillometric blood pressures. *Arch Pediatr Adolesc Med.* 2001;155:50-53.
21. Midgley PC, Wardhaugh B, Macfarlane C, et al. Blood pressure in children aged 4-8 years: comparison of Omron HEM 711 and sphygmomanometer blood pressure measurements. *Arch Dis Child.* 2009;94:955-958.
22. Flynn JT, Pierce CB, Miller ER, et al. Reliability of resting blood pressure measurement and classification using an oscillometric device in children with chronic kidney disease. *J Pediatr.* 2012;160:434-440.
23. Cohen DL, Townsend RR. Should all patients have ambulatory blood pressure monitoring performed to validate the diagnosis of hypertension? *J Clin Hypertens.* 2015;17:412-413.
24. Swartz SJ, Srivaths PR, Croix B, Feig Dl. Cost effectiveness of ambulatory blood pressure monitoring in the initial evaluation of hypertension in children. *Pediatrics.* 2008;122:1177-1181.
25. Davis ML, Ferguson MA, Zachariah JP. Clinical predictors and impact of ambulatory blood pressure monitoring in pediatric hypertension referrals. *J Am Soc Hypertens.* 2014;8:660-667.
26. Sorof JM, Portman RJ. White coat hypertension in children with elevated casual blood pressures. *J Pediatr.* 2000;137:493-497.
27. Matsuoka S, Kawamura K, Honda M, Awazu M. White coat effect and white coat hypertension in pediatric patients. *Pediatr Nephrol.* 2002;17:950-953.
28. Wühl E, Hadtstein C, Mehls O, et al. Home, clinic, and ambulatory blood pressure monitoring in children with chronic renal failure. *Pediatr Res.* 2004;55:492-497.
29. Salgado CM, Jardim PC, Viana JK, et al. Home blood pressure in children and adolescents: a comparison with office and ambulatory blood pressure measurements. *Acta Pædiatr.* 2011;100:e163-e168.
30. Flynn J, Daniels SR, Hayman LL, et al. Update: ambulatory blood pressure monitoring in children and adolescents: a scientific statement from the American Heart Association. *Hypertension.* 2014;63:1116-1135.
31. Flynn J, Zhang Y, Solar-Yohay S, Shi V. Clinical and demographic characteristics of children with hypertension. *Hypertension.* 2012;60:1047-1054.
32. Wyszynska T, Cichocka E, Wieteska-Klimczak A, et al. A single center experience with 1025 children with hypertension. *Acta Pædiatrica.* 1992;81:244-246.
33. Flynn JT, Alderman MH. Characteristics of children with primary hypertension seen at a referral center. *Pediatr Nephrol.* 2005;20:961-966.
34. Kapur G, Ahmed M, Pan C, et al. Secondary hypertension in overweight and stage 1 hypertensive children: a Midwest Pediatric Nephrology Consortium report. *J Clin Hypertens (Greenwich).* 2010;12:34-39.
35. Blowey DL, Duda PJ, Stokes P, Hall M. Incidence and treatment of hypertension in the neonatal intensive care unit. *J Am Soc Hypertens.* 2011;5:478-483.
36. Sahu R, Pannu H, Yu R, et al. Systemic hypertension requiring treatment in the neonatal intensive care unit. *J Pediatr.* 2013;163:84-88.
37. Dionne JM, Abitbol CL, Flynn JT. Hypertension in infancy: diagnosis, management and outcome. *Pediatr Nephrol.* 2012;27:17-32. Erratum in: *Pediatr Nephrol.* 2012;27:159-160.
38. Cruickshank JK, Mzayek F, Liu L, et al. Origins of the "black/white" difference in BP. Roles of birth weight, postnatal growth, early blood pressure, and adolescent body size. The Bogalusa Heart Study. *Circulation.* 2005;111:1932-1937.
39. Rostand SG, Cliver SP, Goldenberg RL. Racial disparities in the association of foetal growth retardation to childhood blood pressure. *Nephrol Dial Transplant.* 2005;20:1592-1597.
40. Steinthorsdottir SD, Eliasdottir SB, Indridason OS, et al. The relationship between body weight and blood pressure in childhood: a population-based study. *Am J Hypertens.* 2013;26:76-82.
41. Burney B, Oliva R, Zorn KC, Bakris G. Hypertension following kidney injury. *J Clin Hypertens.* 2010;12:727-730.
42. McQuire C, Hassiotis A, Harrison B, Pilling S. Pharmacological interventions for challenging behavior in children with intellectual disabilities: a systematic review and meta-analysis. *BMC Psychiatry.* 2015;15:303.
43. Sowinski H, Karpawich PP. Management of a hyperactive teen and cardiac safety. *Pediatr Clin North Am.* 2014;61:81-90.
44. Grossman E, Messerli FH. Drug-induced hypertension: an unappreciated cause of secondary hypertension. *Am J Med.* 2012;125:14-22.
45. Li AM, Au CT, Ng C, et al. A 4-year prospective follow-up study of childhood OSA and its association with BP. *Chest.* 2014;145:1255-1263.
46. Hartzell K, Avis K, Lozano D, Feig D. Obstructive sleep apnea and periodic limb movement disorder in a population of children with hypertension and/or nocturnal nondipping blood pressures. *J Am Soc Hypertens.* 2016;10:101-107.
47. Khoury PR, Mitsnefes M, Daniels SR, Kimball TR. Age-specific reference intervals for indexed left ventricular mass in children. *J Am Soc Echocardiography.* 2009;22:709-714.
48. Hanevold C, Waller J, Daniels S, et al. The effects of obesity, gender, and ethnic group on left ventricular hypertrophy and geometry in hypertensive children: a collaborative study of the International Pediatric Hypertension Association. *Pediatrics.* 2004;113:328-333. Erratum in: *Pediatrics.* 2005;115:1118.
49. Brady TM, Fivush B, Flynn JT, Parekh R. Ability of blood pressure to predict left ventricular hypertrophy in children with primary hypertension. *J Pediatr.* 2008;152:73-78, 78.e1.
50. Tullus K. Renal artery stenosis: is angiography still the gold standard in 2011? *Pediatr Nephrol.* 2011;26:833-837.
51. Vehaskari VM. Heritable forms of hypertension. *Pediatr Nephrol.* 2009;24:1929-1937.
52. Weise M, Merke DP, Pacak K, et al. Utility of plasma free metanephrines for detecting childhood pheochromocytomas. *J Clin Endocrinol Metab.* 2002;87:1955-1960.
53. Ferguson MA, Flynn JT. Treatment of pediatric hypertension: lessons learned from recent clinical trials. *Curr Cardiovasc Risk Rep.* 2014;8:399.
54. Reinehr T, Andler W. Changes in the atherogenic risk factor profile according to degree of weight loss. *Arch Dis Child.* 2004;89:419-422.
55. Expert Panel on Integrated Guidelines for Cardiovascular Health and Risk Reduction in Children and Adolescents; National Heart, Lung, and Blood Institute. Expert panel on integrated guidelines for cardiovascular health and risk reduction in children and adolescents: summary report. *Pediatrics.* 2011;128(Suppl 5):S213-S256.
56. Kalarchian MA, Levine MD, Arslanian SA, et al. Family-based treatment of severe pediatric obesity: randomized, controlled trial. *Pediatrics.* 2009;124:1060-1068.
57. Farpour-Lambert NJ, Aggoun Y, et al. Physical activity reduces systemic blood pressure and improves early markers of atherosclerosis in pre-pubertal obese children. *J Am Coll Cardiol.* 2009;54:2396-2406.
58. García-Hermoso A, Saavedra JM, Escalante Y. Effects of exercise on resting blood pressure in obese children: a meta-analysis of randomized controlled trials. *Obes Rev.* 2013;14:919-928.

59. Jackson SL, King SM, Zhao L, Cogswell ME. Prevalence of excess sodium intake in the United States—NHANES, 2009-2012. *MMWR Morb Mortal Wkly Rep.* 2016;64:1393-1397.

60. He FJ, Marrero NM, MacGregor GA. Salt intake is related to soft drink consumption in children and adolescents: a link to obesity? *Hypertension.* 2008;51:629-634.

61. He FJ, MacGregor GA. Importance of salt in determining blood pressure in children: meta-analysis of controlled trials. *Hypertension.* 2006;48:861-869.

62. Mu JJ, Liu ZQ, Liu WM, et al. Reduction of blood pressure with calcium and potassium supplementation in children with salt sensitivity: a 2-year double-blinded placebo-controlled trial. *J Hum Hypertens.* 2005;19:479-483.

63. Appel LJ, Brands MW, Daniels SR, et al. Dietary approaches to prevent and treat hypertension: a scientific statement from the American Heart Association. *Hypertension.* 2006;47:296-308.

64. Couch SC, Saelens BE, Levin L, et al. The efficacy of a clinic-based behavioral nutrition intervention emphasizing a DASH-type diet for adolescents with elevated blood pressure. *J Pediatr.* 2008;52:494-501.

65. Dionne JM. Evidence-based guidelines for the management of hypertension in children with chronic kidney disease. *Pediatr Nephrol.* 2015;30:1919-1927.

66. Thompson M, Dana T, Bougatsos C, et al. Screening for hypertension in children and adolescents to prevent cardiovascular disease. *Pediatrics.* 2013;131:490-525.

67. Chaturvedi S, Lipszyc DH, Licht C, et al. Pharmacological interventions for hypertension in children. *Cochrane Database Syst Rev.* 2014;2:CD008117.

68. Flynn JT, Tullus K. Severe hypertension in children and adolescents: pathophysiology and treatment. *Pediatr Nephrol.* 2009;24:1101-1112. Erratum in *Pediatr Nephrol.* 2012;27:503-504.

69. Singh D, Akingbola O, Yosypiv I, El-Dahr S. Emergency management of hypertension in children. *Int J Nephrol.* 2012;2012:420247.

70. Bender SR, Fong MW, Heitz S, Bisognano JD. Characteristics and management of patients presenting to the emergency department with hypertensive urgency. *J Clin Hypertens (Greenwich).* 2006;8:12-18.

71. Webb TN, Shatat IF, Miyashita Y. Therapy of acute hypertension in hospitalized children and adolescents. *Curr Hypertens Rep.* 2014;16:425.

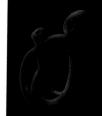

SECTION IV

RISK STRATIFICATION

18 The Natural History of Untreated Hypertension

Elvira O. Gosmanova and William C. Cushman

Our knowledge about the natural history of untreated hypertension is mainly based on historical information from a relatively short duration of time (1900s to 1970s). During that period, there was a significant evolution in the understanding of the health-related impact of elevated blood pressure (BP) and in developing new antihypertensive medications (Fig. 18.1) that solidified the awareness of the adverse association between untreated hypertension and cardiovascular morbidity and mortality. Therefore, from the early 1970s, it was no longer ethical to conduct observational studies or hypertensive clinical trials that included hypertensive individuals with untreated diastolic hypertension. Similarly, isolated systolic hypertension could not be left untreated starting in the 1990s.

The diagnosis of hypertension in ancient times was based on analysis of arterial pulse and it has been known for millennia that "hard pulse disease" (what we now call hypertension) is a major risk factor for apoplexy or the modern diagnosis of stroke, and usually resulted in untimely individual death.[1] The first scientific reports about the association of hardening pulse with end-organ damage appeared in the early 19th century when Bright published a case series illustrating patients with hardening pulse, elevated blood urea, dropsy with albuminuria, and histological findings of left ventricular hypertrophy and hardening of the kidneys.[2] However, these patients likely comprised a heterogeneous group with various etiologies of renal disease, and elevated blood pressure in many cases was secondary as a result of renal disease itself. Forty years later Mohamed described histologic findings of nephrosclerosis in individuals with hardening pulse that he believed were independent from primary renal disease; this was the first suggestion that hypertension itself can result in kidney damage.[3] Subsequently, Gull and Sutton described hypertensive left ventricular hypertrophy, and Gowers reported retinal hypertensive changes.[4,5] The development of a method for indirect BP measurement was the next crucial step in understanding of effects of elevated BP. The first sphygmomanometer was invented by Samuel Siegfried Karl Ritter von Basch in 1881 and later improved by Scipione Riva-Rocci in 1896.[6] However, the Riva-Rocci method allowed only measurement of systolic blood pressure (SBP) through palpation of the pulse obliteration pressure. Systolic and diastolic blood pressure (DBP) differentiation and measurements became possible after Nikolai Korotkoff introduced auscultation of sounds into existing sphygmomanometric technique in 1905.[7] This method allowed for routine accurate BP measurement and enabled the development of average age-specific BP charts and understanding of the relationship of different levels of BP and patient-related outcomes.

Early scientific reports from the 1910s to 1930s described hypertension as a disease with two variants. It was noted that many individuals with elevated BP, usually in the outpatient setting, were asymptomatic and had little abnormal physical and laboratory findings.[8] This type of hypertension was considered to be "benign" and not requiring any treatment and many prominent physicians continued to advocate until the early 1950s that elevation of blood pressure was a physiologic response to maintain adequate blood flow to vital organs in the setting of aging vasculature. The second type of hypertension, which was often referred as malignant or accelerated hypertension, was mainly observed in the hospital setting when patients typically presented with markedly elevated BP (SBP in upper 200s and lower 300s, and DBP above 120 mm Hg) and suffering terminal complications of hypertension such as stroke, heart failure, papilledema, and renal failure. Only these extreme elevations in blood pressure were considered to require treatment, which at that time was mostly symptomatic because of a lack of other definitive therapies. The thresholds for abnormal BP were slowly decreasing, but remained much higher than what is accepted today. For example, the recommended BP levels for intervention were suggested as higher than 200/100 and 180/110 in two respected cardiology textbooks in the 1940s.[8] The 1950 edition of Harrison's Internal Medicine textbook still advocated that asymptomatic hypertension should not be treated.[9]

One of the best case illustrations of natural history of untreated hypertension was written by one of the earliest hypertension treatment advocates, Dr. Marvin Moser, and described the medical history of the 32nd United States President, Franklin Roosevelt.[8] It was first noted that Mr. Roosevelt suffered moderate BP elevations in the mid 1930s. Untreated hypertension in his case progressed from moderate elevations, 160/90s mm Hg, to a higher level (>180/110 mm Hg) over a 7-year period. This was associated with the sharp deterioration of Mr. Roosevelt's health and the development of progressive heart failure and his untimely death (likely from stroke) in less than 1 year.

In this chapter we will review the important, although generally older, information from epidemiologic studies and clinical trials that led to the clear and inescapable conclusion that elevated BP is associated with adverse cardiovascular and

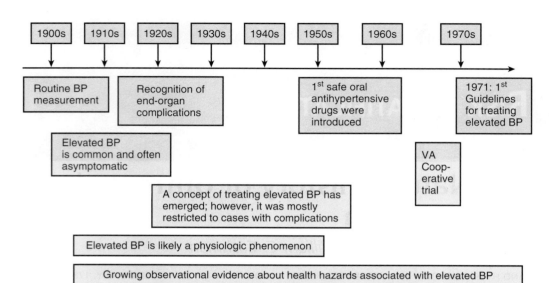

FIG. 18.1 Schematic model of the evolution of understanding and approaches to hypertension in the 20th century.

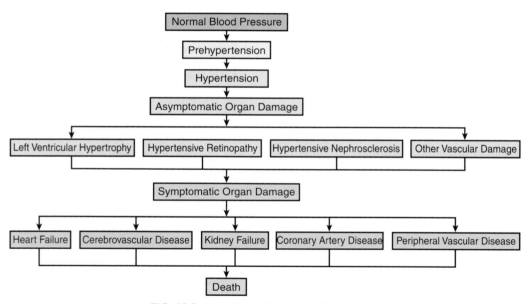

FIG. 18.2 Schematic model of untreated hypertension.

renal outcomes. Fig. 18.2 depicts the framework of the discussion, which broadly characterizes the progression of prehypertension to hypertension to target organ damage to adverse clinical events, and finally to death.

PREHYPERTENSION AND HYPERTENSION

Hypertension is typically preceded by a gradual rise in BP from normal values into the prehypertensive range. Prehypertension is defined as SBP 120 to 139 mm Hg and/or DBP 80 to 89 mm Hg.[10] Because hypertension is mostly asymptomatic, unless BP is measured regularly, it is often not possible to detect when these transitions occur. However, there are several indirect and direct observations supporting gradual progression of elevated BP. First, it was known from series of life insurance reports conducted from the 1920s through the 1960s and later confirmed by the National Health Examination Survey (NHES 1960 to 1962) and three separate Health and Nutrition Examination Survey (NHANES 1 to 3) that average SBP and DBP tends to increase with aging.[11] NHANES 1[12] was conducted in 1971 to 1974, when hypertension treatment was still not uniform and it showed that the

mean SBP at age 18 increased by 0.2 mm Hg per year until age 35, and after that the rise in mean SBP accelerates to an average 0.8 mm Hg per year. Although males aged 18 to 44 have higher mean SBP compared with females, with the difference in mean SBP up to 9 mm Hg, the rate of mean SBP rise per year among females in the 18 to 44 years age group exceeds the rates of the mean SBP rise in males, leading to "equalization" of mean SBP at around age 55. After the age of 55, the mean SBP in females starts to exceed the mean SBP in males by as much as 4 to 6 mm Hg. The mean DBP in males increases with aging; however, the rate of DBP increase is less pronounced as compared with SBP. In contrast to the mean SBP, the mean DBP in females rises in ages 18 to 64 and then remains stable thereafter. In addition, the mean DBP in men exceeds the mean of DBP in females until age 54 and becomes similar after age 55. As average BP rises with age, the proportion of individuals with prehypertension and hypertension increases with age as well. The prevalence of SBP 140 or higher and/or DBP 90 or higher mm Hg at age 18 to 34 in males and females is 13.8% and 6.3%, respectively, and increases to 65% and 74%, respectively, in the 65 to 74 age group (NHANES 1971 to 1974).

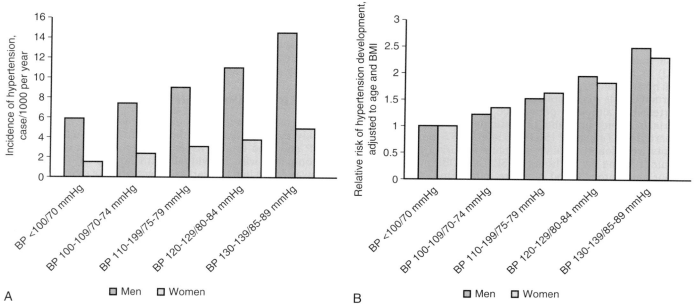

FIG. 18.3 Incidence of hypertension among adolescents with normal baseline blood pressure or prehypertension during 17 years of follow-up. *BP,* Blood pressure. *(From Tirosh A, Afek A, Rudich A, et al. Progression of normotensive adolescents to hypertensive adults: a study of 26,980 teenagers.* Hypertension. *2010;56:203-209.)*

Several prospective cohort studies looked at rates of progression of normotension and prehypertension to hypertension. The Framingham Heart Study (FHS) was initiated in 1948 and included 5209 men and women aged 30 to 62 years who were subsequently followed for over 30 years.[13] During an average of 26 years of follow-up, 23.6% and 36.2% of men and women with normal BP (defined as DBP <85 mm Hg) at baseline developed hypertension (defined as DBP ≥95 mm Hg) as compared with 54.2% and 60.6% of men and women with prehypertension (defined as DBP 85 to 89 mm Hg) at baseline. In the age-adjusted analysis, the presence of prehypertension was associated with a 3.4-fold increased risk of subsequent hypertension in both men and women, as compared with normal BP at baseline.[13] The metabolic Life Style and Nutrition Assessment in Young Adults prospective cohort study evaluated the development of hypertension in 26,980 adolescents with mean age 17.4 years.[14] Overall, 12.4% of young adults with normal BP (BP <120/80 mm Hg) and 17.1% of young adults with prehypertension (BP 120 to 139/80 to 89 mm Hg) developed hypertension during a maximum of 17 years of follow-up with the incidence of hypertension among men being four-fold higher as compared with women (Fig. 18.3A). In a Cox regression analysis adjusted for age and body mass index (BMI), the cumulative incidence of hypertension gradually increased for each 10/5 mm Hg BP increase from baseline BP less than 100/70 mm Hg with no evidence for a threshold (Fig. 18.3B). In a more modern investigation, the Trial of Preventing Hypertension (TROPHY), during 2-year and 4-year follow-ups, 40% and 60% of individuals, respectively, with prehypertension developed sustained hypertension.[15] There is a consistent pattern among nonmodifiable (increasing age, African-American race) and modifiable (weight) risks factors that are shown to accelerate the conversion rates of prehypertension to hypertension.

UNTREATED HYPERTENSION AND SUBCLINICAL TARGET ORGAN DAMAGE

Left Ventricular Hypertrophy

The FHS demonstrated substantially higher risk of future clinical coronary heart disease in individuals with electrocardiographic (ECG) or echocardiographic left ventricular hypertrophy (LVH).[16,17] In early series of hypertensive patients (before the advent of drug therapy), ECG LVH was very commonly found at diagnosis (usually ~40% to 60% were affected), and a much higher prevalence was found during follow-up. Janeway, in his 1912 report, demonstrated that in patients with median SBP between 200 and 220 mm Hg LVH based on physical examination was present in 75.7% of patients.[18] The majority of patients with LVH (81%) had mild to moderate LVH on physical examination (defined as presence of one or two of the following three findings: enlarged area of cardiac percussion, downward displacement of cardiac apex, and upward lifting of cardiac impulse). However, severe LVH (defined as presence of the all three findings) was found in 22.8% of patients who died during follow-up, as compared with 7.8% of patients who were still alive (*p* < 0.001). In a series of 500 consecutive hypertensive patients (mean age 32 years) without target organ damage at baseline, Perera[19] reported in 1955 that during 20 years of average follow-up, 59% to 74% of patients developed LVH (detected by electrocardiogram or chest radiograph, respectively), after which they lived only 6 or 8 more years (on average). LVH was shown to correlate with levels of systolic and diastolic BP.[20,21] Another strong piece of evidence supporting the relationship between elevated BP and LVH comes from clinical trials, such as the Losartan Intervention For Endpoint (LIFE) reduction study, which showed that antihypertensive drug therapy reduces LVH, which in turn was associated with reduction in cardiovascular events.[22] Overall, LVH is more closely related to systolic rather than diastolic BP. It has been observed that patients with untreated isolated systolic hypertension had similar significant LVH as compared with patients with combined (elevation of both systolic and diastolic BP) hypertension despite 12 mm Hg lower mean BP in patients with isolated systolic hypertension.[23]

Albuminuria

Urinary albumin excretion (UAE) exceeding normal values (≥30 mg of albumin per gram of creatinine or ≥30 mg per 24 hours) in patients with hypertension is considered a marker of widespread endothelial dysfunction and is associated with other asymptomatic organ damage such as LVH, carotid intima thickness, hypertensive retinopathy, and higher risk of symptomatic cardiovascular disease (CVD).[24,25] Abnormal UAE is also associated with a higher risk of progression of renal dysfunction and the development of end-stage renal disease (ESRD) in patients with hypertension (HTN).[26,27] UAE, even within normal range, positively correlated with levels of BP.[28,29] Abnormal UAE is a common finding in patients with untreated hypertension, although prevalence varies across different cohorts. In a study involving 127 patients with untreated stage 1 hypertension (mean BP 150.1 ± 16.9/96.7 ± 8.5 mm Hg), 24.4% patients were found to have microalbuminuria (urine microalbumin ≥ 30 mg per 24 hours).[30] SBP and DBP measured by 24-hour ambulatory blood pressure monitoring (ABPM) best correlated with the presence of microalbuminuria.[30] Another study found even higher prevalence of microalbuminuria in up to 40% of untreated individuals with stage 1 hypertension.[31] However, a study involving a larger number (787) of untreated hypertensive individuals found lower rates of abnormal UAE at 6.7%.[32] Microalbuminuria in hypertensive individuals is associated with a faster rate of glomerular filtration rate (GFR) decline as compared with normal UAE. In a study involving 141 hypertensive individuals followed for 7 years, an adjusted analysis showed the rate of estimated GFR (eGFR) decline was faster in patients with microalbuminuria than was in those with normal UAE (decrease of 12.1 ± 2.77 mL per min versus 7.1 ± 0.88 mL per min, $p < 0.03$, respectively).[25]

Retinal Microvascular Changes

Among asymptomatic target organ damage, retinal microvascular changes are by far the most common finding in patients with untreated hypertension. Hypertensive retinopathy was evident by nonmydriatic retinography in up to 85% of 437 untreated hypertensive individuals.[33] In comparison, LVH is typically found in up to 44% of patients, followed by carotid intima thickness in 21.8%, microalbuminuria in 14.6%, and elevated serum creatinine (SCr) concentration in 11% of patients with untreated hypertension at the time of diagnosis.[34] Historically, hypertensive retinopathy played a very important role in the assessment of target organ damage in the era before antihypertensive drugs were available, but its incidence and progression have been reduced since the advent of antihypertensive therapy.[35] Papilledema or grade IV hypertensive retinopathy, the hallmark of malignant hypertension, was strongly associated with mortality in individuals with untreated hypertension.[36] However, even the lower grades of hypertensive retinopathy carry important prognostic implications and are associated with increased all-cause mortality and stroke.[37,38]

UNTREATED HYPERTENSION AND MORTALITY

As soon as routine BP measurements became available, it was quickly evident that individuals with even a mild elevation in BP and who remain asymptomatic suffered earlier death as compared with individuals with normal BP. Theodore C. Janeway published the earliest description of mortality among 458 individuals with hypertension in 1913.[18] His cohort was restricted to patients with SBP higher than 165 mm Hg; therefore, excluding observations in individuals with milder BP elevations, Janeway noted that 21.8% of patients died within 1 year of diagnosis of hypertension and the 5-year mortality rate was 42.5%. The median SBP in survivors was 200 mm Hg as compared with a median SBP of 220 mm Hg in individuals who died. The most common causes of death were cardiac insufficiency (32.6%), uremia (25%), cerebral apoplexy (15.8%), and angina (5.4%). Janeway analyzed the relationship of BP to the cause of death and found that patients dying from angina had the lowest median SBP, in the 175 to 180 mm Hg range; whereas patients dying from heart failure and uremia had a median SBP in the 215 to 220 mm Hg range. A higher median SBP was associated with death from cerebral apoplexy (225 to 230 mm Hg) and pulmonary edema (245 to 250 mm Hg). The median age of 50 to 59 years was similar in men and women dying from cardiac insufficiency and uremia, whereas median age of death from stroke was 10 years earlier in men (50 to 59 years), as compared with women (60 to 69 years).

The life insurance industry was the champion in detecting and reporting the adverse association between elevated levels of BP and mortality on a large population level, although analysis included a disproportionally higher number of middle-aged employed men. The Medical Impairment Study of 1929[39] involved information about approximately 1,200,000 policyholders and reported that the observed over-expected (O/E) mortality rates in all age groups (24 to ≥65 years) with SBP greater than 5 mm Hg over age-specific average SBP was 1.74, even though the average BP levels were below 140/90 mm

TABLE 18.1 All-Cause Mortality and Cardiac and Renal Outcomes in the Build and Blood Pressure Study 1959 and the Build and Blood Pressure Study 1971 to 1974

	BLOOD PRESSURE 138/83 TO 147/92 mm Hg	BLOOD PRESSURE 148/93 TO 167/97 mm Hg	BLOOD PRESSURE 168/93 TO 177/102 mm Hg
All-Cause Mortality (Excess Over the Standard)			
Build and Blood Pressure Study 1959	48%	Not reported	137%
Build and Blood Pressure Study 1971 to 1974	42%	93%	119%
Death From CAD (Excess Over the Standard)			
Build and Blood Pressure Study 1959	61%	Not reported	140%
Build and Blood Pressure Study 1971 to 1974	51%	137%	59%
Death From Cerebral Hemorrhage (Excess Over the Standard)			
Build and Blood Pressure Study 1959	131%	Not reported	480%
Build and Blood Pressure Study 1971 to 1974	62%	140%	321%
Death From Coronary Heart Disease (Excess Over the Standard)			
Build and Blood Pressure Study 1959	Not reported	Not reported	Not reported
Build and Blood Pressure Study 1971 to 1974	136%	312%	258%
Death From Renal Disease (Excess Over the Standard)			
Build and Blood Pressure Study 1959	160%	Not reported	350%
Build and Blood Pressure Study 1971 to 1974	21%	23%	250%

CAD, Coronary artery disease.

Hg. The O/E mortality ratio was further increased to 2.05, 2.65, and 3.84 in individuals with SBP 25 to 34, 34 to 45, and greater than 45 mm Hg above age-specific averages, respectively. The causes of death could not be evaluated in the whole group of individuals with elevated BP; however, a limited sample of 200 individuals with BP above average showed that the incidence of cerebrovascular death and coronary heart disease were 3.5 and 2.75 times higher than average, respectively. The findings of increased mortality with increasing BP levels were corroborated with minor differences in the Build and Blood Pressure Study of 1959 and 1971 to 1974.[40,41] In addition, the later two studies also demonstrated a gradual increase in O/E mortality with increases above average DBP. It was also possible to more granularly assess causes of death among hypertensive individuals. Individuals with a BP in range of 138/83 to 147/92 and 148/93 to 167/97 mm Hg experienced markedly higher than standard all-cause mortality, coronary artery disease, cerebral hemorrhage, hypertensive heart disease, and renal disease (Table 18.1).

John Fry published similar observations from the cohort of 704 individuals with untreated hypertension who were followed between 1949 and 1969.[42] The diagnosis of hypertension in his study was based on DBP of 100 or higher mm Hg. There was an inverse relation in the O/E death rates and age until age 70. Hypertensive individuals aged 30 to 39, 40 to 49, 50 to 59, 60 to 69, and older than 70 were 7.5, 4.9, 2.2, 1.15, 0.9 times more likely to die, as compared with corresponding ages in normotensive counterparts. Similar to Janeway's report, the most common causes of death were cardiac death (about 50%) and cerebrovascular death (25%).

The Veterans Administration (VA) Cooperative Trial investigating the role of lowering BP with antihypertensive medications in never-treated individuals with DBP 90 or higher mm Hg, had a control arm with placebo and no active treatment received, which provided important information about the natural history of untreated hypertension.[43,44] The results of that study were reported for two separate cohorts. The first manuscript described outcomes among 143 individuals with DBP between 115 and 129 mm Hg and randomized to antihypertensive treatment versus a placebo control group.[43] At the baseline, the average age of participants was 51 years and mean BP was 187/121 mm Hg. During an average of 15.7 months of follow-up, 27 major adverse CVD events occurred in untreated patients, including 4 deaths (3 from abdominal aortic aneurism catastrophe and 1 sudden death). The remaining events included accelerated hypertension with grade 3 and 4 hypertensive retinopathy, congestive heart failure (CHF), cerebrovascular accident (CVA), coronary artery disease (CAD), and 2 cases of renal failure. In contrast, in the treated group BP dropped from baseline 186/121 mm Hg to 143/91 mm Hg during 20.7 months of follow-up. There were no deaths and only 1 CVA in the treated group. The second cohort included 380 individuals with DBP between 90 and 114 mm Hg who were randomized to the active treatment arm (186 patients) or placebo (194 patients).[44] The average age of patients in the control group was 50.5 years and the mean BP was 162/104 mm Hg. During 3.9 years of follow-up, SBP and DBP increased by 4.2 mm Hg and 1.2 mm Hg, respectively, on placebo. Additionally, 20 patients (10.3%) developed persistently elevated DBP greater than 124 mm Hg. A total of 19 patients died in the control group. There were a total of 56 morbid events in the control group: 20 (10.3%) patients experienced cerebrovascular events, 11 (5.7%) patients had congestive heart failure, 13 (6.7%) patients had coronary artery disease events, and 3 (1.6%) patients experienced progressive renal disease. In contrast, BP fell in the treated patients from a mean baseline BP of 165/105 mm Hg by 27.2/17.4 mm Hg; 8 deaths were observed during an average of 3.7 years of follow-up (relative risk [RR] 0.44, $p < 0.001$). The number of morbid events was also significantly reduced with hypertension

treatment. CVA events occurred in 5 (2.7%) (RR 0.26, $p = 0.003$) and CAD in 5 (2.7%) (RR 0.40, $p = 0.066$) of treated patients, and no CHF or renal events were observed. Overall, the treatment of hypertension resulted in a 70% reduction of combined outcomes of all-cause mortality, uncontrolled hypertension, and morbid events among individuals with baseline DBP between 90 and 114 mm Hg. Of note, adverse events were more pronounced in untreated patients with higher baseline BP. For example, adverse events occurred in 15.3% of patients with SBP lower than 165 mm Hg, as compared with 42.7% in patients with baseline SBP 165 or higher mm Hg. Similarly, adverse events were higher in patients with higher baseline DBP: 25% of patients with baseline DBP 90 to 104 mm Hg had morbid events, compared with 31.8% of patients with DBP 105 to 114 mm Hg. It is not surprising, therefore, that the effect of BP reduction was also more pronounced in those with a higher baseline BP. For example, in patients with baseline SBP less than 165 mm Hg or DBP 90 to 104 mm Hg, the reduction in morbid events with hypertension treatment was 40% and 35%, respectively. A more pronounced effect of hypertension treatment was seen in patients with baseline SBP 165 or higher mm Hg or DBP between 105 and 114 mm Hg, where the reduction in morbid events with hypertension treatment was 64% and 75%, respectively. These data strongly support that high cardiovascular and renal complications and mortality are directly attributed to the elevated BP. Additionally, the outcomes of untreated hypertension varied with age in the VA Cooperative Trial.[45] Patients aged older than 60 years were more likely to die, have CVA or CHF; whereas patients younger than 50 years were more likely to develop progressive hypertension with DBP greater than 124 mm Hg or renal failure. However, the incidence of CAD did not appear to vary with age.

The Multiple Risk Factor Intervention Trial (MRFIT) evaluated the relationship between levels of systolic and diastolic BP and fatal coronary heart disease (CHD) among 356,222 men aged 35 to 57 years screened for, but not entered into, the randomized trial. During 6 years of follow-up there was a strong graded relationship between levels of SBP from less than 115 mm Hg to 175 or higher mm Hg and of DBP from less than 75 mm Hg to 115 or higher mm Hg.[46] The finding of an adverse association between isolated systolic HTN and CHD mortality is also an important contribution of this study.

The latest and perhaps one of the most powerful evidence of the relationship of elevated blood pressure and vascular mortality came with the publication of the Prospective Study Collaboration in 2002, which included information about causes of death among close to 1 million participants (958,074) from 61 individual prospective observational studies of BP and mortality.[47] Using time-dependent correlation, this meta-analysis demonstrated that usual (or long-term average) SBP and DBP strongly and directly correlated with stroke, ischemic heart disease, and other vascular-related mortality rates (Fig.18.4). In ages 40 to 69 years (irrespective of gender) each difference of 20 mm Hg in SBP or 10 mm Hg in DBP over BP 115/75 mm Hg was associated with over a two-fold increase in stroke death rates, two-fold increase in ischemic heart disease death rates, and other vascular death rates. Although proportional differences in death rates are lower in persons aged older than 80, given the higher incidence of vascular events, the annual difference in absolute risks of vascular death are greater in older age.

UNTREATED HYPERTENSION AND CLINICAL CARDIOVASCULAR DISEASE

It is important to highlight that it may be difficult to discern pure effect of untreated hypertension on CVD, as patients with elevated BP often have other concomitant cardiovascular risk factors. Nevertheless, similar to all-cause mortality, there is undisputable observational evidence supporting a direct link

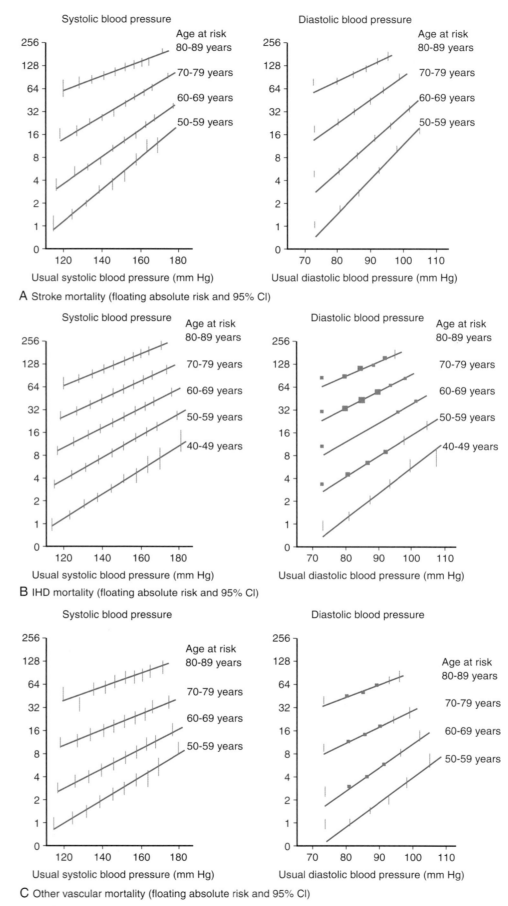

FIG. 18.4 Cardiovascular mortality rates in each decade of age versus usual blood pressure at the start of that decade. (A) Stroke mortality rate in each decade of age versus usual blood pressure at the start of each decade. (B) Ischemic heart disease mortality rate in each decade of age versus usual blood pressure at the start of each decade. (C) Other vascular mortality rate in each decade of age versus usual blood pressure at the start of each decade. (*Adapted from Lewington S, Clarke R, Qizilbash N, Peto R, Collins R, Prospective Studies Collaboration. Age-specific relevance of usual blood pressure to vascular mortality: a meta-analysis of individual data for one million adults in 61 prospective studies. Lancet. 2002;360:1903-1913.*)

between untreated hypertension and CVD. In addition, the improvement of cardiovascular outcomes by antihypertensive treatment further strengthens the association between CVD and hypertension.

Coronary Heart Disease

Although, CHD prevalence varies by age, number, and severity of total risk factors and geographic regions, hypertension is by far the most important hazard for CHD because of its high population-wide prevalence.[48] Overall, the incidence of nonfatal CHD events is up to two-fold higher than fatal CHD events. There have been reported differences among those studied early as to whether systolic or diastolic, or pulse pressure (PP) correlates better with CHD. A detailed analysis of the FHS demonstrated that the association between different BP measures varies at different ages.[49] For example, in persons younger than 50 years, every 10 mm Hg rise in SBP clearly predicted CHD events (hazard ratio [HR] 1.14, 95% confidence interval [CI] 1.06 to 1.24). In the same age group, DBP was an even stronger predictor of future CHD (HR 1.34, 95% CI 1.18 to 1.51, for every 10 mm Hg increment); whereas the association between PP and CHD was not significant. Among persons 50 to 59 and older than 59 years, only SBP (HR 1.08, $p = 0.01$ and 1.17, $p < 0.001$ for the two age categories, respectively) and PP (1.11, $p = 0.02$ and 1.24, $p < 0.001$, for the two age categories, respectively) predicted future CHD.[49] Similarly, MRFIT showed independent associations for both SBP and DBP at baseline with subsequent CHD mortality, although SBP was a stronger predictor than DBP.[50]

Given the strong relationship between BP and CHD, BP has been incorporated into CHD risk calculators. For example, the Third Report of the National Cholesterol Education Program (NCEP) calculator indicated that an untreated SBP greater than 160 mm Hg does not increase the 10-year risk of CHD in a very young and low-risk man or woman, but does increase the risk by 16% in an older woman with other risk factors. In high-risk people, an untreated SBP between 140 and 159 mm Hg increases the 10-year risk of CHD by more than 6% (in a man) or more than 13% (in a woman).[51] More recently, the 2013 American College of Cardiology/American Heart Association (ACC/AHA) Guideline on the Assessment of Cardiovascular Risk[52] stated that in non-Hispanic White adults aged 45 to 50 treated hypertension or untreated SBP 160 or higher mm Hg or DBP 100 or higher mm Hg is a major risk factor for CHD and translates into lifetime risk of CHD of 39% to 50%. Untreated SBP 140 to 160 mm Hg or DBP 90 to 100 mm Hg, and SBP 120 to 139 mm Hg or DBP 80 to 89 mm Hg, even in the absence of diabetes and smoking, carry 39% to 46% and 26% to 36% lifetime risk of CHD, respectively.[52]

Additional proof for the association between elevated BP and CHD comes from hypertension treatment clinical trials with placebo or no treatment arms. Fig. 18.5 shows, on the x-axis, the wide range of absolute risk for CHD (calculated as CHD events per 1000 patient-years of follow-up) across 26 clinical trials with a placebo/no treatment arm, in which each randomized arm included at least 50 subjects who experienced a CHD event (CHD death or nonfatal myocardial infarction). The absolute risk of a CHD event varied greatly in these studies, probably because they enrolled widely different populations. The number of CHD events prevented (per 1000 patient-years of treatment) significantly correlated ($r = 0.74$, $p < 0.001$) with the absolute risk of CHD events in the untreated group (i.e., those with an unaltered natural history of untreated hypertension). This relationship has important economic implications, as those at highest absolute risk derive the most benefit from therapy. The correlation was unchanged when only the 15 trials that used no active drug therapy in the placebo group were analyzed separately ($r = 0.72$, $p < 0.001$).

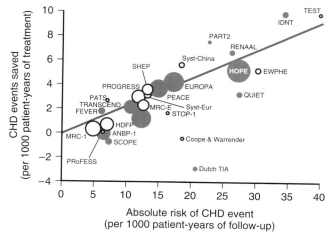

FIG. 18.5 Correlation between the absolute risk of a coronary heart disease (CHD) and the number of CHD events prevented per 1000 patient-years of treatment. Correlation ($r = 0.74$, $p < 0.001$ unweighted, or $r = 0.78$, $p < 0.001$, weighted for number of events) between the absolute risk of a CHD event (calculated per 1000 patient-years of follow up) in 26 clinical trials involving placebo or no treatment only (open circles, $n = 15$) or placebo or no treatment atop other antihypertensive drugs, and the number of CHD events prevented per 1000 patient-years of treatment. The values on the x-axis denote the wide variability of the natural history of (untreated) hypertension in control groups in clinical trials. The circles are drawn encompassing an area proportional to the number of CHD events in the trial. *ADVANCE*, Action in Diabetes and Vascular disease: preterAx and diamicroN Controlled Evaluation; *ANBP-1*, Australian National Blood Pressure trial no. 1; *Coope & Warrender*, Coope and Warrender study; *Dutch TIA*, Dutch Transient Ischemic Attack trial; *EUROPA*, EUropean Reduction Of cardiac events with Perindopril in stable coronary Artery disease; *EWPHE*, European Working Party on Hypertension in the Elderly; *FEVER*, Felodipine EVEnt Reduction trial; *HDFP*, Hypertension Detection and Follow-up Program; *HOPE*, Heart Outcomes Prevention Evaluation; *IDNT*, Irbesartan Diabetes Nephropathy Trial; *MRC-E*, Medical Research Council Trial in Older Patients; *MRC-1*, Medical Research Council Trial (in mild hypertension); *PART2*, Prevention of Atherosclerosis with Ramipril Trial no. 2; *PATS*, Post-stroke Antihypertensive Treatment Study; *PEACE*, Prevention of Events with Angiotensin-Converting Enzyme inhibition; *PROGRESS*, Perindopril pROtection aGainst REcurrent Stroke Study; *PRoFESS*, Prevention Regimen For Effectively avoiding Second Strokes; *QUIET*, QUinapril Ischemic Events Trial; *RENAAL*, Reduction of Endpoints in Non-Insulin Dependent Diabetes Mellitus with the Angiotensin II Antagonist Losartan trial; *SCOPE*, Study on COgnition and Prognosis in the Elderly; *SHEP*, Systolic Hypertension in the Elderly Program; *STOP*, Swedish Trial in Old Patients with hypertension no. 1; *Syst-China*, Systolic hypertension in China trial; *Syst-Eur*, Systolic hypertension in Europe trial; *TEST*, TEnormin after Stroke and TIA; *TRANSCEND*, Telmisartan RaNdomised assessment Study in aCe-iNtolerant subjects with cardiovascular Disease.

Stroke

The association between hard pulse disease and apoplexy was known for millennia. This correlation was unequivocally confirmed with the institution of routine BP measurements and further strengthened by data from antihypertensive clinical trials demonstrating reduction in stroke rates with improved BP control. Overall, 80% to 87% of strokes related to hypertension are ischemic, 10% are hemorrhagic, and the remaining are subarachnoid hemorrhage. In a study conducted in the era of untreated hypertension (study initiated 1965) and involving 2772 individuals aged 65 to 74 years, the incidence of any stroke and ischemic stroke progressively increased with increasing baseline SBP and DBP during 3 years of follow-up.[53] For example, age-adjusted, sex-adjusted, and race-adjusted rates of new total and ischemic strokes were 47/1000 and 11/1000, respectively, in individuals with SBP less than130 mm Hg, 57/1000 and 19/1000, respectively, in individuals with SBP 130 to 143 mm Hg, 65/1000 and 20.5/1000, respectively, in individuals with SBP 144 to 179 mm Hg, and further rose to 135/1000 and 36/1000, respectively, in individuals with SBP 180 or higher mm Hg. The age-adjusted, sex-adjusted, and race-adjusted rates of new total and ischemic strokes in relationship to baseline DBP were 50.5/1000 and 22.5/1000, respectively, in individuals with DBP less than 75 mm Hg, 76/1000 and 49/1000, respectively, in individuals with DBP 75 to 84 mm Hg, 79/1000 and 45/1000, respectively, in individuals with

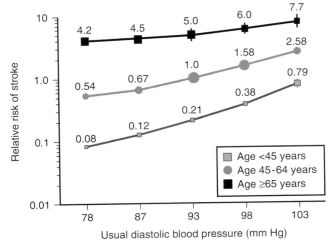

FIG. 18.6 The relationship of fatal or nonfatal stroke with usual diastolic blood pressure and age. Relative risk of fatal or nonfatal stroke in 448,415 persons followed for an average of 13 years, during which time 13,397 fatal or nonfatal strokes were observed. The normalized relative risk of 1.0 was assigned to the middle-aged (45 to 64 years old) individuals with usual diastolic blood pressure of 91 mm Hg. Note the exponential scale on the y-axis. Symbols encompass area in proportion to the number of strokes for each group; standard deviations are shown when they extend beyond the symbol. *(Data from Cholesterol, diastolic blood pressure, and stroke: 13,000 strokes in 450,000 people in 45 prospective cohorts. Prospective studies collaboration. Lancet. 1995;346(8991-8992):1647-1653.)*

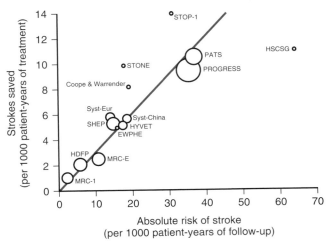

FIG. 18.7 Correlation between the absolute risk of stroke and the number of stroke events prevented per 1000 patient-years of treatment. Correlation ($r = 0.76$, $p < 0.001$ unweighted, or $r = 0.82$, $p < 0.001$, weighted for number of strokes) between the absolute risk of stroke (calculated per 1000 patient-years of follow up) in 15 clinical trials involving effective antihypertensive therapy versus placebo or no treatment, and the number of strokes prevented per 1000 patient-years of treatment. The values on the x-axis denote the wide, 28-fold variability of the natural history of (untreated) hypertension progressing to stroke in control groups in clinical trials. The circles are drawn encompassing an area proportional to the number of strokes in the trial. The acronyms of the trials are identical to those in Fig. 5, with the addition of the following: *HSCSG*, Hypertension-Stroke Cooperative Study Group; *HYVET*, Hypertension in the Very Elderly Trial; *STONE*, Shanghai Trial Of Nifedipine in the Elderly.

DBP 85 to 94 mm Hg, and further rose to 95/1000 and 69/1000, respectively, in individuals with DBP 95 or higher mm Hg.[53]

Multiple studies and meta-analyses found similar positive associations between increasing levels of BP and stroke risks.[54] For each 10 mm Hg increase in usual DBP, the risk of stroke increased by 84%. The effect was particularly pronounced in younger people, although a significant trend also exists up to 80 years of age. There were no significant differences between men or women, although in African Americans the trend was even stronger. Similarly, the FHS showed that during a 36-year follow-up of the original FHS cohort, hypertension (defined then as BP ≥160/95 mm Hg) was associated with a highly significant 3.8-fold age-adjusted biennial risk of stroke for men (12.4 versus 3.3 events per 100) and a 2.6-fold increase for women (6.2 versus 2.4 events per 100). Interestingly, in the FHS, the absolute risk for stroke was about 3.5-fold lower in hypertensive men and women than for CHD; the increment for CHD over stroke in nonhypertensive men was about 6.8-fold, and in women about four-fold.

Fig. 18.6 summarizes the findings regarding the relationship of fatal or nonfatal stroke with BP and age.[55] A 1990 meta-analysis of the effects of antihypertensive drug therapy showed nearly all of the expected reduction in stroke (−46% ± 2%), as compared with the expected improvement based on epidemiologic studies (42% ± 6%).[56] The reduction in stroke events with hypertension treatment was especially pronounced in earlier trials because of the presence of a placebo arm as a comparator group and partially as a result of much higher levels of BP in enrolled participants.

In the VA Cooperative Trial that included 143 individuals with DBP between 115 and 129 mm Hg who were randomized to antihypertensive treatment versus a control group receiving no treatment (placebo), there were four strokes and one transient ischemic attack among men assigned to placebo, and only one nondebilitating stroke in the actively treated group.[43] Although this was not analyzed separately at the time, there was an impressive 81% relative risk reduction for stroke or transient ischemic attack in that study. In the second VA Cooperative Trial that enrolled patients with DBPs between 90 and 114 mm Hg, there was a significant reduction in stroke (20 versus 5, relative risk reduction 74%, 95%

CI, 32% to 90%).[44] The U.S. Public Health Service Cooperative study, which enrolled 389 "mildly" hypertensive people, also reported a reduction in stroke risk (6 versus 1, $p = 0.13$); however, its results did not reach statistical significance possibly from confounding by treatment crossovers attributed to uncontrolled hypertension in many originally assigned to placebo patients and small sample size.[57]

Fig. 18.7 shows the large variability in stroke risk (along the x-axis) for individuals enrolled in 15 trials comparing effective antihypertensive drug therapy with only placebo or no treatment in the control group. Trials that experienced very little BP difference between the two randomized groups (e.g., trials in which either other antihypertensive drugs were allowed, or beta-blockers were given to normotensive people) were excluded from this analysis. The highest-risk patients were those with a previous history of neurologic events (e.g., Perindopril Protection Against Recurrent Stroke Study [PROGRESS], Poststroke Antihypertensive Treatment Study [PATS], Hypertension-Stroke Cooperative Study Group) or with advanced age (e.g., Swedish Trial in Old Patients with Hypertension [STOP-1]). In these high-risk people, antihypertensive drug therapy is quite effective and even cost-effective in preventing a stroke, as shown by the corresponding values on the y-axis (strokes prevented per 1000 patient-years of treatment). On the contrary, very low-risk people, such as those in the first Medical Research Council trial on mild hypertension, had only one stroke prevented for every 850 patients treated for a year.

Heart Failure

Persistently elevated BP is the major risk factor for heart failure, and in the classic paradigm of hypertensive heart disease the development of heart failure starts with elevated BP leading to LVH with concentric hypertrophy that is later followed by dilated or "burnt out" left ventricle.[58] In early reports of untreated patients with very high BPs (SBP >200 mm Hg), the signs of heart failure were common. For example, in his 1912 report of 870 untreated individuals with median BP 200 to 220 mmHg, Janeway observed that 42.7%, 11.3%, and 3.0% of these individuals experienced dyspnea, lower extremity edema, and pulmonary edema, respectively.[18] Additionally, Janeway attributed 32.6% of all deaths in his cohort to progressive heart failure.

The FHS provided strong evidence that hypertension is the major risk factor for heart failure.[59] Among 5192 men and women during 16 years of follow up, 55% of individuals who developed heart failure (HF) had hypertension, and both SPB and DBP had a strong graded relationship to the development of heart failure. Compared with SBP, neither DBP nor PP was a better predictor of new heart failure. Heart failure carried a poor prognosis with 50% of patients dying within 5 years of the onset of symptoms. The lifetime risk for heart failure in the Framingham Offspring Study[60] was 21% for men and 20.3% for women at 40 years of age, but it doubled if the baseline BP (in 1971) was 160/90 or higher mm Hg, as opposed to less than 140/90 mm Hg. These data may have been confounded by antihypertensive treatment (which was widely available in Framingham beginning in the mid-1960s), so the natural history of untreated hypertension might result in a different lifetime risk.

Further proof of the direct relationship between untreated hypertension and heart failure comes from clinical trials of antihypertensive medications. In the VA Cooperative Trial of hypertension treatment among individuals with DBP 115 or higher mm Hg, during a mean 15.7 months of follow up, no heart failure events were observed in the treated group as compared with two episodes in the placebo group.[43] In the other VA Cooperative Trial cohort among individuals with DBP 90 to 114 mm Hg, during an average 3.9 years of follow up 11 episodes of heart failure occurred in the 194 patients originally given placebo, and heart failure did not occur in the drug-treated group.[44] This corresponds to a significant relative risk reduction of 95% (95% CI: 20% to 99%). Interestingly, heart failure events overall were infrequently reported in clinical trials that compared active antihypertensive drugs with placebo/no treatment, although many of these trials did not include HF in their primary outcomes. The largest number of newly diagnosed patients (150) with HF were seen in the Systolic Hypertension in the Elderly Program (SHEP),[61] in which 102 of 2371 patients originally given placebo developed heart failure over an average of 4.5 years of follow up (or roughly 24 events/1000 patient-years of follow up). In comparison, the group given chlorthalidone (and atenolol or reserpine, if needed) enjoyed a relative risk reduction of 52%. A recent meta-analysis of 222,851 participants from 43 individual randomized controlled trials (RCTs) showed that every 10 mm Hg reduction in SBP was associated with a 28% reduction in the risk of heart failure (RR 0.72, 95% CI 0.67 to 0.78).[62]

Note that in the era of hypertension treatment the overall incidence of heart failure is actually rising. Between 1970 and 1974 and 1990 and 1994, age-adjusted and gender-adjusted incidence of heart failure increased by 14% (95% CI 2 to 28%). This rise was mainly seen in older adults.[63] It is possible that antihypertensive therapy retards the development of heart failure without fully eliminating its risk.

Hypertension and Renal Disease

The link between hypertension and renal dysfunction was first suggested in the 19th century before routine BP measurements were available. In the era of untreated hypertension, most observations linking elevated BP and renal disease came from individually hospitalized patients with malignant hypertension.[36] The combination of malignant hypertension and uremia typically carried a grave prognosis with more than 90% of patients dying within 1 year of the diagnosis of renal dysfunction.[64]

Overall, there is ample evidence linking elevated BP and ESRD, the terminal stage of chronic kidney disease (CKD).[65-67] Nonetheless, there are fewer studies that investigated the association between BP and earlier manifestations of renal disease in individuals with untreated hypertension, because

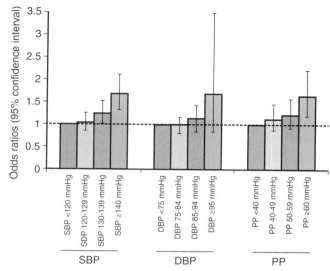

FIG. 18.8 The association between baseline measurement of blood pressure and the development of renal dysfunction during 14 years of follow up. *DBP,* Diastolic blood pressure; *PP,* pulse pressure; *SBP,* systolic blood pressure. *(Adapted from Schaeffner ES, Kurth T, Bowman TS, Gelber RP, Gaziano JM. Blood pressure measures and risk of chronic kidney disease in men.* Nephrol Dial Transplan. *2008;23:1246-1251.)*

monitoring of albuminuria and creatinine were not included in earlier observational studies. Therefore, we mostly rely on the information from later cohort studies when at least some participants were already receiving antihypertensive therapy, as well as from RCTs that included placebo and antihypertensive treatment arms.

The Clue Study was an observational study based on a community cancer screening program that enrolled 1399 mostly Caucasian participants aged 45 to 60 years in 1974 (mean standard deviation [SD]) BP 131(16)/83(10) mm Hg and followed these individuals for the development of elevated SCr between 1986 and 1989.[68] There was a linear association between levels of both systolic and diastolic BP in 1974 and SCr at the 1986 to 1989 follow-up period. Overall, age-adjusted, gender-adjusted, and lean-body-mass-adjusted association was stronger for DBP (change in SCr for each 20 mm Hg increase in DBP was 1.9 μmol/L [95% CI 0.4 to 3.4]) than for SBP (change in SCr for each 20 mm Hg increase in SBP was 0.9 μmol/L [95% CI –0.1 to 1.9]). Individuals with DBP within third and fourth quartiles were at two-fold and three-fold, respectively, higher risk for the development of abnormal SCr (SCr >115 μmol/L [1.31mg/dL] for males and 97 μmol/L [1.10 mg/dL for females]) during 12 to 15 years of follow up, as compared with individuals whose DBP was in the first quartile. Similarly, individuals with SBP in the fourth quartile had 2.2-fold higher risk of developing abnormal SCr, as compared with SBP in the first quartile.

The Physician Health Study (PHS)[69] evaluated the association between baseline BP and the development of renal dysfunction defined as eGFR less than 60 mL per minute per 1.73m[2] among 8093 participants aged 40 to 84 years old. At baseline, 26.5%, 63.1%, and 10.4% had SBP in normal (<120 mm Hg), prehypertensive (120 to 139 mm Hg), and hypertensive range (≥140 mm Hg) range, respectively. During 14 years of follow up, there was a graded and statistically significant increase in risk of the development of renal dysfunction with rising SBP and PP. The association between DBP and renal outcome was also present; however, it did not reach statistical significance (Fig. 18.8).

The results of secondary analysis of the SHEP[70] study among 2181 men and women aged 65 and older were essentially similar. The adjusted RR (95% CI) of the development of renal dysfunction defined as SCr increase by more than 0.4 mg per dL over a 5-year period were 2.44 (1.67 to 3.56), 1.29 (0.87

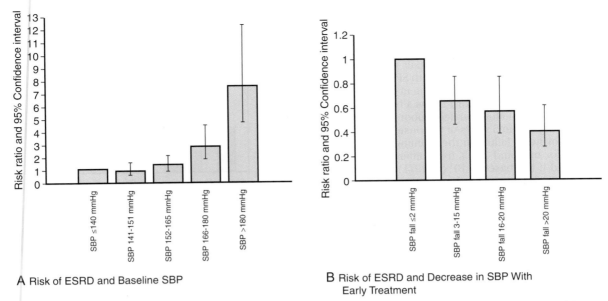

FIG. 18.9 The association between baseline measurements of blood pressure and the development of end-stage renal disease during 13.9 years of follow up. *SBP,* Systolic blood pressure. *(Adapted from Perry HM, Jr., Miller JP, Fornoff JR, et al. Early predictors of 15-year end-stage renal disease in hypertensive patients. Hypertension. 1995;25(4 Pt 1):587-594.)*

to 1.91), and 1.80 (1.21 to 2.66) for the highest versus lowest quartiles of SBP, DBP, and PP, respectively.

Among 10,940 patients in the Hypertension Detection and Follow-Up Program,[71] 99 in the Stepped Care group, and 101 in the Referred Care group developed renal insufficiency defined as SCr 2.0 or higher mg per dL, and a 25% increment over the baseline value during average follow up of 5 years. Although, the incidence of renal insufficiency increased with higher baseline DBP, this association did not reach statistical significance. Overall, in most of the clinical trials that had a placebo or no treatment group, renal failure and renal insufficiency were uncommon, because nearly all studies used an opt-out threshold, with all patients whose BP exceeded a very high level (typically 200/120 mm Hg) being removed from their originally assigned treatment arm and given open-label effective antihypertensive drugs.

The data from the MRFIT and the Hypertension Clinics in the U.S. Department of Veterans Affairs Medical System consistently showed a significant correlation of both SBP and DBP with the future risk of ESRD.[66,67] Among 332,544 participants aged 35 to 47 years in the MRFIT study, 814 (0.25%) developed ESRD during 16 years of follow up. In an analysis adjusted to baseline variables (demographic, comorbidities, and baseline SCr and proteinuria), there was a strong, graded association with both SBP and DBP.[66] The adjusted risk of ESRD for those with BP 210/120 or higher mm Hg was 22.1 times the risk for those with BP less than 120/80 mm Hg. In the VA Hypertension Screening and Treatment Program (HSTP), 11,912 men (mean [SD] age 52.5 [10.2] years, mean [SD] BP 154.3[19.0]/100.8 [9.8] mm Hg) were followed from 1974 to 1976 for an average of 13.9 years, and 245 (2.1%) of participants developed ESRD.[67] In the adjusted analysis for baseline demographic and clinical variables, there was a significant association between ESRD risk and pretreatment SBP (Fig.18.9). Additionally, the risk of ESRD was significantly reduced with successful reduction in BP during early treatment.

SUMMARY

Elevated BP is a strong, graded, and continuous risk factor for major adverse cardiovascular disease and mortality, as well as renal disease. The natural history of untreated hypertension varies in different age groups and can be modified by

degrees of BP elevation, life style factors, drug treatment for hypertension, and by the presence of additional risk factors. Nevertheless, hypertension, because of its high prevalence, is considered to be the major risk factor for all-cause mortality, cardiovascular morbidity and mortality, and ESRD. Although, treatment of hypertension does not eradicate all of its associated complications, therapeutic reduction of BP is associated with a decline in the risk of most cardiovascular events, in proportion to the individual's absolute risk before treatment. This is the major reason for advocating treatment of all risk factors, and for focusing attention on at least lifestyle treatment of individuals with prehypertension, who may well benefit from preventing or postponing a transition to frank hypertension.

References

1. Esunge PM. From blood pressure to hypertension: the history of research. *J Royal Society Med.* 1991;84:621.
2. R. B. Tabular view of the morbid appearances in 100 cases connected with albuminous urine. *Guy's Hosp Rep.* 1836;1:338-379.
3. Mahomed FA. The etiology of Bright's disease and the prealbuminuric stage. *Med Chir Trans.* 1874;57:197-228.
4. Gull WW, Sutton HG. On the pathology of the morbid state commonly called chronic Bright's disease with contracted kidney, ("Arterio-capillary fibrosis."). *Med Chir Trans.* 1872;55:273-330.
5. Gowers WR. The state of the arteries in Bright's disease. *BMJ.* 1876;2:743-745.
6. Riva-Rocci S. *Gazz Med Torino.* 1896;47:981-1001.
7. Korotkoff NS. *Izvestuya Imperatorskoi Voenno-Meditsinkoy Akademii (Rep Imper Mil-Med Acca St Peterburg).* 1905;11:365-367.
8. Moser M. Historical perspectives on the management of hypertension. *J Clin Hypertens.* 2006;8(8 Suppl 2):15-20. quiz 39.
9. Harrison TR. *Principles of Internal Medicine.* New York, NY: Blakiston Division, 1950.
10. Chobanian AV, Bakris GL, Black HR, et al. The Seventh Report of the Joint National Committee on prevention, detection, evaluation, and treatment of high blood pressure: the JNC 7 report. *JAMA.* 2003;289:2560-2572.
11. Burt VL, Cutler JA, Higgins M, et al. Trends in the prevalence, awareness, treatment, and control of hypertension in the adult US population. Data from the health examination surveys, 1960 to 1991. *Hypertension.* 1995;26:60-69.
12. US Health and Nutrition Examination Survey, 1971-1974. Advance data, vital health statistics of the National Center of Health Statistics. 1976;1.
13. Leitschuh M, Cupples LA, Kannel W, Gagnon D, Chobanian A. High-normal blood pressure progression to hypertension in the Framingham Heart Study. *Hypertension.* 1991;17:22-27.
14. Tirosh A, Afek A, Rudich A, et al. Progression of normotensive adolescents to hypertensive adults: a study of 26,980 teenagers. *Hypertension.* 2010;56:203-209.
15. Julius S, Nesbitt SD, Egan BM, et al. Feasibility of treating prehypertension with an angiotensin-receptor blocker. *N Engl J Med.* 2006;354:1685-1697.
16. Kannel WB, Gordon T, Castelli WP, Margolis JR. Electrocardiographic left ventricular hypertrophy and risk of coronary heart disease. The Framingham study. *Ann Intern Med.* 1970;72:813-822.
17. Levy D, Garrison RJ, Savage DD, Kannel WB, Castelli WP. Prognostic implications of echocardiographically determined left ventricular mass in the Framingham Heart Study. *N Engl J Med.* 1990;322:1561-1566.
18. Janeway TC. A clinical study of hypertensive cardiovascular disease. *Arch Intern Med.* 1913;12:755-798.
19. Perera GA. Hypertensive vascular disease; description and natural history. *J Chronic Dis.* 1955;1:33-42.

20. Feola M, Boffano GM, Procopio M, Reynaud S, Allemano P, Rizzi G. Ambulatory 24-hour blood pressure monitoring: correlation between blood pressure variability and left ventricular hypertrophy in untreated hypertensive patients. *J Ital Cardiol*. 1998;28:38-44.
21. Levy D, Anderson KM, Savage DD, Kannel WB, Christiansen JC, Castelli WP. Echocardiographically detected left ventricular hypertrophy: prevalence and risk factors. The Framingham Heart Study. *Ann Intern Med*. 1988;108:7-13.
22. Dahlof B, Devereux RB, Kjeldsen SE, et al. Cardiovascular morbidity and mortality in the Losartan Intervention For Endpoint reduction in hypertension study (LIFE): a randomised trial against atenolol. *Lancet*. 2002;359:995-1003.
23. Papademetriou V, Devereux RB, Narayan P, et al. Similar effects of isolated systolic and combined hypertension on left ventricular geometry and function: the LIFE Study. *Am J Hypertens*. 2001;14(8 Pt 1):768-774.
24. Pontremoli R, Leoncini G, Ravera M, et al. Microalbuminuria, cardiovascular, and renal risk in primary hypertension. *J Am Soc Nephrol*. 2002;13(Suppl 3):S169-S172.
25. Bigazzi R, Bianchi S, Baldari D, Campese VM. Microalbuminuria predicts cardiovascular events and renal insufficiency in patients with essential hypertension. *J Hypertens*. 1998;16:1325-1333.
26. Chua DC, Bakris GL. Is proteinuria a plausible target of therapy? *Curr Hypertens Rep*. 2004;6:177-181.
27. Peterson JC, Adler S, Burkart JM, et al. Blood pressure control, proteinuria, and the progression of renal disease. The Modification of Diet in Renal Disease Study. *Ann Intern Med*. 1995;123:754-762.
28. Gerber LM, Shmukler C, Alderman MH. Differences in urinary albumin excretion rate between normotensive and hypertensive, white and nonwhite subjects. *Arch Intern Med*. 1992;152:373-377.
29. Parving HH, Mogensen CE, Jensen HA, Evrin PE. Increased urinary albumin-excretion rate in benign essential hypertension. *Lancet*. J1974;1:1190-1192.
30. Redon J, Liao Y, Lozano JV, Miralles A, Pascual JM, Cooper RS. Ambulatory blood pressure and microalbuminuria in essential hypertension: role of circadian variability. *J Hypertens*. 1994;12:947-953.
31. Bigazzi R, Bianchi S, Campese VM, Baldari G. Prevalence of microalbuminuria in a large population of patients with mild to moderate essential hypertension. *Nephron*. 1992;61:94-97.
32. Pontremoli R, Sofia A, Ravera M, et al. Prevalence and clinical correlates of microalbuminuria in essential hypertension: the MAGIC Study. Microalbuminuria: a genoa investigation on complications. *Hypertension*. 1997;30:1135-1143.
33. Cuspidi C, Meani S, Salerno M, et al. Retinal microvascular changes and target organ damage in untreated essential hypertensives. *J Hypertens*. 2004;22:2095-2102.
34. Papazafiropoulou A, Skliros E, Sotiropoulos A, et al. Prevalence of target organ damage in hypertensive subjects attending primary care: C.V.P.C. study (epidemiological cardiovascular study in primary care). *BMC Fam Pract*. 2011;12:75.
35. Wong TY, Klein R, Klein BE, Tielsch JM, Hubbard L, Nieto FJ. Retinal microvascular abnormalities and their relationship with hypertension, cardiovascular disease, and mortality. *Surv Ophthalmol*. 2001;46:59-80.
36. Keith NM, Wagener HP, Kernohan, JW. The syndrome of malignant hypertension. *Arch Int Med*. 1928;41:141-188.
37. Wong TY, Klein R, Couper DJ, et al. Retinal microvascular abnormalities and incident stroke: the Atherosclerosis Risk in Communities Study. *Lancet*. 2001;358:1134-1140.
38. Wong TY, Klein R, Nieto FJ, et al. Retinal microvascular abnormalities and 10-year cardiovascular mortality: a population-based case-control study. *Ophthalmology*. 2003;110:933-940.
39. The Actuarial Society of America and the Association of Life Insurance Medical Directors: medical Impairment Study, 1929. New York, NY. 1931.
40. Build and Blood Pressure Study. *Society of Actuaries. vol I and II*. 2nd ed. Chicago, IL. 1959.
41. New Build and Blood Pressure Study 1971-1974. *Record of Society of Actuaries*. 1978;4:847-866.
42. Fry J. Natural history of hypertension. A case for selective non-treatment. *Lancet*. 1974;2:431-433.
43. Effects of treatment on morbidity in hypertension. Results in patients with diastolic blood pressures averaging 115 through 129 mm Hg. *JAMA*. 1967;202:1028-1034.
44. Effects of treatment on morbidity in hypertension. II. Results in patients with diastolic blood pressures averaging 90 through 114 mm Hg. *JAMA*. 1970;213:1143-1152.
45. Effects of treatment on morbidity in hypertension. 3. Influence of age, diastolic pressure, and prior cardiovascular disease; further analysis of side effects. *Circulation*. 1972;45:991-1004.
46. Stamler J, Neaton JD, Wentworth DN. Blood pressure (systolic and diastolic) and risk of fatal coronary heart disease. *Hypertension*. 1989;13(5 Suppl):I2-12.
47. Lewington S, Clarke R, Qizilbash N, Peto R, Collins R, Prospective Studies C. Age-specific relevance of usual blood pressure to vascular mortality: a meta-analysis of individual data for one million adults in 61 prospective studies. *Lancet*. 2002;360:1903-1913.
48. Stokes J, 3rd Kannel WB, Wolf PA, D'Agostino RB, Cupples LA. Blood pressure as a risk factor for cardiovascular disease. The Framingham Study–30 years of follow-up. *Hypertension*. 1989;13(5 Suppl):I13-I18.
49. Franklin SS, Larson MG, Khan SA, et al. Does the relation of blood pressure to coronary heart disease risk change with aging? The Framingham Heart Study. *Circulation*. 2001;103:1245-1249.
50. Neaton JD. Wentworth D. Serum cholesterol, blood pressure, cigarette smoking, and death from coronary heart disease. Overall findings and differences by age for 316,099 white men. Multiple Risk Factor Intervention Trial Research Group. *Arch Int Med*. 1992;152:56-64.
51. Expert Panel on Detection E, Treatment of High Blood Cholesterol in A. Executive Summary of The Third Report of The National Cholesterol Education Program (NCEP) Expert Panel on Detection, Evaluation, And Treatment of High Blood Cholesterol In Adults (Adult Treatment Panel III). *JAMA*. 16 2001;285:2486-2497.
52. Goff DC Jr, Lloyd-Jones DM, Bennett G, et al. American College of Cardiology/American Heart Association Task Force on Practice Guidelines. 2013 ACC/AHA guideline on the assessment of cardiovascular risk: a report of the American College of Cardiology/American Heart Association Task Force on Practice Guidelines. *Circulation*. 2014;129(25 Suppl 2):S49-73.
53. Shekelle RB, Ostfeld AM, Klawans HL, Jr. Hypertension and risk of stroke in an elderly population. *Stroke*. 1974;5:71-75.
54. Voko Z, Bots ML, Hofman A, Koudstaal PJ, Witteman JC, Breteler MM. J-shaped relation between blood pressure and stroke in treated hypertensives. *Hypertension*. 1999;34:1181-1185.
55. Cholesterol, diastolic blood pressure, and stroke: 13,000 strokes in 450,000 people in 45 prospective cohorts. Prospective studies collaboration. *Lancet*. 1995;346:1647-1653.
56. Collins R, Peto R, MacMahon S, et al. Blood pressure, stroke, and coronary heart disease. Part 2, Short-term reductions in blood pressure: overview of randomised drug trials in their epidemiological context. *Lancet*. 1990;335:827-838.
57. Smith WM. Treatment of mild hypertension: results of a ten-year intervention trial. *Circulation Res*. 1977;40(5 Suppl 1):I98-105.
58. Drazner MH. The progression of hypertensive heart disease. *Circulation*. 2011;123:327-334.
59. Kannel WB, Castelli WP, McNamara PM, McKee PA, Feinleib M. Role of blood pressure in the development of congestive heart failure. The Framingham study. *New Eng J Med*. 1972;287:781-787.
60. Lloyd-Jones DM, Larson MG, Leip EP, et al. Lifetime risk for developing congestive heart failure: the Framingham Heart Study. *Circulation*. 2002;106:3068-3072.
61. Kostis JB, Davis BR, Cutler J, et al. Prevention of heart failure by antihypertensive drug treatment in older persons with isolated systolic hypertension. SHEP Cooperative Research Group. *JAMA*. 1997;278:212-216.
62. Ettehad D, Emdin CA, Kiran A, et al. Blood pressure lowering for prevention of cardiovascular disease and death: a systematic review and meta-analysis. *Lancet*. 2015;387:957-967.
63. Barker WH, Mullooly JP, Getchell W. Changing incidence and survival for heart failure in a well-defined older population, 1970-1974 and 1990-1994. *Circulation*. 2006;113:799-805.
64. Whelton PK, Klag MJ. Hypertension as a risk factor for renal disease. Review of clinical and epidemiological evidence. *Hypertension*. 1989;13(5 Suppl):I19-27.
65. Hsu CY, McCulloch CE, Darbinian J, Go AS, Iribarren C. Elevated blood pressure and risk of end-stage renal disease in subjects without baseline kidney disease. *Arch Int Med*. 2005;165:923-928.
66. Klag MJ, Whelton PK, Randall BL, et al. Blood pressure and end-stage renal disease in men. *N Engl J Med*. 1996;334:13-18.
67. Perry HM, Jr., Miller JP, Fornoff JR, et al. Early predictors of 15-year end-stage renal disease in hypertensive patients. *Hypertension*. 1995;25(4 Pt 1):587-594.
68. Perneger TV, Nieto FJ, Whelton PK, Klag MJ, Comstock GW, Szklo M. A prospective study of blood pressure and serum creatinine. Results from the 'Clue' Study and the ARIC Study. *JAMA*. 1993;269:488-493.
69. Schaeffner ES, Kurth T, Bowman TS, Gelber RP, Gaziano JM. Blood pressure measures and risk of chronic kidney disease in men. *Nephrol Dial Transplant*. 2008;23:1246-1251.
70. Young JH, Klag MJ, Muntner P, Whyte JL, Pahor M, Coresh J. Blood pressure and decline in kidney function: findings from the Systolic Hypertension in the Elderly Program (SHEP). *J Am Soc Nephrol*. 2002;13:2776-2782.
71. Shulman NB, Ford CE, Hall WD, et al. Prognostic value of serum creatinine and effect of treatment of hypertension on renal function. Results from the hypertension detection and follow-up program. The Hypertension Detection and Follow-up Program Cooperative Group. *Hypertension*. 1989;13(5 Suppl):180-I93.

For many years, clinicians have used diastolic blood pressure as the main risk indicator in hypertensive patients. However, several developments have caused a paradigmatic shift in our thinking about hypertension as a risk factor. First of all, the recognition from epidemiological studies that systolic pressure is a much stronger predictor of future cardiovascular events than diastolic pressure. Secondly, many studies have shown that pulse pressure is independently associated with cardiovascular risk and an increased pulse pressure is mainly related to an elevated systolic pressure. Finally, with the aging of the world's population more emphasis has been put on a more slowly evolving form of hypertension that is predominately systolic in nature and primarily affects middle-aged and older persons.

Currently, isolated systolic hypertension (ISH) is defined as a systolic blood pressure of 140 mm Hg or above together with a diastolic blood pressure below 90 mm Hg.[1] It has become the most common and the most difficult form of hypertension to treat successfully, and hence a public health problem of major proportion. The purpose of this chapter is to provide a better understanding of ISH and how to treat it effectively.

EPIDEMIOLOGY OF ISOLATED SYSTOLIC HYPERTENSION

The longitudinal data from the Framingham Heart Study clearly indicate that systolic blood pressure (SBP) continues to rise with age whereas diastolic blood pressure (DBP) increases in young adulthood, but levels off at age 50 to 55 years only to decrease after age 60 to 65 years.[2] As a corollary, pulse pressure (PP), defined as the difference between SBP and DBP, increases after age 50 to 55 years. Normotensives who reach the age of 65 years have a 90% lifetime risk of developing hypertension (and almost exclusively of the ISH subtype) if they live another 20 to 25 years.[3]

Studies on the prevalence of ISH in untreated populations have yielded inconsistent results, which may, at least in part, be explained by differences in age, gender distribution, and in definition of ISH across the various surveys. Surely, when one takes a systolic pressure above 160 mm Hg as the criterion for ISH, then the condition is virtually nonexistent in younger people. However, with the currently accepted threshold of 140 mm Hg the situation may be different. In the Chicago Heart Association Detection Project in Industry Study, for instance, the prevalence of ISH in participants between 18 and 49 years of age was about 25% in men and 13% in women.[4] These prevalence rates are higher than those found in several other studies and may well be related to comorbid conditions such as obesity.

In persons above age 60, ISH usually is found in a quarter to a third of the population.[5] Of particular interest are the data from the National Health and Nutrition Examination Survey (NHANES) program. In the third survey (NHANES III, 1988 to 1994) it was found that ISH is the predominant form of hypertension above age 50 years, constituting 60% to 90% of all cases of uncontrolled hypertension.[6] Recently, Liu and coworkers analyzed the data from six cycles of NHANES surveys from 1999 to 2010.[5] Interestingly, they found that the overall prevalence of untreated ISH had decreased from 9.4% in 1999 to 2004 to 8.5% in 2005 to 2010, a highly significant difference (p = 0.0025; Fig. 19.1). In participants aged 60 years and above there was an even more pronounced fall in the prevalence of ISH from 34% to 25% ($p < 0.0001$). Consistent with previous reports the prevalence of ISH was greater in females than in males, most likely because blood pressure tends to rise more steeply with age in older women than in men. Nevertheless, also in women the prevalence of ISH has decreased over time. Finally, in non-Hispanic blacks, a group with a very high risk of developing ISH, there were also fewer cases during the last examination. This positive trend in the United States may be seen as a reflection of public health measures and better treatment of hypertensive patients. However, such a development is not seen globally. In Korea, for instance, a similar program as NHANES found that, although the proportion of untreated hypertensive patients had remained relatively constant from 1998 to 2012, ISH is becoming more prevalent attributed to the rapid aging of the population.[7] Also in China, ISH has risen significantly over the last 20 years.[8] Thus, the problem of ISH may be particularly relevant in the Asian-Pacific region.

A question that comes up frequently is whether in older people ISH develops de novo, that is, as a separate disease, or that it is a naturally occurring stage in the hypertensive process. In the Framingham study, the conversion from untreated or poorly controlled diastolic hypertension at a younger age to ISH later in life did occur in about 40% of patients but, as illustrated in Fig. 19.2, the majority of people acquired ISH without going through a stage of elevated DBP.[9]

The Campania Salute Network study set out to determine which factors could predict the transition from systolic-diastolic hypertension toward ISH.[10] In 7801 hypertensive patients who were free of cardiovascular or severe chronic kidney disease, ISH developed in 21% over an average period of 55 months. Independent predictors of incident ISH were older age, female gender, higher baseline SBP, lower DBP, longer duration of hypertension, higher cardiac mass, greater arterial stiffness, and higher intima-media thickness of the carotid artery. These predictors were independent of antihypertensive treatment, obesity, diabetes, and fasting glucose. This suggests that ISH is a sign of aggravation of the atherosclerotic disease already evident by the target organ damage.[10]

The age-related changes in PP suggest an interaction between vascular aging and the development of systolic hypertension. Indeed, participants in the Framingham Heart Study who were followed from age 30 to 84 years in the absence of antihypertensive therapy and with a mean baseline blood pressure of 110/70 mm Hg at 30 years of age had no rise in PP from age 30 to 55 years of age.[2] However, this group of subjects did show a significant rise in PP and fall in DBP after 60 years of age, presumably caused by an increase in large artery stiffness secondary to aging. In contrast, participants

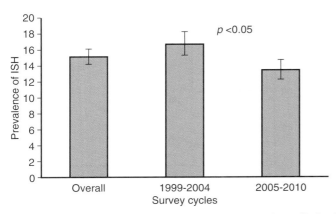

FIG. 19.1 Prevalence and 95% confidence intervals for the prevalence of isolated systolic hypertension in untreated adults. Based on the NHANES (National Health and Nutrition Examination Survey) 1999 to 2010 data. *(From Liu X, Rodriguez CJ, Wang K. Prevalence and trends of isolated systolic hypertension among untreated adults in the United States. J Am Soc Hypertens. 2015;9:197-205.)*

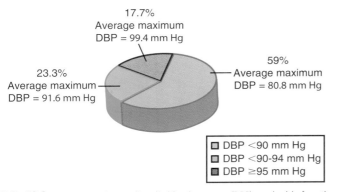

FIG. 19.2 Average maximum diastolic blood pressure (DBP) reached before the development of isolated systolic blood pressure for those who reached a DBP of less than 90 mm Hg, from 90 to 94 mm Hg, and 95 or higher mm Hg, respectively, in the Framingham Heart Study. *(Based on Franklin SS, Pio JR, Wong ND, et al. Predictors of new-onset diastolic and systolic hypertension: the Framingham Heart Study. Circulation. 2005;111:1121-1127.)*

with a mean baseline blood pressure of 130/84 mm Hg at 30 years of age demonstrated a steeper rise in PP and a steeper fall in DBP after age 60 than was observed in the other group, again in the absence of antihypertensive therapy. This divergent, rather than parallel tracking pattern suggests a linkage between hypertension left untreated and subsequent acceleration of large artery stiffness and the development or worsening of ISH.

PATHOPHYSIOLOGICAL FEATURES OF ISOLATED SYSTOLIC HYPERTENSION

Some Considerations About Etiology

Normally, the conduit vessels (the aorta and the carotid, brachial, iliac, and femoral arteries) will substantially buffer the pressure rise, which results from the ejection of blood by the left ventricle (Windkessel function). They can do so by virtue of a high elastin content. During systole, the aortic wall is stretched so that it can accommodate the stroke volume and at the same time increase elastic tensile energy. At late-systole and during the diastolic phase this accumulated energy recoils the aorta and pushes, as it were, the amount of blood that has not yet been directed forward into the peripheral vasculature. This way, a continuous flow is ensured. The structural basis for this mechanism lies primarily in the medial and adventitial layers of the vessel wall.[11] During normal aging, changes in the composition and the structure of the media lead to generalized

arterial stiffening. This process needs to be distinguished from intimal changes, which may occur simultaneously and which form the basis of atherosclerotic lesions. Although our information about the age-related pathological changes in the arterial wall of humans, for obvious reasons, is limited, there is agreement that with time the elastin in the wall in the larger vessels nearby the heart decreases. In fact, elastin becomes thinner and fragmented and then is degraded and replaced by collagen, which is much stiffer.[11] Why this happens, is not entirely clear. Some have suggested that it is a matter of fatigue failure as a result of repetitive cyclic loading.[12] Indeed, by the time a person reaches age 55 years the heart has contracted about 2 billion times and the elastic protein in the central conduit vessels may well show signs of wear and tear at that time.

Another possibility is that calcification of the media plays a role in the stiffening of the larger arteries. The mechanisms of this mineralization process are very complex and involve an array of biochemical substances.[11] Because most of the data on this process stem from animal and cellular studies and are not derived directly from human material these mechanisms will not be discussed in detail here. Nevertheless, it is likely that a combination of biochemical derangements and calcification contribute to a state of progressive arterial stiffening.

Despite an enormous body of evidence that links loss of elasticity and calcification via increased arterial stiffness to the development of de novo ISH, absolute proof that these are causally related to each other is still lacking. However, several clinical observations speak in favor of such a connection. For instance, elongation of the aorta or aortic unfolding as it is commonly called, is an age-related radiological change in the aorta, which is supposed to result from the loss of elastic material. With modern radiological techniques it has been possible to show that at least in normotensive people the ascending part of the thoracic aorta, the site of greatest pressure dampening, increases almost two-fold in length between 20 and 80 years of age.[13] Interestingly, the aortic diameter does not change that much so that it seems longitudinal strain during the cardiac cycle is greater than circumferential strain.[14] Of note, even in these normotensives the degree of lengthening correlated positively with measures of arterial stiffness as well as with the height of aortic systolic and pulse pressure.[13] Thus, it is not unreasonable to assume that in susceptible individuals this will end in systolic hypertension.

A second line of evidence is provided by epidemiological observations, which indicate that people with diabetes (both type 1 and type 2) run a greater risk of developing ISH and sooner than those without diabetes.[15,16] Conversely, the prevalence of type 2 diabetes is high in patients with ISH.[17] It is also known that increased arterial stiffness is already apparent in the phase of impaired glucose tolerance.[18] Most likely, this is related to the accumulation of advanced glycation end-products, which stiffen the aorta. Thirdly, ISH becomes more prevalent in conditions that are associated with a tendency to increased calcification such as renal insufficiency[19-21] and osteoporosis.[22-24] Finally, aortic calcification, as measured by quantitative high-resolution computed tomography imaging at the ascending, descending, and abdominal aorta, correlates with aortic stiffness and with the severity of ISH in patients who are otherwise apparently healthy.[25]

Taken together, these observations are consistent with the view that loss of elastin and/or calcification in the proximal aorta cause or contribute to arterial stiffness and the development of ISH.

Hemodynamics

When discussing hemodynamics in ISH it is essential to make a distinction between central hemodynamics and arterial stiffness. Central (or systemic) hemodynamics comprises intravascular pressure, cardiac output (CO), and total peripheral resistance (TPR). Although cross-sectional studies in normotensives suggest that an age-related rise in blood pressure is as a result of an increase in TPR, longitudinal investigations hardly show any changes in either pressure or CO or TPR over time.[26] In patients with hypertension hemodynamic changes with age are more pronounced. Cardiac output falls by about 15% over a period of 10 to 20 years caused by a reduction in stroke volume without significant changes in heart rate. The almost parallel rise in SBP, DBP, and mean arterial pressure (MAP) up to age 50 to 55 years can best be explained by the increase in peripheral vascular resistance.[2,26]

The consequence of diminished elasticity of the aorta and the larger vessels is loss of the Windkessel function and, hence, less dampening of the pulsatility. This will result in a greater rise in systolic pressure and in pulse pressure. Another sequela is that the pressure wave now travels much faster along the stiffened arterial system than it used to do when the system was still more elastic. Because of the high resistance in the microcirculation the forward moving pressure wave is reflected, thus causing a retrograde pressure wave, which amplifies the former.[27] Although this sequence of events fairly well explains the rise in SBP and the widening of PP with advancing age, it is less easy to understand why DBP falls. A commonly held view is that with age-related stiffening of the aorta, there is a greater peripheral runoff of stroke volume during systole. With less blood remaining in the aorta at the beginning of diastole, and with diminished elastic recoil, DBP decreases and the diastolic decay curve becomes steeper. Although this may be true for the ones who develop ISH de novo, it remains enigmatic why those patients who initially exhibited elevated diastolic pressures and a high TPR would lower their DBP.

Whatever the precise mechanisms, the blood pressure pattern of ISH with wide PP, from age 50 to 55 onward, is best explained by a predominance of large artery stiffness. The rise in PP is both a marker for large artery stiffness and a measure of vascular aging. In fact, untreated hypertension can accelerate the rate of vascular aging by as many as 15 to 20 years as illustrated in Fig. 19.3. Thus, although increased PVR probably initiates essential hypertension, acceleration of large artery stiffness is the driving force leading to the development of ISH with a steeper rise of SBP after 50 years of age and a fall in DBP as compared with normotensive people.[2] Beyond 60 years of age, increased central arterial stiffness and forward wave amplitude (rather than increased TPR, MAP, and early wave augmentation) become the dominant hemodynamic factors in both normotensive and hypertensive individuals.[28] At that point, cardiac workload and myocardial oxygen demand during ventricular ejection will progressively increase and cardiac output may decline further. Ultimately, with no or inadequate treatment left ventricular failure may ensue.

Arterial Wave Reflection, Central Blood Pressure, Pressure Amplification, and Pulse Wave Velocity

The morphology of any pulse wave results from the summation of incident (forward-traveling) and reflected (backward-traveling) pressure waves (Fig. 19.4).[27] Timing depends on both pulse wave velocity (PWV) and distance to the predominant or "effective" reflecting site. As has been known for a long time, the summation of the incident pressure wave with the reflected wave produces in young healthy adults a normal phenomenon of pressure amplification from the aorta to the brachial artery, resulting in a higher SBP and PP at the distal brachial artery as compared with the proximal ascending aortic site.[29] The degree to which amplification occurs can be quantified as the augmentation index (AIx). A marked increase

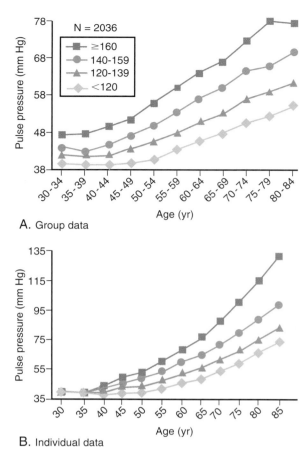

FIG. 19.3 Pulse pressure by age. Group-averaged data (A) and averaged individual regression analysis (B) for all subjects with deaths, myocardial infarction, and chronic heart failure excluded. Curves plotted based on blood pressure predicted values at 5-year age intervals by systolic blood pressure groupings. *(Adapted from Franklin SS, Gustin WT, Wong ND, Larson MG, Weber MA, Kannel WB, Levy D. Hemodynamic patterns of age-related changes in blood pressure. The Framingham Heart Study. Circulation. 1997;96:308-315.)*

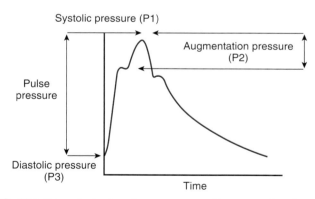

FIG. 19.4 Schematic drawing of a pressure wave with augmentation of systolic pressure by a reflected wave. The augmentation index is the ratio of the augmentation pressure to pulse pressure. *(From Laurent S, Cockcroft J, Van Bortel L, et al. Expert consensus document on arterial stiffness: methodological issues and clinical applications. Eur Heart J. 2006;27:2588-2605.)*

in stiffness or impedance at the reflecting site generates a larger reflected wave and can add to a greater augmentation index.

Importantly, central SBP and PP, augmentation index, and pressure amplification are all influenced by arterial stiffness without necessarily being an accurate measurement of arterial stiffness itself. Indeed, all these variables are determined primarily by the speed of wave travel, the sites of reflectance, the amplitude of the reflected wave, and left ventricular ejection and contractility.[30] On the other hand, aortic PWV is a well-defined surrogate for arterial stiffness that can be determined from pulse transit time and the distance traveled by the pulse between the common carotid and femoral arteries (CF-PWV). Aortic PWV increases with aging[31] and the development of ISH,[32] and therefore is a sensitive indicator of physiologic stiffness after the age of 50 to 60 years. By that time, the fall in DBP and the rapid widening of PP become surrogate indicators of central arterial stiffening. At that age, however, aortic stiffness (measured by CF-PWV) reaches and then exceeds peripheral arterial stiffness, measured by carotid-to-brachial PWV.[28] As a result, reflection at this interface is reduced with reflecting sites shifting distally. This impedance matching at the proximal reflecting sites leads to reduced reflectance and therefore increased transmission of pulsatility distally, with a resultant increase in brachial artery PP and the development of ISH.[28]

TARGET ORGAN DAMAGE IN ISOLATED SYSTOLIC HYPERTENSION

Should increased arterial stiffness be considered as a cause or a consequence of the elevated pulse pressure? Data from the Baltimore Longitudinal Study of Aging (BLSA) demonstrate a greater arterial stiffness at baseline predicted a larger increase in systolic blood pressure with aging as well as the incidence of hypertension,[33] whereas a higher SBP at baseline was associated with a greater increase in stiffness over time.[34] Thus, it is a vicious cycle and any attempt to detect a starting point is bound to fail.[35]

The organ that is closest to the site of the stiffened aorta is of course the heart and it is not surprising, therefore, that this organ gets most of the complications of ISH. In fact, the increased PP may even be a surrogate marker for several possible cardiac abnormalities, which all originate from the underlying increased central arterial stiffness and wave reflection. Increased aortic pulsatile afterload is a major factor in the development of left ventricular hypertrophy (LVH) with increased coronary blood flow requirements.[36] In addition, increased turbulent flow leads to endothelial dysfunction with a greater propensity for coronary atherosclerosis and for rupture of unstable atherosclerotic plaques.

The rise in SBP and the fall in DBP in elderly persons with ISH could result in a coronary supply/demand imbalance and myocardial ischemia. The decline in DBP, however, rarely falls to the critical level (<60 mm Hg) required to disturb coronary flow autoregulation.[37] Thus, it is unlikely that the reduction in DBP that occurs in most individuals with ISH compromises coronary perfusion. Nonetheless, there is a potential imbalance between systolic demand and coronary supply. Furthermore, cardiac ejection into the stiff arterial system results in more coronary perfusion during the systolic period, making the heart more vulnerable to changes in SBP and systolic heart function. In addition to arterial stiffening, the left ventricle itself develops systolic stiffness, perhaps as an adaptive change to facilitate cardiac ejection and to maintain matched coupling of heart to arteries. The combination of an elevated cardiac afterload and a compromised left ventricle will ultimately lead to heart failure.

Importantly, the increase in forward wave amplitude that leads to the development of ISH also increases transmission of pulsatility to the microcirculation of the brain and kidneys. This can stimulate local hypertrophy, remodeling, and rarefaction. This, in turn, will lead to a further rise in TPR and blood pressure and enhanced burden on the heart. In addition, endothelial function in stiffened vessels is impaired and this may accelerate the development of atherosclerotic lesions.[11] All these abnormalities markedly increase the cardiovascular risk profile of patients with ISH.

CARDIOVASCULAR RISK IN PERSONS WITH ISOLATED SYSTOLIC HYPERTENSION

Risk of Coronary Heart Disease

Numerous population-based investigations confirm that ISH is a significant risk factor for cardiovascular complications. In Framingham, a cohort consisting of 1924 men and women between 50 and 79 years of age at baseline was followed up for 20 years.[38] When Framingham was started none of the participants had any clinical evidence of coronary heart disease (CHD) or were receiving any antihypertensive drugs. In this population, CHD risk was inversely correlated with DBP at any level of SBP greater than 120 mm Hg, suggesting that pulse pressure is an important component of CHD risk in persons with ISH (Fig. 19.5). There was a greater increase in CHD risk with increments in PP for a given SBP than with increments in SBP with a constant PP. These observations are consistent with the premise that in people above age 50 years the risk of CHD events is more closely related to the pulsatile stress of elastic artery stiffness during systole (as reflected by a rise in PP) than to the steady-state stress of resistance during diastole (as reflected by a parallel rise in SBP and DBP).

The increased risk is not only apparent in people over age 65 years but also in younger people. The Chicago Heart Association Detection Project in Industry Study followed 27,000 people who originally were 18 to 49 years over an average period of 31 years. In this population CHD mortality was significantly increased in those who had ISH at baseline.[4]

It should be emphasized that ISH is not always a significant predictor of coronary events. A meta-analysis of eight treatment trials involving ISH patients failed to show an association with coronary events although other outcome measures were associated.[39] The lack of an association with coronary complications in this analysis may be attributed to the threshold for diagnosis of ISH that was set at a systolic pressure of 160 mm Hg. If there were also more coronary events in the 140 to 160 mm Hg range, this could have diluted any difference between those with and without ISH.

A recent survey in a Mongolian cohort of almost 2600 adults in China also could not convincingly show an increased risk of cardiovascular disease in individuals with ISH either. Although the hazard ratio, adjusted for age and gender as well as other cardiovascular risk factors was 2.00, this failed to

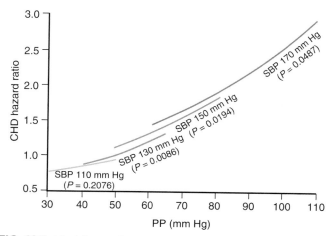

FIG. 19.5 Joint influence of systolic blood pressure (SBP) and pulse pressure (PP) on coronary heart disease (CHD) risk. CHD hazard ratios (HRs) were determined from the level of PP within SBP groups. HRs were set to a reference value of 1.0 for SBP of 130 mm Hg and PP of 50 mm Hg and are plotted for SBP values of 110, 130, 150, and 170 mm Hg, respectively. Probability values were for β coefficients for this model. All estimates were adjusted for age, sex, and body mass index, number of cigarettes smoked per day, glucose intolerance, and total cholesterol/high-density lipoproteins. *(From Franklin SS, Khan SA, Wong ND, Larson MG, Levy D. Is pulse pressure useful in predicting risk for coronary heart Disease? The Framingham Heart Study. Circulation. 1999;100:354-360.)*

reach statistical significance.[40] In all likelihood, methodological differences and perhaps ethnic characteristics underlie this discrepancy with other studies.

Risk of Cerebrovascular Disease

As early as 1980, information was available from the Framingham study that ISH could increase the risk of cerebrovascular complications by a factor of two to four relative to normotensive people.[41,42] This was corroborated in a follow-up study among 2636 Californian adults aged 60 years or older, of whom 6.3% had isolated systolic hypertension at baseline.[43] At that time ISH was still defined as a systolic blood pressure 160 or higher mm Hg and a diastolic blood pressure less than 90 mm Hg. After a 6.4-year follow-up of this cohort, males (but not females) with isolated systolic hypertension had an excess risk of death from stroke, even after adjustment for age and other covariates.[43] At the same time, reports from Europe started to appear that highlighted the unfavorable prognosis of ISH.[44,45] Since then various clinical studies have confirmed that ISH predisposes to cerebrovascular disease and stroke.[39,46-48]

The data from the Framingham study on stroke incidence in relation to blood pressure suggest that the risk associated with isolated systolic hypertension is independent of the height of diastolic pressure. Although diastolic pressure is related to stroke incidence as well, the diastolic component adds little to risk assessment and even appears unrelated to stroke incidence in men with ISH.[42]

Except for stroke, cognitive impairment may be aggravated by ISH. Indeed, the Baltimore Longitudinal Study on Aging showed that elevated PP and PWV were related to cognitive impairment, based on decline in verbal and nonverbal memory test scores in nondemented middle-aged individuals.[49] Although cognitive impairment has not been specifically linked to ISH, the data from Baltimore at least suggest that such a relationship may exist.

Vascular Complications

Subclinical abnormalities such as diastolic dysfunction or an increased intima-media thickness (IMT) of the carotid artery also occur in conjunction with ISH.[50,51] A recent study from Greece evaluated IMT in patients with so-called masked ISH.[52] This condition was defined as an office pressure below 140 mm Hg systolic and 90 mm Hg diastolic with an average SBP 135 or higher mm Hg and DBP less than 85 mm Hg on 24-hour ambulatory monitoring. In these patients the IMT was significantly higher than in other forms of masked hypertension. An increased carotid IMT is a biomarker for atherosclerotic disease, not only in the cerebral vasculature but also elsewhere in the body. Indeed, compared with a normotensive group, patients with ISH also have more evidence of carotid stenosis, especially when diastolic BP is below 75 mm Hg.[53] In the Rotterdam Study, an increased IMT was even associated with future cerebrovascular and cardiovascular events.[54]

Peripheral vascular complications are frequently seen in patients with ISH as well, although these could easily be considered as manifestations of underlying atherosclerosis.[55] In the prospective Women's Health Study the incidence of peripheral arterial disease was three-fold to four-fold higher in those with ISH (SBP ≥ 140 mm Hg, DBP < 90 mm Hg) than in normotensive women.[56] Obviously, this study had several limitations, yet it fits with other observations.[57] Taken together, both carotid and lower extremity arterial disease seem to be prevalent abnormalities in patients with ISH,[55] but the cause-and-effect relationship remains to be determined.

A similar problem concerns the role of the kidney. There is no doubt that impaired renal function increases arterial stiffness and that the prevalence of ISH increases stepwise with the stages of chronic kidney disease.[20] Whether the opposite

is also true, is less easy to define. In one cross-sectional study, renal hemodynamics (renal plasma flow, glomerular filtration rate) were inversely related to pulse pressure in patients with ISH but, after correction for age, the relationship persisted only in persons above 60 years of age (Fig. 19.6).[58] Although this suggests that ISH is detrimental for the kidney in elderly patients, it does not rule out the alternative possibility that a subtle decline in kidney function initiated or aggravated loss of arterial elasticity, which in turn accounted for the development of ISH.

A prospective observation comes from the Systolic Hypertension in the Elderly Program (SHEP).[59] This study showed that both SBP and PP at baseline were significantly associated with a decline in renal function over time. Again, the data do not allow definite conclusions about the prime mover; in addition, it is almost impossible to exclude an effect of age.

Other Aspects

Although some uncertainty remains about the relative importance of the various components of blood pressure in predicting risk, most data prognostically suggest no difference

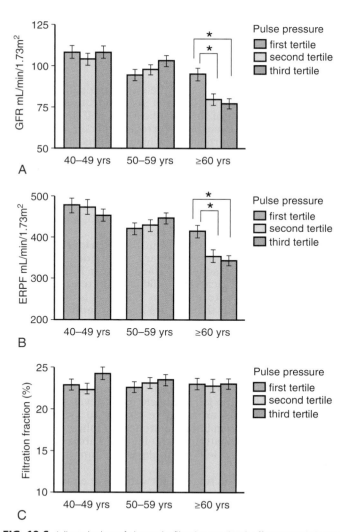

FIG. 19.6 Adjusted values of glomerular filtration rate (GFR), effective renal plasma flow (ERPF) and filtration fraction (FF) according to tertiles of pulse pressure in three age categories. All patients had isolated systolic hypertension, defined as an SBP 140 or higher mm Hg and a DBP less than 90 mm Hg. (*From Verhave JC, Fesler P, du Cailar G, Ribstein J, Safar ME, Mimran A. Elevated pulse pressure is associated with low renal function in elderly patients with isolated systolic hypertension. Hypertension. 2005;45:586-591.*)

between PP and SBP. Thus, SBP is probably the best overall single predictor of CVD risk because it includes elements of both increased resistance and stiffness. It is important to know that risk relates not only to office pressures but also to noninvasive 24-hour blood pressure (Fig. 19.7)[60] and home blood pressure measurements.[61,62]

Although both brachial artery SBP and PP are powerful indicators of risk in patients with isolated systolic hypertension, the heart only sees central blood pressure, that is, SBP and PP in the ascending aorta and the carotid artery, and it is precisely this pressure that determines cardiac afterload and hence cardiac risk. Although in younger people brachial artery pressure may exceed central pressure, there is a lesser or even no difference between the two at higher ages.[36] Although central pressure has little, if any, superiority over brachial pressure in predicting events, the augmentation index and aortic pulse wave velocity have predictive value independent of peripheral pressures.[63,64] In a French-Italian study in nursing home residents aged 80 years or older, risk was even stronger related to pulse pressure amplification than to blood pressure.[65]

TREATMENT OF ISOLATED SYSTOLIC HYPERTENSION

Evidence From Trials

In 1991, the Systolic Hypertension in the Elderly Program (SHEP) study established that older patients with ISH benefited from treatment.[66] Later on, the Syst-Eur and Syst-China trials corroborated these findings.[67,68] The positive results are probably well maintained over a prolonged period of time.[69] The HYpertension in the Very Elderly Trial (HYVET), an intervention trial involving the very old (from 80 to 105 years of age at baseline) included patients with sustained SBP of 160 or higher mm Hg, of whom one-third had ISH.[70] Although no results have been reported for the subgroup with ISH, the trial did show substantial benefit from treatment. Table 19.1 summarizes the main results of these four trials.[71]

There is some evidence from Syst-Eur that active treatment protects against dementia,[72,73] but this was less clear in the SHEP-trial.[66,74] Likewise, incident dementia was not reduced by treatment in the Hypertension in the Very Elderly Trial Cognitive Function Assessment (HYVET-COG).[75]

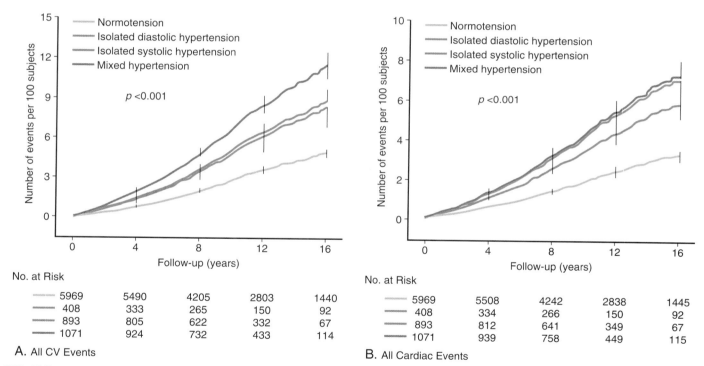

FIG. 19.7 Incidence of composite cardiovascular (CV) endpoints (A) and fatal combined with nonfatal cardiac events (B) in four categories of ambulatory blood pressure. Incidence was standardized to sex distribution and mean age in the whole study population. *(From Li Y, Wei FF, Thijs L, et al. International Database on Ambulatory blood pressure in relation to Cardiovascular Outcomes I. Ambulatory hypertension subtypes and 24-hour systolic and diastolic blood pressure as distinct outcome predictors in 8341 untreated people recruited from 12 populations. Circulation. 2014;130:466-474.)*

TABLE 19.1 Effects of Antihypertensive Treatment in Patients With Isolated Systolic Hypertension

	HYVET	SHEP	SYST-EUR	SYST-CHINA	SPRINT
Mean treatment BP reduction, SBP/DBP (mm Hg)	−29/−13	−27/−9	−23/−7	−20/−5	−15/−7
Stroke, % reduction	−30%	−32%	−42%	−38%	−38%
Coronary disease, % reduction	−23%[a]	−27%	−30%	+6%	−22%[a]
Heart failure, % reduction	−64%	−55%	−29%	−58%	−33%

HYVET, SHEP, Syst-Eur, and Syst-China, Outcome in actively treated group versus placebo; *SPRINT,* outcome in intensively treated group versus standard treatment.
[a]Only myocardial infarction.
(Modified and extended from Burney BO, Bakris GL. Hypertension and its management in the elderly. Semin Nephrol. 2009;29:604-609.)
BP, Blood pressure; *DBP,* diastolic blood pressure; *SBP,* systolic blood pressure.

Unanswered Questions

The major placebo-controlled trials of hypertension in older persons with ISH have recruited patients with a systolic blood pressure at entry of 160 or higher mm Hg. However, the current definition takes 140 mm Hg as the cutoff level so there is still a need for studies to test the benefit of lowering blood pressure in patients with ISH and an SBP between 140 and 160 mm Hg.

Another issue is to what level blood pressure can safely be reduced. Only prospective trials can establish whether a treatment-induced J-curve exists. One trial that comes close was the Valsartan in Elderly Isolated Systolic Hypertension Study (VALISH). In this trial more than 3000 patients between 70 and 85 years of age with ISH (SBP > 160 mm Hg, DBP < 90 mm Hg) were randomized to either strict (target SBP < 140 mm Hg) or moderate control (target SBP ≥ 140 to <150 mm Hg).[76] After a follow-up period of nearly three years, fewer patients in the group with strict control experienced the composite primary endpoint. Although the difference was small and not statistically significant,[76] the trial showed at least that it was safe to lower blood pressure below 140 mm Hg in this population.

Another relevant study is the Systolic Blood Pressure Intervention Trial (SPRINT).[77] This trial recruited high-risk hypertensive patients with a systolic blood pressure of 130 to 180 mm Hg and randomized them to standard treatment (SBP target of 140 mm Hg) or intensive treatment (SBP < 120 mm Hg). The average DBP at baseline was 78 mm Hg, so that there must have been a substantial proportion of patients with ISH. The results showed overwhelming benefit in the group with intensive treatment, suggesting that it is both beneficial and safe to lower blood pressure to such a low level.[77]

Still, some concern exists with respect to renal function. In the Syst-Eur trial, active treatment did not influence average serum creatinine or calculated creatinine clearance and even reduced the incidence of mild renal dysfunction and proteinuria.[78] Conversely, in the SPRINT study[77] significantly more patients from the intensive-treatment group experienced a decrease in estimated glomerular filtration rate of 30% or more to a value of less than 60 mL per minute per 1.73 m[2].

Finally, there is the issue of frailty. There is some concern that frail patients benefit less from antihypertensive treatment,[79] although no evidence for such an effect was found in the HYVET study.[80] However, patients who enter a clinical trial tend to be healthier than their peers.[81] Indeed, a study in frail nursing home residents suggested that antihypertensive therapy may even enhance mortality.[82] Overall, hypertensive patients who are functionally independent are best treated in the same way as younger patients but there is insufficient evidence that frail polymedicated octogenarians benefit much from treatment.[83]

WHICH ANTIHYPERTENSIVE TREATMENT FOR ISOLATED SYSTOLIC HYPERTENSION?

In older patients lifestyle measures should always form part of an antihypertensive regimen[84] although their efficacy has not been very well established. A re-analysis of salt reduction trials did provide evidence, however, that even in ISH a modest decrease in salt intake may lower systolic blood pressure by approximately 10 mm Hg.[85] However, in most cases this will not be enough to control the blood pressure and additional pharmacotherapy will be necessary.[86]

The issue of which drug class is best suited to start with in patients with ISH remains controversial. Prognostic benefit can only be ascribed to those drugs that have been used in large placebo-controlled outcome trials. For ISH, this means chlorthalidone and/or atenolol (SHEP), nitrendipine and/or enalapril and/or hydrochlorothiazide (Syst-Eur), captopril (Syst-China), and perhaps also indapamide and/or perindopril (HYVET). If one takes a more liberal standpoint, this translates into diuretics, beta-blockers, calcium channel blockers, and angiotensin-converting enzyme (ACE) inhibitors: in short four of the five major classes of antihypertensive drugs. There is no such prognostic evidence in patients with ISH for the angiotensin II receptor, type 1 (AT1)-receptor blockers. Nevertheless, a substudy of the LIFE (Losartan Intervention For Endpoint reduction in hypertension study) trial in patients with ISH and electrocardiographically documented left ventricular hypertrophy demonstrated a greater benefit incurred by losartan with or without hydrochlorothiazide than by atenolol with or without this diuretic.[87] We should keep in mind, however, that the majority of patients in all these trials required combination therapy of at least two drugs.[84] Therefore, it is useful to compare different treatment regimens. This was done in the Avoiding Cardiovascular events through Combination Therapy in Patients Living with Systolic Hypertension (ACCOMPLISH) trial, which compared morbidity and mortality among 11,506 high-risk men and women (average age, 68 years) randomized with one of two initial combination regimens: a calcium channel blocker (amlodipine) plus an ACE-inhibitor (benazepril) versus a diuretic (hydrochlorothiazide) plus the same ACE-inhibitor.[88] Both regimens reduced blood pressure nearly equally to less than 130/80 in almost 80% of patients but there was a 20% greater reduction in cardiovascular morbidity and mortality endpoints in the benazepril/amlodipine arm compared with the other one.[88] In addition, renal function was better preserved with benazepril/amlodipine.[84]

Presently, several antihypertensive drug combinations are compared head-to-head in patients with ISH with regard to their blood pressure lowering potential. This may yield no or minor differences[89] but will provide us with useful information about which type of drugs are worthwhile to use as long as no further outcome data are available.

A recent development in the treatment of hypertension, in particular resistant hypertension, is that of renal denervation.[90,91] Briefly, a radiofrequency-catheter (or variant) is advanced into the renal artery and the autonomic nerve fibers, which run along the renal artery, are ablated. This will lead to a reduction in overall sympathetic activity and hence blood pressure. The true value of this technique, however, has not yet been fully established and in any case the effect seems to be less pronounced in patients with ISH.[92]

SHOULD WE TARGET BLOOD PRESSURE OR ARTERIAL STIFFNESS?

Our classic approach to the treatment of hypertension is to employ drugs, which lower the pressure. In the case of ISH this may not be enough and we may have to look for therapies that are able to lessen arterial stiffness. Manisty and coworkers performed a meta-analysis of the comparative effects of different classes of antihypertensive drugs on central and brachial pressure and augmentation index as observed in 24 randomized trials.[93] Although sample sizes were small, they found that all classes of drugs reduced brachial and central pressure as compared with placebo with a slightly greater effect on brachial pressure. They further found that beta-blockers and diuretics had a lesser effect on central than on brachial pressures whereas other monotherapies had equal effects. This would imply that beta-blockers are less favorable drugs to use. However, given the limited sample sizes these data must still be interpreted with some caution.

Several other trials have shown that a variety of antihypertensive agents are able to reduce PWV but it remains enigmatic whether or not this is entirely independent from their effect on blood pressure.[94] There is one meta-analysis of individual data from 15 randomized trials that has suggested such an independent effect.[95]

Antihypertensive drugs with vasodilator properties will decrease large artery stiffness upstream by diminishing intramural pressure and decreasing the stretch on elastic arteries.[96] However, to date there is still no evidence that arterial stiffness is reversible and the available antihypertensive agents will at most ameliorate stiffness but not reverse it.

Nitrates have sometimes been recommended for use in patients with ISH. Indeed, in doses that do not affect peripheral vascular resistance, they can decrease early wave reflection, reduce central PP, and hence lower left ventricular load on the heart, even without causing a significant change in arterial stiffness. Whether or not that translates into a better prognosis, though, remains to be seen.[94]

SUMMARY

Once considered an inconsequential part of the aging process, the development of ISH is now seen as a late manifestation of increased arterial stiffness in the middle-aged and older population. Its inherent increased risk for vascular events highlights the importance of its control. There is overwhelming evidence that pharmacologic treatment of ISH reduces cardiovascular events in the elderly. Paradoxically, ISH remains more difficult to control than diastolic hypertension and we still do not know which type of drug is preferable in this regard.

References

1. 2013 esh/esc guidelines for the management of arterial hypertension. *J Hypertens.* 2013;31:1281-1357.
2. Franklin SS, Gustin Wt, Wong ND, et al. Hemodynamic patterns of age-related changes in blood pressure. The Framingham Heart Study. *Circulation.* 1997;96:308-315.
3. Vasan RS, Beiser A, Seshadri S, et al. Residual lifetime risk for developing hypertension in middle-aged women and men: The Framingham Heart Study. *JAMA.* 2002;287:1003-1010.
4. Yano Y, Stamler J, Garside DB, et al. Isolated systolic hypertension in young and middle-aged adults and 31-year risk for cardiovascular mortality: the Chicago Heart Association Detection Project in Industry study. *J Am Coll Cardiol.* 2015;65:327-335.
5. Liu X, Rodriguez CJ, Wang K. Prevalence and trends of isolated systolic hypertension among untreated adults in the United States. *J Am Soc Hypertens.* 2015;9:197-205.
6. Franklin SS, Jacobs MJ, Wong ND, L'Italien GJ, Lapuerta P. Predominance of isolated systolic hypertension among middle-aged and elderly us hypertensives: analysis based on National Health and Nutrition Examination Survey (NHANES) III. *Hypertension.* 2001;37:869-874.
7. Kim NR, Kim HC. Prevalence and Trends of Isolated Systolic Hypertension among Korean Adults: the Korea National Health and Nutrition Examination Survey, 1998-2012. *Korean Circ J.* 2015;45:492-499.
8. Qi SF, Zhang B, Wang HJ, et al. Prevalence of hypertension subtypes in 2011 and the trends from 1991 to 2011 among Chinese adults. *J Epidemiol Community Health.* 2016;70:444-451.
9. Franklin SS, Pio JR, Wong ND, et al. Predictors of new-onset diastolic and systolic hypertension: the Framingham Heart Study. *Circulation.* 2005;111:1121-1127.
10. Esposito R, Izzo R, Galderisi M, et al. Identification of phenotypes at risk of transition from diastolic hypertension to isolated systolic hypertension. *J Hum Hypertens.* 2016;30:392-396.
11. Greenwald SE. Ageing of the conduit arteries. *J Pathol.* 2007;211:157-172.
12. O'Rourke MF. Pulsatile arterial haemodynamics in hypertension. *Aust N Z J Med.* 1976;6(Suppl 2):40-48.
13. Sugawara J, Hayashi K, Yokoi T, Tanaka H. Age-associated elongation of the ascending aorta in adults. *JACC Cardiovasc Imaging.* 2008;1:739-748.
14. O'Rourke M, Farnsworth A, O'Rourke J. Aortic dimensions and stiffness in normal adults. *JACC Cardiovasc Imaging.* 2008;1:749-751.
15. Ronnback M, Fagerudd J, Forsblom C, Pettersson-Fernholm K, Reunanen A, Groop PH, Finnish Diabetic Nephropathy Study G. Altered age-related blood pressure pattern in type 1 diabetes. *Circulation.* 2004;110:1076-1082.
16. Ko GT, Cockram CS, Chow CC, et al. Effects of body mass index, plasma glucose and cholesterol levels on isolated systolic hypertension. *Int J Cardiol.* 2005;101:429-433.
17. Franklin SS, Chow VH, Mori AD, Wong ND. The significance of low dbp in us adults with isolated systolic hypertension. *J Hypertens.* 2011;29:1101-1108.
18. Li CH, Wu JS, Yang YC, Shih CC, Lu FH, Chang CJ. Increased arterial stiffness in subjects with impaired glucose tolerance and newly diagnosed diabetes but not isolated impaired fasting glucose. *J Clin Endocrinol Metab.* 2012;97:E658-662.
19. Cheng LT, Chen HM, Tang LJ, et al. The study of aortic stiffness in different hypertension subtypes in dialysis patients. *Hypertens Res.* 2008;31:593-599.
20. Cheng LT, Gao YL, Gu Y, et al. Stepwise increase in the prevalence of isolated systolic hypertension with the stages of chronic kidney disease. *Nephrol Dial Transplant.* 2008;23:3895-3900.
21. Tomiyama H, Tanaka H, Hashimoto H, et al. Arterial stiffness and declines in individuals with normal renal function/early chronic kidney disease. *Atherosclerosis.* 2010;212:345-350.
22. Sprini D, Rini GB, Di Stefano L, Cianferotti L, Napoli N. Correlation between osteoporosis and cardiovascular disease. *Clin Cases Miner Bone Metab.* 2014;11:117-119.
23. Cappuccio FP, Meilahn E, Zmuda JM, Cauley JA. High blood pressure and bone-mineral loss in elderly white women: a prospective study. Study of osteoporotic fractures research group. *Lancet.* 1999;354:971-975.
24. Schulz E, Arfai K, Liu X, Sayre J, Gilsanz V. Aortic calcification and the risk of osteoporosis and fractures. *J Clin Endocrinol Metab.* 2004;89:4246-4253.
25. McEniery CM, McDonnell BJ, So A, et al. Anglo-Cardiff Collaboration Trial I. Aortic calcification is associated with aortic stiffness and isolated systolic hypertension in healthy individuals. *Hypertension.* 2009;53:524-531.
26. Omvik P, Lund-Johansen P. Hemodynamics of hypertension. In: Mancia G, Grassi G, Redon J, eds. *Manual of hypertension of the European Society of Hypertension.* Boca Raton, FL: CRC Press; 2014:101-114.
27. Laurent S, Cockcroft J, Van Bortel L, et al. European Network for Non-invasive Investigation of Large Arteries. Expert consensus document on arterial stiffness: methodological issues and clinical applications. *Eur Heart J.* 2006;27:2588-2605.
28. Mitchell GF, Parise H, Benjamin EJ, et al. Changes in arterial stiffness and wave reflection with advancing age in healthy men and women: the framingham heart study. *Hypertension.* 2004;43:1239-1245.
29. Kroeker EJ, Wood EH. Comparison of simultaneously recorded central and peripheral arterial pressure pulses during rest, exercise and tilted position in man. *Circ Res.* 1955;3:623-632.
30. Laurent S, Safar M. Large artery damage: measurement and clinical importance. In: Mancia G, Grassi G, Redon J, eds. *Manual of hypertension of the European Society of Hypertension.* Boca Raton, FL: CRC Press; 2014:191-202.
31. Reference Values for Arterial Stiffness Collaboration. Determinants of pulse wave velocity in healthy people and in the presence of cardiovascular risk factors: 'establishing normal and reference values'. *Eur Heart J.* 2010;31:2338-2350.
32. Verwoert GC, Franco OH, Hoeks AP, et al. Arterial stiffness and hypertension in a large population of untreated individuals: the Rotterdam Study. *J Hypertens.* 2014;32:1606-1612. discussion 1612.
33. Najjar SS, Scuteri A, Shetty V, et al. Pulse wave velocity is an independent predictor of the longitudinal increase in systolic blood pressure and of incident hypertension in the Baltimore Longitudinal Study of Aging. *J Am Coll Cardiol.* 2008;51:1377-1383.
34. AlGhatrif M, Strait JB, Morrell CH, et al. Longitudinal trajectories of arterial stiffness and the role of blood pressure: the Baltimore Longitudinal Study of Aging. *Hypertension.* 2013;62:934-941.
35. AlGhatrif M, Lakatta EG. The conundrum of arterial stiffness, elevated blood pressure, and aging. *Curr Hypertens Rep.* 2015;17:12.
36. Giannattasio C, Laurent S. Central blood pressure. In: Mancia G, Grassi G, Redon J, eds. *Manual of hypertension of the European Society of Hypertension.* Boca Raton, FL: CRC Press; 2014:257-268.
37. Somes GW, Pahor M, Shorr RI, Cushman WC, Applegate WB. The role of diastolic blood pressure when treating isolated systolic hypertension. *Arch Intern Med.* 1999;159:2004-2009.
38. Franklin SS, Khan SA, Wong ND, Larson MG, Levy D. Is pulse pressure useful in predicting risk for coronary heart disease? The Framingham heart study. *Circulation.* 1999;100:354-360.
39. Staessen JA, Gasowski J, Wang JG, et al. Risks of untreated and treated isolated systolic hypertension in the elderly: meta-analysis of outcome trials. *Lancet.* 2000;355:865-872.
40. Li H, Kong F, Xu J, Zhang M, Wang A, Zhang Y. Hypertension subtypes and risk of cardiovascular diseases in a Mongolian population, inner Mongolia, China. *Clin Exp Hypertens.* 2016;38:39-44.
41. Kannel WB, Dawber TR, McGee DL. Perspectives on systolic hypertension. The Framingham study. *Circulation.* 1980;61:1179-1182.
42. Kannel WB, Wolf PA, McGee DL, Dawber TR, McNamara P, Castelli WP. Systolic blood pressure, arterial rigidity, and risk of stroke. The Framingham study. *JAMA.* 1981;245:1225-1229.
43. Garland C, Barrett-Connor E, Suarez L, Criqui MH. Isolated systolic hypertension and mortality after age 60 years. A prospective population-based study. *Am J Epidemiol.* 1983;118:365-376.
44. Ambrosio GB, Zamboni S, Pilotto L, Dal Palu C. Isolated systolic hypertension in the community. Data from a population survey and hypertension register in Northern Italy. *Clin Exp Hypertens A.* 1982;4:1133-1150.
45. Forette F, de la Fuente X, Golmard JL, Henry JF, Hervy MP. The prognostic significance of isolated systolic hypertension in the elderly. Results of a ten year longitudinal survey. *Clin Exp Hypertens A.* 1982;4:1177-1191.
46. Staessen J, Amery A, Fagard R. Isolated systolic hypertension in the elderly. *J Hypertens.* 1990;8:393-405.
47. Petrovitch H, Curb JD, Bloom-Marcus E. Isolated systolic hypertension and risk of stroke in Japanese-American men. *Stroke.* 1995;26:25-29.
48. Domanski MJ, Davis BR, Pfeffer MA, Kastantin M, Mitchell GF. Isolated systolic hypertension. Prognostic information provided by pulse pressure. *Hypertension.* 1999;34:375-380.
49. Waldstein SR, Rice SC, Thayer JF, Najjar SS, Scuteri A, Zonderman AB. Pulse pressure and pulse wave velocity are related to cognitive decline in the Baltimore Longitudinal Study of Aging. *Hypertension.* 2008;51:99-104.
50. Psaty BM, Furberg CD, Kuller LH, et al. Isolated systolic hypertension and subclinical cardiovascular disease in the elderly. Initial findings from the cardiovascular health study. *JAMA.* 1992;268:1287-1291.
51. Bots ML, Hofman A, de Bruyn AM, de Jong PT, Grobbee DE. Isolated systolic hypertension and vessel wall thickness of the carotid artery. The Rotterdam Elderly Study. *Arterioscler Thromb.* 1993;13:64-69.
52. Manios E, Michas F, Stamatelopoulos K, et al. Association of isolated systolic, isolated diastolic, and systolic-diastolic masked hypertension with carotid artery intima-media thickness. *J Clin Hypertens (Greenwich).* 2015;17:22-26.
53. Sutton-Tyrrell K, Alcorn HG, Wolfson Jr SK, Kelsey SF, Kuller LH. Predictors of carotid stenosis in older adults with and without isolated systolic hypertension. *Stroke.* 1993;24:355-361.
54. Bots ML, Hoes AW, Koudstaal PJ, Hofman A, Grobbee DE. Common carotid intima-media thickness and risk of stroke and myocardial infarction: the Rotterdam study. *Circulation.* 1997;96:1432-1437.
55. Sutton KC, Wolfson Jr SK, Kuller LH. Carotid and lower extremity arterial disease in elderly adults with isolated systolic hypertension. *Stroke.* 1987;18:817-822.
56. Powell TM, Glynn RJ, Buring JE, Creager MA, Ridker PM, Pradhan AD. The relative importance of systolic versus diastolic blood pressure control and incident symptomatic peripheral artery disease in women. *Vasc Med.* 2011;16:239-246.
57. Safar ME, Priollet P, Luizy F, et al. Peripheral arterial disease and isolated systolic hypertension: the ATTEST study. *J Hum Hypertens.* 2009;23:182-187.
58. Verhave JC, Fesler P, du Cailar G, Ribstein J, Safar ME, Mimran A. Elevated pulse pressure is associated with low renal function in elderly patients with isolated systolic hypertension. *Hypertension.* 2005;45:586-591.
59. Young JH, Klag MJ, Muntner P, Whyte JL, Pahor M, Coresh J. Blood pressure and decline in kidney function: findings from the systolic hypertension in the elderly program (shep). *J Am Soc Nephrol.* 2002;13:2776-2782.
60. Li Y, Wei FF, Thijs L, et al. Ambulatory hypertension subtypes and 24-hour systolic and diastolic blood pressure as distinct outcome predictors in 8341 untreated people recruited from 12 populations. *Circulation.* 2014;130:466-474.
61. Hozawa A, Ohkubo T, Nagai K, et al. Prognosis of isolated systolic and isolated diastolic hypertension as assessed by self-measurement of blood pressure at home: the Ohasama study. *Arch Intern Med.* 2000;160:3301-3306.
62. Niiranen TJ, Rissanen H, Johansson JK, Jula AM. Overall cardiovascular prognosis of isolated systolic hypertension, isolated diastolic hypertension and pulse pressure defined with home measurements: the Finn-home study. *J Hypertens.* 2014;32:518-524.

63. Vlachopoulos C, Aznaouridis K, O'Rourke MF, Safar ME, Baou K, Stefanadis C. Prediction of cardiovascular events and all-cause mortality with central haemodynamics: a systematic review and meta-analysis. *Eur Heart J.* 2010;31:1865-1871.

64. Ben-Shlomo Y, Spears M, Boustred C, et al. Aortic pulse wave velocity improves cardiovascular event prediction: an individual participant meta-analysis of prospective observational data from 17,635 subjects. *J Am Coll Cardiol.* 2014;63:636-646.

65. Benetos A, Gautier S, Labat C, et al. Mortality and cardiovascular events are best predicted by low central/peripheral pulse pressure amplification but not by high blood pressure levels in elderly nursing home subjects: the PARTAGE (predictive values of blood pressure and arterial stiffness in institutionalized very aged population) study. *J Am Coll Cardiol.* 2012;60:1503-1511.

66. SHEP Cooperative Research Group. Prevention of stroke by antihypertensive drug treatment in older persons with isolated systolic hypertension. Final results of the systolic hypertension in the elderly program (shep). *JAMA.* 1991;265:3255-3264.

67. Staessen JA, Fagard R, Thijs L, et al. Randomised double-blind comparison of placebo and active treatment for older patients with isolated systolic hypertension. *Lancet.* 1997;350:757-764.

68. Liu L, Wang JG, Gong L, Liu G, Staessen JA, for the Systolic Hypertension in China (Syst-China) Collaborative Group. Comparison of active treatment and placebo in older Chinese patients with isolated systolic hypertension. *J Hypertens.* 1998;16:1823-1829.

69. Patel AB, Kostis JB, Wilson AC, Shea ML, Pressel SL, Davis BR. Long-term fatal outcomes in subjects with stroke or transient ischemic attack: fourteen-year follow-up of the systolic hypertension in the elderly program. *Stroke.* 2008;39:1084-1089.

70. Beckett NS, Peters R, Fletcher AE, et al. Treatment of hypertension in patients 80 years of age or older. *N Engl J Med.* 2008;358:1887-1898.

71. Burney BO, Bakris GL. Hypertension and its management in the elderly. *Semin Nephrol.* 2009;29:604-609.

72. Forette F, Seux ML, Staessen JA, et al. The prevention of dementia with antihypertensive treatment: new evidence from the systolic hypertension in europe (syst-eur) study. *Arch Intern Med.* 2002;162:2046-2052.

73. Forette F, Seux ML, Staessen JA, et al. Prevention of dementia in randomised double-blind placebo-controlled systolic hypertension in Europe (Syst-Eur) trial. *Lancet.* 1998;352:1347-1351.

74. Staessen JA, Richart T, Birkenhager WH. Less atherosclerosis and lower blood pressure for a meaningful life perspective with more brain. *Hypertension.* 2007;49:389-400.

75. Peters R, Beckett N, Forette F, et al. Incident dementia and blood pressure lowering in the hypertension in the very elderly trial cognitive function assessment (hyvet-cog): a double-blind, placebo controlled trial. *Lancet Neurol.* 2008;7:683-689.

76. Ogihara T, Saruta T, Rakugi H, et al. Target blood pressure for treatment of isolated systolic hypertension in the elderly: valsartan in elderly isolated systolic hypertension study. *Hypertension.* 2010;56:196-202.

77. Group SR, Wright JT, Jr., Williamson JD, et al. randomized trial of intensive versus standard blood-pressure control. *N Engl J Med.* 2015;373:2103-2116.

78. Voyaki SM, Staessen JA, Thijs L, et al. Follow-up of renal function in treated and untreated older patients with isolated systolic hypertension. Systolic Hypertension in Europe (Syst-Eur) Trial Investigators. *J Hypertens.* 2001;19:511-519.

79. Muller M, Smulders YM, de Leeuw PW, Stehouwer CD. Treatment of hypertension in the oldest old: a critical role for frailty? *Hypertension.* 2014;63:433-441.

80. Warwick J, Falaschetti E, Rockwood K, et al. No evidence that frailty modifies the positive impact of antihypertensive treatment in very elderly people: an investigation of the impact of frailty upon treatment effect in the hypertension in the very elderly trial (HYVET) study, a double-blind, placebo-controlled study of antihypertensives in people with hypertension aged 80 and over. *BMC Med.* 2015;13:78.

81. Bulpitt CJ, Beckett NS, Peters R, et al. Baseline characteristics of participants in the hypertension in the very elderly trial (HYVET). *Blood Press.* 2009;18:17-22.

82. Benetos A, Labat C, Rossignol P, et al. Treatment with multiple blood pressure medications, achieved blood pressure, and mortality in older nursing home residents: the PARTAGE study. *JAMA Intern Med.* 2015;175:989-995.

83. Benetos A, Rossignol P, Cherubini A, et al. Polypharmacy in the aging patient: management of hypertension in octogenarians. *JAMA.* 2015;314:170-180.

84. Oliva RV, Bakris GL. Management of hypertension in the elderly population. *J Gerontol A Biol Sci Med Sci.* 2012;67:1343-1351.

85. He FJ, Markandu ND, MacGregor GA. Modest salt reduction lowers blood pressure in isolated systolic hypertension and combined hypertension. *Hypertension.* 2005;46:66-70.

86. Weinberger MH. Salt restriction in the treatment of isolated systolic and combined hypertension: is that enough? *Hypertension.* 2005;46:31-32.

87. Kjeldsen SE, Dahlof B, Devereux RB, et al. Effects of losartan on cardiovascular morbidity and mortality in patients with isolated systolic hypertension and left ventricular hypertrophy: a losartan intervention for endpoint reduction (life) substudy. *JAMA.* 2002;288:1491-1498.

88. Jamerson K, Weber MA, Bakris GL, et al. Benazepril plus amlodipine or hydrochlorothiazide for hypertension in high-risk patients. *N Engl J Med.* 2008;359:2417-2428.

89. Modesti PA, Omboni S, Taddei S, et al. Zofenopril or irbesartan plus hydrochlorothiazide in elderly patients with isolated systolic hypertension untreated or uncontrolled by previous treatment: a double-blind, randomized study. *J Hypertens.* 2015.

90. Krum H, Schlaich M, Whitbourn R, et al. Catheter-based renal sympathetic denervation for resistant hypertension: a multicentre safety and proof-of-principle cohort study. *Lancet.* 2009;373:1275-1281.

91. Krum H, Schlaich M, Sobotka P, Scheffers I, Kroon AA, de Leeuw PW. Novel procedure- and device-based strategies in the management of systemic hypertension. *Eur Heart J.* 2011;32:537-544.

92. Ewen S, Ukena C, Linz D, et al. Reduced effect of percutaneous renal denervation on blood pressure in patients with isolated systolic hypertension. *Hypertension.* 2015;65:193-199.

93. Manisty CH, Hughes AD. Meta-analysis of the comparative effects of different classes of antihypertensive agents on brachial and central systolic blood pressure, and augmentation index. *Br J Clin Pharmacol.* 2013;75:79-92.

94. Fok H, Cruickshank JK. Future treatment of hypertension: shifting the focus from blood pressure lowering to arterial stiffness modulation? *Curr Hypertens Rep.* 2015;17:67.

95. Ong KT, Delerme S, Pannier B, et al. Aortic stiffness is reduced beyond blood pressure lowering by short-term and long-term antihypertensive treatment: a meta-analysis of individual data in 294 patients. *J Hypertens.* 2011;29:1034-1042.

96. Nichols WW, O'Rourke MF. *Mcdonald's blood flow in arteries: theoretical, experimental and clinical principles.* London: Arnold; 1998.

20 Assessment of Target Organ Damage

Christian Ott and Roland E. Schmieder

Hypertension-induced cardiovascular (CV) morbidity and mortality is caused by structural and functional alterations of the brain, heart, eyes, kidneys, and vasculature. Importantly, these hypertensive target organ damage (TOD) can be detected in an early subclinical stage, that is, as an asymptomatic and reversible stage of disease before fatal and nonfatal CV events occur. The classical score systems used to estimate the total CV risk do not take TOD into account because these score systems are only valid in hypertensive patients without TOD. Once TOD, even intermediate, has developed (e.g., decreased estimated glomerular filtration rate [GFR], left ventricular hypertrophy [LVH]), these conditions are by far overwriting any risk prediction from the CV risk factor scores. TOD represents an intermediate stage in the CV, cerebrovascular, and renal continuum and its progression depends on both the duration and severity of high blood pressure (BP). Although there is no doubt that arterial hypertension has an independent relationship on several TODs, the individual impact of hypertension is diverse. Hence, this chapter mainly addresses TODs with arterial hypertension being the most important attributable risk factor.

From a therapeutic perspective it is essential to treat hypertension at a stage when TOD changes are reversible, and to be aggressive to achieve BP control rapidly.

A variety of techniques are available nowadays to diagnose TOD in different organs but with differences in sensitivity and specificity. TOD can be routinely assessed in the clinical work up, but the applicability is limited depending on the availability of the various techniques and the reimbursement strategy of health care systems. The clinical importance of TOD is also underlined by the fact that TOD requires not only more aggressive and immediate drug therapy, but also by the clear perspective to reduce TOD and the associated risk. Thus, regression of TOD is clinically a useful tool for evaluation of the efficacy of antihypertensive treatment in individual patients. Therefore this chapter also emphasizes the consequences of TOD regression by antihypertensive treatment, and attempts to establish whether or not changes of TOD have related prognostic significance.

TARGET ORGAN *"BRAIN"*

In general, the brain is highly vulnerable to the deleterious effects of elevated BP and represents the classic target organ of BP-induced damage. Arterial hypertension, beyond its well-known effect to cause clinical (ischemic and hemorrhagic) stroke, is also associated with the risk of asymptomatic (subclinical) brain damage, such as cerebral small vessel disease (SVD). Widespread use of magnetic resonance imaging (MRI) applied to search for cerebrovascular and brain damage has limited availability (in some countries) and high costs in the evaluation of hypertensive patients, although silent brain infarction should be searched for in all hypertensive subjects with disturbances, cognitive impairment, and, particularly, memory loss.

Stroke

Stroke incidence has declined by over 40% in the past 4 decades in high-income countries, but over the same period, incidence has doubled in low-income and middle-income countries.[1] Because age is one of most important risk factors for stroke it has been proposed that aging of the world population implies a growing number of persons at risk.[2] The decline of stroke incidence in high-income countries is also thought to be related to better CV risk management. In Western countries about 80% of strokes are ischemic and the remaining 20% are hemorrhagic. This distinction between hemorrhagic and ischemic stroke is critical for stroke management and treatment decisions.

The main mechanisms causing ischemic stroke are thrombosis and embolism. Atherosclerosis is the most common feature, and a plaque rupture causes downstream ischemic stroke. Pathological conditions causing thrombotic ischemic stroke are high-grade stenosis of the internal carotid artery, fibromuscular dysplasia (FMD), arteritis (i.e., giant cell and Takayasu), and vascular dissection. Embolic stroke may occur as a result of embolization from a variety of sources (e.g., left atrium, mitral valve disease, atherothrombotic plaques in the aortic area), but the most common underlying cause is atrial fibrillation.

Multiple infarct locations (in different vascular beds) suggest the heart (and aorta) as the origin of the embolism. Ischemic stroke can be subdivided according the TOAST (Trial of Org 10172 in Acute Stroke Treatment) classification,[3] which is based on clinical symptoms as well as results of further investigations (Box 20.1).

Prognostic Value of Change

In primary and secondary prevention of stroke, antihypertensive treatment represents a cornerstone of treatment options. A continuous relationship between BP and the occurrence of stroke has been documented[4] and, conversely, clinical trials and meta-analyses have revealed that lowering BP results in a substantially reduced risk of stroke in both primary and secondary prevention.[5,6]

Small Vessel Disease

It has to be taken into account that the terminology and definitions for SVD varies between studies (e.g., white matter lesions, -hyperintensity, -changes, -disease). Hence, the STandards for ReportIng Vascular changes in nEuroimaging (STRIVE) have proposed MRI-terminology and lesion findings (Fig. 20.1).[7]

White Matter Hyperintensity

Among all subtypes of SVD, white matter hyperintensity (WMH) is the most prevalent lesion in the general population. About every second patient in their forties,[8] and more than 90% aged over 80 years of age have WMH.[9]

Hypertension is considered to be an important risk factor for both WMH volume and progression.[10] Importantly,

189

BOX 20.1 TOAST Classification of Ischemic Stroke

1. Large Artery Atherosclerosis (Embolus/Thrombosis)
Features:
1. Clinical: cortical or brainstem or cerebellar dysfunction
2. Imaging: cortical, cerebellar, brainstem, or subcortical infarct greater than 1.5 cm on computed tomography (CT) or magnetic resonance imaging (MRI)
3. Test: stenosis (greater than 50%) or occlusion of a major brain artery or branch cortical artery evidenced by duplex ultrasound imaging or arteriography.

2. Cardioembolism (High Risk/Medium Risk)
Features:
1. Clinical: cortical, brainstem or cerebellar dysfunction or the evidence of a previous transient ischemic attack or stroke in more than one vascular territory
2. Imaging: cortical, cerebellar, brainstem, or subcortical infarct greater than 1.5 cm on CT or MRI
3. Test major cardiac source of emboli (e.g.,):
   a. mechanical prosthetic valve
   b. atrial fibrillation
   c. left atrial/atrial appendage thrombus
   d. left ventricular thrombus
   e. dilated cardiomyopathy
   f. akinetic left ventricular apex
   g. atrial myxoma
   h. infective endocarditis

3. Small-Vessel Occlusion (Lacunae)
Features:
1. Clinical: lacunar syndromes without evidence of cortical or brainstem or cerebellar dysfunction (a history of diabetes mellitus or hypertension supports the clinical diagnosis)
2. Imaging: normal CT/MRI examination or a relevant subcortical or brainstem infarct smaller than 1.5 cm
3. Test: potential cardiac sources for embolism should be absent, and evaluation of the large extracranial arteries should not demonstrate a stenosis of greater than 50% in an ipsilateral artery.

4. Stroke of Other Determined Etiology
Blood tests or arteriography should reveal one of the following unusual causes of stroke
   a. nonatherosclerotic vasculopathies
   b. hypercoagulable states
   c. hematologic disorders
   Patients in this group should have clinical and CT/MRI findings of an acute ischemic stroke, regardless of the size or location.

5. Stroke of Undetermined Etiology
   a. two or more causes identified
   b. negative evaluation
   c. incomplete evaluation

(Adapted from Reference 3.)

a systematic review and meta-analysis revealed that WMH predicts a three-fold increased risk of stroke, and double increased risk of both dementia and mortality.[9]

Prognostic Value of Change

Increasing evidence suggests that BP control may reduce the course of WMH progression.[11] Moreover, it was shown that uncontrolled patients with untreated hypertension had significantly more WMH progression than subjects with uncontrolled treated hypertension and controlled treated hypertension. These data indirectly suggest that antihypertensive therapy may prevent WML progression in the hypertensive population.[12] However, until today, there is not a single study demonstrating that decrease of WMH induced by effective antihypertensive therapy is associated with improved prognosis (Table 20.1).

Microbleeds

Similarly, aging and hypertension are independently associated with cerebral microbleeds (MB).[13,14] Importantly, higher BP (e.g., odds ratio [OR] 2.69; 95% confidence interval [CI], 1.40 to 5.21 per standard deviation [SD] increase for 24-hour BP) was associated with new development of MB.[15] Presence of MB is associated with increased risk of incident intracerebral hemorrhage, in particular in patients on anticoagulation therapy. Presence of MB increased the risk of both hemorrhagic and ischemic stroke in patients after ischemic stroke.[16] Studies revealed that MB is associated with increased risk of stroke-related death as well as all-cause and CV mortality.[17,18]

Prognostic Value of Change

Although the magnitude of BP elevation is associated with the occurrence of MB, effective BP reduction had surprisingly no clear impact on MB progression during follow-up.[15]

Small Subcortical Infarcts

Small subcortical infarcts (SSI), historically commonly called "lacunar stroke," are primarily located in the motor and sensory pathways and explain the clinical symptoms despite lacunar size. Only half of SSI are detected on computed tomography (CT), but at least 70% are visible on diffusion-weighted MRI. Although pathogenetic mechanisms between hypertension and SSI are largely unknown, the prevalence of hypertension is highest in patients with SSI compared with any other subtype of ischemic stroke.[19] The presence and progression of SSI is an independent risk factor for cerebrovascular disease and impairment of cognitive function.[20,21]

Prognostic Value of Change

In the recently published "Secondary Prevention of Small Subcortical Stroke (SPS3)" trial, a systolic BP target of less than 130 mm Hg was accompanied by a nonsignificant reduction in all stroke, disabling or fatal, but with a significant reduction of intracerebral hemorrhagic stroke compared with a systolic BP target of 130 to 149 mm Hg.[22] In the European Society of Hypertension/European Society of Cardiology (ESH/ESC) guidelines BP reduction less than 140/90 mm Hg is recommended for primary and secondary stroke prevention, but no specific recommendation is made for WMH, MB, and SSI.[23]

Lacunes

Previous SSI, silent brain infarction (SBI), and hemorrhage (territory of one penetrating arteriole) are vascular causes of lacunes, but shrunk striatocapsular strokes may also form a lacunar-like cavity. Although an association between BP and incident lacunes was seen in patients without baseline documentation, higher BP did not contribute to lesion progression in patients with already severe findings at baseline.[24]

Prognostic Value of Change

Because SBI increases the risk of stroke up to five times, indirect evidence based on a small Japanese study demonstrates that BP control reduced the risk of SBI.[25] Whether or not such a reduction of SBI is related to improved survival remains to be proven.

Perivascular Space

The fluid-filled space surrounding the path of penetrating arteries is named perivascular space (PVS). In the Northern Manhattan Study it was recently shown that dilated PVS is more common in patients with higher peripheral pulse pressure (PP) and systolic BP, the pulsatile components of BP.[26]

Prognostic Value of Change

Compared with normotensive patients, uncontrolled hypertensive patients during follow-up were at increased risk

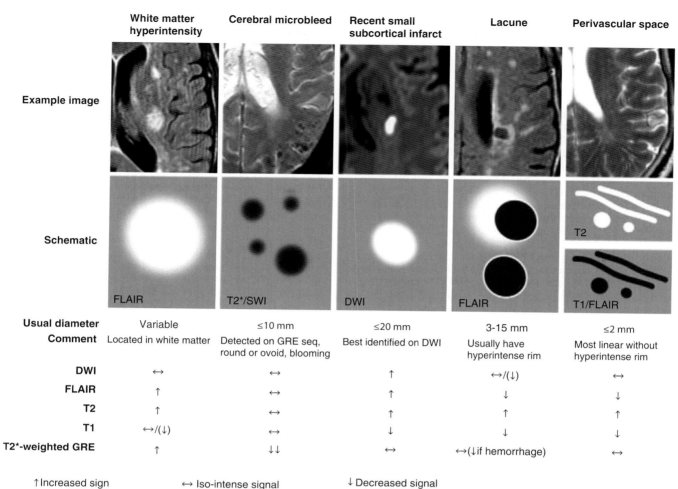

	White matter hyperintensity	Cerebral microbleed	Recent small subcortical infarct	Lacune	Perivascular space
Usual diameter	Variable	≤10 mm	≤20 mm	3-15 mm	≤2 mm
Comment	Located in white matter	Detected on GRE seq, round or ovoid, blooming	Best identified on DWI	Usually have hyperintense rim	Most linear without hyperintense rim
DWI	↔	↔	↑	↔/(↓)	↔
FLAIR	↑	↔	↑	↓	↓
T2	↑	↔	↑	↑	↑
T1	↔/(↓)	↔	↓	↓	↓
T2*-weighted GRE	↑	↓↓	↔	↔(↓if hemorrhage)	↔

↑ Increased sign   ↔ Iso-intense signal   ↓ Decreased signal

FIG. 20.1 Recommendation by STandards for ReportIng Vascular changes in nEuroimaging (STRIVE) for magnetic resonance imaging terminology and lesion findings related to vascular brain injury. *(Adapted from Reference 7.)*

TABLE 20.1 Prognostic Significance of Treatment-Induced Changes of (Asymptomatic) Target Organ Damage

TARGET ORGAN DAMAGE	SENSITIVITY FOR CHANGES	TIME OF CHANGE	PROGNOSTIC SIGNIFICANCE OF CHANGES
Brain			
Small vessel disease	No data	No data	No data
Heart			
LVH			
ECG	Low	>6 months	Yes
Echo	Moderate	>6 months	Yes
MRI	High	>6 months	No data
Eye			
Qualitative signs	Low–high	Weeks–months	No data
Quantitative signs	No data	No data	No data
Kidney			
eGFR	Moderate	Month–years	Yes
Albuminuria	High	Weeks–months	Yes
Vasculature			
IMT	Very low	>12 months	No
PWV	High	Weeks–months	Limited data
Central BP	High	Days–weeks	No data

BP, Blood pressure; *ECG,* electrocardiogram; *Echo,* echocardiography; *eGFR,* estimated glomerular filtration rate; *IMT,* intima-media thickness; *LVH,* left ventricular hypertrophy; *MRI,* magnetic resonance imaging; *PWV,* pulse wave velocity.

of dilated PVS.[26] Studies analyzing whether an increase or decrease of PVS bears any prognostic information are missing.

Dementia

The link between hypertension and the incidence and prevalence of dementia is well established. Hypertension is either a causal risk factor or an indirect promoter of dementia. Studies assessing the midlife BP (measured between 40 and 65 years) revealed a relationship between higher midlife BP and risk of incident vascular dementia. Of note, however, no clear association with late-life BP and the development and prevalence of dementia was found.[27] Regarding both main subtypes of dementia, namely Alzheimer disease and vascular dementia, there was a clear association for hypertension and vascular dementia (e.g., Hiyasama study: hazard ratio [HR]: 10.07 [3.25 to 31.25] for BP range 160 to 179/100 to 109 mm Hg versus normal BP range [<130/85 mm Hg]), but less clear for Alzheimer disease (e.g., Hiyasama study: HR 1.05 [0.50 to 2.22] BP range 160 to 179/100 to 109 mm Hg versus normal BP range [<130/85 mm Hg]).[27] In contrast, Launer et al.[28] observed a significant relation between hypertension and Alzheimer disease (OR 4.47 [1.53 to 13.09] for diastolic blood pressure [DBP] ≥ 95 mm Hg versus 80 to 89 mm Hg), supporting the hypothesis that vascular factors cause or at least accelerate Alzheimer disease.[29]

Alzheimer disease and vascular dementia may often coexist and thus, misclassification may happen (e.g., vascular dementia or a mixed dementia rather than Alzheimer disease).[30]

Although not directly recommended in most guidelines, the cognitive assessment instruments, particularly in patients with increased risk or based on clinical assumptions, may reasonably be part of routine clinical work up of hypertensive patients. Different screening questionnaires are available, such as the Mini-Mental State Examination (MMSE), the Informant Questionnaire on Cognitive Decline in the Elderly (IQCODE), and the Montreal Cognitive Assessment (MoCA) (Screening for cognitive impairment in older adults: and evidence update for the U.S: Preventive Services Task Force, 2013. www.ahrq.gov.).

Although MMSE is the most widely used test (including five sections, namely orientation, registration, attention and calculation, recall and language), it cannot evaluate executive function and cognitive impairment only with low sensitivity. The MoCA, which incorporates subtests for executive function and psychomotor speed (often impaired in cognitive impairment), is specially designed for detecting mild cognitive impairment.[31] Compared with MMSE, the MoCA test showed remarkably improved sensitivity and specificity for cognitive impairment (18% versus 90%).[32] Moreover, sensitivity of detecting cognitive impairment was greater with MoCA than with MMSE in patients with acute transient ischemic attack or minor stroke, even when other neurologic deficits were not evident.[33]

Prognostic Value of Change

Longitudinal observational studies found benefits of BP reduction for the risk of incident vascular dementia, but results are uncertain with respect to BP reduction and Alzheimer disease. Longer duration of BP reduction was associated with less risk of dementia.[34,35] In contrast, pooled analysis with meta-regression technique of large-scale randomized controlled trials (mainly active treatment versus placebo) revealed that risk of cognitive impairment was not clearly reduced by active treatment, probably attributed to the relatively short treatment duration of 2 to 5 years.[36] It remains to be proven whether or not improvement or stabilization in the MoCA score (by BP reduction) is associated with improved neurologic outcome, cognitive impairment, and risk of stroke and mortality. Nevertheless, despite the lack of clear evidence, BP lowering is thought to decrease or stop the process and progression of dementia.

TARGET ORGAN "HEART"

Longstanding hypertension leads to LVH modified by various pathogenetic factors and, if untreated, to congestive heart failure (CHF).

Left Ventricular Hypertrophy

Initially, LVH occurs as an adaptive process to the pressure-load imposed on the heart to reduce wall stress and maintain LV pump function and ejection fraction (EF). As a consequence, wall thickness increases on the expanses of the LV internal diameter and relative wall thickness (ratio of wall thickness [RWT] to LV internal diameter) increases as well, so-called concentric pattern of LVH. Over time, LV remodeling processes aggravate, hypertrophied muscle fibers become thickened and shortened, and perivascular and interstitial collagen content increases, ultimately resulting in LV dilation, so-called pattern of eccentric LVH. However, only a small portion of left ventricular mass (LVM) variation are explained by BP (only 10% with office systolic BP over 30 years and up to 25% with 24-hour ambulatory BP), and solid evidence is available that several nonhemodynamic factors (e.g., body mass index,[37] dietary salt intake,[38] genetic factors,[39] activation of the sympathetic nervous system,[40] and renin-angiotensin-system [RAS][41]) determines the development as well as the degree of LVM (Fig. 20.2).

Several methods, with different sensitivity and specificity are available for the assessment of LVH in hypertension. From some decades ago, epidemiological studies have revealed that LVH is one of the independent risk factors determining prognosis of hypertensive patients.[42] Both clinical and epidemiological studies have shown that LVH, irrespective of whether assessed by electrocardiogram (ECG) or echocardiography, is associated with a several-fold increase in CV and all-cause mortality.[43] Interestingly, LVH diagnosed by ECG and by echocardiography does not encompass the same entity; that is, they reflect different pathogenetic aspects related to LVH adaptive process because LVH by ECG and by echocardiography are independently associated with mortality.[44]

Electrocardiography

In hypertension guidelines, ECG is recommended as the primary diagnostic tool to detect LV remodeling and LVH,[23] and in a recent analysis of 26 studies, the role of ECG as a first-line examination for identifying subclinical cardiac organ damage has been highlighted.[45]

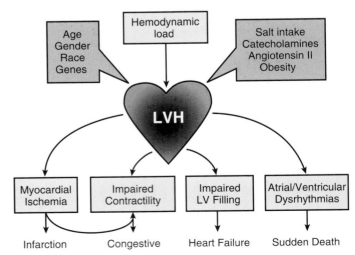

FIG. 20.2 Determinants of left ventricular hypertrophy (LVH) and consecutive cardiovascular (CV) complications.

There are several criteria for detecting LVH by ECG based on voltage and in part, repolarization patterns and/or QRS duration. The most common criteria are (modified) Sokolow-Lyon index as $S_{V1} + R_{V5} > 3,5$ mV and the Cornell product criteria ($S_{V3} + R_{aVL}$ * QRS-duration >244 mV*ms) (Table 20.2).[46] In obese patients the Cornell product[47] and, if left anterior fascicular block is evident, other criteria (e.g., Siii + max. R/S any lead >30 mV men [>28 mV women]; for details see Hancock et al.[48]) may be preferred, because voltage, repolarization pattern, and QRS duration may be differently affected as a result of these conditions.

Regardless of used criteria, the sensitivity in detecting LVH is at best about 50% to 60%, but of high specificity (about 85% to 90%).[48,49] Nevertheless, a 12-lead ECG should be performed in all hypertensive patients, because other signs of hypertensive damage to the heart and/or CV complications (e.g., atrial fibrillation) can be detected. Notably, there is evidence that new-onset of atrial fibrillation must be considered as TOD[50] and specific antihypertensive therapy is recommended.[51]

Echocardiography

Echocardiography is more sensitive than ECG in detecting LVH and is the gold standard for quantifying cardiac structural and functional changes of the LV in hypertensive patients. Echocardiographic evaluation allows quantitative measurements of interventricular septum wall thickness (IVST), left ventricular internal diameter (LVID), and posterior wall thickness (PWT) in diastole (d) and systole (s). LVM is calculated under the assumption of a prolate ellipsoid shape of the LV according a mathematical formula of the American Society of Echocardiography (LVM = $0.8 \times (1.04 [(LVIDd + PWTd + IVSTd)^3 - (LVIDd)^3] + 0.6g)$.[52] A normalization of LVM for various body constitutions is necessary to avoid underestimation and overestimation, and the indexation to height 1.7 ($g/m^{1.7}$) appears to be best, although the standard index based on body surface area (BSA) is still used in clinical practice.[53] More recently, data from the Echocardiographic Normal Ranges Meta-Analysis of the Left Heart (EchoNoRMAL) project suggest that different allometric power for BSA and height should be applied according to gender and ethnic group,[54] but these complex algorithms have not found general acceptances. Calculation of RWT (as 2 × PWTd/LVIDd) with its cut-off value of 0.42 permits the classification of concentric (RWT > 0.42) or eccentric (RWT ≤ 0.42) hypertrophy as well as concentric remodeling (normal LVM, but RWT > 0.42). This is of importance because the patterns of LVH are differently associated with CV risk, with concentric LVH to have the greatest risk.[55-57] Finally, it needs to be stressed that echocardiography offers the opportunity to assess additional information on anatomy and function of the heart as well as valves and thereby allows the diagnosis of other hypertensive-related TOD, such as CHF with reduced or preserved EF and coronary heart disease among others.

Magnetic Resonance Imaging

It has been proposed that MRI is the new "gold-standard" for noninvasive evaluation of LVH,[58] but the low availability and high cost clearly argue against this claim and has to be refuted.[23] Nevertheless, MRI should be considered in patients with poor echocardiographic quality. Notably, MRI enables an answer regarding LVH pattern and its cause.[58] Detailed protocols[59] and reference values (partly given in Table 20.2) have been published.[60]

Prognostic Value of Change

It was repeatedly shown that regression of LVH, irrespective of whether assessed by ECG or echocardiography, conferred an improvement of associated CV risk.[61-63] In the echocardiographic substudy of the LIFE trial, LVM reduction of one standard deviation (i.e., 25 g/m^2) results in a 20% decrement of the primary endpoint (death, nonfatal MI, and stroke).[62] For a single patient, it is proposed that LVM changes of 10% to 15% may have clinical significance.[64] A meta-analysis directly comparing regression of LVH among different antihypertensive classes revealed that RAS blockers (angiotensin-converting enzyme [ACE] inhibitor or angiotensin receptor blocker [ARB]) and calcium channel blocker (CCB) exhibited the most pronounced effect, which was found to be superior to those of beta-blockers and diuretics.[65] Subsequently, a more recently published meta-analysis confirmed that RAS blockers are better able to reduce LVH than beta-blockers.[66] Nevertheless, achievement of BP control is the most important target in obtaining LV reduction.[67] Interestingly, besides the rapidly proven relationship that LVM reduction results in less CV events, regression of LVH in hypertensive patients still has an adverse CV prognosis compared to those who never had LVH; that is, the CV prognosis improves but is still elevated after reduction of LVM.[68]

Heart Failure

Epidemiological studies have shown that hypertension is the most frequent underlying cause of CHF. Notably, in a large proportion of patients, antihypertensive drugs (ACE inhibitor, ARB, aldosterone-antagonist, beta-blocker, diuretic), and angiotensin receptor Neprilysin inhibitor are now standard of care not only to lower afterload but also to counteract neuroendocrine stimulation (inherent in CHF).

Heart Failure With Preserved Ejection Fraction

Alterations in LV relaxation and filling pattern are main features of diastolic dysfunction in hypertension, which may precede alteration in systolic dysfunction. Diastolic dysfunction, often associated with LV remodeling and concentric LVH, may result in clinical symptoms of CHF, although EF is preserved (HFpEF). The diagnosis of HFpEF is challenging because it is largely based on the exclusion of other noncardiac causes of symptoms suggestive of CHF.

TABLE 20.2 Cut-Off Values of Noninvasive Common Parameters Used in the Assessment of (Asymptomatic) Target Organ Damage of the Heart

Electrocardiography		
Sokolow-Lyon Index	$S_{V1} + R_{V5}$	>3,5 mV
Cornell voltage criteria	$S_{V3} + R_{aVL}$	>2,8 mV
QRS duration product	(Cornell voltage * QRS-duration)	>244mV*ms
Echocardiography		
LV mass (BSA, g/m^2)		>95 (♀)/>115 (♂)
LV mass index (height$^{1.7}$, $g/m^{1.7}$)		>60 (♀)/>81 (♂)
Type		
• Concentric	(LVH and) RWT	>0.42
• Eccentric	(LVH and) RWT	≤0.42
• Concentric remodeling	(no LVH) RWT	>0.42
Magnetic Resonance Imaging		
LV mass (BSA, g/m^2) (without papillary muscle mass)[145]		>85 (♀)/>108 (♂)
LV mass (BSA, g/m^2) (with papillary muscle mass)[146]		>89 (♀)/>112 (♂)

BSA, Body surface area; *LV*, left ventricular; *LVH*, left ventricular hypertrophy; *RWT*, relative wall thickness.

Both diagnosis and grading of diastolic dysfunction is based on Doppler tissue analysis (E/e' ratio), preferably assessed at septal and lateral mitral annulus. Additional indicators of impaired diastolic filling are the ratio between transmitral peak early and late filling velocity (E/A ratio) and atrial size, an indicator of diastolic dysfunction.[69,70] Of all Doppler parameters, the E/e' ratio has been shown to be the strongest predictor of first cardiac events in hypertensive patients independent of LVM and RWT.[71] Likewise, left atrial (LA) enlargement, reflecting increased left ventricular filling pressure, indexed by volume (LAVi >34 mL/m^2), is also predictive of CHF and mortality.[72]

Heart Failure With Reduced Ejection Fraction

Global alteration of LV systolic function is the key diagnostic criteria of heart failure with reduced EF (HfrEF) whose two major underlying diseases are nowadays hypertension and coronary artery disease. Two-dimensional echocardiography using the modified Simpson method (average of apical four- and two-chamber views) is the traditional measurement of systolic LV function, and EF above 55% is defined as normal, between 55% and 45% as moderate, and below 35% as severe LV systolic dysfunction.

Nowadays, three-dimensional technology allows frame-by-frame detection of the endocardial surface from real-time three-dimensional datasets. An improved accuracy and reproducibility of three-dimensional measurements of LV volumes and LVEF compared with two-dimensional have been demonstrated by using independent reference technique (e.g., MRI).[73]

Prognostic Value of Change

Prevention of CHF represents the largest benefit that is associated with the use of BP-lowering drugs.[74] A meta-analysis of major interventional randomized trials comprising patients with hypertension has revealed that not only BP reduction but also the used class of antihypertensive drugs are related to decreased incidence of CHF.[75] In contrast, only a few studies have investigated the effect of BP reduction in patients already suffering from CHF and up-to-date, no efficacious therapy have been identified for HFpEF.[76] On the contrary, a sub-analyis of the I-PRESERVE study showed that HFpEF patients hospitalized for any reason, and especially for HF, were at increased risk for subsequent death.[77] Randomized controlled trials have mainly enrolled patients with HFrEF. Efficacious therapies for treating HFrEF in hypertensive patients are the preferential use of ACEs, ARBs, beta-blockers, diuretic, and aldosterone-antagonists.[78]

TARGET ORGAN *"EYE"*

For decades, direct ophthalmoscopic examination using the traditional four-grade classification system with increasing severity was regarded as part of standard work up of hypertensive patients.[79] In contrast, nowadays, its clinical usefulness in current clinical practice has been questioned because of its unreliable reproducibility, particularly in the low-grade retinopathy (grade 1 and 2).[80] Only for advanced grades, characterized by hemorrhages and exudates (grade 3) and papilla edema (grade 4), the assessment has been found to be reliable.[81] Hence, routine funduscopic examination is no longer recommended.[23]

The ability to digitize retinal photographs allows the assessment of outer arteriolar and venular diameter, and subsequently the arteriole-to-venule ratio (AVR) can be calculated.[82] In the last 2 decades, several large-scale, population-based studies assessing retinal photographs were conducted, including patients with and without hypertension. There is good evidence, that retinal alterations precede the development of hypertension,[83] and in a population-based cohort comprising 1572 children aged 6 to 8 years, each 10 mm Hg increase of systolic BP was associated with arteriolar narrowing by 2.08 μm (95 % CI: 1.38 to 2.79, $p < 0.0001$), indicating that effects of elevated BP manifest early in life.[84]

There is an ambiguous picture about the CV risk and associated arteriolar and venular diameter. In some studies arteriolar narrowing and venular widening were associated with incident stroke, whereas in the Rotterdam Study, only an association of venular widening was found.[85] In latter study, venular widening was also associated with cerebral infarction and intracerebral hemorrhages, but not arteriolar narrowing.[86] These conflicting results of the individual components with respect to prognostic indications of arteriolar and venular diameter have to be taken into account when interpreting individual AVR findings in hypertensive patients. An altered AVR can be attributed to single and concomitant changes of the individual components overall. The AVR did not enter routine clinical practice.

New technologies (e.g., scanning laser Doppler flowmetry [SLDF]) assessing the wall-to-lumen ratio (WLR) of retinal arterioles, and hence measuring directly the vascular remodeling are currently under investigation.[87] In a small cross-sectional study AVR was not able to discriminate between patients with cerebral damage and normotensive as well as hypertensive patients. In contrast, WLR was significantly higher and could therefore discriminate between patients with cerebrovascular event compared with both normotensive controls and hypertensive patients without cerebrovascular damage.[88]

Prognostic Value of Change

In several studies antihypertensive therapy, and hence BP reduction, resulted in disappearance of severe (grade 3 and 4) hypertensive retinopathy.[89,90] In contrast, data on improvement or disappearance of quantitative retinal signs (e.g., arteriolar narrowing) are much less clear. Moreover, no data are available on whether treatment-induced regression of retinal alterations is related with reduction of CV events. No prospective study is yet available analyzing treatment changes of retinal alterations assessed with SLDF and its associated prognostic value.

TARGET ORGAN *"KIDNEY"*

There is a strong association, and vicious circle, between arterial hypertension, chronic kidney disease (CKD), and CV disease.[91] Moreover, the presence of elevated albuminuria is an independent risk factor for CV events,[92] but it also predicts progression of CKD.[93] Hence, hypertension-induced renal damage is based on both reduced estimated glomerular filtration rate (eGFR) and elevated urinary albumin excretion (i.e., albuminuria), and hence both should be simultaneously assessed (Fig. 20.3).

Estimated Glomerular Filtration Rate

In general, eGFR declines with age after the thirties, with a progressive loss of 1% per year. In contrast, annual loss in untreated hypertensive patients is up to 4 to 8 mL/min.[94] However, it is of crucial importance to understand the physiology and, hence, pitfalls of renal function assessment using eGFR. Although, indexing eGFR to body surface area (i.e., mL/min per 1.73 m^2) reduces variation, equation of eGFR is affected by numerous circumstances (e.g., dietary protein intake, muscle mass, pregnancy, and several drugs). Several equations for eGFR have been introduced, which require in part more or less information. Although not requiring more information (age, gender, ethnicity, and serum creatinine concentration), the CKD-EPI equation performed better at higher GFRs (approximately >60 mL/min per 1.73 m^2) whereas both CKD-EPI and the MDRD Study equation performed reliably at lower GFRs. These facts are of importance because in CKD stage 3 or higher (<60 mL/min per 1.73 m^2) CV risk is most pronounced.

				Persistent albuminuria categories Description and range		
				A1 Normal to mildly increased	**A2** Moderately increased	**A3** Severely increased
				<30 mg/g <3 mg/mmol	30–300 mg/g 3–30 mg/mmol	>300 mg/g >30 mg/mmol
GFR categories (mL/min/1.73 m²) Description and range	**G1**	Normal or high	≥90			
	G2	Mildly decreased	60–89			
	G3a	Mildly to moderately decreased	45–59			
	G3b	Moderately to severely decreased	30–44			
	G4	Severely decreased	15–29			
	G5	Kidney failure	<15			

FIG. 20.3 Prognosis of chronic kidney disease (CKD) by estimated glomerular filtration rate (eGFR) and albuminuria category. *(Adapted from Reference 95.)*

The 2012 "Kidney Disease Improving Global Outcome" (KDIGO) clinical practice guidelines for evaluation and management of CKD recommend the 2009 CKD-EPI creatinine equation for initial assessment.[95] Alternative creatinine-based GFR estimating equations are acceptable if they have been shown to improve accuracy of GFR estimates compared with the 2009 CKD-EPI creatinine equation. Importantly, the 2009 CKD-EPI creatinine equation for reporting eGFR has replaced the MDRD in countries (e.g., France) as well as laboratory providers (Quest and Labcorp).[96]

Prognostic Value of Change

It has to be taken into account that initiation/intensification of antihypertensive therapy, in particular with RAS blockers, may induce a drop in eGFR. Although a reduction of 10 (–20)% is often considered as clinically relevant, this initial reduction of eGFR may not be interpreted as sign of progressive renal deterioration, but rather reflects the decrement of RAS activity and hence may result in long-term protection.[97]

A patient-based meta-analysis of 1.7 million participants (35 cohorts in the CKD Prognosis Consortium) found that declines in eGFR smaller than doubling of serum creatinine concentration occurred more commonly than doubling of serum creatinine concentration, but were also strongly and consistently associated with the risk of end-stage renal disease (ESRD) and mortality, supporting consideration of lesser declines in eGFR (such as a 30% reduction over 2 years).[98] In another cohort, however, after adjustment for the last measured eGFR, decline in eGFR per se was no longer associated with increased risk of acute myocardial infarction or stroke.[99] Thus, these results demonstrate the importance of monitoring the change in eGFR over time to monitor CV risk during follow-up. In a hypertensive study population comprising 4940 patients, the decrease of eGFR is associated, even in treated hypertensive subjects, with all-cause and CV mortality.[100]

Albuminuria

Albumin excretion measured from 24-hour collection with simultaneous assessment of total creatinine excretion (verifying a well-conducted sampling) may be best, but nowadays, albumin-to-creatinine ratio (UACR) taken ideally in the first morning spot-urine sample is recommended.[95,101,102]

Albuminuria is divided into microalbuminuria (also referring to moderately increased; category A2 [KDIGO]) defined by UACR from 30 to 300 mg/g creatinine (or equivalent amount over 24 hours) and macroalbuminuria (also referring to severely increased; category A3 [KDIGO]) defined by UACR greater than 300 mg/g creatinine. Although guidelines define a threshold for abnormal albuminuria, it should be taken into account that albuminuria is linearly or even exponentially and without threshold associated with CV mortality, even after adjustment for CV risk factors and eGFR.[92,103]

Prognostic Value of Change

A recent study demonstrated that an increment of albuminuria at any time during antihypertensive treatment was related to an increased CV risk.[104] Data from the ONTARGET program, including 23,480 patients with vascular disease, showed that overall a reduction in albuminuria of 50% or more translated into a 15% decrease of all-cause mortality compared with those with lesser changes in albuminuria, even after adjustment for baseline albuminuria, BP, and other confounding factors.[105] Recently, the analysis was expanded demonstrating that albuminuria over time was a better parameter than glucose status and BP control in predicting mortality and both CV and renal outcomes in patients at a high CV risk.[106] In a meta-regression and a meta-analysis it was confirmed that changes in albuminuria indicate renal and CV prognosis.[107,108]

TARGET ORGAN *"SMALL AND LARGE ARTERIES"*

Carotid Intima-Media Thickness

Population-based studies (e.g., Vobarno study) have shown that systolic BP is the major determinant of intima-media thickness (IMT) increment, particularly in arterial hypertension.[109] For high-resolution ultrasound examination of carotid IMT (double-line pattern on both walls) and presence of plaques (focal structure encroaching into the arterial lumen of at least 0.5 mm or 50% of the surrounding IMT value or demonstrates a thickness >1.5 mm as measured from the media-adventitia interface to the intima-lumen interface),[110] the carotid artery should be divided in three segments: the common carotid artery (CCA), the carotid bifurcation (bulb), and the internal carotid artery (ICA). However, measurement and reproducibility of IMT in CCA is better than bulb and ICA.[111] It is proposed that IMT at the bulb reflects primarily atherosclerosis and at the CCA vascular hypertrophy. Both IMT and plaques have been shown to be predictive for CV events.[112]

A value of IMT greater than 0.9 mm for abnormalities is stated in the recent guidelines (ESH/ESC 2013),[23] although in both middle-aged (1.16 mm)[113] and elderly patients (1.06 mm)[114] higher threshold values were reported.

Prognostic Value of Change

In a large prospective study although baseline carotid IMT and plaques are important, added risks of CV outcomes in a treated hypertensive population (independent of BP and traditional risk factors), treatment-induced IMT changes have failed to prove a significant predictive role for any type of CV outcome.[115]

Pulse Wave Velocity

Arterial stiffness results primarily from arteriosclerosis (disease of the media) rather than from atherosclerosis (disease of the intima). In principle, loss of compliance results in an increased faster travel of pulse waves. Measurement of (carotid-femoral) pulse wave velocity (PWV) is the gold standard for noninvasive assessment of arterial stiffness.[116] PWV is usually measured by the foot-to-foot velocity method from various waveforms, often obtained at the right CCA and the right femoral artery, and the time delay (Δt) between the feet of the two waveforms. The true anatomical distance traveled by the pressure wave is about 20% shorter than the direct measured carotid-to-femoral distance (D), which is also the underlying cause of the adjustment of threshold value of 10 m/s (instead of 12m/s).[117] Hence, PWV is calculated by $D(\times 0.8)/\Delta t$.

Arterial stiffness in general and aortic stiffness in particular can be considered as a measure of the cumulative long-lasting burden of all identified and nonidentified CV risk factors with aging on the arterial tree. Nonmodifiable factors such as age, gender,[118] genetic markers,[119] but also level of BP, high-salt-intake,[120] or metabolic abnormalities[121] have been proposed to modulate impact on vascular structural remodeling, and hence CV risk.

An independent predictive value of PWV has been demonstrated after adjusting for classical CV risk factors (e.g., including brachial BP), and the additive value of PWV above/beyond a combination of traditional risk factors (e.g., FRS).[122,123] An increase in PWV of 1 m/s results in an age-adjusted, sex-adjusted, and risk factor-adjusted increment of 14% in total CV events and 15% in CV mortality.[124] More recently (and practicable) it was shown that a change in PWV of 1 m/s leads to a 7% increase of HR for CV events for nonsmoking, nondiabetic, normotensive, and normolipidemic, 60-year-old men.[125] Moreover, a reclassification into both higher and lower risk categories is possible.[125,126] Thus the damage to the arterial wall, reflecting the integrated damage has been proposed as a "hypertensive disease marker."[127]

Notably, measurement of PWV is not recommended by the American College of Cardiology Foundation/American Heart Association (ACCF/AHA) guidelines for the assessment of CV risk in asymptomatic adults.[128]

Prognostic Value of Change

BP reduction passively unloads the stiff components of the aortic wall, and thus, reduces PWV (i.e., arterial stiffness). Moreover, long-term antihypertensive therapy (usually years are required) may result in arterial remodeling, and hence in reduction of arterial stiffness per se (i.e., beyond BP reduction). Indeed, it was shown that long-term reduction of arterial stiffness (PWV) was only slightly explained by the mean BP reduction, but this analysis is less conclusive because no adjustment for systolic BP has been made, which is closely related to PWV velocity. Notably, only patients were investigated in which a significant treatment-induced BP reduction before the PWV measurement were observed.[129] Currently, there is only one small study in ESRD demonstrating that the absence of PWV reduction in response to BP reduction was a strong independent predictor of all-cause (2.59 [95% CI, 1.51 to 4.43]) and CV mortality (2.35 [95% CI, 1.23 to 4.41]).[130]

Central Blood Pressure and Pulse Pressure

Pulse pressure (PP) is a valid and widely applicable proxy for arterial stiffness.[116] An office PP greater than 60 mm Hg in the elderly is an acknowledged marker of TOD influencing prognosis, and hence used for stratification of total CV risk.[23]

Nowadays, not only peripheral BP but also central pressure recording can be assessed noninvasively in daily practice by pressure waveforms. Using different approaches (e.g., validated transfer function), aortic pressure waveform and hence, aortic central pressure can be calculated. Central pressures do not correspond to brachial pressures, and increases with aging accelerated by diverse factors (Fig. 20.4). Reference values based on 45,436 subjects out of 82,930 (77 studies in 53 centers) were reported and central systolic BP was stratified by brachial BP.[131] However, remember that brachial BP is necessary to calibrate central pressures. Hence, all recommendations of correct measurement and limitations of peripheral (brachial) BP have to be taken into account.

Pathophysiologically, central pressure in the aorta, which is actually the perfusion pressure to key organs, rather than the pressure in the arm, may provide more relevant prognostic information. Indeed, several studies have shown that central BP is more strongly related to TOD-like LVM compared with peripheral BP.[132-134] Confirming this, a systemic review and meta-analysis have shown that central compared with peripheral (brachial) systolic BP and PP, respectively, was more strongly associated with TOD-like LVM (12 studies, n = 6341), carotid IMT (7 studies, n = 6136) and PWV (14 studies, n = 3699), but not with albuminuria (4 studies, n = 3718).[135] Moreover, former studies also revealed that central BP more accurately predicts all-cause and CV mortality compared with peripheral BP,[132-134] and in the Conduit Artery Function Evaluation (CAFE) study a Cox proportional-hazards modeling showed that cPP was significantly associated with a post hoc-defined composite outcome (total CV events/procedures and development of renal impairment).[136] Notably, in a small study it was shown that regression of LVM (with antihypertensive treatment) was more strongly linked to central than brachial BP.[137] In meta-analyses the added value of central PP versus brachial PP regarding clinical events just failed formal significance ($p = 0.057$).[138] However, not all large studies were included (e.g., studies demonstrating significant independent predictive value for central PP) and findings were based on published summary statistics and not individual patient data.[139,140]

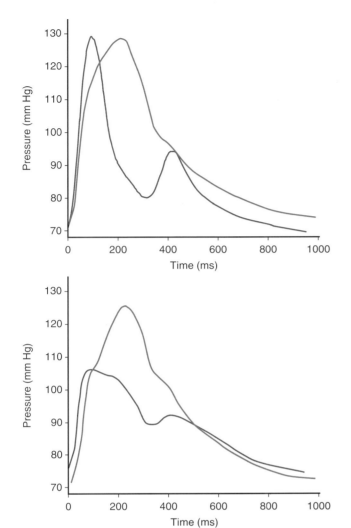

FIG. 20.4 Radial (top) and corresponding aortal (bottom) pressure waveform in a young person (blue) and an old person (green).

Prognostic Value of Change

Studies are lacking on whether reduction of central BP is related to improved CV events. Although the CAFE study revealed that the amlodipine-based was more effective than an atenolol-based regime to lower central BP, despite similar reductions of brachial BP, superiority cannot be claimed because at baseline no central BP was measured, and hence no change in central BP could be related to prognostic data.[136]

A prospective, open-label, blinded endpoint study in hypertensive patients tended to find a greater LVM decrease in the group with central BP-guided hypertension management as opposed to the group with practical usual care, despite significant medication withdrawal in the central BP guided hypertension management group.[141] However, no study with incident hard endpoints has been carried out analyzing the prognostic value of change in central pressure.

SUMMARY

In general, based on availability, cost and clinical significance, assessment of LVM, albuminuria and eGFR are the minimal requirements to search for asymptomatic hypertensive TOD (e.g., ESH/ESC class I recommendation with evidence level B).[23] Until now, data are evident showing that any of four TOD (LVH, microalbuminuria, carotid plaques, and increased

PWV) predict CV mortality independently of SCORE (Systemic COronary Risk Evaluation) classification.[142-144] In the follow-up, LVM (either by ECG or echocardiography), eGFR and albuminuria should also be assessed because changes of these TOD markers reflect effective antihypertensive therapy, and indicate reduced CV risk.

References

1. Ferri CP, Schoenborn C, Kalra L, et al. Prevalence of stroke and related burden among older people living in Latin America, India and China. *J Neurol Neurosurg psychiatry.* 2011;82:1074-1082.
2. Di Carlo A. Human and economic burden of stroke. *Age Aging.* 2009;38:4-5.
3. Adams Jr HP, Bendixen BH, Kappelle LJ, et al. Classification of subtype of acute ischemic stroke. Definitions for use in a multicenter clinical trial. TOAST. Trial of Org 10172 in Acute Stroke Treatment. *Stroke.* 1993;24:35-41.
4. Lewington S, Clarke R, Qizilbash N, Peto R, Collins R. Age-specific relevance of usual blood pressure to vascular mortality: a meta-analysis of individual data for one million adults in 61 prospective studies. *Lancet.* 2002;360:1903-1913.
5. Law MR, Morris JK, Wald NJ. Use of blood pressure lowering drugs in the prevention of cardiovascular disease: meta-analysis of 147 randomised trials in the context of expectations from prospective epidemiological studies. *BMJ.* 2009;338:b1665.
6. Ettehad D, Emdin CA, Kiran A, et al. Blood pressure lowering for prevention of cardiovascular disease and death: a systematic review and meta-analysis. *Lancet.* 2016;387:957-967.
7. Wardlaw JM, Smith EE, Biessels GJ, et al. Neuroimaging standards for research into small vessel disease and its contribution to ageing and neurodegeneration. *Lancet Neurol.* 2013;12:822-838.
8. Wen W, Sachdev PS, Li JJ, Chen XH, Anstey KJ. White matter hyperintensities in the forties: their prevalence and topography in an epidemiological sample aged 44-48. *Hum Brain Mapp.* 2009;30:1155-1167.
9. Debette S, Markus HS. The clinical importance of white matter hyperintensities on brain magnetic resonance imaging: systematic review and meta-analysis. *BMJ.* 2010;341:c3666.
10. Debette S, Seshadri S, Beiser A, et al. Midlife vascular risk factor exposure accelerates structural brain aging and cognitive decline. *Neurology.* 2011;77:461-468.
11. Godin O, Tzourio C, Maillard P, Mazoyer B, Dufouil C. Antihypertensive treatment and change in blood pressure are associated with the progression of white matter lesion volumes: the Three-City (3C)-Dijon Magnetic Resonance Imaging Study. *Circulation.* 2011;123:266-273.
12. Verhaaren BF, Vernooij MW, de Boer R, et al. High blood pressure and cerebral white matter lesion progression in the general population. *Hypertension.* 2013;61:1354-1359.
13. Cordonnier C, Al-Shahi Salman R, Wardlaw J. Spontaneous brain microbleeds: systematic review, subgroup analyses and standards for study design and reporting. *Brain.* 2007;130(Pt 8):1988-2003.
14. Poels MM, Vernooij MW, Ikram MA, et al. Prevalence and risk factors of cerebral microbleeds: an update of the Rotterdam scan study. *Stroke.* 2010;41(10 Suppl):S103-S106.
15. Klarenbeek P, van Oostenbrugge RJ, Rouhl RP, Knottnerus IL, Staals J. Higher ambulatory blood pressure relates to new cerebral microbleeds: 2-year follow-up study in lacunar stroke patients. *Stroke.* 2013;44:978-983.
16. Charidimou A, Kakar P, Fox Z, Werring DJ. Cerebral microbleeds and recurrent stroke risk: systematic review and meta-analysis of prospective ischemic stroke and transient ischemic attack cohorts. *Stroke.* 2013;44:995-1001.
17. Altmann-Schneider I, Trompet S, de Craen AJ, et al. Cerebral microbleeds are predictive of mortality in the elderly. *Stroke.* 2011;42:638-644.
18. Akoudad S, Ikram MA, Koudstaal PJ, Hofman A, van der Lugt A, Vernooij MW. Cerebral microbleeds and the risk of mortality in the general population. *Eur J Epidemiol.* 2013;28:815-821.
19. Vemmos KN, Takis CE, Georgilis K, et al. The Athens stroke registry: results of a five-year hospital-based study. *Cerebrovasc Dis.* 2000;10:133-141.
20. Vermeer SE, Hollander M, van Dijk EJ, Hofman A, Koudstaal PJ, Breteler MM. Silent brain infarcts and white matter lesions increase stroke risk in the general population: the Rotterdam Scan Study. *Stroke.* 2003;34:1126-1129.
21. Vermeer SE, Prins ND, den Heijer T, Hofman A, Koudstaal PJ, Breteler MM. Silent brain infarcts and the risk of dementia and cognitive decline. *N Engl J Med.* 2003;348:1215-1222.
22. Group SPSS, Benavente OR, Coffey CS, et al. Blood-pressure targets in patients with recent lacunar stroke: the SPS3 randomised trial. *Lancet.* 2013;382:507-515.
23. Mancia G, Fagard R, Narkiewicz K, et al. 2013 ESH/ESC Guidelines for the management of arterial hypertension: the Task Force for the management of arterial hypertension of the European Society of Hypertension (ESH) and of the European Society of Cardiology (ESC). *J Hyperten.* 2013;31:1281-1357.
24. van Dijk EJ, Prins ND, Vrooman HA, Hofman A, Koudstaal PJ, Breteler MM. Progression of cerebral small vessel disease in relation to risk factors and cognitive consequences: rotterdam Scan study. *Stroke.* 2008;39:2712-2719.
25. Sugiyama T, Lee JD, Shimizu H, Abe S, Ueda T. Influence of treated blood pressure on progression of silent cerebral infarction. *J Hypertens.* 1999;17:679-684.
26. Gutierrez J, Elkind MS, Cheung K, Rundek T, Sacco RL, Wright CB. Pulsatile and steady components of blood pressure and subclinical cerebrovascular disease: the Northern Manhattan Study. *J Hypertens.* 2015;33:2115-2122.
27. Ninomiya T, Ohara T, Hirakawa Y, et al. Midlife and late-life blood pressure and dementia in Japanese elderly: the Hisayama study. *Hypertension.* 2011;58:22-28.
28. Launer LJ, Ross GW, Petrovitch H, et al. Midlife blood pressure and dementia: the Honolulu-Asia aging study. *Neurobiol Aging.* 2000;21:49-55.
29. de la Torre JC. Is Alzheimer's disease a neurodegenerative or a vascular disorder? Data, dogma, and dialectics. *Lancet Neurol.* 2004;3:184-190.
30. Power MC, Weuve J, Gagne JJ, McQueen MB, Viswanathan A, Blacker D. The association between blood pressure and incident Alzheimer disease: a systematic review and meta-analysis. *Epidemiology.* 2011;22:646-659.
31. Hachinski V, Iadecola C, Petersen RC, et al. National Institute of Neurological Disorders and Stroke-Canadian Stroke Network vascular cognitive impairment harmonization standards. *Stroke.* 2006;37:2220-2241.
32. Ismail Z, Rajji TK, Shulman KI. Brief cognitive screening instruments: an update. *Int J Geriatr Psychiatry.* 2010;25:111-120.
33. Sivakumar L, Kate M, Jeerakathil T, Camicioli R, Buck B, Butcher K. Serial montreal cognitive assessments demonstrate reversible cognitive impairment in patients with acute transient ischemic attack and minor stroke. *Stroke.* 2014;45:1709-1715.
34. in't Veld BA, Ruitenberg A, Hofman A, Stricker BH, Breteler MM. Antihypertensive drugs and incidence of dementia: the Rotterdam Study. *Neurobiol Aging.* 2001;22:407-412.

35. Peila R, White LR, Masaki K, Petrovitch H, Launer LJ. Reducing the risk of dementia: efficacy of long-term treatment of hypertension. *Stroke*. 2006;37:1165-1170.
36. Anderson C, Teo K, Gao P, et al. Renin-angiotensin system blockade and cognitive function in patients at high risk of cardiovascular disease: analysis of data from the ONTARGET and TRANSCEND studies. *Lancet Neurol*. 2011;10:43-53.
37. Lauer MS, Anderson KM, Levy D. Separate and joint influences of obesity and mild hypertension on left ventricular mass and geometry: the Framingham Heart Study. *J Am Coll Cardiol*. 1992;19:130-134.
38. Schmieder RE, Messerli FH, Garavaglia GE, Nunez BD. Dietary salt intake. A determinant of cardiac involvement in essential hypertension. *Circulation*. 1988;78:951-956.
39. Deschepper CF, Boutin-Ganache I, Zahabi A, Jiang Z. In search of cardiovascular candidate genes: interactions between phenotypes and genotypes. *Hypertension*. 2002;39(2 Pt 2):332-336.
40. Schlaich MP, Kaye DM, Lambert E, Sommerville M, Socratous F, Esler MD. Relation between cardiac sympathetic activity and hypertensive left ventricular hypertrophy. *Circulation*. 2003;108:560-565.
41. Schmieder RE, Langenfeld MR, Friedrich A, Schobel HP, Gatzka CD, Weihprecht H. Angiotensin II related to sodium excretion modulates left ventricular structure in human essential hypertension. *Circulation*. 1996;94:1304-1309.
42. Levy D, Garrison RJ, Savage DD, Kannel WB, Castelli WP. Prognostic implications of echocardiographically determined left ventricular mass in the Framingham Heart Study. *N Engl J Med*. 1990;322:1561-1566.
43. Vakili BA, Okin PM, Devereux RB. Prognostic implications of left ventricular hypertrophy. *Am Heart J*. 2001;141:334-341.
44. Sundstrom J, Lind L, Arnlov J, Zethelius B, Andren B, Lithell HO. Echocardiographic and electrocardiographic diagnoses of left ventricular hypertrophy predict mortality independently of each other in a population of elderly men. *Circulation*. 2001;103:2346-2351.
45. Cuspidi C, Rescaldani M, Sala C, Negri F, Grassi G, Mancia G. Prevalence of electrocardiographic left ventricular hypertrophy in human hypertension: an updated review. *J Hypertens*. 2012;30:2066-2073.
46. Levy D, Salomon M, D'Agostino RB, Belanger AJ, Kannel WB. Prognostic implications of baseline electrocardiographic features and their serial changes in subjects with left ventricular hypertrophy. *Circulation*. 1994;90:1786-1793.
47. Okin PM, Jern S, Devereux RB, Kjeldsen SE, Dahlof B. Effect of obesity on electrocardiographic left ventricular hypertrophy in hypertensive patients: the losartan intervention for endpoint (LIFE) reduction in hypertension study. *Hypertension*. 2000;35(1 Pt 1):13-18.
48. Hancock EW, Deal BJ, Mirvis DM, et al. AHA/ACCF/HRS recommendations for the standardization and interpretation of the electrocardiogram: part V: electrocardiogram changes associated with cardiac chamber hypertrophy: a scientific statement from the American Heart Association Electrocardiography and Arrhythmias Committee, Council on Clinical Cardiology; the American College of Cardiology Foundation; and the Heart Rhythm Society. Endorsed by the International Society for Computerized Electrocardiology. *J Am Coll Cardiol*. 2009;53:992-1002.
49. Pewsner D, Juni P, Egger M, Battaglia M, Sundstrom J, Bachmann LM. Accuracy of electrocardiography in diagnosis of left ventricular hypertrophy in arterial hypertension: systematic review. *BMJ*. 2007;335:711.
50. Chrispin J, Jain A, Soliman EZ, et al. Association of electrocardiographic and imaging surrogates of left ventricular hypertrophy with incident atrial fibrillation: MESA (Multi-Ethnic Study of Atherosclerosis). *J Am Coll Cardiol*. 2014;63:2007-2013.
51. Schneider MP, Hua TA, Bohm M, Wachtell K, Kjeldsen SE, Schmieder RE. Prevention of atrial fibrillation by Renin-Angiotensin system inhibition a meta-analysis. *J Am Coll Cardiol*. 2010;55:2299-2307.
52. Lang RM, Bierig M, Devereux RB, et al. Recommendations for chamber quantification. *Eur J Echocardiography*. 2006;7:79-108.
53. Chirinos JA, Segers P, De Buyzere ML, et al. Left ventricular mass: allometric scaling, normative values, effect of obesity, and prognostic performance. *Hypertension*. 2010;56:91-98.
54. Poppe KK, Doughty RN, Whalley GA. Redefining normal reference ranges for echocardiography: a major new individual person data meta-analysis. *Eur Heart J Cardiovasc Imaging*. 2013;14:347-348.
55. Muiesan ML, Salvetti M, Monteduro C, et al. Left ventricular concentric geometry during treatment adversely affects cardiovascular prognosis in hypertensive patients. *Hypertension*. 2004;43:731-738.
56. Verdecchia P, Schillaci G, Borgioni C, et al. Adverse prognostic significance of concentric remodeling of the left ventricle in hypertensive patients with normal left ventricular mass. *J Am Coll Cardiol*. 1995;25:871-878.
57. Cuspidi C, Meani S, Negri F, et al. Indexation of left ventricular mass to body surface area and height to allometric power of 2.7: is the difference limited to obese hypertensives? *J Human Hypertens*. 2009;23:728-734.
58. Maceira AM, Mohiaddin RH. Cardiovascular magnetic resonance in systemic hypertension. *J Cardiovasc Magn Reson*. 2012;14:28.
59. Kramer CM, Barkhausen J, Flamm SD, Kim RJ, Nagel E. Standardized cardiovascular magnetic resonance (CMR) protocols 2013 update. *J Cardiovasc Magn Reson*. 2013;15:91.
60. Maceira AM, Prasad SK, Khan M, Pennell DJ. Normalized left ventricular systolic and diastolic function by steady state free precession cardiovascular magnetic resonance. *J Cardiovasc Magn Reson*. 2006;8:417-426.
61. Okin PM, Devereux RB, Jern S, et al. Regression of electrocardiographic left ventricular hypertrophy during antihypertensive treatment and the prediction of major cardiovascular events. *JAMA*. 2004;292:2343-2349.
62. Devereux RB, Wachtell K, Gerdts E, et al. Prognostic significance of left ventricular mass change during treatment of hypertension. *JAMA*. 2004;292:2350-2356.
63. Okin PM. Serial evaluation of electrocardiographic left ventricular hypertrophy for prediction of risk in hypertensive patients. *J Electrocardiol*. 2009;42:584-588.
64. de Simone G, Muiesan ML, Ganau A, et al. Reliability and limitations of echocardiographic measurement of left ventricular mass for risk stratification and follow-up in single patients: the RES trial. Working Group on Heart and Hypertension of the Italian Society of Hypertension. Reliability of M-mode Echocardiographic Studies. *J Hypertens*. 1999;17(12 Pt 2):1955-1963.
65. Klingbeil AU, Schneider M, Martus P, Messerli FH, Schmieder RE. A meta-analysis of the effects of treatment on left ventricular mass in essential hypertension. *Am J Med*. 2003;115:41-46.
66. Fagard RH, Celis H, Thijs L, Wouters S. Regression of left ventricular mass by antihypertensive treatment: a meta-analysis of randomized comparative studies. *Hypertension*. 2009;54:1084-1091.
67. Miller AB, Reichek N, St John Sutton M, et al. Importance of blood pressure control in left ventricular mass regression. *J Am Soc Hypertens*. 2010;4:302-310.
68. Angeli F, Reboldi G, Poltronieri C, Stefanetti E, Bartolini C, Verdecchia P. The prognostic legacy of left ventricular hypertrophy: cumulative evidence after the MAVI study. *J Hypertens*. 2015;33:2322-2330.
69. Nagueh SF, Appleton CP, Gillebert TC, et al. Recommendations for the evaluation of left ventricular diastolic function by echocardiography. *Eur Soc Cardiology*. 2009;10:165-193.
70. Mor-Avi V, Lang RM, Badano LP, et al. Current and evolving echocardiographic techniques for the quantitative evaluation of cardiac mechanics: ASE/EAE consensus statement on methodology and indications endorsed by the Japanese Society of Echocardiography. *J Am Soc Echocardiogr*. 2011;24:277-313.
71. Sharp AS, Tapp RJ, Thom SA, et al. Tissue Doppler E/E′ ratio is a powerful predictor of primary cardiac events in a hypertensive population: an ASCOT substudy. *Eur Heart J*. 2010;31:747-752.
72. Abhayaratna WP, Seward JB, Appleton CP, et al. Left atrial size: physiologic determinants and clinical applications. *J Am Coll Cardiol*. 2006;47:2357-2363.
73. Jenkins C, Bricknell K, Hanekom L, Marwick TH. Reproducibility and accuracy of echocardiographic measurements of left ventricular parameters using real-time three-dimensional echocardiography. *J Am Coll Cardiol*. 2004;44:878-886.
74. Turnbull F. Effects of different blood-pressure-lowering regimens on major cardiovascular events: results of prospectively-designed overviews of randomised trials. *Lancet*. 2003;362:1527-1535.
75. Turnbull F, Neal B, Algert C, et al. Effects of different blood pressure-lowering regimens on major cardiovascular events in individuals with and without diabetes mellitus: results of prospectively designed overviews of randomized trials. *Arch Int Med*. 2005;165:1410-1419.
76. Yancy CW, Jessup M, Bozkurt B, et al. 2013 ACCF/AHA guideline for the management of heart failure: executive summary: a report of the American College of Cardiology Foundation/American Heart Association Task Force on practice guidelines. *Circulation*. 2013;128:1810-1852.
77. Carson PE, Anand IS, Win S, et al. The hospitalization burden and post-hospitalization mortality risk in heart failure with preserved ejection fraction: results from the I-PRESERVE Trial (Irbesartan in Heart Failure and Preserved Ejection Fraction). *JACC Heart Fail*. 2015;3:429-441.
78. McMurray JJ, Adamopoulos S, Anker SD, et al. ESC Guidelines for the diagnosis and treatment of acute and chronic heart failure 2012: the Task Force for the Diagnosis and Treatment of Acute and Chronic Heart Failure 2012 of the European Society of Cardiology. Developed in collaboration with the Heart Failure Association (HFA) of the ESC. *Eur Heart J*. 2012;33:1787-1847.
79. 1999 World Health Organization-International Society of Hypertension Guidelines for the Management of Hypertension. Guidelines Subcommittee. *J Hypertens*. 1999;17:151-183.
80. Dimmitt SB, West JN, Eames SM, Gibson JM, Gosling P, Littler WA. Usefulness of ophthalmoscopy in mild to moderate hypertension. *Lancet*. 1989;1:1103-1106.
81. van den Born BJ, Hulsman CA, Hoekstra JB, Schlingemann RO, van Montfrans GA. Value of routine funduscopy in patients with hypertension: systematic review. *BMJ*. 2005;331:73.
82. Hubbard LD, Brothers RJ, King WN, et al. Methods for evaluation of retinal microvascular abnormalities associated with hypertension/sclerosis in the Atherosclerosis Risk in Communities Study. *Ophthalmology*. 1999;106:2269-2280.
83. Ding J, Wai KL, McGeechan K, et al. Retinal vascular caliber and the development of hypertension: a meta-analysis of individual participant data. *J Hypertens*. 2014;32:207-215.
84. Mitchell P, Cheung N, de Haseth K, et al. Blood pressure and retinal arteriolar narrowing in children. *Hypertension*. 2007;49:1156-1162.
85. Ikram MK, de Jong FJ, Bos MJ, et al. Retinal vessel diameters and risk of stroke: the Rotterdam Study. *Neurology*. 2006;66:1339-1343.
86. Wieberdink RG, Ikram MK, Koudstaal PJ, Hofman A, Vingerling JR, Breteler MM. Retinal vascular calibers and the risk of intracerebral hemorrhage and cerebral infarction: the Rotterdam Study. *Stroke*. 2010;41:2757-2761.
87. Harazny JM, Raff U, Welzenbach J, et al. New software analyses increase the reliability of measurements of retinal arterioles morphology by scanning laser Doppler flowmetry in humans. *J Hypertens*. 2011;29:777-782.
88. Baleanu D, Ritt M, Harazny J, Heckmann J, Schmieder RE, Michelson G. Wall-to-lumen ratio of retinal arterioles and arteriole-to-venule ratio of retinal vessels in patients with cerebrovascular damage. *Invest Ophthalmol Vis Sci*. 2009;50:4351-4359.
89. Bock KD. Regression of retinal vascular changes by antihypertensive therapy. *Hypertension*. 1984;6(6 Pt 2):III158-III162.
90. Strachan MW, McKnight JA. Images in clinical medicine. Improvement in hypertensive retinopathy after treatment of hypertension. *N Engl J Med*. 2005;352:e17.
91. Mahmoodi BK, Matsushita K, Woodward M, et al. Associations of kidney disease measures with mortality and end-stage renal disease in individuals with and without hypertension: a meta-analysis. *Lancet*. 2012;380:1649-1661.
92. Matsushita K, van der Velde M, Astor BC, et al. Association of estimated glomerular filtration rate and albuminuria with all-cause and cardiovascular mortality in general population cohorts: a collaborative meta-analysis. *Lancet*. 2010;375:2073-2081.
93. Gansevoort RT, Correa-Rotter R, Hemmelgarn BR, et al. Chronic kidney disease and cardiovascular risk: epidemiology, mechanisms, and prevention. *Lancet*. 2013;382:339-352.
94. Bakris GL, Williams M, Dworkin L, et al. Preserving renal function in adults with hypertension and diabetes: a consensus approach. National Kidney Foundation Hypertension and Diabetes Executive Committees Working Group. *Am J Kidney Dis*. 2000;36:646-661.
95. KDIGO 2012 Clinical Practice Guideline for the Evaluation and Management of Chronic Kidney Disease. *Kidney Int Suppl*. 2013;3:1-150.
96. Levey AS, Inker LA, Matsushita K, et al. GFR decline as an end point for clinical trials in CKD: a scientific workshop sponsored by the National Kidney Foundation and the US Food and Drug Administration. *Am J Kidney Dis*. 2014;64:821-835.
97. Holtkamp FA, de Zeeuw D, Thomas MC, et al. An acute fall in estimated glomerular filtration rate during treatment with losartan predicts a slower decrease in long-term renal function. *Kidney Int*. 2011;80:282-287.
98. Coresh J, Turin TC, Matsushita K, et al. Decline in estimated glomerular filtration rate and subsequent risk of end-stage renal disease and mortality. *JAMA*. 2014;311:2518-2531.
99. Turin TC, Jun M, James MT, Tonelli M, Coresh J, Manns BJ, Hemmelgarn BR. Magnitude of rate of change in kidney function and future risk of cardiovascular events. *Int J Cardiol*. 2016;202:657-665.
100. Chowdhury EK, Langham RG, Ademi Z, et al. Rate of change in renal function and mortality in elderly treated hypertensive patients. *Clin J Am Soc Nephrol*. 2015;10:1154-1161.
101. Gansevoort RT, Verhave JC, Hillege HL, et al. The validity of screening based on spot morning urine samples to detect subjects with microalbuminuria in the general population. *Kidney Int Suppl*. 2005;94:S28-S35.
102. Witte EC, Lambers Heerspink HJ, de Zeeuw D, Bakker SJ, de Jong PE, Gansevoort R. First morning voids are more reliable than spot urine samples to assess microalbuminuria. *J Am Soc Nephrol*. 2009;20:436-443.
103. van der Velde M, Matsushita K, Coresh J, et al. Lower estimated glomerular filtration rate and higher albuminuria are associated with all-cause and cardiovascular mortality. A collaborative meta-analysis of high-risk population cohorts. *Kidney Int*. 2011;79:1341-1352.
104. Pascual JM, Rodilla E, Costa JA, Garcia-Escrich M, Gonzalez C, Redon J. Prognostic value of microalbuminuria during antihypertensive treatment in essential hypertension. *Hypertension*. 2014;64:1228-1234.

105. Schmieder RE, Mann JF, Schumacher H, et al. Changes in albuminuria predict mortality and morbidity in patients with vascular disease. *J Am Soc Nephrol.* 2011;22:1353-1364.

106. Schmieder RE, Schutte R, Schumacher H, et al. Mortality and morbidity in relation to changes in albuminuria, glucose status and systolic blood pressure: an analysis of the ONTARGET and TRANSCEND studies. *Diabetologia.* 2014;57:2019-2029.

107. Heerspink HJ, Kropelin TF, Hoekman J, de Zeeuw D. Drug-Induced Reduction in Albuminuria Is Associated with Subsequent Renoprotection: A Meta-Analysis. *J Am Soc Nephrol.* 2015;26:2055-2064.

108. Savarese G, Dei Cas A, Rosano G, et al. Reduction of albumin urinary excretion is associated with reduced cardiovascular events in hypertensive and/or diabetic patients. A meta-regression analysis of 32 randomized trials. *Int J Cardiol.* 2014;172:403-410.

109. Muiesan ML, Pasini G, Salvetti M, et al. Cardiac and vascular structural changes. Prevalence and relation to ambulatory blood pressure in a middle-aged general population in northern Italy: the Vobarno Study. *Hypertension.* 1996;27:1046-1052.

110. Touboul PJ, Hennerici MG, Meairs S, et al. Mannheim carotid intima-media thickness and plaque consensus (2004-2006-2011). An update on behalf of the advisory board of the 3rd, 4th and 5th watching the risk symposia, at the 13th, 15th and 20th European Stroke Conferences, Mannheim, Germany, 2004, Brussels, Belgium, 2006, and Hamburg, Germany, 2011. *Cerebrovasc Dis.* 2012;34:290-296.

111. Pignoli P, Tremoli E, Poli A, Oreste P, Paoletti R. Intimal plus medial thickness of the arterial wall: a direct measurement with ultrasound imaging. *Circulation.* 1986;74:1399-1406.

112. Lorenz MW, Markus HS, Bots ML, Rosvall M, Sitzer M. Prediction of clinical cardiovascular events with carotid intima-media thickness: a systematic review and meta-analysis. *Circulation.* 2007;115:459-467.

113. O'Leary DH, Polak JF, Kronmal RA, Manolio TA, Burke GL, Wolfson Jr SK. Carotid-artery intima and media thickness as a risk factor for myocardial infarction and stroke in older adults. Cardiovascular Health Study Collaborative Research Group. *N Engl J Med.* 1999;340:14-22.

114. Zanchetti A, Bond MG, Hennig M, et al. Calcium antagonist lacidipine slows down progression of asymptomatic carotid atherosclerosis: principal results of the European Lacidipine Study on Atherosclerosis (ELSA), a randomized, double-blind, long-term trial. *Circulation.* 2002;106:2422-2427.

115. Zanchetti A, Hennig M, Hollweck R, et al. Baseline values but not treatment-induced changes in carotid intima-media thickness predict incident cardiovascular events in treated hypertensive patients: findings in the European Lacidipine Study on Atherosclerosis (ELSA). *Circulation.* 2009;120:1084-1090.

116. Laurent S, Cockcroft J, Van Bortel L, et al. Expert consensus document on arterial stiffness: methodological issues and clinical applications. *Eur Heart J.* 2006;27:2588-2605.

117. Van Bortel LM, Laurent S, Boutouyrie P, et al. Consensus document on the measurement of aortic stiffness in daily practice using carotid-femoral pulse wave velocity. *J Hypertens.* 2012;30:445-448.

118. Mitchell GF, Parise H, Benjamin EJ, et al. Changes in arterial stiffness and wave reflection with advancing age in healthy men and women: the Framingham Heart Study. *Hypertension.* 2004;43:1239-1245.

119. Laurent S, Boutouyrie P, Lacolley P. Structural and genetic bases of arterial stiffness. *Hypertension.* 2005;45:1050-1055.

120. Safar ME, Temmar M, Kakou A, Lacolley P, Thornton SN. Sodium intake and vascular stiffness in hypertension. *Hypertension.* 2009;54:203-209.

121. Scuteri A, Najjar SS, Muller DC, et al. Metabolic syndrome amplifies the age-associated increases in vascular thickness and stiffness. *J Am Coll Cardiol.* 2004;43:1388-1395.

122. Boutouyrie P, Tropeano AI, Asmar R, et al. Aortic stiffness is an independent predictor of primary coronary events in hypertensive patients: a longitudinal study. *Hypertension.* 2002;39:10-15.

123. Mattace-Raso FU, van der Cammen TJ, Hofman A, et al. Arterial stiffness and risk of coronary heart disease and stroke: the Rotterdam Study. *Circulation.* 2006;113:657-663.

124. Vlachopoulos C, Aznaouridis K, Stefanadis C. Prediction of cardiovascular events and all-cause mortality with arterial stiffness: a systematic review and meta-analysis. *J Am Coll Cardiol.* 2010;55:1318-1327.

125. Ben-Shlomo Y, Spears M, Boustred C, et al. Aortic pulse wave velocity improves cardiovascular event prediction: an individual participant meta-analysis of prospective observational data from 17,635 subjects. *J Am Coll Cardiol.* 2014;63:636-646.

126. Mitchell GF, Hwang SJ, Vasan RS, et al. Arterial stiffness and cardiovascular events: the Framingham Heart Study. *Circulation.* 2010;121:505-511.

127. Laurent S, Alivon M, Beaussier H, Boutouyrie P. Aortic stiffness as a tissue biomarker for predicting future cardiovascular events in asymptomatic hypertensive subjects. *Ann Med.* 2012;44(Suppl 1):S93-S97.

128. Greenland P, Alpert JS, Beller GA, et al. 2010 ACCF/AHA guideline for assessment of cardiovascular risk in asymptomatic adults: a report of the American College of Cardiology Foundation/American Heart Association Task Force on Practice Guidelines. *J Am Coll Cardiol.* 2010;56:e50-e103.

129. Ait-Oufella H, Collin C, Bozec E, et al. Long-term reduction in aortic stiffness: a 5.3-year follow-up in routine clinical practice. *J Hypertens.* 2010;28:2336-2341.

130. Guerin AP, Blacher J, Pannier B, Marchais SJ, Safar ME, London GM. Impact of aortic stiffness attenuation on survival of patients in end-stage renal failure. *Circulation.* 2001;103:987-992.

131. Herbert A, Cruickshank JK, Laurent S, et al. Establishing reference values for central blood pressure and its amplification in a general healthy population and according to cardiovascular risk factors. *Eur Heart J.* 2014;35:3122-3133.

132. Roman MJ, Devereux RB, Kizer JR, et al. Central pressure more strongly relates to vascular disease and outcome than does brachial pressure: the Strong Heart Study. *Hypertension.* 2007;50:197-203.

133. Wang KL, Cheng HM, Chuang SY, et al. Central or peripheral systolic or pulse pressure: which best relates to target organs and future mortality? *J Hypertens.* 2009;27:461-467.

134. Huang CM, Wang KL, Cheng HM, et al. Central versus ambulatory blood pressure in the prediction of all-cause and cardiovascular mortalities. *J Hypertens.* 2011;29:454-459.

135. Kollias A, Lagou S, Zeniodi ME, Boubouchairopoulou N, Stergiou GS. Association of central versus brachial blood pressure with target-organ damage: systematic review and meta-analysis. *Hypertension.* 2016;67:183-190.

136. Williams B, Lacy PS, Thom SM, et al. Differential impact of blood pressure-lowering drugs on central aortic pressure and clinical outcomes: principal results of the Conduit Artery Function Evaluation (CAFE) study. *Circulation.* 2006;113:1213-1225.

137. de Luca N, Asmar RG, London GM, O'Rourke MF, Safar ME, Investigators RP. Selective reduction of cardiac mass and central blood pressure on low-dose combination perindopril/indapamide in hypertensive subjects. *J Hypertens.* 2004;22:1623-1630.

138. Vlachopoulos C, Aznaouridis K, O'Rourke MF, Safar ME, Baou K, Stefanadis C. Prediction of cardiovascular events and all-cause mortality with central haemodynamics: a systematic review and meta-analysis. *Eur Heart J.* 2010;31:1865-1871.

139. Williams B, Lacy PS. Central haemodynamics and clinical outcomes: going beyond brachial blood pressure? *Eur Heart J.* 2010;31:1819-1822.

140. McEniery CM, Cockcroft JR, Roman MJ, Franklin SS, Wilkinson IB. Central blood pressure: current evidence and clinical importance. *Eur Heart J.* 2014;35:1719-1725.

141. Sharman JE, Marwick TH, Gilroy D, et al. Randomized trial of guiding hypertension management using central aortic blood pressure compared with best-practice care principal findings of the BP GUIDE study. *Hypertension.* 2013;62:1138-1145.

142. Sehestedt T, Jeppesen J, Hansen TW, et al. Risk prediction is improved by adding markers of subclinical organ damage to SCORE. *Eur Heart J.* 2010;31:883-891.

143. Sehestedt T, Jeppesen J, Hansen TW, et al. Thresholds for pulse wave velocity, urine albumin creatinine ratio and left ventricular mass index using SCORE, Framingham and ESH/ESC risk charts. *J Hypertens.* 2012;30:1928-1936.

144. Volpe M, Battistoni A, Tocci G, et al. Cardiovascular risk assessment beyond Systemic Coronary Risk Estimation: a role for organ damage markers. *J Hypertens.* 2012;30:1056-1064.

145. Edvardsen T, Rosen BD, Pan L, et al. Regional diastolic dysfunction in individuals with left ventricular hypertrophy measured by tagged magnetic resonance imaging—the Multi-Ethnic Study of Atherosclerosis (MESA). *Am Heart J.* 2006;151:109-114.

146. Drazner MH, Dries DL, Peshock RM, et al. Left ventricular hypertrophy is more prevalent in blacks than whites in the general population—The Dallas Heart Study. *Hypertension.* 2005;46:124-129.

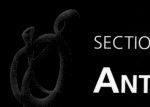

SECTION V

ANTIHYPERTENSIVE THERAPY

21 Diet and Blood Pressure

Lawrence J. Appel

Elevated blood pressure (BP) remains an extraordinarily common and important risk factor for cardiovascular (CV) and renal diseases throughout the world.[1] According to the 2011-2012 National Health and Nutrition Examination Survey (NHANES), around 70 million adult Americans (29%) have hypertension (a systolic BP ≥ 140 mm Hg, a diastolic BP ≥ 90 mm Hg, or are being treated with antihypertensive medication),[2] and at least as many Americans have prehypertension (systolic BP of 120 to 139 mm Hg or diastolic BP of 80 to 89 mm Hg, not on medication). Regrettably, the prevalence of hypertension remains essentially unchanged for the past 2 decades, and control rates remain low, at about 53%.[3]

Systolic BP progressively rises with age, such that hypertension becomes almost ubiquitous among the elderly. As a result of the age-related rise in systolic BP, around 90% of adult Americans will develop hypertension over their lifetime.[4] Elevated BP afflicts both men and women. African Americans, on average, have higher BP than non-African Americans, as well as an increased risk of BP-related disease, particularly stroke and kidney disease.

Blood pressure is a strong, consistent, continuous, independent and etiologically relevant risk factor for CV and renal disease.[5] Importantly, there is no evidence of a BP threshold, that is, the risk of CV disease increases progressively throughout the range of BP, including in the prehypertensive range.[6] It has been estimated that almost a third of BP-related deaths from coronary heart disease (CHD) occur in individuals with BP in the nonhypertensive range. Accordingly, prehypertensive individuals not only have a high probability of developing hypertension, but also carry an excess risk of CV disease compared with those with a normal BP (systolic BP < 120 mm Hg and diastolic BP < 80 mm Hg).[7] About 54% of strokes and 47% of ischemic heart disease events worldwide have been attributed to an elevated BP.[8]

Elevated BP results from environmental factors (including dietary factors), genetic factors, and interactions among these factors. Of the environmental factors that affect BP (diet, physical inactivity, toxins, and psychosocial factors), diet likely has the predominant role in BP homeostasis. Well-established dietary modifications that lower BP are a reduced sodium intake, weight loss, moderation of alcohol consumption (among those who drink excessively), and healthy dietary patterns, specifically, dietary approaches to stop hypertension (DASH)-style diets, vegetarian diets, and to a lesser extent, Mediterranean-style diets.

In nonhypertensive individuals, dietary changes that lower BP have the potential to prevent hypertension and reduce the risk of BP-related CV disease. Indeed, even an apparently small BP reduction, if applied broadly to an entire population, could have an enormous, beneficial impact. For example, it has been estimated that a 3 mm Hg average reduction in systolic BP could lead to an 8% reduction in stroke mortality and a 5% reduction in mortality from CHD (see Fig. 21.1).[9] In uncomplicated stage I hypertension (systolic BP 140 to 159 mm Hg or diastolic BP 90 to 99 mm Hg), dietary changes can serve as first-line therapy before antihypertensive medication. Among hypertensive individuals who are already on medication, dietary changes can further lower BP and make it possible to reduce the number and doses of medications. In general, the magnitude of BP reduction from dietary changes is greater in hypertensive individuals than in nonhypertensive individuals.

Although dietary changes lower BP, there is considerably less evidence on whether dietary changes blunt the age-related rise in systolic BP. On average, systolic BP rises by around 0.6 mm Hg per year. Efforts to prevent this age-associated rise in systolic BP hold the greatest promise as a means to prevent elevated BP and curb the epidemic of BP-related disease. Unfortunately, even the longest diet-BP intervention trials have lasted less than 5 years. Whether the BP reductions observed in these trials have merely shifted the age-associated rise in BP curve downward, without a change in slope (Fig. 21.2A) or actually reduced its slope (Fig. 21.2B) cannot be determined. Still, evidence from migration studies, ecologic studies, and most recently observational analyses of trial data,[10] suggest that dietary factors should reduce the rise in systolic BP with age.

The objective of this chapter is to synthesize evidence on the relationship of diet and BP. The summary of evidence and corresponding recommendations largely reflect previous reviews.[11,12] Table 21.1 provides a summary of this evidence, whereas Table 21.2 provides a summary of recommendations.

DIETARY FACTORS THAT REDUCE BLOOD PRESSURE

Weight Loss

Weight is directly associated with BP. The importance of this relationship is reinforced by the high and increasing prevalence of obesity throughout the world. In the United States,

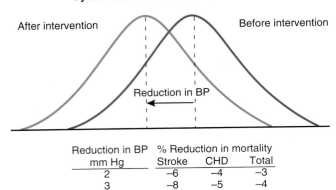

Systolic Blood Pressure Distributions

After intervention

Before intervention

Reduction in BP

Reduction in BP	% Reduction in mortality		
mm Hg	Stroke	CHD	Total
2	−6	−4	−3
3	−8	−5	−4
5	−14	−9	−7

FIG. 21.1 Estimated effects of population-wide shifts in systolic blood pressure on mortality. *BP,* Blood pressure; *CHD,* congestive heart disease. *(Adapted with permission, Stamler R. Implications of the INTERSALT study. Hypertension. 1991;17[1 Suppl]:I16-120.).*

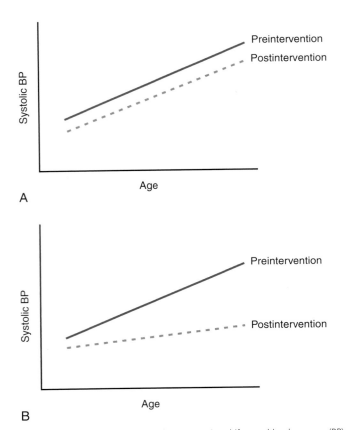

FIG. 21.2 A, Model in which a dietary intervention shifts age-blood pressure (BP) curve downward without affecting slope. B, Model in which a dietary intervention that shifts age-BP curve downward and reduces its slope.

around 69% of adults have a body mass index (BMI) 25 kg/m² or higher and therefore are classified as either overweight or obese; around 35% of adults are obese (BMI ≥ 30 kg/m²).[13] Likewise, among infants, toddlers, children and adolescents, the prevalence of high weight persists, with scant evidence of any improvement.

Weight loss lowers BP. Reductions in BP occur before, and even without, attainment of a desirable body weight. In a meta-analysis of 25 trials, an average weight loss of 5.1 kg reduced systolic BP by a mean of 4.4 mm Hg and diastolic BP by a mean of 3.6 mm Hg.[14] In subgroup analyses, BP reductions were greater in those who lost more weight. Within trial,

TABLE 21.1 A Summary of the Evidence on the Effects of Dietary Factors and Dietary Patterns on Blood Pressure

	HYPOTHESIZED EFFECT	EVIDENCE
Weight	direct	++
Sodium chloride (Salt)	direct	++
Potassium	inverse	++
Magnesium	inverse	+/−
Calcium	inverse	+/−
Alcohol	direct	++
Fat		
Saturated fat	direct	+/−
Omega-3 polyunsaturated fat	inverse	++
Omega-6 polyunsaturated fat	inverse	+/−
Monounsaturated fat	inverse	+
Protein		
Total protein	uncertain	+
Vegetable protein	inverse	+
Animal protein	uncertain	+/−
Carbohydrate	uncertain	+/−
Fiber	inverse	+
Cholesterol	direct	+/−
Vitamin C	uncertain	+/−
Dietary Patterns		
Vegetarian diets	inverse	++
DASH diet	inverse	++
Mediterranean	inverse	+

Key to evidence:
+/−, Limited or equivocal evidence; +, suggestive evidence, typically from observational studies and some clinical trials; ++, persuasive evidence, typically from clinical trials.
(Reproduced with permission from Appel LJ, Brands MW, Daniels SR, et al. Dietary approaches to prevent and treat hypertension: a Scientific Statement from the American Heart Association. Hypertension. 2006;47:296-308.)

dose-response analyses[15] and observational studies, also provide evidence that greater weight loss leads to greater BP reduction. However, given the potential for huge reductions in weight, a linear dose response relationship is unlikely.

Other research has documented that modest weight loss, with or without sodium reduction, can prevent hypertension by around 20% among overweight, nonhypertensive individuals, and can facilitate the reduction of the number and doses of medications. Behavioral intervention trials have uniformly achieved short-term weight loss, primarily through a reduction in energy intake. In several instances, substantial weight loss has also been maintained over 3 or more years.[16-18] Regular physical activity is well-recognized as a critical factor in sustaining weight loss. Whether or not weight loss can blunt the age-related rise in systolic BP is uncertain. In one of the longest weight loss trials, those individuals who sustained a greater than 10-pound weight loss achieved a lower BP that nonetheless rose over time (see Fig. 21.3).[19]

In aggregate, available evidence strongly supports weight reduction as an effective approach to prevent and treat hypertension.

Reduced Salt (Sodium Chloride) Intake

On average, as dietary sodium intake rises, so does BP. Available types of evidence include animal studies,

TABLE 21.2 Diet-Related Lifestyle Recommendations That Lower Blood Pressure

LIFESTYLE MODIFICATION	RECOMMENDATION
Weight loss	For overweight or obese persons, lose weight, ideally attaining a body mass index < 25 kg/m² For nonoverweight persons, maintain desirable body mass index < 25 kg/m²
Reduced sodium intake	Lower sodium intake as much as possible, with a goal of no more than 2300 mg/day in the general population and no more than 1500 mg/day in blacks, middle- and older-aged persons, and individuals with hypertension, diabetes, or chronic kidney disease
Dietary pattern	Consume a dietary approach to stop hypertension (DASH)-style dietary pattern rich in fruits and vegetables (8 to 10 servings/day), rich in low-fat dairy products (2 to 3 servings/day), and reduced in saturated fat and cholesterol. Vegetarian diets and to a lesser extent, Mediterranean style diets, are effective options
Increased potassium intake	Increase potassium intake to 4.7 gm/day, which is also the level provided in the DASH diet
Moderation of alcohol intake	For those who drink alcohol, consume ≤ 2 alcoholic drinks/day (men) and ≤ 1 alcohol drinks/day (women)[a]

[a]One alcoholic drink is defined as 12 oz of regular beer, 5 oz of wine (12% alcohol), or 1.5 oz of 80 proof distilled spirits.
(Reproduced with permission from Appel LJ, Brands MW, Daniels SR, et al. Dietary approaches to prevent and treat hypertension: a Scientific Statement from the American Heart Association. Hypertension. 2006;47:296-308.)

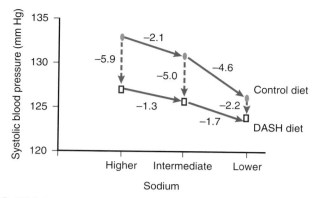

FIG. 21.4 Mean systolic blood pressure changes in the DASH-Sodium trial. The sample size was 412, 59% were prehypertensive, and 57% were African American. Solid lines display the effects of sodium reduction in the two diets; hatched lines display the effects of the DASH diet at each sodium level. *DASH*, Dietary approach to stop hypertension. *(Adapted with permission from Sacks FM, Svetkey LP, Vollmer WM, et al. Effects on blood pressure of reduced dietary sodium and the dietary approaches to stop hypertension (DASH) diet. DASH-sodium collaborative research group. N Engl J Med. 2001;344:3-10).*

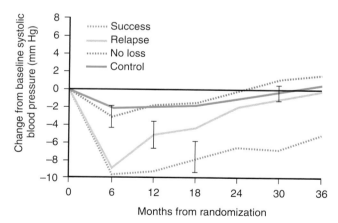

FIG. 21.3 Mean systolic blood pressure change in the Trials of Hypertension Prevention (TOHP2) in 4 groups of participants: (1) those assigned to weight loss group who successfully maintained weight loss, (2) those assigned to weight loss group who lost weight but experienced relapse, (3) those assigned to weight loss group who never lost weight, and (4) control group. *(Reprinted with permission from Stevens VJ, Obarzanke E, Cook NR, et al. Long-term weight loss and changes in blood pressure. Results of the Trials of Hypertension Prevention, Phase II. Ann Intern Med. 2001;134:1-11).*

epidemiologic studies, dose-response trials, and meta-analyses of trials. To date, over 100 randomized trials have been performed. In one of the most recent meta-analyses,[20] a reduction in sodium intake of 2.3 grams per day lowered systolic BP by 3.8 in adults; larger BP reductions occurred in older rather than younger persons, African Americans compared with whites, and hypertensive individuals compared with normotensive individuals. In a small but well-done trial of patients with medication-treated, resistant hypertension, reducing

sodium intake by around 4.5 grams per day lowered systolic/diastolic BP by 22.7/9.1 mm Hg.[21]

The most persuasive evidence on the effects of sodium intake on BP comes from rigorously controlled, dose-response studies.[22,23] Each of these trials tested at least three sodium levels, and each documented statistically significant, direct, progressive, dose-response relationships. The largest of these trials, the DASH Sodium trial, tested the effects of three different sodium intakes separately in two diets: the DASH diet (see subsequent section) and a control diet more typical of what Americans usually eat. As estimated from 24-hour urine collections, the three sodium levels (termed lower, intermediate, and higher) provided 65, 107, and 142 mmol of sodium per day, respectively (corresponding to 1.5, 2.5, and 3.3 g per day).

The main results of this trial are displayed in Fig. 21.4. The BP response to sodium reduction, although direct and progressive, was nonlinear. Decreasing sodium intake by approximately 0.9 grams per day (40 mmol/day) caused a greater BP reduction when the starting sodium intake was below 100 mmol per day than when it was above this level. In subgroup analyses of this trial,[24,25] a reduced sodium intake significantly lowered BP in each of the major subgroups studied (i.e., African American, non-African American, men, women). Importantly, sodium reduction significantly lowered BP in nonhypertensive individuals on both diets.

In addition to lowering BP, trials have documented that a reduced sodium intake can prevent hypertension (relative risk reduction of ~20% with or without concomitant weight loss), can lower BP even in the setting of BP-lowering medications,[26] and can improve hypertension control. In observational studies, a reduced sodium intake is associated with a blunted age-related rise in systolic BP. Several observational studies have explored the relationship of sodium intake with CV disease. These reports have been notable for their inconsistent and occasionally paradoxical results,[27,28] which likely result from methodological limitations, particularly, the potential for reverse causality and the challenge of accurately estimating usual sodium intake.[29]

To date, few trials have reported the effects of a reduced sodium intake on clinical CV events.[26,27,30] Two trials tested reduced sodium lifestyle interventions, and one trial assessed the effects of a reduced sodium/high potassium salt substitute. In each, there was a 21% to 41% reduction in clinical CV disease events in those who received the reduced sodium intervention (significant reduction in 2 studies[27,30]). A fourth trial with few CVD outcomes had a null result. In a meta-analysis of these trials, there was a 20% reduction in CVD outcomes.[31] Hence, direct evidence from trials, albeit limited, is consistent with indirect evidence on the health benefits of sodium reduction.[32]

Similar to other interventions, the BP response to changes in dietary sodium intake is heterogeneous. Despite attempts to classify individuals in research studies as salt sensitive and salt resistant, the change in BP in response to a change in sodium intake is not binary.[33] Rather, the change in BP from a reduced sodium intake has a continuous distribution, that is, individuals have greater or lesser degrees of BP reduction. In general, the extent of BP reduction as a result of reduced sodium intake is greater in African Americans, middle-aged and older-aged persons, and individuals with hypertension and likely those with diabetes or kidney disease. These groups tend to have a less responsive renin-angiotensin-aldosterone system.[34] It has been hypothesized that sodium sensitivity is a phenotype that reflects subclinical kidney dysfunction.[35] As discussed later, genetic and dietary factors also influence the response to sodium. The rise in BP for a given increase in sodium is blunted in the setting of either the DASH diet or a high dietary potassium intake.

A reduced sodium intake should have other beneficial effects that are independent of its effects on BP. Potential benefits include a reduced risk of subclinical CVD (i.e., left ventricular hypertrophy, ventricular fibrosis, and diastolic dysfunction), kidney damage, gastric cancer, and disordered mineral metabolism (i.e., increased urinary calcium excretion, potentially leading to osteoporosis).[36] Specifically, in cross-sectional studies, left ventricular (LV) mass is directly related to sodium intake, and one small trial in the early 1990s documented that sodium reduction can reduce LV mass.

Importantly, there is no convincing or consistent evidence of harm from a reduced sodium intake. Although some sodium intake is essential, there is no evidence that inadequate sodium intake is a public health problem. Extreme sodium reduction to less than 20 mmol per day might adversely affect blood lipids and insulin resistance; however, moderate sodium reduction has no such effects.[37,38] A potential adverse effect of a reduced sodium intake is an increase in plasma renin activity (PRA) and uric acid. However, in contrast to the well-accepted benefits of BP reduction, the clinical relevance of modest rises in PRA and uric acid as a result of sodium reduction and other antihypertensive therapies is uncertain. In fact, thiazide diuretics, a class of antihypertensive drug therapies that raises PRA and uric acid substantially reduces CV disease risk.[39]

Available evidence supports population-wide sodium reduction, as recommended by the U.S. Dietary Guidelines for Americans and numerous other organizations. Current dietary guidelines recommend an upper limit of 2300 mg per day in the general population and an upper limit of 1500 mg per day for African American, middle-aged and older-aged persons, and individuals with hypertension, diabetes, or chronic kidney disease (CKD); together these groups represent well over 50% of U.S. adults.[40] In this setting, the American Heart Association set 1.5 gm (65 mmol) of sodium per day as the recommended upper limit of intake for all Americans.[41] Survey data indicate that most children and adults exceed this limit.

In summary, available data strongly support current, population-wide recommendations to lower sodium intake. Consumers should choose foods low in sodium and limit the amount of sodium added to food. However, because over 75% of consumed sodium comes from processed foods, any meaningful strategy to reduce sodium intake must involve food manufacturers and restaurants. Recent guidelines have recommended that the food industry should progressively reduce the sodium added to foods by 50% over the next 10 years.[42] In the absence of meaningful reductions in sodium intake through voluntary recommendations, a recent Institute of Medicine (IOM) report has recommended a national approach, implemented through the United States Food and Drug Administration (FDA), to accomplish population-wide reductions in sodium intake.[43]

Increased Potassium Intake

High potassium intake is associated with lower BP. Available evidence includes animal studies, observational studies, clinical trials, and meta-analyses of these trials. Although data from individual trials have typically been inconsistent, several meta-analyses have each documented a significant inverse relationship between potassium intake and BP in hypertensive patients and equivocal effects in nonhypertensive individuals.[44] In one meta-analysis, a net increase in urinary potassium excretion of 2 gm per day (50 mmol/day) was associated with average systolic and diastolic BP reductions of 4.4 and 2.5 mm Hg in hypertensive individuals, and 1.8 and 1.0 in nonhypertensive persons. Increased potassium has beneficial effects on BP in the setting of a low potassium intake (e.g., 1.3 to 1.4 gm/day, or 35 to 40 mmol/day), or a much higher intake (e.g., 3.3 gm/day, or 84 mmol/day).[45] Importantly, increased potassium intake reduces BP to a greater extent in African Americans compared with whites, and therefore may be a valuable tool to reduce health disparities related to the prevalence of elevated BP and its complications.

Because a high intake of potassium can be achieved through diet and because potassium contained in foods is also accompanied by a variety of other nutrients, the preferred strategy to increase potassium intake is to consume foods, such as fruits and vegetables that are rich in potassium. In the DASH trial, the two groups that increased fruit and vegetable consumption both lowered BP.[46] The DASH diet provides around 4.7 grams per day (120 mmol/day) of potassium. Another trial documented that increased fruit and vegetable intake lowers BP, but it did not specify the amount of potassium that was provided.[47]

Potassium and sodium interact such that the effects of potassium on BP depend on the concurrent intake of sodium and vice versa. Specifically, an increased intake of potassium has greater BP-lowering effects in the setting of a higher sodium intake and lesser BP effects when sodium intake is already low. Conversely, the BP reduction from a lower sodium intake is greatest when potassium intake is also low. In one trial, a high potassium intake (120 mmol/day) blunted the pressor response to increased sodium intake in nonhypertensive African-American men and to a lesser extent in non-African Americans (see Fig. 21.5).[48] A 2 × 2 factorial trial, conducted in Australia, tested the effects of reduced sodium intake and increased potassium intake, alone or together, on BP in 212 hypertensives; in this trial, a reduced sodium intake lowered BP to the same extent as an increased potassium intake; however, the combination did not further lower BP. Overall, available data are consistent with subadditive effects of reduced sodium intake and increased potassium intake on BP.

The dearth of dose-response studies precludes a firm recommendation for a specific level of potassium intake to lower BP. However, an IOM committee set the recommended potassium intake level at 4.7 grams per day (120 mmol/day).[49] This level is similar to the average total potassium intake in clinical trials, the highest dose in the one available dose-response trial, and the potassium content of the DASH diet.[46]

In the generally healthy population with normal kidney function, a potassium intake from foods above 4.7 grams per day (120 mmol/day) poses no risk because excess potassium is readily excreted. However, in individuals whose urinary potassium excretion is impaired, an intake less than 4.7 grams per day (120 mmol/day) is appropriate, because of adverse cardiac effects (dysrhythmias) from hyperkalemia. Common drugs that impair potassium excretion are angiotensin-converting enzyme inhibitors, angiotensin receptor blockers, nonsteroidal

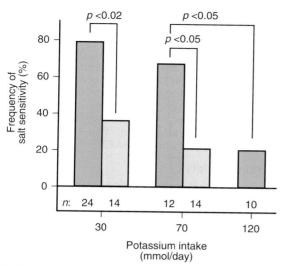

FIG. 21.5 Prevalence of sodium sensitivity in normotensive individuals (African Americans, blue bars; whites, light brown bars) at three levels of potassium intake. Sodium sensitivity is defined by a sodium-induced increase in mean arterial pressure of at least 3 mm Hg. *(Reprinted with permission from Morris RJ Jr, Sebastian A, Forman A, et al. Normotensive salt sensitivity: effects of race and dietary potassium. Hypertension. 1999;33:18-23).*

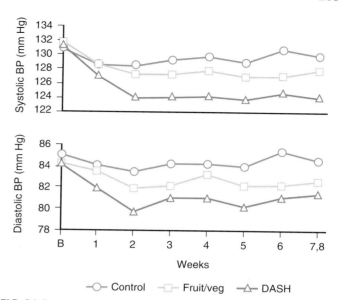

FIG. 21.6 Blood pressure (BP) by week during the dietary approach to stop hypertension (DASH) feeding study in three diets (control diet, fruits and vegetables diet, and the 'DASH diet'. *(Adapted with permission from Appel LJ, Moore TJ, Obarzanek E, et al. A clinical trial of the effects of dietary patterns on blood pressure. DASH collaborative research group. N Engl J Med. 1997;336:1117-1124).*

antiinflammatory drugs (NSAIDs), and potassium-sparing diuretics. Medical conditions associated with impaired renal excretion of potassium include diabetes, CKD, end-stage renal disease, severe heart failure, and adrenal insufficiency. Elderly individuals are at increased risk of hyperkalemia. Available evidence is insufficient to identify the level of kidney function at which individuals with CKD are at risk for hyperkalemia from a high dietary intake of potassium. In this setting, namely, patients with advanced CKD, that is, stage 3 or 4, an expert panel set a wide range of recommended potassium intake of between 2000 and 4000 mg per day.[50]

Moderation of Alcohol Consumption

Observational and experimental studies have documented a direct, dose-response relationship between alcohol intake and BP, particularly as the intake of alcohol increases above two drinks per day.[51] This relationship is independent of potential confounders such as age, obesity, and sodium intake.[52] Although some studies have shown that the alcohol-BP relationship also extends into the "light drinking" range, that is, at or below two drinks per day, this is the range in which alcohol may reduce the risk of coronary heart disease.

A meta-analysis of 15 randomized trials reported that decreased alcohol consumption (median reduction in self-reported alcohol intake of 76%, range 16% to 100%) lowered BP by 3.3/2.0 mm Hg.[51] Reductions were similar in nonhypertensives and hypertensives, and the relationship appeared dose-dependent.

In aggregate, available evidence supports moderation of alcohol intake (among those who drink) as an effective strategy to lower BP. The prevailing consensus is that alcohol consumption should be limited to no more than two alcoholic drinks per day in men and to no more than 1 alcoholic drink per day in women and lighter weight persons [one drink is defined as 12 oz. of regular beer, 5 oz. of wine (12% alcohol), and 1.5 oz. of 80 proof distilled spirits].

Dietary Patterns

Vegetarian Diets

Certain dietary patterns, particularly vegetarian diets, have been associated with low BP. In industrialized countries, where elevated BP is extremely commonplace, individuals who consume a vegetarian diet have markedly lower BP than nonvegetarians. Some of the lowest BPs observed in industrialized countries have been documented in strict vegetarians living in Massachusetts. Vegetarians may also experience a slower, age-related rise in BP.

Several aspects of a vegetarian lifestyle might affect BP. These lifestyle factors include nondietary factors (e.g., physical activity), established dietary risk factors (e.g., sodium, potassium, weight, alcohol), and other aspects of a vegetarian diet (e.g., high fiber, no meat). To a limited extent, observational studies have controlled for the well-established dietary determinants of BP. For instance, in a study of Seventh Day Adventists, analyses were adjusted for weight but not dietary sodium or potassium intake.[53] In a recent meta-analysis of 7 trials and 32 cohort studies, vegetarian diets were associated with lower systolic BP (mean net difference of −6.9 mm Hg) and diastolic BP (mean net difference of −4.7 mm Hg) compared with omnivorous diets.[54]

The Dietary Approaches to Stop Hypertension Diet

The DASH trial was a randomized feeding study that tested the effects of three diets on BP.[46] The most effective diet, now termed the DASH diet, emphasized fruits, vegetables, and low-fat dairy products; included whole grains, poultry, fish and nuts; and was reduced in fats, red meat, sweets, and sugar-containing beverages. It was rich in potassium, magnesium, calcium and fiber, and reduced in total fat, saturated fat and cholesterol; it was also slightly increased in protein. Among all participants, the DASH diet significantly lowered BP by a mean of 5.5/3.0 mm Hg, each net of control. The BP-lowering effects of the diets were rapid, occurring within only 2 weeks (see Fig. 21.6).

In subgroup analyses,[46] the DASH diet significantly lowered BP in all major subgroups (men, women, African Americans, non-African Americans, hypertensives, and nonhypertensives). However, the effects of the DASH diet in the African-American participants were striking (mean net BP reductions of 6.9/3.7 mm Hg) and were significantly greater than corresponding reductions in white participants (net BP reductions of 3.3/2.4 mm Hg). The effects in hypertensive individuals (net BP reductions of 11.6/5.3 mm Hg) have obvious clinical

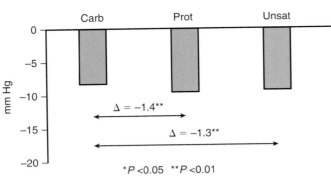

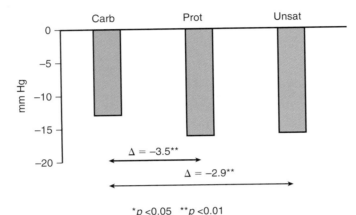

FIG. 21.7 Effects of three healthy dietary patterns tested in the OmniHeart feeding study on systolic blood pressure [Carb (similar to the dietary approach to stop hypertension diet), Prot (rich in protein, about half from plant sources), Unsat (rich in monounsaturated fat)] in all participants (A) and in hypertensive participants (B). *(Reprinted with permission from Appel LJ, Brands MW, Daniels SR, et al. Dietary approaches to prevent and treat hypertension: a Scientific Statement from the American Heart Association. Hypertension. 2006;47:296-308).*

significance. The corresponding effects in nonhypertensive individuals (3.5/2.2 mm Hg) have major public health importance (see Fig. 21.1). In a subsequent trial that enrolled a similar population,[22] the DASH diet significantly lowered BP at each of three sodium levels (see Fig. 21.4), and the combination of the DASH diet with sodium reduction resulted in the lowest level of BP.

The issue of whether modifying macronutrient content might improve the DASH diet was tested in a third trial, OmniHeart.[55] This feeding study tested 3 variants of the DASH diets (a diet rich in carbohydrate [58% of total calories] and similar to the original DASH diet, a second rich in protein [about half from plant sources], and a third diet rich in unsaturated fat [predominantly monounsaturated fat]). In several respects, each diet was similar to the original DASH diet; each was reduced in saturated fat, cholesterol, and sodium, and rich in fruit, vegetables, fiber, and potassium at recommended levels. Although each diet lowered systolic BP (see Fig. 21.7), substituting some of the carbohydrate (approximately 10% of total kcal) with either protein (about half from plant sources) or with unsaturated fat (mostly monounsaturated fat) further lowered BP.

Speculation about the effective components of DASH-style diets has been considerable. The diet that emphasized fruits and vegetables resulted in BP reductions that were approximately half of the total effect of the DASH diet (see Fig. 21.6). Fruits and vegetables are rich in potassium, magnesium, fiber, and many other nutrients. Of these nutrients, potassium is

best established to lower BP, particularly in hypertensives and in African Americans. In view of the additional BP reduction from the DASH diet beyond that of the fruits and vegetables diet, some other aspect(s) of the DASH diet further lowered BP. Compared with the fruits and vegetables diet, the DASH diet had more vegetables, low-fat dairy products, and fish, and was lower in red meat, sugar, and refined carbohydrates.

The DASH diet is safe and broadly applicable to the general population. However, because of its relatively high potassium, phosphorus and protein content, this diet is not recommended for persons with advanced CKD.[50]

Mediterranean Diets

Mediterranean diet is a general descriptive term applied to diets consumed in several regions close to the Mediterranean Sea. Typically, these diets are rich in plant foods (fruit, vegetables, breads, other forms of cereals, potatoes, beans, nuts, and seeds). Fruit is the typical daily dessert, and olive oil is the principal source of fat. Dairy products (mostly cheese and yogurt), fish and poultry are consumed in low to moderate amounts, zero to four eggs consumed weekly, red meat consumed in low amounts, and wine is consumed in low to moderate amounts, usually with meals. This diet is low in saturated fat (≤7% to 8% of energy) but moderate to high in total fat, ranging from less than 25% to more than 40% of energy. Such a diet is similar to the DASH-style diet, termed UNSAT, tested in the OmniHeart trial.[55]

In observational studies, Mediterranean diets are associated with a reduced risk of CV disease and other degenerative conditions.[56] In a major trial, PREDIMED (Prevención con Dieta Mediterránea), advice to consume a Mediterranean diet coupled with supplemental foods (either extra virgin olive oil or mixed nuts) reduced the risk of CV disease, particularly stroke, an outcome that largely reflects BP.[57] Still, the effects of a Mediterranean-style diet on BP appear to be modest, that is, net reductions in systolic and diastolic BP less than 2 mm Hg, in a meta-analysis of 6 trials.[58]

DIETARY FACTORS WITH LIMITED OR UNCERTAIN EFFECTS

Fish Oil Supplementation

Several predominantly small trials, and meta-analyses of these trials have documented that high-dose, omega-3 polyunsaturated fatty acid (commonly termed 'fish oil') supplements can reduce BP in hypertensive individuals.[59] In nonhypertensive individuals, BP reductions tend to be small or nonsignificant. In some analyses, the effects appear to be dose-dependent, with BP reductions occurring at relatively high doses of fish oil, namely, 3 grams per day or more. In hypertensive individuals, average BP reductions were 2.6/1.5 mm Hg. Side effects, including a fishy taste and belching, are common. In view of these side effects and the high dose required to lower BP, fish oil supplements cannot be routinely recommended to lower BP.

Fiber

Fiber consists of the indigestible components of food from plants. Evidence from observational studies and several trials suggests that increased fiber intake may reduce BP. Over 20 trials of fiber supplementation have been conducted. Most did not have BP as their primary outcome, and many had a multicomponent intervention. Also differences in definition and classification of fiber have complicated interpretation of trial findings. Two meta-analyses estimated the impact of fiber supplements on BP,[60,61] and both noted net systolic and diastolic BP reductions less than 2 mm Hg, often nonsignificant. Overall, data are insufficient to recommend supplemental fiber or an increased intake of dietary fiber alone to lower BP.

Calcium and Magnesium

Evidence that increased dietary calcium intake might lower BP comes from a variety of sources including animal studies, observational studies, trials, and meta-analyses. In a 1995 meta-analysis of 23 observational studies, Cappuccio et al. noted an inverse association between dietary calcium intake and BP.[62] However, the effect size was relatively small, and there was evidence of publication bias and heterogeneity across studies. Subsequent meta-analyses of randomized trials documented modest reductions in BP of 0.9 to 1.4/0.2 to 0.8 mm Hg from calcium supplementation (400 to 2000 mg/day).[63] The level of dietary calcium intake may affect the pressor response to sodium. In three small trials, calcium supplementation mitigated the effects of a high sodium intake on BP.

Evidence implicating magnesium as a major determinant of BP is inconsistent. In observational studies, often cross-sectional, a common finding is an inverse association between dietary magnesium and BP, a relationship seen in a pooled analysis of 29 observational studies. However, in a meta-analysis of 20 randomized clinical trials, there was no clear effect of increased magnesium intake on BP.[64]

Overall, evidence is insufficient to recommend either supplemental calcium or magnesium to lower BP.

Intake of Fats Other Than n-3 Polyunsaturated Fatty Acids

Total fat includes saturated fat, omega-3 polyunsaturated fat, omega-6 polyunsaturated fat, and monounsaturated fat. Early studies focused on the effects of total fat intake on BP. However, there is a plausible biological basis to hypothesize that certain types of fat (e.g., omega-3 polyunsaturated fat) might lower BP and that other types of fat (e.g., saturated fat) might raise it.

Saturated Fat

Several observational studies and a few trials have assessed the effects of saturated fat on BP. In the vast majority, including two prospective observational studies, the Nurses Health Study and the Health Professionals Follow-up Study, saturated fat intake was not associated with incident hypertension. In the few available clinical trials, diet interventions focused on reducing saturated fat had no effect on BP. Because most trials tested diets that were simultaneously reduced in saturated fat and increased in polyunsaturated fat, the absence of a BP effect also suggests no benefit from polyunsaturated fat.

Omega-6 Polyunsaturated Fat Intake

Dietary intake of omega-6 polyunsaturated fat (mainly linoleic acid in western diets) has little or no effect on BP. In an overview of cross-sectional studies that correlated BP with tissue or blood levels of omega-6 polyunsaturated fat, there was no apparent relationship. Prospective observational studies and clinical trials have likewise been unsupportive.

Monounsaturated Fat Intake

Although the earliest trials did not support a relationship between monounsaturated fat and BP, subsequent trials have shown that diets rich in monounsaturated fats modestly lower BP.[65] However, an increase in monounsaturated fat is commonly linked with a reduction in the amount of carbohydrate consumed, potentially with a change in the type of carbohydrate as well.[66] Hence, it remains unclear whether the effects of increased monounsaturated fat intake reflect an increase in this nutrient and/or a decrease in carbohydrate intake or change in the type of carbohydrate, per se.

Carbohydrate

Both amount and type of carbohydrate may affect BP, but the evidence is uncertain. Worldwide, many populations that eat carbohydrate-rich, low-fat diets have low BP levels compared with Western countries. However, the results of observational studies have been inconsistent. In small early trials, increasing carbohydrate by reducing total fat typically did not reduce BP. In the OmniHeart feeding trial, partial substitution of carbohydrate with either protein (about half from plant sources) or monounsaturated fat lowered BP.[55] In a subsequent trial, a high glycemic compared with low glycemic index diet had no significant effect on BP.[67]

An emerging but inconclusive body of evidence suggests that increased intake of added sugars might raise BP. Studies include animal studies in which rats are fed high doses of fructose, acute ingestion studies in which humans are fed high doses of different sugars, and more recently epidemiologic studies. In cross-sectional studies, higher sugar-sweetened beverage intake has been associated with elevated BP in adolescents. In prospective observational studies, consumption of more than one soft drink per day significantly increased the odds of developing high BP.[68] In post-hoc analyses of a completed trial, there was a direct association between reductions in sugar-sweetened beverage intake with reductions in BP.[69] Nonetheless, results from randomized trials in humans are inconsistent.[70] Overall, additional research is warranted before making recommendations about the amount and type of carbohydrate as a means to lower BP.

Cholesterol

Few studies have examined the BP effects of dietary cholesterol. In the observational analyses of the Multiple Risk Factor Intervention Trial, there were significant, direct relationships between cholesterol intake (mg/day) and both systolic and diastolic BP. The Keys score was also associated with diastolic BP, but not systolic BP. In longitudinal analyses from the Western Electric Study, there were significant positive relationships of change in systolic BP over 8 years with dietary cholesterol, as well as the Keys score.[60] Despite these reports, the paucity of evidence precludes any firm conclusion about a relationship between dietary cholesterol and BP.

Protein Intake

An extensive, and generally consistent, body of evidence from observational studies has documented inverse associations between BP and protein intake, particularly protein from plants. Two major observational studies, the International Study on Macronutrients and Blood Pressure (INTERMAP) and the Chicago Western Electric Study, have documented significant inverse relationships between protein intake and BP.[71,72] In these studies, protein from plant sources was associated with lower BP, whereas protein from animal sources had no significant effect.

In contrast to the large volume of evidence from observational studies, few trials have examined the effects of increased protein intake on BP. Two trials documented that increased protein intake from soy supplements can reduce BP. In one trial, supplemental soy protein (total of 25% kcal protein, 12.5% from soy) lowered average 24-hour BP by 5.9/2.6 mm Hg in hypertensive individuals. In a large trial conducted in the Peoples Republic of China, supplemental soy protein, which increased total protein intake from 12% to 16% kcal, lowered average BP by 4.3/2.7 mm Hg, net of a control group which received supplemental carbohydrate. A meta-analysis of 40 trials documented that supplementation of diet with protein, compared with carbohydrate, significantly lowered systolic BP by 1.8 mm Hg and diastolic BP by 1.2 mm Hg, with no difference in effects from animal and vegetable protein.[73]

In aggregate, clinical trials and observational studies support the hypothesis that an increased intake of protein from plants can lower BP. However, further evidence is needed before recommendations can be made.

Vitamin C

Laboratory studies, depletion-repletion studies, and observational studies suggest that increased vitamin C intake and higher vitamin C levels are associated with lower BP. A large number of randomized trials, often with small samples, have tested whether or not vitamin C supplements lower BP. A 2012 meta-analysis of these trials suggested that supplementation of diet with vitamin C might lower BP.[74] At this time, it remains unclear whether an increased intake or supplementation of diet with vitamin C lowers BP.

GENE-DIET INTERACTIONS

A substantial and increasing body of evidence has documented that genetic factors affect BP levels and the BP response to dietary changes. Most of the available research has focused on genetic factors that influence the BP response to dietary sodium intake. Several genotypes that affect BP have been identified, and most influence the renin-angiotensin-aldosterone axis or renal sodium handling. In a line of research that has focused on Mendelian diseases associated with either high or low BP, six genes associated with higher BP and eight genes associated with lower BP have been identified.[75] Of considerable importance is the fact that each of these genes regulates renal sodium handling; mutations that increase net sodium chloride reabsorption raise BP, whereas mutations that lower sodium chloride reabsorption reduce BP.

A few trials have examined the interactive effects of specific genotypes and the BP response to dietary changes. In three trials, genetic variation of the angiotensinogen gene modified the BP response to changes in sodium intake in whites,[23] and the BP responses to weight change, and the DASH diet.[76] Polymorphism of the α-adducin gene also appears to affect the BP response to sodium chloride.[77] Lastly, angiotensin–converting-enzyme insertion-deletion (ACE I/D) polymorphism may also affect the BP response to weight change.[78]

EFFECTS OF MULTIPLE DIETARY CHANGES

Despite the potential for large BP reductions from simultaneously implementing multiple dietary changes, few trials have examined the combined effects of multicomponent interventions. In general, multicomponent intervention trials have documented subadditivity, that is, the BP effect of interventions with two or more components is less than the sum of BP reductions from interventions that implement each component alone. Despite subadditivity, the BP effects of multicomponent interventions are often large and clinically relevant. One small, but well controlled trial tested the effects of a comprehensive program of supervised exercise with provision of prepared meals to accomplish weight loss, sodium reduction, and the DASH diet; participants were medication-treated hypertensive adults. The program substantially lowered daytime ambulatory BP by 12.1/6.6 mm Hg, net of control.[79] Subsequently, a behavioral intervention trial, PREMIER, tested the effects of the major lifestyle recommendations (weight loss, sodium reduction, increased physical activity, and the DASH diet).[80] In nonhypertensives, mean BP reductions were 9.2/5.8 mm Hg (3.1/2.0 mm Hg, net of control). In hypertensive individuals, none of whom were on medication, corresponding BP reductions were 14.2/7.4 mm Hg (6.3/3.6 mm Hg, net of control).

BEHAVIORAL INTERVENTIONS TO ACCOMPLISH LIFESTYLE MODIFICATION

Numerous behavioral intervention trials have tested the BP effects of dietary change. Several theories and models have informed the design of these trials, including social cognitive theory, self-applied behavior modification techniques, "behavioral self-management," the relapse prevention model, and the trans-theoretical, or stages-of-change model. Application of these theories and models typically leads to a common intervention approach that emphasizes behavioral skills training, self-monitoring, self-regulation, and motivational interviewing. Often these studies enrolled motivated individuals, selected in part because of their self-reported readiness to change. Further, these studies relied on skilled therapists, often health educators or dietitians. At least for weight loss trials, characteristic findings result in successful behavior change over the short-term, usually 6 months or less, and then subsequent recidivism. The limited long-term success of these intensive intervention programs highlights the importance of environmental and policy changes that facilitate adoption of desirable lifestyle changes broadly across whole populations.

SPECIAL POPULATIONS

Children

The problem of elevated BP begins early in life, perhaps in utero. Numerous observational studies have documented that BP tracks from childhood into adulthood.[81] Hence, efforts to reduce BP in children and prevent the age-related rise in BP seem prudent. The importance of efforts to reduce BP in children is highlighted by evidence that BP levels and the prevalence of obesity in children and adolescents have increased between NHANES surveys conducted in 1988 to 1994 and 1999 to 2000.[82] The importance of sodium reduction in children is highlighted by a meta-analysis of trials in children, in whom reduced dietary sodium interventions lowered BP.[83] In addition, observational studies have documented that U.S. children have BP levels that exceed BP levels of middle-aged adults in populations exposed to a low sodium diet.[84]

Otherwise, evidence on the effects of dietary factors on BP in children is limited and has methodologic limitations, including small sample size, suboptimal BP measurements, and limited dietary contrast. Accordingly, the BP effects of diet in children and adolescents is extrapolated from studies conducted in adults. Such extrapolations are reasonable, because elevated BP is a chronic condition resulting from the insidious rise in BP throughout childhood and adulthood.

Older-Aged Persons

Dietary strategies should be especially beneficial as adults age. The age-related rise in BP is particularly prominent in middle-aged and older-aged persons, and the incidence of BP-related CV disease is especially high in older-aged persons. Although most diet-BP trials were conducted in middle-aged persons, several were conducted in older-aged individuals. Other trials have presented results stratified by age. Several important findings emerge. First, evidence is remarkably consistent that older-aged persons can make and sustain dietary changes, specifically dietary sodium reduction and weight loss.[85] Second, BP reduction from dietary interventions is greater in older-aged persons in comparison to middle-aged individuals.[24] Third, because of high attributable risk associated with elevated BP in the elderly, the beneficial effects of dietary changes on BP should reduce CV risk substantially.

African Americans

In comparison with whites, African Americans have higher BP, and are at greater risk of BP-related complications, especially stroke and kidney disease. As documented previously, in well-controlled efficacy trials, African Americans achieve greater BP reduction than whites from several nonpharmacologic therapies, specifically, sodium reduction, increased potassium intake, and the DASH diet. The potential benefits of modifying these dietary factors is amplified because survey data indicate that, on average, African Americans consume high levels of sodium whereas their potassium intake, on average, is less than that of whites.[49] In this setting, the potential benefits of dietary change are substantial and should provide a means to reduce racial disparities in BP and its CV and renal complications.[86]

Health Care Providers

The clinician's office can be a powerful setting to advocate and accomplish lifestyle change. Through advice and by example, physicians can have a powerful influence on their patients' willingness to make lifestyle changes. Although behavioral counseling is usually beyond the scope of many office practices, simple assessments and provision of advice is typically feasible (e.g., calculation of body mass index). The success of physician-directed, office-based attempts to achieve lifestyle changes is dependent upon several factors, including the skills of the physician and staff, available resources, organizational structure of the office, and the availability of algorithms that incorporate locally available resources. The Center for Medicare and Medicaid Services (CMS) recently decided to cover intensive behavioral therapy for weight control interventions delivered in the primary care setting; however, available data are more persuasive for interventions delivered by nonphysicians in settings other than the medical office.[87]

Individualized, physician-directed efforts should be guided, in large part, by the patient's willingness to adopt lifestyle changes. Motivated patients should be referred to a skilled dietitian, health educator, or behavioral change program, because success in clinical trials has typically required frequent visits and other contacts. Even without the assistance of ancillary personnel and programs, health care providers should routinely encourage lifestyle modification.

SUMMARY

A compelling body of evidence supports the concept that multiple dietary factors affect BP. Dietary changes that effectively lower BP are weight loss, reduced sodium intake, increased potassium intake, moderation of alcohol intake (among those who drink), and DASH-style and vegetarian dietary patterns. Other dietary factors may also affect BP, but the effects are small and/or the evidence uncertain.

In view of the increasing levels of BP in children and adults and the continuing epidemic of BP-related CV and renal diseases, efforts to reduce BP in both nonhypertensive and hypertensive individuals are warranted. Such efforts will require individuals to change behavior and society to make environmental changes that encourage such changes. The challenge to health care providers, researchers, government officials, and the general public is developing and implementing effective clinical and public health strategies that lead to sustained dietary changes among individuals and more broadly among populations.

References

1. Kearney PM, Whelton M, Reynolds K, Muntner P, Whelton PK, He J. Global burden of hypertension: analysis of worldwide data. *Lancet.* 2005;365:217-223.
2. Nwankwo T, Yoon SS, Burt V, Gu Q. Hypertension among adults in the United States: National Health and Nutrition Examination Survey, 2011-2012. *NCHS Data Brief.* 2013:1-8.
3. Whelton PK. The elusiveness of population-wide high blood pressure control. *Annu Rev Public Health.* 2015;36:109-130.
4. Vasan RS, Beiser A, Seshadri S, Larson MG, Kannel WB, D'Agostino RB, et al. Residual lifetime risk for developing hypertension in middle-aged women and men: The Framingham Heart Study. *JAMA.* 2002;287:1003-1010.
5. Chobanian AV, Bakris GL, Black HR, et al. Seventh Report of the Joint National Committee on Prevention, Detection, Evaluation, and Treatment of High Blood Pressure. *Hypertension.* 2003:1206-52.
6. Lewington S, Clarke R, Qizilbash N, Peto R, Collins R. Age-specific relevance of usual blood pressure to vascular mortality: a meta-analysis of individual data for one million adults in 61 prospective studies. *Lancet.* 2002;360:1903-1913.
7. Vasan RS, Larson MG, Leip EP, et al. Impact of high-normal blood pressure on the risk of cardiovascular disease. *N Engl J Med.* 2001;345:1291-1297.
8. Lawes CM, Vander Hoorn S, Rodgers A. Global burden of blood-pressure-related disease, 2001. *Lancet.* 2008;371:1513-1518.
9. Stamler R. Implications of the INTERSALT study. *Hypertension.* 1991;17(1 Suppl):I16-120.
10. Sacks FM, Campos H. Dietary therapy in hypertension. *N Engl J Med.* 2010;362:2102-2112.
11. Appel LJ, Giles TD, Black HR, et al. ASH position paper: dietary approaches to lower blood pressure. *J Am Soc Hypertens.* 2010;4:79-89.
12. Appel LJ, Brands MW, Daniels SR, Karanja N, Elmer PJ, Sacks FM. Dietary approaches to prevent and treat hypertension: a scientific statement from the American Heart Association. *Hypertension.* 2006;47:296-308.
13. Ogden CL, Carroll MD, Kit BK, Flegal KM. Prevalence of childhood and adult obesity in the United States, 2011-2012. *JAMA.* 2014;311:806-814.
14. Neter JE, Stam BE, Kok FJ, Grobbee DE, Geleijnse JM. Influence of weight reduction on blood pressure: a meta-analysis of randomized controlled trials. *Hypertension.* 2003;42:878-884.
15. Stevens VJ, Obarzanek E, Cook NR, et al. Long-term weight loss and changes in blood pressure: results of the Trials of Hypertension Prevention, phase II. *Ann Intern Med.* 2001;134:1-11.
16. Wing RR. Long-term effects of a lifestyle intervention on weight and cardiovascular risk factors in individuals with type 2 diabetes mellitus: four-year results of the Look AHEAD trial. *Arch Intern Med.* 2010;170:1566-1575.
17. Svetkey LP, Stevens VJ, Brantley PJ, et al. Comparison of strategies for sustaining weight loss: the weight loss maintenance randomized controlled trial. *JAMA.* 2008;299:1139-1148.
18. Knowler WC, Barrett-Connor E, Fowler SE, et al. Reduction in the incidence of type 2 diabetes with lifestyle intervention or metformin. *N Engl J Med.* 2002;346:393-403.
19. Stevens VJ, Obarzanek E, Cook NR, et al. Long-term weight loss and changes in blood pressure: results of the Trials of Hypertension Prevention, phase II. *Ann Intern Med.* 2001;134:1-11.
20. Mozaffarian D, Fahimi S, Singh GM, et al. Global sodium consumption and death from cardiovascular causes. *N Engl J Med.* 2014;371:624-634.
21. Pimenta E, Gaddam KK, Oparil S, et al. Effects of dietary sodium reduction on blood pressure in subjects with resistant hypertension: results from a randomized trial. *Hypertension.* 2009;54:475-481.
22. Sacks FM, Svetkey LP, Vollmer WM, et al. Effects on blood pressure of reduced dietary sodium and the Dietary Approaches to Stop Hypertension (DASH) diet. DASH-Sodium Collaborative Research Group. *N Engl J Med.* 2001;344:3-10.
23. Johnson AG, Nguyen TV, Davis D. Blood pressure is linked to salt intake and modulated by the angiotensinogen gene in normotensive and hypertensive elderly subjects. *J Hypertens.* 2001;19:1053-1060.
24. Vollmer WM, Sacks FM, Ard J, et al. Effects of diet and sodium intake on blood pressure: subgroup analysis of the DASH-sodium trial. *Ann Intern Med.* 2001;135:1019-1028.
25. Bray GA, Vollmer WM, Sacks FM, et al. A further subgroup analysis of the effects of the DASH diet and three dietary sodium levels on blood pressure: results of the DASH-Sodium Trial. *Am J Cardiol.* 2004;94:222-227.
26. Appel LJ, Espeland MA, Easter L, Wilson AC, Folmar S, Lacy CR. Effects of reduced sodium intake on hypertension control in older individuals: results from the Trial of Nonpharmacologic Interventions in the Elderly (TONE). *Arch Intern Med.* 2001;161:685-693.
27. Cook NR, Cutler JA, Obarzanek E, et al. Long term effects of dietary sodium reduction on cardiovascular disease outcomes: observational follow-up of the trials of hypertension prevention (TOHP). *BMJ.* 2007;334:885-888.
28. O'Donnell M, Mente A, Rangarajan S, et al. Urinary sodium and potassium excretion, mortality, and cardiovascular events. *N Engl J Med.* 2014;371:612-623.
29. Cobb LK, Anderson CA, Elliott P, et al. Methodological issues in cohort studies that relate sodium intake to cardiovascular disease outcomes: a science advisory from the American Heart Association. *Circulation.* 2014;129:1173-1186.
30. Chang HY, Hu YW, Yue CS, et al. Effect of potassium-enriched salt on cardiovascular mortality and medical expenses of elderly men. *Am J Clin Nutr.* 2006;83:1289-96.
31. He FJ, MacGregor GA. Salt reduction lowers cardiovascular risk: meta-analysis of outcome trials. *Lancet.* 2011;378:380-382.
32. Strazzullo P, D'Elia L, Kandala NB, Cappuccio FP. Salt intake, stroke, and cardiovascular disease: meta-analysis of prospective studies. *BMJ.* 2009;339:b4567.
33. Obarzanek E, Proschan MA, Vollmer WM, et al. Individual blood pressure responses to changes in salt intake: results from the DASH-Sodium trial. *Hypertension.* 2003;42:459-467.
34. He FJ, Markandu ND, MacGregor GA. Importance of the renin system for determining blood pressure fall with acute salt restriction in hypertensive and normotensive whites. *Hypertension.* 2001;38:321-325.
35. Johnson RJ, Herrera-Acosta J, Schreiner GF, Rodriguez-Iturbe B. Subtle acquired renal injury as a mechanism of salt-sensitive hypertension. *N Engl J Med.* 2002;346:913-923.
36. Frohlich ED. The salt conundrum: a hypothesis. *Hypertension.* 2007;50:161-166.
37. He FJ, MacGregor GA. Effect of modest salt reduction on blood pressure: a meta-analysis of randomized trials. Implications for public health. *J Hum Hypertens.* 2002;16:761-770.
38. Harsha DW, Sacks FM, Obarzanek E, et al. Effect of dietary sodium intake on blood lipids: results from the DASH-sodium trial. *Hypertension.* 2004;43:393-398.
39. Psaty BM, Lumley T, Furberg CD, et al. Health outcomes associated with various antihypertensive therapies used as first-line agents: a network meta-analysis. *JAMA.* 2003;289:2534-2544.
40. Application of lower sodium intake recommendations to adults—United States, 1999-2006. *MMWR Morb Mortal Wkly Rep.* 2009;58:281-283.
41. Lloyd-Jones DM, Hong Y, Labarthe D, et al. Defining and setting national goals for cardiovascular health promotion and disease reduction: the American Heart Association's strategic Impact Goal through 2020 and beyond. *Circulation.* 2010;121:586-613.
42. Havas S, Dickinson BD, Wilson M. The urgent need to reduce sodium consumption. *JAMA.* 2007;298:1439-1441.
43. Institute of Medicine (U.S.) Committee on Strategies to Reduce Sodium Intake, Henney JE, Taylor CL, Boon CS. Strategies to reduce sodium intake in the United States. Washington, D.C.: National Academies Press; 2010.
44. Geleijnse JM, Kok FJ, Grobbee DE. Blood pressure response to changes in sodium and potassium intake: a metaregression analysis of randomised trials. *J Hum Hypertens.* 2003;17:471-480.

45. Naismith DJ, Braschi A. The effect of low-dose potassium supplementation on blood pressure in apparently healthy volunteers. *Br J Nutr*. 2003;90:53-60.

46. Appel LJ, Moore TJ, Obarzanek E, et al. A clinical trial of the effects of dietary patterns on blood pressure. DASH Collaborative Research Group. *N Engl J Med*. 1997;336:1117-1124.

47. John JH, Ziebland S, Yudkin P, Roe LS, Neil HA. Effects of fruit and vegetable consumption on plasma antioxidant concentrations and blood pressure: a randomised controlled trial. *Lancet*. 2002;359:1969-1974.

48. Morris RC, Jr., Sebastian A, Forman A, Tanaka M, Schmidlin O. Normotensive salt sensitivity: effects of race and dietary potassium. *Hypertension*. 1999;33:18-23.

49. Institute of Medicine (U.S.). Panel on Dietary Reference Intakes for Electrolytes and Water. DRI, dietary reference intakes for water, potassium, sodium, chloride, and sulfate. Washington, D.C.: National Academies Press; 2005.

50. K/DOQI clinical practice guidelines on hypertension and antihypertensive agents in chronic kidney disease. *Am J Kidney Dis*. 2004;43(5 Suppl 1):S1-290.

51. Xin X, He J, Frontini MG, Ogden LG, Motsamai OI, Whelton PK. Effects of alcohol reduction on blood pressure: a meta-analysis of randomized controlled trials. *Hypertension*. 2001;38:1112-1117.

52. Okubo Y, Miyamoto T, Suwazono Y, Kobayashi E, Nogawa K. Alcohol consumption and blood pressure in Japanese men. *Alcohol*. 2001;23:149-156.

53. Armstrong B, van Merwyk AJ, Coates H. Blood pressure in Seventh-day Adventist vegetarians. *Am J Epidemiol*. 1977;105:444-449.

54. Yokoyama Y, Nishimura K, Barnard ND, et al. Vegetarian diets and blood pressure: a meta-analysis. *JAMA Intern Med*. 2014;174:577-587.

55. Appel LJ, Sacks FM, Carey VJ, et al. Effects of protein, monounsaturated fat, and carbohydrate intake on blood pressure and serum lipids: results of the OmniHeart randomized trial. *JAMA*. 2005;294:2455-2464.

56. Sofi F, Abbate R, Gensini GF, Casini A. Accruing evidence on benefits of adherence to the Mediterranean diet on health: an updated systematic review and meta-analysis. *Am J Clin Nutr*. 2010;92:1189-1196.

57. Estruch R, Ros E, Salas-Salvado J, et al. Primary prevention of cardiovascular disease with a Mediterranean diet. *N Engl J Med*. 2013;368:1279-1290.

58. Nordmann AJ, Suter-Zimmermann K, Bucher HC, et al. Meta-analysis comparing Mediterranean to low-fat diets for modification of cardiovascular risk factors. *Am J Med*. 2011;124:841-851.e2.

59. Campbell F, Dickinson HO, Critchley JA, Ford GA, Bradburn M. A systematic review of fish-oil supplements for the prevention and treatment of hypertension. *Eur J Prev Cardiol*. 2013;20:107-120.

60. Streppel MT, Arends LR, van't Veer P, Grobbee DE, Geleijnse JM. Dietary fiber and blood pressure: a meta-analysis of randomized placebo-controlled trials. *Arch Intern Med*. 2005;165:150-156.

61. Whelton SP, Hyre AD, Pedersen B, Yi Y, Whelton PK, He J. Effect of dietary fiber intake on blood pressure: a meta-analysis of randomized, controlled clinical trials. *J Hypertens*. 2005;23:475-481.

62. Cappuccio FP, Elliott P, Allender PS, Pryer J, Follman DA, Cutler JA. Epidemiologic association between dietary calcium intake and blood pressure: a meta-analysis of published data. *Am J Epidemiol*. 1995;142:935-945.

63. Allender PS, Cutler JA, Follmann D, Cappuccio FP, Pryer J, Elliott P. Dietary calcium and blood pressure: a meta-analysis of randomized clinical trials. *Ann Intern Med*. 1996;124:825-831.

64. Jee SH, Miller ER, 3rd, Guallar E, Singh VK, Appel LJ, Klag MJ. The effect of magnesium supplementation on blood pressure: a meta-analysis of randomized clinical trials. *Am J Hypertens*. 2002;15:691-696.

65. Ferrara LA, Raimondi AS, d'Episcopo L, Guida L, Dello Russo A, Marotta T. Olive oil and reduced need for antihypertensive medications. *Arch Intern Med*. 2000;160:837-842.

66. Shah M, Adams-Huet B, Garg A. Effect of high-carbohydrate or high-cis-monounsaturated fat diets on blood pressure: a meta-analysis of intervention trials. *Am J Clin Nutr*. 2007;85:1251-1256.

67. Sacks FM, Carey VJ, Anderson CA, et al. Effects of high vs low glycemic index of dietary carbohydrate on cardiovascular disease risk factors and insulin sensitivity: the OmniCarb randomized clinical trial. *JAMA*. 2014;312:2531-2541.

68. Dhingra R, Sullivan L, Jacques PF, et al. Soft drink consumption and risk of developing cardiometabolic risk factors and the metabolic syndrome in middle-aged adults in the community. *Circulation*. 2007;116:480-488.

69. Chen L, Caballero B, Mitchell DC, et al. Reducing consumption of sugar-sweetened beverages is associated with reduced blood pressure: a prospective study among United States adults. *Circulation*. 2010;121:2398-2406.

70. Visvanathan R, Chen R, Horowitz M, Chapman I. Blood pressure responses in healthy older people to 50 g carbohydrate drinks with differing glycaemic effects. *Br J Nutr*. 2004;92:335-340.

71. Elliott P, Stamler J, Dyer AR, Appel L, Dennis B, Kesteloot H, et al. Association between protein intake and blood pressure: the INTERMAP Study. *Arch Intern Med*. 2006;166:79-87.

72. Stamler J, Liu K, Ruth KJ, Pryer J, Greenland P. Eight-year blood pressure change in middle-aged men: relationship to multiple nutrients. *Hypertension*. 2002;39:1000-1006.

73. Rebholz CM, Friedman EE, Powers LJ, Arroyave WD, He J, Kelly TN. Dietary protein intake and blood pressure: a meta-analysis of randomized controlled trials. *Am J Epidemiol*. 2012;176(Suppl 7):S27-43.

74. Juraschek SP, Guallar E, Appel LJ, Miller ER, 3rd. Effects of vitamin C supplementation on blood pressure: a meta-analysis of randomized controlled trials. *Am J Clin Nutr*. 2012;95:1079-1088.

75. Lifton RP, Wilson FH, Choate KA, Geller DS. Salt and blood pressure: new insight from human genetic studies. *Cold Spring Harb Symp Quant Biol*. 2002;67:445-450.

76. Svetkey LP, Moore TJ, Simons-Morton DG, et al. Angiotensinogen genotype and blood pressure response in the Dietary Approaches to Stop Hypertension (DASH) study. *J Hypertens*. 2001;19:1949-1956.

77. Grant FD, Romero JR, Jeunemaitre X, et al. Low-renin hypertension, altered sodium homeostasis, and an alpha-adducin polymorphism. *Hypertension*. 2002;39:191-196.

78. Kostis JB, Wilson AC, Hooper WC, et al. Association of angiotensin-converting enzyme DD genotype with blood pressure sensitivity to weight loss. *Am Heart J*. 2002;144:625-629.

79. Miller ER 3rd, Erlinger TP, Young DR, et al. Results of the Diet, Exercise, and Weight Loss Intervention Trial (DEW-IT). *Hypertension*. 2002;40:612-618.

80. Appel LJ, Champagne CM, Harsha DW, et al. Effects of comprehensive lifestyle modification on blood pressure control: main results of the PREMIER clinical trial. *JAMA*. 2003;289:2083-2093.

81. Dekkers JC, Snieder H, Van Den Oord EJ, Treiber FA. Moderators of blood pressure development from childhood to adulthood: a 10-year longitudinal study. *J Pediatr*. 2002;141:770-779.

82. Muntner P, He J, Cutler JA, Wildman RP, Whelton PK. Trends in blood pressure among children and adolescents. *JAMA*. 2004;291:2107-2113.

83. He FJ, MacGregor GA. Importance of salt in determining blood pressure in children: meta-analysis of controlled trials. *Hypertension*. 2006;48:861-869.

84. Appel LJ. At the tipping point: accomplishing population-wide sodium reduction in the United States. *J Clin Hypertens (Greenwich)*. 2008;10:7-11.

85. Whelton PK, Appel LJ, Espeland MA, et al. Sodium reduction and weight loss in the treatment of hypertension in older persons: a randomized controlled trial of nonpharmacologic interventions in the elderly (TONE). TONE Collaborative Research Group. *JAMA*. 1998;279:839-846.

86. Erlinger TP, Vollmer WM, Svetkey LP, Appel LJ. The potential impact of nonpharmacologic population-wide blood pressure reduction on coronary heart disease events: pronounced benefits in African-Americans and hypertensives. *Prev Med*. 2003;37:327-333.

87. Wadden TA, Butryn ML, Hong PS, Tsai AG. Behavioral treatment of obesity in patients encountered in primary care settings: a systematic review. *JAMA*. 2014;312:1779-1791.

Diuretics are one of the most important classes of drugs used in hypertension.[1,2] In simplistic terms, the basic premise for their use is that they reduce extracellular fluid volume and increase sodium excretion, which leads to reductions in blood pressure. Historically, the degree of efficacy in lowering blood pressure was considered directly proportional to the dose. Diuretics have been used in hypertension for 60 years and they are now appreciated as a much more complex class of drugs, and their role in therapy continues to evolve.[3-5] Previous guidelines endorsed them as first-line therapy,[6] whereas the most recent 2014 Hypertension Guidelines suggested they were now one of five drug classes acceptable as initial agents.[7] Regardless of where and when they are employed, it is universally agreed that diuretics remain a mainstay in the pharmacologic management of hypertension.

This chapter will initially focus on thiazides (hydrochlorothiazide [HCTZ], indapamide, metolazone), and thiazide-like (chlorthalidone) agents because they account for the vast majority of diuretic use in primary hypertension and are the only diuretic agents to demonstrate efficacy in reducing hypertensive-related morbidity and mortality.

Loop diuretics (bumetanide, furosemide, or torsemide) have a more specialized role in hypertension, particularly for patients with kidney disease, low glomerular filtration rate, or with accompanying edematous disorders. Potassium-sparing diuretics (especially spironolactone) have been shown to be effective for patients with resistant or difficult to control blood pressure. These agents will also be briefly discussed in this chapter.

PHARMACOLOGY

Thiazides and Thiazide-Like Diuretics

These diuretics act primarily within the early distal convoluted tubule to reduce the reabsorption of sodium and chloride. Thiazide and thiazide-like diuretics must be secreted into the renal tubule, which is reduced with significant renal impairment. Although some antihypertensive activity remains even in the presence of significant renal impairment,[8-10] most clinicians switch to loop diuretics when glomerular filtration rate (GFR) is less than 20 to 30 mL/min.[6,11] The exact GFR threshold at which efficacy is lost is not well studied, and the switch to loop diuretics is based largely on the theory that there is a ceiling effect of thiazides in chronic kidney disease (CKD) that is controlled by several factors, including the reduced delivery of filtered solute and drug to the distal tubule site of action, and the fact that only a small amount of sodium reabsorption occurs in the distal tubule even under normal circumstances. Chlorthalidone, perhaps because of its long-acting nature, has been shown to remain effective at usual doses in patients with uncontrolled hypertension and chronic kidney disease and may be a preferred choice in this setting.[12,13]

Thiazide, thiazide-like and loop diuretics (below) all result in initial volume depletion which then stimulates the renin, aldosterone, angiotensin system (RAAS). Sodium depletion can also lead to increased serum aldosterone. In extreme cases, these effects can lead to a decreased antihypertensive effect and in some cases resistant hypertension. Diuretics are more effective when given first in a regimen rather than second, probably because they prime the RAAS.[14] These effects make the addition of a RAAS blocker an attractive combination to improve blood pressure (BP) control.[15,16]

Hydrochlorothiazide (HCTZ) is the most commonly prescribed thiazide diuretic.[17] However, chlorthalidone use has increased in recent years in large part because of its longer duration of action and indirect evidence suggesting it may be superior to HCTZ in reducing morbidity from hypertension.[18,19] Better outcomes with chlorthalidone are plausible as a result of differences in the pharmacokinetic properties of these two agents.[3,20] Chlorthalidone has a much longer duration of action, and is nearly twice as potent as HCTZ (Table 22.1).[3] Chlorthalidone is different from other diuretics because it heavily compartmentalizes into red blood cells by binding to carbonic anhydrase and then slowly "backleaks" into serum.[21] This backleaking leads to an equilibrium between the amount of drug bound to carbonic anhydrase in the red blood cell compartment and the amount of free drug available in the plasma compartment. This theorized depot effect presumably results in a prolonged, low-level diuresis which sustains its antihypertensive action and mitigates the rebound antinatiuretic period occurring when the plasma level of the diuretic falls below the threshold for diuresis.[21,22]

Table 22.1 compares the pharmacokinetics and pharmacodynamics of the most commonly used diuretics. The comparative antihypertensive effects of equivalent doses of chlorthalidone and HCTZ has only recently been examined. Ernst et al. compared 50 mg of HCTZ with 25 mg of chlorthalidone in how each influenced both office and 24-hour ambulatory BP monitoring values. In spite of similar reductions in clinic BP, 24-hour monitoring revealed a significantly lower nighttime BP with chlorthalidone even though the dose of HCTZ was twice that of chlorthalidone.[23] Peterzan et al. performed a meta-analysis and found that the estimated dose of bendroflumethiazide, chlorthalidone, or HCTZ to reduce systolic BP by 10 mm Hg was 1.4, 8.6, and 26.4 mg, respectively, and there was no evidence of a difference in maximum reduction of systolic BP (SBP) by high doses of different thiazides.[24] Potency series for diastolic BP, serum potassium, and urate were similar to those seen for SBP. Their data suggests that chlorthalidone is three times as potent as HCTZ. These and other data also indicate that HCTZ should ideally be given twice daily compared with once daily with chlorthalidone.

Potassium-Sparing Agents

Potassium-sparing agents can be divided into those that antagonize aldosterone (spironolactone and eplerenone) and those independent of aldosterone (amiloride and triamterene). The latter are in the class of epithelial sodium channel blockers.

TABLE 22.1 Pharmacokinetics and Pharmacodynamics of Diuretics

DRUG	PERCENT ABSORBED	ONSET (HOURS)	PEAK (HOURS)	HALF-LIFE (HOURS)	DURATION (HOURS)	EVIDENCE-BASED DOSE[a] (MG/DAY)	NUMBER OF DOSES PER DAY[b]
Thiazide-Like							
Bendroflumethiazide	90-100	2	4	3-4	6-12	10	1
Chlorthalidone	65	2-3	2-6	45-60	48-72	12.5-25	1
Hydrochlorothiazide	65-75	2	4-6	8-15	12-16	25-50	1-2
Indapamide	90	1-2	2	15-20	24-36	1.25	1
Potassium-Sparing							
Amiloride	20	2	6-10	6-9	24	5-10	1
Eplerenone	70	1-2	2	4-6	24	25-50	1
Spironolactone	90	24-48	48-72	48-72	24-36[c]	12.5-50	1
Triamterene	>80	2-4	6-8	3	12-16	100-200	2
Loop							
Bumetanide	72-96	0.5-1	1-2	1-2	4-6	0.5-2	1-2
Furosemide	10-100	0.5-1	6-8	1.5-2	6-8	40-80	2
Torsemide	80	0.5-1	1-2	3.5	6-8	5-10	1-2

(Adapted from refs 3, 7, 23, 25, 31)
[a]Only the thiazide-like agents have been demonstrated to reduce morbidity and mortality.
[b]Daily doses for a sustained antihypertensive effect
[c]For canrenone (active metabolite)

Potassium-sparing agents are not primary monotherapies for hypertension; however, they have been used to counter the potassium wasting effects, and/or the increases in aldosterone following the use of other diuretics. More recently, amiloride and spironolactone have been shown to be highly effective at achieving better blood pressure when combined with other agents for patients with resistant or difficult to control blood pressure.[15,16] This latter effect makes these agents particularly important for the small percentage of patients who cannot achieve BP control despite the use of multiple medications.

All of the agents in this class inhibit sodium absorption in the distal tubule and the collecting duct. With the reduction in sodium/potassium ATPase, potassium secretion is reduced. This effect can lead to hyperkalemia and further limit use in patients with reduced renal function and in some with heart failure.[1] These agents also reduce the excretion of calcium and magnesium.

Spironolactone has two active metabolites, 7α-thiomethylspirolactone and canrenone. These metabolites result in a slow onset of action and a very long half-life. Spironolactone has been shown to cause impressive reductions in SBP (20 to 30 mm Hg) when combined with other agents for patients with resistant or difficult to control blood pressure.[15,16,25-27] This latter effect makes these agents particularly important for the small percentage of patients, including African Americans, who often cannot achieve BP control despite the use of multiple medications.[28] One randomized, crossover study evaluated spironolactone, doxazosin, and bisoprolol in 335 subjects with uncontrolled hypertension despite maximal doses of 3 medications.[29] The average reduction in home SBP by spironolactone was significantly greater than placebo (-8.70 mm Hg [95% confidence interval {CI} -9.72 to -7.69]; $p < 0.0001$), or compared with doxazosin (-4.03 [-5.04 to -3.02]; $p < 0.0001$) or bisoprolol (-4.48 [-5.50 to -3.46]; $p < 0.0001$). Although spironolactone has not been shown to lower morbidity or mortality in hypertension, it did reduce mortality 30% when added to standard therapy for patients with heart failure (HF).[30]

Eplerenone is an mineralocorticoid receptor antagonist with greater selectivity for the aldosterone receptor and less for androgen and progesterone receptors leading to less gynecomastia than with spironolactone.[31] Eplerenone is a weak diuretic but it has antihypertensive effects similar to angiotensin converting-enzyme (ACE)-inhibitors and calcium channel blockers (CCBs).[32,33] Eplerenone has also been shown to be effective for patients with resistant hypertension.[34-36] Eplerenone reduced morbidity and mortality in patients with a recent myocardial infarction (MI) and left ventricular dysfunction or HF, as well as in systolic HF and mild symptoms.[37,38]

Finerenone is another mineralocorticoid receptor antagonist currently being evaluated in clinical trials. It appears to cause less hyperkalemia than spironolactone or eplerenone, especially in patients with chronic kidney disease. One study evaluated finerenone in doses of 7.5, 10, 15, and 20 mg daily in patients with diabetes and high or very high albuminuria.[39] There was a dose-dependent reduction in urine albumin-to-creatinine ratio with finerenone at 90 days compared with baseline with 7.5, 10, 15, and 20 mg per day groups (7.5 mg/day, 0.79 [90% CI, 0.68 to 0.91; $p = 0.004$]; 0.76 [90% CI, 0.65 to 0.88; $p = 0.001$]; 0.67 [90% CI, 0.58 to 0.77; $p < 0.001$]; 0.62 [90% CI, 0.54 to 0.72; $p < 0.001$], respectively). The secondary outcome discontinuation as a result of hyperkalemia was not observed in the placebo and finerenone 10 mg per day groups, whereas the incidences in the finerenone 7.5, 15, and 20 mg per day groups were 2.1%, 3.2%, and 1.7%, respectively. These investigators concluded that the use of finerenone in diabetic patients with nephropathy, many of whom received RAAS-blocking therapy, reduced the urinary albumin-creatinine ratio with minimal risk of hyperkalemia.

Amiloride is actively secreted in the proximal tubule and blocks sodium excretion. Amiloride is cleared extensively by the kidney and accumulates in patients with CKD and can cause hyperkalemia. If amiloride therapy is needed in patients with CKD, the dose should be reduced or the dosing frequency decreased. Amiloride was compared with spironolactone in blacks who still had uncontrolled hypertension despite a diuretic and calcium channel blocker. The addition of these drugs resulted in reductions in systolic and diastolic blood pressures (mm Hg) that were, respectively, 9.8 and 3.4 for amiloride ($p < 0.001$) and 4.6 ($p = 0.006$) and 1.8 for spironolactone ($p = 0.07$).[28] These authors concluded that treatment with either amiloride or spironolactone provided an additional reduction in blood pressure in blacks already receiving conventional antihypertensive therapy. Amiloride alone or in combination with HCTZ was evaluated to determine their effects on serum potassium and glucose.[40] These investigators found that equipotent doses on BP of the combination of amiloride with hydrochlorothiazide prevented glucose intolerance and improved BP control compared with monotherapy with either drug alone.

Triamterene is a weak antihypertensive so it is typically combined with HCTZ to minimize hypokalemia and hypomagnesemia.[41] Triamterene is metabolized to an active metabolite and both accumulate in patients with CKD. Triamterene would rarely be necessary in CKD but if used the dosage should be reduced to prevent hyperkalemia. Triamterene is a potential nephrotoxin, and is associated with formation of crystals, nephrolithiasis, and interstitial nephritis. It can cause acute kidney injury (AKI) when given with other potentially nephrotoxic drugs, such as nonsteroidal antiinflammatory agents, perhaps as a result of increased renal vascular resistance and reduced renal blood flow.[41]

Loop Diuretics

Loop diuretics primarily act on the ascending limb of the loop of Henle to inhibit sodium and chloride reabsorption. Furosemide is historically the most commonly prescribed loop diuretic. However, furosemide has erratic absorption and unpredictable bioavailability.[1,42] Bumetanide and torsemide have more predictable absorption and longer durations of action, and may be preferred over furosemide.[1]

Loop diuretics are not a primary therapy in uncomplicated hypertensive patients and thus do not have the same evidence as thiazides in lowering hypertensive-related morbidity and mortality. Loop diuretics are relatively weak antihypertensive agents.[6] The pharmacologic basis for this lies primarily in their short duration of action; when the blood level falls below the diuretic threshold, it prompts a compensatory period of postdose sodium retention that is a natural response designed to mitigate extracellular fluid loss. Other adaptive responses contribute, but the net result limits their antihypertensive effect. Loop diuretics have an important role in hypertensive patients who have chronic kidney disease and/or accompanying edematous disorders such as heart failure, and nephrotic syndrome. In these situations, thiazides may have more limited antihypertensive efficacy and may result in inadequate diuresis of the underlying edema. In some isolated situations, loops can be considered for use in combination with a thiazide in a therapeutic strategy known as sequential nephron blockade, but the risks of electrolyte imbalances and hypoperfusion necessitate use of these combinations only in rare circumstances.

CLINICAL TRIALS

Previous U.S. guidelines had suggested that diuretics were the preferred drug class for the initial treatment of hypertension.[6] However, the 2014 National Guideline Committee did not feel there was sufficient evidence to suggest that diuretics be preferred and, instead, listed them as one of five preferred drug classes.[7]

Several thiazide-type diuretics and/or other agents in combination with diuretics have been studied as initial therapy (Table 22.2).[43-48] It is interesting to observe that of the trials with neutral or negative results, HCTZ was used,[49-53] whereas those with more favorable outcomes used chlorthalidone.[20,54-58] The HCTZ studies with favorable outcomes typically used doses of 50 mg daily or more and frequently administered HCTZ twice daily. Several of the modern diuretic trials establishing the role of diuretic therapy in hypertension are further discussed later.

An interesting finding was reported by investigators conducting the Multiple Risk Factor Intervention Trial (MRFIT).[20] Patients were randomized to either special intervention (SI) or usual care (UC). The initial therapy for hypertensive patients in the SI group was either HCTZ or chlorthalidone in a dose range of 50 to 100 mg without specification on frequency of dosing. Of note, the choice of diuretic was made locally by the clinic staff. The study followed 8012 men for 6.9 years and found a trend in favor of the SI group compared with the UC group but the difference was not statistically significant.[20] However, 6 years into the trial the investigators observed that in the nine clinics predominantly using HCTZ, the mortality rate was 44% *higher* in the SI group compared with the UC group.[20] The opposite was true in the six clinics that predominantly used chlorthalidone, where mortality in the SI group was more favorable compared with the UC group. As a result, the MRFIT Data Safety Monitoring Board changed the protocol to exclusively use chlorthalidone (daily maximum dose of 50 mg) in the SI group. In the clinics initially using HCTZ, that had a 44% *higher* mortality in the SI group, the trend reversed after the protocol change and they then had a 28% *lower* risk compared with UC at the end of the study (p = 0.04 comparing coronary heart disease [CHD] mortality at the two time periods).

The MRFIT investigators proposed several possible explanations for the finding that mortality was more favorable in the SI group at 10.5 years but not at 6.9 years of follow-up including: a possible time delay in risk reduction that required longer follow-up to observe the effect or, alternatively, that the change in the protocol to switch to chlorthalidone produced the more favorable effect observed toward the end of the trial. Our comparative trial (discussed below) between HCTZ and chlorthalidone showing better 24-hour BP control with chlorthalidone may be one explanation for the MRFIT study findings that has been endorsed by other investigators.[18,23,59]

Several studies have compared thiazide-type diuretics with other drug classes, including ALLHAT, the Second Australian National Blood Pressure Study (ANBP2), and the Avoiding Cardiovascular Events in Combination Therapy in Patients Living with Systolic Hypertension (ACCOMPLISH) trial.[49,53,57] The ALLHAT was a randomized, double-blind, active-controlled antihypertensive treatment trial in 42,418 patients assigned to a chlorthalidone, an ACE-inhibitor (lisinopril), a CCB (amlodipine), or an alpha blocker (doxazosin).[57] The doxazosin arm was terminated early after 3.3 years of follow-up when higher rates of heart failure were observed when compared with chlorthalidone. After an average of 4.9 years of follow-up, chlorthalidone was at least as beneficial as the comparator drugs in lowering BP and preventing cardiovascular (CV) and renal outcomes and was superior for preventing HF (versus each comparator arm), combined CV events (versus α-blocker and ACE-inhibitor arms), and stroke (versus ACE inhibitor [African Americans only] and α-blocker).[57]

The ANBP2 was an open-label trial in 6083 subjects treated with either diuretic-based therapy (primarily HCTZ) or ACE inhibitor (enalapril recommended).[49] Cardiovascular events were lower in the ACE group (relative risk [RR], 0.89; 95% CI, 0.79 to 1.00) but this difference was right at the threshold of statistical significance (p = 0.05). Differences between this study and ALLHAT were that the latter had far more African Americans and 8 times as many CV events compared with ANBP2. Because ANBP2 was an open-label study with agents selected by the individual practitioners, it is not possible to determine if evidence-based doses of HCTZ were used.

The ACCOMPLISH trial included 11,462 high-risk patients and was stopped early after an average of 42 months of follow-up. Amlodipine/benazepril had an RR of 0.8 (95% CI, 0.72 to 0.90; p = 0.0002) for major fatal and nonfatal CV events when compared with HCTZ/benazepril despite nearly identical office BPs. This study has been criticized because the composite

TABLE 22.2 Selected Clinical Trials Using Thiazide-Type Diuretic-Based Therapy

TRIAL (YEAR PUBLISHED)	REGIMEN[a]	POPULATION	OUTCOME
	CLINICAL TRIALS WITH HYDROCHLOROTHIAZIDE-BASED REGIMENS		
Oslo Hypertension Study (1982)[51]	Hydrochlorothiazide (HCTZ) 50 mg/day (36%), HCTZ 50 mg/day + propranolol 320 mg/day (26%), HCTZ 50 mg/day + methyldopa 1000 mg/day (20%), or other drugs (18%) compared with no treatment	Men aged 40-49 years (406 treated and 379 untreated); Blood pressure (BP) (baseline): 156/97 mm Hg; 17/10 mm Hg reduction (systolic blood pressure/diastolic blood pressure [SBP/DBP]) vs. untreated	More noncoronary events in untreated ($p < 0.001$); more coronary events in treated (14) compared with untreated (3). ($p < 0.01$)
European Working Party on High Blood Pressure in the Elderly (EWPHBPE) (1985)[111]	HCTZ 25-50 mg + triamterene 50-100 mg; methyldopa 500-2000 mg could be added, compared with placebo	840 patients over 60 years blood pressure (BP; baseline): 183/101 mm Hg; BP (active treatment): 148/85 mm Hg; BP (placebo): 167/90 mm Hg	Cardiovascular (CV) mortality reduced 27% ($p = 0.037$), cardiac mortality 38% ($p = 0.036$) in active treatment group; no change in total mortality ($p = 0.41$)
Medical Research Council (MRC) (1992)[50]	HCTZ 25-50 mg + amiloride 2.5-5 mg vs. atenolol 50 mg vs. placebo	4396 patients 65-74 years BP (baseline): 185/91 mm Hg; BP (diuretic): 150/78 mm Hg; BP (atenolol): 152/78 mm Hg	31% fewer strokes ($p = 0.04$) in HCTZ group, 44% fewer coronary events ($p = 0.0009$), and 35% fewer CV events ($p = 0.0005$) compared with placebo. No significant reductions in outcomes for atenolol group.
Multicenter Isradipine Diuretic Atherosclerosis Study (MIDAS) (1996)[112]	HCTZ 12.5-25 mg BID vs. Isradipine 2.5-5 mg two times daily; open label enalapril could be added	883 patients; mean age = 58 years. BP with HCTZ decreased from 149/96 mm Hg to 130/82 mm Hg; BP with isradipine decreased from 151/97 mm Hg to 135/84 mm Hg	Fewer major vascular events (3.2% vs. 5.7%, $p = 0.07$) and fewer nonmajor vascular events (5.2% vs. 9.1%, $p = 0.02$) with HCTZ than isradipine
International Nifedipine GITS Study (INSIGHT) (2000)[88]	HCTZ 25-50 mg + amiloride 50-100 mg vs. nifedipine GITS 30-60 mg and atenolol or enalapril could be added	6321 patients aged 55-80 years; similar BP decline in both groups from 173/99 mm Hg to 138/82 mm Hg	No difference overall in combined (primary and secondary) endpoints. However, there were more fatal myocardial infarctions (16 vs. 5, odds ratio [OR] 3.2, $p = 0.017$) and nonfatal heart failure (24 vs. 11, OR 2.2, $p = 0.028$) with nifedipine compared with the diuretic.
Second Australian National Blood Pressure Study (ANBP-2) (2003)[49]	Randomized to either HCTZ or enalapril (doses were adjusted by family practitioner and not reported)	6083 patients aged 65 to 84 years: BP (baseline) 168/91 mm Hg; BP (HCTZ): 144/81 mm Hg; BP (enalapril): 145/81 mm Hg	Significantly fewer CV events or deaths in enalapril group compared with HCTZ (hazard ratio [HR] = 0.89, $p = 0.05$).
Avoiding Cardiovascular Events through Combination Therapy in Patients Living with Systolic Hypertension (ACCOMPLISH) (2008)[53]	Randomized to amlodipine 5-10 mg + benazepril 20-40 mg or benazepril 20-40 mg + HCTZ 12.5-25 mg	11,462 patients ≥ 55 years: SBP ≥ 160 mm Hg	Relative risk (RR) 0.8 (0.72-0.90) for composite of CV mortality/morbidity for amlodipine-benazepril group vs. benazepril-HCTZ group ($p = 0.0002$)
Trials With Chlorthalidone-Based Regimens			
Hypertension Detection and Follow-up Program (HDFP) (1979)[54]	Stepped care (SC) using chlorthalidone as Step 1 compared with regular care (RC) consisting of multiple regimens and doses	10,940 patients age 30-69 years; BP (baseline): 159/101 mm Hg; reported DBP only: RC 89 mm Hg; SC 84 mm Hg	17% lower mortality in SC than RC groups ($p < 0.01$). Total stroke was lower in the SC than RC groups ($p < 0.01$).
Multiple Risk Factor Intervention Trial (MRFIT) (1990)[20]	Randomized to special intervention (SI) or usual care (UC). Step 1 included either HCTZ or chlorthalidone (50-100 mg daily). Mid-study protocol changed HCTZ to chlorthalidone.	8012 hypertensive men; BP (baseline): 141/91 mm Hg; BP (UC group): 130/86 mm Hg; BP (SI group): 122/81 mm Hg	Mortality reduced 36% ($p = 0.07$) and coronary heart disease (CHD) reduced 50% ($p = 0.0001$) in SI group vs. UC. Early mortality was 44% higher in SI clinics using HCTZ vs. UC but was 28% lower following a change from HCTZ to chlorthalidone ($p = 0.04$ comparing the two time periods)
Systolic Hypertension in the Elderly (SHEP) (1991)[56]	Randomized to chlorthalidone 12.5-25 mg and could add atenolol 25 mg or reserpine 0.05 mg vs. placebo	4736 patients, mean age 72 years; BP (baseline): 170/76 mm Hg; BP (chlorthalidone): 144/68 mm Hg; BP (placebo): 155/71 mm Hg	Significant reduction in stroke for chlorthalidone compared with placebo (RR = 0.64, $p = 0.0003$); 32% fewer combined nonfatal and fatal CV events in chlorthalidone group. Heart failure reduced 54% in chlorthalidone group compared with placebo.

Study	Regimen	Patient Characteristics/BP	Results
Verapamil in Hypertension and Atherosclerosis Study (VHAS)[113]	Chlorthalidone 25 mg (707 patients) vs. verapamil slow release 240 mg daily (707 patients) Captopril 25 mg daily could be added to either regimen	1414 patients mean age 53.9 years; BP (baseline): 169/102 mm Hg; BP reduced by −29/17 mm Hg (chlorthalidone) and −28/17 mm Hg (verapamil)	After 2 years of follow-up; no difference in fatal plus nonfatal events 43 vs. 42.
Treatment of Mild Hypertension Study (TOMHS) (1998)[114]	Randomized to chlorthalidone 15-30 mg/day (136 patients), acebutolol 400 mg/day (132 patients), doxazosin 1-2 mg/day (134 patients), amlodipine 5 mg/day (131 patients), or enalapril 5 mg/day (135 patients) vs. placebo; chlorthalidone could be added to placebo if nutritional-hygienic intervention did not control BP	Men and women 45 to 69 years of age; BP (baseline): 140/91 mm Hg; largest reduction in systolic BP in chlorthalidone group (−17.7 mm Hg)	Rate of all clinical events was 11.1% in combined active treatments vs. 16.2% for placebo (p = 0.03); no consistent differences among active treatments for LV mass, lipid levels, or other outcomes
Antihypertensive and Lipid-lowering Treatment to Prevent Heart Attack Trial (ALLHAT) (2002)[57]	Randomized to chlorthalidone 12.5-25 mg, lisinopril 10-40 mg, amlodipine 2.5-10 mg, or doxazosin 2-8 mg	42,424 patients over 55 years; BP (baseline): 146/84 mm Hg; BP (chlorthalidone): 134/75 mm Hg; BP (amlodipine) 135/75 mm Hg; BP (lisinopril) 136/75 mm Hg	Doxazosin arm discontinued because of significantly higher stroke (p = 0.04), heart failure (p = <0.001), or combined CVD (p < 0.001) compared with chlorthalidone. No differences in primary outcome for lisinopril or amlodipine compared with chlorthalidone. Higher risk of heart failure with amlodipine (RR = 1.38) or lisinopril (RR = 1.19) compared with chlorthalidone. Combined CVD (RR = 1.10) and stroke (RR = 1.15) were higher with lisinopril than chlorthalidone.
Treatment of Isolated Systolic Hypertension (SHELL) (2003)[115]	Chlorthalidone 12.5-25 mg vs. lacidipine 4-6 mg daily. Fosinopril 10 mg daily or other ACE inhibitor could be added.	1882 subjects, mean age 72 years and baseline BP 178/87 mm Hg; BP after 32 months was reduced −37/8 mm Hg with chlorthalidone vs. −38/8 mm Hg with lacidipine	Composite primary endpoint hazard ratio (HR) = 1.01 (0.75-1.36, p = 0.94). All-cause mortality 122 chlorthalidone vs. 145 lacidipine HR = 1.23 (0.97-1.57, p = 0.09).

Clinical Trial With Indapamide-Based Regimen

Hypertension in the Very Elderly Trial (HYVET) (2008)[60]	Indapamide sustained release 1.5 mg could add perindopril 2-4 mg vs. placebo	3845 subjects age ≥80 years (mean 83.5 years) with SBP >160 mm Hg and DBP 90-110 mm Hg	Fatal or nonfatal CV events 33.7/1000 person years for indapamide versus 50.6 for indapamide (p < 0.01, HR 0.66 [0.53-0.82])

Clinical Trials With Bendroflumethiazide-Based Regimens

Metoprolol Atherosclerosis Prevention in Hypertensives (MAPHY) (1988)[52]	Metoprolol vs. HCTZ 50 mg daily or bendroflumethiazide 5 mg daily	1609 men aged 40-64 years BP (baseline): 167/107; BP (treatment): 142/89	Metoprolol treated subjects had significantly lower CV mortality (p = 0.012), CHD mortality (p = 0.048), stroke mortality (p = 0.043), or total mortality (p = 0.28) compared with diuretics
Medical Research Council (MRC) trial (1985)[116]	Bendroflumethiazide 10 mg vs. propranolol 240 mg daily or vs. placebo	17,354 subjects, mean age 35-64 years with SBP < 200 mm Hg and DBP < 90 mm Hg	No difference between drugs in combined CV events, coronary events and mortality.

a Starting and end-titration dose range given for diuretic used.

(Adapted from Carter and Carter BL, Sica DA. Strategies to improve the cardiovascular risk profile of thiazide-type diuretics as used in the management of hypertension. Expert Opin Drug Saf. 2007;6:583-594; Ernst ME, Grimm RH Jr. Thiazide diuretics: 50 years and beyond. Curr Hypertens Rev. 2008;4:256-265.)

endpoint did not include HF, which is a critical hypertension endpoint found to be reduced by 505 to 68% in diuretic-based regimens.[56,57,60] There are other design features that may help explain differences between ALLHAT and ACCOMPLISH trials. First, benazepril does not have consistent 24-hour BP coverage.[61] Because both ACCOMPLISH arms included benazepril, the comparison is essentially between HCTZ and amlodipine. The study used HCTZ in suboptimal doses of only 12.5 to 25 mg once daily, which at best has only an 8- to 15-hour duration of action.[7] As displayed in Table 22.2 and recommended by national guidelines, the HCTZ dose should be twice as high and perhaps given twice daily. Amlodipine is one of the longest acting antihypertensives with a half-life of 38 to 50 hours and provides definitive 24-hour coverage.[61] One explanation is that HCTZ did not provide sufficient 24-hour BP coverage. However, the ACCOMPLISH investigators subsequently reported that in a subset of subjects who received 24-hour BP monitoring, the BP values were similar in the two arms.[62]

An indapamide-based regimen has been shown to lower hypertension-related mortality. The Hypertension in the Very Elderly Trial (HYVET) was a randomized, double-blind, placebo-controlled study that compared sustained release indapamide (1.5 mg) with or without perindopril (2 to 4 mg) to placebo in 3845 patients over the age of 80 years.[60] The target BP was less than 150/80 mm Hg and at 21 years there was a 21% reduction in all-cause death (95% CI, 4 to 35; $p = 0.02$), a 39% reduction in fatal stroke (95% CI, 1 to 62; $p = 0.05$), a 64% reduction in fatal and nonfatal HF (95% CI, 42 to 78; $p < 0.001$), and a 34% reduction in any CV event (95% CI, 18 to 47; $p < 0.001$). The use of long-acting compounds (sustained-release indapamide and perindopril) would suggest that nighttime BP may have been effectively reduced and led to such positive outcomes.

These and other studies suggest that diuretics are particularly effective in the elderly and African-American patients. For these reasons, it is often necessary to add a thiazide-type diuretic, or loop agent in the presence of moderate CKD, to achieve good BP control in these populations.

The studies described above led the members of the 2014 national BP guideline committee to conclude that the scientific evidence suggests that thiazide-type diuretics, ACE inhibitors, and CCBs are equally effective as initial therapy.[7] There is also insufficient evidence to suggest chlorthalidone is different from HCTZ on critical CV endpoints. However, when all of the diuretic-based outcome trials are examined, those that used chlorthalidone have all been significantly different from placebo or other therapy.[3,18,61] Studies that used HCTZ have had mixed results, with approximately half finding benefit and half finding either no benefit or inferior results to other drug therapy. For these reasons, we and other experts believe that chlorthalidone is the preferred thiazide diuretic.[21] If HCTZ is used, it should be given twice daily. The only time when HCTZ once daily can be justified is within a combination regimen that clearly has 24-hour BP coverage, ideally demonstrated by ambulatory BP monitoring in each specific patient.

Loop diuretics and potassium-sparing agents have not been studied to evaluate their effects on morbidity or mortality. Therefore, loop diuretics should not be selected unless renal function is so poor, or edema so significant, that thiazide-type diuretics are ineffective. Potassium-sparing agents should not be used alone and would generally be reserved for cases where they can be combined with a thiazide-type diuretic.

PLACE OF DIURETICS IN MULTIDRUG THERAPY

The most recent antihypertensive guidelines indicated that thiazide-type diuretics did not provide unique benefits concerning morbidity or mortality when compared with ACE inhibitors, ARBs, or CCBs.[7] Therefore, there is no compelling reason that a diuretic needs to be the initial agent used for hypertension. However, it is clear that hypertension is much more difficult to control if a diuretic, especially a thiazide-type agent, is not in the regimen. Therefore, it is generally advisable that a thiazide-type diuretic be the first or second drug in a multidrug regimen. There is, however, evidence that initiating therapy with HCTZ with subsequently adding atenolol resulted in a 3 to 4 mm Hg greater reduction in SBP than starting with atenolol perhaps because of a priming effect of HCTZ on the RAAS.[14] Although this BP difference may be modest, it could lead to better controlled BP in many patients.

DIURETIC DOSING

The comparative antihypertensive effects of "equivalent" doses of chlorthalidone and HCTZ have only recently been examined. Ernst et al. compared 50 mg of HCTZ with 25 mg of chlorthalidone in how each influenced both office and 24-hour ambulatory BP monitoring values. In spite of similar reductions in clinic BP, 24-hour monitoring revealed a significantly lower nighttime BP with chlorthalidone at half the dose of hydrochlorothiazide.[23] Monotherapy with chlorthalidone is more effective than HCTZ, especially at lowering BP throughout the entire 24-hour treatment interval. These data do not imply that HCTZ is a poor antihypertensive per se or that it is necessarily inferior to chlorthalidone when used in an appropriate combination regimen. However, outcome studies that favored HCTZ-based therapy over nondiuretic agents used higher doses and often used the drug twice daily. Therefore, doses of chlorthalidone should be 12.5 to 25 mg *once daily* whereas the appropriate evidence-based dose for hydrochlorothiazide to achieve similar BP control is likely 12.5 to 25 mg *twice daily*. These are significant differences in dosage that must be considered before appropriate interpretations of the clinical trials comparing thiazides with other classes can be made. At equivalent doses, the metabolic effects, especially hypokalemia, are similar between these two diuretics.[23,24,63,64] However, the more widespread availability of antihypertensive combinations that include HCTZ makes it difficult to use chlorthalidone unless individual agents are selected.

Loop diuretics have not been studied to evaluate their ability to reduce morbidity and mortality so they should be reserved for patients who cannot take thiazide-type diuretics. Table 22.1 displays typical doses for these agents. Furosemide is short-acting, and when used for hypertension it should be prescribed twice daily for a more sustained antihypertensive effect and minimize the postdose antinatriuretic period. Bumetanide and torsemide are labeled for once daily dosing but the half-life of both suggests that twice daily dosing may be necessary to achieve a sustained antihypertensive effect. Additionally, torsemide has an aldosterone reducing effect which causes less kaliuresis than other diuretics and may be beneficial in heart failure but there are no randomized trials to confirm these potential benefits in humans.[65]

Potassium-sparing agents are typically dosed in combination with thiazide diuretics to mitigate potassium and magnesium excretion and not for their antihypertensive efficacy. They are rarely used as monotherapies and their dosing is regulated through the specific combination tablet they are contained within (e.g., triamterene/HCTZ 12.5/25 mg). Newer research has discovered the role of low doses of aldosterone antagonists such as spironolactone as add-on therapy in patients with resistant hypertension. For resistant hypertension, the initial dose should be 12.5 to 25 mg once daily with a maximum of 50 mg daily.[15,16] One study used doses up to 100 mg daily but those doses may cause more hyperkalemia and gynecomastia.[16]

Eplerenone is another aldosterone antagonist that has more selectivity for aldosterone receptors and less affinity for androgen and progestin receptors than spironolactone.[31] Given the traditional cost differences between the two agents, it is unclear whether the safety and efficacy profile of eplerenone constitute clinically significant advancements over spironolactone.

ADVERSE EFFECTS OF DIURETICS

Hypokalemia and Hyperkalemia

Hypokalemia is a common, dose-related effect of thiazide and loop diuretics and is usually defined as a serum potassium below 3.5 mEq/L. Serum potassium reaches a nadir within 3 to 5 days of initiation of therapy and averages about 0.4 mEq/L with doses equivalent to HCTZ 25 mg daily. It was commonly believed that chlorthalidone causes more hypokalemia than HCTZ. A meta-analysis of 137 studies using 12.5 to 25 mg of these two drugs found a reduction of 0.36 mEq/L for HCTZ and 0.45 mEq/L with chlorthalidone.[64] However, studies with chlorthalidone had a greater reduction in BP, so at equipotent doses, the reductions in serum potassium were similar. Reductions with furosemide are less (0.3 mEq/L) but it is not as effective in lowering BP compared with thiazide-like diuretics.[24,66]

Hypokalemia can be prolonged or more difficult to reverse in the face of a high sodium diet, metabolic alkalosis or hyperaldosteronism. In contrast, hypokalemia can be reversed or minimized when patients restrict excess sodium, and/or are treated with potassium supplements, potassium sparing diuretics, or ACE inhibitors.[67,68]

There are conflicting data regarding adverse cardiac effects of diuretic-induced hypokalemia, in part, related to the difficulty extrapolating cellular potassium from serum potassium levels. There are also questions about the relative contributions of hypokalemia versus hypomagnesemia to these adverse events.[69,70] Various studies have found increased ventricular ectopy[71] or increased ventricular fibrillation in acute MI when patients have hypokalemia on admission.[72] The risk of CV events following diuretic-induced hypokalemia is more common in patients with left ventricular hypertrophy, HF, or myocardial ischemia.[66,73] Mortality was increased in patients with HF and low serum potassium and magnesium.[70] Data from the Systolic Hypertension in Elderly (SHEP) trial found that although CV events were reduced with diuretic therapy compared with placebo, those who develop hypokalemia did not receive such benefit.[74]

The risk of CV events is dose related and much more common with HCTZ or chlorthalidone doses from 25 to 100 mg daily.[75] The fact that higher doses of thiazide-type diuretics were used in the past likely minimized the benefit of these drugs on CV events. Using evidence-based doses should optimize the benefit to risk with these agents, and the historical concern about diuretics increasing the risk for CV events has now been largely dismissed (Table 22.1).

In addition to concerns about CV events, use of potassium supplementation to reverse hypokalemia can also improve BP by reducing mean arterial pressure by 5.5 mm Hg.[67] Maintaining serum potassium has also been reported to minimize diuretic-induced hyperglycemia (see below).[76] Maintain serum potassium above 3.5 mEq/L and perhaps closer to 4.0 mEq/L, which can be done with potassium supplementation or with the combination of thiazide-type diuretic with potassium sparing diuretic. The risk of cardiac arrest among patients receiving combined thiazide and K+-sparing diuretic therapy was lower than a thiazide alone, with the risk of an event increasing significantly as the dose of HCTZ increased from 25 to 100 mg/day.[75] However, potassium sparing diuretics can cause significant hyperkalemia, especially in elderly patients and/or those with reduced GFR; concomitant therapy with potassium supplements, ACE inhibitors, ARBs, nonsteroidal antiinflammatory drugs (NSAIDs), or heparin; or conditions such as metabolic acidosis or hyporeninemic hypoaldosteronism.[77]

Hyponatremia

Hyponatremia is more common with thiazide-type diuretics than with loop diuretics.[78] Although this adverse event is uncommon, it can be serious.[78,79] Diuretic-induced hyponatremia can develop acutely or gradually.[78] It is more common in elderly women, but other risk factors include dehydration, low sodium intake, or diminished ability to excrete free water.

Treatment for mild, asymptomatic diuretic-induced hyponatremia (typically 125 to 135 mEq/L) can be accomplished by: restricting water intake, restoring K+ losses if present, withholding diuretics, or converting thiazide to loop diuretic therapy.[80] Symptomatic hyponatremia (typically <125 mEq/L) calls for intensive therapy but it should not be corrected rapidly because of an increased risk for osmotic demyelinating syndrome. Hyponatremia complicated by seizures or other neurologic sequelae is a medical emergency. The risks of ongoing hyponatremia must be weighed against those of too rapid a correction. Serum sodium should not to be corrected by more than 0.5 mEq/L/hour during the first 24 hours. Treatment should be slowed or discontinued once a serum sodium of approximately 125 to 130 mEq/L has been attained. Hyponatremia that has occurred for more than several days can be treated less aggressively. Selective vasopressin-2 receptor antagonists (e.g., tolvaptan) have been used for hyponatremia in patients with heart failure or volume overload but the use in diuretic-induced hyponatremia is not recommended.[81]

Hypomagnesemia

Therapy with thiazide or loop diuretics typically decreases plasma magnesium concentration by 5% to 10%, but reductions can be more severe in some patients. Up to 50% of patients have cellular magnesium depletion regardless of normal serum concentrations. Hypomagnesemia occurs more often in the elderly, and in those receiving continuous high-dose diuretic therapy (such as HF patients) which may increase mortality.[70,82] Hypomagnesemia often occurs with hypokalemia, hyponatremia, and/or hypocalcemia. Although potassium-sparing diuretics can diminish the magnesuria that accompanies thiazide and/or loop diuretic use, they cannot fully correct serum sodium or calcium unless the underlying magnesium deficit is corrected.[83]

Hypomagnesemia can also be suspected from characteristic electrocardiogram that can include a prolongation of the QT and/or PR intervals, widening of the QRS complex, ST-segment depression, low amplitude T-waves, supraventricular arrhythmias, or ventricular tachyarrhythmias. Hypomagnesemia may cause nonspecific mental status changes and/or neuromuscular irritability. Tetany is a classic manifestation of magnesium deficiency but it is uncommon. Less specific signs such as tremor, muscle twitching, peculiar limb movements, focal seizures, generalized convulsions, delirium, or coma are observed more often.[83]

Serum magnesium is not routinely monitored but should definitely be considered in patients with hypokalemia. Diuretic-related hypomagnesemia should be treated because correction may reduce BP, prevent arrhythmias, and/or prevent or resolve coexisting electrolyte or neuromuscular symptoms. In mild deficiency states, magnesium balance can often be reestablished by limiting contributing factors (decreasing diuretic dose and/or sodium intake) and letting dietary magnesium correct the deficit.

Parenteral magnesium is the most efficient way to correct hypomagnesemia and is preferred in urgent settings. Total body magnesium deficits are typically in the order of 1 to 2 mEq/kg body weight in patients with magnesium depletion. Typical treatment involves giving 2 grams of magnesium sulfate (16.3 mEq) intravenously over 30 minutes, followed by a constant infusion providing between 32 and 64 mEq/day until the estimated deficit is corrected.

A variety of magnesium preparations are available orally. Magnesium oxide is not very water-soluble and has a significant cathartic effect; thus, it has an unpredictable influence on magnesium concentrations. Magnesium gluconate is the preferred oral preparation because this salt is water-soluble and causes minimal diarrhea. Magnesium carbonate has low water-solubility and is not as effective as the gluconate in correcting hypomagnesemia. Oral magnesium is not recommended in urgent situations. The intramuscular route is painful and should only be used when intravenous access is not readily available.[83]

Hyperuricemia

Thiazide-type diuretics use the same anion transporter as urate. They reduce renal urate clearance attributed to increased tubular reabsorption following extracellular fluid depletion and competition for tubular secretion. Serum uric acid increased from a baseline of 5.5 mg/dL at baseline to 6.8 mg/dL after six weeks of treatment with HCTZ 25 mg.[84] The Verapamil in Hypertension and Atherosclerosis Study (VHAS) found that 10.8% of subjects developed hyperuricemia with chlorthalidone 25 mg daily compared with 3.9% with verapamil ($p < 0.01$).[85] Because this is a dose-related effect, higher doses have increased serum uric acid by even more but gout is not usually precipitated unless the patient has a tendency to gout. Diuretics increased serum urate levels from 6.3 to 7.1 mg/dL and the hazard ratio for gout was 1.44 in a population-based study in adults with hypertension.[86]

The HAPPY (Heart Attack Primary Prevention in Hypertension) trial found 3.6% of subjects who received the diuretic developed gout compared with 3.0% with the beta-blocker ($p > 0.2$).[87] In the Medical Research Council (MRC) trial (Table 22.2), there were significantly more withdrawals for gout (2.6%) compared with the beta-blocker (0.3%) or placebo (0.16%) ($p < 0.001$). Gout occurred in 2.1% of diuretic-treated compared with 1.3% taking nifedipine in the INSIGHT (Intervention as a Goal in Hypertension Treatment) trial (Table 22.2).[88]

Although diuretic use is a risk factor for incident gout, their use in patients with a history of gout is not an absolute contraindication. Likewise, the patient with hypertension treated with a diuretic who has a gout attack does not necessarily have to discontinue the diuretic or avoid future use. The decision about continuing a diuretic really depends on the severity (and frequency, if recurrent) of the gout attack, the level of uric acid following resolution, and the degree of difficulty obtaining BP control.[89] Lifestyle modifications should always be employed because hypertension and gout are overlapping diseases.

METABOLIC ABNORMALITIES

Hyperglycemia

Clinical trials and observational studies have found undesirable metabolic biochemical effects during diuretic treatment compared with other drugs, including hyperglycemia.[76,90-95] Diuretic-induced increases in serum glucose levels are small (3 to 4 mg/dL) compared with other therapies and may attenuate over time. In ALLHAT, the odds ratio for developing new-onset diabetes at 2 years was lower with lisinopril (0.55 [CI, 0.43 to 0.70]) or amlodipine (0.73 [CI, 0.58 to 0.91]) when compared with chlorthalidone ($p < 0.01$).[96] However, by 6 years the odds ratios for lisinopril was 0.86 (0.40 to 1.86) and for amlodipine was 0.96 (0.58 to 1.90) compared with chlorthalidone but these differences were no longer significant. Additionally, diuretic-based therapy still afforded similar or superior CV benefits compared with lisinopril or amlodipine, even in patients with diabetes.[97-99]

Risk factors for hyperglycemia and new-onset diabetes mellitus with thiazides include baseline glucose, abdominal obesity, hypokalemia, and pretherapy glucose and triglyceride values.[84,100] Interestingly, the relationship between thiazide-induced hyperglycemia and hypokalemia has been well described since the 1950s.[76,101]

A systematic analysis of the literature found a significant correlation between the degree of hypokalemia and increases in serum glucose.[76] Of interest, the mean reduction of serum potassium in study arms that did not add potassium supplements was -0.37 mEq/L with an increase in plasma glucose of 6.01 mg/dL. However, in study arms that did provide potassium supplements, the mean reduction in serum potassium was -0.23 mEq/L with a resulting increase in plasma glucose of only 3.26 mg/dL. These authors concluded that there is a clear and significant association between serum potassium and diuretic-induced hyperglycemia. They recommended that serum potassium be maintained at approximately 4.0 mEq/L. This analysis resulted in a working group from the National Heart, Lung, and Blood Institute to recommend additional research into these and other mechanisms for thiazide-induced hyperglycemia.[95] The likely mechanism for this association is that potassium is essential for beta cell secretion of insulin. An analysis of SHEP data found that during year 1 of the study but not later, each 0.5-mEq/L decrease in serum potassium was independently associated with a 45% higher adjusted diabetes risk (95% CI: 24% to 70%; $p < 0.001$).[102] However, a smaller study was unable to find an association between thiazide-induced hypokalemia and the development of hyperglycemia.[103]

Because patients with diabetes still receive CV benefit, it is important to continue thiazide-type diuretics even if diabetes develops. Potassium supplementation or the use of potassium-sparing agents may, but not always, modify the effect on glucose. Although evidence-based doses of thiazides should be used (Table 22.1), reductions in the dose may improve glucose homeostasis.

Hyperlipidemia

Thiazide-type and loop diuretics all cause a dose-dependent increase in total cholesterol, low density lipoprotein (LDL) cholesterol, and triglycerides.[104,105] An analysis of 474 clinical trials in over 65,000 participants found that diuretics increased cholesterol levels only 0.13 mmol/L, were greater at higher doses, 0.25 mmol/L, and that African Americans had a cholesterol that was 0.13 mmol/L greater than non-African Americans.[106]

Total and LDL cholesterol were reduced in all the drug classes in TOMHS (Treatment of Mild Hypertension Study), but the reduction was not as great with chlorthalidone compared with the other agents.[104] In addition, the effect at 1 year was no longer present at 4 years. Weight loss with a low fat diet and increased exercise reversed any deleterious effect from the diuretic.

Therefore, the effect on lipids is relatively small especially when current lower evidence-based doses are used. The effect of diuretics on lipids can be overcome with weight loss and exercise, and the high prevalence of statin background therapy in hypertensive patients makes this a relatively inconsequential effect.

Other Adverse Effects

Impotence

Many men refuse to take diuretics or discontinue them because of impotence that includes erectile dysfunction and difficulty ejaculating. However, this problem is more common with hypertension, especially as blood pressure is reduced and in those with diabetes. Even so, the MRC trial found men reported study withdrawal because of impotence much more often with the diuretic (2%), compared with the beta-blocker (1%) or placebo (0.02%).[50]

Problems with sexual interest, erection, and orgasm in TOMHS were greater among men receiving chlorthalidone, compared with those given placebo or atenolol.[107] Weight loss improved chlorthalidone-induced sexual dysfunction and the significant early increase in sexual dysfunction with chlorthalidone (compared with other drugs) was not present at 4 years.

The mechanism for impotence with thiazides is unclear, but these drugs may have a direct effect on vascular smooth muscle cells and/or decrease the response to catecholamines. Patients with diuretic-related impotence can respond favorably to sildenafil without an associated additional increase in BP.

Impotence and decreased libido are more frequent with spironolactone. Gynecomastia, another fairly frequent complication of spironolactone therapy, is typically bilateral and may be associated with mastodynia. The sexual side effects of spironolactone have been attributed to its inhibiting the binding of dihydrotestosterone to androgen receptors, thus leading to an increased clearance of testosterone. Eplerenone is more selective than spironolactone and may be less likely to produce these sexual side effects.[31]

Drug Allergy

Thiazides and furosemide may cause photosensitivity dermatitis which is more common with HCTZ but these findings may simply be because they are the most commonly used agents. Diuretics may occasionally cause a more serious generalized dermatitis or necrotizing vasculitis. A small degree of cross-sensitivity exists with diuretics and other sulfonamide-based drugs, but the increased risk appears primarily the result of the patient's underlying propensity for atopy rather than a specific chemical cross-reactivity.[108]

In cases of significant concern (e.g., previous sulfa reaction resulted in laryngeal edema, or anaphylaxis) patients can receive ethacrynic acid. Severe necrotizing pancreatitis is a rare, life-threatening complication of thiazide therapy. Acute allergic interstitial nephritis with fever, rash, and eosinophilia may also occur. The latter adverse effect is insidious and may result in permanent renal failure if the drug is not discontinued.

ADVERSE DRUG INTERACTIONS

The types of drug interactions with diuretics was previously reviewed.[109] A beneficial interaction is the combination of a loop diuretic with a thiazide-type diuretic, especially metolazone, when insufficient diuresis occurs with a loop agent alone. However, this can result in a profound and extensive diuresis and must be monitored carefully to avoid serious electrolyte disturbances and the potential to critically reduce perfusion to vital organs. Diuretics and bile acid sequestrant administration should be separated by several hours to avoid binding of the diuretic. NSAIDs can antagonize the effects of diuretics and predispose diuretic-treated patients to a generally reversible form of renal failure. Acetaminophen or salsalate can be used instead. Plasma lithium concentrations can increase substantially with thiazide therapy as a result of the associated increase in the tubular reabsorption of lithium that is handled similarly to sodium. However, some diuretics with significant carbonic anhydrase inhibitory activity (e.g., thiazides, chlorthalidone, furosemide) can increase lithium clearance, thus leading to a decrease in blood levels. Whole-blood lithium levels should be closely monitored in patients receiving lithium and diuretics.

Loop diuretics (particularly high-dose) can cause ototoxicity, and can potentiate aminoglycoside nephrotoxicity. Diuretics increase the risk of digitalis toxicity if hypokalemia develops. Because triamterene may cause nephrotoxicity, it should be used cautiously, if at all, with nonsteroidal antiinflammatory drugs, which may increase adverse effects on the kidney.

PRACTICAL CONSIDERATIONS

In primary or uncomplicated hypertension, the two diuretic agents with the most evidence are HCTZ and chlorthalidone. Based on its favorable pharmacokinetic profile, and long history of success in clinical trials, we suggest chlorthalidone as a preferred option because it achieves better 24-hour BP control with no increase in hypokalemia when compared with equivalent doses of HCTZ.[23] A low dose should be selected initially (chlorthalidone 6.25 to 12.5 mg *once daily* or HCTZ 12.5 mg *twice daily*) and then increased to chlorthalidone 25 mg *once daily*. This dosing with chlorthalidone can be challenging because 25 mg is the lowest strength commercially available. When we conducted our trial using 12.5 mg chlorthalidone, one of us (MEE) used a tablet splitter to carefully cut the 25-mg tablets in half, which can be done fairly accurately.[23] Tablet splitting can be a challenge for some patients but a family member or some pharmacies will do this if requested. Not many patients will require a dose of 6.25 mg daily but this might be needed as an initial, temporary dose in some elderly subjects before a dose escalation. To achieve a daily dose of 6.25 mg, we recommend every other day dosing of one-half of a 25-mg tablet, which is feasible because of the extremely long half-life of chlorthalidone.

If HCTZ is used, the optimal dose would be 25 mg *twice daily* if it is used as monotherapy. HCTZ once daily is best used in combination with other drugs with 24-hour durations of action. Indapamide 1.25 to 2.5 mg once daily is also an acceptable option based on the impressive results in HYVET.[60]

Patients should be counseled to adhere to a low salt, high potassium diet. Potassium supplements or potassium-sparing diuretics should be added if baseline serum potassium values are below 4.0 mmol/L. With hypokalemia or uncontrolled hypertension, either amiloride or low-dose spironolactone should be added as they are very effective in patients with resistant hypertension and to increase serum potassium.[15,28,95] An antihypertensive regimen can be designed to minimize hypokalemia with addition of an ACE inhibitor.[68,110]

SUMMARY

Thiazide-type diuretics are one of the most important antihypertensive classes and are a foundational piece of most successful antihypertensive drug regimens. Thiazide diuretics are one of the preferred antihypertensive classes for therapy of hypertension according to treatment guidelines. If they are not the initial agent, they should clearly be added when BP is difficult to control because they provide synergy in lowering blood pressure to nearly all other antihypertensive classes. Careful attention to dosing and individual patient characteristics can ensure that adverse effects remain minimal and easily manageable.

References

1. Sica DA, Carter B, Cushman W, Hamm L. Thiazide and loop diuretics. *J Clin Hypertens (Greenwich)*. 2011;13:639-643.
2. Ernst ME, Moser M. Use of diuretics in patients with hypertension. *N Engl J Med*. 2009;361:2153-2164.
3. Carter BL, Ernst ME, Cohen JD. Hydrochlorothiazide versus chlorthalidone: evidence supporting their interchangeability. *Hypertension*. 2004;43:4-9.
4. Cutler JA, Davis BR. Thiazide-type diuretics and beta-adrenergic blockers as first-line drug treatments for hypertension. *Circulation*. 2008;117:2691-2704; discussion 2705.
5. Messerli FH, Bangalore S, Julius S. Risk/benefit assessment of beta-blockers and diuretics precludes their use for first-line therapy in hypertension. *Circulation*. 2008;117:2706-2715; discussion 2715.
6. Chobanian AV, Bakris GL, Black HR, et al. Seventh report of the Joint National Committee on prevention, detection, evaluation, and treatment of high blood pressure. *Hypertension*. 2003;42(6):1206-1252.
7. James PA, Oparil S, Carter BL, et al. 2014 evidence-based guideline for the management of high blood pressure in adults: report from the panel members appointed to the Eighth Joint National Committee (JNC 8). *JAMA*. 2014;311:507-520.

8. Dussol B, Moussi-Frances J, Morange S, Somma-Delpero C, Mundler O, Berland Y. A randomized trial of furosemide vs hydrochlorothiazide in patients with chronic renal failure and hypertension. *Nephrol Dial Transplant*. 2005;20:349-353.

9. Dussol B, Moussi-Frances J, Morange S, Somma-Delpero C, Mundler O, Berland Y. A pilot study comparing furosemide and hydrochlorothiazide in patients with hypertension and stage 4 or 5 chronic kidney disease. *J Clin Hypertens (Greenwich)*. 2012;14:32-37.

10. Knauf H, Mutschler E. Diuretic effectiveness of hydrochlorothiazide and furosemide alone and in combination in chronic renal failure. *J Cardiovasc Pharmacol*. 1995;26:394-400.

11. Chapter 2: lifestyle and pharmacological treatments for lowering blood pressure in CKD ND patients. *Kidney Int Suppl (2011)*. 2012;2:347-356.

12. Agarwal R, Sinha AD, Pappas MK, Ammous F. Chlorthalidone for poorly controlled hypertension in chronic kidney disease: an interventional pilot study. *Am J Nephrol*. 2014;39:171-182.

13. Cirillo M, Marcarelli F, Mele AA, Romano M, Lombardi C, Bilancio G. Parallel-group 8-week study on chlorthalidone effects in hypertensives with low kidney function. *Hypertension*. 2014;63:692-697.

14. Johnson JA, Gong Y, Bailey KR, et al. Hydrochlorothiazide and atenolol combination antihypertensive therapy: effects of drug initiation order. *Clin Pharmacol Ther*. 2009;86:533-539.

15. Chapman N, Dobson J, Wilson S, et al. Effect of spironolactone on blood pressure in subjects with resistant hypertension. *Hypertension*. 2007;49:839-845.

16. de Souza F, Muxfeldt E, Fiszman R, Salles G. Efficacy of spironolactone therapy in patients with true resistant hypertension. *Hypertension*. 2010;55:147-152.

17. Ernst ME, Lund BC. Renewed interest in chlorthalidone: evidence from the Veterans Health Administration. *J Clin Hypertens (Greenwich)*. 2010;12:927-934.

18. Dorsch MP, Gillespie BW, Erickson SR, Bleske BE, Weder AB. Chlorthalidone reduces cardiovascular events compared with hydrochlorothiazide: a retrospective cohort analysis. *Hypertension*. 2011;57:689-694.

19. Roush GC, Holford TR, Guddati AK. Chlorthalidone compared with hydrochlorothiazide in reducing cardiovascular events: systematic review and network meta-analyses. *Hypertension*. 2012;59:1110-1117.

20. Mortality after 10 1/2 years for hypertensive participants in the Multiple Risk Factor Intervention Trial. *Circulation*. 1990;82:1616-1628.

21. Sica DA. Chlorthalidone: has it always been the best thiazide-type diuretic? *Hypertension*. 2006;47:321-322.

22. Ernst ME, Grimm RH Jr. Thiazide diuretics: 50 years and beyond. *Curr Hypertens Rev*. 2008;4:256-65.

23. Ernst ME, Carter BL, Goerdt CJ, et al. Comparative antihypertensive effects of hydrochlorothiazide and chlorthalidone on ambulatory and office blood pressure. *Hypertension*. 2006;47:352-358.

24. Peterzan MA, Hardy R, Chaturvedi N, Hughes AD. Meta-analysis of dose-response relationships for hydrochlorothiazide, chlorthalidone, and bendroflumethiazide on blood pressure, serum potassium, and urate. *Hypertension*. 2012;59:1104-1109.

25. Trewet CL, Ernst ME. Resistant hypertension: identifying causes and optimizing treatment regimens. *South Med J*. 2008;101:166-173.

26. Engbaek M, Hjerrild M, Hallas J, Jacobsen IA. The effect of low-dose spironolactone on resistant hypertension. *J Am Soc Hypertens*. 2010;4:290-294.

27. Vaclavik J, Sedlak R, Plachy M, et al. Addition of spironolactone in patients with resistant arterial hypertension (ASPIRANT): a randomized, double-blind, placebo-controlled trial. *Hypertension*. 2011;57:1069-1075.

28. Saha C, Eckert GJ, Ambrosius WT, et al. Improvement in blood pressure with inhibition of the epithelial sodium channel in blacks with hypertension. *Hypertension*. 2005;46:481-487.

29. Williams B, MacDonald TM, Morant S, et al. Spironolactone versus placebo, bisoprolol, and doxazosin to determine the optimal treatment for drug-resistant hypertension (PATHWAY-2): a randomised, double-blind, crossover trial. *Lancet*. 2015;386:2059-2068.

30. Pitt B, Zannad F, Remme WJ, et al. The effect of spironolactone on morbidity and mortality in patients with severe heart failure. Randomized Aldactone Evaluation Study Investigators. *N Engl J Med*. 1999;341:709-717.

31. Zillich AJ, Carter BL. Eplerenone—a novel selective aldosterone blocker. *Ann Pharmacother*. 2002;36:1567-1576.

32. Williams GH, Burgess E, Kolloch RE, et al. Efficacy of eplerenone versus enalapril as monotherapy in systemic hypertension. *Am J Cardiol*. 2004;93:990-996.

33. White WB, Duprez D, St Hillaire R, et al. Effects of the selective aldosterone blocker eplerenone versus the calcium antagonist amlodipine in systolic hypertension. *Hypertension*. 2003;41:1021-1026.

34. Calhoun DA, White WB. Effectiveness of the selective aldosterone blocker, eplerenone, in patients with resistant hypertension. *J Am Soc Hypertens*. 2008;2:462-468.

35. Karns AD, Bral JM, Hartman D, Peppard T, Schumacher C. Study of aldosterone synthase inhibition as an add-on therapy in resistant hypertension. *J Clin Hypertens (Greenwich)*. 2013;15:186-192.

36. Dahal K, Kunwar S, Rijal J, et al. The Effects of Aldosterone Antagonists in Patients With Resistant Hypertension: A Meta-Analysis of Randomized and Nonrandomized Studies. *Am J Hypertens*. 2015;28:1376-1385.

37. Pitt B, Remme W, Zannad F, et al. Eplerenone, a selective aldosterone blocker, in patients with left ventricular dysfunction after myocardial infarction. *N Engl J Med*. 2003;348:1309-1321.

38. Zannad F, McMurray JJ, Krum H, et al. Eplerenone in patients with systolic heart failure and mild symptoms. *N Engl J Med*. 2011;364:11-21.

39. Bakris GL, Agarwal R, Chan JC, et al. Effect of Finerenone on Albuminuria in Patients With Diabetic Nephropathy: A Randomized Clinical Trial. *JAMA*. 2015;314:884-894.

40. Brown MJ, Williams B, Morant SV, et al. Effect of amiloride, or amiloride plus hydrochlorothiazide, versus hydrochlorothiazide on glucose tolerance and blood pressure (PATHWAY-3): a parallel-group, double-blind randomised phase 4 trial. *Lancet Diabetes Endocrinol*. 2016;4:136-147.

41. Sica DA, Gehr TW. Triamterene and the kidney. *Nephron*. 1989;51:454-461.

42. Murray MD, Haag KM, Black PK, Hall SD, Brater DC. Variable furosemide absorption and poor predictability of response in elderly patients. *Pharmacotherapy*. 1997;17:98-106.

43. Spiers DR, Wade RC. Double-blind parallel study of a combination of chlorthalidone 50 mg and triamterene 50 mg in patients with mild and moderate hypertension. *Curr Med Res Opin*. 1996;13:409-415.

44. Hort JF, Wilkins HM. Changes in blood pressure, serum potassium and electrolytes with a combination of triamterene and a low dose of chlorthalidone. *Curr Med Res Opin*. 1991;12:430-440.

45. Multiclinic comparison of amiloride, hydrochlorothiazide, and hydrochlorothiazide plus amiloride in essential hypertension. Multicenter Diuretic Cooperative Study Group. *Arch Intern Med*. 1981;141:482-486.

46. Myers MG. Hydrochlorothiazide with or without amiloride for hypertension in the elderly. A dose-titration study. *Arch Intern Med*. 1987;147:1026-1030.

47. Kohvakka A, Salo H, Gordin A, Eisalo A. Antihypertensive and biochemical effects of different doses of hydrochlorothiazide alone or in combination with triamterene. *Acta Med Scand*. 1986;219:381-386.

48. Larochelle P, Logan AG. Hydrochlorothiazide-amiloride versus hydrochlorothiazide alone for essential hypertension: effects on blood pressure and serum potassium level. *Can Med Assoc J*. 1985;132:801-805.

49. Wing LM, Reid CM, Ryan P, et al. A comparison of outcomes with angiotensin-converting–enzyme inhibitors and diuretics for hypertension in the elderly. *N Engl J Med*. 2003;348:583-592.

50. Medical Research Council trial of treatment of hypertension in older adults: principal results. MRC Working Party. *BMJ*. 1992;304:405-412.

51. Leren P, Helgeland A. Oslo Hypertension Study. *Drugs*. 1986;31(Suppl 1):41-45.

52. Wikstrand J, Warnold I, Olsson G, Tuomilehto J, Elmfeldt D, Berglund G. Primary prevention with metoprolol in patients with hypertension. Mortality results from the MAPHY study. *JAMA*. 1988;259:1976-1982.

53. Jamerson K, Bakris GL, Dahlof B, Pitt B, Velazquez EJ, Weber MA, for the ACCOMPLISH Investigators. Avoiding cardiovascular events through combination therapy in patients living with systolic hypertension. Results presented at American College of Cardiology, Chicago, Ill. March 2008.

54. Five-year findings of the hypertension detection and follow-up program. I. Reduction in mortality of persons with high blood pressure, including mild hypertension. Hypertension Detection and Follow-up Program Cooperative Group. *JAMA*. 1979;242:2562-2571.

55. Five-year findings of the hypertension detection and follow-up program. III. Reduction in stroke incidence among persons with high blood pressure. Hypertension Detection and Follow-up Program Cooperative Group. *JAMA*. 1982;247:633-638.

56. Prevention of stroke by antihypertensive drug treatment in older persons with isolated systolic hypertension. Final results of the Systolic Hypertension in the Elderly Program (SHEP). SHEP Cooperative Research Group. *JAMA*. 1991;265:3255-3264.

57. Major outcomes in high-risk hypertensive patients randomized to angiotensin-converting enzyme inhibitor or calcium channel blocker vs diuretic: The Antihypertensive and Lipid-Lowering Treatment to Prevent Heart Attack Trial (ALLHAT). *JAMA*. 2002;288:2981-2997.

58. Anonymous. Major cardiovascular events in hypertensive patients randomized to doxazosin vs chlorthalidone: the antihypertensive and lipid-lowering treatment to prevent heart attack trial (ALLHAT). ALLHAT Collaborative Research Group.[comment]. *JAMA*. 2000;283:1967-1975.

59. Grimm R. Diuretics are preferred over angiotensin II-converting enzyme inhibitors for initial therapy of uncomplicated hypertension. *Am J Kidney Dis*. 2007;50:188-196.

60. Beckett NS, Peters R, Fletcher AE, et al. Treatment of hypertension in patients 80 years of age or older. *N Engl J Med*. 2008;358:1887-1898.

61. Ernst ME, Carter BL, Basile JN. All thiazide-like diuretics are not chlorthalidone: putting the ACCOMPLISH study into perspective. *J Clin Hypertens (Greenwich)*. 2009;11:5-10.

62. Jamerson KA, Devereux R, Bakris GL, et al. Efficacy and duration of benazepril plus amlodipine or hydrochlorothiazide on 24-hour ambulatory systolic blood pressure control. *Hypertension*. 2011;57:174-179.

63. Carter BL, Sica DA. Strategies to improve the cardiovascular risk profile of thiazide-type diuretics as used in the management of hypertension. *Expert Opin Drug Saf*. 2007;6:583-594.

64. Ernst ME, Carter BL, Zheng S, Grimm RH, Jr. Meta-analysis of dose-response characteristics of hydrochlorothiazide and chlorthalidone: effects on systolic blood pressure and potassium. *Am J Hypertens*. 2010;23:440-446.

65. Goodfriend TL, Ball DL, Oelkers W, Bahr V. Torsemide inhibits aldosterone secretion in vitro. *Life Sci*. 1998;63:PL45-50.

66. Macdonald JE, Struthers AD. What is the optimal serum potassium level in cardiovascular patients? *J Am Coll Cardiol*. 2004;43:155-161.

67. Kaplan NM, Carnegie A, Raskin P, Heller JA, Simmons M. Potassium supplementation in hypertensive patients with diuretic-induced hypokalemia. *N Engl J Med*. 1985;312:746-749.

68. Weinberger MH. Influence of an angiotensin converting-enzyme inhibitor on diuretic-induced metabolic effects in hypertension. *Hypertension*. 1983;5(5 Pt 2):III132-138.

69. Kafka H, Langevin L, Armstrong PW. Serum magnesium and potassium in acute myocardial infarction. Influence on ventricular arrhythmias. *Arch Intern Med*. 1987;147:465-469.

70. Dargie HJ, Cleland JG, Leckie BJ, Inglis CG, East BW, Ford I. Relation of arrhythmias and electrolyte abnormalities to survival in patients with severe chronic heart failure. *Circulation*. 1987;75(5 Pt 2):IV98-107.

71. Holland OB, Nixon JV, Kuhnert L. Diuretic-induced ventricular ectopic activity. *Am J Med*. 1981;70:762-768.

72. Nordrehaug JE, von der Lippe G. Hypokalaemia and ventricular fibrillation in acute myocardial infarction. *Br Heart J*. 1983;50:525-529.

73. Sica DA, Struthers AD, Cushman WC, Wood M, Banas JS, Jr., Epstein M. Importance of potassium in cardiovascular disease. *J Clin Hypertens (Greenwich)*. 2002;4:198-206.

74. Franse LV, Pahor M, Di Bari M, Somes GW, Cushman WC, Applegate WB. Hypokalemia associated with diuretic use and cardiovascular events in the Systolic Hypertension in the Elderly Program.[comment]. *Hypertension*. 2000;35:1025-1030.

75. Siscovick DS, Raghunathan TE, Psaty BM, et al. Diuretic therapy for hypertension and the risk of primary cardiac arrest. *N Engl J Med*. 1994;330:1852-1857.

76. Zillich AJ, Garg J, Basu S, Bakris GL, Carter BL. Thiazide diuretics, potassium, and the development of diabetes: a quantitative review. *Hypertension*. 2006;48:219-224.

77. Sica DA, Hess M. Pharmacotherapy in congestive heart failure: aldosterone receptor antagonism: interface with hyperkalemia in heart failure. *Congest Heart Fail*. 2004;10:259-264.

78. Mann SJ. The silent epidemic of thiazide-induced hyponatremia. *J Clin Hypertens (Greenwich)*. 2008;10:477-484.

79. Chow KM, Szeto CC, Wong TY, Leung CB, Li PK. Risk factors for thiazide-induced hyponatraemia. *QJM*. 2003;96:911-917.

80. Fadel S, Karmali R, Cogan E. Safety of furosemide administration in an elderly woman recovered from thiazide-induced hyponatremia. *Eur J Intern Med*. 2009;20:30-34.

81. Elhassan EA, Schrier RW. Hyponatremia: diagnosis, complications, and management including V2 receptor antagonists. *Curr Opin Nephrol Hypertens*. 2011;20:161-168.

82. Martin BJ, Milligan K. Diuretic-associated hypomagnesemia in the elderly. *Arch Intern Med*. 1987;147:1768-1771.

83. Sica DA, Frishman WH, Cavusoglu E. Magnesium, potassium, and calcium as potential cardiovascular disease therapies. In: Frishman W, Sica DA, eds. Cardiovascular Pharmacotherapeutics. Minneapolis, MN: Cardiotext; 2012:177-188.

84. Cooper-DeHoff RM, Wen S, Beitelshees AL, et al. Impact of abdominal obesity on incidence of adverse metabolic effects associated with antihypertensive medications. *Hypertension*. 2010;55:61-68.

85. Zanchetti A, Rosei EA, Dal Palu C, Leonetti G, Magnani B, Pessina A. The Verapamil in Hypertension and Atherosclerosis Study (VHAS): results of long-term randomized treatment with either verapamil or chlorthalidone on carotid intima-media thickness. *J Hypertens*. 1998;16:1667-1676.

86. McAdams DeMarco MA, Maynard JW, Baer AN, et al. Diuretic use, increased serum urate levels, and risk of incident gout in a population-based study of adults with hypertension: the Atherosclerosis Risk in Communities cohort study. *Arthritis Rheum.* 2012;64:121-129.

87. Wilhelmsen L, Berglund G, Elmfeldt D, et al. Beta-blockers versus diuretics in hypertensive men: main results from the HAPPHY trial. *J Hypertens.* 1987;5:561-572.

88. Brown MJ, Palmer CR, Castaigne A, et al. Morbidity and mortality in patients randomised to double-blind treatment with a long-acting calcium-channel blocker or diuretic in the International Nifedipine GITS study: intervention as a Goal in Hypertension Treatment (INSIGHT). *Lancet.* 2000;356:366-372.

89. Handler J. Managing hypertensive patients with gout who take thiazide. *J Clin Hypertens (Greenwich).* 2010;12:731-735.

90. Amery A, Berthaux P, Bulpitt C, et al. Glucose intolerance during diuretic therapy. Results of trial by the European Working Party on Hypertension in the Elderly. *Lancet.* 1978;1:681-683.

91. Murphy MB, Lewis PJ, Kohner E, Schumer B, Dollery CT. Glucose intolerance in hypertensive patients treated with diuretics; a fourteen-year follow-up. *Lancet.* 1982;2:1293-1295.

92. Pollare T, Lithell H, Berne C. A comparison of the effects of hydrochlorothiazide and captopril on glucose and lipid metabolism in patients with hypertension. *N Engl J Med.* 1989;321:868-873.

93. Savage PJ, Pressel SL, Curb JD, et al. Influence of long-term, low-dose, diuretic-based, antihypertensive therapy on glucose, lipid, uric acid, and potassium levels in older men and women with isolated systolic hypertension: The Systolic Hypertension in the Elderly Program. SHEP Cooperative Research Group. *Arch Int Med.* 1998;158:741-751.

94. Tweeddale MG, Ogilvie RI, Ruedy J. Antihypertensive and biochemical effects of chlorthalidone. *Clin Pharmacol Ther.* 1977;22(5 Pt 1):519-527.

95. Carter BL, Einhorn PT, Brands M, et al. Thiazide-induced dysglycemia: call for research from a working group from the national heart, lung, and blood institute. *Hypertension.* 2008;52:30-36.

96. Barzilay JI, Davis BR, Cutler JA, et al. Fasting glucose levels and incident diabetes mellitus in older nondiabetic adults randomized to receive 3 different classes of antihypertensive treatment: a report from the Antihypertensive and Lipid-Lowering Treatment to Prevent Heart Attack Trial (ALLHAT). *Arch Intern Med.* 2006;166:2191-2201.

97. Phillips RA. New-onset diabetes mellitus less deadly than elevated blood pressure? Following the evidence in the administration of thiazide diuretics. *Arch Intern Med.* 2006;166:2174-2176.

98. Whelton PK, Barzilay J, Cushman WC, et al. Clinical outcomes in antihypertensive treatment of type 2 diabetes, impaired fasting glucose concentration, and normoglycemia: Antihypertensive and Lipid-Lowering Treatment to Prevent Heart Attack Trial (ALLHAT). *Arch Intern Med.* 2005;165:1401-1409.

99. Curb JD, Pressel SL, Cutler JA, et al. Effect of diuretic-based antihypertensive treatment on cardiovascular disease risk in older diabetic patients with isolated systolic hypertension. Systolic Hypertension in the Elderly Program Cooperative Research Group.[comment][erratum appears in *JAMA* 1997 May 7;277:1356]. *JAMA.* 1996;276:1886-1892.

100. Mariosa LS, Ribeiro-Filho FF, Batista MC, et al. Abdominal obesity is associated with potassium depletion and changes in glucose homeostasis during diuretic therapy. *J Clin Hypertens (Greenwich).* 2008;10:443-449.

101. Carter BL, Basile J. Development of diabetes with thiazide diuretics: the potassium issue. *J Clin Hypertens (Greenwich).* 2005;7:638-640.

102. Shafi T, Appel LJ, Miller ER, 3rd, Klag MJ, Parekh RS. Changes in serum potassium mediate thiazide-induced diabetes. *Hypertension.* 2008;52:1022-1029.

103. Smith SM, Anderson SD, Wen S, et al. Lack of correlation between thiazide-induced hyperglycemia and hypokalemia: subgroup analysis of results from the pharmacogenomic evaluation of antihypertensive responses (PEAR) study. *Pharmacotherapy.* 2009;29:1157-1165.

104. Grimm RH, Jr., Flack JM, Grandits GA, et al. Long-term effects on plasma lipids of diet and drugs to treat hypertension. Treatment of Mild Hypertension Study (TOMHS) Research Group. *JAMA.* 1996;275:1549-1556.

105. Lakshman MR, Reda DJ, Materson BJ, Cushman WC, Freis ED. Diuretics and beta-blockers do not have adverse effects at 1 year on plasma lipid and lipoprotein profiles in men with hypertension. Department of Veterans Affairs Cooperative Study Group on Antihypertensive Agents. *Arch Intern Med.* 1999;159:551-558.

106. Kasiske BL, Ma JZ, Kalil RS, Louis TA. Effects of antihypertensive therapy on serum lipids. *Ann Intern Med.* 1995;122:133-141.

107. Grimm RH, Jr., Grandits GA, Prineas RJ, et al. Long-term effects on sexual function of five antihypertensive drugs and nutritional hygienic treatment in hypertensive men and women. Treatment of Mild Hypertension Study (TOMHS). *Hypertension.* 1997;29(1 Pt 1):8-14.

108. Strom BL, Schinnar R, Apter AJ, et al. Absence of cross-reactivity between sulfonamide antibiotics and sulfonamide nonantibiotics. *N Engl J Med.* 2003;349:1628-1635.

109. The sixth report of the Joint National Committee on prevention, detection, evaluation, and treatment of high blood pressure. *Arch Intern Med.* 1997;157:2413-2446.

110. Simunic M, Rumboldt Z, Ljutic D, Sardelic S. Ramipril decreases chlorthalidone-induced loss of magnesium and potassium in hypertensive patients. *J Clin Pharmacol.* 1995;35:1150-1155.

111. Amery A, Birkenhager W, Brixko P, et al. Mortality and morbidity results from the European Working Party on High Blood Pressure in the Elderly trial. *Lancet.* 1985;1:1349-1354.

112. Borhani NO, Mercuri M, Borhani PA, et al. Final outcome results of the Multicenter Isradipine Diuretic Atherosclerosis Study (MIDAS). A randomized controlled trial. *JAMA.* 1996;276:785-791.

113. Rosei EA, Dal Palu C, Leonetti G, Magnani B, Pessina A, Zanchetti A. Clinical results of the Verapamil in Hypertension and Atherosclerosis Study. VHAS Investigators. *J Hypertens.* 1997;15:1337-1344.

114. Neaton JD, Grimm RH, Jr., Prineas RJ, et al. Treatment of mild hypertension study. Final results. Treatment of mild hypertension study research group. *JAMA.* 1993;270:713-724.

115. Malacco E, Mancia G, Rappelli A, et al. Treatment of isolated systolic hypertension: the SHELL study results. *Blood Press.* 2003;12:160-167.

116. MRC trial of treatment of mild hypertension: principal results. Medical Research Council Working Party. *BMJ (Clin Res Ed).* 1985;291:97-104.

23 | Peripheral Adrenergic Blockers

Orit Barrett and Talya Wolak

THE SYMPATHETIC NERVOUS SYSTEM IN HYPERTENSION

The notion that sympathetic fibers are found on the vascular wall and when stimulated cause vasoconstriction was proposed in 1840.[1] The activity of these fibers is one of the components that control peripheral vascular resistance.[2] Hyperactivity of the sympathetic nervous system is well described not only in hypertensive patients, but also in subjects at risk of progressing to hypertension,[3] namely normotensive individuals with a family history of hypertension[4,5] and those with white-coat hypertension.[6]

The high adrenergic drive in hypertensive patients is attributed to: (1) enhanced spillover rate from neuroeffective junctions and the resulting augmented norepinephrine secretion from sympathetic nerve terminals[7]; (2) impaired vagal tone and reduced parasympathetic activity[8]; and (3) increased central adrenergic drive and peripheral sympathetic nerve traffic to the skeletal muscle circulation.[9]

In patients with sustained hypertension, the high sympathetic drive is demonstrated in all subgroups of the hypertensive population: males, females, diabetics, and those with metabolic syndrome, young and old.[3] Furthermore, the degree of the sympathetic drive has a positive correlation with the severity of hypertension[10] and with hypertensive complications, especially left ventricular hypertrophy.[11]

ALPHA ADRENERGIC RECEPTORS

The alpha adrenergic receptors (α-ARs) are activated by the catecholamines epinephrine and norepinephrine. Alpha and beta ARs are divided into subclasses: α₁-AR–α₁A-AR, α₁B-AR, and α₁D-AR; α₂-AR–α₂A-AR, α₂B-AR, and α₂C-AR; and β-AR–β₁-AR, β₂-AR, and β₃-AR. Most of the cells in the human body express at least one of the nine AR subclasses. The α-ARs are composed of α₁-*ARs* and α₂-*ARs*. The α₁-*ARs* are postsynaptic. Their activation results in norepinephrine release and vasoconstriction. The α₂-*ARs* are located in the presynaptic and postsynaptic areas. When located presynaptically, they inhibit norepinephrine release, whereas when located postsynaptically, they increase norepinephrine release and mediate vasoconstriction and venoconstriction.[12]

ALPHA₁-ADRENERGIC RECEPTORS: ORGAN DISTRIBUTION AND ACTIVITY

α₁-ARs are expressed in various organs, including the brain, heart, liver, kidney, prostate, spleen, and blood vessels. Activation of the α₁-AR mediates modulation of neurotransmission as well as regulation of the cardiovascular system and metabolism.[13]

Systemic Blood Vessels

All α₁-ARs play a role in the regulation of vascular tone. However, the most major contribution to vascular tone is made by the α₁A-AR and α₁D-AR subclasses; α₁A-ARs are located in distributing arteries (the mesenteric and renal arteries) and α₁D-ARs are located in large conducting arteries (the aorta, the carotid), as well in the coronary arteries. The expression of the α₁B-AR subclass is minor in the vascular structure, but is increased in older individuals (>65 years).[14-17]

Cerebral Circulation

The cerebral arteries are richly innervated with sympathetic nerve fibers.[18] The adrenergic modulation of cerebral blood flow is delicate and complex. The complexity of sympathetic cerebral vascular autoregulation is further demonstrated by studies using an α-AR vasopressor/agonist. An infusion of phenylephrine (a selective α1-adrenergic vasopressor) resulted in an increase in systemic blood pressure and blood flow velocity in the middle cerebral artery, but a decrease in frontal lobe oxygenation.[19] Using norepinephrine resulted in an even more prominent effect on cerebral vascular autoregulation, secondary to increases in systemic blood pressure; there is a decrease in both middle cerebral artery mean flow velocity and cerebral oxygenation.[20] The blockade of α₁-AR, on the other hand, also disrupts cerebral autoregulation, mainly during hypotension[21] and exercise.[22]

Alpha₁-Adrenergic Receptors and the Heart

Various in-vitro and animal studies demonstrate the role of α₁-ARs as being cardioprotective. α₁-ARs are involved in the inhibition of myocyte apoptosis, the enhancement of protein synthesis, the improvement of glucose metabolism, and cardiac contractility.[23] The heart contains all three subclasses of α₁-ARs: α₁A-AR and α₁B-AR are found mainly in the myocytes,[24] whereas α₁D-ARs are located in the coronaries.[25] Myocardial α₁-ARs have an important role in normal postnatal growth of the heart, and possess protective effects during chronic stress, including heart failure. In the heart failure setting, the abundance of α₁-ARs and their function is intact or increased, in contrast to β-ARs, which decline in abundance and function.[24] These experimental findings might shed light on the observation that in large-scale human clinical trials, the use of α₁-AR antagonists was associated with an increased incidence of heart failure.[26] Although the blockade of β-AR is beneficial in left ventricular dysfunction, the blockade of α₁-ARs probably abolishes their compensatory effect in heart failure.

Alpha₁-Adrenergic Receptor Blockers: Metabolic Effects

α₁-AR blocker therapy has been associated with significantly favorable effects on serum lipid profile. Decreases in total cholesterol (about 5%), low-density lipoprotein (LDL) cholesterol (about 5%), and triglycerides (about

5%), and increases in high-density lipoprotein (HDL) cholesterol (about 4%) are typical.[26-28] These changes occur soon after patients begin therapy and are sustained as long as the drug is continued. They are expressed in multiple mechanisms, including: (1) an increase in the number of LDL cholesterol receptors and lipoprotein lipase activity; (2) a decrease in the synthesis of both LDL cholesterol and very-low-density lipoprotein cholesterol; and (3) a reduction in the absorption of dietary cholesterol.[29,30] In addition, oxidation of LDL-cholesterol can be inhibited by two different hydroxylated metabolites of doxazosin. Similarly, treatment with an α_1-AR blocker is found to have favorable effects on insulin sensitivity in hypertensive patients.[31-34]

In the Antihypertensive and Lipid-Lowering [to prevent] Heart Attack Trial (ALLHAT) trial, as found in previous studies, a significant reduction ($p < 0.001$) in mean fasting glucose was noted in patients who received doxazosin (from 122 mg/dL initially to 117 mg/dL at 4 years), whereas patients treated with chlorthalidone experienced an increase from 123 mg/dL at baseline to 125 mg/dL at 4 years.[27] A Japanese study from 2009 found a significant beneficial effect on insulin resistance (evaluated by homeostatic model assessment-insulin resistance [HOMA-IR]) when an α_1-AR blocker was added to patients' antihypertensive regimen (compared with patients in whom no change was made in their existing treatment). In multivariate analysis, change in HOMA-IR was found to be independently and significantly associated with morning BP (beta = 0.15, $p = 0.016$)[35] (Table 23.1). The metabolic effects of α_1-AR blocker therapy may be most relevant in hypertensive patients with diabetes mellitus and/or metabolic syndrome. For this population, treatment with an α_1-AR blocker is associated with lower serum lipids and improved glycemic control and endothelial function.[36,37] A recently published study found that the use of α_1-AR blockers for the treatment of hypertension resulted in a significantly lower incidence of new-onset diabetes mellitus in women with coronary heart disease.[38]

Alpha₁-Adrenergic Receptors Blockers and Cancer

Quinazoline, a compound made up of two fused six-member simple aromatic rings, displays hypotensive and anticancer activities. The α_1-AR blockers prazosin, doxazosin, and terazosin are quinazoline-based drugs.[39]

α_1-AR blockers were found to have antitumor efficacy through the induction of apoptosis in benign and malignant prostate cells,[17] to reduce tumor growth and suppressed tumor vascularization in a xenograft model of human ovarian cancer,[40] and to suppress the migration of prostate cancer, breast cancer, and glioma cells,[41] as well as to inhibit both benign and malignant prostate cell growth by down regulating the expression of androgen receptors.[42] These data support the use of quinazoline-based α_1-AR blockers as safe antihypertensive medications in patients with malignancies.

CLINICAL INDICATIONS AND ADVERSE EFFECTS

The α_1-AR blockers available as antihypertensive medications include: prazosin, terazosin, and doxazosin. Alfuzosin, silodosin, and tamsulosin are uroselective, and thus reserved for benign prostatic hyperplasia (BPH) and lower urinary tract symptoms (LUTS)[43] (Table 23.2).

Hypertension

From the second half of the 20th century and until the beginning of the current century (2000), α_1-AR blockers were widely used and considered safe and effective antihypertensive medications. Their blood-pressure-lowering effect was supported by numerous clinical trials published from the mid-1970s that demonstrated a dose-dependent lowering of BP much greater in comparison to placebo,[44] and found that their antihypertensive properties were not affected by patients' age, race, or plasma renin activity. α_1-AR blockers were used either as monotherapy or in combination with other antihypertensive

TABLE 23.1 Alpha-Adrenergic Receptors-Mediated Medications

	DRUG NAME	DOSE ADMINISTRATION	HALF-LIFE	OTHER CLINICAL INDICATIONS	SPECIAL CONSIDERATIONS
α_1-AR blockers	Prazosin	2-20 mg/day Every 8-12 hours	3 hours	PTSD nightmares and sleep disruption. BPH, Raynaud phenomenon	
	Terazosin	1-5 mg/day Every 24 hours	12 hours	BPH	Increased risk for hypotension with PDE-5-inhibitors
	Doxazosin	1-16 mg/day Every 24 hours	20 hours	BPH, ureteral calculi expulsion	Increased risk for hypotension with PDE-5-inhibitors
α_2-AR agonists	Clonidine	Oral: 0.1-0.2 mg Every 12 hours Patch 0.1-0.3/24 hours Applied every 7 days	16 hours	Nicotine withdrawal, Tourette syndrome, pain management (epidural infusion), ADHD	
	Methyldopa	Oral: 250 mg-3gr Every 8-12 hours IV: 250-1000 mg 6-8 hours	24-48 hours		
Non selective-AR blockers	Phenoxybenzamine	20-40 mg every 8-12 hours	24 hours		Preoperative pheochromocytoma
	Phentolamine (used only IV)	5 mg	20 min		Pheochromocytoma Before and during surgery.

ADHD, Attention-deficit/hyperactivity disorder; AR, adrenergic receptors; BPH, benign prostatic hyperplasia; IV, intravenous; PDE, phosphodiesterase; PTSD, posttraumatic stress disorder.

ANTIHYPERTENSIVE THERAPY V

TABLE 23.2 α₁-AR Blockers Therapy: Statistically Significant Benefits and Adverse Events Form Clinical Trials

REF.	METHODS AND AIMS	RESULTS	ADVERSE EVENTS
26	• A randomized, double-blind, active-controlled clinical trial • Evaluation of the incidence of CVD in patients with hypertension and at least one other CHD risk factor who are receiving first-line treatment with either doxazosin or chlorthalidone • A total of 24,335 patients were included.	• Doxazosin showed inferiority in lowering BP compared with chlorthalidone.	• Doxazosin was associated with higher risk of stroke and combined CVD. • Doubled risk for HF • Higher RR for angina coronary revascularization
72	• A double-blind, placebo-controlled, crossover trial • Assessment of the efficacy of an "add-on" therapy with spironolactone, bisoprolol, doxazosin, or placebo on BP-control, in patients with resistant HTN • Of 335 randomized patients, 314 had follow-up and were included in the intention-to-treat analysis	• Doxazocin is less effective in lowering BP compared with spironolactone, especially in patients with low plasma renin levels.	
89	• A 3-month multicenter, randomized, open-label study • Evaluation of efficacy on BP and safety, with treatment of either alfuzosin as monotherapy or alfuzosin combined with an antihypertensive agent, in patients with clinical diagnosis of BPH/LUTS, with or without ongoing treatment with antihypertensive medication. • 335 patients aged ≥ 45 years were included.	• In normotensive patients or those with controlled HTN, treatment with alfuzosin is effective and well tolerated in patients with BPH/LUTS, with or without antihypertensive medications. • Improvement in IPSS and in IPSS-quality of life scores	• In patients with uncontrolled or untreated hypertension, alfuzosin, alone or combined with antihypertensive therapy, was associated with undesired decreases of systolic and diastolic BP. • The most common side effect of monotherapy/combined therapy were headache (1.47% and 2.14%, respectively), dizziness/postural dizziness (5.88% and 4.28%, respectively), hypotension/postural hypotension (0.74% and 1.43%, respectively), and syncope (0% and 1.43%, respectively). • Sexual function-related adverse events (1.47% and 1.43%, respectively)
35	• Randomized study • Evaluation of the effect of "add-on" treatment with doxazosin (compared with no change in antihypertensive treatment) on insulin resistance in patients with morning hypertension • 611 treated hypertensive patients with morning hypertension were randomized	• Reduced insulin resistance evaluated by HOMA-IR • Reduced morning SBP • Correlation between the change in insulin resistance and the change in morning BP was relatively weak.	

BP, Blood pressure; *BPH,* benign prostatic hyperplasia; *CHD,* coronary heart disease; *CVD,* cardiovascular disease; *HF,* heart failure; *HOMA-IR,* homeostatic model assessment-insulin resistance; *HTN,* hypertension; *LUTS,* lower urinary tract; *RR,* relative risk; *SBP,* systolic blood pressure.

drugs.[45-49] The ALLHAT was the first double-blind, randomized, multicenter, federally funded long-term clinical trial to evaluate doxazosin, an α₁-AR blocker, as an initial antihypertensive therapy to prevent cardiovascular (CV) events.[50] The ALLHAT assessed four different classes of first-line antihypertensive medications (angiotensin-converting enzyme inhibitors [ACE-I], calcium antagonists, α₁-AR blockers, and thiazide-like diuretics), comparing the incidence of CV events in high-risk hypertensive subjects aged 55 years or older. In 2000, the National Heart, Lung, and Blood Institute ordered the prompt discontinuation of the α₁-AR blocker doxazosin arm of ALLHAT because not only did doxazosin show inferiority in lowering BP compared with chlorthalidone, but, more importantly, it was associated with a 25% greater incidence of combined cardiovascular disease (CVD) outcomes. A major component of this treatment difference regarding CVD outcomes was a two-fold increase in risk of heart failure (HF) with doxazosin, which remains highly significant, with a 66% increase in risk even after considering only hospitalized or fatal incidents of HF. The differential effect of treatment on HF was consistently observed in each of the prespecified subgroups (age, gender, race/ethnicity, and diabetic status) (Table 23.2).

Significant adverse trends were also observed for other secondary endpoints, including stroke and combined coronary heart disease.[26,51] Additional analyses confirm the findings of excess HF with doxazosin treatment.[27,52-57] Following publication of the ALLHAT, much debate was generated regarding its study design (withdrawal of diuretics, which might have

unmasked the symptoms of HF, in participants who were on antihypertensive therapy before randomization) and the validity of HF diagnosis in the study.[58-61] Nevertheless, this study was the major driving force for the change in hypertension guidelines. Following its publication, clinical recommendations against the use of α₁-AR blockers as first-line agents for hypertension treatment were released, and the use of α₁-AR blockers as antihypertensive drugs declined dramatically worldwide.[62]

During the post-ALLHAT era, although α₁-AR blockers were not positioned in the first line of antihypertensive treatment, a number of studies (The African American Study of Kidney Disease and Hypertension [AASK][63] and the Reduction of Endpoints in Non-Insulin-Dependent Diabetes with the Angiotensin II Antagonist Losartan [RENAAL][64] study) demonstrated the benefit of α₁-AR blockers in lowering BP in uncontrolled hypertensive patients. α₁-AR blockers were useful as "add-on" antihypertensive drugs.

Observational analysis of data from the multicenter, international, randomized Anglo-Scandinavian Cardiac Outcomes Trail (ASCOT), conducted on individuals with hypertension and an additional CV risk factor (but no history of coronary heart disease), showed that third-line α₁-AR blocker gastrointestinal therapeutic system (GITS) therapy is both safe and effective in lowering BP, with a mean BP reduction of almost 12/7 mm Hg achieved in all patients. Exposure to doxazosin did not appear to be associated with excess risk of HF or other adverse CV outcomes.[28] Although favorable results with α₁-AR blocker treatment,

TABLE 23.3 **Summary of Current Guidelines**

GUIDELINE	YEAR	SUMMARY OF RECOMMENDATIONS
The American Eight Joint National Committee of Prevention, Detection, Evaluation and Treatment of High Blood Pressure (JNC-8)	2014	• α-blockers are not recommended as first-line therapy because initial therapy with α_1-blockers resulted in adverse combined cardiovascular, HF, and cerebrovascular outcomes. • α-blockers are not listed as an optional treatment for resistant HTN.
The European Society of Hypertension and European Society of Cardiology (ESH/ESC)	2013	• The α_1-blocker doxazosin should be considered for the treatment of resistant HTN (class IIa) (level B).
The British National Institute for Health and Clinical Excellence (NICE)	2011	• α-blocker can be used as a fourth-line treatment for hypertension.
The Canadian Hypertension Education Program Recommendations (CHEP)	2015	• α-blockers are not recommended as first-line therapy for uncomplicated HTN or as monotherapy (grade A). • For uncontrolled BP with a combination of 2 or more first-line agents, or if there are adverse effects, α-blockers may be added (grade D).

BP, Blood pressure; *HF,* heart failure; *HTN,* hypertension.

including BP control and beneficial metabolic effects,[31,61] were shown in the ASCOT study and similar studies,[65] they failed to convince medical panels to change the previously determined guidelines. The eight joint national committees of prevention, detection, evaluation, and treatment of high blood pressure (JNC-8) carried on the same strict approach adopted by the JNC-7, according to which α_1-AR blockers have no place in recommended treatment.[66,67]

The European guidelines, published in 2013 by the European Society of Hypertension and European Society of Cardiology (ESH/ESC), stated that α_1-AR blockers are effective antihypertensive agents and can be employed for combination treatment with diuretics, β-blockers, calcium channel blockers, ACE inhibitors, and/or angiotensin receptor blockers, primarily as part of a multiple-drug combination or for the treatment of resistant hypertension.[68] The Canadian Hypertension Education Program Recommendations (CHEP), published in 2015, took the same approach as the ESH/ESC guidelines, recommending the use of α_1-AR blockers as an optional third-line treatment in multidrug regimens,[69] whereas, in the latest British guidelines, published in 2011 by the National Institute for Health and Clinical Excellence (NICE), α_1-AR blockers are located lower on the treatment tree, as a fourth-line therapeutic option[70] (Table 23.3).

According to the aforementioned guidelines, the main use of α_1-AR blockers is as an "add-on" agent in hypertension treatment regimens. When treating patients with resistant hypertension, clinicians are faced with the question of which add-on treatment, an aldosterone antagonist or an α_1-AR blocker, is best. In 2012, a retrospective study aimed to answer this question was performed. The investigators assessed the efficacy of a mechanism-based algorithm for the treatment of resistant HTN. The study included 27 patients with resistant HTN, who, based on clinical judgment, using the clues of volume excess and neurogenic hypertension, received one of three therapeutic interventions: (1) strengthening of the diuretic regimen, usually by means of a potassium-sparing agent; (2) combination therapy that included both an α-blocker and a β-blocker; or (3) both of these two interventions. Study findings indicate that BP control in resistant hypertension can be achieved by two very different treatment options, and that the key to success is logical drug selection, achieved by identifying the patients most or least likely to respond to each treatment.[71]

The PATHWAY-2 trial examined the same issue but prospectively. This randomized, double-blind, controlled, crossover study, with 285 participants, compared different active drug treatments: spironolactone, doxazosin, bisoprolol, and a placebo, as "add-on" fourth-line treatments for resistant hypertension. The intention-to-treat analyses demonstrate that spironolactone was significantly more effective in achieving blood pressure control relative to placebo, bisoprolol, and doxazosin (all *p* < 0.0001). The superiority of spironolactone was seen particularly in patients with lower plasma renin levels[72] (Table 23.2).

These two studies highlight the significance of personalized medicine in hypertensive patients. Usually when a hypertensive patient needs a fourth drug for blood pressure control, clinical judgment is needed to evaluate whether he will enjoy volume reduction (aldosterone blockade will be effective) or whether sympathetic blockade with α_1-AR blockers will be more useful.[73] Another trial that examined the cardiac safety of α_1-AR blockers in hypertensive patients demonstrated the importance of the personalized medicine approach. This study included more than 19,000 hypertensive patients, and evaluated the effect of α_1-AR blockers on cardiac outcome in patients who had previously undergone single-photon emission computed tomography myocardial perfusion imaging (SPECT MPI) testing, which accurately evaluates the reversibility of cardiac perfusion defects (ischemia). Study results showed that α_1-AR blockers are safe as antihypertensive therapy in patients with a mild degree or any extent of fixed cardiac ischemia. However, in patients with more substantial (moderate to severe) ischemia, treatment with doxazosin for HTN was associated with increased risk of adverse cardiac outcomes (cardiac death and MI) (hazard ratio [HR] 1.5; 95% confidence incidence [CI], 1.14 to 1.98).[74] This study supports results of previous studies that demonstrate the efficacy and safety of α_1-AR blocker treatment in combination regimens, even in the presence of mild to moderate heart failure.[65,75]

Recently, the Randomized Trial of Intensive versus Standard Blood-Pressure Control (the "SPRINT" trial) demonstrated that in nondiabetic patients at high risk for cardiovascular events, targeting a systolic blood pressure of less than 120 mm Hg, as compared with less than 140 mm Hg, resulted in lower rates of fatal and nonfatal major cardiovascular events and death from any cause. To achieve the desired blood pressure target, α_1-AR blockers were included in the medical regimen in both arms of the study: 10.3% of patients in the intensive group and 5.5% of patients in the standard group. There were fewer cardiovascular events in the intensive care group and the incidence of heart failure was 38% lower.[76] This recent landmark trial confirms the safety of α_1-AR blockers as add-on medications in high-risk cardiovascular patients. According to the above data, α_1-AR blockers are not in the first line to treat hypertension, but they can be used as add-on medications in hypertensive patients with resistant hypertension who did not achieve their blood pressure target under treatment with ACE-I/angiotensin-receptor blockers, calcium channel blockers, and diuretics. They are mainly effective in patients with evidence of high sympathetic drive.

α_2-AR agonists: The α_2-AR agonists are central sympatholytic drugs and are covered in detail in Chapter 26. These drugs reduce blood pressure by activating the presynaptic α_2-AR in the rostral ventrolateral medulla, causing a decrease in central and peripheral sympathetic nerve activity, resulting in a reduction in heart rate, myocardial contractility, and peripheral resistance. The α_2-AR agonists used as antihypertensive medications are clonidine, methyldopa, guanfacine, and guanabenz.[43,76] Clonidine, an α_2-AR agonist medication used to treat hypertension, produces its pharmacologic effect in the central nervous system not only by interacting with the α_2-AR receptors, but also by activating the central imidazoline receptors.[77] Imidazoline receptor-1(I-1) is found upstream from the α_2-AR. The I-1 receptors suppress sympathetic outflow at postganglionic sympathetic neurons.[78]

Cardiac Safety

During the 1970s Prazosin (a frequently used α_1-AR blocker) was found to relieve heart failure and pulmonary congestion as a result of reduced preload and afterload. It also reduced left ventricular filling pressure and systemic vascular resistance, improved cardiac index, cardiac efficiency of stroke work, and myocardial oxygen consumption index.[79,80] However, a decade later, in the Veterans Administration Cooperative Study (V-HEFT I), conducted on 642 heart failure patients, Prazosin failed to improve survival compared with a placebo, whereas a combination treatment of isosorbide dinitrate with hydralazine reduced mortality.[81] Later, in the ALLHAT study, the α_1-AR blocker doxazosin was excluded primarily because of an increase in heart failure events in this study arm.[26] However, when an α_1-AR blocker is used as an add-on medication, it can have beneficial cardiac effects. Ikeda et al. showed that the α_1-AR blocker doxazosin as an "add-on" therapy not only improved BP control, but was also associated with decreases in left ventricular mass index (LVMI) ($p < 0.001$), relative wall thickness ($p < 0.001$), and insulin resistance (evaluated by the HOMA-IR) ($p < 0.001$).[82]

The prospective, randomized, open-label, blinded-evaluation CARDHIAC (CARduran en pacientes Diabéticos con HIpertensi'on Arterial no Controlada) study found that in type II diabetes mellitus patients, a significant reduction in LVMI ($p = 0.001$) was associated with doxazosin treatment, but not with atenolol treatment.[83] Reduced LVMI may contribute to a more favorable pattern of ventricular geometry, which may provide further CV benefits in hypertensive individuals. New evidence from recent studies further demonstrates that α_1-AR blockers might have a favorable cardiac influence. In a multicenter, randomized study published in 2015, urapidil (an α_1-AR blocker and 5-HT1A receptor agonist) was compared with nitroglycerin (NG) for treatment of heart failure complicated by hypertension and DM in elderly patients. The study results demonstrated the superiority of urapidil in controlling systolic BP compared with NG ($p < 0.05$). Moreover, treatment with urapidil was associated with higher ejection fraction (t = 2.206, $p < 0.05$), cardiac index (t = 2.206, $p < 0.05$ and t= 3.13, $p < 0.05$), and left end-diastolic volume (t = -3.014, $p < 0.05$), but lower N-terminal pro-B-type natriuretic peptide (NT-proBNP) levels (t = 2.206, $p < 0.05$) in comparison with NG treatment.[84]

Taken together, the results of the landmark ALLHAT trial and the later studies might lead to the conclusion that α_1-AR blocker are not recommended as the initial drug of choice to treat hypertension. However, at the same time it should be remembered that they have beneficial effects on cardiac outcome, including heart failure, when taken as part of a multidrug antihypertensive regimen. This favorable effect is probably attributed to improved blood pressure control, the leading factor that prevents diastolic dysfunction.

Benign Prostatic Hyperplasia/Lower Urinary Tract Symptoms and Hypertension

The use of α_1-AR blockers for the treatment of symptomatic BPH and LUTS has been adequately studied and found to be effective for this indication.[85-87]

Pharmacologically, α_1-AR blockers bind to the highly concentrated α_1-AR present in the prostate, bladder and neck, leading to relaxation of the smooth muscle and thereby reducing resistance to urine flow.[88] Because of their frequent use in the elderly population, which also suffers from hypertension, their efficacy and safety profile in hypertensive patients with BPH/LUTS is important.

Findings from a multicenter, prospective, comparative cohort study showed that treatment of BPH/LUTS with the uroselective α_1-AR blocker alfuzosin alone in combination with antihypertensive therapy is effective and has only a marginal effect on blood pressure in normotensive patients and in patients with controlled hypertension. In patients with untreated or uncontrolled hypertension, a significant decrease in systolic and diastolic BP was documented, with a mean 12-week reduction of -11.3 mm Hg in systolic BP and -5.1 mm Hg in diastolic BP in the untreated hypertension subgroup and mean decreases in systolic and diastolic BP of -9.9 mm Hg and -2.9 mm Hg, respectively, in the uncontrolled hypertension subgroup (both $p < 0.001$). The author concluded that although it is safe and effective to start treatment with uroselective α_1-AR blockers in normotensive and controlled hypertensive patients without further evaluation, patients with untreated or uncontrolled hypertension should undergo careful evaluation before the initiation of treatment with uroselective α_1-AR blockers for BPH/LUTS[89] (Table 23.2).

Pheochromocytoma

Pheochromocytoma treatment is extensively covered in Chapter 15. Before surgery, adequate blood pressure control is needed to avoid a hypertensive crisis during surgery and improve morbidity and mortality outcomes. Although there is no consensus regarding the preferred drugs for preoperative blood pressure control, initial treatment with α-AR blockers is widely accepted, with a preference for the nonselective α-blocker phenoxybenzamine. Other selective α_1-AR blockers, such as prazosin, terazosin, and doxazosin, can also be used although high-dose doxazosin is preferred over the shorter acting agents to reduce the risk of breakthrough during catecholamine surges. Despite preoperative alpha blockade, hemodynamic liability can still occur intraoperatively, especially during tumor manipulation.[90,91] This fact was confirmed in a recently published retrospective study, in which 48 patients with pheochromocytoma were treated with doxazosin in the perioperative setting. Results from this study showed that adrenergic blockage by selective α_1-AR blockers did not fully prevent intraoperative hypertensive crisis, but was associated with short episodes without major cardiovascular complication.[92]

Adverse Effects

Large placebo-controlled studies showed very slight decreases in hemoglobin, hematocrit, leukocyte count, serum total protein, and albumin levels, which were generally attributed to mild fluid retention and resultant hemodilution. Prolonged treatment (e.g., as in either ALLHAT[26] or ASCOT[28]) has not led to any long-term concerns about these parameters. Changes in serum potassium levels were minor and inconclusive in several studies. Elevation in plasma creatinine level was apparent, but had no clinical significance.

During trials against placebo, the following symptoms occurred in more than 5% of the α_1-AR blocker-treated hypertensive population: dizziness, headache, fatigue/malaise,

TABLE 23.4 Alpha₁-Adrenergic Receptors Blocker: Common Adverse Effects

	DIZZINESS	HEADACHE	FATIGUE/MALAISE
Doxazosin	19%	14%	12%
Prazosin	10%	8%	8%
Terazosin	19%	16%	11%

TABLE 23.5 Complications Associated With Alpha₁-Adrenergic Receptors Blocker Therapy

Hip Fracture

RESULTS	STUDY GROUP	REF.
• Adverse events were more frequent during the four consecutive months after treatment with α_1-AR blockers was initiated, compared with the time before drug initiation (1.82 vs 0.02 events per 10,000 person-days). Higher risk for adverse effects was seen in patients with prior initiation of other antihypertensive medication.	• A cohort of 53,824 men with a medical office-generated diagnosis code for LUTS/BPH	97
• α_1-AR blockers and hip fracture was found in men who were treated with α_1-AR blockers for cardiovascular disease (adjusted OR 2.8, 95% CI: 1.4-5.4), but not when provided for men with a diagnosis of BPH (adjusted OR 1.0, 95% CI: 0.4-2.5).	• The UK General Practitioners Research; case-control study including 4571 cases in each arm	98
• Incident rate ratio of hip/femur fractures within the first 21 days after exposure to α_1-AR blocker treatment was 1.36 ($p = 0.017$, 95% CI: 1.06-1.74), compared with the unexposed period.	• Taiwan's National Health Insurance claims database data on 5875 elderly patients without hypertension	99

Cerebral Hypoperfusion and Ischemic Stroke

RESULTS	STUDY GROUP	REF.
• An increased risk of ischemic stroke during the first 21 days following treatment initiation with α_1-AR blockers was found among the whole study population (adjusted IRR 1.40, 95% CI, 1.22-1.61), with more substantial risk in patients without any other antihypertensive treatment (adjusted IRR 2.11, 95% CI, 1.73-2.57). Patients with underlying hypertension appeared to be tolerant of the first dose effect of α_1-AR blockers.	• National Health Insurance claims database of Taiwan, information on 7502 men (mean age 71) case series study.	100

α_1-AR, Alpha₁-adrenergic receptors; BPH, benign prostatic hyperplasia; CI, confidence interval; IRR, incidence rate ratio; LUTS, lower urinary tract; OR, odds ratio; UK, United Kingdom.

and palpitations (Table 23.4). α_1-AR blockers should be used in the evening, preferably before bedtime, increasing the likelihood that patients will remain recumbent for several hours, and thus reducing the risk of syncope. This practice should be recommended especially for the first dose, when vascular dilatation and reduced venous return are the most significant. This "first-dose phenomenon" often attenuates with time, but may reappear with rapid increases in dosage or reinitiation of treatment after therapy interruption. Doxazosin GITS appears to have a lower risk of this problem, probably because doxazosin is released slowly from the tablet.[93] This enables the administration of a therapeutic dose at the initiation of therapy, and eliminates the need for multiple dose titrations.

Hip fracture, cerebral hypoperfusion, and ischemic stroke are severe adverse events that are associated with syncope and dizziness. Several large-scale observational studies examined the possible association of α_1-AR blocker therapy with these complications (summarized in Table 23.5).

Another rare but severe complication of α_1-AR blocker use is intraoperative floppy iris syndrome (IFIS). This is an ophthalmologic complication that occurs during cataract extraction, and is associated with intraoperative complications that may lead to poor postoperative outcomes. This syndrome complicates approximately 1% of patients who undergo surgical intervention for cataract. The syndrome's pathophysiological basis is thought to be related to the loss of dilator muscle tone, which occurs as a result of blockage of postsynaptic α_1-AR that predominates in the iris dilator smooth muscle, leading to pupil contraction.[94] IFIS may complicate patients treated with all types of α_1-AR blockers, but it is most strongly associated with the uroselective α_1-AR blocker tamsulosin.[95,96]

Only a small number of drug-drug interactions with α_1-AR blocker are of clinical importance. Hypotension can be precipitated or exacerbated when an α_1-AR blocker is coadministered with any phosphodiesterase type 5 inhibitor (PDE5 inhibitor), although only tadalafil and vardenafil are specifically contraindicated in this setting. Verapamil and α_1-AR blockers may produce more orthostatic hypotension and dizziness than either drug alone. Postmenopausal women with pelvic relaxation syndrome can experience urinary incontinence resulting from α_1-AR blocker mediated relaxation of the bladder outlet; this can also occur in more unusual types of bladder dysfunction in either gender.

References

1. Parati G, Esler M. The human sympathetic nervous system: its relevance in hypertension and heart failure. *Eur Heart J.* 2012;33:1058-1066.
2. Charkoudian N, Joyner MJ, Johnson CP, Eisenach JH, Dietz NM, Wallin BG. Balance between cardiac output and sympathetic nerve activity in resting humans: role in arterial pressure regulation. *J Physiol.* 2005;568(Pt 1):315-321.
3. Mancia G, Grassi G. The autonomic nervous system and hypertension. *Circ Res.* 2014;114:1804-1814.
4. Horikoshi Y, Tajima I, Igarashi H, Inui M, Kasahara K, Noguchi T. The adreno-sympathetic system, the genetic predisposition to hypertension, and stress. *Am J Med Sci.* 1985;289:186-191.
5. Yamada Y, Miyajima E, Tochikubo O, et al. Impaired baroreflex changes in muscle sympathetic nerve activity in adolescents who have a family history of essential hypertension. *J Hypertens Suppl.* 1988;6:S525-S528.
6. Smith PA, Graham LN, Mackintosh AF, Stoker JB, Mary DA. Sympathetic neural mechanisms in white-coat hypertension. *J Am Coll Cardiol.* 2002;40:126-132.
7. Grassi G. Assessment of sympathetic cardiovascular drive in human hypertension: achievements and perspectives. *Hypertension.* 2009;54:690-697.
8. Julius S, Pascual AV, London R. Role of parasympathetic inhibition in the hyperkinetic type of borderline hypertension. *Circulation.* 1971;44:413-418.
9. Floras JS, Hara K. Sympathoneural and haemodynamic characteristics of young subjects with mild essential hypertension. *J Hypertens.* 1993;11:647-55.
10. Smith PA, Graham LN, Mackintosh AF, Stoker JB, Mary DA. Relationship between central sympathetic activity and stages of human hypertension. *Am J Hypertens.* 2004;17:217-22.
11. Burns J, Sivananthan MU, Ball SG, Mackintosh AF, Mary DA, Greenwood JP. Relationship between central sympathetic drive and magnetic resonance imaging-determined left ventricular mass in essential hypertension. *Circulation.* 2007;115:1999-2005.

12. Michelotti GA, Price DT, Schwinn DA. Alpha 1-adrenergic receptor regulation: basic science and clinical implications. *Pharmacol Ther.* 2000;88:281-309.

13. Cotecchia S. The alpha1-adrenergic receptors: diversity of signaling networks and regulation. *J Recept Signal Transduct Res.* 2010;30:410-419.

14. Rokosh DG, Simpson PC. Knockout of the alpha 1A/C-adrenergic receptor subtype: the alpha 1A/C is expressed in resistance arteries and is required to maintain arterial blood pressure. *Proc Natl Acad Sci USA.* 2002;99: 9474-8479.

15. Tanoue A, Nasa Y, Koshimizu T, et al. The alpha(1D)-adrenergic receptor directly regulates arterial blood pressure via vasoconstriction. *J Clin Invest.* 2002;109:765-775.

16. Rudner XL, Berkowitz DE, Booth JV, et al. Subtype specific regulation of human vascular alpha(1)-adrenergic receptors by vessel bed and age. *Circulation.* 1999;100:2336-2343.

17. Gradinaru I, Babaeva E, Schwinn DA, Oganesian A. Alpha1a-adrenoceptor genetic variant triggers vascular smooth muscle cell hyperproliferation and agonist induced hypertrophy via EGFR transactivation pathway. *PloS One.* 2015;10. e0142787.

18. Edvinsson L. Neurogenic mechanisms in the cerebrovascular bed. Autonomic nerves, amine receptors and their effects on cerebral blood flow. *Acta Physiol Scand Suppl.* 1975;427:1-35.

19. Ogoh S, Sato K, Fisher JP, Seifert T, Overgaard M, Secher NH. The effect of phenylephrine on arterial and venous cerebral blood flow in healthy subjects. *Clin Physio Funct Imaging.* 2011;31:445-451.

20. Brassard P, Seifert T, Secher NH. Is cerebral oxygenation negatively affected by infusion of norepinephrine in healthy subjects? *Br J Anaesth.* 2009;102:800-805.

21. Ogoh S, Brothers RM, Eubank WL, Raven PB. Autonomic neural control of the cerebral vasculature: acute hypotension. *Stroke.* 2008;39:1979-1987.

22. Purkayastha S, Saxena A, Eubank WL, Hoxha B, Raven PB. alpha1-Adrenergic receptor control of the cerebral vasculature in humans at rest and during exercise. *Exp Physiol.* 2013;98:451-461.

23. Jensen BC, O'Connell TD, Simpson PC. Alpha-1-adrenergic receptors in heart failure: the adaptive arm of the cardiac response to chronic catecholamine stimulation. *J Cardiovasc Pharmacol.* 2014;63:291-301.

24. Jensen BC, Swigart PM, De Marco T, Hoopes C, Simpson PC. {alpha}1-Adrenergic receptor subtypes in nonfailing and failing human myocardium. *Circ Heart Failure.* 2009;2:654-663.

25. Jensen BC, Swigart PM, Laden ME, DeMarco T, Hoopes C, Simpson PC. The alpha-1D Is the predominant alpha-1-adrenergic receptor subtype in human epicardial coronary arteries. *J Am Coll Cardiol.* 2009;54:1137-1145.

26. Major cardiovascular events in hypertensive patients randomized to doxazosin vs chlorthalidone: the antihypertensive and lipid-lowering treatment to prevent heart attack trial (ALLHAT). ALLHAT Collaborative Research Group. *JAMA.* 2000;283:1967-1975.

27. Antihypertensive, Lipid-Lowering Treatment to Prevent Heart Attack Trial Collaborative Research G. Diuretic versus alpha-blocker as first-step antihypertensive therapy: final results from the Antihypertensive and Lipid-Lowering Treatment to Prevent Heart Attack Trial (ALLHAT). *Hypertension.* 2003;42:239-246.

28. Chapman N, Chang CL, Dahlof B, et al. Effect of doxazosin gastrointestinal therapeutic system as third-line antihypertensive therapy on blood pressure and lipids in the Anglo-Scandinavian Cardiac Outcomes Trial. *Circulation.* 2008;118:42-48.

29. Hirano T, Yoshino G, Kashiwazaki K, Adachi M. Doxazosin reduces prevalence of small dense low density lipoprotein and remnant-like particle cholesterol levels in nondiabetic and diabetic hypertensive patients. *Am J Hypertens.* 2001;14(9 Pt 1):908-13.

30. Kinoshita M, Shimazu N, Fujita M, et al. Doxazosin, an alpha1-adrenergic antihypertensive agent, decreases serum oxidized LDL. *Am J Hypertens.* 2001;14:267-270.

31. Maheux P, Facchini F, Jeppesen J, et al. Changes in glucose, insulin, lipid, lipoprotein, and apoprotein concentrations and insulin action in doxazosin-treated patients with hypertension. Comparison between nondiabetic individuals and patients with non-insulin-dependent diabetes mellitus. *Am J Hypertens.* 1994;7:416-424.

32. Huupponen R HR, Lehtonen A, Vähätalo M. Effect of doxazosin on insulin sensitivity in hypertensive non-insulin dependent diabetic patients. *Eur J Clin Pharmacol.* 1992;43:365.

33. Hobbs FR, Khan T, Collins B. Doxazosin versus bendrofluazide: a comparison of the metabolic effects in British South Asians with hypertension. *Br J Gen Pract.* 2005;55:437-443.

34. Derosa GDG, Cicero AFG, D'Angelo A, et al. Synergistic effect of doxazosin and acarbose in improving metabolic control in patients with impaired glucose tolerance. *Clin Drug Invest.* 2006;26:529.

35. Shibasaki S, Eguchi K, Matsui Y, et al. Adrenergic blockade improved insulin resistance in patients with morning hypertension: the Japan Morning Surge-1 Study. *J Hypertens.* 2009;27:1252-1257.

36. Dell'Omo G, Penno G, Pucci L, et al. The vascular effects of doxazosin in hypertension complicated by metabolic syndrome. *Coron Artery Dis.* 2005;16:67-73.

37. Inukai T, Inukai Y, Matsutomo R, et al. Clinical usefulness of doxazosin in patients with type 2 diabetes complicated by hypertension: effects on glucose and lipid metabolism. *J Int Med Res.* 2004;32:206-213.

38. Liou YS, Chen HY, Tien L, Gu YS, Jong GP. Antihypertensive drug use and new-onset diabetes in female patients with coronary artery disease: a population-based longitudinal cohort study. *Medicine.* 2015;94:e1495.

39. Patane S. Insights into cardio-oncology: Polypharmacology of quinazoline-based alpha1-adrenoceptor antagonists. *World J Cardiol.* 2015;7:238-242.

40. Park MS, Kim BR, Dong SM, Lee SH, Kim DY, Rho SB. The antihypertension drug doxazosin inhibits tumor growth and angiogenesis by decreasing VEGFR-2/Akt/mTOR signaling and VEGF and HIF-1alpha expression. *Oncotarget.* 2014;5:4935-4944.

41. Patane S. Is there a role for quinazoline-based alpha (1)-adrenoceptor antagonists in cardio-oncology? *Cardiovasc Drugs Ther.* 2014;28:587-588.

42. Liu CM, Lo YC, Tai MH, et al. Piperazine-designed alpha 1A/alpha 1D-adrenoceptor blocker KMUP-1 and doxazosin provide down-regulation of androgen receptor and PSA in prostatic LNCaP cells growth and specifically in xenografts. *Prostate.* 2009;69:610-623.

43. McComb MN, Chao JY, Ng TM. Direct Vasodilators and Sympatholytic Agents. *J Cardiovasc Pharmacol Ther.* 2016;21:3-19.

44. Heran BS, Galm BP, Wright JM. Blood pressure lowering efficacy of alpha blockers for primary hypertension. *Cochrane Database Syst Rev.* 2009;(4):CD004643.

45. Fukiyama K, Omae T, Iimura O, et al. A double-blind comparative study of doxazosin and prazosin in the treatment of essential hypertension. *Am Heart J.* 1991;121(1 Pt 2):317-322.

46. Sega R, Marazzi ME, Bombelli M, et al. Comparison of the new alpha 1-blocker alfuzosin with propranolol as first-line therapy in hypertension. *Pharmacol Res.* 1991;24:41-52.

47. Itskovitz HD. Alpha 1-blockade for the treatment of hypertension: a megastudy of terazosin in 2214 clinical practice settings. *Clin Ther.* 1994;16:490-504.

48. Neaton JD, Grimm RH Jr., Prineas RJ, et al. Treatment of mild hypertension study. final results. treatment of mild hypertension study research group. *JAMA.* 1993;270:713-724.

49. Os I, Stokke HP. Effects of doxazosin in the gastrointestinal therapeutic system formulation versus doxazosin standard and placebo in mild-to-moderate hypertension. Doxazosin Investigators' Study Group. *J Cardiovasc Pharmacol.* 1999;33:791-797.

50. Davis BR, Cutler JA, Gordon DJ, et al. Rationale and design for the Antihypertensive and Lipid Lowering Treatment to Prevent Heart Attack Trial (ALLHAT). ALLHAT Research Group. *Am J Hypertens.* 1996;9(4 Pt 1):342-360.

51. Morlock R, Goodwin B, Gomez Rey G, Eaddy M. Clinical progression, acute urinary retention, prostate-related surgeries, and costs in patients with benign prostatic hyperplasia taking early versus delayed combination 5alpha-reductase inhibitor therapy and alpha-blocker therapy: a retrospective analysis. *Clin Ther.* 2013;35:624-633.

52. Piller LB, Davis BR, Cutler JA, et al. Validation of heart failure events in the Antihypertensive and Lipid Lowering Treatment to Prevent Heart Attack Trial (ALLHAT) participants assigned to doxazosin and chlorthalidone. *Curr Control Trials Cardiovasc Med.* 2002;3:10.

53. Davis BR, Cutler JA, Furberg CD, et al. Relationship of antihypertensive treatment regimens and change in blood pressure to risk for heart failure in hypertensive patients randomly assigned to doxazosin or chlorthalidone: further analyses from the Antihypertensive and Lipid-Lowering treatment to prevent Heart Attack Trial. *Ann Int Med.* 2002;137(5 Part 1):313-320.

54. Einhorn PT, Davis BR, Massie BM, et al. The Antihypertensive and Lipid Lowering Treatment to Prevent Heart Attack Trial (ALLHAT) Heart Failure Validation Study: diagnosis and prognosis. *Am Heart J.* 2007;153:42-53.

55. Davis BR, Kostis JB, Simpson LM, et al. Heart failure with preserved and reduced left ventricular ejection fraction in the antihypertensive and lipid-lowering treatment to prevent heart attack trial. *Circulation.* 2008;118:2259-2267.

56. Grimm RH, Davis BR, Piller LB, et al. Heart failure in ALLHAT: did blood pressure medication at study entry influence outcome? *J Clin Hypertens.* 2009;11:466-474.

57. Davis BR, Piller LB, Cutler JA, et al. Role of diuretics in the prevention of heart failure: the Antihypertensive and Lipid-Lowering Treatment to Prevent Heart Attack Trial. *Circulation.* 2006;113:2201-2210.

58. Poulter N, Williams B. Doxazosin for the management of hypertension: implications of the findings of the ALLHAT trial. *Am J Hypertens.* 2001;14(11 Pt 1):1170-2.

59. Messerli FH. Implications of discontinuation of doxazosin arm of ALLHAT. Antihypertensive and Lipid-Lowering Treatment to Prevent Heart Attack Trial. *Lancet.* 2000;355:863-864.

60. Furberg CD, Psaty BM, Pahor M, Alderman MH. Clinical implications of recent findings from the Antihypertensive and Lipid-Lowering Treatment To Prevent Heart Attack Trial (ALLHAT) and other studies of hypertension. *Ann Int Med.* 2001;135:1074-1078.

61. Chapman N, Chen CY, Fujita T, et al. Time to re-appraise the role of alpha-1 adrenoceptor antagonists in the management of hypertension? *J Hypertens.* 2010;28:1796-1803.

62. Stafford RS, Furberg CD, Finkelstein SN, Cockburn IM, Alehegn T, Ma J. Impact of clinical trial results on national trends in alpha-blocker prescribing, 1996-2002. *JAMA.* 2004;291:54-62.

63. Wright JT, Bakris G, Greene T, et al. Effect of blood pressure lowering and antihypertensive drug class on progression of hypertensive kidney disease: results from the AASK trial. *JAMA.* 2002;288:2421.

64. Bakris GL, Weir MR, Shanifar S, et al. Effects of blood pressure level on progression of diabetic nephropathy: results from the RENAAL study. *Arch Int Med.* 2003;163:1555.

65. Spoladore R, Roccaforte R, Fragasso G, et al. Safety and efficacy of doxazosin as an "add-on" antihypertensive therapy in mild to moderate heart failure patients. *Acta Cardiol.* 2009;64:485-491.

66. Lenfant C, Chobanian AV, Jones DW, Roccella EJ. Joint National Committee on the Prevention, Detection, Evaluation, and Treatment of High Blood Pressure. Seventh report of the Joint National Committee on the Prevention, Detection, Evaluation, and Treatment of High Blood Pressure (JNC 7): resetting the hypertension sails. *Hypertension.* 2003;41:1178-1179.

67. James PA, Oparil S, Carter BL, et al. 2014 evidence-based guideline for the management of high blood pressure in adults: report from the panel members appointed to the Eighth Joint National Committee (JNC 8). *JAMA.* 2014;311:507-520.

68. ESH/ESC Task Force for the Management of Arterial Hypertension. 2013 Practice guidelines for the management of arterial hypertension of the European Society of Hypertension (ESH) and the European Society of Cardiology (ESC): ESH/ESC Task Force for the Management of Arterial Hypertension. *J Hypertens.* 2013;31:1925-1938.

69. Daskalopoulou SS, Rabi DM, Zarnke KB, et al. The 2015 Canadian Hypertension Education Program recommendations for blood pressure measurement, diagnosis, assessment of risk, prevention, and treatment of hypertension. *The Can J Cardiol.* 2015;31:549-568.

70. Ritchie LD, Campbell NC, Murchie P. New NICE guidelines for hypertension. *BMJ.* 2011;343. d5644.

71. Mann SJ, Parikh NS. A simplified mechanistic algorithm for treating resistant hypertension: efficacy in a retrospective study. *J Clin Hypertens.* 2012;14:191-197.

72. Williams B, MacDonald TM, Morant S, et al. Spironolactone versus placebo, bisoprolol, and doxazosin to determine the optimal treatment for drug-resistant hypertension (PATHWAY-2): a randomised, double-blind, crossover trial. *Lancet.* 2015;386:2059-2068.

73. Brown MJ. Personalised medicine for hypertension. *BMJ.* 2011;343. d4697.

74. Wolak T, Toledano R, Novack V, Sharon A, Shalev A, Wolak A. Doxazosin to treat hypertension: it's time to take it personally—a retrospective analysis of 19,495 patients. *J Hypertens.* 2014;32:1132-1137. discussion 7.

75. Zaca F, Benassi A, Bolzani R, Stefanio C. Comparative effects of doxazosin and carvedilol on clinical status and left ventricular function in hypertensive patients with mild heart failure. *High Blood Press Cardiovasc Preven.* 2004;12:37-44.

76. Vongpatanasin W, Kario K, Atlas SA, Victor RG. Central sympatholytic drugs. *J Clin Hypertens.* 2011;13:658-661.

77. Lowry JA, Brown JT. Significance of the imidazoline receptors in toxicology. *Clin Toxicol.* 2014;52:454-469.

78. Head GA, Burke SL. I1 imidazoline receptors in cardiovascular regulation: the place of rilmenidine. *Am J Hypertens.* 2000;13(6 Pt 2):89S-98S.

79. Miller RR, Awan NA, Maxwell KS, Mason DT. Sustained reduction of cardiac impedance and preload in congestive heart failure with the antihypertensive vasodilator prazosin. *N Engl J Med.* 1977;297:303-307.

80. Awan NA, Miller RR, DeMaria AN, Maxwell KS, Neumann A, Mason DT. Efficacy of ambulatory systemic vasodilator therapy with oral prazosin in chronic refractory heart failure. Concomitant relief of pulmonary congestion and elevation of pump output demonstrated by improvements in symptomatology, exercise tolerance, hemodynamics and echocardiography. *Circulation.* 1977;56:346-354.

81. Cohn JN, Archibald DG, Ziesche S, et al. Effect of vasodilator therapy on mortality in chronic congestive heart failure. Results of a Veterans Administration Cooperative Study. *N Engl J Med.* 1986;314:1547-1552.

82. Ikeda T, Gomi T, Shibuya Y, Shinozaki S, Suzuki Y, Matsuda N. Add-on effect of bedtime dosing of the alpha(1)-adrenergic receptor antagonist doxazosin on morning hypertension and left ventricular hypertrophy in patients undergoing long-term amlodipine monotherapy. *Hypertens Res.* 2007;30:1097-1105.

83. Barrios V, Escobar C, Tomas JP, Calderon A, Echarri R. Comparison of the effects of doxazosin and atenolol on target organ damage in adults with type 2 diabetes mellitus and hypertension in the CARDHIAC study: a 9-month, prospective, randomized, open-label, blinded-evaluation trial. *Clin Therap.* 2008;30:98-107.

84. Yang W, Zhou YJ, Fu Y, et al. A multicenter, randomized, trial comparing urapidil and nitroglycerin in multifactor heart failure in the elderly. *Am J Med Sci.* 2015;350:109-115.

85. Roehrborn CG. Efficacy of alpha-Adrenergic receptor blockers in the treatment of male lower urinary tract symptoms. *Rev Urol.* 2009;11(Suppl 1):S1-S8.

86. Cantrell MA, Bream-Rouwenhorst HR, Hemerson P, Magera JS, Jr. Silodosin for benign prostatic hyperplasia. *Ann Pharmacother.* 2010;44:302-310.

87. Milani S, Djavan B. Lower urinary tract symptoms suggestive of benign prostatic hyperplasia: latest update on alpha-adrenoceptor antagonists. *BJU Int.* 2005;95(Suppl 4):29-36.

88. Chapple CR. Alpha-adrenergic blocking drugs in bladder outflow obstruction: what potential has alpha 1-adrenoceptor selectivity? *Br J Urol.* 1995;76(Suppl 1):47-55.

89. Zhang LTZLT, Lee SW, Park K, et al. Multicenter, prospective, comparative cohort study evaluating the efficacy and safety of alfuzosin 10 mg with regard to blood pressure in men with lower urinary tract symptoms suggestive of benign prostatic hyperplasia with or without antihypertensive medications. *Clin Interv Aging.* 2015;10:277.

90. Kinney MA, Warner ME, vanHeerden JA, et al. Perianesthetic risks and outcomes of pheochromocytoma and paraganglioma resection. *Anesth Analg.* 2000;91:1118-1123.

91. Ahmed A. Perioperative management of pheochromocytoma: anaesthetic implications. *J Pak Med Ass.* 2007;57:140-146.

92. Conzo G, Musella M, Corcione F, et al. Role of preoperative adrenergic blockade with doxazosin on hemodynamic control during the surgical treatment of pheochromocytoma: a retrospective study of 48 cases. *Am Surg.* 2013;79:1196-1202.

93. Lund-Johansen P, Kirby RS. Effect of doxazosin GITS on blood pressure in hypertensive and normotensive patients: a review of hypertension and BPH studies. *Blood Press Suppl.* 2003;1:5-13.

94. Santaella RM, Destafeno JJ, Stinnett SS, Proia AD, Chang DF, Kim T. The effect of alpha1-adrenergic receptor antagonist tamsulosin (Flomax) on iris dilator smooth muscle anatomy. *Ophthalmology.* 2010;117:1743-1749.

95. Chadha V, Borooah S, Tey A, Styles C, Singh J. Floppy iris behaviour during cataract surgery: associations and variations. *Br J Ophthalmol.* 2007;91:40-42.

96. Blouin MC, Blouin J, Perreault S, Lapointe A, Dragomir A. Intraoperative floppy-iris syndrome associated with alpha1-adrenoreceptors: comparison of tamsulosin and alfuzosin. *J Cataract Refract Surg.* 2007;33:1227-1234.

97. Chrischilles E, Rubenstein L, Chao J, Kreder KJ, Gilden D, Shah H. Initiation of nonselective alpha1-antagonist therapy and occurrence of hypotension-related adverse events among men with benign prostatic hyperplasia: a retrospective cohort study. *Clinical Ther.* 2001;23:727-743.

98. Souverein PC, Van Staa TP, Egberts AC, De la Rosette JJ, Cooper C, Leufkens HG. Use of alpha-blockers and the risk of hip/femur fractures. *J Int Med.* 2003;254:548-554.

99. Lai CL, Kuo RN, Chen HM, Chen MF, Chan KA, Lai MS. Risk of hip/femur fractures during the initiation period of alpha-adrenoceptor blocker therapy among elderly males: a self-controlled case series study. *Br J Clin Pharmacol.* 2015;80:1208-1218.

100. Lai CL, Kuo RN, Chen HM, Chen MF, Chan KA, Lai MS. Risk of ischemic stroke during the initiation period of α-blocker therapy among older men. *CMAJ.* 2016;188:255-260.

24 Renin Angiotensin Aldosterone System Blockers

Shigeru Shibata and Toshiro Fujita

The renin angiotensin aldosterone (RAA) system plays a central role in regulating cardiovascular and renal functions, and is a key component of the blood pressure homeostasis system in humans. Renal hypoperfusion triggers the production and release of renin from the juxtaglomerular cells, converting angiotensinogen to the decapeptide angiotensin I (angiotensin [1-10]). In the next step, the dipeptidyl-carboxyl peptidase angiotensin-converting enzyme (ACE) cleaves angiotensin I into angiotensin II (angiotensin [1-8]). Angiotensin II binds to the G protein-coupled receptor, angiotensin type 1 receptor (AT1R), and increases blood pressure by facilitating vascular constriction and by increasing sodium reabsorption in the kidney. Angiotensin II also stimulates the production of the steroid hormone aldosterone, the final product of the RAA cascade. The lipophilic hormone aldosterone passes through the plasma membrane of the target cells and binds to the nuclear receptor, mineralocorticoid receptor (MCR), in the cytoplasm of renal tubular cells. The aldosterone-MCR complex translocates into the nucleus and regulates the transcription of target genes, resulting in the upregulation of electrolyte flux pathways in the kidney. There are four classes of pharmacological agents that can block the RAA system; these are ACE inhibitors, angiotensin II receptor blockers (ARBs), renin inhibitors, and MCR antagonists.

ANGIOTENSIN-CONVERTING ENZYME INHIBITORS

ACE, also known as kininase II, is a metalloprotease with zinc at its active center. Besides the well-known role in converting angiotensin I (Ang I) to angiotensin II (Ang II), it promotes the degradation of bradykinin. Therefore, ACE positively controls the RAA system (which increases vasoconstriction, extracellular volume, and blood pressure) and negatively controls the kinin-kallikrein-bradykinin system (which promotes vasodilation). There are membrane-bound and soluble forms ACE. Membrane-bound ACE is an ectoenzyme, anchoring to the plasma membrane with the C-terminal hydrophobic portion.[1,2] The membrane-bound ACE is present in various tissues including the blood vessels, heart, kidneys, adrenal gland, and brain. The soluble form, which lacks the C-terminal anchor residues, is present in the plasma. ACE inhibitors affect both plasma and tissue ACE, blocking the generation of Ang II and suppressing the degradation of bradykinin.

Pharmacology of Angiotensin-Converting Enzyme Inhibitors

ACE inhibitors are classified according to the chemical structure of the site of binding (sulfhydryl, phosphinyl, carboxyl) to the active center of ACE. Captopril (the first ACE inhibitor to be developed) and alacepril (available in Japan) have a sulfhydryl moiety. ACE inhibitors with the sulfhydryl group may have properties different from those of other ACE inhibitors,

such as antioxidative action, although the clinical relevance remains unknown. This sulfhydryl group may also be involved in adverse events such as skin eruptions. Captopril has a short half-life of about two hours, and needs to be administered three times a day (Table 24.1). Alacepril produces captopril by releasing a phenylalanine after being deacetylated. ACE inhibitors with a carboxyl or phosphinyl moiety have a longer half-life, and are effective with a single daily dose. Fosinopril is unique in that it has a phosphinyl moiety at the ACE binding site. With the exception of captopril and lisinopril, ACE inhibitors are prodrugs that are metabolized into their active forms when absorbed from the intestinal tract. As for the route of elimination, trandolapril, fosinopril, benazepril, and temocapril are metabolized by both the liver and kidney; other ACE inhibitors are renally excreted, and serum levels can be elevated in subjects with reduced kidney function.

Mechanisms of Action

The antihypertensive effects of ACE inhibitors can involve the inhibition of both Ang II production and bradykinin degradation. The diverse actions of Ang II include vascular smooth muscle cell contraction, secretion of aldosterone from the adrenal cortex, and the direct effects on renal tubules to increase Na-Cl reabsorption. Bradykinin, a polypeptide composed of nine amino acids, acts on the bradykinin B1 and B2 G protein-coupled receptors, and induces the production of prostacyclin and nitric oxide in the vascular endothelium, resulting in vasodilation. ACE inhibitors increase Ang I by blocking its conversion to Ang II. This may result in the increased formation of Ang(1-7) by ACE2, a homologue of ACE, and stimulate the Mas G protein-coupled receptors.[3,4] The Ang(1-7)-Mas receptor system regulates vascular tone and acts to antagonize AT1R signaling. These effects may also play a role, although their clinical relevance has not been demonstrated.

The importance of tissue ACE activity is confirmed by an animal model that expresses ACE lacking the C-terminal region.[5] In this model, ACE is catalytically active but is entirely secreted from the cells. The mice exhibit significant plasma ACE activity with no tissue ACE activity, resulting in profound hypotension. ACE inhibitors are capable of antagonizing plasma as well as tissue ACE; however, the extent of the ACE inhibiting activity may vary depending on the tissues. For example, a single oral dose of lisinopril suppressed plasma ACE activity at 4 hours but not at 24 hours.[6] In contrast, the same dose of lisinopril continued to inhibit ACE through 24 hours in the kidney.[6]

Blood Pressure-Lowering Effect and Combination With Other Antihypertensives

ACE inhibitors lower both systolic and diastolic blood pressure in hypertensive patients, and are recommended as a first-line therapy in the Eighth Report of the Joint National Committee

TABLE 24.1 Angiotensin-Converting Enzyme Inhibitors: Dosage Strengths and Treatment Guidelines

DRUG	TRADE NAME (IN UNITED STATES)	USUAL TOTAL DOSE AND/OR RANGE—HYPERTENSION (FREQUENCY/DAY)	USUAL TOTAL DOSE AND/OR RANGE—HEART FAILURE (FREQUENCY/DAY)
Benazepril	Lotensin	20-40 (1)	Not FDA approved for heart failure
Captopril	Capoten	12.5-100 (2-3)	18.75-150 (3)
Enalapril	Vasotec	5-40 (1-2)	5-40 (2)
Fosinopril	Monopril	10-40 (1)	10-40 (1)
Lisinopril	Prinivil, Zestril	2.5-40 (1)	5-20 (1)
Moexipril	Univasc	7.5-30 (1)	Not FDA approved for heart failure
Perindopril	Aceon	2-16 (1)	Not FDA approved for heart failure
Quinapril	Accupril	5-80 (1)	10-40 (1-2)
Ramipril	Altace	2.5-20 (1)	10 (2)
Trandolapril	Mavik	1-8 (1)	1-4 (1)

FDA, United States Food and Drug Administration.

on Prevention, Detection, Evaluation, and Treatment of High Blood Pressure (JNC 8).[7] Unlike Ca^{2+} channel blockers (CCBs) and other antihypertensives, ACE inhibitors reduce vascular resistance but have little effect on heart rate. The increase in the heart rate in response to postural change is usually maintained during treatment with ACE inhibitors, and the frequency of orthostatic hypotension is low. ACE inhibitors also inhibit both central and peripheral sympathetic nerve activation by Ang II.

Although ACE inhibitors are generally effective in the treatment of hypertension, its efficacy seems weaker in the African-American hypertensive population. In the Antihypertensive and Lipid-Lowering Treatment to Prevent Heart Attack Trial (ALLHAT), thiazide diuretics were superior to lisinopril in suppressing stroke and cardiovascular events in African Americans.[8] The antihypertensive effects of ACE inhibitors also tend to be weaker in patients with a high salt intake[9] presumably because of the suppressed RAA system. Conversely, as a result of the compensatory activation of RAA system, the combination with a thiazide diuretic enhances the effect of ACE inhibitors. The Perindopril Protection Against Recurrent Stroke Study (PROGRESS) showed that combining an ACE inhibitor perindopril with a thiazide indapamide provides a synergistic antihypertensive effect, and that the combination of the two drugs is effective in preventing stroke recurrence.[10]

Combination with a Ca^{2+} channel blocker (CCB) is also effective in controlling blood pressure. The Anglo-Scandinavian Cardiac Outcomes Trial-Blood Pressure Lowering Arm (ASCOT-BPLA) showed that combining an ACE inhibitor perindopril with a CCB amlodipine was superior to the combination of atenolol and bendroflumethiazide in preventing cardiovascular events.[11] In the Avoiding Cardiovascular Events in Combination Therapy in Patients Living with Systolic Hypertension (ACCOMPLISH) trial,[12] combining benazepril with amlodipine offered superior antihypertensive effects and suppression of the onset of cardiovascular events as compared with combination with hydrochlorothiazide in high-risk hypertensive patients, and also suppressed the progression of kidney damage. However, in the Gauging Albuminuria Reduction with Lotrel in Diabetic Patients with Hypertension (GUARD) study, antialbuminuric effect of combining benazepril with amlodipine was inferior to the combination with hydrochlorothiazide in diabetic patients.[13]

Combining ACE inhibitors and angiotensin receptor blockers (ARBs) has been reported to increase adverse events such as acute kidney damage and hyperkalemia in several clinical trials, including the Ongoing Telmisartan Alone and in Combination with Ramipril Global Endpoint Trial (ONTARGET)

and the Veterans Affairs Nephropathy in Diabetes (VA NEPHRON-D) study.[14,15] Currently, combining these drugs is not recommended.

End-Organ Effects and Clinical Trials

Cardiac Effects

Heart Failure and Left Ventricular Dysfunction After Myocardial Infarction

ACE inhibitors reduce preload and afterload, and increase the cardiac output without increasing the heart rate. ACE inhibitors can also inhibit chronic activation of the tissue renin angiotensin system involved in the pathogenesis of left ventricular (LV) dysfunction.

The Cooperative North Scandinavian Enalapril Survival Study (CONSENSUS) was the first to show that combining ACE inhibitors with other medications for heart failure reduces the risk of death.[16] In this trial, the ACE inhibitor enalapril significantly inhibited the progression of heart failure and death in patients with New York Heart Association (NYHA) class IV heart failure. Following this trial, the Studies of Left Ventricular Dysfunction (SOLVD) treatment trial showed that enalapril reduces all-cause mortality in NYHA class II and III cases,[17] verifying the prognosis-improving effects of ACE inhibitors in these patient groups as well. The SOLVD prevention trial also compared enalapril with a placebo in patients with LV dysfunction (ejection fraction < 35%) who had no prior history of heart failure,[18] and showed that enalapril significantly reduces cardiovascular mortality. These clinical trials have had a major impact on the management of chronic heart failure by showing the efficacy of long-acting ACE inhibitors.

ACE inhibitors also improve the prognosis of reduced systolic function after myocardial infarction. The Survival And Ventricular Enlargement (SAVE) trial evaluated whether or not beginning captopril administration early after the onset of LV dysfunction following acute myocardial infarction (AMI) improves the long-term prognosis.[19] The study showed that when compared with a placebo, captopril significantly reduced total and cardiovascular mortality, and suppressed the progression to severe heart failure and the recurrence of AMI. Usefulness in reduced systolic function after MI has been consistently shown for other ACE inhibitors, such as ramipril, lisinopril, trandolapril, and zofenopril.[20-23] In the CONSENSUS II trial, which evaluated the efficacy of early administration of enalapril for patients after AMI, the use of the ACE inhibitor did not reduce overall mortality.[24] In this study, intravenous administration of enalapril within 24 hours after MI resulted in hypotensive (<90 mm Hg) episodes in 12% (placebo 3%; $p < 0.001$), and the timing and amount of ACE inhibitor administration possibly affected the results. Given these data, initiation of oral ACE inhibitors is recommended in patients with stable hemodynamics after MI, especially if LV function has been reduced. However, the optimal dose and timing are unknown, and hemodynamic parameters need to be monitored to prevent excessive lowering of blood pressure. Because several ACE inhibitors have been consistently found to benefit survival, their effect on cardiac dysfunction following MI is likely to be the class effect. In the Perindopril in Elderly People with Chronic Heart Failure (PEP-CHF) trial, the clinical efficacy of the ACE inhibitor in diastolic heart failure patients with preserved systolic function (HFpEF) was not observed on the primary endpoint of combined all-cause mortality and unexpected hospitalization for heart failure, despite significant improvements in functional class and six-minute walk distance.[25]

Atherosclerotic Vascular Disease

The Heart Outcomes Prevention Evaluation (HOPE) study investigated the protective effects of ramipril in patients with preserved LV function who had evidence of vascular disease or diabetes with one other risk factor for cardiovascular disease.[26] In this trial, the ACE inhibitor significantly suppressed the incidence of primary endpoint, which was the composite of cardiovascular death, myocardial infarction, and stroke. A majority of patients in this study had a systolic blood pressure of 140 mm Hg or lower, and changes in blood pressure caused by therapeutic intervention were modest at 2 to 3 mm Hg, indicating that ACE inhibitors have an action independent of blood pressure. The suggested mechanisms include the improvement in vascular endothelial function via Ang II inhibition and bradykinin induction, or an improvement in fibrinolytic balance by suppressing plasminogen activator inhibitor and inducing tissue plasminogen activator (tPA). Similarly, The European Trial on Reduction of Cardiac events with Perindopril in Stable Coronary Artery Disease (EUROPA) study showed that in patients with stable coronary artery diseases, perindopril suppressed primary endpoint (cardiovascular death, myocardial infarction, or cardiac arrest).[27] However, in the Prevention of Events with Angiotensin-Converting Enzyme inhibition (PEACE) study, which included patients with stable coronary artery disease with preserved ejection fraction, adding trandolapril did not reduce cardiovascular events.[28] In this study, 70% of patients had already received lipid-lowering therapy and 72% had already received revascularization. Therefore, uncertainty remains about the protective effects of ACE inhibitors in the lower risk group.

Renal Effects

ACE inhibitors exert renoprotective actions by antagonizing the various injurious effects of Ang II, most importantly by lowering the intraglomerular pressure and improving hyperfiltration through the dilatation of renal efferent arterioles. The Ramipril Efficacy In Nephropathy (REIN) trial tested the protective effects of an ACE inhibitor ramipril in patients with decreased glomerular filtration rate (GFR) or overt proteinuria, and showed that the ACE inhibitor reduces the risk of end-stage kidney disease.[29] In the post hoc analysis, the rate of GFR decline (delta GFR) was compared within three tertiles of basal GFR. The study showed that Ramipril decreased delta GFR by 22%, 22%, and 35% in the lowest, middle, and highest tertiles, respectively, demonstrating that the renoprotective effects of ACE inhibitors do not depend on the stage of the chronic kidney disease (CKD).[30]

The United States Food and Drug Administration (FDA) has approved captopril for the treatment of type 1 diabetic nephropathy, based on the study showing that captopril inhibits the progression of nephropathy in type 1 diabetes.[31] The African American Study of Kidney Disease and Hypertension (AASK) study, which evaluated the usefulness of ACE inhibitors in African Americans with hypertensive kidney damage, reported that ramipril can have a protective effect in slowing GFR decline compared with amlodipine or metoprolol, especially in patients with proteinuria (Uprot/Cr >0.22), whereas strict control of blood pressure did not slow progression of kidney disease in this population.[32]

On the basis of the above evidence, the JNC 8 recommends ACE inhibitors (and ARBs) as first-line treatment for hypertension complicated by CKD at ages 18 years and up, for all races, irrespective of whether the patient has diabetes or not.[7]

Diabetes

ACE inhibitors are preferably used in patients with hypertension and diabetes, based on the evidence that these agents effectively reduce blood pressure and that they prevent the progression of atherosclerotic complications. Unlike diuretics or beta-blockers, ACE inhibitors do not decrease insulin sensitivity. Rather, some studies show that these agents may have favorable effects on glycemic control. In the Diabetes Reduction Assessment with ramipril and rosiglitazone Medication (DREAM) study, which included patients with fasting hyperglycemia or impaired glucose tolerance, ramipril promoted the regression to normal glycemia (the onset of diabetes was not prevented by the ACE inhibitor).[33] A meta-analysis published in 2011 also reported that ACE inhibitors and ARBs reduce the new onset of diabetes.[34] Notably, the 5-year treatment of valsartan, an angiotensin receptor blocker, along with lifestyle modification, in patients with impaired glucose tolerance and cardiovascular disease or risk factors led to a decrease of 14% in the incidence of diabetes but did not reduce the rate of cardiovascular events.[35]

Adverse Effects and Important Drug Interactions

A decrease in GFR associated with the use of ACE inhibitors is usually functional and reversible, and discontinuing ACE inhibitors returns serum creatinine to baseline levels. Nonetheless, patients with renal artery stenosis and other causes of renal hypoperfusion (e.g., hypovolemia and congestive heart failure), those taking nonsteroidal antiinflammatory drugs (NSAIDs), cyclosporine, or vasoconstrictor agents, and subjects with CKD have increased risk of having progressive deterioration of kidney function with ACE inhibitors (Fig. 24.1). The combined use of ACE inhibitors with mineralocorticoid receptor antagonists or other potassium-sparing diuretics increases the risk of hyperkalemia and necessitates careful monitoring of serum K^+ levels and kidney function.

The use of ACE inhibitors in pregnant women is contraindicated because they cause oligohydramnios and congenital anomalies, such as fetal limb deformities, growth retardation, and renal dysfunction (Table 24.2). A dry cough is observed in 20% to 30% of cases and is particularly frequent in Asian people. This is attributed to the enhanced activity of bradykinin; the symptom resolves quickly by discontinuing the ACE inhibitors. ACE inhibitors may improve airway sensitivity and have been reported to reduce the risk of pneumonia in elderly people with hypertension,[36] likely via the inhibition of bradykinin and substance P degradation.

Though rare, angioneurotic edema is a serious adverse effect, which is reported to occur in 0.1% to 0.2% of patients taking an ACE inhibitor. The actual incidence may be higher given that the Omapatrilat Cardiovascular Treatment versus Enalapril (OCTAVE) study reported angioedema in 86 of 12,634 cases (0.68%).[37] Angioneurotic edema is commonly seen in the face and upper respiratory tract, but can also involve the intestine in some cases, causing gastrointestinal symptoms including abdominal pain and diarrhea. Combined use of dipeptidyl peptidase 4 (DPP-4) inhibitors may increase the risk of angioneurotic edema.[38]

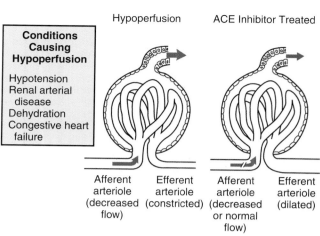

FIG. 24.1 Schematic illustration of settings in which angiotensin-converting enzyme (ACE) inhibitor and angiotensin receptor blocker (ARB) may worsen renal function. Conditions causing renal hypoperfusion include systemic hypotension, high-grade renal artery stenosis, extracellular fluid volume contraction (simplified as "dehydration"), and administration of vasoconstrictor agents (nonsteroidal antiinflammatory drugs or cyclosporine, not shown), and heart failure. These conditions typically increase renin secretion and Ang II production. Ang II constricts the efferent arteriole to a greater extent than the afferent arteriole, such that glomerular hydrostatic pressure and the glomerular filtration rate (GFR) can be maintained despite hypoperfusion. *(Adapted with permission from Schoolwerth AC, Sica DA, Ballermann BJ, Wilcox CS. Renal considerations in angiotensin converting enzyme inhibitor therapy: a statement for healthcare professionals from the Council on the Kidney in Cardiovascular Disease and the Council for High Blood Pressure Research of the American Heart Association. Circulation. 2001;104:1985-1991.)*

TABLE 24.2 Congenital Anomalies Associated With the Use of Angiotensin-Converting Enzyme Inhibitors or Angiotensin Receptor Blockers in Early Pregnancy

	ACE INHIBITORS	ARBS (N [%])
Central nervous system	9 (20.9)	1 (8.3)
Cardiovascular system	8 (18.6)	1 (8.3)
Renal-urologic system	5 (11.6)	5 (41.7)
Skeletal	4 (9.3)	1 (8.3)
Pulmonary	0	1 (8.3)
Gastrointestinal	3 (7.0)	0
Other	9 (20.9)	0
Not specified	5 (11.6)	1 (8.3)
Total	43 (100)	12 (100)

(Reports from the UK Medicine and Healthcare Products Regulatory Agency [Yellow Card system]. Adapted from Karthikeyan VJ, Ferner RE, Baghdadi S, et al. Are angiotensin-converting enzyme inhibitors and angiotensin receptor blockers safe in pregnancy: a report of ninety-one pregnancies. J Hypertens. 2011;29:396-399.) ACE, Angiotensin-converting enzyme; ARB, angiotensin receptor blockers.

The use of ACE inhibitors is contraindicated in patients undergoing dialysis using acrylonitrile membranes, and those receiving immunoadsorption therapy using a dextran-sulfate or tryptophan-immobilized polyvinyl alcohol column, because the concomitant use can cause anaphylactoid reactions as a result of excessive activation of the kinin-kallikrein-bradykinin system.

ANGIOTENSIN II RECEPTOR BLOCKERS

The AT1R is predominantly expressed in the heart, kidneys, blood vessels, brain, and adrenal glands, and is involved in multiple functions including cardiomyocyte and vascular smooth muscle contraction, aldosterone biosynthesis, release of catecholamines from the nerve endings, and Na-Cl reabsorption in the kidney. Ang II and AT1R also act to promote cell growth and proliferation, thereby accelerating target organ dysfunction. ARBs or "sartans" inhibit these actions of Ang II by binding to AT1R. About 20% to 30% of systemic Ang II is produced via an alternative pathway rather than through ACE, such as through chymases, but ARBs also block these signals at the receptor level. The degradation of bradykinin by ACE is not inhibited, and coughing and angioedema occur much less frequently than ACE inhibitors.

Pharmacology of Angiotensin II Receptor Blockers

The use of saralasin (1-sar-8-ala-angiotensin II) in subjects with elevated plasma renin activity has provided evidence that the agents that block binding of Ang II to angiotensin receptor may be used to treat hypertension, although saralasin itself has low bioavailability. Subsequently, researchers at Takeda found that benzimidazoles (compound CV-2198 and CV-2961) have an AT1R inhibitory effect, and scientists at DuPont finally developed the first ARB losartan based on the structure of these lead compounds. Currently, eight ARBs are commercially available, and all have a high affinity for AT1R (Table 24.3). The interactions between ARBs and the receptor are hydrophobic bonds between the phenyl group and AT1R, and an ionic interaction between the acidic moiety and AT1R, representing a common mechanism. Losartan has a biphenyl moiety and an acidic tetrazole group; candesartan, valsartan, irbesartan, and olmesartan all have a backbone similar to losartan. In telmisartan, the tetrazole has been substituted with a carboxyl group; in azilsartan, the tetrazole is replaced by the 5-oxo 1,2,4 oxadiazole group. In eprosartan, the biphenyl tetrazole has been substituted with benzoic acid.

Each ARB has different characteristics in terms of absorption, metabolism, and half-life. Losartan has a short half-life of 2 hours, but is metabolized into EXP-3174, which is an active metabolite with a half-life of 6 to 9 hours. Telmisartan, the longest-acting ARB, has a half-life of 24 hours. The half-lives of the other ARBs are in between these extremes. The pharmacological activity of ARBs is affected by the half-life as well as by the dissociation from the receptor. Off rate of ARBs from the receptor is generally low, and their antihypertensive effects can last longer than the half-life.

Candesartan cilexetil and olmesartan medoxomil are prodrugs with improved bioavailability and are completely hydrolyzed and converted into candesartan and olmesartan, respectively, during absorption. Azilsartan medoxomil (available in the Unites States and in Europe) is the prodrug of azilsartan (available in Japan); the former is absorbed in the gastrointestinal tract and is metabolized into azilsartan by ester hydrolysis. The excretion route varies among ARBs; telmisartan and irbesartan are metabolized predominantly by the liver, whereas other ARBs are excreted by both hepatic and renal routes. Clinically, there are no reliable measurements for Ang II inhibition and the optimal dose is determined by the antihypertensive effects, changes in GFR, and serum K^+ levels. Serum aldosterone levels may be used but they are also affected by serum K^+ and ACTH.

Among the ARBs, losartan has a unique property in increasing uric acid excretion, thereby decreasing serum uric acid levels. Losartan can inhibit uric acid reabsorption in the proximal tubules by binding to URAT1 (urate transporter 1). Indeed, several clinical studies have shown that losartan lowers serum uric acid levels, and at least some of the organ-protective effects of losartan may originate from this action.[39] The American College of Rheumatology Guidelines for Management of Gout include losartan as a uricosuric agent, although this is an off-label use. Among the other ARBs, irbesartan and telmisartan also can have a URAT1-inhibiting

TABLE 24.3 Pharmacologic Properties of Angiotensin II Receptor Blockers Available in the United States

PARAMETER	LOSARTAN POTASSIUM	VALSARTAN	IRBESARTAN	CANDESARTAN CILEXETIL	TELMISARTAN	EPROSARTAN	OLMESARTAN MEDOXOMIL	AZILSARTAN MEDOXOMIL
U.S. Trade Name	Cozaar	Diovan	Avapro	Atacand	Micardis	Teveten	Benicar	Edarbi
Manufacturer/Marketer	Merck & Co., Inc., Generic	Novartis Pharmaceuticals Corporation	Bristol-Myers Squibb/Sanofi-Aventis Partnership	AstraZeneca, L.P.	Boehringer Ingleheim	Abbott Laboratories	Daiichi Sankyo Inc.	Takeda Pharmaceuticals US
Doses available	50, 100	40, 80, 160, 320	75, 150, 300	4, 8, 16, 32	40, 80	400, 600	5, 20, 40	40, 80
Usual initial dose (mg/day)	50	80	150	8	40	600	20	40
Dosing frequency (per day)	1-2	1	1	1-2	1	1-2	1	1
Oral bioavailability	33%	23%	60%-80%	15%	42%-58%	13%	26%	60%
Prodrug?	Yes	No	No	Yes	No	No	Yes	Yes
Active metabolite?	EXP3174	No	No	Candesartan	No	No	Olmesartan	Azilsartan
Plasma elimination half-life (hour)	1.5-2.0 (or 6-9, for EXP3174)	6	11-15	5-9	24	5-9	12-15	11
Renal/hepatic elimination (%)	10/90 (or 50/50 for EXP3174)	30/70	1/99	60/40	1/99	30/70	10/90 (age-dependent)	55/42
Trough/peak ratio (at dose, in mg)	58-78 (50-100)	69-76 (80-160)	>60 (≥150)	80 (8-16)	≥97 (20-80)	67 (600)	57-70 (5-80)	~70 (80)
Dose Adjustment for:								
eGFR <30 mL/min/1.73 m²	No	Caution	Caution	Caution	No	No	No	No
Hepatic impairment	Yes, decrease by 50%	Caution	No	No	Caution	No	No	No
Dialyzable	No	No	No	No	No	No	Uncertain	No
FDA-Approved for:								
Hypertension	Yes	Yes	Yes	Yes	Yes	Yes	Yes	Yes
Severe hypertension	Yes	No	No	No	No	No	No	No
Prevention of ESRD in type 2 diabetic nephropathy	Yes	No	Yes	No	No	No	No	No
Prevention of progression of type 2 diabetic nephropathy	Yes	No	Yes	No	No	No	No	No
Heart failure in patients intolerant of ACE inhibitors	No	Yes	No	Yes	No	No	No	No
Heart failure	No	Yes	No	Yes	No	No	No	No
Prevention of stroke in hypertensive patients with left ventricular hypertrophy	Yes	No	No	No	No	No	No	No
Prevention of cardiovascular events in "high-risk" hypertensives	No	No	No	No	Yes (80-mg dose, in ACE-intolerant patients)	No	No	No
Available in combination with	HCTZ	HCTZ, amlodipine, aliskiren, HCTZ + amlodipine	HCTZ	HCTZ	HCTZ, amlodipine	HCTZ	HCTZ, amlodipine, HCTZ + amlodipine	Chlorthalidone

ACE, Angiotensin-converting enzyme; eGFR, estimated glomerular filtration rate; ESRD, end-stage renal disease; FDA, United States Food and Drug Administration; HCTZ, hydrochlorothiazide.

action in vitro, but it is not clear whether or not these ARBs have a clinically significant uric acid-lowering action. Other drug effects include activation of peroxisome proliferator-activated receptor γ (PPARγ) and an inverse agonist action, but the clinical significance of these effects has not been established.

Mechanisms of Action

Inhibition of AT1R signaling is a central mechanism of the antihypertensive action of ARBs. In addition to ACE, Ang II is produced via alternative pathways, such as via chymases ("Ang II escape"), but ARBs block binding of Ang II to AT1R regardless of the source. AT1R is found in the heart, kidneys, blood vessels, brain, adrenal glands, and elsewhere; clinically, it is unclear which organ is responsible for the antihypertensive effects of ARBs. However, basic research using tissue-specific AT1R knockout animals has shown the importance of AT1R in the renal tubules and vascular smooth muscle. Proximal tubular cell-specific AT1R knockout in mice decrease blood pressure through increased urinary sodium excretion.[40] Similarly, vascular smooth muscle cell-specific AT1R knockout mice show reduced blood pressure caused by increased renal blood flow and natriuresis.[41]

Stimulation of AT2R and Ang(1-7)/Mas receptor signaling may also contribute to the depressor effects of ARBs. ARBs increase plasma Ang II levels via a negative feedback mechanism, which results in either binding to AT2R or the formation of Ang(1-7) by ACE2, a homologue of ACE. Ang(1-7) then binds to the Mas receptor, a G protein-coupled receptor. Generally, these two pathways have actions to counteract AT1R signaling. In an animal model, systemic infusion of Compound 21, a selective AT2 receptor agonist, induces natriuresis and lowers blood pressure in angiotensin II-infused rat.[42] ACE2-deficient mice show increased blood pressure,[43] although this is associated with increased Ang II accumulation in the kidney. Clinically, the contribution of AT2R signaling and Ang(1-7)/Mas receptor axis in patients taking ARBs has not been fully elucidated.

Blood Pressure-Lowering Effect and Combination With Other Antihypertensives

ARBs are one of the four classes of antihypertensive agents recommended in the general hypertensive population in JNC 8 except in African Americans.[7] Similar to ACE inhibitors, combined use of ARBs with thiazide diuretics enhances blood pressure-lowering effects, because ARBs suppress compensatory activation of the RAA system during thiazide treatment. Combined treatment with ARBs and CCBs is also useful in blood pressure control. In the Reduction of Endpoints in NIDDM with the Angiotensin II Antagonist Losartan (RENAAL) study, which investigated the effectiveness of losartan in type 2 diabetes and diabetic nephropathy, 80% of subjects received CCBs.[44] Single-pill triple-combinations of ARBs, CCBs, and diuretics (valsartan or olmesartan/amlodipine/hydrochlorothiazide) are also in clinical use.

Use of ACE inhibitors and ARBs together in the same patient is not recommended. In The ONTARGET trial, the combination therapy of ramipril and telmisartan was not effective in suppressing primary effects, but did significantly increase adverse events including kidney damage, hyperkalemia, and symptomatic hypotension.[14] The Aliskiren Trial in Type 2 Diabetes Using Cardio-Renal Endpoints (ALTITUDE) trial, which examined the effects of combining the renin inhibitor aliskiren with an ACE inhibitor or ARB, also found that there was no suppression of cardiovascular events, whereas hyperkalemia and other adverse events were increased.[45]

Neprilysin Inhibitor and Angiotensin II Receptor Blockers

LCZ696, a novel compound composed of valsartan and sacubitril, an inhibitor of neprilysin, a neutral endopeptidase (NEP), provides simultaneous neprilysin inhibition and AT1R blockade. Both the greater increase of natriuretic peptides and reduction of aldosterone with LCZ696 over valsartan is consistent with the simultaneous blockade of the AT1-receptor and enhancement of the NEP system. These results support further development of LCZ696 for the management of cardiovascular diseases. The Prospective Comparison of ARNI with ACEI to Determine Impact on Global Mortality and Morbidity in Heart Failure (PARADIGM-HF) trial showed that LCZ696 was superior to enalapril in reducing the rates of death from cardiovascular causes or hospitalization for heart failure and death from any cause among patients with heart failure and a reduced ejection fraction (HFrEF).[46] In the Prospective Comparison of ARNI with ARB on Management of Heart Failure with Preserved Ejection Fraction (PARAMOUNT) study, LCZ696 reduced NT-proBNP and left atrial size in HFpEF patients, each powerful predictors of outcome in heart failure,[47] although the outcomes studied are surrogate endpoints and larger trials testing the effect of LCZ696 on morbidity and mortality in patients with heart failure and a preserved ejection fraction (HFpEF) may be needed.

End-Organ Effects and Clinical Trials
Cardiac Effects

Given that ARBs and ACE inhibitors block the RAA system at distinct levels, the cardioprotective effects of ARBs have been evaluated in large-scale clinical trials. The Losartan Intervention For Endpoint reduction (LIFE) study is a double-blind, randomized trial comparing the effects of the ARB losartan and the β-blocker atenolol on blood pressure in patients presenting with LV hypertrophy on electrocardiography.[48] In this study, the losartan group had a significantly reduced occurrence of the primary endpoint, a composite of cardiovascular death, nonfatal MI, and stroke. However, in the breakdown of mortality rates, the effect of preventing the primary endpoint was mainly derived from stroke prevention (-25%; $p = 0.0010$), and the effect of suppressing the onset of MI, which was expected in light of the established effects of ACE inhibitors on heart failure, was largely equivalent to that of atenolol ($p = 0.49$).

The Losartan Heart Failure Survival (ELITE-II) trial, which compared the efficacy of the ARB losartan and the ACE inhibitor captopril in patients with symptomatic heart failure, found that losartan was better tolerated, but that the two did not show a significant difference in overall mortality.[49] The Optimal Trial in Myocardial Infarction with Angiotensin II Antagonist Losartan (OPTIMAAL) trial, comparing losartan and captopril in heart failure after MI, did not find a significant difference but did show a tendency for mortality to be higher in the losartan group (18% versus 16%; $p = 0.07$).[50]

The Valsartan Heart Failure Trial (Val-HeFT) investigated the efficacy of valsartan in heart failure when added to standard therapy including an ACE inhibitor and beta-blocker.[51] The addition of valsartan was not associated with a decrease in overall mortality, and reduced only the combined endpoint of mortality and morbidity, such as hospitalization for heart failure and receipt of intravenous inotropic or vasodilator therapy. Subgroup analysis showed an overall mortality-improving effect in patients not taking an ACE inhibitor. However, administering valsartan was associated with increased mortality in patients who were taking both an ACE inhibitor and a beta-blocker.[51]

The Candesartan in Heart failure: Assessment of moRtality and Morbidity (CHARM) trial investigated whether or not candesartan reduces mortality and complications in chronic heart failure, and was composed of the following: CHARM-Alternative, evaluating the effects in cases where ACE inhibitor were not tolerated; CHARM-Added, investigating combined use of candesartan and an ACE inhibitor; and CHARM-Preserved, investigating the efficacy in heart failure with ejection fraction greater than 40%.[52] Of these, CHARM-Alternative showed that candesartan suppresses cardiovascular death and exacerbation of heart failure in cases that are intolerant of ACE inhibitors (33% versus 40%; p = 0.0004).[53] In the CHARM-Added study, with a mean follow-up period of 41 months, candesartan significantly reduced the incidence of the primary endpoint (composite of cardiovascular death or hospital admission for congestive heart failure) as well as cardiovascular mortality, as compared with a placebo.[54] Unlike the results of the Val-HeFT study,[51] it was reported that the candesartan group had a reduced incidence of the primary endpoint, even in cases taking both an ACE inhibitor and a β-blocker. In the CHARM-Preserved study, however, treatment with candesartan was associated with a nonsignificant reduction in the primary endpoint of cardiovascular death or heart failure hospitalizations in patients with preserved systolic function (HFpEF).[55] In the I-PRESERVE study,[56] irbesartan did not improve the outcomes of HFpEF patients. These results are compatible with those of studies using ACE inhibitors.

The VALsartan In Acute myocardial iNfarcTion (VALIANT) trial investigated the efficacy (noninferiority) of valsartan, captopril, or combination therapy in AMI patients with complicating LV systolic failure or heart failure.[57] The trial found that overall mortality was equivalent in the valsartan and captopril groups, and showed that valsartan is noninferior to captopril. Combined use, however, was found to increase adverse events.

The ONTARGET trial investigated whether the ARB telmisartan is as effective as the ACE inhibitor ramipril in patients at high risk for cardiovascular events, and whether the combined use of the two is more effective than ramipril monotherapy if noninferiority is observed.[14] The trial found no difference in efficacy between ramipril and telmisartan in the occurrence of the primary endpoints (cardiovascular death, MI, stroke, heart failure hospitalization), showing the noninferiority of the ARB over the ACE inhibitor. In the combination therapy group, however, there was no effect in reducing the primary endpoints and the treatment was associated with an increase in adverse events such as hypotension, fainting, and renal dysfunction. Therefore, the combined use of ACE inhibitors and ARBs did not provide an additional cardioprotective effect, but rather increased adverse events attributed to excessive inhibition of the RAA system.

Renal Effects

ARBs exert a renoprotective effect by antagonizing the efferent arteriole-contracting action of Ang II and improving hyperfiltration. The JNC 8 recommends ARBs and ACE inhibitors as first-line treatment for hypertension complicated by CKD at ages 18 years and up for all races.[7] Among the ARBs, losartan and irbesartan have FDA approval for preventing the progression of type 2 diabetes; they are based on the results of the Irbesartan Type II Diabetic Nephropathy Trial (IDNT) and RENAAL.

The IDNT investigated the renoprotective effects of irbesartan in 1715 patients with hypertension complicated by type 2 diabetes, proteinuria at more than 900 mg per day, and elevated serum creatinine (mean 1.67 mg/dL).[58] The subjects were randomly assigned to irbesartan, amlodipine, or placebo group, and the blood pressure was controlled to a target of 135/85 mm Hg or less. The mean blood pressure during the study period was 140/77 mm Hg in the irbesartan group, 141/77 mm Hg in the amlodipine group, and 144/80 mm Hg in the placebo group. The mean follow-up period was 2.6 years, during which the risk of the primary composite endpoint (composed

of doubling of the baseline serum creatinine concentration, the development of end-stage renal disease [ESRD], or death from any cause) was reduced by 23% (p = 0.006) as compared with the amlodipine group. These results are independent of differences in antihypertensive action, thus showing that irbesartan has a protective effect beyond blood pressure.

The RENAAL study investigated the renoprotective effects of losartan in patients with type 2 diabetes, proteinuria of more than 500 mg per day, and elevated serum creatinine, and who were taking antihypertensive medications (primary endpoints were the same for the IDNT).[44] A total of 1513 subjects with a mean creatinine level of 1.8 mg/dL were divided into a losartan group and a placebo group; after a mean follow-up of 3.4 years, the losartan group had significantly fewer primary endpoints (16% risk reduction; p = 0.02) and ESRD (28% risk reduction; p = 0.002). The blood pressure was similar in the two groups, at 140/74 mm Hg in the losartan group and 142/74 mm Hg in the placebo group, respectively (p = 0.59), again suggesting a blood pressure-independent effect.

The Randomized Olmesartan and Diabetes Microalbuminuria Prevention (ROADMAP) study investigated the efficacy of olmesartan for type 2 diabetes patients with cardiovascular risk factors.[59] This study showed that olmesartan suppresses the onset of microalbuminuria, but an increase in fatal cardiovascular events was observed in the olmesartan group. The reason for the increased cardiovascular events is unclear.

The combined use of ARBs and ACE inhibitors does not seem to provide additional benefit compared with monotherapy in patients with chronic kidney disease, which is consistent with the finding in heart failure. In the ONTARGET trial, the incidence of the primary endpoint, which was the composite of end-stage kidney disease, creatinine doubling, or death was equivalent between telmisartan and ramipril groups; the primary endpoint was significantly increased in those who received both agents.[60] In Olmesartan Reducing Incidence of End Stage Renal Disease in Diabetic Nephropathy Trial (ORIENT), olmesartan did not improve renal outcome in Asian diabetic patients with overt nephropathy who received ACE inhibitors, and was associated with higher incidence of cardiovascular death.[61] Combination therapy with lisinopril and losartan, as compared with the monotherapy of lisinopril, was associated with the increased risk of hyperkalemia and acute kidney injury, and did not provide a significant benefit with respect to renal nor cardiovascular outcomes despite the significant reduction of albuminuria in patients with diabetic nephropathy.[15] This discrepancy indicates that albuminuria is not an appropriate surrogate of renal progression, but recent meta-analysis data of 21 clinical studies show the positive correlation between the reduction of residual albuminuria and the inhibition of progression to ESRD.[62]

Adverse Effects and Important Drug Interactions

ARB administration is contraindicated in pregnant women because its use is associated with congenital anomalies (Table 24.2). Similar to ACE inhibitors, ARBs may cause a rapid decline in renal function in those who have renal hypoperfusion, such as renal artery stenosis.

Most ARBs are metabolized by the liver, and there are reports of liver dysfunction associated with the use of ARBs. GFR and serum K^+ need to be monitored in CKD patients, especially those taking potassium-sparing diuretics (e.g., mineralocorticoid receptor antagonists). A nonproductive cough, the most common adverse effect of ACE inhibitors, is much less common with ARBs (Fig. 24.2).

Generally, ARBs have few drug interactions; however, the combined use of telmisartan and digoxin can elevate the peak and trough digoxin concentration by about 50% and 13%, respectively.[63] Frequent monitoring of digoxin concentration is recommended when telmisartan is used in those taking digoxin.

RENIN INHIBITOR

Renin is a specific aspartyl protease that regulates the production of Ang I from angiotensinogen. Plasma angiotensinogen levels are at least 1000 times higher than Ang I and Ang II, and renin activity is the rate-limiting step of Ang II production. As illustrated by the renovascular hypertension and malignant hypertension, abnormal renin activity is a major cause of hypertension. Given that ACE inhibitors and ARBs do not inhibit renin activity, and that their use is instead associated with an increase in renin and Ang I as a result of a negative feedback mechanism (Table 24.4), a search for compounds that inhibit renin has been an area of intensive investigation. Although several approaches such as angiotensinogen analogs, renin prosegment analogs, and peptide-like renin inhibitors were tested, they were not suitable for clinical application because of low bioavailability or half-life issues. Based on the crystal structure of renin, researchers at Ciba-Geigy discovered aliskiren (CGP 50536 B), a nonpeptide, orally active compound that specifically binds to the active center of renin. Aliskiren is the only renin inhibitor currently available for clinical use.

Pharmacology of Renin Inhibitor

Aliskiren has a high affinity for the active form of renin (IC50 = 0.6 mmol/L). Although the bioavailability is low, aliskiren is virtually unmetabolized in the body and has a half-life of 20 to 45 hours, which is the longest among all the antihypertensive agents; it takes 5 to 8 days to achieve steady-state levels in the plasma. The main route of excretion is biliary, and 10% to 20% of absorbed aliskiren is excreted in an unchanged form in the urine. Aliskiren is not metabolized by cytochrome P450, and has not been found to interact with warfarin, lovastatin, and atenolol. Aliskiren (and likely the new renin inhibitor VTP-27999) is characterized by the high accumulation in the kidneys[64]; the concentration in the renal tissue is tens of times higher than the plasma concentration. Levels in the kidney remain high for several days or weeks after drug cessation.

Mechanisms of Action

Renin is synthesized as preprorenin from the renin gene, and the N-terminal signal sequence is cleaved in the endoplasmic reticulum to be converted to prorenin. A prosegment composed of 43 amino acids blocks the active site in prorenin, making it incapable to associate with its substrate angiotensinogen (termed "closed conformation"). Renal juxtaglomerular cells have an enzyme that cleaves the prosegment, producing renin from prorenin (proteolytic activation); the renin is then released into the kidney tissue and blood. Prorenin is also produced extrarenally and secreted into the systemic circulation. Prorenin itself does not have an activity to cleave angiotensinogen; however, the binding to (pro)renin receptor (PRR) present in various tissues causes structural changes, producing "open conformation" that associates with the substrate.

Aliskiren inhibits Ang I production in the plasma and tissues by binding to renin (and also to "open-conformation" prorenin). Of the RAA system inhibitors, only the renin inhibitor reduces renin activity and Ang I (Table 24.4). Aliskiren reduces plasma renin activity (PRA) but not active renin concentration (ARC), because the monoclonal antibodies used for ARC measurement recognize the aliskiren-renin complex.

Blood Pressure Lowering Effect, Combination With Other Antihypertensives, and Clinical Trials

Aliskiren effectively inhibits renin activity in the plasma and in the kidney. The potent blood pressure lowering effects and the adverse effects (hypotension, hyperkalemia, and kidney damage) represent two sides of the same coin. Aliskiren may be used in those that are not tolerable to ACE inhibitors and ARBs, or in hypertensive patients with consistently high plasma renin activity.

Several clinical studies evaluated the effects of aliskiren. The ALTITUDE trial investigated the addition of aliskiren to conventional therapy (including ACE inhibitors or ARBs) in

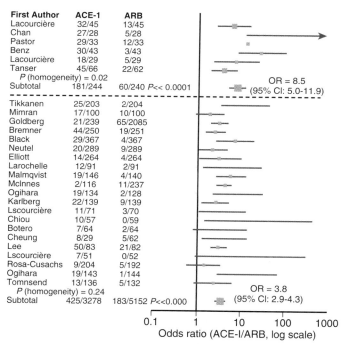

FIG. 24.2 Meta-analysis of cough in comparative studies of angiotensin II receptor blockers (ARBs) and angiotensin-converting enzyme (ACE) inhibitors. The six studies at the top of the figure involved patients with a known history of ACE-inhibitor–associated cough; the 21 studies at the bottom involved patients that were not preselected in this way. In both analyses, there is a significantly higher frequency of cough with ACE inhibitors than with ARBs.

TABLE 24.4 Effects of Inhibitors of the Renin Angiotensin Aldosterone Systems on Enzymes, Substrates and End-Products

	PRA	ARC	ANG I	ANG II	ALDOSTERONE	BRADYKININ
Renin inhibitor	↓	↑	↓	↓	↓	NA
ACE inhibitors	↑	↑	↑	↓	↓	↑
ARBs	↑	↑	↑	↑	↓	NA
MCR antagonists	↑	↑	↑	↑	↑	NA

(Adapted and modified from Staessen JA, Li Y, Richart T. Oral renin inhibitors. Lancet. 2006:368:1449-1456.)
ACE, Angiotensin-converting enzyme; ARBs, angiotensin II receptor blockers; ARC, active renin concentration; MCR, mineralocorticoid receptor; NA, not addressed; PRA, plasma renin activity.

high-risk type 2 diabetes patients.[45] The primary endpoint was a composite of cardiovascular death, nonfatal MI, nonfatal stroke, hospitalization attributed to heart failure, and onset of a renal event. The study found that aliskiren had no additional effect in reducing the incidence of the primary endpoint, and was instead associated with an increase in adverse events, including hyperkalemia and hypotension. Based on these data, the FDA announced that aliskiren should not be used in diabetic patients with an ACE inhibitor or ARB treatment.

The Aliskiren Trial on Acute Heart Failure Outcomes (ASTRONAUT) study investigated the usefulness of administering aliskiren in addition to standard therapy in patients with heart failure.[65] The result showed that there was no difference between the groups in cardiovascular death or hospitalization as a result of heart failure. In this study, 80% or more of patients were taking an ACE inhibitor or ARB at baseline, and the aliskiren group again exhibited an increase in hyperkalemia, hypotension, and kidney damage.

The addition of aliskiren to a diuretic can have an additive blood pressure-lowering effect similar to ACE inhibitors and ARBs. The Aliskiren and the Calcium Channel Blocker Amlodipine Combination as an Initial Treatment Strategy for Hypertension (ACCELERATE) study reported that the combined use of amlodipine with aliskiren is effective in early control of blood pressure.[66] It is not known whether these combinations improve long-term prognosis.

Adverse Effects and Drug Interactions

Similar to ACE inhibitors and ARBs, aliskiren is contraindicated in pregnant women and patients with bilateral renal artery stenosis or unilateral renal artery stenosis in a single kidney. Suppressing the RAA system can cause hyperkalemia, hypotension, and kidney damage; the risk is especially high in diabetic patients taking ACE inhibitors or ARBs, and in CKD patients.

Combined use with itraconazole or cyclosporine may increase the plasma concentration of aliskiren.[67,68] This seems to be associated with the inhibition of P-glycoprotein-mediated excretion by these agents; in a basic research using P-glycoprotein knockout mice, the area under the curve of aliskiren was elevated by nearly seven times that of the wild type mice.[69] Therefore, the use of aliskiren should be avoided in patients who are taking itraconazole or cyclosporine.

MINERALOCORTICOID RECEPTOR (MCR) ANTAGONISTS

Aldosterone is a steroid hormone that is synthesized from cholesterol in the adrenal gland. CYP11B2, the key enzyme that regulates the conversion of corticosterone to 18-hydroxycorticosterone and aldosterone, is specifically present in the zona glomerulosa cells of the adrenal cortex, ensuring the selective production of aldosterone in these cells. During extracellular volume depletion, angiotensin II binds to AT1R receptor in the zona glomerulosa cells, which inhibits K+ channels such as the inwardly rectifying K+ channel Kir3.4 (encoded by *KCNJ5* gene), resulting in membrane depolarization. This triggers Ca^{2+} influx through voltage-gated Ca^{2+} channels, and upregulates CYP11B2 expression. The production of aldosterone is also regulated *via* angiotensin II-independent mechanisms, including hyperkalemia and ACTH stimulation.

Mineralocorticoid receptor (MCR) belongs to the nuclear receptor superfamily, which regulates the transcription of target genes in response to ligand binding. In the apo state, MCR is present in the cytoplasm and complexes with chaperon proteins including heat shock protein 90. Upon binding with aldosterone, the holoreceptor translocates to the nucleus, and binds to the hormone responsive elements in the promoters of target DNA to control gene transcription. Mineralocorticoid receptor antagonists (MCRAs) competitively block the

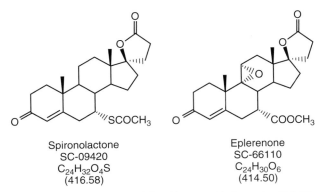

FIG. 24.3 Chemical structures of the aldosterone blockers spironolactone and eplerenone. (*Adapted from Garthwaite SM, McMahon EG. The evolution of aldosterone antagonists. Mol Cell Endocrinol. 2004:217:27-31.*)

TABLE 24.5 Comparison of Spironolactone and Eplerenone Selectivity at Human Steroid Receptors

	EPLERENONE (μM)	SPIRONOLACTONE (μM)
MCR (IC50)	0.081	0.002
AR (IC50)	4.827	0.013
GR (IC50)	>100	2.899
PR (IC50)	>100	2.619

AR, Androgen receptor; GR, glucocorticoid receptor; MCR, mineralocorticoid receptor; PR, progesterone receptor.
(*Adapted from Garthwaite SM, McMahon EG. The evolution of aldosterone antagonists. Mol Cell Endocrinol. 2004:217:27-31.*)

formation of the aldosterone-MCR complex and inhibit biological action of aldosterone and MCR.

Pharmacology of Mineralocorticoid Receptor Antagonists

There are currently two MCRAs that are available, spironolactone and eplerenone (Fig. 24.3). Spironolactone was first approved by the FDA in 1960 for the control of hypertension, edema, and primary aldosteronism. Although spironolactone has a high affinity for MCR, it also binds to other receptors such as androgen and progesterone receptors, exhibiting significant antiandrogenic and progestogenic activity especially at higher doses (more than 100 mg). Development of highly selective MCRAs has been challenging as a result of the conserved structure of the steroid receptors. In 1987, scientists at Ciba-Geigy discovered that 9-11-α-epoxy derivatives of spironolactone have a high selectivity for MCR, and eplerenone was brought to market in 2002, 42 years after the introduction of spironolactone.

Spironolactone and eplerenone are both synthetic steroids that competitively inhibit the binding of ligand to MCR. The affinity of eplerenone for MCR is around 40 times lower than that of spironolactone. However, eplerenone rarely causes gynecomastia and other sexual side effects because it exhibits high specificity towards the MCR (Table 24.5).[70]

Spironolactone binds to plasma proteins and has a short plasma half-life (approximately 1.5 hours). It is converted to two active metabolites, 7α-thiomethylspironolactone (TMS) and canrenone (which is also commercially available as a diuretic in Europe). These two metabolites have longer plasma half-lives, 13.8 hours for TMS and 16.5 hours for canrenone, respectively. Spironolactone is metabolized by the liver, and pharmacokinetic studies on cirrhotic patients revealed a significant increase in the half-life of spironolactone and its active metabolites.[71] Unlike spironolactone, eplerenone is not converted into any active metabolites, and its plasma half-life is approximately 3 to 4 hours. Eplerenone is moderately (50%) plasma protein-bound, and is metabolized in the liver by CYP3A4 (Cytochrome P450 3A4).

Mechanism of Action

Aldosterone and MCR control fluid and electrolyte homeostasis in the body. High levels of MCR are present in the distal nephron of the kidney, where the fine tuning of the total amount of salt reabsorption occurs. Unlike thiazide and loop diuretics, MCRAs do not directly inhibit the activity of an electrolyte transporter at the plasma membrane. Instead, they modulate the synthesis and degradation of multiple electrolyte flux mediators by counteracting the effects of aldosterone. Because of this nature, the natriuretic effect of MCRAs occurs relatively slowly. In principal cells, MCR regulates transcription of *SGK1* (encoding Ser/Thr kinase SGK1) and *SCNN1A* (encoding ENaC, the epithelial Na+ channel). SGK1 phosphorylates ubiquitin ligase NEDD4-2 (neuronal precursor cell expressed developmentally downregulated 4-2), resulting in its inactivation and decreased degradation of ENaC.[72] Aldosterone and MCR also regulate the expression of Na-Cl cotransporter NCC in distal convoluted tubules and pendrin, the Cl^-/HCO_3^- exchanger in intercalated cells.[73-75] These effects of aldosterone are antagonized by MCRAs. In addition to the epithelial cells of the renal tubules and colon, MCR is present in a variety of tissues and organs, modulating diverse cellular processes. MCR signaling accelerates end-organ damage by promoting tissue oxidative stress, hypertrophy, inflammation, and fibrosis.[76-78] These effects are also blocked by MCRAs.

Blood Pressure-Lowering Effect and Combination With Other Antihypertensives

MCRAs reduce blood pressure by inhibiting Na-Cl reabsorption in the distal nephron, and also by reducing vascular myogenic tone. In one study, a mean dose of 96.5 mg of spironolactone decreased systolic/diastolic blood pressure by 18/10 mm Hg.[79] Spironolactone dose above 150 mg had no additional effect on the blood pressure, but was associated with the increased incidence of gynecomastia.[79] In resistant hypertension, spironolactone at a dose of 25 mg in combination with other antihypertensives (diuretics and ACE inhibitors or ARB) reduced the blood pressure effectively by 20 to 25 mm Hg.[80] The antihypertensive effect of eplerenone seems to be less than that of spironolactone at the same dose, although the incidence of gynecomastia or mastodynia was significantly less with the use of eplerenone.[81] The antihypertensive effect of eplerenone is reported to be equal in African Americans and white persons, and is superior to an ARB losartan in the African-American population.[82] In JNC 8, the use of MCRAs is a preferable option for treatment-resistant hypertension patients who are taking three or more antihypertensive medications.[7] Given the good evidence that MCRAs protect against left ventricular dysfunction, they are especially indicated for hypertension with chronic heart failure.

End-Organ Effects and Clinical Trials

Cardiac Effects

Spironolactone and eplerenone are approved for the treatment of heart failure and left ventricular dysfunction in the U.S. based on the results of a series of clinical studies including RALES (Randomized Aldactone Evaluation Study),[83] EPHESUS (Eplerenone Post-Acute Myocardial Infarction Heart Failure Efficacy and Survival Study),[84] and EMPHASIS-HF (Eplerenone

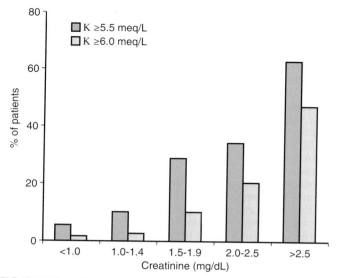

FIG. 24.4 The incidence of hyperkalemia associated with the use of spironolactone in subjects with normal and decreased kidney function. The risk of hyperkalemia increased to more than 20% when serum creatinine levels are 1.5 mg/dL or above. *(Adapted from Shah KB, Rao K, Sawyer R, Gottlieb SS. The adequacy of laboratory monitoring in patients treated with spironolactone for congestive heart failure. JACC. 2005;46:845-849.)*

in Mild Patients Hospitalization and Survival Study in Heart Failure).[85] RALES is a landmark study evaluating the protective effects of low-dose spironolactone in heart failure.[83] A total of 1663 patients with decreased ejection fraction (<35%) treated with ACE inhibitors and loop diuretics were enrolled in the study. After a mean follow-up of 24 months, the study was terminated early because the interim analysis determined that spironolactone was efficacious. The study demonstrated that the addition of spironolactone to standard therapy was associated with 30% decline in the all-cause mortality. Gynecomastia or breast pain was observed in 10% of the patients in the spironolactone group, as compared with the 1% of the patients in the placebo group.

The incidence of hyperkalemia was minimal in the RALES study. Nevertheless, the risk of serum K+ elevation with the use of spironolactone should not be underestimated, given that CKD patients with serum creatinine levels of more than 2.5 mg/dL were excluded in RALES, and that the serum K+ levels were carefully monitored during the course of the study. In a retrospective study using the Veterans Affairs Information System Technology and Architecture (VISTA) database, the use of spironolactone in heart failure was associated with hyperkalemia (defined as 5.5 mEq/L or higher) in 15% of the 551 patients enrolled (among whom 86% were taking ACEI or ARB).[86] In this study, the authors noted that even a modest increase in creatinine concentration increased the incidence of hyperkalemia (Fig. 24.4).

The EPHESUS study evaluated the efficacy of adding 25 to 50 mg eplerenone to standard therapy in 6632 patients with acute MI complicated with left ventricular dysfunction (ejection fraction of 40% or lower) and heart failure.[84] Similar to the RALES study, eplerenone reduced the risk of total mortality (relative risk 0.85; *p* = 0.008). Serious hyperkalemia (6.0 mEq/L or higher) was observed in 5.5% of the subjects in the eplerenone group and 3.9% of the subjects in the placebo group (*p* = 0.008). The risk of hypokalemia (less than 3.5 mEq/L) was significantly higher in the placebo group. Subsequently, the EMPHASIS-HF study, involving 2737 patients with NYHA class II and an ejection fraction of no more than 35%, demonstrated that the primary outcome (composite of death from cardiovascular causes or hospitalization for heart failure) occurred significantly less in the eplerenone group than in the placebo group (18.3% versus 25.9%; $p < 0.001$).[85] In summary, these studies show that eplerenone has protective effects against chronic heart failure with decreased ejection fraction, similar to the result seen with spironolactone. Whether or not MCRAs can be protective in heart failure with preserved ejection fraction has not been known. In the TOPCAT (Treatment of Preserved Cardiac Function Heart Failure with an Aldosterone Antagonist) study, eplerenone treatment was neutral in patients with symptomatic heart failure and preserved ejection fraction (>45%, mean ejection fraction of 56%).[87] Interestingly, the subanalysis of the TOPCAT study showed the benefit of spironolactone in patients recruited from the U.S. but not in the other half of patients from Russia/Georgia; and the U.S. patients were associated with the decreased blood pressure and the increased serum potassium and creatinine concentrations, whereas those in Russia/Georgia were associated without changes in blood pressure, serum potassium or creatinine, suggesting the importance of hemodynamic change in the beneficial effect of the MCRAs.[88]

Renal Effects

Several randomized trials have shown that MCRAs reduce proteinuria in CKD patients, although the efficacy on renal hard endpoint (i.e., the incidence of end-stage kidney disease) remains to be determined. In the EVALUATE study, eplerenone, at a small dose of 50 mg, ameliorated albuminuria in nondiabetic CKD patients who had hypertension and were already on ACE inhibitors or ARB treatment.[89] The study participants had normal to mild reduction of GFR, and the use of eplerenone was associated with the significantly increased levels of plasma potassium; however, none of the participants presented severe hyperkalemia, defined as a potassium concentration greater than 5.6 mEq/L. Similarly, the treatment with finerenone (BAY 94-8862), a nonsteroidal MCR antagonist under development of Bayer, induced dose-dependent reduction of albuminuria in patients with diabetic nephropathy and moderately reduced GFR.[90] In both studies, antialbuminuric effects of the MCR blockers are associated with significant reductions of blood pressure and GFR, despite no correlation of changes in albuminuria by the MCRAs to those in blood pressure nor GFR. The importance of natriuresis in the antihypertensive effect of MCRAs is indicated by a recent study showing the negative correlation between baseline PRA and spironolactone-induced reduction of blood pressure in patients with drug-resistant hypertension.[91] However, experimental studies have suggested that, in addition to the effect on blood pressure, the protective effects of MCRAs can be attributed to the prevention of the hyperfiltration, amelioration of the renal inflammation, and the favorable effects on glomerular filtration barrier integrity. Importantly, the treatment of spironolactone reduced cardiovascular outcomes in patients receiving dialysis, without increasing the risk of hyperkalemia.[92]

There are several studies showing the antiproteinuric effect of MCRAs in diabetic nephropathy. Because of the risk of potential hyperkalemia, eplerenone is contraindicated in diabetic patients with proteinuria. Using finerenone with possibly lesser incidence of hyperkalemia than spironolactone and eplerenone, there are two ongoing phase III clinical studies evaluating the efficacy in diabetic nephropathy (FIGARO-DKD and FIDELIO-DKD).

Adverse Effects and Important Drug Interactions

Use of MCRAs (both spironolactone and eplerenone) is associated with the increase in serum K^+ levels, because aldosterone increases urinary K^+ secretion in exchange for Na^+ reabsorption in principal cells of the collecting duct. MCRAs may increase serum creatinine, which is presumably as a result of the amelioration of hyperfiltration. These effects are more likely to occur in patients with reduced kidney function, and who also receive ACE inhibitors or ARBs. Serum K^+ and creatinine levels should be monitored when MCRAs are used in such patients.

Spironolactone has an affinity for androgen receptor and progesterone receptor and its use is associated with male gynecomastia and mastodynia, especially at a higher dose. Eplerenone is metabolized by CYP3A4 and the concomitant administration of CYP3A4 inhibitors, including ketoconazole, itraconazole, and clarithromycin, is contraindicated. Other less potent CYP3A4 inhibitors (erythromycin, verapamil, and fluconazole) can also increase the serum concentration of eplerenone, and therefore it is recommended to reduce the starting dose of eplerenone in patients who are already receiving these medications.

References

1. Dzau VJ, Bernstein K, Celermajer D, et al. The relevance of tissue angiotensin-converting enzyme: manifestations in mechanistic and endpoint data. *Am J Cardiol.* 2001;88:1L-20L.
2. Woodman ZL, Oppong SY, Cook S, et al. Shedding of somatic angiotensin-converting enzyme (ACE) is inefficient compared with testis ACE despite cleavage at identical stalk sites. *Biochemic J.* 2000;347(Pt 3):711-718.
3. Donoghue M, Hsieh F, Baronas E, et al. A novel angiotensin-converting enzyme-related carboxypeptidase (ACE2) converts angiotensin I to angiotensin 1-9. *Circ Res.* 2000;87:E1-9.
4. Santos RA, Simoes e Silva AC, Maric C, et al. Angiotensin-(1-7) is an endogenous ligand for the G protein-coupled receptor Mas. *Proc Natl Acad Sci USA.* 2003;100:8258-8263.
5. Esther CR, Marino EM, Howard TE, et al. The critical role of tissue angiotensin-converting enzyme as revealed by gene targeting in mice. *J Clin Invest.* 1997;99:2375-2385.
6. Sakaguchi K, Chai SY, Jackson B, et al. Inhibition of tissue angiotensin converting enzyme. Quantitation by autoradiography. *Hypertension.* 1988;11:230-238.
7. James PA, Oparil S, Carter BL, et al. 2014 evidence-based guideline for the management of high blood pressure in adults: report from the panel members appointed to the Eighth Joint National Committee (JNC 8). *JAMA.* 2014;311:507-520.
8. ALLHAT officers and coordinators for the ALLHAT collaborative research group. The Antihypertensive and Lipid-Lowering Treatment to Prevent Heart Attack Trial. Major outcomes in high-risk hypertensive patients randomized to angiotensin-converting enzyme inhibitor or calcium channel blocker vs diuretic: The Antihypertensive and Lipid-Lowering Treatment to Prevent Heart Attack Trial (ALLHAT). *JAMA.* 2002;288:2981-2997.
9. Heerspink HJ. Therapeutic approaches in lowering albuminuria: travels along the renin-angiotensin-aldosterone-system pathway. *Adv Chronic Kidney Dis.* 2011;18:290-299.
10. Group PC. Randomised trial of a perindopril-based blood-pressure-lowering regimen among 6,105 individuals with previous stroke or transient ischaemic attack. *Lancet.* 2001;358:1033-1041.
11. Dahlof B, Sever PS, Poulter NR, et al. Prevention of cardiovascular events with an antihypertensive regimen of amlodipine adding perindopril as required versus atenolol adding bendroflumethiazide as required, in the Anglo-Scandinavian Cardiac Outcomes Trial-Blood Pressure Lowering Arm (ASCOT-BPLA): a multicentre randomised controlled trial. *Lancet.* 2005;366:895-906.
12. Jamerson K, Weber MA, Bakris GL, et al. Benazepril plus amlodipine or hydrochlorothiazide for hypertension in high-risk patients. *N Engl J Med.* 2008;359:2417-2428.
13. Bakris GL, Toto RD, McCullough PA, et al. Effects of different ACE inhibitor combinations on albuminuria: results of the GUARD study. *Kidney Int.* 2008;73:1303-1309.
14. Investigators O, Yusuf S, Teo KK, et al. Telmisartan, ramipril, or both in patients at high risk for vascular events. *N Engl J Med.* 2008;358:1547-1559.
15. Fried LF, Emanuele N, Zhang JH, et al. Combined angiotensin inhibition for the treatment of diabetic nephropathy. *N Engl J Med.* 2013;369:1892-1903.
16. Effects of enalapril on mortality in severe congestive heart failure. Results of the Cooperative North Scandinavian Enalapril Survival Study (CONSENSUS). The CONSENSUS Trial Study Group. *N Engl J Med.* 1987;316:1429-1435.
17. Effect of enalapril on survival in patients with reduced left ventricular ejection fractions and congestive heart failure. The SOLVD Investigators. *N Engl J Med.* 1991;325:293-302.
18. Effect of enalapril on mortality and the development of heart failure in asymptomatic patients with reduced left ventricular ejection fractions. The SOLVD Investigattors. *N Engl J Med.* 1992;327:685-691.
19. Pfeffer MA, Braunwald E, Moye LA, et al. Effect of captopril on mortality and morbidity in patients with left ventricular dysfunction after myocardial infarction. Results of the survival and ventricular enlargement trial. The SAVE Investigators. *N Engl J Med.* 1992;327:669-677.
20. Effect of ramipril on mortality and morbidity of survivors of acute myocardial infarction with clinical evidence of heart failure. The Acute Infarction Ramipril Efficacy (AIRE) Study Investigators. *Lancet.* 1993;342:821-828.
21. GISSI-3: effects of lisinopril and transdermal glyceryl trinitrate singly and together on 6-week mortality and ventricular function after acute myocardial infarction. Gruppo Italiano per lo Studio della Sopravvivenza nell'infarto Miocardico. *Lancet.* 1994;343:1115-1122.
22. Kober L, Torp-Pedersen C, Carlsen JE, et al. A clinical trial of the angiotensin-converting-enzyme inhibitor trandolapril in patients with left ventricular dysfunction after myocardial infarction. Trandolapril Cardiac Evaluation (TRACE) Study Group. *N Engl J Med.* 1995;333:1670-1676.
23. Ambrosioni E, Borghi C, Magnani B. The effect of the angiotensin-converting-enzyme inhibitor zofenopril on mortality and morbidity after anterior myocardial infarction. The Survival of Myocardial Infarction Long-Term Evaluation (SMILE) Study Investigators. *N Engl J Med.* 1995;332:80-85.
24. Swedberg K, Held P, Kjekshus J, et al. Effects of the early administration of enalapril on mortality in patients with acute myocardial infarction. Results of the Cooperative New Scandinavian Enalapril Survival Study II (CONSENSUS II). *N Engl J Med.* 1992;327:678-684.
25. Cleland JG, Tendera M, Adamus J, et al. The perindopril in elderly people with chronic heart failure (PEP-CHF) study. *Eur Heart J.* 2006;27:2338-2345.
26. Yusuf S, Sleight P, Pogue J, et al. Effects of an angiotensin-converting-enzyme inhibitor, ramipril, on cardiovascular events in high-risk patients. The Heart Outcomes Prevention Evaluation (HOPE) Study Investigators. *N Engl J Med.* 2000;342:145-153.

27. Fox KM, Investigators EUtOrocewPiscAd. Efficacy of perindopril in reduction of cardiovascular events among patients with stable coronary artery disease: randomised, double-blind, placebo-controlled, multicentre trial (the EUROPA study). *Lancet.* 2003;362:782-788.
28. Braunwald E, Domanski MJ, Fowler SE, et al. Angiotensin-converting-enzyme inhibition in stable coronary artery disease. *N Engl J Med.* 2004;351:2058-2068.
29. Ruggenenti P, Perna A, Gherardi G, et al. Renal function and requirement for dialysis in chronic nephropathy patients on long-term ramipril: REIN follow-up trial. Gruppo Italiano di Studi Epidemiologici in Nefrologia (GISEN). Ramipril Efficacy in Nephropathy. *Lancet.* 1998;352:1252-1256.
30. Ruggenenti P, Perna A, Remuzzi G, et al. ACE inhibitors to prevent end-stage renal disease: when to start and why possibly never to stop: a post hoc analysis of the REIN trial results. Ramipril Efficacy in Nephropathy. *J Am Soc Nephrol.* 2001;12:2832-2837.
31. Lewis EJ, Hunsicker LG, Bain RP, et al. The effect of angiotensin-converting-enzyme inhibition on diabetic nephropathy. The Collaborative Study Group. *N Engl J Med.* 1993;329:1456-1462.
32. Wright JT Jr., Bakris G, Greene T, et al. Effect of blood pressure lowering and antihypertensive drug class on progression of hypertensive kidney disease: results from the AASK trial. *JAMA.* 2002;288:2421-2431.
33. Investigators DT, Bosch J, Yusuf S, et al. Effect of ramipril on the incidence of diabetes. *N Engl J Med.* 2006;355:1551-1562.
34. Tocci G, Paneni F, Palano F, et al. Angiotensin-converting enzyme inhibitors, angiotensin II receptor blockers and diabetes: a meta-analysis of placebo-controlled clinical trials. *Am J Hypertens.* 2011;24:582-590.
35. Group NS, McMurray JJ, Holman RR, et al. Effect of valsartan on the incidence of diabetes and cardiovascular events. *N Engl J Med.* 2010;362:1477-1490.
36. Caldeira D, Alarcao J, Vaz-Carneiro A, et al. Risk of pneumonia associated with use of angiotensin converting enzyme inhibitors and angiotensin receptor blockers: systematic review and meta-analysis. *BMJ.* 2012;345:e4260.
37. Kostis JB, Packer M, Black HR, et al. Omapatrilat and enalapril in patients with hypertension: the Omapatrilat Cardiovascular Treatment vs. Enalapril (OCTAVE) trial. *Am J Hypertens.* 2004;17:103-111.
38. Brown NJ, Byiers S, Carr D, et al. Dipeptidyl peptidase-IV inhibitor use associated with increased risk of ACE inhibitor-associated angioedema. *Hypertension.* 2009;54:516-523.
39. Miao Y, Ottenbros SA, Laverman GD, et al. Effect of a reduction in uric acid on renal outcomes during losartan treatment: a post hoc analysis of the reduction of endpoints in non-insulin-dependent diabetes mellitus with the Angiotensin II Antagonist Losartan Trial. *Hypertension.* 2011;58:2-7.
40. Gurley SB, Riquier-Brison AD, Schnermann J, et al. AT1A angiotensin receptors in the renal proximal tubule regulate blood pressure. *Cell Metab.* 2011;13:469-475.
41. Sparks MA, Stegbauer J, Chen D, et al. Vascular type 1A angiotensin II receptors control BP by regulating renal blood flow and urinary sodium excretion. *J Am Soc Nephrol.* 2015;26:2953-2962.
42. Kemp BA, Howell NL, Gildea JJ, et al. AT(2) receptor activation induces natriuresis and lowers blood pressure. *Circ Res.* 2014;115:388-399.
43. Gurley SB, Allred A, Le TH, et al. Altered blood pressure responses and normal cardiac phenotype in ACE2-null mice. *J Clin Invest.* 2006;116:2218-2225.
44. Brenner BM, Cooper ME, de Zeeuw D, et al. Effects of losartan on renal and cardiovascular outcomes in patients with type 2 diabetes and nephropathy. *N Engl J Med.* 2001;345:861-869.
45. Parving HH, Brenner BM, McMurray JJ, et al. Cardiorenal end points in a trial of aliskiren for type 2 diabetes. *N Engl J Med.* 2012;367:2204-2213.
46. McMurray JJ, Packer M, Desai AS, et al. Angiotensin-neprilysin inhibition versus enalapril in heart failure. *N Engl J Med.* 2014;371:993-1004.
47. Jhund PS, Claggett B, Packer M, et al. Independence of the blood pressure lowering effect and efficacy of the angiotensin receptor neprilysin inhibitor, LCZ696, in patients with heart failure with preserved ejection fraction: an analysis of the PARAMOUNT trial. *Eur J Heart Fail.* 2014;16:671-677.
48. Dahlof B, Devereux RB, Kjeldsen SE, et al. Cardiovascular morbidity and mortality in the Losartan Intervention For Endpoint reduction in hypertension study (LIFE): a randomised trial against atenolol. *Lancet.* 2002;359:995-1003.
49. Pitt B, Poole-Wilson PA, Segal R, et al. Effect of losartan compared with captopril on mortality in patients with symptomatic heart failure: randomised trial—the Losartan Heart Failure Survival Study ELITE II. *Lancet.* 2000;355:1582-1587.
50. Dickstein K, Kjekshus J. Group OSCotOS. Effects of losartan and captopril on mortality and morbidity in high-risk patients after acute myocardial infarction: the OPTIMAAL randomised trial. Optimal Trial in Myocardial Infarction with Angiotensin II Antagonist Losartan. *Lancet.* 2002;360:752-760.
51. Cohn JN, Tognoni G. Valsartan Heart Failure Trial I. A randomized trial of the angiotensin-receptor blocker valsartan in chronic heart failure. *N Engl J Med.* 2001;345:1667-1675.
52. Pfeffer MA, Swedberg K, Granger CB, et al. Effects of candesartan on mortality and morbidity in patients with chronic heart failure: the CHARM-Overall programme. *Lancet.* 2003;362:759-766.
53. Granger CB, McMurray JJ, Yusuf S, et al. Effects of candesartan in patients with chronic heart failure and reduced left-ventricular systolic function intolerant to angiotensin-converting-enzyme inhibitors: the CHARM-Alternative trial. *Lancet.* 2003;362:772-776.
54. McMurray JJ, Ostergren J, Swedberg K, et al. Effects of candesartan in patients with chronic heart failure and reduced left-ventricular systolic function taking angiotensin-converting-enzyme inhibitors: the CHARM-Added trial. *Lancet.* 2003;362:767-771.
55. Yusuf S, Pfeffer MA, Swedberg K, et al. Effects of candesartan in patients with chronic heart failure and preserved left-ventricular ejection fraction: the CHARM-Preserved Trial. *Lancet.* 2003;362:777-781.
56. Massie BM, Carson PE, McMurray JJ, et al. Irbesartan in patients with heart failure and preserved ejection fraction. *N Engl J Med.* 2008;359:2456-2467.
57. Pfeffer MA, McMurray JJ, Velazquez EJ, et al. Valsartan, captopril, or both in myocardial infarction complicated by heart failure, left ventricular dysfunction, or both. *N Engl J Med.* 2003;349:1893-1906.
58. Lewis EJ, Hunsicker LG, Clarke WR, et al. Renoprotective effect of the angiotensin-receptor antagonist irbesartan in patients with nephropathy due to type 2 diabetes. *N Engl J Med.* 2001;345:851-860.
59. Haller H, Ito S, Izzo JL Jr., et al. Olmesartan for the delay or prevention of microalbuminuria in type 2 diabetes. *N Engl J Med.* 2011;364:907-917.
60. Mann JF, Schmieder RE, McQueen M, et al. Renal outcomes with telmisartan, ramipril, or both, in people at high vascular risk (the ONTARGET study): a multicentre, randomised, double-blind, controlled trial. *Lancet.* 2008;372:547-553.
61. Imai E, Chan JC, Ito S, et al. Effects of olmesartan on renal and cardiovascular outcomes in type 2 diabetes with overt nephropathy: a multicentre, randomised, placebo-controlled study. *Diabetologia.* 2011;54:2978-2986.
62. Heerspink HJ, Kropelin TF, Hoekman J, et al. Drug-induced reduction in albuminuria is associated with subsequent renoprotection: a meta-analysis. *J Am Soc Nephrol.* 2015;26:2055-2064.
63. Stangier J, Su CA, Hendriks MG, et al. The effect of telmisartan on the steady-state pharmacokinetics of digoxin in healthy male volunteers. *J Clin Pharmacol.* 2000;40(12 Pt 1):1373-1379.
64. Te Riet L, van Esch JH, Roks AJ, et al. Hypertension: renin-angiotensin-aldosterone system alterations. *Circ Res.* 2015;116:960-975.
65. Gheorghiade M, Bohm M, Greene SJ, et al. Effect of aliskiren on postdischarge mortality and heart failure readmissions among patients hospitalized for heart failure: the ASTRONAUT randomized trial. *JAMA.* 2013;309:1125-1135.
66. Brown MJ, McInnes GT, Papst CC, et al. Aliskiren and the calcium channel blocker amlodipine combination as an initial treatment strategy for hypertension control (ACCELERATE): a randomised, parallel-group trial. *Lancet.* 2011;377:312-320.
67. Tapaninen T, Backman JT, Kurkinen KJ, et al. Itraconazole, a P-glycoprotein and CYP3A4 inhibitor, markedly raises the plasma concentrations and enhances the renin-inhibiting effect of aliskiren. *J Clin Pharmacol.* 2011;51:359-367.
68. Rebello S, Compain S, Feng A, et al. Effect of cyclosporine on the pharmacokinetics of aliskiren in healthy subjects. *J Clin Pharmacol.* 2011;51:1549-1560.
69. Tsukimoto M, Ohashi R, Torimoto N, et al. Effects of the inhibition of intestinal P-glycoprotein on aliskiren pharmacokinetics in cynomolgus monkeys. *Biopharm Drug Dispos.* 2015;36:15-33.
70. Garthwaite SM, McMahon EG. The evolution of aldosterone antagonists. *Mol Cell Endocrinol.* 2004;217:27-31.
71. Sungaila I, Bartle WR, Walker SE, et al. Spironolactone pharmacokinetics and pharmacodynamics in patients with cirrhotic ascites. *Gastroenterology.* 1992;102:1680-1685.
72. Kamynina E, Staub O. Concerted action of ENaC, Nedd4-2, and Sgk1 in transepithelial Na(+) transport. *Am J Physiol Renal Physiol.* 2002;283:F377-387.
73. Kim GH, Masilamani S, Turner R, et al. The thiazide-sensitive Na-Cl cotransporter is an aldosterone-induced protein. *Proc Natl Acad Sci USA.* 1998;95:14552-14557.
74. Verlander JW, Hassell KA, Royaux IE, et al. Deoxycorticosterone upregulates PDS (Slc26a4) in mouse kidney: role of pendrin in mineralocorticoid-induced hypertension. *Hypertension.* 2003;42:356-362.
75. Shibata S, Rinehart J, Zhang J, et al. Mineralocorticoid receptor phosphorylation regulates ligand binding and renal response to volume depletion and hyperkalemia. *Cell Metab.* 2013;18:660-671.
76. Fraccarollo D, Berger S, Galuppo P, et al. Deletion of cardiomyocyte mineralocorticoid receptor ameliorates adverse remodeling after myocardial infarction. *Circulation.* 2011;123:400-408.
77. Shibata S, Fujita T. Mineralocorticoid receptors in the pathophysiology of chronic kidney diseases and the metabolic syndrome. *Mol Cell Endocrinol.* 2012;350:273-280.
78. Ayuzawa N, Nagase M, Ueda K, et al. Rac1-Mediated Activation of Mineralocorticoid Receptor in Pressure Overload-Induced Cardiac Injury. *Hypertension.* 2016;67:99-106.
79. Jeunemaitre X, Chatellier G, Kreft-Jais C, et al. Efficacy and tolerance of spironolactone in essential hypertension. *Am J Cardiol.* 1987;60:820-825.
80. Nishizaka MK, Zaman MA, Calhoun DA. Efficacy of low-dose spironolactone in subjects with resistant hypertension. *Am J Hypertens.* 2003;16(11 Pt 1):925-930.
81. Parthasarathy HK, Menard J, White WB, et al. A double-blind, randomized study comparing the antihypertensive effect of eplerenone and spironolactone in patients with hypertension and evidence of primary aldosteronism. *J Hypertens.* 2011;29:980-990.
82. Flack JM, Oparil S, Pratt JH, et al. Efficacy and tolerability of eplerenone and losartan in hypertensive black and white patients. *J Am Coll Cardiol.* 2003;41:1148-1155.
83. Pitt B, Zannad F, Remme WJ, et al. The effect of spironolactone on morbidity and mortality in patients with severe heart failure. Randomized Aldactone Evaluation Study Investigators. *N Engl J Med.* 1999;341:709-717.
84. Pitt B, Remme W, Zannad F, et al. Eplerenone, a selective aldosterone blocker, in patients with left ventricular dysfunction after myocardial infarction. *N Engl J Med.* 2003;348:1309-1321.
85. Zannad F, McMurray JJ, Krum H, et al. Eplerenone in patients with systolic heart failure and mild symptoms. *N Engl J Med.* 2011;364:11-21.
86. Shah KB, Rao K, Sawyer R, et al. The adequacy of laboratory monitoring in patients treated with spironolactone for congestive heart failure. *J Am Coll Cardiol.* 2005;46:845-849.
87. Pitt B, Pfeffer MA, Assmann SF, et al. Spironolactone for heart failure with preserved ejection fraction. *N Engl J Med.* 2014;370:1383-1392.
88. Pfeffer MA, Claggett B, Assmann SF, et al. Regional variation in patients and outcomes in the Treatment of Preserved Cardiac Function Heart Failure With an Aldosterone Antagonist (TOPCAT) trial. *Circulation.* 2015;131:34-42.
89. Ando K, Ohtsu H, Uchida S, et al. Anti-albuminuric effect of the aldosterone blocker eplerenone in non-diabetic hypertensive patients with albuminuria: a double-blind, randomised, placebo-controlled trial. *Lancet Diab Endocrinol.* 2014;2:944-953.
90. Bakris GL, Agarwal R, Chan JC, et al. Effect of Finerenone on Albuminuria in Patients With Diabetic Nephropathy: A Randomized Clinical Trial. *JAMA.* 2015;314:884-894.
91. Williams B, MacDonald TM, Morant S, et al. Spironolactone versus placebo, bisoprolol, and doxazosin to determine the optimal treatment for drug-resistant hypertension (PATHWAY-2): a randomised, double-blind, crossover trial. *Lancet.* 2015;386:2059-2068.
92. Matsumoto Y, Mori Y, Kageyama S, et al. Spironolactone reduces cardiovascular and cerebrovascular morbidity and mortality in hemodialysis patients. *J Am Coll Cardiol.* 2014;63:528-536.

25 Calcium Channel Blockers

Alun Hughes

Calcium channel blockers (CCB) have extensive therapeutic applications. Three CCB were listed in the forty most commonly used prescriptions and over-the-counter drugs in the Slone Survey of Recent Medication Use by the adult ambulatory population of the United States in 1998 to 1999.[1] Over the period 2001 to 2010 approximately 20% of hypertensive adults in the United States reported taking a CCB,[2] with amlodipine being the most prescribed drug.[3]

This chapter will focus on this class of medications in relation to systemic arterial hypertension. The use of CCB in combination therapy for hypertension is dealt with in Chapter 27. Uses of CCB in other conditions including angina pectoris and ischemic heart disease, cardiac arrhythmias, congestive heart failure, pulmonary hypertension, migraine, Reynaud disease, obstetrics, and neurological diseases will not be covered, except to the extent that the coexistence of these conditions may influence the selection of this class of agents in hypertension. Consideration will also be restricted to clinically-used drugs that act selectively on voltage-gated calcium channels (VGCC). Consequently this chapter will not cover nonselective agents (e.g., piperazines, benzothiazinones, pyrazines, and indole sulfones) that are sometimes included in some CCB classification systems.[4,5]

CALCIUM AND CELLS

Under resting conditions the cell membrane is highly impermeable to Ca^{2+} ions and there is a considerable electrochemical gradient for Ca^{2+} entry as a result of the negative cell membrane potential and the steep concentration gradient of Ca^{2+} across the cell membrane. Ingress and efflux of Ca^{2+} into and out of the cell depends on a number of specialized channels, exchangers and transporters,[6] and changes in the concentration of intracellular Ca^{2+} resulting from changes in net permeability to Ca^{2+} play a major role in cell physiology from fertilization to cell death.[6]

MOLECULAR BIOLOGY AND PHYSIOLOGY OF VOLTAGE-GATED CALCIUM CHANNELS

VGCC comprise a large family of transmembrane proteins that play an important role in Ca^{2+} entry into many cell types. Brief histories of their discovery and the key personalities involved have been published.[7,8] As their name implies the gating of VGCC is sensitive to the cell membrane potential and depolarization is associated with an increase in probability of the channel adopting a conformation that allows Ca^{2+} permeation (an 'open state'). VGCC are considered to exist in at least four distinct conformational states: resting, partially activated, open, and inactivated[9]; and CCB can modify transition between channel states (see later). Under physiological conditions an open VGCC will allow more than 10^6 Ca^{2+} ions to pass per second, while maintaining extremely high selectivity for Ca^{2+} ions.[10] The high selectivity of VGCC is attributed to four glutamate residues in the channel pore that act as a selectivity filter.[11]

Voltage-Gated Calcium Channel Subtypes

VGCC were originally subdivided into subtypes based on their electrophysiological characteristics.[12] Six main categories have been described: L (Long-lasting), T (Transient), N (Neither T nor L, or Neuronal), P (Purkinje cells), Q (after P), and R (Remaining, or Resistant, or after Q), each with many subtypes. More recently classification has been refined on the basis of the molecular biology of the α1 subunits (Table 25.1).[12,13]

Typically, VGCC consist of three subunits (α1, β, α2δ) (Fig. 25.1); in skeletal muscle an additional subunit is present (γ subunit).[14] The α1 subunit forms the core of the channel and is responsible for Ca^{2+} permeation. It consists of four homologous domains (domains I-IV), each composed of six membrane-spanning α-helices (S1-S6). S4 is thought to act as the voltage sensor.[13] Other auxiliary subunits (Table 25.2) influence channel anchorage, trafficking, gating, and inactivation behavior, and may also associate with other channels or proteins influencing their function.[14,15]

Voltage-Gated Calcium Channels in Cardiac and Smooth Muscle

L-type calcium channels ($Ca_V1.2$) are the predominant subtype present in cardiac and smooth muscle,[14] but other subtypes (P/Q-type VGCC [$Ca_V2.1$][16]; T-type VGCC [$Ca_V3.1$ and $Ca_V3.2$][17,18]) coexist and contribute to cardiovascular function, albeit with seemingly minimal roles in overall blood pressure control.[19-21] Conditional knockout of $Ca_V1.2$ in smooth muscle in the mouse markedly reduced blood pressure and abolished myogenic tone consistent with a major functional role for this channel subtype.[19] Conversely knockout of $Ca_V3.1$ or $Ca_V3.2$ (T-type VGCC) had no effect on blood pressure,[20,21] although atrioventricular conduction was delayed and resting heart rate was decreased by knockout of $Ca_V3.1$.[20] Despite the lack of effect on blood pressure, evidence from knockout mice suggests Cav3.1 participates in neointima formation following vascular injury,[20] whereas Cav3.2 participates in pressure-induced and angiotensin II-induced cardiac hypertrophy.[22] $Ca_V2.1$ (P/Q-type VGCC) and $Ca_V3.1$ (T-type VGCC) are present in the arterial vasculature and may play a role in the regulation of renal vascular resistance.[23] L-type and P/Q-type VGCCs are present and play a functional role in preglomerular arteries, whereas T-type VGCCs are present in both afferent and efferent arterioles.[22,24]

All genes for VGCC subunits can undergo alternative splicing[14]; for example the $Ca_V1.2$ gene contains 55 exons, of which 19 exons can undergo alternative splicing, potentially yielding 2^{19} combinations.[25] Variable splicing gives rise to ion channels with discernibly different gating characteristics, differing affinities for CCB and, in some cases, pathological consequences.[14] VGCC behavior is modulated by a wide range of intracellular signaling mechanisms, with cyclic guanosine monophosphate-dependent protein kinase, cyclic adenosine

TABLE 25.1 Voltage-Gated Calcium Channel Types, α1 Subunits, Physiological Function, and Inherited Diseases

Ca²⁺ CURRENT	α1 SUBUNIT	GENE	CHROMOSOME	SPECIFIC BLOCKER	FUNCTION	INHERITED DISEASES
L-type	Ca_V1.1	CACNA1S	1q31-32	DHP	Excitation-contraction coupling in skeletal muscle, gene transcription	Hypokalemic periodic paralysis
	Ca_V1.2	CACNA1C	12p13.3	DHP	Excitation-contraction coupling in cardiac and smooth muscle, endocrine secretion, neuronal Ca²⁺ transients in cell bodies and dendrites, enzyme regulation, gene transcription	Timothy syndrome; cardiac arrhythmia with developmental abnormalities and autism spectrum disorders
	Ca_V1.3	CACNA1D	3p14.3	DHP	Cardiac pacemaking, endocrine secretion, Ca²⁺ transients in cell bodies and dendrites, auditory transduction	
	Ca_V1.4	CACNA1F	Xp11.23	DHP	Visual transduction	Stationary night blindness
P/Q-type	Ca_V2.1	CACNA1A	19p13.1	ω-CTx-GVIA	Neurotransmitter release, dendritic Ca²⁺ transients	
N-type	Ca_V2.2	CACNA1B	9q34	ω-agatoxin	Neurotransmitter release, dendritic Ca²⁺ transients	
R-type	Ca_V2.3	CACNA1E	1q25.31	SNX-482	Neurotransmitter release, dendritic Ca²⁺ transients	Familial hemiplegic migraine cerebellar ataxia
T-type	Ca_V3.1	CACNA1G	17q22		Pacemaking and repetitive firing	
	Ca_V3.2	CACNA1H	16p13.3		Pacemaking and repetitive firing	Absence seizures
	Ca_V3.3	CACNA1I	22q13			

(Modified from Catterall WA. Voltage-gated calcium channels. Cold Spring Harb Perspect Biol. 2011; 3[8].)
ω-CTx-GVIA, ω-conotoxin-GVIA from the cone snail *Conus geographus*; *DHP*, dihydropyridine; *SNX-482*, a synthetic version of a peptide toxin from the tarantula *Hysterocrates gigas*.

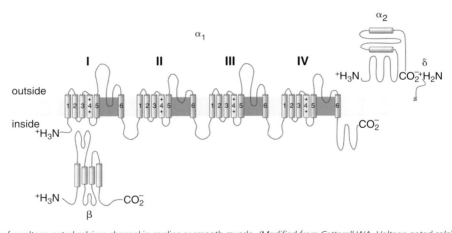

FIG. 25.1 Subunit structure of a voltage-gated calcium channel in cardiac or smooth muscle. *(Modified from Catterall WA. Voltage-gated calcium channels. Cold Spring Harb Perspect Biol. 2011; 3[8].)*

monophosphate-dependent protein kinase, and protein kinase C playing important roles in mediating the effect of inotropic and chronotropic stimuli on the heart and vasomotor influences on the vasculature.[14,26]

DRUGS ACTING ON L-TYPE VOLTAGE-GATED CALCIUM CHANNELS

Dihydropyridines

1,4 dihydropyridines (DHP) are the most commonly used type of CCB in hypertension.[3] DHP act by binding to a site that is formed by amino acid residues in two adjacent S6 segments plus the intervening S5 segment (Fig. 25.1).

They gain access to this site from the extracellular side of the membrane,[27] possibly via a sidewalk pathway similar to that postulated for local anesthetics.[28] DHP bind preferentially to the open/inactivated state of the VGCC and binding results in modification of channel gating. All DHP used clinically act by promoting transition of VGCC into a nonconducting inactivated state as envisaged by the "modulated receptor" hypothesis.[29] Agonist forms of DHP also exist, although they have no clinical role. Agonist DHP bind to the same region of the VGCC as antagonist DHP (although they may not have identical molecular targets[27]) and increase the likelihood of the channel adopting a long open state that occurs only rarely under normal conditions.[30] In some cases (e.g., [S]-BAY K 8644 and [R]-BAY K 8644), enantiomers of the same chemical entity

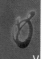
TABLE 25.2 Voltage-Gated Calcium Channel Accessory Subunits

SUBUNIT	FORMS	GENE	CHROMOSOME	FUNCTION
$\alpha_2\delta$	$Ca_V\alpha_2\delta$-1	CACNA2D1	7q21-q22	Membrane trafficking of α_1 subunit, increase in current amplitude, activation/inactivation kinetics, voltage dependence of activation
	$Ca_V\alpha_2\delta$-2	CACNA2D2	3p21.3	Increase in current amplitude
	$Ca_V\alpha_2\delta$-3	CACNA2D3	3p21.1	Increase in current density, voltage dependence of activation, steady state inactivation
	$Ca_V\alpha_2\delta$-4	CACNA2D4	12p13.33	Increase in current amplitude
β	$Ca_V\beta1$	CACNB1	17q21-q22	Membrane trafficking of α_1 subunit, targeting of $\alpha_1 1.1$ to triads, increase in current amplitude, activation/inactivation kinetics
	$Ca_V\beta2$	CACNB2	10p12	Membrane trafficking of α_1 subunit, increase in current amplitude activation/inactivation kinetics, targeting of $\alpha_1 1.4$ in retina
	$Ca_V\beta3$	CACNB3	12q13	Membrane trafficking of α_1 subunit, increase in current amplitude, activation/inactivation kinetics
	$Ca_V\beta4$	CACNB4	2q22-q23	Membrane trafficking of α_1 subunit, increase in current amplitude, activation/inactivation kinetics
γ[a]	$Ca_V\gamma1$	CACNG1	17q24	Inhibitory effect, activation/inactivation kinetics
	$Ca_V\gamma6$	CACNG6	19q13.4	Reduction of current amplitude

[a]Total of 8 γ subunits have been identified but only $\gamma1$ and $\gamma6$ are considered to be subunits of voltage-gated calcium channels.
(Modified from Arikkath J, Campbell KP. Auxiliary subunits: essential components of the voltage-gated calcium channel complex. Curr Opin Neurobiol. 2003;13:298-307.)

TABLE 25.3 Classification of Dihydropyridines Into First, Second, and Third Generation

FIRST GENERATION	SECOND GENERATION		THIRD GENERATION[b]
	Novel Formulation (IIa)	New Chemical Entity (IIb)	
Nifedipine	Nifedipine SR/GITS	Benidipine	Amlodipine
Nicardipine	Felodipine ER[a]	Felodipine[a]	Azelnidipine
	Nicardipine SR	Isradipine	Clevidipine
		Nilvadipine	Efonidipine
		Nimodipine	Lacidipine
		Nisoldipine	Lercanidipine
		Nitrendipine	Manidipine

[a]Felodipine may be classified as either a IIa or a IIb agent.
[b]In some classifications clevidipine, lercanidipine, and lacidipine are referred to as fourth-generation dihydropyridines.
(Table modified from Toyo-Oka T, Nayler WG. Third generation calcium entry blockers. Blood Press. 1996;5:206-208.)
GITS, Gastrointestinal therapeutic system; ER, extended-release; SR, sustained-release.

act as agonist and antagonist, respectively, and agonists can be converted to antagonists or vice versa following site-specific mutation of the channel or by modified experimental conditions.[5]

The mechanism by which DHP reduce Ca^{2+} entry has been studied extensively. A recent model suggests that DHP stabilize an impermeable state which binds a single Ca^{2+} ion.[27] The preferential binding of DHP to channels in the open or inactivated state means that the affinity of DHP is influenced by the membrane potential (i.e., voltage dependence). DHP show higher affinity for VGCC under more depolarized conditions because in these conditions the probability of the open or inactivated state is favored. The voltage-dependence of DHP partially explains why these drugs act preferentially on VGCC in vascular smooth muscle compared with cardiac muscle because vascular smooth muscle cells generally maintain a more depolarized membrane potential than cardiac myocytes.[31] However, other factors also contribute to the preferential action of DHP on the vasculature. These factors include the lower DHP sensitivity of $Ca_V1.3$ and $Ca_V1.4$ subtypes in the heart, and the higher expression of splice variants of $Ca_V1.2$ in vascular smooth muscle that show greater affinity for DHP.[32]

DHP can be further subclassified into first-, second-, and third-generation agents. Initially this was based on the sequence of drug development, however just because a drug is developed later does not necessarily imply superiority.[33] A more recent and persuasive classification is based on the pharmacokinetic and pharmacodynamic properties of DHP (Table 25.3).[34] Other classifications based on vascular: cardiac selectivity and duration of action have also been proposed.[33]

Phenylalkylamines

Verapamil, a member of the phenylalkylamine (PAA) subclass of CCB (other members of this subclass include gallopamil and tiapamil) was the first CCB to be discovered and is the only member of this subclass to be widely used in hypertension.[35] Verapamil binds to amino acids in the S6 segments in domains III and IV of the $\alpha1$ subunit of the VGCC.[36] The PAA binding site overlaps with the site to which DHP bind (Fig. 25.2) and binding of verapamil may result in allosteric modulation of DHP binding.[36]

Unlike DHP, verapamil gains access to its binding site *via* an intracellular route and shows preferential binding to channels in the open state.[37] Verapamil therefore displays frequency-dependence or use-dependence, that is, its binding is favored by frequent repetitive opening of VGCC. This accounts for the efficacy of verapamil in the treatment of supraventricular arrhythmias, and the more pronounced cardiac effects of verapamil compared with DHP. Unlike DHP, verapamil slows the heart rate after chronic use in hypertension, an effect that is more marked during exercise.[38] Nevertheless verapamil has minimal effects on cardiac output due to a compensatory increase in stroke volume, and blood pressure lowering is attributable to a reduction in systemic vascular resistance.[38]

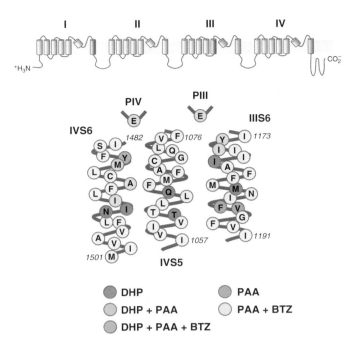

FIG. 25.2 Segments and amino acids in segments interacting with calcium channel blockers. Interactions with dihydropyridines (DHP; red), phenylakylamines (PAA; purple), PAA + benzothiazepines (PAA + BTZ; yellow), DHP+PAAs (orange) and all three blocker classes, DHP + PAAs + BTZs (green) are shown. The IS6 segment contributes significantly to high affinity binding of DHP to the smooth muscle L-type channel. Numbering of amino acids is according to the $Ca_v1.2b$ sequence. *(Modified from Lacinova L. Voltage-dependent calcium channels. Gen Physiol Biophys. 2005; 24(Suppl 1):1-78.)*

Benzothiazipines

Diltiazem, is the only example of the benzothiazepine subclass of CCB used clinically. Diltiazem inhibition of VGCC is effected by binding to amino acid residues located in segments IIIS6, IVS6.[39] Some, but not all, of these amino acids are also involved in binding of DHP and PAAs (Fig. 25.2). Verapamil and diltiazem do not compete with one another for binding,[36] although they can both modulate DHP binding.[40] Diltiazem, similar to verapamil, inhibits VGCC in a frequency and use-dependent manner, although the use-dependence of diltiazem is less prominent than for verapamil[37] and its cardiodepressant effects are less marked.[38,41] Despite its cardiodepressant activity, diltiazem lowers blood pressure by a reduction in systemic vascular resistance.[42]

Pharmacokinetics and Drug Interactions

The pharmacokinetics of the first-generation DHP and the non-DHP, verapamil and diltiazem are relatively similar.[43] They are almost completely absorbed after oral administration and primarily eliminated by hepatic metabolism, but their bioavailability ranges between 10% and 60% because of differences in first-pass metabolism.[44] The duration of action of first-generation DHP and immediate-release formulations of verapamil and diltiazem is quite short, making them less than ideal in the treatment of hypertension. Immediate-release formulations of first- and shorter-acting second-generation DHP (e.g., nifedipine, nicardipine, nimodipine, nitrendipine) had rapid onsets of action which were associated with tachycardia mediated by baroreflex activation.[45,46] This phenomenon may explain cases of angina pectoris following nifedipine.[47] In a case-control study in 1995 Psaty et al. reported that the use of short-acting CCB, especially in high doses, was associated with an increased risk of myocardial infarction.[48] A subsequent meta-analysis based on

TABLE 25.4 Pharmacokinetics of Selected Calcium Channel Blockers Used in Hypertension

DRUG	HALF-LIFE, HOURS	T_{max}, HOURS	REFERENCE
Amlodipine	35-50	6-12	57
Clevidipine[a,b]	0.25 (i.e., ~15 mins)	0.03-0.06 (i.e., 2-4 mins)	160
Felodipine	20-25	2-8	57
Isradipine	8-12	1.5	57
Lacidipine	6-19	1-2[c]	161,162
Lercanidipine	2-5	1.5-3	162,163
Nicardipine	1-4	1-2	57
Nifedipine GITS	2	6	57
Nisoldipine	6-19	1-2	57
Diltiazem	2.5	6-11	164
Verapamil	4.5-12	4-6	164

Drugs chosen are calcium channel blockers approved for use in hypertension in the United States, Europe, or United Kingdom.
[a]Indicated for the reduction of blood pressure by the Federal Drugs Agency when oral therapy is not feasible or not desirable.
[b]Approved for use to lower blood pressure in adults preparing for surgery, undergoing surgery, or immediately after surgery by Medicines & Healthcare products Regulatory Agency.
[c]Despite a relatively short plasma half-life, lacidipine has a long duration of action, probably because of its high lipophilicity.
GITS, Gastrointestinal therapeutic system; T_{max}, time taken to reach maximum concentration.

16 secondary-prevention randomized clinical trials (RCTs) found a significant adverse effect on total mortality, largely attributable to RCTs that used 80 mg or more of nifedipine per day.[49] Although controversial,[50] these findings and others led to calls to avoid short-acting DHP.[51] A consensus view is that these short-acting formulations have no place even in hypertension management, even in the emergency setting[51] and that long-acting drugs in once daily formulations are preferable.[52]

Subsequently modified-release formulations of nifedipine were developed to achieve a slower onset and more prolonged duration of action; a once daily use of such formulations reduces tachycardia and attains 24-hour levels of blood pressure control and peak-to-trough ratios that are similar to newer generation CCB.[53] Newer generation CCB have slow onset and longer duration of action allied to greater preferential effects on the vasculature (vascular/cardiac ratios >100)[54] and are not associated with much if any reflex tachycardia.[46,54] The pharmacokinetic properties of selected CCB are summarized in Table 25.4.

CCB have many important interactions with other drugs.[43] Some arise from pharmacodynamic interactions; for example, beta-blockers and verapamil should not be used simultaneously because of their additive negative inotropic and chronotropic effects on the heart.[3] The combination of dantrolene and verapamil has also been reported to result in hyperkalemia and myocardial depression, probably because hyperkalemia enhances the cardiodepressant effects of verapamil.[55] Other interactions may be attributed to pharmacokinetic effects; for example, verapamil and diltiazem increase digoxin levels probably by decreasing renal and extrarenal clearance.[43] Verapamil and diltiazem also increase levels of cyclosporine, carbamazepine, phenytoin, prazosin, and theophylline.[43] Verapamil and diltiazem are metabolized by CYP3A4, therefore inducers (e.g., rifampin) and inhibitors (e.g., erythromycin, itraconazole, cimetidine) are likely to result respectively in decreased and increased plasma levels of these two CCB.[43] Grapefruit juice, which contains flavonoids that inhibit gut

TABLE 25.5 Inhibition of Non-L-Type Voltage-Gated Calcium Channels by Calcium Channel Blockers

CHANNEL SUBTYPE	DRUG	REFERENCES
N	Amlodipine, barnidipine, benidipine, cilnidipine, nicardipine	165-167
P/Q	Amlodipine, barnidipine, benidipine, nicardipine (equivocal or inconsistent evidence for cilnidipine and nimodipine)	165-167
T-type	Barnidipine, benidipine, isradipine, efonidipine, manidipine, nicardipine, niguldipine, nisoldipine (equivocal or inconsistent evidence for amlodipine, felodipine, nimodipine, and nitrendipine)	65,66,168

Drugs listed achieve 50% or greater inhibition (IC$_{50}$) for the channel subtype at concentrations that overlap with, or are not more than three-fold less than their IC$_{50}$ for L-type calcium channels.
Inconsistent evidence may result from experimental and methodological differences between studies, differences between expressed and native channels, or differences between splice variants.

CYP3A4 increases the oral bioavailability of several CCB, with the most marked effect on felodipine.[56] In addition, verapamil inhibits P-glycoprotein–mediated drug transport, which may alter the intestinal absorption of several drugs and affect their distribution into peripheral tissues and the central nervous system.[57]

Caution should be exercised in using CCB in patients with liver disease because their metabolism may be reduced leading to higher plasma concentrations and potential toxicity. In general lower starting and maintenance doses of CCB should be used in hepatic impairment.[58] Dose modification for most CCB is not usually required in renal insufficiency,[59] although verapamil may be an exception.[58]

Actions on Non-L-Type (N-Type, P/Q-Type, and T-Type) Voltage-Gated Calcium Channels

The three major classes of CCB were originally identified on the basis of their blocking effects on L-type VGCC. Other (non-L-type) VGCC were considered to be relatively insensitive to DHP.[60] More recently, however, several CCB have been found to inhibit N-type and P/Q-type and/or T-type VGCC at concentrations that overlap with or are close to those that inhibit L-type VGCC (Table 25.5). Blockade of N-type VGCC could result in more pronounced sympatho-inhibitory effects,[61,62] or inhibitory effects on aldosterone release.[62] Inhibitory actions on P/Q-type VGCC could augment vasodilator effects, particularly in the renal circulation.[23] Inhibition of T-type VGCC could lessen reflex tachycardia, reduce aldosterone secretion, and contribute to renal protective effects.[63] Differences between first- and second/third-generation DHP have been attributed in part to such differences in pharmacodynamics with second/third-generation agents tending to possess a more mixed inhibitory profile on VGCC,[64] although as discussed above differences in pharmacokinetics are also likely to be clinically important.

Recently other CCB have been developed with the aim of having preferential or equipotent effects on non-L-type VGCC. These include mebefradil (Ro 40-5967), a benzimidazolyl-substituted tetraline derivative, which showed selectivity for T-type over L-type VGCC,[65] but also affected other channels[66] and was withdrawn as a result of risks from drug-drug interactions.[67] Efonidipine, a third-generation DHP, shows a slight selectivity for T-type VGCC,[65] but is probably best regarded as a mixed blocker of L-type and T-type VGCC.[68]

Ancillary Actions

Some CCB may possess ancillary actions unrelated to their ability to block VGCC. Several DHP, including amlodipine, benidipine, nisolidipine, nitrendipine, and nifedipine (the latter inconsistently) have been reported to increase endothelial nitric oxide release in vitro and/or in vivo.[69,70] This property seems unrelated to a drug's ability to block VGCC as it is displayed by VGCC agonists, such as BAY 8644 and the inactive enantiomer, (R)-amlodipine.[69,70] It may be related to the presence of nitric oxide (NO) donor furoxans in DHP,[71] antioxidant properties,[70] or disruption of cell membrane caveolae.[72] The antioxidant properties of some DHP have also been proposed to contribute to antiatherosclerotic actions of CCB,[70] but as with other ancillary actions whether or not these effects should influence selection of CCB in clinical practice remains to be established.

CALCIUM CHANNEL BLOCKERS IN THE MANAGEMENT OF HYPERTENSION

Blood Pressure Lowering and Hemodynamic Actions

Although they were originally envisaged as antianginal and antiarrhythmic agents,[8] CCB have been used as hypotensive agents since the late 1970s.[73] All CCB lower blood pressure when given acutely and following chronic administration,[74] and the maximum blood pressure lowering effects of the various subclasses of CCB are similar.[75] All CCB lower blood pressure as a consequence of arterial vasodilation, although there are some differences between CCB subclasses with respect to regional blood flow.[74] CCB do possess modest venodilator actions,[76] but have minimal effects on total venous capacitance.[77] This may explain why orthostatic hypotension is not especially common with CCB therapy compared with other vasodilators.[78] There is evidence that CCB are more effective compared with angiotensin-converting enzyme (ACE) inhibitors or beta-blockers in people of African heritage,[79,80] or individuals with low plasma renin levels.[81]

Effective blood pressure reduction over 24 hours is a desirable feature of any antihypertensive agent,[82] and newer generation CCB and prolonged release formulations provide sustained blood pressure control. A recent systematic review[83] of 16 RCTs of DHP (2768 participants; drugs studied: amlodipine, lercanidipine, manidipine, nifedipine, and felodipine [once daily] and nicardipine [administered twice daily]) reported that all these CCB lowered blood pressure by a relatively similar amount each hour over the course of 24 hours.

Longer term variability in blood pressure (i.e., over periods of months or years) has also been proposed as a risk factor for cardiovascular disease,[84] particularly stroke.[85] CCB have been reported to be the most effective antihypertensive class in reducing this long-term variability.[86] The extent to which this contributes to their beneficial effects on cardiovascular (CV) outcomes in hypertension is uncertain.

Differences in antihypertensive efficacy on aortic (central) and brachial (peripheral) blood pressure may also influence CV outcomes in hypertension.[87] A recent meta-analysis[88] indicated that CCB lowered central and peripheral blood pressures to similar extents, unlike diuretics and beta-blockers which were less effective in lowering central blood pressure.

CCB decrease renal vascular resistance and consequently renal blood flow is maintained despite reductions in blood pressure.[89] Typically, CCB also increase glomerular filtration rate[24] and, unlike most other arterial vasodilators (e.g., hydralazine and minoxidil), cause a modest natriuresis, which is partly as a result of inhibition of tubular reabsorption of sodium.[89]

Effects on Target Organ Damage in Hypertension

Left Ventricular Hypertrophy

Left ventricular hypertrophy (LVH) and abnormal left ventricular geometry is associated with an increased incidence of CV events independent of blood pressure,[90] and individuals who show regression of LVH during antihypertensive therapy have better CV outcomes than those who do not.[91]

A number of RCTs have examined the ability of CCB to induce regression of LVH in comparison with other antihypertensive agents. In the Effects of Amlodipine and Lisinopril on LV Mass and Diastolic Function (ELVERA) study, amlodipine was as effective as lisinopril in reducing LV mass index in 166 newly diagnosed hypertensive individuals over 2 years of treatment.[92] The Prospective Randomized Enalapril Study Evaluating Regression of Ventricular Enlargement (PRESERVE) study showed similar regression of LVH by nifedipine gastrointestinal therapeutic system (GITS) or enalapril in 235 patients over 1 year of treatment.[93] A substudy of the European Lacidipine Study on Atherosclerosis (ELSA) reported no significant difference in LV mass index reduction in 174 patients treated with lacidipine or atenolol after 4 years of treatment.[94] A substudy of the ASCOT trial also found no difference in LV mass regression following treatment of 536 participants with either amlodipine-based or atenolol-based therapy for an average of 3.5 years.[95] A meta-analysis of 80 RCTs, 146 active treatment arms (3767 patients), and 17 placebo arms (346 patients) found significant differences between antihypertensive agents in their ability to cause regression of left ventricular mass index, with CCB and ACE inhibitors being more effective than beta-blockers.

Arterial Stiffness

Increased arterial stiffness (higher pulse wave velocity [PWV] or reduced arterial compliance) plays a key role in the age-dependent increase in pulse pressure[96] and isolated systolic hypertension (ISH),[96,97] and predicts cardiovascular events independently of blood pressure.[98] Central pulse pressure and augmentation index, although related to arterial compliance and wave reflection, should not be interpreted as direct measures of arterial stiffness.[99] Interpreting the effect of antihypertensive agents on arterial stiffness is complicated by its inherent pressure-dependence[100,101]; hence blood pressure reduction should inherently reduce arterial stiffness.[99] Consequently the reductions in PWV observed following administration of CCB[102-105] may simply be a consequence of blood pressure lowering. There is, however, some evidence that antihypertensive agents can reduce arterial stiffness beyond that expected simply on the basis of the reduction in mean arterial pressure.[106] A study comparing valsartan plus hydrochlorothiazide with amlodipine in 131 patients with type 2 diabetes, pulse pressure 60 mm Hg or higher and raised albumin excretion rate found a greater reduction in PWV for valsartan/hydrochlorothiazide than amlodipine (difference = –0.9 m/s [95% confidence interval {CI} –1.4 to –0.3]; p = 0.002) despite similar reductions in brachial and central pulse pressure. However, a recent meta-analysis found no evidence of difference in the ability of individual antihypertensive agents to reduce PWV, although the number of eligible studies was small and confidence limits were wide.[107] Whether or not CCB can reduce PWV through mechanisms unrelated to blood pressure reduction therefore remains uncertain.

Renal Function and Progression of Kidney Disease

Blood pressure lowering is associated with diminished urinary protein excretion and reduced progression of nephropathy in patients with chronic kidney disease (see also Chapter 33). In the Systolic Hypertension in Europe (Syst-Eur) trial[108] patients randomized to nitrendipine had a 64% lower incidence of mild renal dysfunction and a 33% lower incidence of new proteinuria than those randomized to placebo.[109]

Several RCTs have compared CCB with other antihypertensive regimens and reported renal functional outcomes. In INSIGHT[110] there was a lower incidence of impaired renal function in patients treated with nifedipine than a diuretic (1.8% versus 4.6%, p < 0.0001), ALLHAT[111] reported higher estimated glomerular filtration rate (eGFR) with amlodipine than chlortalidone (75.1 versus. 70.0 mL/min/1.73m²; p = 0.001) or lisinopril (75.1 versus 70.7 mL/min/1.73 m²), and no significant difference in the incidence of end-stage renal disease (ESRD) when analysis was restricted to patients with reduced renal function at baseline.[112] VALUE[113] also reported no difference in renal outcomes with amlodipine or valsartan. However, in an RCT that recruited African-American hypertensive patients with nondiabetic nephropathy, amlodipine was associated with a greater decline in eGFR than ramipril, especially in those with significant proteinuria.[114] A recent meta-analysis of 26 trials (152,290 participants), including 30,295 individuals with reduced estimated glomerular filtration rate, found little evidence of a difference between drug classes for the prevention of cardiovascular events in chronic kidney disease.[115]

A meta-analysis indicates that non-DHP may have more favorable effects on proteinuria and the progression of kidney disease than DHP despite similar hypotensive effects.[109] New generation DHP that additionally block non-L-type VGCC may improve renal function more than classical DHP, although evidence related to specific drugs is limited. A meta-analysis[116] of 24 studies (1696 participants) that compared T-type CCB (efonidipine, azelnidipine, benidipine, manidipine, nilvadipine) to L-type CCB (amlodipine or nifedipine) or to renin-angiotensin system (RAS) antagonists found that proteinuria (mean difference = –0.73 [95% CI –0.88, –0.57]; p < 10^{-5}), protein-to-creatinine ratio (mean difference = –0.22 [95% CI –0.41, –0.03]; p = 0.02), and urinary albumin-to-creatinine ratio (mean difference = –55.38 [95% CI –86.67, –24.09]; p = 0.0005) were reduced when T-type CCB were compared with L-type CCB despite similar blood pressure reductions. The effects of T-type CCB did not significantly differ from RAS antagonists in terms of blood pressure or renal measures. A multi-center, open-labeled, and randomized trial comparing cilnidipine, an L/N-type blocker, with amlodipine in 339 participants found a significant reduction in urinary protein-to-creatinine ratio with no difference in blood pressure after 12 months of treatment.[117]

Cognitive Function and Dementia

The association between blood pressure and cognitive function and dementia is complex and seems to be modified by age.[118] There is reasonably convincing evidence that elevated blood pressure in mid-life (40 to 64 years) is associated with subsequent impaired cognitive function or dementia.[118] However, evidence that antihypertensive treatment (usually initiated in later life) can prevent this is unconvincing,[119] and relatively few RCTs have looked at cognitive function or dementia as an outcome. In Syst-Eur,[120] which included participants 60 years of age or older with systolic hypertension and without dementia at baseline, nitrendipine treatment (with enalapril and/or hydrochlorothiazide added if necessary) was associated with a 50% reduction in incident dementia (vascular and Alzheimer) over a median 2-year follow-up compared with placebo. At present this study remains the only RCT examining the effect of CCB on dementia. A meta-analysis of all data including observational studies was unable to provide clear evidence either way regarding the effects of CCB on cognitive function and dementia.[121] Further clinical trials are required to definitively establish whether or not CCB have benefits for cognitive function and prevention of dementia.

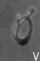

Major Clinical Outcomes

There have been numerous RCTs examining the effect of CCB on major cardiovascular outcomes (e.g., myocardial infarction, stroke, angina, coronary revascularization, congestive heart failure, and peripheral arterial disease) in hypertension. Relevant RCTs are shown in Table 25.6. In the majority of these trials treatment was initiated with a CCB or comparator and other agents were added as necessary to achieve target blood pressure (Table 25.7); in some, CCB or comparator was added to existing antihypertensive therapy. These studies have convincingly established that CCB are effective in reducing cardiovascular events compared with placebo, and that they have broadly similar effects on outcomes to other major classes of antihypertensive agents (diuretics, beta-blockers, angiotensin-converting enzyme inhibitors, and angiotensin receptor blockers). Studies have been conducted in the elderly,[122,123] patients with stable coronary heart disease,[124,125] and some non-European/Caucasian ethnic groups[111,123,126] and so have reasonably wide applicability. These conclusions are supported by recent meta-analyses of data from RCTs. The Blood Pressure Lowering Treatment Trialists' Collaboration undertook a prospectively designed meta-analysis of placebo-controlled RCTs of calcium antagonists (two trials, 5520 patients mostly with hypertension) and showed strong evidence of cardiovascular benefit of CCB: a 28% (95% CI 13, 41) reduction in major cardiovascular events, with similar magnitude reductions in coronary heart disease, stroke, heart failure, and cardiovascular death.[127] A subsequent meta-analysis[128] that included 27 RCTs (175,634 individuals) confirmed that CCB reduced major cardiovascular events by 24% and provided evidence that the risk of major cardiovascular events (pooled fatal and nonfatal myocardial infarction, stroke, cardiovascular death, heart

TABLE 25.6 Trials Comparing Antihypertensive Treatment Initiated With a Calcium Channel Blocker With (A) Placebo; (B) Diuretic/Beta-Blocker; (C) Angiotensin Converting Enzyme Inhibitor or Angiotensin Receptor Blocker

(A)

Trial	Agents Compared (1 vs. 2)	ΔSBP/DBP, mm Hg (1 vs. 2)	Primary Outcome Difference
STONE[169]	Nifedipine SR vs. placebo	−9/−6	−62% (p < 0.001) [CV events]
Syst-Eur[122]	Nitrendipine vs. placebo	−10/−4.5	−42% (p = 0.003) [stroke]
Syst-China[123]	Nitrendipine vs. placebo	−9/−3	−38% (p = 0.01) [stroke]
ACTION-HT[124]	Nifedipine GITS vs. placebo	−6.6/−3.5	−13% (p = 0.02) [CV events]
CAMELOT[125]	Amlodipine vs. placebo	−5.5/−3.1	−31% (p = 0.003) [CV events]
FEVER[145]	Felodipine vs. placebo	−4.2/−2.1	−27% (p = 0.002) [stroke]

(B)

Trial	Agents Compared (1 vs. 2)	ΔSBP/DBP, mmHg (1 vs. 2)	Primary Outcome Difference
STOP-2[170]	Felodipine or isradipine vs. Atenolol or pindolol or HCTZ	+2/<1	−3% (p = 0.7) [CV death]
NICS-EH[126]	Nicardipine vs. trichlormethiazide	0/+2%	−3% (p > 0.9) [CV events]
NORDIL[171]	Diltiazem vs. β-blocker or diuretic	+3/<1	0% (p > 0.9) [CV events]
INSIGHT[110]	Nifedipine GITS vs. HCTZ + amiloride	<1/<1	+11% (p = 0.35) [CV events]
ALLHAT[111]	Amlodipine vs. chlortalidone	+1/<1	−2% (p = 0.65) [cardiac events]
CONVINCE[143]	COER-verapamil vs. HCTZ or atenolol	<1/<1	+2% (p = 0.77) [CV events]
SHELL[172]	Lacidipine vs. chlortalidone	−1/	+1% (p > 0.9) [CV events]
INVEST[144]	Verapamil vs. atenolol	<1/<1	−2% (p = 0.57) [CV events]
ASCOT[173]	Amlodipine vs. atenolol	−2.7/−1.9	−10% (p = 0.1)ᵃ [CV events]

(C)

Trial	Agents Compared (1 vs. 2)	ΔSBP/DBP, mm Hg (1 vs. 2)	Primary Outcome Difference
STOP-2[170]	Felodipine ER or isradipine vs. enalapril or lisinopril	<1/<1	−4% (p = 0.67) [CV death]
JMIC-B[174]	Nifedipine vs. ACEi	−2/−2	+5% (p = 0.86) [cardiac events]
ALLHAT[175]	Amlodipine vs. lisinopril	−1.5/1.1	0% (p = 0.85) [cardiac events]
CAMELOT[125]	Amlodipine vs. enalapril	<1/<1	−19% (p = 0.1) [CV events]
VALUE[147]	Amlodipine vs. valsartan	−2.6/−1.6	−4% (p = 0.49) [cardiac events]
MOSES[176]	Nitrendipine vs. eprosartan	−1.5/<1	+31% (p = 0.03) [CV events]

ᵃStudy was stopped prematurely after 5.5 years' median follow-up as a result of higher mortality and worse outcomes on several other secondary effects in those randomized to atenolol-based regimen compared with the amlodipine-based regimen.
p Values are those reported for the primary outcome as defined in the study.
(Modified from Zanchetti A. Calcium channel blockers in hypertension. In: Black HR, Elliott WJ, eds. Hypertension: A Companion to Braunwald's Heart Disease. Philadelphia: Saunders Elsevier; 2007: 268-285.)
ACEi, Angiotensin-converting enzyme inhibitor; CV, cardiovascular; ER, extended-release; GITS, gastrointestinal therapeutic system; HCTZ, hydrochlorothiazide; ΔSBP, difference in systolic blood pressure; ΔDBP, difference in diastolic blood pressure.
Trial acronyms: ACTION-HT, A Coronary Disease Trial Investigating Outcomes with Nifedipine GITS—Hypertensive Cohort; ALLHAT, Antihypertensive and Lipid Lowering Treatment to Prevent Heart Attack Trial; ASCOT, Anglo-Scandinavian Cardiac Outcomes Trial; CAMELOT, Comparison of Amlodipine versus Enalapril to Limit Occurrences of Thrombosis; CONVINCE, Controlled Onset Verapamil Investigation of Cardiovascular Endpoints; FEVER, Felodipine Event Reduction; INSIGHT, International Nifedipine GITS Study, Intervention as a Goal in Hypertension Treatment; INVEST, International Verapamil SR/Trandolapril study; JMIC-B, Japan Multicenter Investigation for Cardiovascular Disease-B; MOSES, Morbidity and Mortality After Stroke, Eprosartan Compared with Nitrendipine for Secondary Prevention Study; NICS-EH, National Intervention Cooperative Study in Elderly Hypertensives; NORDIL, Nordic Diltiazem Trial; SHELL, Systolic Hypertension in the Elderly Lacidipine Trial; STONE, Shanghai Trial on Nifedipine in the Elderly; STOP-2, Swedish Trial in Old Patients with Hypertension-2; Syst-Eur, Systolic Hypertension in Europe; Syst-China, Systolic Hypertension in China; VALUE, Valsartan Antihypertensive Long-Term Use Evaluation.

failure) was similar between CCB and non-CCB drugs (beta-blockers, diuretics, angiotensin converting enzyme inhibitors, and angiotensin receptor blockers). Compared with other antihypertensive medications, CCB were associated with a modestly lower risk of stroke (odds ratio [OR] 0.86 [95% CI 0.82, 0.90]), similar risks of coronary heart disease and a modestly increased risk of heart failure (OR 1.17 [95% CI 1.11, 1.24]). A more recent meta-analysis[129] based on 18 RCTs (141,807 participants) compared individual classes of antihypertensive agent (Fig. 25.3). This analysis found that all-cause mortality was not different between first-line CCB and any other first-line antihypertensive classes. Compared with beta-blockers, CCB reduced total cardiovascular events, cardiovascular mortality, and stroke but were associated with increased total cardiovascular events and congestive heart failure events compared with diuretics. CCB also reduced stroke compared with ACE inhibitors and reduced stroke and myocardial infarction compared with ARBs, but increased congestive heart failure events compared with ACE inhibitors or ARBs. The other evaluated outcomes did not differ significantly.

Safety of Calcium Channel Blockers

Adverse Effects

Many of the adverse effects of CCB are a consequence of vasodilation and are typically dose dependent.[130,131] Vasodilator side effects tend to be more common with DHP than verapamil or diltiazem,[131] but non-DHP are more commonly associated with cardiac and gastrointestinal side effects (particularly constipation with verapamil).[131] Table 25.8 lists some common adverse effects observed in some large RCTs comparing a CCB with other antihypertensive agents. In addition to vasodilator effects CCB can be associated with gingival hyperplasia; this underrecognized adverse effect has been reported to occur in 14% to 83% of patients treated with nifedipine, and it appears to be less common with other CCB (~4%).[132]

DHP are associated with headache, dizziness or lightheadedness, flushing, hypotension, and peripheral edema in between 10% and 20% of patients.[133] Peripheral edema occurs in around 10% of patients,[130] is more common in women,[134] and leads to withdrawal of about 2% of participants in RCTs.[130] CCB-induced edema is believed to be secondary to increased capillary pressure because of precapillary arterial and arteriolar vasodilatation without equivalent postcapillary vasodilatation. Edema is less common when lipophilic or non-DHP CCB are used.[130,135] Diuretics may not relieve this edema,[136] but ACE inhibitors and, perhaps to a lesser extent, other inhibitors of the RAS may reduce or prevent CCB-induced edema.[137] These effects of RAS inhibition may be attributed to venodilation and an amelioration of elevated capillary pressures.[138]

Vasodilator side effects are less common with verapamil and diltiazem,[41,139] but constipation is more common and is more frequent for verapamil than diltiazem.[41] In a meta-analysis of 7 double-blind RCTs (1999 participants) verapamil use was associated with constipation in 13% compared with 2% of patients receiving placebo. Dizziness (6% versus 2%), and back pain (3% versus 1%) were also increased by verapamil.

CCB are generally considered metabolically neutral[140] and a network meta-analysis of 22 clinical trials with 143,153 participants without diabetes at randomization indicated that incidence of diabetes with CCB was less than with diuretics and beta-blockers, similar to placebo, and greater than ACE inhibitors or ARB (Fig. 25.4).[141]

Serious alarms over associations between CCB use and cancer were raised by a cohort study in the 1990s[142] but large RCTs[110,111,143-145] and a recent meta-analysis[146] have not borne out this concern. Similarly, RCTs[111,143,144] do not suggest a clinically important increase in risk of gastrointestinal bleeding in patients receiving CCB.

TABLE 25.7 Drugs Combined as Second Agent With Calcium Channel Blockers in Major Controlled Randomized Trials

TRIAL	CALCIUM CHANNEL BLOCKER	ADDED AGENT
Syst-Eur[19]	Nitrendipine	ACEi: Enalapril
Syst-China[20]	Nitrendipine	ACEi: Captopril
VHAS[46]	Verapamil	ACEi: Captopril
HOT[45]	Felodipine	ACEi: Any (enalapril in United States)
NORDIL[26]	Diltiazem	ACEi: Any
INVEST[31]	Verapamil	ACEi: Trandolapril
ASCOT[32]	Amlodipine	ACEi: Perindopril
HOT[45]	Felodipine	BB: Any
STOP-2[24]	Felodipine or Isradipine	BB: Any
INSIGHT[27]	Nifedipine	BB: Atenolol
ALLHAT[28]	Amlodipine	BB: Atenolol
ELSA[52]	Lacidipine	D: Hydrochlorothiazide
CONVINCE[29]	Verapamil	D: Hydrochlorothiazide
VALUE[34]	Amlodipine	D: Hydrochlorothiazide
FEVER[23]	Felodipine	D: Hydrochlorothiazide[a]

[a]Hydrochlorothiazide as background drug to all patients.
(Modified from Zanchetti A. Calcium channel blockers in Hypertension. In: Black HR, Elliott WJ, eds. Hypertension: A Companion to Braunwald's Heart Disease. Philadelphia: Saunders Elsevier; 2007: 268-285.)
ACEi, Angiotensin-converting enzyme inhibitor; BB, β-blocker; D, diuretic.
For trial acronyms, see Table 25.1 and the text.

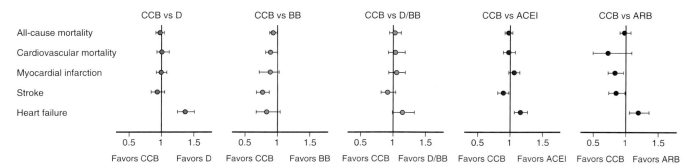

FIG. 25.3 Meta-analysis of randomized clinical trials comparing outcomes of blood pressure lowering using calcium channel blockers (CCB) with regimens based on diuretics (D), beta-blockers (BB), diuretics and beta-blockers (D/BB), where a diuretic, a beta-blocker or both were used but could not be analyzed separately, angiotensin-converting enzyme inhibitors (ACEi), or angiotensin receptor blockers (ARB). The circles indicate the risk ratios and the bars the 95% confidence intervals. (Redrawn from data Chen N, Zhou M, Yang M, et al. Calcium channel blockers versus other classes of drugs for hypertension. Cochrane Database Syst Rev 2010;(8):Cd003654.)

TABLE 25.8 Major Adverse Effects Reported in Some Randomized Trials Comparing Calcium Channel Blockers With Other Antihypertensive Medications

ADVERSE EFFECT	VHAS[177] CCB D	NORDIL[171] CCB D/BB p	INVEST[144] CCB BB p	INSIGHT[110] CCB D p	STOP-2[170] CCB D/BB ACEi	ASCOT[173] CCB BB p	VALUE[147] CCB ARB p
Edema	— —	— —	— —	28 4.3 <0.0001	25.5 8.5 8.7	23 6 <0.0001	**32.9** 14.9 <0.0001
Headache	3.1 3.4	**8.5** 5.7 <0.001	— —	12 9.2 0.0002	10.0 5.7 7.7	— —	12.5 14.7 <0.0001
Flushing	— —	— —	— —	4.3 2.3 <0.0001	9.7 1.6 2.2	— —	— —
Palpitations	— —	— —	— —	2.5 2.7 NS	7.9 2.9 5.3	— —	— —
Bradycardia	— —	— —	0.66 **1.26** <0.01	— —	1.4 3.7 0.8	0.4 6 <0.0001	— —
Dyspnea	— —	2.9 3.9 0.006	0.73 1.01 0.03	— —	8.5 11.8 7.3	6 10 <0.0001	— —
Dizziness	3.5 3.1	9.3 8.9 NS	1.37 1.34 NS	8.0 **10.0** 0.006	24.5 **27.8** 27.7	12 16 <0.0001	14.3 **16.5** <0.0001
Syncope	— —	— —	1.73 0.013 <0.01	1.5 2.8 0.0004	— —	— —	1.0 1.7 <0.0001
Constipation	**13.7** 3.1	— —	— —	— —	— —	— —	— —
Fatigue	4.7 **8.4**	4.4 **6.5** <0.001	— —	— —	— —	8 **16** <0.0001	8.9 9.7 NS
Depression	— —	3.7 3.4 NS	— —	3.09 5.7 0.0009	— —	— —	— —
Cough	— —	5.6 5.4 NS	**1.78** 1.34 0.01	— —	5.7 3.7 **30.1**	19 8 <0.0001	— —

Data are % and p values, where available. Trials and regimens as in Table 25.6. VHAS and STOP-2 did not report significance tests for adverse effects. The numbers in bold indicate the adverse effect with the highest incidence in each trial. In ASCOT, a calcium channel blocker (CCB) was very frequently administered with an angiotensin-converting enzyme inhibitor (ACEi), and the high frequency of cough in the CCB group is likely as a result of the concomitant ACEi.
(Modified from Zanchetti A. Calcium channel blockers in hypertension. In: Black HR, Elliott WJ, eds. Hypertension: A Companion to Braunwald's Heart Disease. Philadelphia: Saunders Elsevier; 2007: 268-285.)
ACEi, Angiotensin-converting enzyme inhibitor; ARB, angiotensin receptor blocker; BB, beta-blocker; CCB, calcium channel blocker; D, diuretic; NS, nonsignificant.

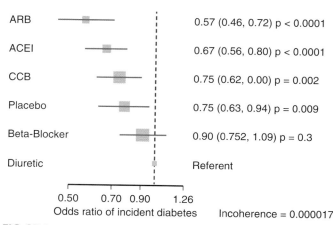

ARB		0.57 (0.46, 0.72) p < 0.0001
ACEI		0.67 (0.56, 0.80) p < 0.0001
CCB		0.75 (0.62, 0.00) p = 0.002
Placebo		0.75 (0.63, 0.94) p = 0.009
Beta-Blocker		0.90 (0.752, 1.09) p = 0.3
Diuretic		Referent

Odds ratio of incident diabetes   Incoherence = 0.000017

FIG. 25.4 Results of network meta-analysis examining the incidence of new diabetes in clinical trials of antihypertensive drugs. Initial diuretic used as referent agent (open box at odds ratio = 1.0). Size of squares (representing the point estimate for each class of antihypertensive drugs) is proportional to number of patients who developed incident diabetes. Horizontal lines indicate 95% confidence intervals. Odds ratios to the left of the vertical line at unity denote a protective effect (compared with initial diuretic). Individual pair-wise comparisons between diuretic versus beta-blocker blocker ($p = 0.30$), placebo versus calcium channel blocker (CCB; $p = 0.72$), angiotensin-converting enzyme inhibitor (ACEi) versus angiotensin receptor blocker (ARB; $p = 0.16$) did not achieve statistical significance. *(Modified from Elliott WJ, Meyer PM. Incident diabetes in clinical trials of antihypertensive drugs: a network meta-analysis. Lancet. 2007; 369:201-207.)*

SPECIAL INDICATIONS AND CONTRAINDICATIONS FOR CALCIUM CHANNEL BLOCKERS

Angina Pectoris

Concerns regarding the possible associations between CCB use and myocardial infarction have been discussed earlier in this chapter ("Pharmacokinetics and Drug Interactions"). CCB are effective in the relief of angina pectoris[124,125,144,147] and are commonly prescribed for this purpose if there are contraindications or adverse reactions to beta-blockers.[148]

Heart Failure

Verapamil and, to a lesser extent, diltiazem can reduce cardiac contractility and slow heart rate and cardiac conduction.[57] These rate-limiting CCB are therefore contraindicated in patients who have severe heart failure with reduced ejection fraction (HFrEF), sick sinus syndrome, broad-complex tachydysrhythmias, and second-degree or third-degree atrioventricular block. Rate-limiting CCB can cause severe conduction disturbances in hypertrophic cardiomyopathy and they should be avoided in patients taking beta-blockers. Nifedipine, although less cardiodepressant than non-DHP, has also been found to have detrimental effects in cardiac failure[149] and should also be avoided. Newer generation CCB, such as amlodipine and felodipine, appear safe in heart failure,[150-152] but confer no benefit in terms of survival.[150-152] Newer generation CCB, such as amlodipine, can be used for the treatment of hypertension in patients with systolic heart failure[153]; however, ACE inhibitors and beta-blockers, both of which improve patient survival in heart failure, are probably a better first choice.[154]

Hypertensive Disorders of Pregnancy

CCB are commonly used in hypertensive disorders of pregnancy.[155] This topic is covered in more detail in Chapter 39.

CONCLUSIONS

CCB are widely used and are likely to remain so for the foreseeable future. They lower blood pressure with a good safety profile and relatively few contraindications. Most national and international guidelines for the management of arterial hypertension[156-159] recommend them as first- or second-line agents in the absence of contraindications.

References

1. Kaufman DW, Kelly JP, Rosenberg L, et al. Recent patterns of medication use in the ambulatory adult population of the United States—The Slone survey. *JAMA.* 2002;287:337-344.
2. Gu Q, Burt VL, Dillon CF, Yoon S. Trends in antihypertensive medication use and blood pressure control among United States adults with hypertension: the National Health And Nutrition Examination Survey, 2001 to 2010. *Circulation.* 2012;126:2105-114.
3. Elliott WJ, Ram CV. Calcium channel blockers. *J Clin Hypertens.* 2011;13:687-689.
4. Vanhoutte PM, Paoletti R. The WHO classification of calcium antagonists. *Trends Pharmacol Sci.* 1987;8:4-5.
5. Zamponi GW. Antagonist binding sites of voltage-dependent calcium channels. *Drug Dev Res.* 1997;42:131-143.
6. Krebs J, Michalak M. *Calcium: A Matter of Life or Death.* 1st ed. Amsterdam; Oxford: Elsevier; 2007.
7. Dolphin AC. A short history of voltage-gated calcium channels. *Br J Pharmacol.* 2006;147(Suppl 1):S56-62.
8. Fleckenstein A. History of calcium antagonists. *Circ Res.* 1983;52(2 Pt 2):I3-16.
9. Bahring R, Covarrubias M. Mechanisms of closed-state inactivation in voltage-gated ion channels. *J Physiol.* 2011;589(Pt 3):461-479.
10. Tsien RW, Hess P, McCleskey EW, Rosenberg RL. Calcium channels: mechanisms of selectivity, permeation, and block. *Annu Rev Biophys Biophys Chem.* 1987;16:265-290.
11. Heinemann SH, Terlau H, Stuhmer W, Imoto K, Numa S. Calcium channel characteristics conferred on the sodium channel by single mutations. *Nature.* 1992;356:441-443.
12. Dolphin AC. A short history of voltage-gated calcium channels. *Br J Pharmacol.* 2006;147 Suppl 1):S56-62.
13. Catterall WA. Voltage-gated calcium channels. *Cold Spring Harb Perspect Biol.* 2011;3(8).
14. Hofmann F, Flockerzi V, Kahl S, Wegener JW. L-type CaV1.2 calcium channels: from in vitro findings to in vivo function. *Physiol Rev.* 2014;94:303-326.
15. Arikkath J, Campbell KP. Auxiliary subunits: essential components of the voltage-gated calcium channel complex. *Curr Opin Neurobiol.* 2003;13:298-307.
16. Hansen PB. New role of P/Q-type voltage-gated calcium channels: from transmitter release to contraction of renal vasculature. *J Cardiovasc Pharmacol.* 2015;65:406-411.
17. Mesirca P, Torrente AG, Mangoni ME. Functional role of voltage gated Ca(2+) channels in heart automaticity. *Front Physiol.* 2015;6:19.
18. Kuo IY, Howitt L, Sandow SL, et al. Role of T-type channels in vasomotor function: team player or chameleon? *Pflugers Arch.* 2014;466:767-779.
19. Moosmang S, Lenhardt P, Haider N, et al. Mouse models to study L-type calcium channel function. *Pharmacol Ther.* 2005;106:347-355.
20. Mangoni ME, Traboulsie A, Leoni AL, et al. Bradycardia and slowing of the atrioventricular conduction in mice lacking CaV3.1/alpha1G T-type calcium channels. *Circ Res.* 2006;98:1422-1430.
21. Chiang CS, Huang CH, Chieng H, et al. The Ca(v)3.2 T-type Ca(2+) channel is required for pressure overload-induced cardiac hypertrophy in mice. *Circ Res.* 2009;104:522-530.
22. Hansen PB. Functional importance of T-type voltage-gated calcium channels in the cardiovascular and renal system: news from the world of knockout mice. *Am J Physiol Regul Integr Comp Physiol.* 2015;308:R227-237.
23. Hansen PB. Functional and pharmacological consequences of the distribution of voltage-gated calcium channels in the renal blood vessels. *Acta Physiol (Oxf).* 2013;207:690-699.
24. Homma K, Hayashi K, Yamaguchi S, Fujishima S, Hori S, Itoh H. Renal microcirculation and calcium channel subtypes. *Curr Hypertens Rev.* 2013;9:182-186.
25. Liao P, Yong TF, Liang MC, Yue DT, Soong TW. Splicing for alternative structures of Cav1.2 Ca2+ channels in cardiac and smooth muscles. *Cardiovasc Res.* 2005;68:197-203.
26. Keef KD, Hume JR, Zhong J. Regulation of cardiac and smooth muscle Ca(2+) channels (Ca(V)1.2a,b) by protein kinases. *Am J Physiol Cell Physiol.* 2001;281:C1743-1756.
27. Tikhonov DB, Zhorov BS. Structural model for dihydropyridine binding to L-type calcium channels. *J Biol Chem.* 2009;284:19006-19017.
28. Tikhonov DB, Bruhova I, Zhorov BS. Atomic determinants of state-dependent block of sodium channels by charged local anesthetics and benzocaine. *FEBS Lett.* 2006;580:6027-6032.
29. Hille B. *Ion Channels of Excitable Membranes.* Sunderland, Mass: Sinauer; 2001.
30. Hess P, Lansman JB, Tsien RW. Different modes of Ca channel gating behaviour favoured by dihydropyridine Ca agonists and antagonists. *Nature.* 1984;311:538-544.
31. Sperelakis N. *Heart Physiology and Pathophysiology.* San Diego, Calif.; London: Academic; 2001.
32. Zamponi GW, Striessnig J, Koschak A, et al. The physiology, pathology, and pharmacology of voltage-gated calcium channels and their future therapeutic potential. *Pharmacol Rev.* 2015;67:821-870.
33. Zanchetti A. Calcium channel blockers in hypertension. In: Black HR, Elliott WJ, eds. *Hypertension: A Companion to Braunwald's Heart Disease.* Philadelphia: Saunders Elsevier; 2007:268-285.
34. Toyo-Oka T, Nayler WG. Third generation calcium entry blockers. *Blood Press.* 1996;5:206-208.
35. Sica DA, Prisant LM. Pharmacologic and therapeutic considerations in hypertension therapy with calcium channel blockers: focus on verapamil. *J Clin Hypertens.* 2007;9:1-22.
36. Catterall WA, Swanson TM. Structural basis for pharmacology of voltage-gated sodium and calcium channels. *Mol Pharmacol.* 2015;88:141-150.
37. Lee KS, Tsien RW. Mechanism of calcium channel blockade by verapamil, D600, diltiazem and nitrendipine in single dialysed heart cells. *Nature.* 1983;302:790-794.
38. Lund-Johansen P, Omvik P. Central hemodynamic changes of calcium antagonists at rest and during exercise in essential hypertension. *J Cardiovasc Pharmacol.* 1987;10(Suppl 1):S139-148.
39. Hockerman GH, Dilmac N, Scheuer T, Catterall WA. Molecular determinants of diltiazem block in domains IIIS6 and IVS6 of L-type Ca(2+) channels. *Mol Pharmacol.* 2000;58:1264-1270.
40. Porzig H, Becker C. Potential-dependent allosteric modulation of 1,4-dihydropyridine binding by d-(cis)-diltiazem and (+/-)-verapamil in living cardiac cells. *Mol Pharmacol.* 1988;34:172-179.
41. Russell RP. Side effects of calcium channel blockers. *Hypertension.* 1988;11(3 Pt 2):Ii42-4.
42. Lund-Johansen P. Clinical use of calcium antagonists in hypertension: update 1986. *J Cardiovasc Pharmacol.* 1987;10(Suppl 10):S29-35.
43. Kirch W, Kleinbloesem CH, Belz GG. Drug interactions with calcium antagonists. *Pharmacol Ther.* 1990;45:109-136.

44. Lydtin H, Trenkwalder P. Chemical structure and pharmacokinetics of calcium antagonists. Calcium Antagonists: Springer Berlin Heidelberg; 1990:16-28.
45. Michalewicz L, Messerli FH. Cardiac effects of calcium antagonists in systemic hypertension. *Am J Cardiol*. 1997;79(10A):39-46. discussion 7–8.
46. Ruzicka M, Leenen FH. Relevance of 24 H blood pressure profile and sympathetic activity for outcome on short- versus long-acting 1,4-dihydropyridines. *Am J Hypertens*. 1996;9:86-94.
47. Jariwalla AG, Anderson EG. Production of ischaemic cardiac pain by nifedipine. *Br Med J*. 1978;1:1181-1182.
48. Psaty BM, Heckbert SR, Koepsell TD, et al. The risk of myocardial infarction associated with antihypertensive drug therapies. *JAMA*. 1995;274:620-625.
49. Furberg CD, Psaty BM, Meyer JV. Nifedipine. Dose-related increase in mortality in patients with coronary heart disease. *Circulation*. 1995;92:1326-1331.
50. Kizer JR, Kimmel SE. The calcium-channel blocker controversy: historical perspective and important lessons for future pharmacotherapies. An international society of pharmacoepidemiology 'hot topic'. *Pharmacoepidemiol Drug Saf*. 2000;9:25-35.
51. Grossman E, Messerli FH, Grodzicki T, Kowey P. Should a moratorium be placed on sublingual nifedipine capsules given for hypertensive emergencies and pseudoemergencies? *JAMA*. 1996;276:1328-1331.
52. Chobanian AV, Bakris GL, Black HR, et al. Seventh report of the Joint National Committee on prevention, detection, evaluation, and treatment of high blood pressure. *Hypertension*. 2003;42:1206-1252.
53. Croom KF, Wellington K. Modified-release nifedipine: a review of the use of modified-release formulations in the treatment of hypertension and angina pectoris. *Drugs*. 2006;66:497-528.
54. Scholz H. Pharmacological aspects of calcium channel blockers. *Cardiovasc Drugs Ther*. 1997;10(Suppl 3):869-872.
55. Rubin AS, Zablocki AD. Hyperkalemia, verapamil, and dantrolene. *Anesthesiology*. 1987;66:246-249.
56. Sica DA. Interaction of grapefruit juice and calcium channel blockers. *Am J Hypertens*. 2006;19:768-773.
57. Abernethy DR, Schwartz JB. Calcium-antagonist drugs. *N Engl J Med*. 1999;341:1447–157.
58. Aronson JK, Dukes MNG. *Meyler's Side Effects of Drugs: The International Encyclopedia of Adverse Drug Reactions and Interactions*. Oxford: Elsevier; 2006.
59. Kappel J, Calissi P. Nephrology: 3. Safe drug prescribing for patients with renal insufficiency. *CMAJ*. 2002;166:473-477.
60. Catterall WA, Striessnig J, Snutch TP, Perez-Reyes E. International Union of Pharmacology. XL. Compendium of voltage-gated ion channels: calcium channels. *Pharmacol Rev*. 2003;55:579-581.
61. Hamada T, Watanabe M, Kaneda T, et al. Evaluation of changes in sympathetic nerve activity and heart rate in essential hypertensive patients induced by amlodipine and nifedipine. *J Hypertens*. 1998;16:111-118.
62. Takahara A. Cilnidipine: a new generation Ca channel blocker with inhibitory action on sympathetic neurotransmitter release. *Cardiovasc Ther*. 2009;27:124-139.
63. Schaffer SW, Li M. *T-type Calcium Channels in Basic and Clinical Science*. Wien: Springer; 2015.
64. Cataldi M, Bruno F. 1,4-dihydropyridines: the multiple personalities of a blockbuster drug family. *Transl Med UniSa*. 2012;4:12-26.
65. Furukawa T, Nukada T, Miura R, et al. Differential blocking action of dihydropyridine Ca2+ antagonists on a T-type Ca2+ channel (alpha1G) expressed in Xenopus oocytes. *J Cardiovasc Pharmacol*. 2005;45:241-246.
66. Heady TN, Gomora JC, Macdonald TL, et al. Molecular pharmacology of T-type Ca2+ channels. *Jpn J Pharmacol*. 2001;85:339-350.
67. SoRelle R. Withdrawal of Posicor from market. *Circulation*. 1998;98:831-832.
68. Ohashi N, Mitamura H, Ogawa S. Development of newer calcium channel antagonists: therapeutic potential of efonidipine in preventing electrical remodelling during atrial fibrillation. *Drugs*. 2009;69:21-30.
69. Berkels R, Taubert D, Rosenkranz A, et al. Vascular protective effects of dihydropyridine calcium antagonists. Involvement of endothelial nitric oxide. *Pharmacology*. 2003;69:171-176.
70. Mason RP, Marche P, Hintze TH. Novel vascular biology of third-generation L-type calcium channel antagonists: ancillary actions of amlodipine. *Arterioscler Thromb Vasc Biol*. 2003;23:2155-2163.
71. Visentin S, Rolando B, Di Stilo A, et al. New 1,4-dihydropyridines endowed with NO-donor and calcium channel agonist properties. *J Med Chem*. 2004;47:2688-2693.
72. Batova S, DeWever J, Godfraind T, et al. The calcium channel blocker amlodipine promotes the unclamping of eNOS from caveolin in endothelial cells. *Cardiovasc Res*. 2006;71:478-485.
73. Guazzi M, Olivari MT, Polese A, et al. Nifedipine, a new antihypertensive with rapid action. *Clin Pharmacol Ther*. 1977;22(5 Pt 1):528-532.
74. Hof RP. Selective effects of different calcium antagonists on the peripheral circulation. *Trends Pharmacol Sci*. 1984;5:100-102.
75. Grossman E, Messerli FH. Calcium antagonists. *Prog Cardiovasc Dis*. 2004;47:34-57.
76. Harada K, Ohmori M, Sugimoto K, et al. Comparison of venodilatory effect of nicardipine, diltiazem, and verapamil in human subjects. *Eur J Clin Pharmacol*. 1998;54:31-34.
77. Oren S, Gossman E, Frohlich ED. Effects of calcium entry blockers on distribution of blood volume. *Am J Hypertens*. 1996;9:628-632.
78. Rutan GH, Hermanson B, Bild DE, Kittner SJ, LaBaw F, Tell GS. Orthostatic hypotension in older adults. The Cardiovascular Health Study. CHS Collaborative Research Group. *Hypertension*. 1992;19(6 Pt 1):508-519.
79. Materson BJ, Reda DJ, Cushman WC. Department of Veterans Affairs single-drug therapy of hypertension study. Revised figures and new data. Department of Veterans Affairs Cooperative Study Group on Antihypertensive Agents. *Am J Hypertens*. 1995;8:189-192.
80. Gupta AK. Racial differences in response to antihypertensive therapy: does one size fits all? *Int J Prev Med*. 2010;1:217-219.
81. Materson BJ, Reda DJ, Cushman WC, et al. Single-drug therapy for hypertension in men. A comparison of six antihypertensive agents with placebo. The Department of Veterans Affairs Cooperative Study Group on Antihypertensive Agents. *N Engl J Med*. 1993;328:914-921.
82. Elliott HL. 24-hour blood pressure control: its relevance to cardiovascular outcomes and the importance of long-acting antihypertensive drugs. *J Hum Hypertens*. 2004;18: 539-543.
83. Ghamami N, Chiang SH, Dormuth C, et al. Time course for blood pressure lowering of dihydropyridine calcium channel blockers. *Cochrane Database Syst Rev*. 2014;8: Cd010052.
84. Diaz KM, Tanner RM, Falzon L, et al. Visit-to-visit variability of blood pressure and cardiovascular disease and all-cause mortality: a systematic review and meta-analysis. *Hypertension*. 2014;64:965-982.
85. Rothwell PM. Limitations of the usual blood-pressure hypothesis and importance of variability, instability, and episodic hypertension. *Lancet*. 2010;375:938-948.
86. Webb AJ, Fischer U, Mehta Z, et al. Effects of antihypertensive-drug class on interindividual variation in blood pressure and risk of stroke: a systematic review and meta-analysis. *Lancet*. 2010;375:906-915.
87. Vlachopoulos C, Aznaouridis K, O'Rourke MF, et al. Prediction of cardiovascular events and all-cause mortality with central haemodynamics: a systematic review and meta-analysis. *Eur Heart J*. 2010;31:1865-1871.
88. Manisty CH, Hughes AD. Meta-analysis of the comparative effects of different classes of antihypertensive agents on brachial and central systolic blood pressure, and augmentation index. *Br J Clin Pharmacol*. 2013;75:79-92.
89. Chan L, Schrier RW. Effects of calcium channel blockers on renal function. *Annu Rev Med*. 1990;41:289-302.
90. Messerli FH, Ketelhut R. Left ventricular hypertrophy: a pressure-independent cardiovascular risk factor. *J Cardiovasc Pharmacol*. 1993;22(Suppl 1):S7-S13.
91. Pierdomenico SD, Cuccurullo F. Risk reduction after regression of echocardiographic left ventricular hypertrophy in hypertension: a meta-analysis. *Am J Hypertens*. 2010;23:876-881.
92. Terpstra WF, May JF, Smit AJ, et al. Long-term effects of amlodipine and lisinopril on left ventricular mass and diastolic function in elderly, previously untreated hypertensive patients: the ELVERA trial. *J Hypertens*. 2001;19:303-309.
93. Devereux RB, Palmieri V, Sharpe N, et al. Effects of once-daily angiotensin-converting enzyme inhibition and calcium channel blockade-based antihypertensive treatment regimens on left ventricular hypertrophy and diastolic filling in hypertension: the prospective randomized enalapril study evaluating regression of ventricular enlargement (preserve) trial. *Circulation*. 2001;104:1248-1254.
94. Agabiti-Rosei E, Trimarco B, Muiesan ML, et al. Cardiac structural and functional changes during long-term antihypertensive treatment with lacidipine and atenolol in the European Lacidipine Study on Atherosclerosis (ELSA). *J Hypertens*. 2005;23:1091-1098.
95. Barron AJ, Hughes AD, Sharp A, et al. Long-term antihypertensive treatment fails to improve E/e' despite regression of left ventricular mass: an Anglo-Scandinavian cardiac outcomes trial substudy. *Hypertension*. 2014;63:252-258.
96. Mitchell GF. Arterial stiffness and hypertension: chicken or egg? *Hypertension*. 2014;64:210-214.
97. Beltran A, McVeigh G, Morgan D, et al. Arterial compliance abnormalities in isolated systolic hypertension. *Am J Hypertens*. 2001;14:1007-1011.
98. Ben-Shlomo Y, Spears M, Boustred C, et al. Aortic pulse wave velocity improves cardiovascular event prediction: an individual participant meta-analysis of prospective observational data from 17,635 subjects. *J Am Coll Cardiol*. 2014;63:636-646.
99. Williams B. Evaluating interventions to reduce central aortic pressure, arterial stiffness and morbidity—mortality. *J Hypertens*. 2012;30(Suppl:S1):3-8.
100. Laurent S, Cockcroft J, Van Bortel L, et al. Expert consensus document on arterial stiffness: methodological issues and clinical applications. *Eur Heart J*. 2006;27:2588-2605.
101. Wolinsky H, Glagov S. Structural basis for the static mechanical properties of the aortic media. *Circ Res*. 1964;14:400-413.
102. London GM, Pannier B, Guerin AP, et al. Cardiac hypertrophy, aortic compliance, peripheral resistance, and wave reflection in end-stage renal disease. Comparative effects of ACE inhibition and calcium channel blockade. *Circulation*. 1994;90:2786-2796.
103. Topouchian J, Asmar R, Sayegh F, et al. Changes in arterial structure and function under trandolapril-verapamil combination in hypertension. *Stroke*. 1999;30:1056-1064.
104. White WB, Duprez D, St Hillaire R, et al. Effects of the selective aldosterone blocker eplerenone versus the calcium antagonist amlodipine in systolic hypertension. *Hypertension*. 2003;41:1021-1026.
105. Mackenzie IS, McEniery CM, Dhakam Z, et al. Comparison of the effects of antihypertensive agents on central blood pressure and arterial stiffness in isolated systolic hypertension. *Hypertension*. 2009;54:409-413.
106. Ong KT, Delerme S, Pannier B, et al. Aortic stiffness is reduced beyond blood pressure lowering by short-term and long-term antihypertensive treatment: a meta-analysis of individual data in 294 patients. *J Hypertens*. 2011;29:1034-1042.
107. Shahin Y, Khan JA, Chetter I. Angiotensin converting enzyme inhibitors effect on arterial stiffness and wave reflections: a meta-analysis and meta-regression of randomised controlled trials. *Atherosclerosis*. 2012;221:18-33.
108. Voyaki SM, Staessen JA, Thijs L, et al. Follow-up of renal function in treated and untreated older patients with isolated systolic hypertension. Systolic Hypertension in Europe (Syst-Eur) Trial Investigators. *J Hypertens*. 2001;19:511-519.
109. Bakris GL, Weir MR, Secic M, et al. Differential effects of calcium antagonist subclasses on markers of nephropathy progression. *Kidney Int*. 2004;65:1991-2002.
110. Brown MJ, Palmer CR, Castaigne A, et al. Morbidity and mortality in patients randomised to double-blind treatment with a long-acting calcium-channel blocker or diuretic in the International Nifedipine GITS study: Intervention as a Goal in Hypertension Treatment (INSIGHT). *Lancet*. 2000;356:366-372.
111. The ALLHAT Officers and Coordinators for the ALLHAT Collaborative Research Group. Major outcomes in high-risk hypertensive patients randomized to angiotensin-converting enzyme inhibitor or calcium channel blocker vs diuretic: The Antihypertensive and Lipid-Lowering Treatment to Prevent Heart Attack Trial (ALLHAT). *JAMA*. 2002;288:2981-2997.
112. Rahman M, Pressel S, Davis BR, et al. Renal outcomes in high-risk hypertensive patients treated with an angiotensin-converting enzyme inhibitor or a calcium channel blocker vs a diuretic: a report from the Antihypertensive and Lipid-Lowering Treatment to Prevent Heart Attack Trial (ALLHAT). *Arch Intern Med*. 2005;165:936-946.
113. Ruilope LM, Zanchetti A, Julius S, et al. Prediction of cardiovascular outcome by estimated glomerular filtration rate and estimated creatinine clearance in the high-risk hypertension population of the VALUE trial. *J Hypertens*. 2007;25:1473-1479.
114. Wright Jr JT, Bakris G, Greene T, et al. Effect of blood pressure lowering and antihypertensive drug class on progression of hypertensive kidney disease: results from the AASK trial. *JAMA*. 2002;288:2421-2431.
115. Ninomiya T, Perkovic V, Turnbull F, et al. Blood pressure lowering and major cardiovascular events in people with and without chronic kidney disease: meta-analysis of randomised controlled trials. *BMJ*. 2013;347:f5680.
116. Li X, Yang MS. Effects of T-type calcium channel blockers on renal function and aldosterone in patients with hypertension: a systematic review and meta-analysis. *PLoS One*. 2014;9:e109834.
117. Fujita T, Ando K, Nishimura H, et al. Antiproteinuric effect of the calcium channel blocker cilnidipine added to renin-angiotensin inhibition in hypertensive patients with chronic renal disease. *Kidney Int*. 2007;72:1543-1549.
118. Kennelly SP, Lawlor BA, Kenny RA. Blood pressure and the risk for dementia: a double edged sword. *Ageing Res Rev*. 2009;8:61-70.
119. McGuinness B, Todd S, Passmore P, Bullock R. Blood pressure lowering in patients without prior cerebrovascular disease for prevention of cognitive impairment and dementia. *Cochrane Database Syst Rev*. 2009;(4):CD004034.
120. Forette F, Seux ML, Staessen JA, et al. Prevention of dementia in randomised double-blind placebo-controlled Systolic Hypertension in Europe (Syst-Eur) trial. *Lancet*. 1998;352:1347-1351.

121. Peters R, Booth A, Peters J. A systematic review of calcium channel blocker use and cognitive decline/dementia in the elderly. *J Hypertens*. 2014;32:1945-1957; discussion 1957–1958.
122. Staessen JA, Fagard R, Thijs L, et al. Randomised double-blind comparison of placebo and active treatment for older patients with isolated systolic hypertension. The Systolic Hypertension in Europe (Syst-Eur) Trial Investigators. *Lancet*. 1997;350:757-764.
123. Liu L, Wang JG, Gong L, et al. Comparison of active treatment and placebo in older Chinese patients with isolated systolic hypertension. Systolic Hypertension in China (Syst-China) Collaborative Group. *J Hypertens*. 1998;16(12 Pt 1):1823-1829.
124. Lubsen J, Wagener G, Kirwan BA, et al. Effect of long-acting nifedipine on mortality and cardiovascular morbidity in patients with symptomatic stable angina and hypertension: the ACTION trial. *J Hypertens*. 2005;23:641-648.
125. Nissen SE, Tuzcu EM, Libby P, et al. Effect of antihypertensive agents on cardiovascular events in patients with coronary disease and normal blood pressure: the CAMELOT study: a randomized controlled trial. *JAMA*. 2004;292:2217-2225.
126. National Intervention Cooperative Study in Elderly Hypertensives Study Group. Randomized double-blind comparison of a calcium antagonist and a diuretic in elderly hypertensives. National Intervention Cooperative Study in Elderly Hypertensives Study Group. *Hypertension*. 1999;34:1129-1133.
127. Neal B, MacMahon S, Chapman N. Blood Pressure Lowering Treatment Trialists Collaboration. Effects of ACE inhibitors, calcium antagonists, and other blood-pressure-lowering drugs: results of prospectively designed overviews of randomised trials. Blood Pressure Lowering Treatment Trialists' Collaboration. *Lancet*. 2000;356:1955-1964.
128. Costanzo P, Perrone-Filardi P, Petretta M, et al. Calcium channel blockers and cardiovascular outcomes: a meta-analysis of 175,634 patients. *J Hypertens*. 2009;27:1136-1151.
129. Chen N, Zhou M, Yang M, et al. Calcium channel blockers versus other classes of drugs for hypertension. *Cochrane Database Syst Rev*. 2010;(8): Cd003654.
130. Makani H, Bangalore S, Romero J, et al. Peripheral edema associated with calcium channel blockers: incidence and withdrawal rate—a meta-analysis of randomized trials. *J Hypertens*. 2011;29:1270-1280.
131. Hedner T. Calcium channel blockers: spectrum of side effects and drug interactions. *Acta Pharmacol Toxicol (Copenh)*. 1986;58(Suppl 2):119-130.
132. Livada R, Shiloah J. Calcium channel blocker-induced gingival enlargement. *J Hum Hypertens*. 2014;28:10-14.
133. Pedrinelli R, Dell'Omo G, Mariani M. Calcium channel blockers, postural vasoconstriction and dependent oedema in essential hypertension. *J Hum Hypertens*. 2001;15:455-461.
134. Sica D. Calcium channel blocker-related periperal edema: can it be resolved? *J Clin Hypertens (Greenwich)*. 2003;5:291-294. 297.
135. Makarounas-Kirchmann K, Glover-Koudounas S, Ferrari P. Results of a meta-analysis comparing the tolerability of lercanidipine and other dihydropyridine calcium channel blockers. *Clin Ther*. 2009;31:1652-1663.
136. van der Heijden AG, Huysmans FT, van Hamersvelt HW. Foot volume increase on nifedipine is not prevented by pretreatment with diuretics. *J Hypertens*. 2004;22:425-430.
137. Makani H, Bangalore S, Romero J, Wever-Pinzon O, Messerli FH. Effect of renin-angiotensin system blockade on calcium channel blocker-associated peripheral edema. *Am J Med*. 2011;124:128-135.
138. Weir MR, Rosenberger C, Fink JC. Pilot study to evaluate a water displacement technique to compare effects of diuretics and ACE inhibitors to alleviate lower extremity edema due to dihydropyridine calcium antagonists. *Am J Hypertens*. 2001;14(9 Pt 1):963-968.
139. Kubota K, Pearce GL, Inman WH. Vasodilation-related adverse events in diltiazem and dihydropyridine calcium antagonists studied by prescription-event monitoring. *Eur J Clin Pharmacol*. 1995;48:1-7.
140. Kasiske BL, Ma JZ, Kalil RS, et al. Effects of antihypertensive therapy on serum lipids. *Ann Intern Med*. 1995;122:133-141.
141. Elliott WJ, Meyer PM. Incident diabetes in clinical trials of antihypertensive drugs: a network meta-analysis. *Lancet*. 2007;369:201-207.
142. Pahor M, Guralnik JM, Ferrucci L, et al. Calcium-channel blockade and incidence of cancer in aged populations. *Lancet*. 1996;348:493-497.
143. Black HR, Elliott WJ, Grandits G, et al. Principal results of the Controlled Onset Verapamil Investigation of Cardiovascular End Points (CONVINCE) trial. *JAMA*. 2003;289:2073-2082.
144. Pepine CJ, Handberg EM, Cooper-DeHoff RM, et al. A calcium antagonist vs a non-calcium antagonist hypertension treatment strategy for patients with coronary artery disease. The International Verapamil-Trandolapril Study (INVEST): a randomized controlled trial. *JAMA*. 2003;290:2805-2816.
145. Liu L, Zhang Y, Liu G, et al. The Felodipine Event Reduction (FEVER) Study: a randomized long-term placebo-controlled trial in Chinese hypertensive patients. *J Hypertens*. 2005;23:2157-2172.
146. Bangalore S, Kumar S, Kjeldsen SE, et al. Antihypertensive drugs and risk of cancer: network meta-analyses and trial sequential analyses of 324,168 participants from randomised trials. *Lancet Oncol*. 2011;12:65-82.
147. Julius S, Kjeldsen SE, Weber M, et al. Outcomes in hypertensive patients at high cardiovascular risk treated with regimens based on valsartan or amlodipine: the VALUE randomised trial. *Lancet*. 2004;363:2022-2031.
148. Fihn SD, Gardin JM, Abrams J, et al. American College of Cardiology F. 2012 ACCF/AHA/ACP/AATS/PCNA/SCAI/STS guideline for the diagnosis and management of patients with stable ischemic heart disease: executive summary: a report of the American College of Cardiology Foundation/American Heart Association task force on practice guidelines, and the American College of Physicians, American Association for Thoracic Surgery, Preventive Cardiovascular Nurses Association, Society for Cardiovascular Angiography and Interventions, and Society of Thoracic Surgeons. *Circulation*. 2012;126:3097-3137.
149. Elkayam U, Amin J, Mehra A, et al. A prospective, randomized, double-blind, crossover study to compare the efficacy and safety of chronic nifedipine therapy with that of isosorbide dinitrate and their combination in the treatment of chronic congestive heart failure. *Circulation*. 1990;82:1954-1961.
150. Packer M, Carson P, Elkayam U, et al. Effect of amlodipine on the survival of patients with severe chronic heart failure due to a nonischemic cardiomyopathy: results of the PRAISE-2 study (prospective randomized amlodipine survival evaluation 2). *JACC Heart Fail*. 2013;1:308-314.
151. Packer M, O'Connor CM, Ghali JK, et al. Effect of amlodipine on morbidity and mortality in severe chronic heart failure. Prospective Randomized Amlodipine Survival Evaluation Study Group. *N Engl J Med*. 1996;335:1107-1114.
152. Cohn JN, Ziesche S, Smith R, et al. Effect of the calcium antagonist felodipine as supplementary vasodilator therapy in patients with chronic heart failure treated with enalapril: V-HeFT III. Vasodilator-Heart Failure Trial (V-HeFT) Study Group. *Circulation*. 1997;96:856-863.
153. de Vries RJ, van Veldhuisen DJ, Dunselman PH. Efficacy and safety of calcium channel blockers in heart failure: focus on recent trials with second-generation dihydropyridines. *Am Heart J*. 2000;139(2 Pt 1):185-194.
154. Hunt SA. ACC/AHA 2005 Guideline Update for the Diagnosis and Management of Chronic Heart Failure in the Adult—Summary Article: A Report of the American College of Cardiology/American Heart Association Task Force on Practice Guidelines (Writing Committee to Update the 2001 Guidelines for the Evaluation and Management of Heart Failure): Developed in Collaboration With the American College of Chest Physicians and the International Society for Heart and Lung Transplantation: Endorsed by the Heart Rhythm Society. *Circulation*. 2005;112:1825-1852.
155. Bateman BT, Hernandez-Diaz S, Huybrechts KF, et al. Patterns of outpatient antihypertensive medication use during pregnancy in a Medicaid population. *Hypertension*. 2012;60:913-920.
156. Mancia G, Fagard R, Narkiewicz K, et al. 2013 ESH/ESC guidelines for the management of arterial hypertension: the Task Force for the Management of Arterial Hypertension of the European Society of Hypertension (ESH) and of the European Society of Cardiology (ESC). *Eur Heart J*. 2013;34:2159-2219.
157. James PA, Oparil S, Carter BL, et al. 2014 evidence-based guideline for the management of high blood pressure in adults: report from the panel members appointed to the Eighth Joint National Committee (JNC 8). *JAMA*. 2014;311:507-520.
158. (UK) NCGC. Hypertension: The Clinical Management of Primary Hypertension in Adults: Update of Clinical Guidelines 18 and 34 (NICE Clinical Guidelines, No. 127). London: Royal College of Physicians (UK), 2011.
159. Shimamoto K, Ando K, Fujita T, et al. Japanese Society of Hypertension Committee for Guidelines for the Management of H. The Japanese Society of Hypertension Guidelines for the Management of Hypertension (JSH 2014). *Hypertens Res*. 2014;37:253-390.
160. Deeks ED, Keating GM, Keam SJ. Clevidipine: a review of its use in the management of acute hypertension. *Am J Cardiovasc Drugs*. 2009;9:117-134.
161. McCormack PL, Wagstaff AJ. Lacidipine: a review of its use in the management of hypertension. *Drugs*. 2003;63:2327-2356.
162. Joint Formulary Committee. British National Formulary (online). London: BMJ Group and Pharmaceutical Press; 2015.
163. Testa R, Leonardi A, Tajana A, et al. Lercanidipine (Rec 15/2375): A novel 1,4-dihydropyridine calcium antagonist for hypertension. *Cardiovasc Drug Rev*. 1997;15:187-219.
164. Sica DA. Calcium channel blocker class heterogeneity: select aspects of pharmacokinetics and pharmacodynamics. *J Clin Hypertens (Greenwich)*. 2005;7(4 Suppl 1):21-26.
165. Diochot S, Richard S, Baldy-Moulinier M, et al. Dihydropyridines, phenylalkylamines and benzothiazepines block N-, P/Q- and R-type calcium currents. *Pflugers Arch*. 1995;431:10-19.
166. Furukawa T, Yamakawa T, Midera T, et al. Selectivities of dihydropyridine derivatives in blocking Ca(2+) channel subtypes expressed in Xenopus oocytes. *J Pharmacol Exp Ther*. 1999;291:464-473.
167. Nimmrich V, Gross G. P/Q-type calcium channel modulators. *Br J Pharmacol*. 2012;167:741-759.
168. Perez-Reyes E, Van Deusen AL, Vitko I. Molecular pharmacology of human Cav3.2 T-type Ca2+ channels: block by antihypertensives, antiarrhythmics, and their analogs. *J Pharmacol Exp Ther*. 2009;328:621-627.
169. Gong L, Zhang W, Zhu Y, et al. Shanghai trial of nifedipine in the elderly (STONE). *J Hypertens*. 1996;14:1237-1245.
170. Hansson L, Lindholm LH, Ekbom T, et al. Randomised trial of old and new antihypertensive drugs in elderly patients: cardiovascular mortality and morbidity the Swedish trial in old patients with hypertension-2 study. *Lancet*. 1999;354:1751-1756.
171. Hansson L, Hedner T, Lund-Johansen P, et al. Randomised trial of effects of calcium antagonists compared with diuretics and beta-blockers on cardiovascular morbidity and mortality in hypertension: the Nordic Diltiazem (NORDIL) study. *Lancet*. 2000;356:359-365.
172. Malacco E, Mancia G, Rappelli A, et al. Treatment of isolated systolic hypertension: the SHELL study results. *Blood Press*. 2003;12:160-167.
173. Dahlof B, Sever PS, Poulter NR, et al. Prevention of cardiovascular events with an antihypertensive regimen of amlodipine adding perindopril as required versus atenolol adding bendroflumethiazide as required, in the Anglo-Scandinavian Cardiac Outcomes Trial-Blood Pressure Lowering Arm (ASCOT-BPLA): a multicentre randomised controlled trial. *Lancet*. 2005;366:895-906.
174. Yui Y, Sumiyoshi T, Kodama K, et al. Japan Multicenter Investigation for Cardiovascular Diseases BSG. Comparison of nifedipine retard with angiotensin converting enzyme inhibitors in Japanese hypertensive patients with coronary artery disease: the Japan Multicenter Investigation for Cardiovascular Diseases-B (JMIC-B) randomized trial. *Hypertens Res*. 2004;27:181-191.
175. Leenen FH, Nwachuku CE, Black HR, et al. Antihypertensive, Lipid-Lowering Treatment to Prevent Heart Attack Trial Collaborative Research G. Clinical events in high-risk hypertensive patients randomly assigned to calcium channel blocker versus angiotensin-converting enzyme inhibitor in the antihypertensive and lipid-lowering treatment to prevent heart attack trial. *Hypertension*. 2006;48:374-384.
176. Schrader J, Luders S, Kulschewski A, et al. Morbidity and Mortality After Stroke, Eprosartan Compared with Nitrendipine for Secondary Prevention: principal results of a prospective randomized controlled study (MOSES). *Stroke*. 2005;36:1218-1226.
177. Rosei EA, Dal Palu C, Leonetti G, et al. Clinical results of the Verapamil in Hypertension and Atherosclerosis Study. VHAS Investigators. *J Hypertens*. 1997;15:1337-1344.

26 Central Sympathetic Agents and Direct Vasodilators

Kazuomi Kario

MECHANISM OF ACTION

Central sympatholytics (e.g., methyldopa, guanabenz, guanfacine, clonidine, moxonidine, and rilmenidine) have a variety of antihypertensive actions[1,2] that result in increased sodium excretion and decreases in the cardiac output, heart rate, total peripheral resistance, and renin release. Central sympatholytics cross the blood-brain barrier and stimulate the imidazoline 1 (I_1) receptors and/or central postsynaptic alpha$_2$ (α_2) adrenoceptors in the brainstem's sympathetic nervous control centers, the rostral ventrolateral medulla (RVLM) and the nucleus tractus solitarii (NTS). As shown in Fig. 26.1, the various central sympatholytics have differing affinities for these two types of receptors. Moxonidine and rilmenidine selectively stimulate the I_1-imidazoline receptors. Methyldopa, guanabenz, and guanfacine selectively stimulate α_2-adrenoceptors more than the I_1-imidazoline receptors, and clonidine nonselectively stimulates both α_2-adrenoceptors and I_1-imidazoline receptors.

Treatment with one of the central sympatholytics that stimulate α_2-adrenoceptors (e.g., methyldopa, clonidine, guanabenz, and guanfacine) is frequently accompanied by adverse effects such as dry mouth, decreased alertness, sedation, and depression. This is because α_2-adrenoceptors are present not only in the RVLM but also in the NTS, nucleus coeruleus, and salivary grands. Treatment with a central sympatholytic that selectively stimulates only I_1-imidazoline receptors (e.g., rilmenidine or moxonidine) results in central adverse effects much less frequently, because the I_1-imidazoline receptors are located almost exclusively in the RVLM.

Perhaps the oldest agent (founded in the 1930s in India) that affects the sympathetic nervous system is reserpine. In contrast, the adrenergic uptake inhibitor reserpine depletes catecholamine storage in both the central and peripheral nervous systems and is associated with many dose-dependent side effects. It is no longer available in the United States.

HEMODYNAMIC EFFECTS

Stimulating the brainstem's central I_1-imidazoline receptors or α_2-adrenoceptors results in several hemodynamic, neurohumoral, and adverse effects, because the stimulation directly inhibits the sympathetic outflow to the heart and blood vessels (Box 26.1).[3] For the main pharmacodynamic effect of compounds in this class to occur, the drugs must pass the blood-brain barrier. As such, there is an implicit time lag between the plasma drug concentration that is achieved and the antihypertensive effect.

The blood pressure (BP)-lowering effect of the central sympatholytics is based on the following: a reduction in norepinephrine; decreased peripheral resistance and decreased cardiac output at rest and during exercise; reduced baroreflex to compensate for the decrease in BP, resulting in relative bradycardia with exaggerated hypotension on standing; decreased plasma levels of aldosterone, angiotensin II, and renin; and preserved glomerular filtration and renal blood flow despite the reduction in BP. However, central sympatholytics often cause fluid retention as overcompensation, and this limits their effectiveness.

CLINICAL APPLICATION

The significant overall effectiveness in reducing BP is a major advantage of the central sympatholytics.[4] They are also useful for treating labile hypertensive patients with associated anxiety, especially when the anxiety is manifested by sympathetic hyperactivity. However, central sympatholytics are currently used less frequently because of their adverse effects, which can be significant. The centrally acting effects of the central sympatholytics (such as depression and sedation) are of particular concern.

Central sympatholytics are also not recommended for use as first-line or second-line monotherapy because they are often less effective in this role and have not been shown in clinical trials to reduce mortality. Moreover, most are associated with a dose-dependent rebound hypertension when abruptly stopped. A combination of a central sympatholytic with a thiazide-type diuretic is often used to manage resistant hypertension and occasionally hypertension in pregnant women, if beta-blockers are contraindicated. In resistant hypertension, these agents are added when combinations of three or more other antihypertensive drugs such as a calcium channel blocker, angiotensin-converting enzyme (ACE) inhibitor, angiotensin receptor blocker (ARB), or diuretic have failed to control blood pressure.

Central sympatholytics can be used safely in individuals with diabetes, with no significant loss of glycemic control. They can also be used safely for individuals with pulmonary diseases such as asthma. Intravenous preparations are available only in certain countries for clonidine and α-methyldopa, and clonidine is the only compound in this class that can be administered via a transdermal delivery system.

The central sympatholytics' quick onset and long duration of action distinguish these drugs. The most rapid onset of action is seen in clonidine, at 30 to 60 minutes.

ADVERSE EFFECTS

The most common adverse effects of the central sympatholytics that stimulate α_2-adrenoceptors are sedation and dry mouth (40%), and these effects are the main reason that the use of central sympatholytics has declined. In addition, the sedative effects of drugs within this class are enhanced by other central nervous system (CNS) depressants such as antihistamines, benzodiazepines, sedative-hypnotics, and ethanol. The central sympatholytics that stimulate I_1-imidazoline receptors do not cause as much sedation and dry mouth, and they are better tolerated by most patients. Dry mouth can be annoying, and the decreased level of saliva can increase an individual's risk of dental caries and periodontal disease (Table 26.1).

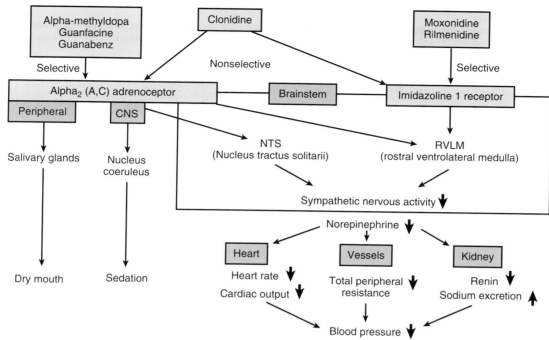

FIG. 26.1 Antihypertensive mechanisms of central sympatholytic agents. Central sympatholytic agents activate α2A and α2C, or imidazoline 1 receptors in the brainstem, resulting in decreases in heart rate, cardiac output, total peripheral resistance, and renin release, and an increase in sodium excretion.

BOX 26.1 Hemodynamic and Adverse Effects of Central Sympatholytics

- Reduction of sympathetic nervous activity reflected in lower norepinephrine
- Decrease in peripheral resistance and cardiac output at rest and during exercise
- Reduced baroreflex to compensate for a decrease in blood pressure (BP), resulting in relative bradycardia with exaggerated hypotension on standing
- Decreased plasma levels of renin, angiotensin II, and aldosterone
- Preserved renal blood flow and glomerular filtration despite BP reduction
- Increase in fluid retention
- Frequent adverse effects such as sedation, depression, decreased alertness, dry mouth

---

THE CENTRAL SYMPATHOLYTICS

The pharmacodynamics, available preparations, daily dosages, contraindications, and adverse effects of the various central sympatholytics are listed in Table 26.1.

Clonidine

Clonidine, the most widely used central sympatholytic.[2,5-8] The onset of action for oral clonidine is 30 to 60 minutes, which is advantageous for hypertensive urgencies. For primary hypertension, clonidine is recommended for use as the fourth or fifth line of therapy. Menopause-associated vasomotor syndrome symptoms such as hot flushes, and sympathetic hyperactivity-related hypertension with restless legs syndrome have all been treated successfully with clonidine. Clonidine has also been shown to be more effective in whites than in African Americans, and in older than in younger African Americans. However, in a blinded, randomized trial with a 2-by-2 factorial design study, it was shown that low-dose clonidine (0.2 mg per

day) did not reduce the rate of the composite outcome (death or nonfatal myocardial infarction) and increase the risk of clinically important hypotension and nonfatal cardiac arrest in patients undergoing noncardiac surgery.[9]

Antihypertensive Effects

Clonidine is easily absorbed. The plasma levels of clonidine peak within 30 to 60 minutes after its oral administration, and its plasma half-life is 6 to 13 hours. The BP reduction peaks at 3 to 5 hours, and the BP-lowering effect lasts 8 to 12 hours. Oral clonidine preparations include 0.1-, 0.2-, and 0.3-mg dosages. Clonidine treatment is often initiated at 0.1 mg 2× per day and then gradually increased to a maximum dose of 2.4 mg per day.

Transdermal (patch) clonidine is particularly effective for treating labile hypertensive patients who need multiple medications, those who cannot take oral medications, and those with prominent early morning BP surges. Transdermal clonidine is available in three preparations: 2.5, 5.0, and 7.5 mg. The best absorption from a clonidine patch is obtained by placing the patch on the chest or upper arm. An optimal transdermal delivery system provides a constant clonidine dose for 7 days, and the peak effect is reached within days 1 to 2 days. The BP-lowering effect of transdermal clonidine lasts 8 to 24 hours after the patch is removed. However, compared with oral clonidine, at equivalent doses transdermal clonidine treatment is more likely to result in a dose-dependent retention of both water and salt.

Adverse Effects

Dry mouth and sedation, the most frequent adverse effects of clonidine treatment, are more common with clonidine than methyldopa, but clonidine does not present a risk of autoimmune hepatic damage as methyldopa does. Other potential adverse effects of clonidine are headache, impotence, and orthostatic hypotension. Known contraindications for clonidine are sick sinus syndrome and second-degree and third-degree atrioventricular (AV) block, because clonidine's depression of sinus and atrioventricular nodal function may result in bradycardia.

ANTIHYPERTENSIVE THERAPY

TABLE 26.1 Central Sympatholytics

DRUG	PREPARATION	PHARMACODYNAMICS	DAILY DOSAGE	ADVERSE EFFECTS	CONTRAINDICATIONS
Clonidine: Oral	0.1 mg 0.2 mg 0.3 mg	Onset: 0.5-1 hour Peak: 3-5 hours Plasma half-life: 12-16 hours Metabolism: liver	Initial: 0.1 mg Range: 0.2-1.2 mg Max.: 1.2 mg usually bid	Sedation, drowsiness, dry mouth, withdrawal syndrome, rebound hypertension (uncommon with doses <1.2 mg qd), headache, bradycardia, orthostatic hypotension, impotence (uncommon; 4%)	Sick sinus syndrome 2nd- and 3rd-degree atrioventricular block
Transdermal	1 (containing 2.5 mg) 2 (containing 5.0 mg) 3 (containing 7.5 mg)	Duration of BP lowering: 1 week	1, 2, 3 once weekly		
Methyldopa	125 mg 250 mg 500 mg	Onset: 2-3 hours Peak: 5 hours Plasma half-life: 12 hours Metabolism: renal	Avg.: 250-300 mg bid Max.: 3000 mg	Sedation, drowsiness, depression, dry mouth, positive Coombs test and anemia, lupuslike syndrome, withdrawal syndrome, rebound hypertension	Active hepatic disease
Guanabenz	4 mg 8 mg	Onset: 1 hour Peak: 4 hours Plasma half-life 6 hours Metabolism: 75% Excretion: renal 80%	Average 16 mg Range 8-48 mg Maximum 48 mg	Sedation, drowsiness, dry mouth, withdrawal syndrome, rebound hypertension, impotence	Pregnancy
Guanfacine	1 mg 2 mg	Onset: 1 hour Peak: 4 hours Plasma half-life: 12 hours Excretion: renal	1 mg at bedtime Maximum 3 mg	Same as clonidine	Allergy to guanfacine

bid, Twice a day; *BP,* blood pressure; *qd,* once a day.

Clonidine treatment is also subject to the risk of the occurrence of rebound syndrome and discontinuation syndrome. When treatment with any antihypertensive drug is abruptly stopped, the discontinuation syndrome may occur at different degrees of severity as follows: a rapid but asymptomatic return of the BP to the patient's pretreatment level, a rebound of the BP with sympathetic hyperactivity symptoms, and the patient's BP overshoots the pretreatment level. The central sympatholytic most frequently cited as resulting in discontinuation syndrome is clonidine (especially at ≥ 1.0 mg), caused by the rapid return of the catecholamine level, which is suppressed by clonidine treatment. Discontinuation syndrome is exacerbated in the presence of a β-blockade, but not in the presence of the α/β adrenergic antagonist labetalol or carvedilol. If discontinuation syndrome is detected in a patient who was treated with clonidine, the clonidine should be restarted, and the symptoms can be expected to quickly resolve.

Rebound hypertension may occur with clonidine transdermal treatment, but it is observed much less frequently than after clonidine oral administration. Skin hypersensitivity (e.g., allergic dermatitis) in response to a clonidine patch occurs in up to 20% of patients, most commonly in white and female patients.

Methyldopa

Methyldopa[6-8,10] is used mainly to treat hypertension in pregnant women. It is not teratogenic and has been shown to produce no fetal adverse effects in utero. Methyldopa treatment maintains uterine perfusion and does not hinder the maternal cardiac output or renal or uterine blood flow. As the α-methylated derivative of dopa (the natural precursor of dopamine and norepinephrine), methyldopa is a suitable alternative to clonidine for patients for whom rebound hypertension or intolerable adverse effects preclude the use of clonidine.

Methyldopa is often used for hypertensive emergencies. It is available as an intravenous formulation (as the parent drug ester) at the typical intravenous dose range (for α-methyldopa) 20 to 40 mg per kg per day in divided doses every 6 hours.

Antihypertensive Effect

A relatively slow onset of action is a feature of methyldopa treatment, and the BP-lowering effect starts approximately 2 to 3 hours after dosing (cf. clonidine's onset at 0.5 to 1.0 hour). At approximately 5 hours after an oral dose of methyldopa, the patient's BP reaches its lowest point, and the effect persists for up to 24 hours. The commonly used initial dose of methyldopa is 250 mg 2× per day, titrated up to 3.0 g at most. In patients with renal insufficiency, this methyldopa dose should be halved.

Methyldopa also effectively reduces supine BP without producing orthostatic hypotension.

Adverse Effects

Methyldopa's adverse effects include sedation and drowsiness, dry mouth, depression, postural hypotension, fluid retention, rebound hypertension, withdrawal syndrome, and various autoimmune reactions including flulike high fever, hepatitis, Coombs-positive hemolytic anemia, and lupuslike syndrome. Between 10% and 20% of patients who are treated with α-methyldopa (≥1 g/d) over a period of several months develop one or more of these adverse events. Occasionally, methyldopa treatment has resulted in drug-induced hepatitis with fever, eosinophilia, and increased transaminase values, but this is a self-limited process that resolves with discontinuation of the methyldopa. It is not necessary to stop methyldopa treatment in asymptomatic patients who become Coombs-positive but do not develop hemolytic anemia.

Guanabenz

The direct central α₂-agonist guanabenz[6-8] acts in the same manner as methyldopa and has similar adverse effects, but it has the advantage of not causing reactive fluid retention. Compared with clonidine, guanabenz treatment is less effective, but it results in rebound hypertension and orthostatic hypotension less frequently. The efficacy of guanabenz in reducing left ventricular hypertrophy in hypertensive patients and in attenuating morning hypertension when administered at nighttime has also been demonstrated.

Antihypertensive Effect

Guanabenz has a 1-hour onset of antihypertensive action. The most commonly used initial dose of guanabenz is 4 mg 2× per day, titrated to a maximum of 64 mg daily. It is eliminated predominantly via hepatic biotransformation. Thus, unlike clonidine, guanabenz dose adjustment is not required in patients with renal failure but is required in those with chronic liver diseases.

Guanabenz has also been shown to reduce total cholesterol levels by 10% to 20%.

Adverse Effects

The potential adverse effects of guanabenz include dry mouth, sedation, drowsiness, and impotence. Guanabenz treatment may also be followed by withdrawal syndrome and rebound hypertension. The adverse effects of guanabenz are essentially the same as those of clonidine.

Guanfacine

Unlike the other members of the class of central sympatholytics, the 17-hour duration of guanfacine's action typically allows it to be dosed once daily.[6-8] It is thought that compared with guanabenz, guanfacine enters the brain more slowly; its antihypertensive effect lasts longer than that of guanabenz. Evening dosing is preferable for guanfacine because its peak effect can be aligned with early-morning catecholamine and BP surges, and the potential sedating effect of guanfacine can play out during sleep. As with other central sympatholytics, the optimal effect of guanfacine can be achieved when it is coadministered with a low-dose diuretic, providing a BP-lowering effect with minimum CNS adverse effects. Patients who are intolerant to clonidine because of it strong sedation effect may benefit from treatment with guanfacine as an alternative.

Adverse Effects

Compared with clonidine, guanfacine has fewer CNS adverse effects and is much less likely to have withdrawal symptoms. The risk of adverse effects from guanfacine treatment increase significantly when doses greater than 1 mg daily are administered.

Imidazoline Receptor Agonists

The imidazoline receptor agonists rilmenidine and moxonidine act on the RVLM's imidazoline receptors.[2] The α_2-adrenergic receptors are less abundant in the RVLM. Moxonidine and rilmenidine effectively suppress sympathetic nervous activity without causing the adverse reactions observed with clonidine or methyldopa treatment such as sedation and dry mouth. In addition, the rebound syndrome caused by clonidine discontinuation has not been observed in cases of moxonidine or rilmenidine treatment.

Moxonidine

Moxonidine therapy effectively reduces BP although it does not reduce the heart rate as clonidine treatment can.[7] Moxonidine's plasma half-life is only 2 to 3 hours, and its extended duration of action suggests prolonged binding to central I_1-imidazoline receptors. The dose of moxonidine must be adjusted according to the patient's glomerular filtration rate (GFR), because moxonidine is extensively cleared by the kidneys.

For example, for patients with moderate renal impairment (i.e., a GFR 30 to 60 mL/min), single-dose moxonidine should not exceed 0.2 mg, and the daily dose should not go beyond 0.4 mg. For patients with severe renal impairment (i.e., a GFR < 30 mL/min), moxonidine should not be used. The same is true of patients with advanced heart failure; in a large cohort of New York Heart Association class II–IV heart failure patients with reduced ejection fraction, a sustained-release form of moxonidine that was force-titrated to 1.5 mg 2× per day was observed to be associated with early increases in morbidity and mortality.

Rilmenidine

For mild-to-moderate hypertension, oral rilmenidine (1 to 2 mg per day) is effective and well-tolerated, alone or in combination with another antihypertensive medication.[7] The most favorable ratio of efficacy to tolerability has been observed with a 1-mg daily dose. Parasympathetic tone is increased by rilmenidine, which may account for its lack of an effect on the heart rate as it works to reduce BP.

CENTRAL AND PERIPHERAL ADRENERGIC INHIBITORS

Reserpine

The only peripheral adrenergic inhibitor that is currently used is reserpine,[5,8] which depletes norepinephrine by blocking the transport of norepinephrine into its storage granules at the site of postganglionic sympathetic nerve endings. Reserpine treatment decreases peripheral vascular resistance because the concentration of neurotransmitters is lower even when sympathetic nerves are stimulated. Catecholamines are also depleted by reserpine treatment, not only in peripheral sympathetic nerves, but also in the brain and other tissues. This CNS effect accounts for the adverse central reactions to reserpine, which include sedation, depression, and nasal congestion. In the myocardium, this may contribute to decreases in the heart rate and cardiac contractility. For drug-resistant hypertension, reserpine is now used as the fourth- or fifth-line drug in multiple-drug regimens.

Antihypertensive Effect

Although reserpine is extremely long-acting, only a relatively mild BP-lowering effect is obtained with reserpine monotherapy (mean BP reduction of 3/5 mm Hg). When administered with a diuretic, reserpine induces a significant regression of left ventricular hypertrophy.

Adverse Effects

When reserpine is used at a low dose, adverse effects are relatively infrequent. The minor adverse effects include nasal congestion. Clinically serious sedation and depression are rare side effects of reserpine treatment.

Direct Vasodilators

Direct vasodilators work by entering the vascular smooth muscle cells, whereas indirect vasodilators prevent the entry of calcium into the smooth muscle cells that initiate vasoconstriction (calcium channel blockers), or they inhibit hormonal vasoconstrictor mechanisms (e.g., ACE inhibitors and ARBs), or they block α-adrenergic receptor-mediated vasoconstriction (α1-blockers).

The vasodilator effect of the direct vasodilators (hydralazine, minoxidil, nitroprusside, and nitroglycerin) differs among large conduit arteries, small branch arteries, arterioles, and veins (Table 26.2). When conduit arteries are relaxed, their compliance increases and systolic and pulse pressures tend to become lower. When small arteries and arterioles are relaxed, wave reflection and systemic vascular resistance are reduced. When veins are relaxed, systemic capacitance is increased and the central venous pressure is lowered. The overall hemodynamic effect of the administration of vasodilators is affected by the balance of these effects of individual drugs, combined with the reflex neurohormonal response.

Minoxidil and hydralazine act by dilating resistance arterioles, thereby reducing peripheral resistance. Baroreflex-mediated venoconstriction occurs, resulting in an increase in the venous return to the heart and direct catecholamine-mediated positive inotropic and chronotropic stimulation of the heart (Fig. 26.2). These two drugs have no dilating effect on the venous side of the circulation.

The direct vasodilator sodium nitroprusside is used to lower BP in hypertensive crises and to treat severe left ventricular failure; it is particularly valuable when a patient's survival is threatened by elevated pressure or severe left ventricular failure.

Nitrates are effective in producing sustained BP reductions when they are added to other antihypertensive regimens, but they are not yet used widely as antihypertensive agents. A recent systematic review demonstrated that when a nitrate and hydralazine were used together in some chronic heart failure trials, morbidity and mortality were reduced.

Hydralazine

The classic direct arteriolar dilator is hydralazine,[11-13] which lowers the total peripheral resistance and BP levels by directly relaxing the smooth muscle cells in the peripheral resistance arteries more than in capacitance veins. Hydralazine's vasodilating action may be mediated in part by its antioxidant action, which inhibits the vascular production of reactive oxygen species (ROS), thereby preventing the development of tolerance to exogenous nitrate, which serves as a source of nitrates.

Although hydralazine treatment significantly lowers BP, its use is limited by immunologic problems and the "pseudotolerance" phenomenon described later (Table 26.3). Hydralazine is currently used only infrequently to treat hypertension, and it is used as part of a multiple-drug regimen on top of other medications. It is usually combined with a sympathetic inhibitor to prevent the reflex activation of baroreflex, and it may be administered with a diuretic agent to prevent the sodium retention caused by reduced renal perfusion pressure. Moreover, given its short half-life of about 4 to 6 hours it must be given at least three times a day and preferably four times a day to maintain BP control over the 24-hour period.

Pregnancy-induced hypertension and eclampsia are the conditions for which hydralazine is most frequently used. Given during pregnancy, hydralazine is not toxic to the fetus.

Because its BP-lowering effect begins within a few minutes and its maximum effect occurs at 15 to 75 minutes after administration, hydralazine is also used for hypertensive emergencies. A parenteral dose of 20 to 40 mg hydralazine that can be repeated every 2 to 4 hours is usually administered. However, in hypertensive crises, hydralazine is not the best choice for patients with aortic dissection (because the hydralazine may increase the stroke volume and extend the dissection) or in patients with coexisting ischemic heart disease because it may worsen ischemia; see Chapter 46.

TABLE 26.2 Vasodilator Drugs for the Management of Hypertension

DRUG	RELATIVE ACTION IN AN ARTERY (A) OR VEIN (V)
Direct:	
Hydralazine	A >> V
Minoxidil	A >> V
Nitroprusside	A + V
Nitroglycerin	V > A
Indirect:	
Calcium channel blockers	A >> V
Angiotensin-converting enzyme inhibitors	A > V
Angiotensin receptor blockers	A >> V
Alpha-blockers	A + V
Alpha1-blockers	A >> V

>>, Much greater than; >, greater than; +, equal or both.

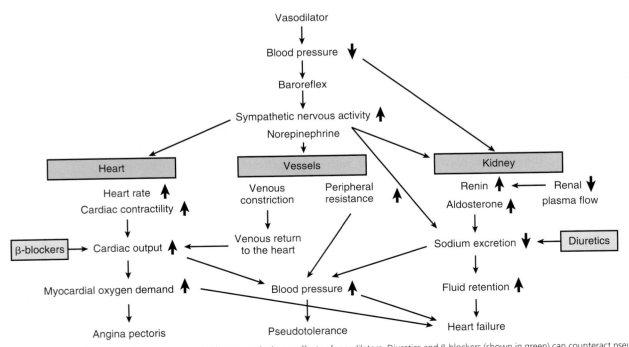

FIG. 26.2 Hemodynamic changes predisposing to pseudotolerance and adverse effects of vasodilators. Diuretics and β-blockers (shown in green) can counteract pseudotolerance when they are used concomitantly with vasodilators as the "standard triple therapy."

Pseudotolerance

The BP-lowering effect of arterial vasodilators tends to wane over time, in a phenomenon called *pseudotolerance*. The prefix *pseudo* is used because the tolerance is attributed not to a loss of the drug's direct BP-lowering effect, but rather to the compensatory mechanisms of BP regulation, that is, those of the renin-angiotensin-aldosterone system and the sympathetic nervous system, and fluid (sodium and water) retention (Fig. 26.2). Following peripheral vasodilation, to compensate for the hemodynamic changes, baroreflex-mediated sympathetic nervous activation increases the heart rate and cardiac output, and increased myocardial oxygen demand develops. Reduced blood flow, reduced renal perfusion pressure, and the sympathetic activation increase the secretion of renin, resulting in a compensatory retention of reactive sodium.

This compensatory sympathetic nervous activation along with the increased fluid retention (cardiac preload) and the increased heart rate may make the use of vasodilator monotherapy in patients with coronary artery disease (CAD) risky. These features may also trigger myocardial ischemia and CAD, and their occurrence helps explain the lesser regression of left ventricular hypertrophy. Hydralazine can be used with a diuretic and a β-blocker or other sympatholytic drug to block the pseudotolerance phenomenon and maintain the efficacy of the vasodilator, in a standard triple therapy. In fact, as a general principle, hydralazine should not be given to patients with cardiac ischemia until after they are on a beta-blocker and diuretic.

Antihypertensive Effect

Hydralazine's plasma half-life is short (approximately 90 minutes) but its clinical effect far outlasts its presence in the blood. Hydralazine may thus be given effectively in a twice-a-day regimen. The most commonly used starting regimen is 10 to 25 mg 2× per day, which can be increased at weekly intervals to the maximum dose of 100 to 200 mg 2× per day. Further BP reduction is not provided by the higher doses, and the use of the higher doses increases the risk of lupuslike syndrome.

Hydralazine is metabolized primarily by N-acetylation in the liver. It also forms hydrazones (i.e., the acetone hydrazone and the pyruvic acid hydrazone), which may contribute to the BP-lowering effect. The rate of this N-acetylation step is determined genetically. This "acetylator status" determines the systemic bioavailability of orally administered hydralazine and, because the patient's response is determined to a large extent by the level of the hydralazine in the blood, the acetylator status also determines the patient's response to the hydralazine. The oral availability of hydralazine has been estimated to be 10% to 30%, depending on the patient's acetylator status. Patients who are rapid acetylators require larger doses than slow acetylators to achieve an equivalent effect. Patients who develop lupuslike syndrome are likely to be slow acetylators and thus exposed to the drug longer.

Adverse Effects

In general, there are three types of adverse effects: (1) reflex sympathetic activation-related, (2) lupuslike syndrome-related, and (3) nonspecific adverse effects.

Adverse effects caused by reflex sympathetic activation include the anticipated tachycardia, palpitation, flashing, fluid retention, and headache, especially in the early days of therapy. Hydralazine may also trigger angina pectoris. However, these adverse effects can frequently be prevented by the concomitant use of a β-blocker. When a β-blocker is contraindicated, central sympatholytics are an alternative choice to reduce the pulse rate. Fluid retention causes not only edema but also pseudotolerance, and these can be prevented by a concomitant use of diuretics. Hydralazine should be avoided or used with caution in patients with a recent history of acute aortic dissection, stroke, coronary artery disease, or heart failure.

Similar to other drugs that are N-acetylated, high doses of hydralazine and long-term uses of hydralazine present a slight risk of lupuslike syndrome, with lupuslike symptoms such as a febrile reaction resembling that seen in systemic lupus erythematosus (SLE) and rheumatoid arthritis. The symptoms of lupuslike syndrome are: arthralgia, sometimes accompanied by pleural and pericardial effusion, splenomegaly, malaise, weight loss, and skin rash. These reactions were dose-dependent; the reactions did not occur in the patients given 50 mg daily, and they occurred in 5.4% of the patients given 100 mg daily and in 10.4% of those given 200 mg daily. The lupuslike reactions developed at approximately 6 to 24 months after the hydralazine therapy was initiated. The reactions were reversible, and when the drug was stopped or the dosage was lowered, a full recovery occurred within weeks.

In contrast to SLE, the hydralazine-induced lupuslike reaction is associated with antibodies directed against single-strand DNA (very high titers) rather than antibodies against the native double-strand DNA. A hydralazine-induced lupuslike reaction is also frequently accompanied by antibodies that are positive to histones, but glomerulonephritis rarely develops.

Other adverse reactions to hydralazine include gastrointestinal problems such as vomiting, nausea, diarrhea, and anorexia. Less common effects are muscle cramps, tremor, and paresthesia. Hydralazine treatment should be avoided in patients with liver damage, as fulminant hepatitis was reported in such patients.

Minoxidil

The direct vasodilator minoxidil[12-15] was introduced in the early 1970s for the treatment of hypertension. Better known for its marketing as a hair restorer, minoxidil opens cardiovascular adenosine triphosphate (ATP)-sensitive potassium

TABLE 26.3 Direct Vasodilators

DRUG	HALF-LIFE	DURATION OF ACTION	INITIAL DOSE	MAINTENANCE DOSE	DOSING FREQUENCY	CLINICAL USE	ADVERSE EFFECTS
Hydralazine	3-7 hours	8-12 hours	10-25 mg	100-200 mg	bid, tid	Pregnancy-associated hypertension Hypertensive emergencies Resistant hypertension	Pseudotolerance angina pectoris flashing, tachycardia, palpitation, headache Lupuslike reaction nausea, vomiting, diarrhea, hepatitis
Minoxidil	3-4 hours	12-72 hours	2.5-5.0 mg	10-40 mg	qd, bid	Severe resistant hypertension with advanced renal disease	Hypertrichosis pericardial effusion

bid, Twice a day; *qd,* once a day; *tid,* three times a day.

channels, which hyperpolarizes the smooth muscle membrane and inhibits the calcium influx through voltage-gated calcium channels. The cytosolic calcium concentration is thus reduced, producing smooth muscle relaxation. Minoxidil also dilates resistance vessels, with little or no action on the venous bed.

The vasodilatory action of minoxidil is stronger and lasts longer compared with that of hydralazine, but the potential adverse effects of minoxidil have limited its clinical use to hypertensive patients who are refractory to all other medications. The treatment of resistant hypertension, especially in patients with advanced renal disease, may be another option for minoxidil, the efficacy of which does not depend on the severity or etiology of the hypertension or the status of the patient's renal function. Prolonged minoxidil treatment can stabilize or improve renal function after an initial decrease in the glomerular filtration rate.

Patients with acute or chronic hypertensive nephrosclerosis have been able to discontinue dialysis based on the sustained BP control they achieved with minoxidil treatment. This beneficial effect was caused primarily by minoxidil's effective BP control rather than a specific renoprotective effect of minoxidil.

Minoxidil is usually administered with both a diuretic and a β-blocker, combined α/β-blocker or a central sympatholytic, because minoxidil increases sympathetic tone and causes significant sodium retention. For refractory edema, it may be necessary to apply a combination of thiazide-type and loop-type diuretics. The tachycardia caused by minoxidil treatment can aggravate myocardial ischemia and, if this is long-standing, left ventricular hypertrophy can develop.

Minoxidil's safety in pregnancy has not been established, but minoxidil is excreted into breast milk and should thus not be used by breastfeeding mothers.

Antihypertensive Effect

Minoxidil for hypertension is usually administered at an initial dose of 2.5 mg to 5 mg, 2× per day or occasionally once daily. Although doses up to 100 mg have been used, the usual maximum daily dose is 50 mg.

The plasma half-life of minoxidil is 2.8 to 4.2 hours, and the plasma protein binding is negligible; its oral absorption is 100%. Minoxidil is metabolized extensively in the liver, along four pathways: glucuronidation (67%), hydroxylation (25%), sulphation, and conversion to an uncharacterized polar compound. The sulphated metabolite of minoxidil is pharmacologically active, and it probably accounts for much of the parent drug's activity.

Adverse Effects

As the most common adverse effect of minoxidil, hirsutism is observed in nearly 80% of patients. The hirsutism begins with the development of fairly fine facial hair, progressing to coarse hair all over the body. The hair disappears gradually after the minoxidil treatment is stopped.

During the first few days of minoxidil treatment, electrocardiographic (ECG) changes are often observed; tachycardia as a result of reflex sympathetic activation may account for these ECG changes, which include T-wave inversion and ST depression but are not associated with cardiac enzyme elevation. In minoxidil-treated patients with ischemic heart disease, angina may be aggravated. Pericardial effusions appear in approximately 3% of minoxidil-treated patients attributed to potent fluid retention and are most common among those with advanced nephropathy or who are on dialysis.

References

1. Izzo JL, Sica DA, Black HR, Hypertension Primar. *The Essentials of High Blood Pressure: Basic Science, Population Science, and Clinical Management.* 4th ed. Philadelphia: Lippincott Williams & Wilkins; 2008.
2. Kaplan NM, Victor RG. *Kaplan's Clinical Hypertension.* 11th ed. Philadelphia: Lippincott Williams & Wilkins; 2014.
3. Saxena PR, Bolt GR. Haemodynamic profiles of vasodilators in experimental hypertension. *Trends Pharmacol Sci.* 1986;7:501-506.
4. Mancia G, Chalmers J, Julius S, et al. *Manual of Hypertension.* London: Churchill Livingstone; 2002.
5. van Zwieten PA. Beneficial interactions between pharmacological, pathophysiological and hypertension research. *J Hypertens.* 1999;17(12 Pt 2):1787-1797.
6. Weber MA. *Hypertension Medicine.* New Jersey: Humana Press; 2001.
7. Sica DA. Centrally acting antihypertensive agents: an update. *J Clin Hypertens (Greenwich).* 2007;9(5):399-405.
8. Vongpatanasin W, Kario K, Atlas SA, Victor RG. Central sympatholytic drugs. *J Clin Hypertens (Greenwich).* 2011;13:658-661.
9. Devereaux PJ, Sessler DI, Leslie K, et al. POISE-2 Investigators. Clonidine in patients undergoing noncardiac surgery. *N Engl J Med.* 2014;370:1504-1513.
10. Henning M, Rubenson A. Evidence that the hypotensive action of methyldopa is mediated by central actions of methylnoradrenaline. *J Pharm Pharmacol.* 1971;23:407-411.
11. Freis ED. Hydralazine in hypertension. *Am Heart J.* 1964;67:133-134.
12. Koch-Weser J. Vasodilator drugs in the treatment of hypertension. *Arch Intern Med.* 1974;133:1017-1027.
13. Cohn JN, McInnes GT, Shepherd AM. Direct-acting vasodilators. *J Clin Hypertens (Greenwich).* 2011;13:690-692.
14. Pettinger WA. Minoxidil and the treatment of severe hypertension. *N Engl J Med.* 1980;303(16):922-926.
15. Sica DA. Minoxidil: an underused vasodilator for resistant or severe hypertension. *J Clin Hypertens.* 2004;6:283-287.

27 Use of Combination Therapies

Hala Yamout and George L. Bakris

Heart disease is the leading cause of death in the United States and hypertension is an important risk factor for cardiovascular (CV) disease.[1] Affecting up to 30% of the population, when hypertension is well controlled it reduces the risk of CV events and death.[2-5] The importance of lowering blood pressure (BP) to reduce CV outcomes is known.[6] BP reduction to levels well below 140/90 mm Hg reduces the risk of heart failure by more than 50%, stroke by 35% to 40%, and myocardial infarction (MI) by 20% to 25%.[3,7]

All international guidelines recommend that BP be reduced to lower than 140/90 mm Hg to decrease the risk of CV events. The most recent Expert Panel Report known as the Joint National Committee (JNC 8) guidelines recommend a goal BP of less than 150/90 mm Hg in those over the age of 60 and less than 140/90 mm Hg in those younger than 60 years, those with diabetes, and/or chronic kidney disease (CKD).[8] Currently only 53% of people with hypertension would meet these criteria[2] based on a target of less than 140/90 mm Hg; based on more recent trial results, if adopted, would make this percentage smaller. The newly published Systolic Blood Pressure Intervention Trial (SPRINT), with more than one-third of the patients being over age 60 years, with 28% being over age 75 years, demonstrated a substantial reduction in heart failure as well as all-cause mortality among those randomized to a BP below 120 mm Hg systolic, using an automated oscillometric device. These patients did not have a history of prior strokes or diabetes.[4]

Given the difficulty in achieving BP goal with one medication, even under controlled conditions in clinical trials where two or more medications are required in more than 50%, the use of single pill combinations in the general population are mandatory (Fig. 27.1). The concept of initial combination therapy is not new because one of the first large clinical trials published in the late 1960s, the Veteran Affairs Cooperative Study, showed reduced morbidity with improved BP control using triple therapy combinations.[9,10]

RATIONALE FOR INITIAL COMBINATION THERAPY

History

The use of combination therapies started in the 1950s, when pills containing reserpine were introduced.[11] This was then followed by availability of several other formulations in the 1960s and 1970s that contained thiazide diuretics, including the triple combination pill of hydralazine and hydrochlorothiazide and reserpine, as well as in combination with potassium-sparing diuretics, beta-blockers, and clonidine.[12,13] In the 1980s, thiazides were combined with angiotensin-converting enzyme (ACE) inhibitors and in the 1990s, a combination of an ACE inhibitor and calcium channel blocker (CCB) was approved (Fig. 27.2).[11,13] Although combination BP lowering therapy was available and proven to reduce BP and mortality in clinical trials, the control of BP with stepwise management was advocated by early guidelines.[14]

The first report favoring combination therapy as an initial approach was seen in 1997 by the JNC VI panel.[15] Since this report, it is clear that initial use of single pill combination therapy is superior to a stepwise approach in controlling hypertension, with 12% more patients at their target BP.[16] Moreover, use of combination therapy improves BP control with fewer adverse events compared with doubling the dose of a single pill. Addition of an antihypertensive agent from a different class is five times more effective in improving BP control than doubling the dose of a single drug[17] (Fig. 27.3). Improvement in BP control occurs when even half the dose of the individual drugs are used in a combination pill compared with full doses of each as monotherapy.[18]

Philosophy and Physiology of Combination Therapy

There are several reasons why BP medications used in combination would allow better management of hypertension.[13,19] First, there are multiple systems that regulate BP and include sympathetic nervous system (SNS), renin-angiotensin system (RAS), and volume modulators from the kidney and heart like natriuretic peptides.[19] It is difficult to determine with certainty which system is dominant in a particular patient and the use of different classes of medications will increase the chance of controlling BP faster and more effectively.[11] Moreover, an increase dose of a single agent is less likely to achieve BP control than adding lower doses of a second agent.

Another reason for using combination therapy is to offset the body's counter-regulatory mechanisms to a particular agent, that is, diuretics used alone can result in relative volume depletion and activate the RAS and to a lesser extent the SNS.[11,13] The use of agents that block these systems, such as ACE inhibitors or beta-blockers, counteract the body's response to diuretics and are complementary to diuretic action to low BP. The use of vasodilators such as hydralazine and minoxidil cause a counter-regulatory activation of the RAS and SNS as well as increase sodium retention. Hence, they are mandated to be used with a beta-blocker and diuretic, making the use of antagonists of these systems additive.[11,13]

MEDICATION ADHERENCE

There are many reasons that only about 50% of hypertensive patients have BP at goal despite the availability of multiple therapies. Two of the most prominent are poor adherence to medication regimens by the patient and therapeutic inertia by physicians.

Medication adherence is a major issue in managing hypertension. Urine screening for medications and their metabolites in those considered to have resistant hypertension, taking approximately six medications a day, showed that about 53% were not adherent to therapy.[20] Of these, 30% were completely nonadherent and 70% were partially adherent, with 82% of the latter taking less than 50% of their prescribed regimen.[20] This was not dependent on the type of antihypertensive medication.

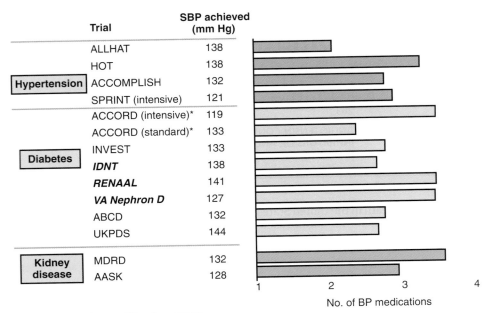

FIG. 27.1 Medications required to achieve blood pressure control in clinical trials.

Bold italic studies-both diabetes and kidney disease outcomes

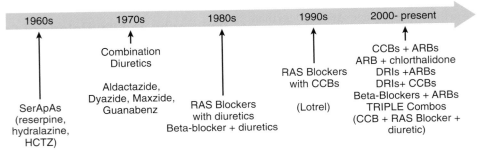

FIG. 27.2 History and evolution of single pill antihypertensive combination therapy.

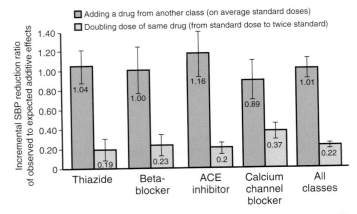

FIG. 27.3 Comparison of observed versus expected effects of a single pill combination versus doubling the dose of an antihypertensive medication. *(From Wald DS, Law M, Morris JK, Bestwick JP, Wald NJ. Combination therapy versus monotherapy in reducing blood pressure: meta-analysis on 11,000 participants from 42 trials. Am J Med. 2009;122:290-300.)*

The evidence for initial use of antihypertensive single pill combinations on outcomes is clear. In addition to the older VA studies already mentioned, the Avoiding Cardiovascular Events through Combination Therapy in Patients Living with Systolic Hypertension (ACCOMPLISH) trial is the most recent CV mortality trial randomizing to two different single pill BP lowering combinations.[16] In this trial, 32% required another drug in addition to the initially randomized single pill dual combination therapy.[21] The Antihypertensive and Lipid-Lowering Treatment to Prevent Heart Attack Trial (ALLHAT) study demonstrated that almost half the patients were on multiple medications by five years.[22] In the International Verapamil-Trandolapril Study (INVEST), the majority (>80%) of the patients required two or more medications to reach goal[23] and in the African American Study of Kidney Disease and Hypertension (AASK) study, an average of three or more antihypertensive agents were needed for the tight BP control group requiring a mean arterial pressure of less than 92 mm Hg[24] (Fig. 27.1).

It is obvious that single pill combination therapy improves adherence by reducing the absolute number of pills and their frequency. The more frequently a medication needs to be taken the lower the probability it is taken, with adherence also dropping from 77% to 55% if four drugs are taken as compared with one.[25] Even when the same two drugs are given as individual pills, adherence rates with combination therapy are significantly higher[26] (Fig. 27.4) and can reduce nonadherence by up to 24%.[24,27]

THERAPEUTIC INERTIA

Therapeutic inertia, or physician inaction in the face of a BP that is above target, is another major reason why hypertension remains poorly controlled. More than 7200 patients studied demonstrated that physicians only made medication changes

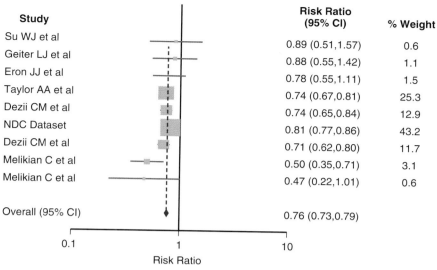

FIG. 27.4 Adherence with single pill combinations compared with free-drug combinations. *(From Bangalore S, Kamalakkannan G, Parkar S, Messerli FH. Fixed-dose combinations improve medication compliance: a meta-analysis. Am J Med. 2007;120:713-719.)*

in 13.1% of visits where BP was above guideline goal, although more recent studies show this has been improving.[28,29] This inaction by physicians is known to have a significant effect on the degree of BP control and accounts for almost 20% of variance in control.[28] It is projected that if medication changes were made in 30% of visits, the proportion of patients reaching BP target would rise from 45.1% to 65.9%.[28] One of the major reasons physician inertia is a problem, is physicians' perception that an uncontrolled patient is actually at target goal.[29]

ADVERSE SIDE EFFECTS

Paradoxically, one of the major reasons taught to avoid combination medications is potential for adverse events. This is antithetical to all published data. All single pill combinations available and approved by the United States Food and Drug Administration (FDA) have demonstrated added BP lowering efficacy with fewer adverse events compared with individual higher dosed components of the combination. Examples of combinations that avoid adverse events include a thiazide diuretic with a potassium-sparing diuretic to avoid hypokalemia.[30] ACE inhibitors induce vasodilation that reduces the incidence of peripheral edema caused by arterial vasodilation of CCBs.[31] Likewise, RAS blockers become more efficacious for BP lowering when used with thiazide-like diuretics and hence, many such combinations exist. Tolerability also improves as combination therapy allows use of lower doses of the individual medications, and using a half standard dose of a drug will only reduce its BP lowering efficacy by 20% but will also reduce the risk of adverse events.[32]

AVAILABLE SINGLE PILL COMBINATIONS

As discussed, there is a key rationale for combining certain classes of antihypertensive agents to reduce BP (Fig. 27.5).[33] Multiple single pill combinations of antihypertensive medications are approved by the FDA and other authorities around the world (Table 27.1).

Renin-Angiotensin System Blockers With Calcium Channel Blockers

Single pill combinations of CCB with RAS blockers such as ACE inhibitors, angiotensin receptor blockers (ARBs), and direct renin inhibitors have been studied. Combinations of RAS

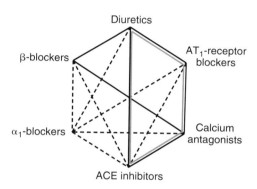

FIG. 27.5 Modification of the European Society of Hypertension illustration of various drug class combinations to lower blood pressure. Solid black lines demonstrate additive effects on blood pressure (BP) lowering; orange lines demonstrate outcome based reduction in either cardiovascular events or kidney disease progression. Dotted lines indicate either no additive effect on BP lowering or benefit in outcome studies. Note renin inhibitors plus diuretics or angiotensin receptor blockers have additive BP reduction but no outcome data. *(From Mancia G, Fagard R, Narkiewicz K, et al. 2013 ESH/ESC practice guidelines for the management of arterial hypertension. Blood Press. 2014;23:3-16.)*

blockers with either thiazide diuretics or CCBs are preferred therapy according to the American Society of Hypertension Consensus Panel Report, given that such combinations reduce mortality with fewer adverse events.[19]

RAS blockers reduce the CCB-induced activation of the RAS and SNS systems that are caused by vasodilatory effect of CCBs.[11] With the activation of the RAS system by CCBs, the antihypertensive effect of RAS blockers is amplified.[11] The use of ACE inhibitors also reduce peripheral edema caused by CCBs[31] and, when used in combination with a nondihydropyridine CCB (i.e., diltiazem or verapamil), there is a synergistic effect on albuminuria reduction.[34]

The combination of ACE inhibitors and CCBs has been established to be superior in reducing BP as compared with its individual monotherapies.[35] The ACCOMPLISH trial was the first trial to study two different single pill combinations on CV and renal outcome. The ACE inhibitor (benazepril) was used in combination with a CCB (amlodipine) or hydrochlorothiazide (thiazide diuretic) in hypertensive patients at high CV risk. Despite similar attained BPs, the trial was terminated early because of a large difference in the primary endpoint of CV events favoring the ACE inhibitor/CCB combination (9.6%

TABLE 27.1 American Society of Hypertension Evidenced-Based Fixed-Dose Antihypertensive Combinations

Preferred	ACE inhibitor/diuretic[a] ARB/diuretic[a] ACE inhibitor/CCB[a] ARB/CCB[a]
Acceptable	Beta-blocker/diuretic[a] CCB (dihydropyridine)/β-blocker CCB/diuretic Renin inhibitor/diuretic[a] Renin inhibitor/ARB[a] Thiazide diuretics/K+ sparing diuretics[a]
Less Effective	ACE inhibitor/ARB ACE inhibitor/β-blocker ARB/β-blocker CCB (nondihydropyridine)/β-blocker Centrally acting agent/β-blocker

[a]SPC available in the United States.
(From Gradman AH, Basile JN, Carter BL, et al. Combination therapy in hypertension. J Am Soc Hypertens. 2010;4:90-98.)
ACE, Angiotensin-converting enzyme; *ARB,* angiotensin receptor blocker; *CCB,* calcium channel blocker.

versus 11.8%, respectively).[21] Further study showed that patients with known coronary artery disease at baseline also had significantly reduced CV events on the ACE inhibitor/CCB combination.[36]

The effect of these combinations on CKD progression, a prespecified secondary endpoint in ACCOMPLISH, demonstrated fewer CKD events (doubling of creatinine or end-stage renal disease) with a slower decline in estimated glomerular filtration rate (eGFR) in the benazepril/amlodipine group.[37]

Many trials have assessed BP lowering ability of various combinations and all have shown additive benefit. The ARB (valsartan) and a CCB (amlodipine) have been studied. Various doses of amlodipine plus valsartan were compared with monotherapy and placebo in those with diastolic BP of 95 to 110 mm Hg.[38] Use of the combination pill resulted in greater reduction of both systolic and diastolic pressures over the monotherapy. The incidence of edema was lower in those on combination therapy.[38]

The combination of aliskiren with the CCB amlodipine has also been compared with the individual component monotherapies. The combination group had significantly lower BPs even when used at half doses[39,40]; however, other studies have shown that the half-dose combination therapy is equivalent to full dose amlodipine.[40]

ANGIOTENSIN-CONVERTING ENZYME INHIBITORS OR ANGIOTENSIN RECEPTOR BLOCKERS WITH DIURETICS

The additive BP lowering effects of an ACE inhibitor or ARB with a thiazide diuretic are well known. The efficacy of the combination comes from their complimentary mechanisms of action because the use of a diuretic activates the RAS system by causing intravascular volume depletion.[19] The combination with RAS blockade is also useful because it reduces the risk of hypokalemia as an adverse effect of thiazide.[41,42]

Multiple trials have shown a significantly greater BP reduction in those on combination ACE inhibitors or ARBs with a thiazide or thiazide-like diuretic (chlorthalidone or indapamide) as compared with monotherapy.[41,43,44] Several outcome studies also show the benefits of these combinations, which include the perindopril protection against recurrent stroke study (PROGRESS). A perindopril-based antihypertensive treatment was compared with placebo in those who have had a history of stroke or transient ischemic attack,[45] with the ACE inhibitor added to indapamide if strict BP control was

needed. The ACE inhibitor/diuretic group was compared with placebo to determine the effect on fatal and nonfatal stroke. The trial revealed a reduced incidence of stroke in the combination group compared with placebo (10% versus 14%, respectively), whereas monotherapy with perindopril was not different from placebo.[45]

In the Hypertension in the Very Elderly Trial (HYVET), patients 80 years old and older were randomized to BP control of less than 150/80 mm Hg using indapamide, with the addition of perindopril if needed, to assess the effect on fatal and nonfatal stroke. The trial was stopped early because of a large difference in outcome between the two groups favoring the treatment group.[46] It is worth noting that this trial also showed that the majority of the groups required more than two medications to reach goal.[46]

COMBINATION RENIN-ANGIOTENSIN SYSTEM BLOCKADE

Direct Renin Inhibitors With Angiotensin Receptor Blockers

Similar to ACE inhibitors/ARB combinations, aliskiren, a direct renin inhibitor, has been tested in combination with a RAS blocking agent. Outcomes studies have also failed to show benefit and suggest harm. The Valsartan Aliskiren Hypertension Diabetes (VIvID) study was performed before an outcome trial to test the antihypertensive efficacy of the aliskiren plus valsartan combination compared with valsartan monotherapy. Patients studied, however, had diabetes and hypertension and good kidney function with a mean baseline eGFR over 80 mL/min/1.73m². Those on the combination pill compared with the monotherapy had a significantly lower BP on both office and ambulatory BP measurements at 8 weeks.[47] There was no significant difference in the adverse effects between the groups. In contrast, the Aliskiren Trial in Type 2 Diabetes Using Cardiorenal Endpoints (ALTITUDE) study evaluated the combination of aliskiren with a RAS blocker on a primary endpoint consisting of combined CV and renal endpoints in diabetic patients with CV disease, CKD, or both with a mean eGFR in the low forties. The study was stopped prematurely because of a significantly higher risk of adverse events and no reduction in primary endpoint among those taking aliskiren in combination with another RAS blocker.[48]

Potassium Sparing Diuretics With Diuretics

Diuretics are extensively discussed in Chapter 22 on diuretics. The combination of a thiazide diuretic with a potassium-sparing diuretic such as amiloride or spironolactone, have been studied given that the latter would reduce the potassium and magnesium wasting associated with thiazide therapy.[49] A significant reduction in risk of cardiac arrest was noted among those receiving a combination thiazide and potassium-sparing diuretic and not in those on potassium supplements.[49]

The use of amiloride in combination with hydrochlorothiazide compared with monotherapy showed significantly better BP control compared with hydrochlorothiazide alone.[50] There was no difference in CV mortality and morbidity in high-risk patients when this combination was compared with CCBs.[51]

Beta-Blockers With Diuretics

The combination of a beta-blocker with thiazide diuretics is highly efficacious[19] because beta-blockers attenuate the activation of the RAS system caused by diuretics and diuretics reduce sodium retention induced by beta-blockers.[11] This would also avoid increasing the dose of thiazide diuretics because doses up to 50 mg of hydrochlorothiazide and 25 mg of chlorthalidone will significantly increase adverse events and only minimally reduce blood pressure (see Chapter 22). The combination of these two agents has been shown to reduce BP more than its individual components.[52]

The effect of this combination on outcomes was studied in The Anglo-Scandinavian Cardiac Outcomes Trial-Blood Pressure Lowering Arm (ASCOT-BPLA), which compared the efficacy of a beta-blocker/thiazide combination with CCB/ACE inhibitor in reducing nonfatal MI and coronary heart disease. In patients with multiple CV risk factors, participants were randomized to a CCB-based therapy with amlodipine, with the addition of perindopril, versus the beta-blocker atenolol adding bendroflumethiazide as required.[53] The trial was stopped early because of favoring the CCB/ACE inhibitor group on primary endpoint as compared with the beta-blockers–based therapy. Blood pressure in the CCB group was lower throughout the trial compared with the beta-blocker group.

Single Pill Triple Combination Therapy

In addition to a single pill with two medications, there are triple-therapy single pill combinations. The benefits of dual therapy, including increased adherence, have been shown with triple therapy as well.[54,55]

The use of triple combination therapy has been available since 1966 and consists of reserpine, hydrochlorothiazide, and hydralazine[13] in the Veterans Affairs Cooperative Study.[9,10,56] Since then, several triple combination therapies have been introduced, many of which consist of a RAS blocker, CCB, and thiazide diuretic.[56]

Although there are no outcome data, there are ample BP studies with single pill triple therapy. One single pill triple therapy combination was tested in the Triple Therapy with Olmesartan Medoxomil, Amlodipine, and Hydrochlorothiazide in Hypertensive Patients (TRINITY) study.[57] A single pill containing the combination of olmesartan 40 mg, amlodipine 10 mg, and hydrochlorothiazide 25 mg, was compared with single pill combinations of its dual components in those with a BP 140/90 or higher mm Hg while on treatment, or 160/90 or less mm Hg off treatment. The triple combination therapy significantly reduced both systolic and diastolic BP compared with dual therapy. This observation was confirmed by 24-hour ambulatory BP monitoring.[58]

The combination of amlodipine with valsartan and hydrochlorothiazide as compared with its dual components has also been evaluated. In more than 4000 patients with a baseline BP of 145/100 or higher mm Hg, there was a greater reduction in BP seen in those on triple therapy as compared with dual therapy.[59] The number of patients reaching blood goal of less than 140/90 mm Hg was greater in the triple therapy group (70.8% versus 44.8%, 48.3%, and 54.1% in the amlodipine/hydrochlorothiazide, valsartan/hydrochlorothiazide, and amlodipine/valsartan groups, respectively). This has also been confirmed by 24-hour ambulatory BP monitoring.[60] The frequency of adverse events was similar across groups. The significant drop in BP in the triple therapy group was evident by the third week of the study, where up to 75% of the overall BP lowering effect of the treatment was already seen.[61]

The triple combination pill of aliskiren/amlodipine/hydrochlorothiazide was also found to reduce overall BP more than its dual components.[62] In those with baseline severe hypertension, defined as a systolic BP 180 or higher mm Hg, BP was reduced by up to 49.5/22.5 mm Hg. Significantly more patients in the triple therapy group also reached a goal BP control as compared with the dual therapy groups. This was also confirmed by 24-hour ambulatory BP monitoring. There was no difference in the incidence of adverse events.

NONAPPROVED COMBINATIONS

Angiotensin-Converting Enzyme Inhibitors With Angiotensin Receptor Blockers

Based on available data from multiple CV outcome studies, it is clear that combinations of ACE inhibitors with ARBs should not be used for BP lowering. The reasons for this are clearly because they do not have additive BP lowering effects and they have uniformly shown higher mortality and morbidity in outcome trials. Therefore, only a brief review is provided. There are two trials that examined this combination on outcomes, The Ongoing Telmisartan Alone and in Combination with Ramipril Global Endpoint Trial (ONTARGET) and the Veterans Affairs Nephropathy in Diabetes (VA NEPHRON-D). ONTARGET evaluated the ARB, telmisartan compared with an ACE inhibitor (ramipril), or the combination of the two agents to prevent CV events in high-risk patients. It found that there was no difference between the two agents on the primary outcome, whereas the combination group had a higher risk of adverse events with no increased benefit.[63] The VA NEPHRON-D evaluated the ARB losartan alone or in combination of ACE inhibitor (lisinopril) on renal outcomes in diabetic nephropathy. The trial was stopped early because of a significantly higher rate of adverse events (hyperkalemia, acute kidney injury) in the combination group.[64]

Renin-Angiotensin System Blockers With Beta-Blockers

The combination of a RAS blocker plus a beta-blocker is not efficacious for lowering BP as other possible combination therapies given the similarity in their mode of action; that is, beta-blockers inhibit renin as a mechanism of BP reduction.[19] Although a post hoc analysis of the Glycemic Effect in Diabetes mellitus: Carvedilol-metoprolol Comparison in Hypertensives (GEMINI) trial, showed that almost 40% of those with hypertension and type 2 diabetes can achieve control when adding carvedilol to an ACE inhibitors or ARBs,[65] a prospective trial. Effect of combining extended-release carvedilol and lisinopril in hypertension (COSMOS) using change in 24-hour ambulatory BP monitoring as primary endpoint, failed to show any additivity of carvedilol to lisinopril on BP reduction.[66]

One possible exception to this rule about BP lowering with a RAS and beta-blockers may be nebivolol, a beta-blocker that stimulates nitric oxide (NO) and is vasodilatory. Results of a trial testing the combination of nebivolol plus the ARB valsartan compared with their monotherapies showed the combination to provide greater reduction in BP with similar risk of adverse events.[67] A similar effect was seen when nebivolol was used in combination with the ACE inhibitor lisinopril as compared with the monotherapies, where more patients reached their target pressure while on the combination treatment.[68] There are no outcome data with this combination and the effects only seen at highest dose of nebivolol.

Diuretics With Calcium Channel Blockers

The combination of CCBs and diuretics is not likely to be as efficacious as other combinations. A direct comparison of chlorthalidone plus nifedipine in combination to the individual agents did not significantly lower BP as compared with nifedipine alone, but combination was better than chlorthalidone.[69] In addition, a separate study examining the effects of nitrendipine plus hydrochlorothiazide to either component showed the combination yielded better BP lowering than either alone.[70] There are no trials evaluating this outcome and, because of the hypokalemia risk, it is not a preferred combination.

Calcium Channel Blockers With Beta-Blockers

Although this single pill combination is approved in certain parts of the world, it is not available in the United States. The combination of CCBs, particularly dihydropyridine CCBs, and beta-blockers would provide additive BP lowering given their respective mechanisms of action. CCBs can diminish the α-adrenergic vasoconstriction caused by beta-blockers, whereas beta-blockers can reduce the SNS activation caused by dihydropyridines.[71] The combination of felodipine and metoprolol significantly lowers BP compared to monotherapy,[71] with the lowest combination dose almost as effective as the highest dose of monotherapy.[72]

Nondihydropyridine CCBs should generally not be used with beta-blockers as they can both affect heart rate and atrioventricular conduction, causing possibly severe bradycardia.[19] In hyperadrenergic states with high pulse rates, however, such combinations are useful.

CONCLUSION

Given the increasing incidence of resistant hypertension and control rates of BP just above the 50% level in the United States, more effective use of an antihypertensive regimen is needed. Clearly, use of single pill combinations has been shown to be associated with better tolerability and fewer side effects as well as better outcomes compared with multiple monotherapy tablets. Thus, single pill combination BP lowering therapy should be preferred among those requiring two or more medications for BP lowering and all those who have a BP 160/100 or higher mm Hg per guidelines. Many combinations have been studied with various results on efficacy and tolerability as well as CV outcomes. The most appropriate regimen for patients should continue to be individualized to their particular cases but should improve tolerability and ability to take medications to reduce their BP and their risk of CV disease and note that the CCB/RAS blocker and RAS blocker/diuretic combinations have the bulk of evidence supporting their use.

References

1. Mozaffarian D, Benjamin EJ, Go AS, et al. Heart disease and stroke statistics-2016 update: a report from the American Heart Association. *Circulation.* 2016;133:e38-60.
2. Yoon SS, Carroll MD, Fryar CD. Hypertension prevalence and control among adults: United States, 2011-2014. *NCHS Data Brief.* 2015;220:1-8.
3. Neal B, MacMahon S, Chapman N. Effects of ACE inhibitors, calcium antagonists, and other blood-pressure-lowering drugs: results of prospectively designed overviews of randomised trials. Blood Pressure Lowering Treatment Trialists' Collaboration. *Lancet.* 2000;356:1955-1964.
4. Wright Jr JT, Williamson JD, Whelton PK, et al. A randomized trial of intensive versus standard blood-pressure control. *N Engl J Med.* 2015;373:2103-2116.
5. Staessen JA, Fagard R, Thijs L, et al. Randomised double-blind comparison of placebo and active treatment for older patients with isolated systolic hypertension. The Systolic Hypertension in Europe (Syst-Eur) Trial Investigators. *Lancet.* 1997;350:757-764.
6. Gradman AH, Parise H, Lefebvre P, Falvey H, Lafeuille MH, Duh MS. Initial combination therapy reduces the risk of cardiovascular events in hypertensive patients: a matched cohort study. *Hypertension.* 2013;61:309-318.
7. Chobanian AV, Bakris GL, Black HR, et al. The seventh report of the Joint National Committee on prevention, detection, evaluation, and treatment of high blood pressure: the JNC 7 report. *JAMA.* 2003;289:2560-2572.
8. James PA, Oparil S, Carter BL, et al. 2014 evidence-based guideline for the management of high blood pressure in adults: report from the panel members appointed to the Eighth Joint National Committee (JNC 8). *JAMA.* 2014;311:507-520.
9. Effects of treatment on morbidity in hypertension. II. Results in patients with diastolic blood pressure averaging 90 through 114 mm Hg. *JAMA.* 1970;213:1143-1152.
10. Effects of treatment on morbidity in hypertension. Results in patients with diastolic blood pressures averaging 115 through 129 mm Hg. *JAMA.* 1967;202:1028-1034.
11. Sica DA. Rationale for fixed-dose combinations in the treatment of hypertension: the cycle repeats. *Drugs.* 2002;62:443-462.
12. Sica D, Gradman AH, Lederballe O, Kolloch RE, Zhang J, Keefe DL. Long-term safety and tolerability of the oral direct renin inhibitor aliskiren with optional add-on hydrochlorothiazide in patients with hypertension: a randomized, open-label, parallel-group, multicentre, dose-escalation study with an extension phase. *Clin Drug Investig.* 2011;31:825-837.
13. Epstein M, Bakris G. Newer approaches to antihypertensive therapy. Use of fixed-dose combination therapy. *Arch Intern Med.* 1996;156:1969-1978.
14. Black HR. Triple fixed-dose combination therapy: back to the past. *Hypertension.* 2009;54:19-22.
15. The sixth report of the Joint National Committee on prevention, detection, evaluation, and treatment of high blood pressure. *Arch Intern Med.* 1997;157:2413-2446.
16. Feldman RD, Zou GY, Vandervoort MK, Wong CJ, Nelson SA, Feagan BG. A simplified approach to the treatment of uncomplicated hypertension: a cluster randomized, controlled trial. *Hypertension.* 2009;53:646-653.
17. Wald DS, Law M, Morris JK, Bestwick JP, Wald NJ. Combination therapy versus monotherapy in reducing blood pressure: meta-analysis on 11,000 participants from 42 trials. *Am J Med.* 2009;122:290-300.
18. Neutel JM, Smith DH, Weber MA. Effect of antihypertensive monotherapy and combination therapy on arterial distensibility and left ventricular mass. *Am J Hypertens.* 2004;17:37-42.
19. Gradman AH, Basile JN, Carter BL, et al. Combination therapy in hypertension. *J Am Soc Hypertens.* 2010;4:90-98.
20. Jung O, Gechter JL, Wunder C, et al. Resistant hypertension? Assessment of adherence by toxicological urine analysis. *J Hypertens.* 2013;31:766-774.
21. Jamerson K, Weber MA, Bakris GL, et al. Benazepril plus amlodipine or hydrochlorothiazide for hypertension in high-risk patients. *N Engl J Med.* 2008;359:2417-2428.
22. Major outcomes in high-risk hypertensive patients randomized to angiotensin-converting enzyme inhibitor or calcium channel blocker vs diuretic: The Antihypertensive and Lipid-Lowering Treatment to Prevent Heart Attack Trial (ALLHAT). *JAMA.* 2002;288:2981-2997.
23. Pepine CJ, Handberg EM, Cooper-DeHoff RM, et al. A calcium antagonist vs a non-calcium antagonist hypertension treatment strategy for patients with coronary artery disease. The International Verapamil-Trandolapril Study (INVEST): a randomized controlled trial. *JAMA.* 2003;290:2805-2816.
24. Wright Jr JT, Bakris G, Greene T, et al. Effect of blood pressure lowering and antihypertensive drug class on progression of hypertensive kidney disease: results from the AASK trial. *JAMA.* 2002;288:2421-2431.
25. Fung V, Huang J, Brand R, Newhouse JP, Hsu J. Hypertension treatment in a medicare population: adherence and systolic blood pressure control. *Clin Ther.* 2007;29:972-984.
26. Dezii CM. A retrospective study of persistence with single-pill combination therapy vs. concurrent two-pill therapy in patients with hypertension. *Manag Care.* 2000;9:2-6.
27. Bangalore S, Kamalakkannan G, Parkar S, Messerli FH. Fixed-dose combinations improve medication compliance: a meta-analysis. *Am J Med.* 2007;120:713-719.
28. Okonofua EC, Simpson KN, Jesri A, Rehman SU, Durkalski VL, Egan BM. Therapeutic inertia is an impediment to achieving the Healthy People 2010 blood pressure control goals. *Hypertension.* 2006;47:345-351.
29. Escobar C, Barrios V, Alonso-Moreno FJ, et al. Evolution of therapy inertia in primary care setting in Spain during 2002-2010. *J Hypertens.* 2014;32:1138-1145.
30. Ernst ME, Moser M. Use of diuretics in patients with hypertension. *N Engl J Med.* 2009;361:2153-2164.
31. Gradman AH, Cutler NR, Davis PJ, Robbins JA, Weiss RJ, Wood BC. Combined enalapril and felodipine extended release (ER) for systemic hypertension. Enalapril-Felodipine ER Factorial Study Group. *Am J Cardiol.* 1997;79:431-435.
32. Law MR, Wald NJ, Morris JK, Jordan RE. Value of low dose combination treatment with blood pressure lowering drugs: analysis of 354 randomised trials. *BMJ.* 2003;326:1427.
33. Mancia G, Fagard R, Narkiewicz K, et al. 2013 ESH/ESC practice guidelines for the management of arterial hypertension. *Blood Press.* 2014;23:3-16.
34. Bakris GL, Weir MR, Secic M, Campbell B, Weis-McNulty A. Differential effects of calcium antagonist subclasses on markers of nephropathy progression. *Kidney Int.* 2004;65:1991-2002.
35. Kuschnir E, Acuna E, Sevilla D, et al. Treatment of patients with essential hypertension: amlodipine 5 mg/benazepril 20 mg compared with amlodipine 5 mg, benazepril 20 mg, and placebo. *Clin Ther.* 1996;18:1213-1224.
36. Bakris G, Briasoulis A, Dahlof B, et al. Comparison of benazepril plus amlodipine or hydrochlorothiazide in high-risk patients with hypertension and coronary artery disease. *Am J Cardiol.* 2013;112:255-259.
37. Bakris GL, Sarafidis PA, Weir MR, et al. Renal outcomes with different fixed-dose combination therapies in patients with hypertension at high risk for cardiovascular events (ACCOMPLISH): a prespecified secondary analysis of a randomised controlled trial. *Lancet.* 2010;375:1173-1181.
38. Philipp T, Smith TR, Glazer R, et al. Two multicenter, 8-week, randomized, double-blind, placebo-controlled, parallel-group studies evaluating the efficacy and tolerability of amlodipine and valsartan in combination and as monotherapy in adult patients with mild to moderate essential hypertension. *Clin Ther.* 2007;29:563-580.
39. Brown MJ, McInnes GT, Papst CC, Zhang J, MacDonald TM. Aliskiren and the calcium channel blocker amlodipine combination as an initial treatment strategy for hypertension control (ACCELERATE): a randomised, parallel-group trial. *Lancet.* 2011;377:312-320.
40. Drummond W, Munger MA, Rafique EM, Maboudian M, Khan M, Keefe DL. Antihypertensive efficacy of the oral direct renin inhibitor aliskiren as add-on therapy in patients not responding to amlodipine monotherapy. *J Clin Hypertens (Greenwich).* 2007;9:742-750.
41. Pool JL, Glazer R, Weinberger M, Alvarado R, Huang J, Graff A. Comparison of valsartan/hydrochlorothiazide combination therapy at doses up to 320/25 mg versus monotherapy: a double-blind, placebo-controlled study followed by long-term combination therapy in hypertensive adults. *Clin Ther.* 2007;29:61-73.
42. McGill JB, Reilly PA. Telmisartan plus hydrochlorothiazide versus telmisartan or hydrochlorothiazide monotherapy in patients with mild to moderate hypertension: a multicenter, randomized, double-blind, placebo-controlled, parallel-group trial. *Clin Ther.* 2001;23:833-850.
43. Owens P, Kelly L, Nallen R, Ryan D, Fitzgerald D, O'Brien E. Comparison of antihypertensive and metabolic effects of losartan and losartan in combination with hydrochlorothiazide—a randomized controlled trial. *J Hypertens.* 2000;18:339-345.
44. Scholze J, Breitstadt A, Cairns V, et al. Short report: ramipril and hydrochlorothiazide combination therapy in hypertension: a clinical trial of factorial design. The East Germany Collaborative Trial Group. *J Hypertens.* 1993;11:217-221.
45. Randomised trial of a perindopril-based blood-pressure-lowering regimen among 6,105 individuals with previous stroke or transient ischaemic attack. *Lancet.* 2001;358:1033-1041.
46. Beckett NS, Peters R, Fletcher AE, et al. Treatment of hypertension in patients 80 years of age or older. *N Engl J Med.* 2008;358:1887-1898.
47. Bakris GL, Oparil S, Purkayastha D, Yadao AM, Alessi T, Sowers JR. Randomized study of antihypertensive efficacy and safety of combination aliskiren/valsartan vs valsartan monotherapy in hypertensive participants with type 2 diabetes mellitus. *J Clin Hypertens (Greenwich).* 2013;15:92-100.
48. Parving HH, Brenner BM, McMurray JJ, et al. Cardiorenal end points in a trial of aliskiren for type 2 diabetes. *N Engl J Med.* 2012;367:2204-2213.
49. Siscovick DS, Raghunathan TE, Psaty BM, et al. Diuretic therapy for hypertension and the risk of primary cardiac arrest. *N Engl J Med.* 1994;330:1852-1857.
50. Brown MJ, Williams B, Morant SV, et al. Effect of amiloride, or amiloride plus hydrochlorothiazide, versus hydrochlorothiazide on glucose tolerance and blood pressure (PATHWAY-3): a parallel-group, double-blind randomised phase 4 trial. *Lancet Diabetes Endocrinol.* 2016;4:136-147.
51. Brown MJ, Palmer CR, Castaigne A, et al. Morbidity and mortality in patients randomised to double-blind treatment with a long-acting calcium-channel blocker or diuretic in the International Nifedipine GITS study: Intervention as a Goal in Hypertension Treatment (INSIGHT). *Lancet.* 2000;356:366-372.

52. Frishman WH, Bryzinski BS, Coulson LR, et al. A multifactorial trial design to assess combination therapy in hypertension. Treatment with bisoprolol and hydrochlorothiazide. *Arch Intern Med*. 1994;154:1461-1468.

53. Dahlof B, Sever PS, Poulter NR, et al. Prevention of cardiovascular events with an antihypertensive regimen of amlodipine adding perindopril as required versus atenolol adding bendroflumethiazide as required, in the Anglo-Scandinavian Cardiac Outcomes Trial-Blood Pressure Lowering Arm (ASCOT-BPLA): a multicentre randomised controlled trial. *Lancet*. 2005;366:895-906.

54. Panjabi S, Lacey M, Bancroft T, Cao F. Treatment adherence, clinical outcomes, and economics of triple-drug therapy in hypertensive patients. *J Am Soc Hypertens*. 2013;7:46-60.

55. Xie L, Frech-Tamas F, Marrett E, Baser O. A medication adherence and persistence comparison of hypertensive patients treated with single-, double- and triple-pill combination therapy. *Curr Med Res Opin*. 2014;30:2415-2422.

56. Gradman AH. Rationale for triple-combination therapy for management of high blood pressure. *J Clin Hypertens (Greenwich)*. 2010;12:869-878.

57. Oparil S, Melino M, Lee J, Fernandez V, Heyrman R. Triple therapy with olmesartan medoxomil, amlodipine besylate, and hydrochlorothiazide in adult patients with hypertension: The TRINITY multicenter, randomized, double-blind, 12-week, parallel-group study. *Clin Ther*. 2010;32:1252-1269.

58. Izzo Jr JL, Chrysant SG, Kereiakes DJ, et al. 24-hour efficacy and safety of Triple-Combination Therapy With Olmesartan, Amlodipine, and Hydrochlorothiazide: the TRINITY ambulatory blood pressure substudy. *J Clin Hypertens (Greenwich)*. 2011;13:873-880.

59. Calhoun DA, Lacourciere Y, Chiang YT, Glazer RD. Triple antihypertensive therapy with amlodipine, valsartan, and hydrochlorothiazide: a randomized clinical trial. *Hypertension*. 2009;54:32-39.

60. Lacourciere Y, Crikelair N, Glazer RD, Yen J, Calhoun DA. 24-Hour ambulatory blood pressure control with triple-therapy amlodipine, valsartan and hydrochlorothiazide in patients with moderate to severe hypertension. *J Hum Hypertens*. 2011;25:615-622.

61. Calhoun DA, Crikelair NA, Yen J, Glazer RD. Amlodipine/valsartan/hydrochlorothiazide triple combination therapy in moderate/severe hypertension: Secondary analyses evaluating efficacy and safety. *Adv Ther*. 2009;26:1012-1023.

62. Lacourciere Y, Taddei S, Konis G, Fang H, Severin T, Zhang J. Clinic and ambulatory blood pressure lowering effect of aliskiren/amlodipine/hydrochlorothiazide combination in patients with moderate-to-severe hypertension: a randomized active-controlled trial. *J Hypertens*. 2012;30:2047-2055.

63. Yusuf S, Teo KK, Pogue J, et al. Telmisartan, ramipril, or both in patients at high risk for vascular events. *N Engl J Med*. 2008;358:1547-1559.

64. Fried LF, Emanuele N, Zhang JH, et al. Combined angiotensin inhibition for the treatment of diabetic nephropathy. *N Engl J Med*. 2013;369:1892-1903.

65. Wright Jr JT, Bakris GL, Bell DS, et al. Lowering blood pressure with beta-blockers in combination with other renin-angiotensin system blockers in patients with hypertension and type 2 diabetes: results from the GEMINI Trial. *J Clin Hypertens (Greenwich)*. 2007;9:842-849.

66. Bakris GL, Iyengar M, Lukas MA, Ordronneau P, Weber MA. Effect of combining extended-release carvedilol and lisinopril in hypertension: results of the COSMOS study. *J Clin Hypertens (Greenwich)*. 2010;12:678-686.

67. Giles TD, Weber MA, Basile J, et al. Efficacy and safety of nebivolol and valsartan as fixed-dose combination in hypertension: a randomised, multicentre study. *Lancet*. 2014;383:1889-1898.

68. Weber MA, Basile J, Stapff M, Khan B, Zhou D. Blood pressure effects of combined beta-blocker and angiotensin-converting enzyme inhibitor therapy compared with the individual agents: a placebo-controlled study with nebivolol and lisinopril. *J Clin Hypertens (Greenwich)*. 2012;14:588-592.

69. Salvetti A, Magagna A, Innocenti P, et al. The combination of chlorthalidone with nifedipine does not exert an additive antihypertensive effect in essential hypertensives: a crossover multicenter study. *J Cardiovasc Pharmacol*. 1991;17:332-335.

70. Massie BM, Tubau JF, Szlachcic J, Vollmer C. Comparison and additivity of nitrendipine and hydrochlorothiazide in systemic hypertension. *Am J Cardiol*. 1986;58:16D-19D.

71. Haria M, Plosker GL, Markham A. Felodipine/metoprolol: a review of the fixed dose controlled release formulation in the management of essential hypertension. *Drugs*. 2000;59:141-157.

72. Frishman WH, Hainer JW, Sugg J. A factorial study of combination hypertension treatment with metoprolol succinate extended release and felodipine extended release results of the Metoprolol Succinate-Felodipine Antihypertension Combination Trial (M-FACT). *Am J Hypertens*. 2006;19:388-395.

Device Therapies

Saif Anwaruddin and Deepak L. Bhatt

Hypertension remains an almost ubiquitous entity as a chronic disease around the world today. Its relevance lies in the fact that it is one of the most common risk factors responsible for cardiovascular morbidity and mortality. It is estimated that there are over 78 million adults in the United States who have hypertension, with African Americans having the highest prevalence of hypertension in the world.[1] Despite the widespread availability of several classes of antihypertensive medications, many patients are not adequately controlled on a medication regimen. The importance of aggressive blood pressure control is well documented in reduction of adverse cardiovascular outcomes. The recently published SPRINT (Systolic Blood Pressure Intervention Trial) demonstrated the reduction in fatal and nonfatal cardiovascular events from more intensive systolic blood pressure reduction in patients at higher cardiovascular risk.[2]

Resistant hypertension is defined as the inability to reduce blood pressure to less than 140/90 mm Hg in patients who are taking maximally tolerated doses of at least three different classes of antihypertensive medications (including a diuretic).[3] The prevalence of resistant hypertension in the hypertensive population varies from 8% to 12%.[4,5] Furthermore, patients with resistant hypertension have higher rates of cardiovascular risk factors and those with higher ambulatory blood pressure monitoring (ABPM) blood pressures are at higher risk of cardiovascular morbidity and mortality[6] (Fig. 28.1). The promise of device-based therapy to treat resistant hypertension has emerged in the past several years with the goal of treating resistant hypertension where medical therapy has been inadequate.[7]

The premise behind treatment of resistant hypertension with device therapy lies in observations that hypertension is mediated by central sympathetic activity. Higher levels of central sympathetic activity, as quantified by muscle sympathetic nerve activity (MSNA), were observed in patients with both essential and borderline hypertension.[8] Furthermore, higher rates of noradrenaline spillover have been observed in hypertensive patients as compared with normotensive patients.[9] Interventions designed to address neurovascular-mediated hypertension seek to interfere with the pathways involved in these processes.

Sympathetic innervation to the kidneys is via a network of efferent noradrenergic nerve fibers to the renal arteries, and afferent fibers from the renal arteries function to return signals to the central nervous system. Stimulation of the efferent fibers of the renal arteries results in renal artery vasoconstriction, increased salt and water uptake, and increased renin production, all of which serve to increase systemic blood pressure. The afferent fibers serve to provide sensory information to the central nervous system so as to help regulate the effects upon the efferent system (Fig. 28.2). The importance of the central nervous system in mediating systemic blood pressure is not limited to the effects of renal innervation, as baroreceptor reflexes are also important in mediating acute blood pressure changes. Chronic elevations in blood pressure can lead to decreased baroreceptor reflex sensitivity. This has also been identified as a target for device based intervention for treatment of resistant hypertension.

RENAL ARTERY SYMPATHETIC DENERVATION

Increased levels of sympathetic activity have been clearly shown to be an underlying feature of many pathologic conditions such as hypertension, but also heart failure, chronic kidney disease, and disorders of blood glucose control.[10-12] Both the afferent and efferent renal innervation has been shown to be important in the regulation of blood pressure. An abundance of preclinical and clinical data have demonstrated the effects of renal artery denervation upon systemic blood pressure. Early surgical experience demonstrated effective blood pressure reduction with surgical sympathectomy and lower associated mortality, although this was balanced, in part, with unpredictable blood pressure results, postoperative complications, prolonged hospital stays, and other serious side effects, such as severe orthostatic hypotension, erectile dysfunction, and incontinence.[13,14] Translating this technique into a viable and safe percutaneous therapy to accomplish renal artery sympathetic denervation for the treatment of resistant hypertension and demonstrating efficacy has been a work in progress. Percutaneous renal artery denervation procedures have been hypothesized to reduce blood pressure while preserving renal homeostatic mechanisms for electrolyte and fluid balance and adrenaline-mediated stress responses.[15]

The advantages of catheter-based techniques for renal denervation (RDN) over a surgical approach include ease of procedure, shorter procedure duration and recovery time, and minimally invasive approach. As such, much enthusiasm has followed the development and evaluation of catheter-based RDN procedures for the potential in treating a disease with enormous public health implications. The Ardian RDN catheter-based system (Medtronic, LLC, Minnesota) consists of a catheter-based delivery catheter and a radiofrequency (RF) generator. After femoral arterial access is obtained, the RDN catheter is delivered to the renal artery under fluoroscopic guidance. The tip of the catheter is placed against the renal artery wall and RF is delivered in four to six different locations throughout each renal artery (Fig. 28.3).[16] Because renal artery innervation is in the adventitial layer, the delivery of RF energy by the catheter tip is designed to ablate the afferent and efferent innervation to the renal artery, understanding that the afferent innervation does not seem to regenerate itself after ablative therapy.

The SYMPLICITY-HTN 1 study was a first in human safety and feasibility study of the Ardian catheter-based system in the treatment of resistant hypertension.[17] A total of 45 patients with resistant hypertension were treated with renal sympathetic denervation and observed for reductions in office blood pressure and renal noradrenaline spillover. The primary study outcome was blood pressure lowering effectiveness and safety. Secondary endpoints included effects on renal function and renal noradrenaline spillover. Mean age of patients undergoing RDN was 58 years and the mean number of antihypertensive drugs they were taking was 4.7. There was a significant reduction of blood pressure postprocedure compared with preprocedure ($p = 0.026$ for systolic and $p = 0.027$ for diastolic). A total of 10 patients from this group were studied to assess effectiveness of RDN using procedural changes in renal adrenaline spillover. In those 10 patients, a 47% mean reduction was noted and the corresponding blood pressure reduction at 6 months was 22/12 mm Hg.

The procedure itself was deemed to be safe. Of the 45 patients, one experienced a renal artery dissection, which was addressed with a renal artery stent and one patient had an access site complication. Short-term renal angiography in 18 patients did not demonstrate any adverse anatomic issues following the procedure. Interestingly, despite the impressive reduction in blood pressures observed, in 13% of the patients RDN had no discernable effect upon blood pressure. A longer-term follow-up on those original 45 patients and an additional 108 treated patients treated with RDN at 19 centers around the world has been published to assess long-term safety and efficacy. The 3-year outcomes on 153 treated patients also demonstrated significant reductions in both systolic and diastolic blood pressures. A 10 or more mm Hg drop in systolic blood pressure was observed in 93% of treated patients at 3 years. Of note, there was no information on medication related changes beyond 12 months in this follow-up study.[17]

The SYMPLICITY HTN-2 study was a prospective randomized multicenter trial examining RDN in 106 patients with resistant hypertension with a primary efficacy endpoint of systolic blood pressure reduction by office-based measurement at 6 months follow-up.[18] At 6 months, there was a significant decrease in systolic and diastolic blood pressure through office-based measurements in the renal denervation group with respect to baseline ($p < 0.0001$). A total of 84% of patients who underwent RDN had a 10 or more mm Hg reduction versus 35% of controls ($p < 0.0001$). There were no serious device or procedure-related complications. Furthermore, there were similar trends noted with both 6 months office-based blood pressure and 24-hour-ABPM in this study.

The SYMPLICITY HTN-3 study was a prospective, randomized, single blinded trial designed to help achieve regulatory approval. The trial sought to examine the safety and efficacy of RDN using the Ardian catheter-based denervation system (Medtronic, LLC) for the treatment of resistant hypertension. The primary endpoint was a change in office-based systolic blood pressure at 6 months and a secondary endpoint of change in average 24-hour ABPM over 6 months. A primary safety endpoint examined was a composite of all-cause mortality, end-stage renal disease, significant embolic events, new renal artery stenosis, renal artery perforation/dissection requiring intervention, vascular complications, or hospitalization secondary to hypertensive crises. Patients between the ages of 18 and 80 years with resistant hypertension who enrolled were randomized in a 2:1 fashion to either RDN versus a sham procedure. In comparison to all prior RDN trials, this trial was designed with a sham procedure, a larger study population, and 24-hour ABPM.[19]

To be eligible for the study, participants had to have a systolic blood pressure (SBP) 160 or higher mm Hg and be on a stable antihypertensive regimen of maximally tolerated doses of at least three drugs, one of which was a diuretic. The patients were required to be stable on this regimen for at least 2 weeks and any postenrollment adjustments in antihypertensive medications would necessitate withdrawal and reenrollment after a 2-week period demonstrating a stable regimen. Specific protocols were established to obtain office-based blood pressures and 24-hour ABPM was performed to document an SBP of 135 or higher mm Hg. Exclusion criteria included hypertension from secondary causes, prior renal artery intervention, and several anatomic criteria for the renal artery.

A total of 535 patients were enrolled in the study across 88 sites in the United States with no differences in baseline characteristics between the randomized groups. For the primary endpoint, there was no significant difference at 6 months between the two groups with regard to office-based blood pressure measurement (-14.13 ± 23.93 mm Hg for RDN versus

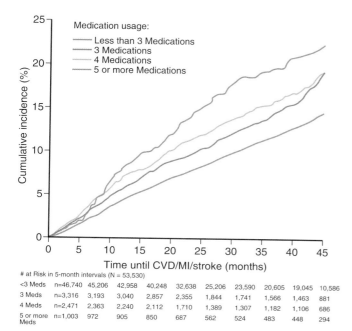

# at Risk in 5-month intervals (N = 53,530)									
<3 Meds	n=46,740	45,206	42,958	40,248	32,638	25,206	23,590	20,605	19,045	10,586
3 Meds	n=3,316	3,193	3,040	2,857	2,355	1,844	1,741	1,566	1,463	881
4 Meds	n=2,471	2,363	2,240	2,112	1,710	1,389	1,307	1,182	1,106	686
5 or more Meds	n=1,003	972	905	850	687	562	524	483	448	294

FIG. 28.1 Cumulative hazard curves for the endpoint of cardiovascular death/myocardial infarction/stroke in patients with nonresistant hypertension (<3 agents, resistant hypertension on 3 agents, resistant hypertension on 4 agents, and resistant hypertension on 5 or more agents [$p < 0.001$]). *(From Kumbhani DJ, Steg PG, Cannon CP, et al. REACH Registry Investigators. Statin therapy and long-term adverse limb outcomes in patients with peripheral artery disease: insights from the REACH registry. Eur Heart J. 2014;35:2864-2872.)*

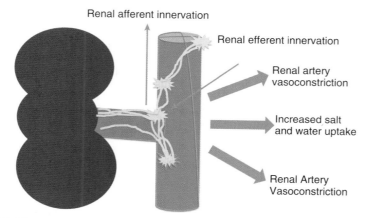

FIG. 28.2 Schematic of the afferent and efferent renal innervation pathways and their actions.

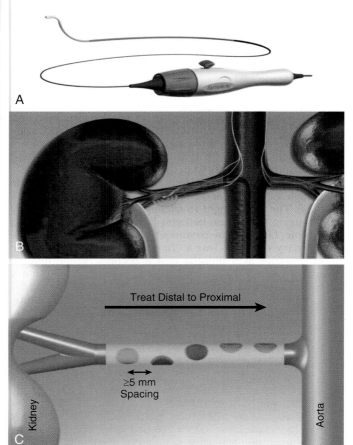

FIG. 28.3 Renal sympathetic denervation using the SYMPLICITY Renal Denervation System. A, The SYMPLICITY catheter is 6 French compatible. B, The catheter features an articulating tip with a radiopaque radiofrequency electrode. C, Four to six 2-minute treatments are delivered per artery. *(From Kandzari DE, Bhatt DL, Sobotka PA, et al. Catheter-based renal denervation for resistant hypertension: rationale and design of the SYMPLICITY HTN-3 Trial. Clin Cardiol. 2012;35:528-535.)*

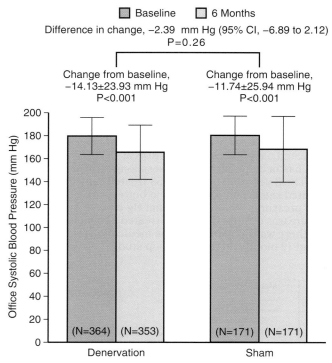

FIG. 28.4 Primary efficacy endpoint of the SYMPLICITY HTN 3 trial. A significant change from baseline to 6 months in office systolic blood pressure was observed in both study groups. The between-group difference (the primary efficacy endpoint) did not meet a test of superiority with a margin of 5 mm Hg. The I bars indicated standard deviations. *(From Bhatt DL, Kandzari DE, O'Neill WW, et al. SYMPLICITY HTN-3 Investigators. A controlled trial of renal denervation for resistant hypertension. N Engl J Med. 2014;370:1393-1401.)*

−11.74 ± 25.94 mm Hg for sham control, difference in change, −2.39 mm Hg; p = 0.26) (Fig. 28.4). With regard to the secondary efficacy endpoint of change from baseline to 6 months in 24-hour average ABPM, there was no significant difference between the two groups (−6.75 ± 15.11 mm Hg for RDN versus −4.79 ± 17.25 mm Hg for sham control, difference in change, −1.96 mm Hg; p = 0.98). The rate of the primary safety endpoint in the trial was 1.4% in the RDN group and 0.6% in the sham-control group (p = 0.67). These results were in direct contrast to the previously reported SYMPLICITY HTN-1 and SYMPLICITY HTN-2 trials. The reasons for the observed differences may have had to do more with the fact that SYMPLICITY HTN-3 was a well-conducted blinded, sham-controlled randomized study which accounted for several biases that prior studies did not.[20]

Similar findings with no further ambulatory or office blood pressure (BP) reductions were observed at 1 year in the SYMPLICITY HTN-3 trial with follow-up data available for most of the denervation patients, non-crossover control subjects, and crossover control subjects.[21] Beyond the trial design and conduct of the study, several other potential reasons for lack of observed response in blood pressure have been suggested. Multivariable analysis of the study population revealed that use of an aldosterone antagonist at baseline was a predictor of increasing 6-month change from baseline in office systolic blood pressure changes, whereas use of a vasodilator was a negative predictor for change in office systolic blood pressure. Furthermore, in the treatment arm, the total number of ablation attempts was a predictor for change in office systolic

blood pressure at 6 months, as was the use of circumferential ablation patterns.[22] This has potentially important implications for the understanding of the effects of RDN and future trial design. Our understanding of the anatomic and physiologic effects of RDN are likely very basic. The anatomy of the afferent and efferent innervation of the renal arteries appears more complex. The mean number of periarterial nerves appears greater in the proximal and midsegments of the renal artery, whereas the nerve distance to arterial lumen was largest in the more proximal segments. There is also a decrease in the amount of afferent fibers from proximal to distal artery and the density of innervation is lowest in the dorsal part of the artery.[23] There may also be value in more distal ablation extending into branches of the main renal artery.[24] This has potentially important implications when designing catheters and for study design. In the SYMPLICITY HTN-3 trial, there was a nonsignificant trend toward lower office and 24-hour ABPM in those patients who had four-quadrant ablations in one or both renal arteries as compared with no four-quadrant ablations. In the SYMPLICTY HTN-3 study, only 19 patients had four-quadrant ablations in both renal arteries, questioning the intensity of treatment in the RDN arm.

User experience may have also influenced the outcome of this study. Data from the Global SYMPLICTY Registry (GSR), an open-label multicenter registry of patients undergoing RDN for hypertension demonstrated a greater drop in both office-based and 24-hour ABPM in those patients from GSR versus SYMPLICTY HTN-3. One of the factors that may be at play is operator experience. The operators in the GSR had more experience in terms of prior cases and the average number of 120 second ablations was greater in the GSR than in SYMPLICTY HTN-3, suggesting that perhaps treatment intensity and operator experience may factor into outcomes.[25]

In addition to procedural variables, classes of antihypertensive medications may have played a role in the outcomes of the study. Again, in a post hoc analysis of the SYMPLICTY HTN-3 data, the effect of vasodilator therapy on African Americans in the sham control in blood pressure reduction was greater than the effect seen on non-African Americans on vasodilator therapy, or on either African Americans or non-African Americans not on vasodilator therapy. Furthermore, there were more African Americans in the trial being prescribed vasodilators than non-African Americans (26.2% of the study population). There was an observed difference in office systolic blood pressure changes in the non-African American subgroup versus the African American subgroup after RDN, whereas no differences were observed in changes in 24-hour ABPM or home systolic blood pressure measurements.[23] A separate analysis of the SYMPLICITY HTN-3 trial demonstrated that there was no differential effect of RDN based on race; however, the larger differences noted in the sham-control group, particularly in African Americans, was believed attributable to changes in medication adherence.[26]

The SYMPLICTY HTN-3 trial serves to illustrate the challenges that persist in carrying out a trial of this magnitude and complexity. Despite the well conducted, sham-controlled, blinded nature of the study, there were still several issues that remain which could explain the lack of treatment effect observed. Furthermore, a standardized treatment algorithm for BP control and evidence of medication adherence among subjects may be needed to account for additional observed differences. Finally, the efficacy and intensity of treatment using RDN not being quantified was likely a weakness of the current study. Future trials need to address issues such as medication classes and adherence, procedural variability, and patient related factors to see if RDN remains a viable treatment option.

Interestingly, the renal denervation for hypertension (DENERHTN) trial[27] used the SYMPLICITY RDN catheter in a prospective, open-label, randomized controlled trial with blinded endpoint evaluation in a multicenter fashion in patients with resistant hypertension. They compared RDN and a standardized stepped-care antihypertensive treatment (SSAHT) with SSAHT alone and found that in 207 patients, RDN and SSAHT decreased ambulatory blood pressure by a modest amount at 6 months, although office-based blood pressures were not significantly reduced. It is unclear as to what impact the sample size and open-label trial design had upon these findings.

The SPYRAL HTN trial (Medtronic) is currently enrolling and will evaluate patients with less severe hypertension than those enrolled in SYMPLICITY HTN-3 for the effectiveness of RDN using the novel SYMPLICITY SPYRAL multielectrode catheter. The trial will enroll 100 patients in each arm in patients with moderate to severe, not resistant, hypertension. In the SPYRAL HTN OFF MED (NCT02439749) arm, the patients will stop antihypertensive medications whereas in the SPYRAL HTN ON MED (NCT02439775) arm, they will continue with their antihypertensive regimen. It is anticipated that specific classes of medications will be used, without needing to achieve maximally tolerated dosages, and that medication adherence will be monitored. The primary efficacy endpoint will be change in 24-hour ABPM at 36 months versus baseline.

The REDUCE HTN:REINFORCE trial (NCT02392351) is also currently enrolling patients with uncontrolled hypertension in a randomized fashion to assess whether or not RDN using the Vessix Reduce Catheter can reduce 24-hour ambulatory systolic blood pressure at 8 weeks in comparison to sham placebo. The EnligHTN Multi-Electrode Denervation System (St Jude Medical, St Paul, Minnesota) is currently under investigation in clinical studies. This device uses an expandable basket with four monopolar radiopaque electrodes and has a CE (Conformite Europeene) mark approval based on the results of EnligHTN-1.[28] The EnligHTN-III trial (NCT01836146) has recently completed enrollment looking to examine the safety and efficacy of the EnligHTN RDN system to treat uncontrolled drug resistant hypertension.

In addition to severe resistant hypertension, RDN has been examined in the context of mild resistant hypertension (SBP 135 to 149 mm Hg, and diastolic 90 to 94 mm Hg).[29] A total of 71 patients were randomized to RDN with the SYMPLICITY catheter versus a sham-control procedure. RDN failed to result in a meaningful reduction in 24-hour systolic blood pressure in the prespecified intention to treat analysis; however, there was a statistically significant reduction in the per protocol analysis.

RDN has also been identified as a therapeutic adjunct in the treatment of heart failure, with the goal of addressing sympathetic overactivation as part of the neurohormonal response. The REACH-Pilot Study was a first-in-man safety study in seven patients using RDN to treat patients with chronic systolic heart failure with a bilateral denervation procedure.[30] The procedure was well tolerated and safe with a resultant increase in 6-minute walk distance at 6 months. The Renal Artery Denervation in Chronic Heart Failure (REACH) Study (NCT01639378) is a prospective, randomized, double-blinded trial examining the safety and efficacy of the SYMPLICITY RDN system in the patients with chronic systolic heart failure.

In addition to RF energy delivered through a catheter, other alternatives are in development for renal artery denervation. Ultrasound energy can be delivered for RDN using noninvasive techniques (Kona Medical, Bellevue, Washington) or intravascularly using a balloon catheter or a separate sound catheter. Guanethidine injections have been carried out using the Bullfrog Microinfusion catheter (Mercator MedSystems, Inc, San Leandro, California). Larger safety and feasibility studies will be ongoing to further evaluate these alternative approaches for RDN.

Although the initial enthusiasm for RDN has waned slightly after the SYMPLICTY HTN-3 trial results, it is clear that our understanding of RDN for the treatment of hypertension has improved. The initial positive results of both the SYMPLICTY HTN-1 and SYMPLICTY HTN-2 studies fueled the enthusiasm for this technology and its role in the management of resistant hypertension. Despite the well-conducted nature of the SYMPLICTY HTN-3 trial, we noted that there were several limitations and confounders that could have influenced the results of the study, including the technology and user experience. It may also be argued that our understanding of the anatomic and physiologic mechanisms behind resistant hypertension is not sophisticated enough. Despite the negative results of the primary trial, there is reason to think that RDN may still be a viable option. As newer devices and trials move forward, it will remain to be seen what role, if any, RDN has to play in the management of hypertensive disease.[31]

BAROREFLEX ACTIVATION THERAPY

Baroreceptors are mechanoreceptors located in the carotid sinuses and the aortic arch, which respond to stretch induced by changes in blood pressure. Acute rises in blood pressure leading to stretch on the carotid baroreceptors send a signal via afferent nerves through the carotid sinus nerve and the glossopharyngeal nerve. These afferent fibers then travel into the medulla of the brain. The efferent innervation affects the heart and blood vessels via both sympathetic and parasympathetic innervation. In the setting of acute increases in blood pressure, afferents are able to fire and send signals to the central nervous system. In the setting of long-standing chronic hypertension, the baroreceptor response diminishes over time.

The principle behind BAT involves resetting the baroreceptor reflex through external stimulation of both carotid sinus baroreceptors using electrodes placed on the carotid sinuses bilaterally and the leads are tunneled subcutaneously and connect to an implantable stimulator placed in the anterior chest

TABLE 28.1 Barostim Trials Currently in Progress

TRIAL	CLINICALTRIALS. GOV NUMBER	STUDY DESIGN	PRIMARY EFFICACY ENDPOINT	DISEASE PROCESS	OTHER ENDPOINTS
NORDIC BAT (Barostim Neo)	NCT02572024	Randomized, double blind, parallel design	Reduction in 24-hour ABPM versus medical therapy	Resistant hypertension	Effects upon arterial and cardiac structure and function
Economic Evaluation (ESTIM-rHTN)	NCT02364310	Open-label, randomized	Cost-effectiveness of Barostim Neo versus medical therapy at 12 months	Resistant hypertension	ABPM at 6 and 12 months
Baroreflex Activation in Heart Failure	NCT01484288	Nonrandomized, single group assignment	Change in sympathetic nervous activity at 6 months	Heart failure	None
Barostim Pivotal Trial	NCT01679132	Randomized	Office-based BP measurement at 6 months postactivation	Resistant hypertension	Safety endpoint related to implant at 30 days, changes in office SBP and ABPM at 12 months
Barostim Neo in the Treatment of Resistant Hypertension	NCT01471834	Nonrandomized, single arm	Change in baseline SBP at 6 months	Resistant hypertension	None
Barostim HOPE4HF	NCT01720160	Randomized	Change from baseline in heart failure parameters at 12 months	Heart failure	Safety endpoints related to system and procedure-related adverse events

ABPM, Ambulatory blood pressure monitoring; *BP,* blood pressure; *SBP,* systolic blood pressure.

wall. Preclinical animal studies demonstrated effectiveness of BAT in reducing mean arterial pressure (MAP) and heart rate. Furthermore, sustained reductions in MAP by reduction in sympathetic activity were not accompanied by increases in plasma renin activity.[32]

In 2007, the results of the feasibility and safety study examining 17 patients with resistant hypertension who underwent the BAT procedure with the Rheos system (CVRx, Inc, Minneapolis, Minnesota) showed significant reductions in systolic blood and diastolic blood pressure and heart rate ($p < 0.0001$ for all) and demonstrated reasonable safety.[33] The DEBuT-HT (device-based therapy in hypertension) study examined 45 patients with resistant hypertension who were treated in a multicenter feasibility study and demonstrated a mean reduction of 33/22 mm Hg at 2 years without any safety issues.[34]

The Rheos Pivotal trial for resistant hypertension was a randomized, double blind, placebo controlled Phase III trial.[35] A total of 265 patients with resistant hypertension were randomized to BAT for the first 6 months versus BAT delayed for 6 months. There were five coprimary endpoints including acute SBP responder rate at 6 months, sustained responder rate at 12 months, procedural safety, device safety, and BAT safety. The study did not meet the acute responder endpoint or the procedural safety endpoint at 6 months; however, it met the other three endpoints including a sustained responder rate at 12 months. Although BAT demonstrated efficacy in reduction of blood pressure, the procedural complications included nerve injury and surgery-related issues. Longer-term follow-up from the Rheos Pivotal study demonstrated sustained reductions in BP over time.[36] Further clinical study will be necessary to define efficacy. Newer devices, such as the second-generation Barostim neo (CVRx, Minneapolis, Minnesota), with a simpler implant procedure, are being evaluated (Table 28.1) and have demonstrated sustained BP reduction with an improved safety profile.[37]

SUMMARY

Hypertension is one of the most widely treated conditions in the world today. In many, it remains an extremely challenging entity to control. Device-based therapy for the treatment of resistant hypertension has been shown to have benefits and limitations. The enthusiasm for RDN has been tempered by the results of the SYMPLICTY HTN-3 trial, but those unanticipated results have provided important lessons about trial design and the procedure itself. Addressing these issues will be the goal of future devices and trials. Our understanding of hypertension as a complex phenotype has been impressed upon us through clinical study. A better understanding of the basic mechanisms at play may lead to more effective interventional therapeutics in this space. It is also possible that in some, the combination of device therapy with medications may be more effective. As the field of interventional therapy of hypertension continues to evolve, our understanding of mechanisms and complexities will hopefully continue to improve.

References

1. Go AS, Mozaffarian D, Roger VL, et al. American Heart Association Statistics Committee and Stroke Statistics Subcommittee. Executive summary: heart disease and stroke statistics—2013 update: a report from the American Heart Association. *Circulation.* 2013;127:143-152.
2. SPRINT Research Group, Wright Jr JT, Williamson JD, et al. A randomized trial of intensive versus standard blood-pressure control. *N Engl J Med.* 2015;373:2103-2116.
3. Calhoun DA, Jones D, Textor S, et al. Resistant hypertension: diagnosis, evaluation, and treatment. A scientific statement from the American Heart Association Professional Education Committee of the Council for High Blood Pressure Research. *Hypertension.* 2008;51:1403-1419.
4. Sarafidis PA, Georgianos P, Bakris GL. Resistant hypertension—its identification and epidemiology. *Nat Rev Nephrol.* 2013;9:51-58.
5. Kumbhani DJ, Steg PG, Cannon CP, et al. REACH Registry Investigators. Statin therapy and long-term adverse limb outcomes in patients with peripheral artery disease: insights from the REACH registry. *Eur Heart J.* 2014;35:2864-2872.
6. Salles GF, Cardoso CR, Muxfeldt ES. Prognostic influence of office and ambulatory blood pressures in resistant hypertension. *Arch Intern Med.* 2008;168:2340-2346.
7. Bhatt DL, Bakris GL. The promise of renal denervation. *Cleve Clin J Med.* 2012;79:498-500.
8. Smith PA, Graham LN, Mackintosh AF, et al. Relationship between central sympathetic activity and stages of human hypertension. *Am J Hypertens.* 2004;17:217-222.
9. Watson RD, Esler MD, Leonard P, Korner PI. Influence of variation in dietary sodium intake on biochemical indices of sympathetic activity in normal man. *Clin Exp Pharmacol Physiol.* 1984;11:163-170.
10. Esler M, Jennings G, Korner P, et al. Assessment of human sympathetic nervous system activity from measurements of norepinephrine turnover. *Hypertension.* 1988;11:3-20.
11. Triposkiadis F, Karayannis G, Giamouzis G, et al. The sympathetic nervous system in heart failure physiology, pathophysiology, and clinical implications. *J Am Coll Cardiol.* 2009;54:1747-1762.
12. Mancia G, Bousquet P, Elghozi JL, et al. The sympathetic nervous system and the metabolic syndrome. *J Hypertens.* 2007;25:909-920.
13. Reginald H, Smithwick MD, Jesse E, Thompson MD. Splanchnicectomy for essential hypertension; results in 1,266 cases. *J Am Med Assoc.* 1953;152:1501-1504.
14. Longland CJ, Gibb WE. Sympathectomy in the treatment of benign and malignant hypertension; a review of 76 patients. *Br J Surg.* 1954;41:382-392.

273

28

Device Therapies

15. Schlaich MP, Sobotka PA, Krum H, Lambert E, Esler MD. Renal sympathetic-nerve ablation for uncontrolled hypertension. *N Engl J Med*. 2009;361:932-934.
16. Kandzari DE, Bhatt DL, Sobotka PA, et al. Catheter-based renal denervation for resistant hypertension: rationale and design of the SYMPLICITY HTN-3 Trial. *Clin Cardiol*. 2012;35:528-535.
17. Krum H, Schlaich M, Whitbourn R, et al. Catheter-based renal sympathetic denervation for resistant hypertension: a multicentre safety and proof-of-principle cohort study. *Lancet*. 2009;373:1275-1281.
18. Symplicity HTN-2 Investigators1, Esler MD, Krum H, et al. Renal sympathetic denervation in patients with treatment-resistant hypertension (The SYMPLICITY HTN-2 Trial): a randomised controlled trial. *Lancet*. 2010;376:1903-1909.
19. Bhatt DL, Kandzari DE, O'Neill WW, et al. SYMPLICITY HTN-3 Investigators. A controlled trial of renal denervation for resistant hypertension. *N Engl J Med*. 2014;370:1393-1401.
20. Howard JP, Shun-Shin MJ, Hartley A, et al. Quantifying the 3 biases that lead to unintentional overestimation of the blood pressure-lowering effect of renal denervation. *Circ Cardiovasc Qual Outcomes*. 2016;9:14-22.
21. Bakris GL, Townsend RR, Flack JM, et al. SYMPLICITY HTN-3 Investigators. 12-month blood pressure results of catheter-based renal artery denervation for resistant hypertension: the SYMPLICITY HTN-3 trial. *J Am Coll Cardiol*. 2015;65:1314-1321.
22. Kandzari DE, Bhatt DL, Brar S, et al. Predictors of blood pressure response in the SYMPLICITY HTN-3 trial. *Eur Heart J*. 2015;36:219-227.
23. Sakakura K, Ladich E, Cheng Q, et al. Anatomic assessment of sympathetic peri-arterial renal nerves in man. *J Am Coll Cardiol*. 2014;64:635-643.
24. Sawlani NN, Bhatt DL. Distal and Tributary Targets: A New Branching Point for Renal Denervation? *J Am Coll Cardiol*. 2015;66:1776-1778.
25. Böhm M, Mahfoud F, Ukena C, et al. GSR Investigators. First report of the Global SYMPLICITY Registry on the effect of renal artery denervation in patients with uncontrolled hypertension. *Hypertension*. 2015;65:766-774.
26. Flack JM, Bhatt DL, Kandzari DE, et al. SYMPLICITY HTN-3 Investigators. An analysis of the blood pressure and safety outcomes to renal denervation in African Americans and Non-African Americans in the SYMPLICITY HTN-3 trial. *J Am Soc Hypertens*. 2015;9:769-779.
27. Azizi M, Sapoval M, Gosse P, et al. Renal Denervation for Hypertension (DENERHTN) investigators. Optimum and stepped care standardised antihypertensive treatment with or without renal denervation for resistant hypertension (DENERHTN): a multicentre, open-label, randomised controlled trial. *Lancet*. 2015;385:1957-1965.
28. Papademetriou V, Tsioufis CP, Sinhal A, et al. Catheter-based renal denervation for resistant hypertension: 12-month results of the EnligHTN I first-in-human study using a multi-electrode ablation system. *Hypertension*. 2014;64:565-572.
29. Desch S, Okon T, Heinemann D, et al. Randomized sham-controlled trial of renal sympathetic denervation in mild resistant hypertension. *Hypertension*. 2015;65:1202-1208.
30. Davies JE, Manisty CH, Petraco R, Barron AJ, et al. First-in-man safety evaluation of renal denervation for chronic systolic heart failure: primary outcome from REACH-Pilot study. *Int J Cardiol*. 2013;162:189-192.
31. Myat A, Redwood SR, Qureshi AC, et al. Renal sympathetic denervation therapy for resistant hypertension: a contemporary synopsis and future implications. *Circ Cardiovasc Interv*. 2013;6:184-197.
32. Lohmeier TE, Irwin ED, Rossing MA, Serdar DJ, Kieval RS. Prolonged activation of the baroreflex produces sustained hypotension. *Hypertension*. 2004;43:306-311.
33. Tordoir JH, Scheffers I, Schmidli J, et al. An implantable carotid sinus baroreflex activating system: surgical technique and short-term outcome from a multi-center feasibility trial for the treatment of resistant hypertension. *Eur J Vasc Endovasc Surg*. 2007;33:414-421.
34. Scheffers IJ, Kroon AA, Schmidli J, et al. Novel baroreflex activation therapy in resistant hypertension: results of a European multi-center feasibility study. *J Am Coll Cardiol*. 2010;56:1254-1258.
35. Bisognano JD, Bakris G, Nadim MK, et al. Baroreflex activation therapy lowers blood pressure in patients with resistant hypertension: results from the double-blind, randomized, placebo-controlled rheos pivotal trial. *J Am Coll Cardiol*. 2011;58:765-773.
36. Bakris GL, Nadim MK, Haller H, et al. Baroreflex activation therapy provides durable benefit in patients with resistant hypertension: results of long-term follow-up in the Rheos Pivotal Trial. *J Am Soc Hypertens*. 2012;6:152-158.
37. Hoppe UC, Brandt MC, Wachter R, et al. Minimally invasive system for baroreflex activation therapy chronically lowers blood pressure with pacemaker-like safety profile: results from the Barostim neo trial. *J Am Soc Hypertens*. 2012;6:270-276.

29 Alternative Approaches for Lowering Blood Pressure

J. Brian Byrd and Robert D. Brook

High blood pressure (BP) is the leading risk factor for global morbidity and mortality.[1] Clinical trials in hypertension have largely focused on the efficacy of oral medications to lower BP and reduce cardiovascular events. However, a variety of other nonpharmacologic treatments have been developed and studied with varying degrees of scientific rigor. The focus of this chapter is to review the BP-lowering efficacy of therapeutic approaches that are alternatives to medications and dietary (or herbal) interventions. The American Heart Association (AHA) recently published in 2013 a comprehensive scientific statement in this regard and highlighted the evidence for, or against, use of these approaches in clinical practice.[2] This chapter summarizes the major conclusions reached by the AHA (Table 29.1) and provides an updated review of randomized clinical trials (RCTs) of at least several weeks' duration and that focus primarily on BP and meta-analyses subsequently published that could substantially impact this field of clinical medicine.

It is important to begin with a cautionary note that many (if not all) of the alternative approaches described in this chapter present several common challenges to researchers. One principal difficulty is the lack of consensus about the appropriate sham or placebo comparator. In principle, a sham or placebo should be similar to the active treatment in all respects (and not be discernable by the study participants), except for the "active ingredient" in the treatment. However, this ideal is not easily implemented or even imagined in many instances. In addition to randomization, gold standard comparators and blinding are crucial elements of robust clinical studies. These elements have not necessarily been successfully achieved in the large variety of studies related to alternative approaches for high BP, even though this review is limited to RCTs and does not involve observational studies. Numerous other potential biases (e.g., cointervention, Hawthorne effect) have often plagued many published trials to date and may thus limit the broader generalization of their findings. Finally, the BP-lowering efficacy of most of the alternative approaches has only been investigated over the short term (few weeks to months) and their benefits in regards to reducing hard cardiovascular events has rarely been evaluated.

Mirroring the AHA scientific statement, we have divided this chapter into four classes of alternative approaches to high BP: behavioral therapies, noninvasive procedures and devices, exercise-based regimens, and other additional noninvasive interventions. Further information and more detailed methodologic descriptions pertaining to the individual approaches can be found in the original AHA scientific statement.

BEHAVIORAL THERAPIES

Meditation

There is a large variety of meditation types, and an appropriate placebo control is difficult to identify for any of them. The "active ingredient(s)" among the various techniques is equally difficult to verify given that these ancient approaches were not specifically formulated with the intent of lowering BP. Thus, it is difficult to design a viable comparator placebo intervention that lacks only the active ingredient (i.e., without changing the entire experience dramatically). Blinding is also problematic, for example, in instructor-led meditation, because either the same instructor must teach two methods (one active and one "placebo") or the instructors must vary. Therefore, these studies often suffer from numerous important limitations. Although acknowledging these inherent shortcomings, numerous meditation approaches have been investigated over the past several decades with respect to their ability to decrease BP.

Transcendental Meditation

One particular form of "mantra-based" meditation, transcendental meditation (TM), has been studied for its effects on a multitude of health-related measures, including high BP. Most studies have compared TM with health education, relaxation, wait-list control, or no treatment. Several attempts have been made to summarize the efficacy of TM in regards to lowering BP. In 2004, a meta-analysis suggested the available studies were of inadequate quality for any conclusion to be drawn. A 2007 review and synthesis of prior and subsequent studies concluded that TM lowered both systolic BP (SBP) and diastolic BP (DBP) compared with progressive muscle relaxation; however, it was not superior to health education.

A few subsequent meta-analyses have concluded that TM lowers systolic and diastolic BP compared with control interventions.[3,4] An important caveat is that meta-analyses necessarily involve many decisions that can unintentionally influence the results, most notably decisions about which studies meet quality standards for inclusion.[5] Thus, the risk of unintentional biases is high. Nevertheless, the most recently published meta-analysis (12 studies; n = 996) to evaluate the effect of TM found evidence for a modest but significant BP-lowering effect (−4.3/2.3 mm Hg) compared with controls.[5] Contrarily, a recent Cochrane review concluded that only two studies could be included in their meta-analysis regarding BP and that excessive trial heterogeneity did not allow for the combining of further data.[6] Therefore, the authors stated that evidence regarding the BP-lowering efficacy of TM should be viewed as "suggestive" at this point in time. Finally, in one of the few long-term trials beyond a few months' duration, BP remained stable (i.e., significantly lower) in the TM group compared with that in participants randomized to health education, in whom systolic BP rose during the 5.4 years of average follow-up.[7] As such, the overall evidence supporting the efficacy of TM in regards to controlling high BP and reducing cardiovascular risk is modest and requires further investigation before reaching firm conclusions (see Table 29.1).

Other Forms of Meditation

The potential BP-lowering efficacy of Zen meditation has also been investigated. A 2007 review and synthesis of data concluded that Zen meditation reduced DBP, but not SBP[8] when compared with repeated BP checks. It should be noted that

TABLE 29.1 2013 American Heart Association Recommendations Regarding Alternative Blood Pressure Lowering Strategies

ALTERNATIVE TREATMENTS	LEVEL OF EVIDENCE[a]	RECOMMENDATION[b]	META-ANALYSES PUBLISHED SINCE THE 2013 SCIENTIFIC STATEMENT	SELECTED TRIALS PUBLISHED SINCE THE 2013 SCIENTIFIC STATEMENT
Behavioral Therapies				
Transcendental meditation	B	IIB	Refs 5,6	
Other meditation techniques	C	III (no benefit)		Ref 9
Biofeedback approaches	B	IIB		
Yoga	C	III (no benefit)	Refs 12-15	Refs 16-20
Other relaxation techniques	B	III (no benefit)		
Noninvasive Procedures or Devices				
Acupuncture	B	III (no benefit)	Refs 24-26	
Device-guided breathing	B	IIA	Refs 35,36	Ref 33
Exercise-Based Regimens				
Dynamic aerobic exercise	A	I		
Dynamic resistance exercise	B	IIA		
Isometric handgrip exercise	C	IIB	Refs 49,50	

[a]A, Data from multiple random controlled studies (RCTs) and/or meta-analyses; B, Data from a single RCT or observational studies; C, Case studies or standard of care.
[b]I, Treatment SHOULD be performed; IIA, It is REASONABLE to perform the treatment; IIB, Treatment can be considered; III, Treatment is not helpful (or harmful) and should not be performed

comparison to repeated BP checks is an appropriate way of controlling for "regression toward the mean." However, it is not equivalent to comparing Zen meditation with a different effective treatment or to the effect of placebo or sham on BP. As such, weaker evidence exists in support of Zen meditation compared with TM for BP-lowering (see Table 29.1). We did not find any RCTs specifically regarding Zen meditation published since the AHA scientific statement.

In contrast to the ancient tradition of Zen meditation, Mindfulness-Based Stress Reduction (MBSR) is a program of contemplative meditation developed in more recent years. The recent HARMONY study was an RCT of MBSR versus wait-list control among 101 adults with untreated stage 1 hypertension. In this well-performed contemporary trial, MBSR did not significantly lower ambulatory BP levels.[9] Moreover, Park et al performed a randomized, controlled crossover trial comparing mindfulness meditation, BP education, and controlled breathing in 15 African Americans with hypertension in the setting of chronic kidney disease. SBP, DBP, mean arterial pressure, heart rate, and muscle sympathetic nerve activity decreased more in the mindfulness meditation condition compared with the BP education control condition. Controlled breathing did not affect these parameters. We identified no other germane RCTs of meditation technique published since the AHA statement.

If one concludes from the preceding data that some forms of meditation lower BP, the question of mechanism of action becomes relevant. This question remains open at the present time; however, it is possible that reductions in sympathetic nervous system activity might be involved. In summary, the AHA scientific statement conferred to TM a Class IIB, level of evidence B recommendation for BP-lowering efficacy. They rated all other forms of meditation a Class III, no benefit, level of evidence C (see Table 29.1). Although some small studies have been published since, our review did not identify RCTs or meta-analyses regarding meditation techniques (other than TM) that alter these conclusions.

Biofeedback Techniques

Biofeedback prototypically involves monitoring of BP and/or one or more putative surrogates for BP or other closely linked cardiovascular parameter (e.g., galvanic skin response, heart rate variability), such that mental states favoring lower BP can be identified and, ideally, recalled and reproduced at will. As with meditation, it is hard to synthesize the trial results into a simple statement of efficacy. The same issues of heterogeneity in study design and biofeedback approaches used, lack of blinding, and lack of consensus about appropriate negative control interventions preclude a simple analysis.

A meta-analysis that included some practitioners of TM is one of two relatively recent meta-analyses reporting that biofeedback does not lower BP.[4,10] Of note, two other systematic reviews reported different conclusions about whether biofeedback reduces BP. The review published in 2003 reported that biofeedback lowers BP more than does nonintervention.[11] In contrast, a 2010 systematic review performed with stricter inclusion criteria reported no effect of biofeedback on hypertension compared with a variety of negative controls.[10]

A few trials have been performed since these meta-analyses were published as outlined by the AHA scientific statement. In one of the most notable studies, 65 participants were randomized to behavioral neurocardiac training (heart rate variability biofeedback) and behavioral relaxation or repetitive visualizations as a control for two months. Daytime (−2.4 mm Hg) and 24-hour (2.1 mm Hg) SBP were reduced by biofeedback with no effect in the control group. Given the mixed results and the large degree of variability between the numerous different biofeedback methodologies, the authors of the AHA Scientific Statement on Alternative Approaches to Lowering Blood Pressure assigned biofeedback a Class IIB, level of evidence B recommendation for lowering BP (see Table 29.1). We did not identify any subsequently published RCTs or meta-analyses devoted to biofeedback that significantly alter this rating.

Yoga

Yoga is practiced in many forms, which may involve quiet contemplation or physically strenuous activity. Several systematic reviews of yoga for hypertension have recently been published since the AHA statement.[12-14] The meta-analyses generally support that the available studies to date are of low quality or suffer from methodologic variations and limitations that do not allow for firm conclusions to be made in regards to the independent BP-lowering efficacy of yoga techniques at the present time. In analyzing 17 RCTs, Posadzki et al concluded that the evidence in favor of an effect on BP was "encouraging but inconclusive." In analyzing seven RCTs with 452 participants, the authors judged the available evidence to be of low quality. With this caveat, they noted that compared with usual care, yoga lowered BP. However, compared with exercise, there was no effect of yoga on SBP or DBP. Another meta-analysis published in 2016 concluded that yoga nonsignificantly reduced SBP by –5.21 mm Hg (95% confidence interval [CI], –8.01 to 2.42) and DBP by –4.98 mm Hg (–7.17 to 2.80).[15]

Unlike many of the other alternative approaches reviewed in this chapter, there has been a recent flurry of RCTs studying the effect of yoga on BP. Wolff randomly assigned primary care patients with hypertension to home-based Kundalini yoga (n = 96) or usual care (n = 95) for 12 weeks.[16] The BP reduction in the yoga group was not different from in the control group. The recent LIMBS (LIfestyle Modification and Blood Pressure Study) trial randomized 137 participants to yoga, BP education, or both.[17] At the end of the 24-week trial, there was no difference in BP lowering between the yoga and control arms. Among the 90 participants who completed the study, the 24-week BPs marginally favored the BP education program over yoga. There was no additive benefit of combining yoga and BP education.

Siu et al randomized 182 patients with metabolic syndrome to yoga or monthly telephone contact for 1 year. There was a trend to greater improvement in SBP in the yoga arm, although this difference was not statistically significant (p = 0.07).[18] In another recent RCT, 171 underactive adults with metabolic syndrome were randomized to yoga or a program of stretching, there was no difference in SBP between the two arms at 6 months or 12 months.[19] Hagins et al randomized 84 participants with prehypertension or stage 1 hypertension to yoga or nonaerobic exercise.[20] There was no significant difference in 24-hour SBP or DBP, daytime SBP or DBP, or nocturnal SBP. The nighttime DBP was marginally different (p = 0.04). In view of the number of analyses performed, there is reason to be concerned that this difference arose by chance. The effect of nonaerobic exercise on hypertension is a relatively unexplored area, so its usefulness as a control intervention is limited. Mechanisms whereby yoga might lower BP are difficult to study rigorously, and we do not yet have satisfactory answers. Despite the variable and occasional positive trend from meta-analyses, numerous limitations exist in regards to the individual trials evaluating the effect of yoga on BP. The more recently published studies have also not provided encouraging findings in regards to BP lowering. Finally, similar to biofeedback, yoga cannot be described as a homogeneous practice. There are many methods involving a variety of different aspects and some practices may be effective, whereas others may not provide the necessary activity (e.g., exercise, breathing, mental state) required to lower BP. The AHA scientific statement concludes that the overall evidence does not support that yoga per se lowers BP (Class III, no benefit, level of evidence C). Based upon the subsequently published RCTs and meta-analysis, we did not find any persuasive evidence to support upgrading the efficacy of yoga at the present time (see Table 29.1). Given the occasionally positive results, further studies would be helpful, in particular if they help to identify the most effective aspects of any practice. The independent actions of yoga per se, beyond the exercise components, also require clarification.

Other Relaxation Techniques

Beyond meditation, biofeedback, and yoga, a broad range of relaxation methods have been studied to see whether they lower BP in the long term. The Hypertension Intervention Pooling Project analyzed the results of 12 RCTs. The authors concluded that relaxation methods reduce DBP by a small amount, but do not reduce SBP. A review in 1991 found that baseline characteristics of patients predicted response to relaxation methods; after controlling for these baseline characteristics, little evidence for a response remained.[21] There was evidence that regression toward the mean, rather than an effect of relaxation, was responsible for decreases in BP. A 1993 review of the literature found that relaxation alone did not reduce BP compared with appropriate sham controls.[22] However, BP appeared to be reduced when compared with no treatment, highlighting again the need for appropriate sham controls. Yet another review in 1994 reported that interventions including more than just stress reduction were more effective than those with stress reduction alone.

A 2008 Cochrane review found that in contrast to poor quality studies, higher quality studies showed relaxation to cause a smaller decrease in BP or even a possible increase in BP.[23] For example, in studies that included a sham control, there was no significant reduction in BP. The authors were unable to determine whether any particular method of relaxation is effective for lowering BP in the long term. We will refrain from speculating about mechanisms because a long-term BP lowering effect of relaxation has not been convincingly demonstrated to exist in the first place. The AHA writing group viewed the data as consistent with a Class III, no benefit, level of evidence B recommendation (see Table 29.1). We found no recent evidence to support altering this conclusion.

OTHER PROCEDURES AND NONINVASIVE DEVICES

Acupuncture

In addition to the approaches described above, a number of other procedures and noninvasive devices have been evaluated for their effects on lowering BP. A prominent alternative approach has been acupuncture. In a 2009 meta-analysis, Lee et al found significant heterogeneity between three major existing randomized trials. SBP was not significantly decreased, and DBP was possibly decreased (effect estimate confidence interval included 0 mm Hg). The authors suggested more rigorous studies are needed to draw strong conclusions about the efficacy of acupuncture to lower BP. The authors of a 2010 meta-analysis concluded that despite a signal for lower BP with acupuncture plus medications compared with sham acupuncture plus medications in heterogeneous trials, more rigorous studies are needed. A 2013 meta-analysis suggested "potential effectiveness" of acupuncture for lowering BP, but the authors felt that higher-quality studies were required.[24] More recent meta-analyses published in 2014[25] and 2015[26] again found evidence that acupuncture lowers BP when combined with antihypertensive medications, but not in the absence of medications (untreated patients).

Certain details of the three major trials that were considered in the meta-analyses are relevant to understanding these findings. Because needle location is important in acupuncture theory, a potentially logical sham control is to place the needles elsewhere. In a single-blind RCT in Germany, 6 weeks of acupuncture lowered 24-hour ambulatory BP compared with sham acupuncture. The effect did not persist at the 3-month and 6-month follow-up visits. Another high-quality study was performed in South Korea comparing acupuncture with nonpenetrating needles as add-on treatment for hypertension. Unfortunately, the results were reported in an unusual way, as three separate comparisons between the two arms. Thus, the likelihood of a false positive result is inflated. There was no difference in between the study arms at 4 weeks; however, at 8 weeks and in the 4 to 8 week interval, BP was lower with real acupuncture. A third, larger high-quality study, the Stop Hypertension with the Acupuncture Research Program (SHARP), was conducted in the United States and included 192 participants with hypertension. The investigators found that acupuncture did not lower BP at 10 weeks compared with invasive sham acupuncture.[27] Acupuncture has been hypothesized to exert effects through mechanotransduction of signals in connective tissues.[28]

The AHA working group had concerns about mixed study results, the variety of acupuncture sites and techniques (with potentially variable ensuing responses), as well as whether or not high-quality acupuncture can be scaled up in countries that lack long-standing traditions in the technique. They noted that acupuncture results in rare minor adverse events. They assigned acupuncture a recommendation of Class III, no benefit, level of evidence (see Table 29.1).[2] Our review of subsequently published trials and meta-analyses does not support any change to this overall recommendation. It remains to be more firmly confirmed if acupuncture can be used as an adjuvant to medications among medically treated hypertensive patients to provide incremental BP-lowering. The results from meta-analyses provide suggestive evidence in this regard, but none of the trials were a priori designed to investigate this specific subgroup and thus these observations could still represent chance findings.

Device-Guided Slow Breathing

Slow deep breathing appears to lower BP at least transiently. Such an approach has also been postulated to have benefits that last weeks or months. A commercially-available device that designed to help users entrain their breathing to a certain cycle has been developed. The device (www.resperate.com) has United States Food and Drug Administration (FDA) clearance "for use as a relaxation treatment for the reduction of stress by leading the user through interactively guided and monitored breathing exercises. The device is indicated for use only as an adjunctive treatment for high BP, together with other pharmacologic and/or nonpharmacologic interventions."[29] Studies of various designs sponsored by the manufacturer have found that the device lowers BP. Some of these studies have only been published in abstract form. However, three randomized trials not sponsored by the manufacturer have not supported this finding.[30-32] A group affiliated with the National Institutes of Health performed an RCT of device-guided breathing (DGB) or passive attention to breathing in 40 participants with hypertension or prehypertension. Resting clinic BP was lower in the device-guided breathing group as was midday ambulatory SBP (in women only). But a more robust estimate "24-hour BP" was not changed by DGB.[32] In the only study we identified published after the AHA statement, DGB was not effective in lowering BP.[33] Forty-eight patient with diabetes and hypertension were enrolled in the trial comparing DGB versus sham (listening to music). After 8 weeks, slow DGB did not lower office SBP or DBP compared with control.

There have been several systematic review and meta-analyses regarding the BP-lowering effect of DGB including positive results in the AHA scientific statement. One meta-analysis including a total of 494 participants from eight trials found that short-term use of DGB significantly lowers SBP and DBP (–3.7/2.5 mm Hg). However, after excluding five trials sponsored by or involving the manufacturer, no effect was found.[34] The authors of two more recent meta-analyses that were more stringent in the included trials (n = 3 to 5 with an active control such as music listening required) for analyses concluded that "treatment with DGB did not significantly lower office BP compared with a sham procedure or music therapy"[35] and "there is no sufficient evidence for recommending device-guided breathing in the treatment of hypertension."[36] There are a variety of small experiments regarding possible mechanisms by which slow breathing could lower BP including contributions of reduction in chemoreceptor sensitivity, changes in autonomic reflexes mediated by pulmonary stretch receptors,

entrainment of central nervous system nuclei, and reduced systemic vascular resistance and total arterial compliance.[2] Based upon the evidence at the time, the AHA scientific statement assigned this DGB a recommendation of Class IIA, level of evidence B for BP-lowering efficacy. However, the results from the one well-performed trial after 2013 and the two subsequent meta-analyses question the overall efficacy of this approach. In light of these findings, further studies are clearly required before making firm recommendations for this treatment in clinical practice.

EXERCISE

A vast number of studies have examined the effect of exercise on BP. For the purposes of this chapter, we will divide exercise into dynamic aerobic or endurance exercise, dynamic resistance exercise, and isometric exercise.

Dynamic Aerobic and Endurance Exercise

Aerobic exercise involves regular body part (e.g., arms or legs) movements that increase workload on the cardiovascular system. It is convenient and useful to think of the intensity of aerobic exercises in metabolic equivalents, or METs. One MET represents the amount of energy used at rest, and two METs is twice that much energy expenditure per unit of time, and so on. Aerobic exercise is widely recommended in contemporary guidelines. However, guidelines also indicate that exercise regimens are contraindicated in patients with unstable cardiovascular conditions, including but not limited to uncontrolled severe hypertension (BP ≥ 180/110 mm Hg). Conditions under which stress testing should be performed before initiation of an exercise regimen have been described.[37]

Meta-analyses and reviews are useful for getting an overall sense of the many studies of aerobic exercise and BP. A 2007 meta-analysis of the effects of endurance exercise on BP found that exercise significantly reduced resting and daytime ambulatory BP.[38] A more recent review (2010) found again that regular aerobic exercise lowered clinical BP.[39] In both the 2007 meta-analysis and the 2010 review, aerobic exercise appeared to reduce BP more in patients with hypertension compared with those without hypertension. Five small studies in women systematically reviewed in 2011 showed a nonsignificant change in BP in response to aerobic interval training of walking. Walking programs appeared to reduce BP in some 9/27 trials reviewed in 2010. Larger trials with increased intensity or frequency of exercise for longer periods tended to be the ones that showed a significant effect.[40] The authors concluded that further high-quality trials are needed. The most comprehensive and latest meta-analysis of all types of exercise clearly demonstrates the ability of aerobic exercise to lower BP within 8 to 12 weeks.[41] In 105 trials, endurance exercise significantly lowered BP by 3.5/2.5 mm Hg. The effect was much larger in patients with preexisting hypertension (–8.3/6.8 mm Hg).

A recent randomized crossover trial of lower-intensity or high-intensity exercise showed decreases in clinical SBP with both types of exercise. However, there was no decrease in mean day or nighttime ambulatory BP with either form of exercise.[42] Aerobic interval training (AIT) combines episodes of high-intensity with episodes of low-intensity aerobic exercise. At least two randomized studies have suggested an advantage of AIT over continuous aerobic exercise.[43,44] Some patients, of course, have limited ability to use their legs, and upper extremity aerobic exercise also has been shown to lower BP.[45]

The question of BP lowering with aerobic exercise in type 2 diabetics has been studied. In the Early Activity in Type 2 Diabetes (ACTID) trial, 593 newly diagnosed diabetics were randomized to use of a pedometer in a program that included intense counseling or standard or intense dietary advice.[46] There was no difference in SBP or DBP after 6 or 12 months, even though the participants using pedometers increased their steps by 17% on average. Whether the exercise was merely of too low a "dose" to be effective is unclear. There may be some male-female differences in BP response to aerobic exercise, with women exhibiting BP lowering with resistance compared with aerobic exercise and men responding similarly to both types of exercise.[47] The 2013 AHA Scientific Statement recommends at least 30 minutes of moderate intensity aerobic exercise per day most days of the week.[2] The authors assigned dynamic aerobic exercise a Class I, level of evidence A recommendation in those for whom it is not contraindicated. Our review of the evidence since 2013, as well as that from another group, confirm these recommendations.[41,48] Whether or not high versus moderate (or interval) intensity training is optimal for BP-lowering as well as other aspects of the dose-response effect (i.e., ideal duration of cumulative exercise per week) and the potential impact of different types of aerobic activity requires further investigation.

Dynamic Resistance Exercise

Dynamic resistance exercise includes activities such as stretching bands or lifting weights. Muscles are shortened and lengthened in the process. A 2011 meta-analysis found a modest, but statistically significant reduction in SBP and DBP in trials that included prehypertensive, or in some cases, hypertensive patients. Unfortunately, the quality of many of the studies was poor. A subsequent meta-analysis focused on trials in which BP was the primary outcome, and it reached a different conclusion, finding no effect of dynamic resistance exercise on BP. There remains some uncertainty about the effectiveness of dynamic resistance exercise to lower BP, and the mechanism by which it could do so is poorly understood. However, the most recent meta-analysis and systematic review of dynamic resistance exercise support that it can lower BP.[48] The overall estimated effect is somewhat less than that observed with aerobic exercise (−1.8/−3.2 mm Hg). The authors of the 2013 AHA Scientific Statement emphasize that no signal for harm was observed in their review of the literature.[2] They assigned dynamic resistance exercise a Class II, level of evidence B recommendation for BP-lowering. A review of the evidence and conclusions reached by others[48] since the AHA statements support performing moderate intensity dynamic exercise (2 to 3 times per week), or adding it to a regimen of aerobic training, for the purposes of lowering BP.

Isometric Resistance Exercise

In this form of exercise, muscles are contracted at a constant tension, but without shortening the muscle's length. Handgrip using a commercial dynamometer or tensing muscles in the leg have been evaluated in various studies. The available small studies have been reviewed and evaluated in several meta-analyses, which have come to similar conclusions that isometric resistance exercise lowers BP.[49,50]

The most recent meta-analysis published after the AHA statement demonstrates that isometric exercise may be even more effective for lowering BP than other exercise modalities. In 11 trials of 302 participants, BP was significantly reduced by 5.2/3.9 mm Hg. As with aerobic training, patients with hypertension had a more robust response. However, several caveats should be noted. First, BP increases during the active tensing of muscles, sometimes in a pronounced manner. Many of the published studies used low-intensity isometric exercise (handgrip at 30% maximum voluntary contraction). Additional large studies are required to evaluate the safety of isometric exercise in patients with hypertension. Although most RCTs investigated the efficacy of 12 to 15 minutes of isometric exercise between 3 to 5 times per week, the optimal intensity, frequency, duration, and muscle groups during exercise require more investigation. Overall, the evidence is supportive of an effect, but there still remains a relative paucity of trials. The AHA scientific statement conferred a level of evidence C with a class of recommendation IIB to isometric exercises. The few trials published since the statement generally support its efficacy for BP-lowering.

SUMMARY

A great variety of adjunctive approaches for BP-lowering have been evaluated over the prior few decades. The AHA scientific statement published in 2013 provides a more complete review and description of the approaches outlined in this chapter as well as other modalities. Overall, our updated review of the published evidence generally supports the prior conclusions (see Table 29.1). Given the hundreds of millions of people impacted by high BP worldwide and the fact that it is the leading risk factor for morbidity and mortality, further studies of these alternative approaches for the management of hypertension are warranted.

References

1. Lim SS, Vos T, Flaxman AD, et al. A comparative risk assessment of burden of disease and injury attributable to 67 risk factors and risk factor clusters in 21 regions, 1990-2010: a systematic analysis for the Global Burden of Disease Study 2010. *Lancet.* 2012;380:2224-2260.
2. Brook RD, Appel LJ, Rubenfire M, et al. Beyond medications and diet: alternative approaches to lowering blood pressure: a scientific statement from the American heart association. *Hypertension.* 2013;61:1360-1383.
3. Anderson JW, Liu C, Kryscio RJ. Blood pressure response to transcendental meditation: a meta-analysis. *Am J Hypertens.* 2008;21:310-316.
4. Rainforth MV, Schneider RH, Nidich SI, et al. Stress reduction programs in patients with elevated blood pressure: a systematic review and meta-analysis. *Curr Hypertens Rep.* 2007;9:520-528.
5. Bai Z, Chang J, Chen C, et al. Investigating the effect of transcendental meditation on blood pressure: a systematic review and meta-analysis. *J Hum Hypertens.* 2015;29:653-662.
6. Hartley L, Mavrodaris A, Flowers N, et al. Transcendental meditation for the primary prevention of cardiovascular disease. *Cochrane Database Syst Rev.* 2014;12:Cd010359.
7. Schneider RH, Grim CE, Rainforth MV, et al. Stress reduction in the secondary prevention of cardiovascular disease: randomized, controlled trial of transcendental meditation and health education in Blacks. *Circ Cardiovasc Qual Outcomes.* 2012;5:750-758.
8. Ospina MB, Bond K, Karkhaneh M, et al. Meditation practices for health: state of the research. *Evid Rep Technol Assess (Full Rep).* 2007:1-263.
9. Blom K, Baker B, How M, et al. Hypertension analysis of stress reduction using mindfulness meditation and yoga: results from the HARMONY randomized controlled trial. *Am J Hypertens.* 2014;27:122-129.
10. Greenhalgh J, Dickson R, Dundar Y. Biofeedback for hypertension: a systematic review. *J Hypertens.* 2010;28:644-652.
11. Nakao M, Yano E, Nomura S, et al. Blood pressure-lowering effects of biofeedback treatment in hypertension: a meta-analysis of randomized controlled trials. *Hypertens Res.* 2003;26:37-46.
12. Cramer H, Haller H, Lauche R, et al. A systematic review and meta-analysis of yoga for hypertension. *Am J Hypertens.* 2014;27:1146-1151.
13. Posadzki P, Cramer H, Kuzdzal A, et al. Yoga for hypertension: a systematic review of randomized clinical trials. *Complement Ther Med.* 2014;22:511-522.
14. Wang J, Xiong X, Liu W. Yoga for essential hypertension: a systematic review. *PLoS ONE.* 2013;8:e76357.
15. Chu P, Gotink RA, Yeh GY, et al. The effectiveness of yoga in modifying risk factors for cardiovascular disease and metabolic syndrome: A systematic review and meta-analysis of randomized controlled trials. *Eur J Prev Cardiol.* 2016;23:291-307.
16. Wolff M, Rogers K, Erdal B, et al. Impact of a short home-based yoga programme on blood pressure in patients with hypertension: a randomized controlled trial in primary care. *J Hum Hypertens.* 2016;30:599-605.
17. Cohen DL, Boudhar S, Bowler A, et al. Blood Pressure Effects of Yoga, Alone or in Combination with Lifestyle Measures: Results of the Lifestyle Modification and Blood Pressure Study (LIMBS). *J Clin Hypertens (Greenwich).* 2016;18:809-816.
18. Siu PM, Yu AP, Benzie IF, et al. Effects of 1-year yoga on cardiovascular risk factors in middle-aged and older adults with metabolic syndrome: a randomized trial. *Diabetol Metab Syndr.* 2015;7:40.
19. Kanaya AM, Araneta MR, Pawlowsky SB, et al. Restorative yoga and metabolic risk factors: the Practicing Restorative Yoga vs. Stretching for the Metabolic Syndrome (PRYSMS) randomized trial. *J Diabetes Complications.* 2014;28:406-412.
20. Hagins M, Rundle A, Consedine NS, et al. A randomized controlled trial comparing the effects of yoga with an active control on ambulatory blood pressure in individuals with prehypertension and stage 1 hypertension. *J Clin Hypertens (Greenwich).* 2014;16:54-62.
21. Jacob RG, Chesney MA, Williams DM, et al. Relaxation therapy for hypertension: Design effects and treatment effects. *Ann Behav Med.* 1991;13:5-17.
22. Eisenberg DM, Delbanco TL, Berkey CS, et al. Cognitive behavioral techniques for hypertension: are they effective? *Ann Intern Med.* 1993;118:964-972.
23. Dickinson H, Campbell F, Beyer F, et al. Relaxation therapies for the management of primary hypertension in adults: a Cochrane review. *J Hum Hypertens.* 2008;22:809-820.
24. Wang J, Xiong X, Liu W. Acupuncture for essential hypertension. *Int J Cardiol.* 2013;169:317-326.
25. Li DZ, Zhou Y, Yang YN, et al. Acupuncture for essential hypertension: a meta-analysis of randomized sham-controlled clinical trials. *Evid Based Complement Alternat Med.* 2014;2014:279478.
26. Zhao XF, Hu HT, Li JS, et al. Is acupuncture effective for hypertension? A systematic review and meta-analysis. *PLoS ONE.* 2015;10:e0127019.
27. Macklin EA, Wayne PM, Kalish LA, et al. Stop Hypertension with the Acupuncture Research Program (SHARP): results of a randomized, controlled clinical trial. *Hypertension.* 2006;48:838-845.
28. Langevin HM, Churchill DL, Cipolla MJ. Mechanical signaling through connective tissue: a mechanism for the therapeutic effect of acupuncture. *FASEB J.* 2001;15:2275-2282.

29. FDA. 510(k) Summary for the InterCure, Ltd. *RESPeRATE*. 2002.
30. Logtenberg SJ, Kleefstra N, Houweling ST, et al. Effect of device-guided breathing exercises on blood pressure in hypertensive patients with type 2 diabetes mellitus: a randomized controlled trial. *J Hypertens*. 2007;25:241-246.
31. Altena MR, Kleefstra N, Logtenberg SJ, et al. Effect of device-guided breathing exercises on blood pressure in patients with hypertension: a randomized controlled trial. *Blood Press*. 2009;18:273-279.
32. Anderson DE, McNeely JD, Windham BG. Regular slow-breathing exercise effects on blood pressure and breathing patterns at rest. *J Hum Hypertens*. 2010;24:807-813.
33. Landman GW, Drion I, van Hateren KJ, et al. Device-guided breathing as treatment for hypertension in type 2 diabetes mellitus: a randomized, double-blind, sham-controlled trial. *JAMA Intern Med*. 2013;173:1346-1350.
34. Mahtani KR, Nunan D, Heneghan CJ. Device-guided breathing exercises in the control of human blood pressure: systematic review and meta-analysis. *J Hypertens*. 2012;30:852-860.
35. Landman GW, van Hateren KJ, van Dijk PR, et al. Efficacy of device-guided breathing for hypertension in blinded, randomized, active-controlled trials: a meta-analysis of individual patient data. *JAMA Intern Med*. 2014;174:1815-1821.
36. van Hateren KJ, Landman GW, Logtenberg SJ, et al. Device-guided breathing exercises for the treatment of hypertension: An overview. *World J Cardiol*. 2014;6:277-282.
37. Pescatello LS, Franklin BA, Fagard R, et al. American College of Sports Medicine position stand. Exercise and hypertension. *Med Sci Sports Exerc*. 2004;36:533-553.
38. Fagard RH, Cornelissen VA. Effect of exercise on blood pressure control in hypertensive patients. *Eur J Cardiovasc Prev Rehabil*. 2007;14:12-17.
39. Cardoso Jr CG, Gomides RS, Queiroz AC, et al. Acute and chronic effects of aerobic and resistance exercise on ambulatory blood pressure. *Clinics (Sao Paulo, Brazil)*. 2010;65:317-325.
40. Lee LL, Watson MC, Mulvaney CA, et al. The effect of walking intervention on blood pressure control: a systematic review. *Int J Nurs Stud*. 2010;47:1545-1561.
41. Cornelissen VA, Smart NA. Exercise training for blood pressure: a systematic review and meta-analysis. *J Am Heart Assoc*. 2013;2:e004473.
42. Cornelissen VA, Arnout J, Holvoet P, et al. Influence of exercise at lower and higher intensity on blood pressure and cardiovascular risk factors at older age. *J Hypertens*. 2009:27753-27762.
43. Guimaraes GV, Ciolac EG, Carvalho VO, et al. Effects of continuous vs. interval exercise training on blood pressure and arterial stiffness in treated hypertension. *Hypertens Res*. 2010;33:627-632.
44. Molmen-Hansen HE, Stolen T, Tjonna AE, et al. Aerobic interval training reduces blood pressure and improves myocardial function in hypertensive patients. *Eur J Prev Cardiol*. 2012;19:151-160.
45. Westhoff TH, Schmidt S, Gross V, et al. The cardiovascular effects of upper-limb aerobic exercise in hypertensive patients. *J Hypertens*. 2008;26:1336-1342.
46. Andrews RC, Cooper AR, Montgomery AA, et al. Diet or diet plus physical activity versus usual care in patients with newly diagnosed type 2 diabetes: the Early ACTID randomised controlled trial. *Lancet*. 2011;378:129-139.
47. Collier SR, Frechette V, Sandberg K, et al. Sex differences in resting hemodynamics and arterial stiffness following 4 weeks of resistance versus aerobic exercise training in individuals with pre-hypertension to stage 1 hypertension. *Biol Sex Differ*. 2011;2:9.
48. Pescatello LS, MacDonald HV, Lamberti L, et al. Exercise for hypertension: A prescription update integrating existing recommendations with emerging research. *Curr Hypertens Rep*. 2015;17:87.
49. Carlson DJ, Dieberg G, Hess NC, et al. Isometric exercise training for blood pressure management: a systematic review and meta-analysis. *Mayo Clin Proc*. 2014;89:327-334.
50. Inder JD, Carlson DJ, Dieberg G, et al. Isometric exercise training for blood pressure management: a systematic review and meta-analysis to optimize benefit. *Hypertens Res*. 2016;39:88-94.

30 Approach to Difficult to Manage Primary Hypertension

Matthew J. Sorrentino and George L. Bakris

Primary, formerly essential, hypertension accounts for about 90% of cases of hypertension. Reduction in systolic and diastolic blood pressure in patients with primary hypertension reduces the risk for cardiovascular (CV) events including myocardial infarction, stroke, and congestive heart failure as well as a reduction in development and progression of chronic kidney disease (CKD). It is important to properly identify individuals with hypertension and document the type of hypertension present. All hypertensive patients should undergo a CV risk assessment. Target organ involvement must be evaluated. A treatment approach can then be formulated that individualizes treatment based on presenting pathophysiologic factors and comorbidities. This chapter will outline the standard evaluation of a patient with primary hypertension and review treatment strategies that can successfully control blood pressure in the vast majority of patients.

DEFINITION OF HYPERTENSION

Hypertension is generally defined as persistent blood pressure readings 140/90 mm Hg or higher, more than 50% of the day obtained under proper measuring conditions. Primary hypertension is persistently elevated blood pressure not found secondary to identifiable causes such as CKD defined as an estimated glomerular filtration rate (eGFR) below 60 mL/min/1.73m^2 or endocrine diseases.

Primary hypertension can be diagnosed in a variety of settings with different patterns of pressure variability (Table 30.1). *White coat hypertension* is defined as a blood pressure measured in a physician's office persistently 140/90 or greater mm Hg, whereas home blood pressure measurements are generally less than 135/85 mm Hg. A stress or alerting reaction may be responsible for the persistently elevated office blood pressure measurements, although a definitive mechanism is unknown. *Masked hypertension* is the inverse of white coat hypertension. Individuals with masked hypertension have office blood pressure measurements of less than 140/90 mm Hg but home or work settings demonstrate 24-hour ambulatory blood pressure measurements consistently elevated. Masked hypertension may be as high as 10% of the population and is associated with increased CV risk and CKD progression. *Isolated systolic hypertension* is defined as a systolic blood pressure consistently 140 mm Hg or higher with a diastolic blood pressure below 90 mm Hg. This pattern of hypertension is relatively common in people over the age of 65 years because of loss of larger artery compliance and is associated with increased CV morbidity. *Resistant hypertension* is defined as elevated blood pressure despite treatment with three appropriate antihypertensive agents at optimal doses with one of the antihypertensive agents being a diuretic appropriate for kidney function. Many patients with resistant hypertension can be successfully treated with an antihypertensive program combining lifestyle and pharmacologic therapy with an understanding of the underlying pathophysiology most likely driving the blood pressure elevation. The following sections will outline diagnostic and treatment strategies for the spectrum of primary hypertensive patients.

HOW TO DIAGNOSE HYPERTENSION

Note that high blood pressure and hypertension are not necessarily the same thing. An increase in blood pressure is a normal physiologic response to exercise and stress. Systemic arterial hypertension is a condition of a persistent nonphysiologic increase in blood pressure. Regulation of blood pressure is complex with interaction between numerous hormonal, neurologic, and local endothelial systems. Imbalance in any of these regulatory systems may be associated with changes in blood pressure. We can consider a blood pressure measurement to be a biomarker for both hypertension and for CV and renal disease. Blood pressure measurements are both prognostic indicators and treatment targets and many clinical trials have shown that reducing persistently elevated blood pressure reduces morbidity and mortality associated with hypertension. The optimal treatment target goal is continuing to be modified as further clinical studies are completed and will likely vary depending on patient comorbidities.

Before a treatment strategy can be implemented, it is important to properly and accurately diagnose hypertension. Evaluation of a patient with hypertension includes a careful review of CV risk factors and assessment of target organ involvement. Elevated blood pressure readings should be recorded using proper technique on at least three separate occasions to establish a persistent elevation in blood pressure unless the pressure is markedly elevated (generally ≥180/110 mm Hg).

TABLE 30.1 Hypertension Definitions

PRIMARY ESSENTIAL HYPERTENSION	BLOOD PRESSURE CONSISTENTLY ≥ 140/90 mm hg
White coat hypertension	Blood pressure ≥ 140/90 mm Hg in the office but normal on home measurements
Masked hypertension	Normal clinic blood pressures, consistently elevated blood pressures on home or ambulatory blood pressure monitoring
Isolated systolic hypertension	Systolic blood pressure ≥ 140 mm Hg, diastolic blood pressure ≤ 90 mm Hg
Resistant hypertension	Elevated blood pressure despite treatment with three appropriate antihypertensive medications at optimal doses with one of the antihypertensive agents being a diuretic

Proper blood pressure measurement technique is crucial to avoid over and under diagnosis of hypertension (see Chapters 4 and 5 for in-depth discussion). Proper blood pressure measurement technique can help eliminate both human error in measuring blood pressure and the reactive component responsible for elevation in blood pressure above the basal blood pressure when an individual is in a relaxed state. If three or more clinic visits document blood pressure readings that are 140/90 or higher mm Hg measured by proper technique, a diagnosis of hypertension can be made. Home blood pressure monitoring or ambulatory monitoring can be used to diagnose hypertension and can be useful for the diagnosis of white coat or masked hypertension.

There are a number of blood pressure measuring devices including the older mercury manometers, aneroid manometers with a dial in the center, and automatic electronic devices. The mercury manometer has been considered the gold standard for blood pressure measurement but because of concerns with mercury toxicity, is largely unavailable. Aneroid manometers are generally accurate but can become inaccurate over time, usually underestimating blood pressure. It has been assumed that automatic electronic blood pressure measurement devices are more accurate by eliminating human error, but are subject to the same inaccuracies in blood pressure measurement if proper technique is not used in obtaining the blood pressure.

HOW TO MEASURE BLOOD PRESSURE

Proper blood pressure measuring technique is crucial for accurate blood pressure readings (see Chapters 4 and 5 for in-depth discussion). Blood pressure is generally measured with a patient sitting comfortably with both feet on the floor and the legs not crossed. As the patient is sitting comfortably, consider factors that may have an impact on the blood pressure measurement such as pain, recent caffeine or tobacco use, recent exercise, or use of certain over-the-counter medications such as nonsteroidal antiinflammatory medications. The clinic setting should be relaxed and quiet (talking can raise blood pressure). The arm wearing the blood pressure cuff should be supported (resting on a table) and relaxed (avoid tensing the muscles). The center of the blood pressure cuff should be at about heart level. Ideally the patient should be relaxed and sitting quietly for a minimum of 5 minutes before a blood pressure check. Multiple blood pressure readings each about 60 seconds between readings should be obtained. The first blood pressure reading is generally discarded. If the next two readings are within 5 mm Hg of each other, the readings can be averaged for the blood pressure measurement. If there is a greater than 5 mm Hg difference, further blood pressure readings are obtained until two readings are within the range. A blood pressure reading should be taken with the cuff over the bare arm and not over clothing. It is recommended to take readings from both arms at least on the first visit to determine if there are significant differences between the two arms. In general, blood pressure is slightly higher in the dominant arm.

Many patients are interested in home blood pressure monitoring. For accurate home blood pressure measurement, proper technique is required the same as in the office. A patient will need to be taught how to properly measure blood pressure and use the home monitoring device. Home blood pressure values tend to be slightly lower than office readings and some recommendations suggest that a persistent blood pressure of more than 135/85 mm Hg at home be considered hypertension. Ambulatory blood pressure monitoring is thought to be accurate and can give information about nocturnal blood pressure and diagnose white coat or masked hypertension. Ambulatory and home blood pressure monitoring correlate well if blood pressure is properly measured.

HYPERTENSION EVALUATION

Patients diagnosed with hypertension should have an evaluation for secondary causes, target organ involvement, and a CV risk assessment. Secondary causes of hypertension should be considered in all individuals with signs and symptoms suggesting a secondary cause such as hypokalemia as well as resistant hypertension. An evaluation of target organ involvement can be individualized depending on the age and physical examination of the patient. Screening laboratory evaluation should include electrolytes and kidney function. An evaluation for microalbuminuria can be considered in patients where there is concern about early kidney involvement or in individuals with other comorbidities that can affect the kidney such as insulin resistance. A cardiac evaluation can be considered if there are signs and symptoms suggesting cardiac disease. An echocardiogram can identify left ventricular hypertrophy and may show signs suggesting ischemic disease. An echocardiogram can measure left ventricular mass and evaluate for both systolic and diastolic dysfunctions.

A hypertension evaluation can help determine an overall general strategy for treatment and may implicate certain hormonal systems involved in the hypertension. A careful evaluation may help determine if a patient is salt sensitive, hyperadrenergic (e.g., high resting heart rate usually >84 beats per minute), has overstimulation of the renin-angiotensin system, or has inappropriate levels of aldosterone. These hypertensive subtypes will be further discussed later.

LIFESTYLE MODIFICATION

Lifestyle modification is the cornerstone of any hypertension treatment strategy. The Joint National Committee on Prevention, Detection, Evaluation, and Treatment of High Blood Pressure seventh report (JNC 7) outlined lifestyle modifications to manage hypertension and the expected blood pressure reduction achievable with each intervention (Table 30.2).[1] A lifestyle modification program may be the initial antihypertensive strategy in patients with borderline or mildly elevated blood pressure and no compelling indications for certain medications or evidence of target organ damage. In addition, a lifestyle program will augment any blood pressure lowering effect achieved by pharmacologic agents. A lifestyle program can gradually improve blood pressure as patients continue to exercise and reduce weight. It is reasonable to try a lifestyle program for 3 to 6 months in low-risk individuals before committing to pharmacologic therapy. In addition, it may be possible to stop certain pharmacologic agents in patients who successfully adhere to a lifestyle program. It is important to note that the efficacy of a lifestyle program is likely proportional to the effort. Small lifestyle changes will only result in minimal blood pressure changes. Finally, a lifestyle program can reduce CV risk independent of the blood pressure lowering effects.

TABLE 30.2 Lifestyle Modifications to Manage Hypertension

MODIFICATION	RECOMMENDATION	SBP REDUCTION
Weight reduction	Maintain normal body weight (BMI 18.5-24.9 kg/m²)	5-20 mm Hg/10 kg weight loss
Adopt DASH eating plan	Consume a diet rich in fruits, vegetables, and low fat dairy products with reduced content of saturated and total fat	8-14 mm Hg
Dietary sodium reduction	Reduce dietary sodium intake to no more than 100 mmol/day (2.4 gm sodium or 6 gm sodium chloride)	2-8 mm Hg
Physical activity	Engage in regular aerobic physical activity such as brisk walking (at least 30 min/day most days of the week)	4-9 mm Hg
Moderation of alcohol consumption	Limit consumption to no more than 2 drinks per day in men and no more than 1 drink per day in women and lighter weight individuals	2-4 mm Hg

BMI, Body mass index; *DASH*, dietary approach to stop hypertension; *SBP*, systolic blood pressure.
(From Chobanian AV, Bakris GL, Black HR, et al. The Seventh Report of the Joint National Committee on prevention, detection, evaluation, and treatment of high blood pressure: the JNC 7 report. JAMA. 2003;289:2560-2572.)

TABLE 30.3 Compelling Indications for Individual Drug Classes

COMPELLING INDICATION	DIURETIC	BB	ACEi	ARB	CCB	ALDO ANT
Heart failure	X	X	X	X		X
Post MI		X	X			XX
High CAD risk	X	X	X		X	
Diabetes	X	X	X	X	X	
CKD			X	X		
Recurrent CVA prevention	X					X

ACEi, Angiotensin converting enzyme inhibitor; *Aldo Ant*, aldosterone antagonist; *ARB*, angiotensin receptor blocker; *BB*, beta-blocker; *CAD*, coronary artery disease; *CCB*, calcium channel blocker, *CKD*, chronic kidney disease; *CVA*, cerebrovascular accident; *MI*, myocardial infarction.
(From Chobanian AV, Bakris GL, Black HR, et al. The Seventh Report of the Joint National Committee on prevention, detection, evaluation, and treatment of high blood pressure: the JNC 7 report. JAMA. 2003;289:2560-2572.)

PHARMACOLOGIC TREATMENT OF HYPERTENSION

Compelling Indications

The choice of pharmacologic agents depends on the presence of target organ involvement and compelling indications for certain medications. The JNC 7 report listed six compelling indications and recommended drugs to both treat hypertension and the clinical condition (Table 30.3).[1] The drug selections for the compelling indications were based on outcome data from clinical trials. It is reasonable to extend the idea of compelling indications to include patients that have similar underlying comorbidities. For example, patients with obesity and insulin resistance may achieve benefit from agents recommended for treatment of blood pressure in diabetes. Moreover, the algorithm by the panel members appointed to the JNC 8 has an evidence-based approach to managing primary hypertension which is meaningful (Fig. 30.1).[2]

Secondary Causes of Hypertension

Secondary causes of hypertension are discussed in detail in Chapters 8 to 11. They should be considered in patients with resistant hypertension, especially those with difficult to treat hypokalemia. The most common secondary cause of hypertension is:

• Primary hyperaldosteronism: These patients generally have no edema secondary to the kidney's ability to escape the effects of aldosterone but typically have inappropriately low serum potassium levels in spite of potassium supplementation off diuretics. The major differential diagnosis

here is high sodium intake with associated pedal edema and easily correctible potassium with supplementation. Less common secondary causes are:

• Renal parenchymal disease: Diagnosed by blood and urine testing and most commonly seen in smokers with high cholesterol values.
• Renovascular hypertension: Consider in patients with renal bruits or known extensive atherosclerotic disease, advancing renal dysfunction, or worsening renal function when treated with an angiotensin-converting enzyme (ACE) inhibitor or angiotensin receptor blocker (ARB).
• Pheochromocytoma: Consider in individuals with labile hypertension and marked hyperadrenergic symptoms.
• Coarctation of the aorta: Diagnosed by measuring arm and leg blood pressures; most commonly seen in young adults and adolescents.

Resistant hypertension is a diagnosis of exclusion and all other causes must be excluded. There are many comorbid conditions that may contribute to resistant hypertension and should be screened for in the appropriate individual. Sleep apnea syndrome is associated with resistant hypertension and with treatment may lead to improved blood pressure response. Patients with insulin resistance have a higher incidence of hypertension. Certain medications may increase blood pressure, cause fluid retention, or interfere with blood pressure lowering agents including nonsteroidal antiinflammatory drugs (NSAIDs). Treating the comorbid conditions or stopping the interfering medications can lead to better blood pressure control.

The Salt-Sensitive Patient

There is a well-known association between sodium intake and hypertension. The International Study of Salt and Blood Pressure (INTERSALT) trial convincingly showed a relationship between salt consumption and blood pressure.[3] It has been observed that certain individuals appear to be more salt sensitive. Salt sensitivity is defined as shifting the dose response curve between a given amount of sodium intake and blood pressure rise. This curve shifts to the left meaning lesser amount of salt is needed to increase blood pressure. People with CKD and those who are older (over 70 years of age) are markedly salt sensitive. African-American patients have a high prevalence of salt sensitivity. Resistant hypertension may be a marker for salt sensitivity. In these individuals, excess sodium intake leads to volume expansion which raises blood pressure.

The initial approach to the salt sensitive volume expanded patient is to reduce sodium intake. Daily sodium intake for adults in the U.S. averages approximately 3400 mg per day and many hypertensive patients have significantly higher intake than average. There remains controversy regarding the recommended daily intake of sodium. The JNC 7 report and

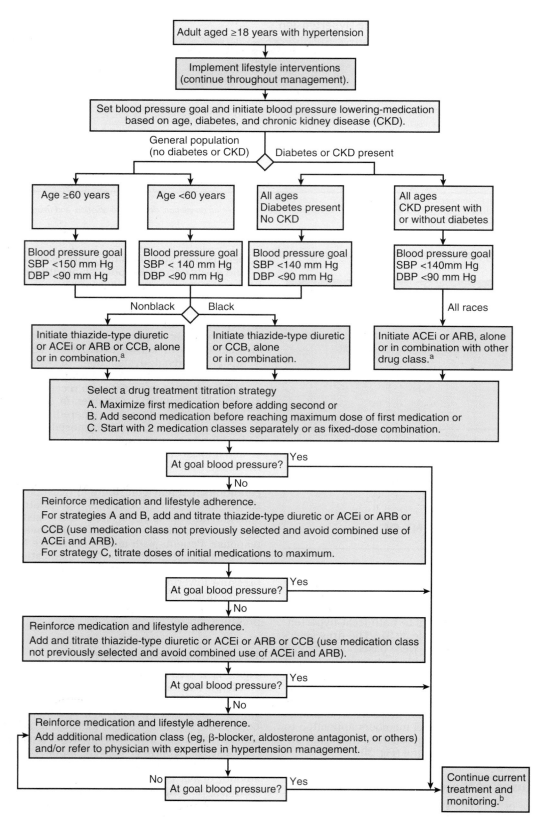

FIG. 30.1 2014 Hypertension guideline management algorithm. [a]ACE inhibitors and ARBs should not be used in combination. [b]If blood pressure fails to be maintained at goal, reenter the algorithm where appropriate based on the current individual therapeutic plan. *ACEi,* Angiotensin-converting enzyme inhibitor; *ARB,* angiotensin receptor blocker; *CCB,* calcium and channel blocker; *DBP,* diastolic blood pressure; *SBP,* systolic blood pressure. *(From James PA, Oparil S, Carter BL, et al. 2014 evidence-based guideline for the management of high blood pressure in adults: report from the panel members appointed to the Eighth Joint National Committee (JNC 8). JAMA. 2014;311:507-520.)*

the Institute of Medicine recommended that the daily intake of sodium should not exceed 2400 mg.[1] The U.S. Dietary Guidelines for Americans (DGA) recommended a sodium intake of less than 1500 mg daily for individuals with hypertension and certain high-risk groups including African Americans, patients with diabetes or kidney disease, and individuals over the age of 50 years.[4] This recommendation remains controversial, however, because certain population studies observed a J-shaped curve with low sodium intake associated with an increased CV mortality.[5] Proposed reasons why a low sodium intake may increase CV mortality include activation of the renin-angiotensin and sympathetic nervous systems with excessive sodium restriction.

Diuretic therapy is the recommended pharmacologic treatment for the volume expanded salt-sensitive individual that cannot reduce blood pressure by diet and salt restriction alone. Many antihypertensive agents become less effective when a patient is volume expanded. The addition of a diuretic can lead to a synergistic effect when combined with an additional agent. It is unlikely that adequate blood pressure control can be achieved without achieving a euvolemic state. Thiazide or thiazide-like diuretics (chlorthalidone and indapamide) are the diuretics of choice, with the thiazide-like diuretics having the best outcome data (see Chapter 18). Hydrochlorothiazide (HCTZ) is a commonly used thiazide diuretic but may not achieve euvolemia in many patients because it has a short half-life and relative lack of efficacy among those with an eGFR less than 45 mL/min/1.73m². Chlorthalidone and indapamide have longer effective half-lives of nearly 72 hours for chlorthalidone and over 24 hours for indapamide and can achieve a more sustained natriuretic effect over hydrochlorothiazide. The thiazide-like diuretics are preferred for many individuals that remain volume expanded on weaker diuretics.

Chlorthalidone is dosed at 12.5 to 25 mg daily; indapamide is dosed at 1.25 to 2.5 mg daily. Because of the long half-life of this agent, every other day or every third day dosing can be considered in sensitive individuals. Chlorthalidone and indapamide are more effective than HCTZ in renal impaired patients down to eGFR of 25 to 30 mL/min/1.73 cm².[6,7]

The Hyperadrenergic Patient

Many patients present with an elevated blood pressure and symptoms of palpitations, a rapid heart rate, headache, fatigue, and diaphoresis. Many patients describe labile blood pressure that may correlate with changes in heart rate. If the symptoms are excessive, a work up for a pheochromocytoma can be considered. A pheochromocytoma can be diagnosed by measuring plasma or a 24-hour urine collection of metanephrines. In most cases this evaluation will be negative for a pheochromocytoma as it accounts for only 0.1% of all secondary hypertension etiologies. These individuals may have abnormalities in adrenergic receptor structure and function that account for differing sensitivities to normal ranges of catecholamines and leads to exaggerated symptoms.

A lifestyle modification program is the initial treatment recommendation in approaching the hyperadrenergic patient. An exercise program can be successful in reducing hyperadrenergic symptoms over time. Submaximal cardiac aerobic exercise most days of the week for a minimum of 30 minutes daily is recommended. Upper body and core exercise are recommended at least two days per week. Patients should avoid stimulants such as caffeine. If a lifestyle modification program is not effective in reducing symptoms and normalizing blood pressure, low-dose beta-blockade can be very effective therapy. Many of these patients will respond very well to lower than average doses of a beta-blocker typically lower than expected to reduce blood pressure in hypertensive patients. Many patients with hyperadrenergic symptoms develop significant fatigue with higher dose beta-blockers which may limit their use.

Atenolol has been a commonly used beta-blocker for treatment of hypertension and works well in the hyperadrenegic patient attributed to minimal blood brain penetrance and a low side effect profile. There has been concern about the efficacy of atenolol as an antihypertensive agent because meta-analyses have suggested that atenolol may be inferior to other antihypertensive medication classes in reducing stroke and mortality.[8] Atenolol, however, should be dosed twice daily in individuals with normal renal function and was likely underdosed in many of the trials represented in the meta-analysis. Data using 24-hour ambulatory blood pressure measurements demonstrate a blood pressure effect of atenolol lasting about 13 hours compared with 23 hours for metoprolol succinate. This may account for as much as a 9 mm Hg difference in early morning blood pressure between these two agents at a time when CV risk is the highest.[9] In addition, beta-blockers with vasodilating activity such as carvedilol may have greater efficacy in lowering blood pressure and therefore may achieve greater risk reduction for CV events.

A subset of hyperadrenegic patients is the patient who has high psychosocial stressors that may be contributing to high blood pressure. Chronic work stress defined as work with high psychologic demands but low decision making has been associated with CV disease thought to be driven in part by an increase in blood pressure as a result of neuroendocrine stimulation.[10] Many patients have observed a significant increase in blood pressure at work compared with measurements taken at home. Ambulatory blood pressure monitoring may be needed to diagnose the work stress-induced elevation in blood pressure. Treatment with a beta-blocker or a rate limiting calcium channel blocker such as verapamil before the shift work can blunt the stress-induced blood pressure elevation. For these individuals, a shorter acting agent may be preferred to avoid hypotension when off work.

Obesity, Inflammation, and the Renin-Angiotensin Activated Patient

Obesity and underlying inflammatory cytokines are associated with an increased risk of CV disease. Visceral or intraabdominal adiposity is more metabolically active than subcutaneous fat accumulation. Visceral adiposity correlates with markers of dyslipidemia, hypertension, insulin resistance and inflammation. Visceral adiposity may contribute to the development of hypertension by releasing free fatty acids and inflammatory mediators into the circulation and change levels of adipocytokines that can lead to endothelial dysfunction. Visceral adipose tissue has also been found to express and secrete factors with endocrine function including proteins of the renin-angiotensin system (RAS) including renin, angiotensinogen, angiotensin I, angiotensin II, and aldosterone.[11] Angiotensin II mediates the effects of the renin-angiotensin system by increasing vasoconstriction and promotes aldosterone secretion and sodium and water reabsorption contributing to an increase in blood pressure.

The release of renin from the kidney is normally a regulated process with negative feedback loops that can reduce renin excretion when renal perfusion is normalized by volume expansion and glomerular afferent arteriole vasoconstriction. The release of RAS hormones from visceral adipose tissue, in contrast, is an unregulated secretion and may lead to chronic overstimulation of the RAS despite volume expansion and an increase in blood pressure.

Overstimulation of the renin-angiotensin syndrome is an important contributor to hypertension in a large number of hypertensive patients especially patients with excess visceral adiposity. Community studies of untreated hypertensive patients suggest that as many as 70% of patients may have medium or high renin levels.[12] In addition, excess amounts of aldosterone produced by visceral and possibly subcutaneous adipocytes may contribute to hypertension in these individuals. For these patients, the renin levels should have been low because the elevated blood pressure and volume expansion should have worked as a negative feedback to the kidney suppressing the production of renin by the juxtaglomerular cells. The medium or high renin levels suggest an abnormality in the negative feedback loop or extrarenal production of renin that is not subjected to a negative feedback mechanism.

It is reasonable to consider visceral adiposity as a compelling indication for the use of an ACE inhibitor or an ARB as first-line therapy for the treatment of hypertension because these patients likely have overstimulation of the RAS system as an underlying pathophysiologic mechanism for hypertension. In addition, patients with visceral adiposity have a higher incidence of developing diabetes mellitus. ACE inhibitors or ARBs may reduce the incidence of diabetes compared with placebo, diuretics, or beta-blockers.[13] In more resistant hypertension cases, the use of a mineralocorticoid antagonist (spironolactone or eplerenone) should be added to the RAS blocker to block the effects of aldosterone.

The Patient With Inappropriately Elevated Aldosterone

Primary hyperaldosteronism is characterized by resistant hypertension, volume expansion, and relative hypokalemia and is the most common secondary cause of hypertension. Many more patients, however, will have aldosterone levels in the upper normal or slightly elevated range not consistent with primary hyperaldosteronism. These patients may be similar to the patients with overstimulation of the renin-angiotensin system because angiotensin II is a major stimulus for release of aldosterone from the adrenal gland. Many of these patients, however, will have low renin because of the volume expansion from the inappropriately elevated aldosterone which suppresses renin release from the kidney. Excess aldosterone as a contributing factor to an increased blood pressure should be considered in hypertensive patients who have resistant hypertension, are retaining fluid or are hypokalemic. Some of these patients may become significantly hypokalemic with diuretic therapy. Consider an inappropriately elevated aldosterone in patients on high-dose RAS blockers that may require potassium supplements or who have low normal or below normal serum potassium levels.

Aldosterone blockade is an effective treatment strategy for patients with resistant hypertension. A treatment approach to resistant hypertension usually begins with a combination of full doses of a RAS blocker, a calcium channel blocker, and a diuretic. In patients who remain volume expanded, changing the diuretic to the longer acting chlorthalidone or indapamide can frequently bring about better blood pressure control. Analysis of participants in the Anglo-Scandinavian Cardiac Outcomes Trial-Blood Pressure Lowering Arm who received spironolactone as a fourth-line antihypertensive agent for uncontrolled blood pressure showed that a mean dose of 25 mg significantly reduced blood pressure by about 22 mm Hg.[14] More recently, the Prevention And Treatment of Hypertension With Algorithm based therapY (PATHWAY-2) trial attempted to determine the optimal drug treatment for patients with resistant hypertension and compared spironolactone with placebo, doxazosin, and bisoprolol.[15] Spironolactone was the most effective blood pressure treatment. The response was shown to be inversely related to plasma renin activity, suggesting that volume expansion from aldosterone excess and excess sodium retention was responsible for the resistant hypertension.

For patients with resistant hypertension that appear to be volume expanded, it is recommended to add spironolactone 25 mg daily. Potassium supplements are usually stopped. For patients with chronic renal insufficiency, 12.5 mg can be used as a starting dose to avoid hyperkalemia. Risk factors for hyperkalemia are an eGFR less than 45 mg/min/1.73[2] and/or a serum potassium of 4.5 mEq/L while on appropriate diuretics for kidney function.[16] These patients should be instructed on low potassium diets because 90% of potassium excretion is by the kidney and only 10% from the gut. Spironolactone can be titrated to diuretic dose of 50 mg daily for further efficacy or if the potassium level remains at levels well below 4.8 mEq/L. A common side effect of spironolactone in men is gynecomastia. Eplerenone is a selective aldosterone antagonist that has much less affinity for androgen and progesterone receptors and avoids the side effects most commonly seen with spironolactone. Eplerenone is not as effective as spironolactone so it is recommended to begin with a 50-mg daily dose.

BLOOD PRESSURE TREATMENT TARGETS

Treatment targets for blood pressure have undergone evolution as newer treatment studies have attempted to define optimal goals in different populations. A treatment target goal of less than 140/90 mm Hg was recommended by earlier JNC guidelines. Epidemiologic studies suggest that further benefit may be achieved with treatment targets as low as less than 120/80 mm Hg.[17] It is important, however, not to extrapolate observational data with treatment studies. A report from the panel members appointed to JNC 8 evaluated major treatment studies in individuals aged 60 years and older and recommended to treat to a blood pressure goal of less than 150/90 mm Hg.[2] The blood pressure arm of the ACCORD trial evaluated the treatment target of less than 120 mm Hg systolic compared with standard therapy with a systolic pressure target of less than 140 mm Hg in high-risk diabetic patients and found no reduction fatal and nonfatal CV events in the lower blood pressure target cohort.[18] There is concern with this conclusion, however, because the ACCORD blood pressure arm was not powered adequately to detect a CV outcome effect at the lower target. In contrast, the SPRINT trial evaluated high CV risk individuals without diabetes and found a significant reduction in cardiac events in patients treated to a target of less than 120 mm Hg systolic compared with less than 140 mm Hg systolic.[19] These studies suggest that blood pressure treatment targets may differ depending on patient characteristics and future guidelines will likely define different targets for different groups.

SUMMARY

Understanding the pathophysiology of essential hypertension can lead to a rational treatment approach to controlling blood pressure. Blood pressure is regulated by multiple systemic and local systems so there is unlikely a single underlying pathophysiologic abnormality responsible for the development of hypertension. A strategy to target the system most likely influencing the increase in blood pressure should be the most successful treatment approach. The salt-sensitive patient should reduce the intake of sodium. Long-acting diuretics such as chlorthalidone and indapamide are more effective than short-acting agents and are more likely to achieve a euvolemic state. The hyperadrenergic patient will respond well to beta-blockade. The viscerally obese patient is likely to have an inappropriately activated renin-angiotensin system and will respond to a strategy using a RAS blocker. Consider inappropriately elevated aldosterone in the volume expanded hypokalemic patient. The resistant hypertensive patient can be effectively treated with a full-dose RAS blocker, a calcium channel blocker, a long-acting diuretic, and an aldosterone blocker. With this approach, the majority of hypertensive patients can be successfully treated without relying on tier two antihypertensive agents such as centrally acting adrenergic agonists and peripheral vasodilators, thereby avoiding side effects of these classes of medications.

References

1. Chobanian AV, Bakris GL, Black HR, et al. The Seventh Report of the Joint National Committee on prevention, detection, evaluation, and treatment of high blood pressure: the JNC 7 report. *JAMA*. 2003;289:2560-2572.
2. James PA, Oparil S, Carter BL, et al. 2014 evidence-based guideline for the management of high blood pressure in adults: report from the panel members appointed to the Eighth Joint National Committee (JNC 8). *JAMA*. 2014;311:507-520.
3. Intersalt: an international study of electrolyte excretion and blood pressure. Results for 24 hour urinary sodium and potassium excretion. Intersalt Cooperative Research Group. *BMJ*. 1988;297:319-328.
4. Strom BL, Anderson CA, Ix JH. Sodium reduction in populations: insights from the Institute of Medicine committee. *JAMA*. 2013;310:31-32.
5. O'Donnell M, Mente A, Rangarajan S, et al. Urinary sodium and potassium excretion, mortality, and cardiovascular events. *N Engl J Med*. 2014;371:612-623.
6. Agarwal R, Sinha AD, Pappas MK, Ammous F. Chlorthalidone for poorly controlled hypertension in chronic kidney disease: an interventional pilot study. *Am J Nephrol*. 2014;39:171-182.
7. Madkour H, Gadallah M, Riveline B, Plante GE, Massry SG. Indapamide is superior to thiazide in the preservation of renal function in patients with renal insufficiency and systemic hypertension. *Am J Cardiol*. 1996;77:23B-25B.
8. Ong HT. Beta blockers in hypertension and cardiovascular disease. *BMJ*. 2007;334:946-949.
9. Sarafidis P, Bogojevic Z, Basta E, Kirstner E, Bakris GL. Comparative efficacy of two different beta-blockers on 24-hour blood pressure control. *J Clin Hypertens (Greenwich)*. 2008;10:112-118.
10. Figueredo VM. The time has come for physicians to take notice: the impact of psychosocial stressors on the heart. *Am J Med*. 2009;122:704-712.
11. Kershaw EE, Flier JS. Adipose tissue as an endocrine organ. *J Clin Endocrinol Metab*. 2004;89:2548-2556.
12. Alderman MH, Cohen HW, Sealey JE, Laragh JH. Plasma renin activity levels in hypertensive persons: their wide range and lack of suppression in diabetic and in most elderly patients. *Am J Hypertens*. 2004;17:1-7.
13. Elliott WJ, Meyer PM. Incident diabetes in clinical trials of antihypertensive drugs: a network meta-analysis. *Lancet*. 2007;369:201-207.
14. Chapman N, Dobson J, Wilson S, et al. Effect of spironolactone on blood pressure in subjects with resistant hypertension. *Hypertension*. 2007;49:839-845.
15. Williams B, MacDonald TM, Morant S, et al. Spironolactone versus placebo, bisoprolol, and doxazosin to determine the optimal treatment for drug-resistant hypertension (PATHWAY-2): a randomised, double-blind, crossover trial. *Lancet*. 2015;386:2059-2068.
16. Lazich I, Bakris GL. Prediction and management of hyperkalemia across the spectrum of chronic kidney disease. *Semin Nephrol*. 2014;34:333-339.
17. Lewington S, Clarke R, Qizilbash N, Peto R, Collins R. Age-specific relevance of usual blood pressure to vascular mortality: a meta-analysis of individual data for one million adults in 61 prospective studies. *Lancet*. 2002;360:1903-1913.
18. Cushman WC, Evans GW, Byington RP, et al. Effects of intensive blood-pressure control in type 2 diabetes mellitus. *N Engl J Med*. 2010;362:1575-1585.
19. Wright Jr JT, Williamson JD, Whelton PK, et al. A randomized trial of intensive versus standard blood-pressure control. *N Engl J Med*. 2015;373:2103-2116.

31 Hypertension in Ischemic Heart Disease

Steven M. Smith and Carl J. Pepine

Hypertension and ischemic heart disease (IHD) are strongly related and the two co-occur frequently, particularly in aging populations. Both conditions cause or contribute to substantial disability and mortality worldwide[1,2] and both are responsible for substantial health care use and economic burden. IHD affects only around 6% of adults in the United States but is the leading proximal cause of death in the U.S. with an age-adjusted mortality rate of around 170 per 100,000 person-years among the general adult population.[3] Moreover, hypertension with IHD is among the most prevalent dyads, and together with hyperlipidemia, the most prevalent triad in our Medicare population.[4]

Numerous pathophysiologic mechanisms contribute to hypertension development (see Chapter 5) and associated organ damage, including IHD. Such mechanisms include sympathetic nervous system and renin angiotensin aldosterone system (RAAS) activation, increased conduit vessel stiffness, endothelial dysfunction, increased inflammatory mediators, hemodynamic changes, and reduced vasodilator reserve or activity. However, hypertension, per se, also directly promotes IHD development through mechanisms that affect the balance of myocardial oxygen supply and demand. For example, any increase in systolic blood pressure (BP) increases myocardial oxygen requirements, whereas more chronic BP elevations promote endothelial injury, resulting in impaired vasodilator (e.g., nitric oxide) release and increased release of inflammatory mediators that promote development of atherosclerosis and vascular occlusion. Oxygen demand can increase because of increased impedance to left ventricular (LV) ejection (e.g., "afterload"), development of LV hypertrophy (LVH) impairing coronary blood flow during diastole, or both, secondary to chronically elevated BP. This combination of limited oxygen supply and increased demand is particularly pernicious and explains, in part, why patients with elevated BP at any level, compared with those without elevated BP, are more likely to develop manifestations of IHD (angina, myocardial infarction [MI], or other major coronary event), and to be at higher mortality risk following an event.

RELATIONSHIP BETWEEN HYPERTENSION AND CORONARY ARTERY DISEASE

Hypertension is well documented as the most prevalent independent risk factor for the development of coronary artery disease (CAD), cardiac failure, stroke, and peripheral arterial disease (PAD). Younger subjects with hypertension (i.e., aged <50 years) often have an increased diastolic BP (DPB), whereas older subjects usually have increased systolic BP (SBP). Accordingly, in younger individuals, DBP is more closely associated with IHD development, whereas SBP is more predictive in those aged 60 years or older.[5] Moreover, in this older age group, DBP is inversely related to CAD development, such that pulse pressure (PP) becomes a strong predictor of CAD risk. Importantly, the risk of CAD-attributable fatal events doubles for every 20-mm Hg increase in SBP or 10-mm Hg increase in DBP between a BP range of 115/75 to 185/115 mm Hg.[6] Thus, patients need not be "hypertensive" by conventional BP thresholds (e.g., >140/90 mm Hg) to be at increased risk of major adverse cardiovascular events.

Arteriosclerotic disease is the consequence of a complex interaction of inflammation, cytokines, free radicals, growth factors, lipids, and endocrine and paracrine factors. Many of these latter substances adversely affect endothelial function and cause, through a common pathway, hypertrophy and reduced compliance of large- and medium-sized arteries and arterioles (Fig. 31.1). Frequently, these changes are present in the vasculature of young individuals before they develop hypertension, especially in the children of hypertensive parents; a finding supporting the notion of a genetic component, but also that hypertension is a consequence of the vasculopathy.[7] Hypertension causes fragmentation and fracture of elastin fibers as well as collagen deposition in arteries, changes that contribute to thickening and stiffening of those arteries. Hypertension also induces endothelial dysfunction, thus reducing many endothelium-dependent functions (e.g., vasodilator capacity, anticoagulation, thrombolysis).

One of the hallmarks of hypertension is stiff arteries. *Compliance* of an artery may be defined as the change of lumen diameter (ΔD), or of cross-sectional area (ΔA) during each cardiac cycle, as a function of the change of distending pressure over one cardiac cycle (ΔP). This change in the distending pressure over one cardiac cycle (ΔP) is the PP. Compliance is thus represented by the slope of $\Delta D/\Delta P$ (or $\Delta A/\Delta P$). In arteriosclerotic disease, ΔD is diminished because of the structural rigidity of the conduit vessels. PP is a function both of the stroke volume, which is usually normal in patients with established or stable hypertension, and of the stiffness of conduit vessels, which is typically increased in hypertension. However, an additional mechanism for increasing PP has been recognized (Fig. 31.2). Pressure and flow waves are generated with each ejection of blood from the LV. The stiffer the large arteries, the greater the pulse wave velocity (PWV). That wave is reflected back from points of discontinuity (branch points) or increased resistance in the arterial tree, particularly at the level of small arteries and arterioles, and the reflected wave returns to the proximal aorta. In younger persons, this reflected wave reaches the aortic valve after closure, leading to a higher DBP, thus *enhancing* coronary perfusion. In older individuals with stiffer conduit vessels, the reflected pressure wave has a greater velocity and may reach the aortic valve before closure, leading to a higher SBP and afterload and a lower DBP, thus *decreasing* coronary perfusion pressure. Importantly, although reflected pressure waves add to the incident pressure wave, reflected flow waves subtract from the incident blood flow wave, thus reducing end-organ blood flow, including coronary blood flow (and cardiac output), renal blood flow, and others. These mechanisms help to explain why older individuals exhibit isolated systolic hypertension, with a normal or low DBP, and elevated PP. Also, why ischemia, heart failure, renal failure, and other associated comorbidities are more prevalent among the elderly. Increased myocardial oxygen *demand* results both from the increased resistance to LV ejection and from LVH. The myocardial oxygen *supply* is diminished, not only because of the atherosclerotic CAD, but also because of the decreased coronary filling pressure associated with the lower-than-normal DBP. This combination of increased oxygen demand and reduced supply in the myocardium of patients with hypertension is particularly problematic because the myocardium, unlike the brain, has relatively fixed oxygen extraction from coronary blood circulation and is unable to adequately compensate for decreased blood flow and oxygen supply.

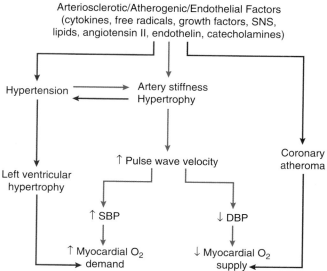

FIG. 31.1 Schematic relationship between hypertension and coronary artery disease. See text for detailed explanation. *DBP,* Diastolic blood pressure; *SBP,* systolic blood pressure; *SNS,* sympathetic nervous system.

PRIMARY PREVENTION OF CORONARY ARTERY DISEASE IN PATIENTS WITH HYPERTENSION

Any increase in BP above 120 mm Hg systolic or 85 mm Hg diastolic is associated with increased risk of developing CAD and mitigating this risk factor is a major goal of primary prevention. Consequently, patients with prehypertension or hypertension should receive guidance on risk-reducing healthy lifestyles, including smoking cessation; management of lipids, diabetes, and weight, as necessary; and a suitable exercise regimen. Daily aspirin reduces the risk of cardiovascular events broadly in at-risk individuals, including those with hypertension, and should be considered in patients at increased risk of developing CAD.[8]

Effective antihypertensive therapy substantially reduces all cardiovascular adverse outcomes. Safely lowering BP is the main goal, which can be accomplished with any number of currently available antihypertensive agents, and most patients will require combination therapy. Whether specific antihypertensive agents exhibit additional benefits, that is, beyond BP-lowering, remains a subject of debate. However, as discussed later, few trials have focused on primary prevention of CAD and existing data do not strongly support any particular agent in preventing CAD development.[9] The optimal BP goal for reducing risk of CAD development is not known. Previous guidelines recommended a goal of less than 130/80 mm Hg for both management of CAD and prevention (in those at high risk),[10] but data supporting this goal, particularly in primary prevention, remain scarce.

Evidence for Antihypertensive Drugs for Primary Prevention of Coronary Heart Disease

Diuretics and Beta-Blockers

Most early clinical trials of antihypertensive therapy used diuretics, beta-blockers, or both and generally found that these agents significantly reduced adverse outcomes,

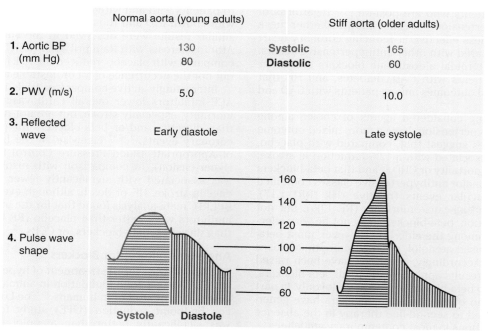

	Normal aorta (young adults)		Stiff aorta (older adults)
1. Aortic BP (mm Hg)	130 80	**Systolic** **Diastolic**	165 60
2. PWV (m/s)	5.0		10.0
3. Reflected wave	Early diastole		Late systole
4. Pulse wave shape	Systole Diastole		

FIG. 31.2 Change in aortic pressure profile resulting from age-related vascular stiffening and increased pulse wave velocity (PWV). 1, Increased systolic blood pressure (SBP) and decreased diastolic blood pressure (DBP) owing to decreased aortic distensibility. 2, Increased PWV as a result of decreased aortic distensibility and increased distal (arteriolar) resistance. 3, Return of the reflected primary pulse to the central aorta in systole rather than in diastole as a result of faster wave travel. 4, Change in aortic pulse wave profile because of early wave reflection. Note the summation of antegrade and retrograde pulse waves to produce a large SBP. This increases LV stroke work and therefore myocardial oxygen demand. Note also the reduction in the diastolic pressure-time (integrated area under the DBP curve). This reduction in coronary perfusion pressure increases the vulnerability of the myocardium to hypoxia. *(Modified from O'Rourke MF. Ageing and arterial function. In: Arterial Function in Health and Disease. New York: Churchill Livingstone; 1982:185-95.)*

especially stroke morbidity and mortality, in all age groups. More recent meta-analyses have shown that, compared with placebo, thiazide diuretic–based therapy reduces relative rates of heart failure (HF) by 41% to 49%, stroke by 29% to 38%, IHD by 14% to 21%, and all-cause death by 10% to 11%.[9,11]

In the Antihypertensive and Lipid Lowering Treatment to Prevent Heart Attack Trial (ALLHAT), among high-risk hypertensive patients, chlorthalidone was superior to lisinopril in preventing stroke, and superior to lisinopril and amlodipine in preventing HF.[12] Importantly, no significant differences were observed among chlorthalidone-treated, lisinopril-treated, or amlodipine-treated patients with regard to combined fatal CAD or nonfatal MI (the primary outcome of the study), combined CAD (fatal CAD, nonfatal MI, coronary revascularization, or hospitalization for angina), or all-cause mortality. However, the so-called "second step" drugs supplied (e.g., atenolol, clonidine, reserpine, hydralazine) were problematic with the possible exception of atenolol. That is, the lack of optimal pharmacologic combination therapy made the results difficult to translate to the clinic, particularly for patients with CAD. In addition, whether thiazide-type diuretics, used at contemporary doses, are equivalent with respect to outcome prevention remains a subject of debate. Recent data suggest that chlorthalidone may reduce cardiovascular events significantly more than hydrochlorothiazide, but at the expense of more hypokalemia and/or hyponatremia.[13,14]

Spironolactone, a steroidal aldosterone antagonist, reduces morbidity and mortality in HF with reduced ejection fraction, with or without CAD[15] and effectively lowers BP in patients with hypertension, including resistant hypertension.[16,17] However, spironolactone has not been studied in prospective clinical trials, with objective outcomes, for the treatment of hypertension, with or without CAD. Eplerenone is a more selective steroidal aldosterone antagonist with lower affinity for androgen, progesterone, and glucocorticoid receptors accounting for its reduced side effect profile (i.e., less gynecomastia in men and dysmenorrhea in women) relative to spironolactone. Eplerenone reduces morbidity and mortality in patients with HF and reduced ejection fraction, and among CAD patients who are post-MI,[18,19] regardless of the presence of hypertension.[19] It is not known whether these agents are more or less effective at reducing coronary heart disease (CHD) compared with other antihypertensive agents. Several newer nonsteroidal aldosterone blockers are under investigation for patients with CAD, diabetes, and HF, that could yield improved outcomes among patients with CAD and hypertension.

Beta-blockers, long considered agents of choice among CAD patients with hypertension, have a more mixed outcome profile. Meta-analyses suggest that, compared with placebo, beta-blockers are associated with a 12% reduction in stroke, but no difference in mortality or CHD,[20] and that beta-blockers are inferior to other major antihypertensive classes combined for major cardiovascular events (relative risk [RR] 1.17), stroke (RR 1.24), and all-cause mortality (RR 1.06), but not HF or CHD.[21] In addition, beta-blockers may not be very effective for BP control among the elderly.[22] However, most beta-blocker trials have used atenolol, often at suboptimal doses or only once daily. Accordingly, questions have been raised over whether these results apply broadly to all beta-blockers, only nonvasodilating beta-blockers, or to atenolol only. In part because of these and other data, beta-blockers have generally been downgraded to second-line therapy in the absence of compelling indications in most contemporary guidelines.

Calcium Channel Blockers

Since the mid-1990s, several trials of calcium channel blockers (CCBs) have been conducted for the primary prevention of cardiovascular complications of hypertension, particularly those related to IHD/CAD. The CCB trials tended to show a significant prevention of stroke, usually compared with placebo or with a diuretic, beta-blocker, or both.[23-28] However, the absolute risk reduction in IHD deaths or nonfatal coronary events with CCBs has been less impressive, and in some cases absent.[29] An extensive meta-analysis by the Blood Pressure Lowering Treatment Trialists' Collaboration (BPLTTC) strongly supports the benefits of CCBs over placebo and for regimens that targeted lower BP goals; however, it found that CCBs, compared with diuretics and/or beta-blockers, significantly lowered stroke risk, but not CAD-related outcomes, and CCBs were associated with a 33% increase in HF.[30] Moreover, CCBs were less effective in preventing CHD and HF than angiotensin converting enzyme (ACE) inhibitors.

Importantly, most of these trials were limited by the inability to determine, with certainty, which patients had preexisting CAD. To this end, the INternational VErapamil SR/trandolapril STudy (INVEST) enrolled only patients with hypertension and documented CAD to evaluate the effects of two different initial pharmacologic combination strategies (a beta-blocker plus hydrochlorothiazide strategy versus a nondihydropyridine CCB [verapamil] plus ACE inhibitor strategy).[31] These INVEST combination strategies yielded excellent BP control (~72% achieving <140/90 mm Hg) with equivalent reductions in all-cause mortality and other major cardiovascular outcomes. Similar risk reduction has also been observed between amlodipine and enalapril in patients with CAD and DBP less than 100 mm Hg.[32] On the basis of the published trials, CCBs may be superior to hydrochlorothiazide in the prevention of coronary events,[33] but not to other antihypertensive agents, particularly chlorthalidone and ACE inhibitors. CCBs also may be modestly superior to other major classes in reducing stroke, but inferior in reducing HF.[21]

Angiotensin-Converting Enzyme Inhibitors

In the Heart Outcomes Prevention Evaluation (HOPE) study, after 4.5 years, ramipril, compared with placebo, was associated with relative risks of 0.74 for death from cardiovascular causes, 0.80 for MI, 0.85 for revascularization procedures, 0.63 for cardiac arrest, and 0.77 for HF.[34] The results were applicable to patients with and without hypertension as well as to those with known IHD and those without CAD at baseline. Broadly similar results were observed in the smaller Prevention of Atherosclerosis with Ramipril Trial (PART-2), where ramipril, compared with placebo, reduced the risk for fatal CAD by 57%, but not the occurrence of MI or unstable angina.[35]

Interestingly, active-comparator trials have suggested that ACE inhibitors lower overall cardiovascular morbidity and mortality, especially stroke, but are not demonstrably better than diuretics and/or beta-blockers for prevention of acute coronary events.[12,36,37] Likewise, in the hypertensive subset of Appropriate Blood Pressure Control in Diabetes (ABCD-Hypertension), in comparison with nisoldipine, perindopril was associated with significantly fewer MIs, but no difference in stroke, HF, or death, although events were few.[38] The BPLTTC meta-analysis found that for the outcome of CAD, ACE inhibitors were better than placebo (RR 0.80), but no better than diuretics, beta-blockers, or CCBs.[30]

Angiotensin Receptor Blockers

The use of ARBs for the treatment of hypertension in patients with CAD has a solid foundation in animal studies and surrogate endpoint studies in humans.[39] The Losartan Intervention For Endpoint reduction (LIFE) study found that losartan was significantly better than atenolol in reducing stroke, but not cardiovascular mortality or MI.[40] In the Valsartan Antihypertensive Long-Term Use Evaluation (VALUE) trial, no significant difference was seen in the primary endpoint (a composite of nine cardiovascular events) between a valsartan-based and an amlodipine-based treatment regimen in high-risk patients.[41] However, this finding is complicated by the fact that nearly all subjects were taking other therapy, mainly diuretics (~25%), other combinations of study drugs (~20%), or no study drug (~25%) by study end, and because amlodipine lowered BP more than valsartan, especially during the early months of treatment.

Somewhat unexpected were the results of Telmisartan Randomised Assessment Study in ACE Intolerant Subjects with Cardiovascular Disease (TRANSCEND) in which telmisartan was no better than placebo, when added to concomitant therapies, in preventing cardiovascular events in ACE-intolerant patients with cardiovascular disease or diabetes, of whom 76% had hypertension.[42] This finding seems to be at odds with the results of HOPE, in which ramipril improved outcomes compared with placebo, given that ACE inhibitors and ARBs have generally been considered equivalent in terms of cardiovascular outcomes. Among the possible reasons for this discrepancy were that in TRANSCEND, compared with HOPE: the incidence of prior CAD and MI was lower; baseline use of other cardiovascular risk–reducing medications was higher; the study may have been underpowered to identify an expected 19% risk reduction; and, hospitalization for HF was included in the composite endpoint.[43] Interestingly, when the primary HOPE composite endpoint, which did not include hospitalization for HF, was assessed in TRANSCEND as a prespecified secondary endpoint, there was a 13% relative risk reduction ($p = 0.068$).[42]

Blood Pressure Targets

The coronary vascular bed, like most others, is capable of autoregulating flow in the face of large changes in perfusion pressure (Fig. 31.3). The relationship of coronary blood flow (F), perfusion pressure (P), and coronary vascular resistance (R) is F∝P/R. In a rigid tube with a fixed resistance, F∝P. The coronary circulation, however, can alter its resistance, such that an increase in P causes coronary vasoconstriction (increased

R), so that, if ventricular work is kept constant, flow remains relatively constant, up to a level at which the vasoconstriction is maximal (the upper limit of coronary vascular autoregulation). Conversely, a fall in P will stimulate vasodilation so that flow remains relatively constant, down to a level of P at which vessels are maximally dilated (the lower limit of coronary vascular autoregulation). Below that limit, any further decline in P will result in decreased flow. Most coronary blood flow occurs in diastole; thus the P referred to here is the mean DBP. The instantaneous coronary flow is a function of DBP, and the total flow per cardiac cycle is proportional to both DBP and the duration of diastole, assessed by the integrated area under the pressure curve during diastole.

Further considerations are the effects of myocardial hypertrophy and exercise. At any given P, coronary reserve is the difference between autoregulated and maximally dilated coronary flow. In Fig. 31.3, curve A_1 represents coronary blood flow over a wide range of perfusion pressures, and the perfusion pressure P_1 is at the lower limit of autoregulation. If the coronary vessels are maximally dilated, a steep, linear pressure-flow relationship exists between pressure and flow (line D_1). The difference between autoregulated and maximally vasodilated flow at any given P represents the coronary flow reserve (R_1). If myocardial hypertrophy is present, total coronary flow is greater, with a higher autoregulatory line (curve A_2) and a rightward shift of the lower limit of autoregulation (point P_2). However, the pressure-flow relation at maximal vasodilation is less steep (line D_2), so that the coronary flow reserve (R_2) at any given P is less. Moreover, the point at which coronary flow reserve is exhausted (point P_2) in the hypertrophied heart will coincide with a higher P than normal (point P_1). Thus, in patients with hypertension and LVH, the lower limit of autoregulation is set at a higher level of P (and therefore DBP), and at any level of P, or DBP, the coronary flow reserve is less than it would be in the normal ventricle.

Given these physiologic considerations, there exists some BP value at the lower limit of coronary vascular autoregulation, below which coronary blood flow is reduced. BP-lowering beyond this point reduces target perfusion and increases risk of adverse cardiovascular outcomes and death. This so-called "J-curve" in the relationship between BP and risk of outcomes continues to be a subject of debate, in part because we do not have very good data about the exact DBP level at which coronary blood flow begins to be reduced in the intact human coronary circulation. In addition, the presence of any significant occlusive coronary atherosclerotic disease will shift the lower limit of autoregulation upward, making patients less tolerant of low DBPs, especially if there is additional myocardial oxygen demand from LVH.

Data from the Framingham study clearly show a demonstrable increase in cardiovascular risk in the general population at DBP less than 80 mm Hg, but only when SBP is higher than 140 mm Hg.[44] This finding makes sense, given that low DBP may reduce coronary perfusion pressure, and higher SBP increases myocardial oxygen demand and may increase intramyocardial wall tension, further limiting perfusion. In patients with occlusive CAD, the perfusion pressure downstream of the stenosis would be even further reduced, and the elevated LV SBP and the presence of LVH would further increase myocardial oxygen demand. These considerations are consistent with epidemiologic data that both PP and presence of LVH are strongly predictive of coronary events.

The Hypertension Optimal Treatment (HOT) trial was designed to prospectively answer the question of whether intensive lowering of DBP would increase cardiovascular events, and it remains one of only large trials to randomly assign patients to more than two BP targets.[8] Only among diabetic patients with the lowest DBP target was the cardiovascular risk the lowest; overall, there was a small increase in major cardiovascular events, MI, and cardiovascular mortality (but

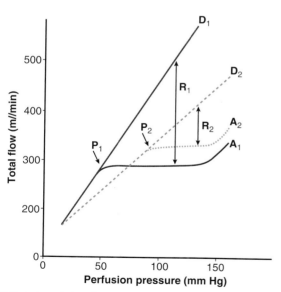

FIG. 31.3 Autoregulation of coronary blood flow and myocardial flow reserve in the presence of LV hypertrophy (LVH). A_1 represents total coronary blood flow over a range of perfusion pressures. P_1 is the lower limit of the autoregulatory range, and D_1 is the pressure-flow relationship in the maximally dilated coronary bed. At any given perfusion pressure, the coronary flow reserve is R_1. A_2, P_2, D_2, and R_2 represent corresponding values in patients with hypertension and LVH. At any given perfusion pressure, coronary flow reserve is less in the hypertensive/hypertrophied hearts, thus increasing the vulnerability of the myocardium to ischemia, especially during exercise or any other situation requiring increased coronary flow. Moreover, the lower limit of coronary autoregulation is shifted to the right (P_1 to P_2) in the hypertensive heart, thereby increasing the vulnerability to a severe drop in perfusion pressure. *(Adapted from Hoffman JIE. A critical view of coronary reserve. Circulation. 1987;75[Suppl I]:I6.)*

not for stroke or renal failure) with DBP 80 or less mm Hg. This finding suggests a unique myocardial susceptibility to low diastolic perfusion pressures because, in contrast to the cerebral circulation, there is maximal oxygen extraction by the myocardium, which therefore cannot compensate for a reduced flow by increasing oxygen extraction. This concept would seem to be supported by the notion that whereas stroke morbidity and mortality is best correlated with the level of mean BP, the best predictor of coronary events seems to be PP. PP is usually greatest in isolated systolic hypertension, in which the DBP is "normal" and often below 80 mm Hg, even before treatment. However, in the elderly with isolated systolic hypertension and low DBP, no J-shaped curve has been described with antihypertensive therapy, even when DBP is reduced from baseline. In addition, a previous meta-analysis suggests that the increased mortality of patients with very low DBP (<65 mm Hg) may be unrelated to antihypertensive treatment and not specific to BP-related events.[45] This evidence highlights the primary argument against the evidence supporting a J-curve at BPs achieved in clinical trial or epidemiologic data; that is, that reverse causality explains the apparent relationship observed in some studies between lower DBP and greater risk of adverse outcomes. In other words, poor health, including poor LV function, leading to a low BP and increased risk of death provide alternative explanations for the J-shaped curve.

Two recent trials are especially noteworthy in the discussion of BP targets. In the Action to Control Cardiovascular Risk in Diabetes (ACCORD) study, 4733 patients with type 2 diabetes were randomly assigned to intensive therapy, targeting an SBP less than 120 mm Hg, or standard therapy, targeting an SBP less than 140 mm Hg, for a mean period of 4.7 years.[46] No significant difference was observed between the two BP target groups in the primary outcome (first occurrence of nonfatal MI, nonfatal stroke, and cardiovascular death), although stroke was modestly reduced (absolute risk reduction, 0.2% per year) at the expense of an increase in treatment-related adverse experiences. The latter led the investigators to conclude that there was no overall advantage to targeting an SBP of less than 120 mm Hg. A recent reanalysis of ACCORD suggests, however, that intensive SBP reduction, with or without intensive glycemic control, was associated with a reduction in the primary outcome, when compared with standard BP and standard glycemic control.[47]

In the Systolic blood PRessure INtervention Trial (SPRINT), more than 9300 patients with hypertension and one or more other cardiovascular risk factor, but without diabetes, were randomly assigned to an intensive SBP goal (<120 mm Hg) or standard SBP goal (<140 mm Hg) for a median of 3.3 years.[48] The trial was ended prematurely on the basis of a 25% lower risk of the primary outcome (first occurrence of MI, other acute coronary syndromes, stroke, HF, or death from cardiovascular causes) and a 27% lower risk of all-cause death in patients treated to an intensive versus standard SBP goal. The risk of HF and death attributed to cardiovascular causes were also lower, the latter being primarily attributable to fewer CHD and sudden cardiac deaths. Serious adverse events, overall, were similar between the treatment arms. Unfortunately, data on the subgroup of patients with prior CAD, MI, or other IHD findings with angina were not provided so it not possible to reach conclusions about lower BP targets in this important subgroup of hypertensive patients. Furthermore, because enrollment targets for women were not met, and the primary outcome was not significantly reduced with the lower BP target among women, it is not possible to reach a conclusion regarding women.

Previous recommendations have specified a goal BP less than 140/90 mm Hg in patients who have no evidence of CAD and proposed that less than 130/80 mm Hg be targeted for those patients without documented CAD, but with high risk for the development of CAD.[10] Given the recent SPRINT trial

results, lower systolic BP goals (i.e., <120 mm Hg) may be considered in patients without CAD, but who are at high risk for developing CAD. However, caution is warranted because such an aggressive goal will require multidrug regimens.[48] Because many of the patients at high risk for developing CAD have isolated systolic hypertension, and thus lower baseline DBP, it seems prudent to lower the DBP slowly and caution is advised in inducing large DBP falls, particularly in patients aged over 60 years.

MANAGEMENT OF HYPERTENSION IN PATIENTS WITH ESTABLISHED CORONARY ARTERY DISEASE

The following sections discuss management of hypertension in various forms of CAD, with a focus on pharmacologic therapy. Pharmacologic recommendations from the 2015 American Heart Association (AHA)/American College of Cardiology (ACC)/American Society of Hypertension (ASH) Scientific Statement are summarized in Table 31.1.

Stable Angina

Hypertension increases the risk of acute coronary events in patients with chronic stable angina because of the enhanced myocardial oxygen demand created by elevations in BP, especially SBP, and LVH, if present. The primary goals of antihypertensive treatment in patients with symptomatic CAD are preventing MI and death and reducing the symptoms of angina and the occurrence of ischemia. In addition to BP control, treatment of risk factors includes smoking cessation, diabetes management, exercise training, lipid management, and weight reduction in obese patients. Antiplatelet agents should also be strongly considered. Other important therapies are short-acting or long-acting nitrates. Antihypertensive therapy roles

TABLE 31.1 Pharmacologic Treatments for Hypertension in Patients With Coronary Artery Disease

DRUG/CLASS	STABLE ANGINA	ACUTE CORONARY SYNDROME	HEART FAILURE
ACE inhibitor or ARB	1[a]	1[a]	1
Diuretic[b]	1	1	1
Beta-blocker	1	1[c]	1[d]
Non-DHP CCB	2	2	
DHP CCB	2	2	
Nitrates	1	2	2
Aldosterone antagonist	2	2	1
Hydralazine/isosorbide dinitrate			2[e]

Numbers represent first-line or second-line therapy, as recommended by the 2015 American Heart Association/American College of Cardiology/American Society of Hypertension Scientific Statement.
[a]Preference given for patients with prior myocardial infarction, left ventricular systolic dysfunction, diabetes, or proteinuric chronic kidney disease.
[b]Chlorthalidone preferred, or loop diuretic (any) in patients with symptomatic heart failure or an estimated glomerular filtration rate less than 30 mL/min^2.
[c]Esmolol intravenously, or metoprolol or bisoprolol orally.
[d]Carvedilol, metoprolol succinate, or bisoprolol.
[e]Hydralazine alone should be avoided in patients with hypertension and ischemic heart disease; data supporting combination hydralazine/isosorbide dinitrate are limited and most patients in clinical trials did not have ischemic coronary artery disease.
(Rosendorff C, Lackland DT, Allison M, et al. Treatment of hypertension in patients with coronary artery disease: A scientific statement from the American Heart Association, American College of Cardiology, and American Society of Hypertension. J Am Coll Cardiol. 2015;65:1998-2038.)
ACE, Angiotensin-converting enzyme; ARB, angiotensin (AT$_2$) receptor blocker; CCB, calcium channel blocker; DHP, dihydropyridine.

are summarized in Table 31.1 and described later. Current AHA/ACC/ASH guidelines recommend beta-blockers, CCBs, and nitrates for angina, whereas cardiovascular risk reduction can be achieved with a variety of antihypertensive agents.[49] Where feasible, a three-drug regimen consisting of a beta-blocker (in patients with prior MI), an ACE inhibitor, or ARB (in patients with prior MI, LV systolic dysfunction, diabetes, or CKD), and a thiazide diuretic (preferably chlorthalidone) can be considered.

A BP goal less than 140/90 mm Hg is currently recommended in patients with stable angina, or, optionally, less than 130/80 mm Hg in selected patients, including those with previous stroke or transient ischemic attack, carotid artery disease, peripheral arterial disease, or abdominal aortic aneurysm.[49] These guidelines were published before the completion of SPRINT, but as only about 20% of patients enrolled in SPRINT had clinical or subclinical cardiovascular disease, it may be premature to extrapolate the SPRINT findings to those with stable angina or the broader IHD population. As discussed previously, excessive lowering of DBP, in particular, may reduce coronary perfusion, thus increasing myocardial ischemia and coronary events. In the HOT trial, in which patients were randomly assigned to three different DBP goals (≤90 mm Hg, ≤85 mm Hg, or, ≤80 mm Hg), a J-curve relationship was noted between DBP and the combined outcome of all MI and silent MI in the subgroup of 3080 patients with IHD at baseline, whereas no such relationship was observed in the much larger subgroup without IHD at baseline (and, indeed, in the overall trial).[50] Data from other population-based and randomized studies (treated essentially as cohort studies) have similarly observed J-curve relationships among patients with atherosclerotic disease.[51-53] However, given the somewhat conflicting data,[32] and the lack of consistency around any particular BP range, it seems prudent to target at least a BP goal less than 140/90 mm Hg, and perhaps less than 130/80 mm Hg, as recommended by the AHA/ACC/ASH guidelines, until more evidence is available in patients with CAD. Higher goals, for example, less than 150/90 mm Hg as recommended in the 2014 "JNC 8" guidelines for patients aged 60 years or older, may be associated with significantly worse outcomes in patients with established CAD.[54]

Beta-Blockers

Beta-blockers are generally considered first-line agents in patients with symptomatic CAD and hypertension. These drugs reduce angina symptoms and lower BP, primarily owing to their negative inotropic and chronotropic effects. The reduced inotropy and heart rate lower myocardial oxygen demand and the slowing of the heart rate prolongs diastolic perfusion time of the coronary arteries, thus enhancing myocardial blood flow. Blood pressure reduction occurs primarily because of reduced cardiac output, and to a lesser extent, through direct renin inhibition at beta-adrenoreceptors on the renal juxtaglomerular apparatus.

Although the benefits of beta-blockers observed in hypertensive and HF populations are presumed to extend to patients with stable CAD, randomized trials in this population are lacking. Most evidence for beta-blocker use comes from post-MI trials performed in the era before modern reperfusion and pharmacologic therapy.[55] This point is especially salient given that, at least in patients with MI, the relative benefits and harms of beta-blockers appear to differ comparing trials performed in the prereperfusion and reperfusion era.[56] Older trial data suggested significant short-term and longer-term (at least to 1 year) mortality benefits with beta-blocker use post-MI. In contradistinction, data from the reperfusion era, in which patients were also on more optimal medical therapy, generally support only short-term benefits of reduced MI recurrence and reduced angina, but negligible mortality benefit and increased risk of HF and cardiogenic shock. In addition, recent data suggest that the benefits of beta-blockers

may be limited in patients with stable CAD, with or without MI. In a recent propensity-matched analysis of more than 44,000 patients with prior MI, CAD without MI, or only risk factors for CAD, beta-blocker use, compared with other therapies, was not associated with a reduced risk of cardiovascular events, among any of the three patient groups.[57] Interestingly, in those with CAD risk factors only, beta-blocker use was actually associated with a marginally greater risk of MI and stroke, compared with other therapies. Similar efficacy between beta-blockers and CCBs is also supported by the INVEST, which found no difference in outcomes comparing a beta-blocker-HCTZ strategy and nondihydropyridine CCB-ACE inhibitor strategy, and a recent meta-analysis.[31,58]

When contraindications to the use of beta-blockers exist, such as significant bronchospastic disease, severe peripheral vascular disease, or severe bradyarrhythmias (e.g., high degree of AV block or sick sinus syndrome), long-acting nondihydropyridine or dihydropyridine (e.g., amlodipine, felodipine, or long-acting nifedipine) CCBs are appropriate alternatives for angina and hypertension. Short-acting dihydropyridine CCBs have the potential to enhance the risk of adverse cardiac events and should be avoided. In general, beta-blockers can be used safely in patients with chronic obstructive pulmonary disease and usually in those with mild bronchospastic disease. In stable LV failure, beta-blockers (ie, carvedilol, metoprolol succinate, or bisoprolol) may be used as a component of the anti-HF therapy, but should be started at a very low dose and titrated slowly to reduce the risk of adverse events.

Calcium Channel Blockers

CCBs, especially dihydropyridine CCBs, decrease peripheral resistance, thus reducing BP and LV wall tension as well as decreasing myocardial oxygen consumption. These drugs also lower coronary resistance, thereby enhancing myocardial oxygen supply, and they are especially useful for coronary spasm, as in variant (Prinzmetal) angina, as well as peripheral artery spasm (Raynaud phenomenon). Nondihydropyridine CCBs have the additional benefit of decreasing heart rate.

Studies of CCBs in patients with CAD, including stable angina, specifically, have generally concluded that CCBs have similar efficacy to beta-blockers on controlling angina and reducing major adverse outcomes, including death.[31,59,60] Meta-analyses with varying inclusion criteria for trials in patients with CAD have confirmed these findings.[61,62] Nevertheless, CCBs generally are recommended as second-line therapy, either as an alternative for patients unable to use a beta-blocker, or as adjunctive therapy when BP remains elevated or when angina persists despite beta-blocker use.[49] The addition of a dihydropyridine CCB to beta-blocker therapy enhances antianginal and antihypertensive efficacy and reduces cardiovascular events.[32] Because of the increased risk of severe bradycardia or heart block if beta-blockers are used together with verapamil or diltiazem, long-acting dihydropyridine CCBs are preferred for combination therapy. Nondihydropyridine CCBs and nifedipine should generally be avoided in patients with LV systolic dysfunction or HF, whereas longer-acting dihydropyridine CCBs are acceptable.

Renin-Angiotensin Aldosterone System Inhibitors

ACE inhibitors are considered first-line therapy in all patients with stable angina and hypertension, unless contraindicated. In the HOPE trial, treatment with ramipril was associated with around a 20% risk reduction in the primary outcome (MI, stroke, or death as a result of cardiovascular causes) among the around 80% of patients with baseline CAD.[34] Similarly, in the European Trial on Reduction of Cardiac Events with Perindopril in Stable Coronary Artery Disease (EUROPA), addition of perindopril to beta-blocker therapy significantly reduced the risk of cardiovascular events and death, without significantly greater risk of adverse effects, among patients with low-risk stable CAD.[63] In the Survival And Ventricular Enlargement (SAVE) trial, the addition of captopril, compared with the addition of placebo, was associated with around a 20% reduction in risk of all-cause and cardiovascular mortality among patients with LV systolic dysfunction (but not overt HF or symptomatic myocardial ischemia) who were 3 to 16 days post-MI.[64] On the basis of these trials, it is reasonable to include an ACE inhibitor in the management of all patients with symptomatic CAD. ARBs can be used in patients who are intolerant of ACE inhibitors. Although evidence supporting their interchangeability in patients with stable angina, per se, are lacking, valsartan has been shown to be noninferior to captopril in preventing all-cause death among patients 0.5 to 10 days post-MI.[65]

Aldosterone antagonists should be prescribed for post-MI patients without significant renal dysfunction (serum creatinine ≥2.5 mg/dL in men and ≥2.0 mg/dL in women) or hyperkalemia (serum potassium ≥5.0 mEq/L), or for those who are already receiving therapeutic doses of an ACE inhibitor (or ARB) and a beta-blocker, have a LVEF 40% or less, and have either DM or HF. Importantly, hyperkalemia is a dose-dependent effect for ACE inhibitors, ARBs, and aldosterone antagonists, and the addition of the latter can increase serum potassium concentration 0.5 or more mEq/L, even at low doses (ie, spironolactone 25 mg once daily).

Acute Coronary Syndromes

Hypertension is common in patients with acute coronary syndrome (ACS), affecting two-thirds of patients with ST-segment elevation MI (STEMI) and between 70% to 80% of patients with non-ST-segment elevation MI (NSTEMI).[49,66] Hypertension management in these patients can be more challenging for several reasons. First, the relationship between BP and outcomes is complex, particularly in the early period following ACS. Previous reports have identified elevated BP as an independent risk factor for mortality post-ACS,[67,68] whereas others have identified elevated BP (up to <200 mm Hg in some cases) on presentation as "protective" against death.[69,70] Substantial elevations in SBP (i.e., approaching and exceeding 200 mm Hg) are hazardous primarily because of their association with intracranial hemorrhage.[71,72] Hemorrhagic stroke risk is especially increased in patients with significantly elevated BP who are given antiplatelet or anticoagulant therapy; thus patients with very elevated SBP must be treated aggressively. However, just as important, several studies have also observed that low BPs, particularly an SBP less than 90 to 100 mm Hg, are much more strongly associated with risk of death than having hypertension or elevated SBP.[69,70,73] Whether or not a patient has a history of hypertension seems to be considerably less important than the actual BP at ACS presentation.[74] Secondly, BPs often fluctuate significantly on ACS presentation (e.g., because of pain), which requires stabilizing the patient before focusing on antihypertensive therapy. Finally, no trials with hard outcomes have prospectively assessed BP lowering in patients with any form of ACS. Thus, BP goals and specific antihypertensive recommendations in this population are largely derived from observational data and trials of antihypertensive therapy assessing benefits independent of BP-lowering.

The goals of therapy for patients with ACS and hypertension are to safely control BP (recognizing that low BP may be prognostically worse than elevated BP), balance myocardial oxygen supply and demand, and prevent subsequent coronary events, disability and death. Data guiding BP targets, either during hospital admission or as an outpatient, are virtually nonexistent and the most recent AHA/ACC/ASH guidelines suggest that "a BP target of less than 130/80 mm Hg at the time of hospital discharge is a reasonable option."[49] Importantly, inpatient BP should be lowered cautiously, particularly in those with only moderately elevated BP, to avoid

significant reduction in SBP (especially to <100 mm Hg). An exaggerated antihypertensive response is not uncommon in patients immediately post-ACS because of vasomotor instability. Likewise, in the outpatient setting, antihypertensive therapy should be initiated cautiously and titrated slowly to avoid substantial reductions in DBP (especially to below 60 mm Hg), particularly in those with isolated systolic hypertension or who otherwise have wide pulse pressures.

The antihypertensive agents with the most compelling evidence for use in patients with hypertension and ACS include beta-blockers, ACE inhibitors, and aldosterone antagonists. Cardioselective beta-blockers absent intrinsic sympathomimetic activity (e.g., metoprolol, atenolol, betaxolol, bisoprolol) should be initiated within 24 hours of symptom onset, or as soon as possible thereafter, in patients who do not have HF, evidence of a low-output state, elevated risk for cardiogenic shock, or other contraindications.[75] Carvedilol, metoprolol succinate, or bisoprolol can be continued in patients with stable HF with reduced systolic function. The most recent AHA/ACC/ASH guidelines recommend continuing beta-blocker therapy for at least 3 years[49]; however, as noted previously, some evidence suggests that the benefits of outpatient beta-blocker therapy occur predominantly in the first year post-MI.[57] These agents reduce infarct size and the occurrence of both sudden cardiac death and subsequent reinfarction. Intravenous beta-blockers should be restricted to those with significant hypertension or tachycardia, ongoing ischemia, and low risk for hemodynamic compromise, and especially avoided in patients with NSTEMI who have risk factors for shock.[49,75]

If beta-blockers are contraindicated, a nondihydropyridine CCB (e.g., verapamil or diltiazem) can be prescribed for angina in patients without significant LV dysfunction. These agents may reduce reinfarction following acute MI (AMI) in patients without LV dysfunction,[76-78] but do not reduce mortality rates in the setting of AMI, and increase mortality in the setting of LV systolic dysfunction or pulmonary edema.[79,80] Verapamil or diltiazem should not be added to beta-blocker therapy because of the risk of bradycardia or heart block. Long-acting dihydropyridine CCBs have not been studied in AMI. Nevertheless, these agents are frequently used as add-on therapy in patients with an AMI when hypertension is not adequately controlled by beta-blockers, ACE inhibitors, and diuretics. Short-acting nifedipine should be avoided in CAD patients, and only used with concomitant heart-rate lowering therapy (i.e., a beta-blocker).[81]

An ACE inhibitor in combination with the beta-blocker is reasonable in most patients with ACS, including any patient with hypertension, as well as in those with normal BP, if the patient has LVEF 40% or less, DM, or CKD. Evidence for the use of ACE inhibitors in NSTEMI or UA are largely extrapolated from the STEMI population, where there is a clear advantage for ACE inhibitors. ACE inhibitor therapy initiated early (0 to 36 hours post-MI) and continued only short-term (4 to 6 weeks) is associated with a reduction in death, regardless of underlying cardiovascular risk.[82] Likewise, in patients with AMI and either HF or LV systolic dysfunction, ACE inhibitor therapy started later (≥3 days following AMI) and continued long-term (≥1 year) is associated with substantial reductions in death, regardless of baseline BP.[83] Importantly, ACE inhibitors should be used cautiously in the acute phase of an MI, especially in those with low SBP (<120 mm Hg) at presentation, in whom critical hypotension or renal dysfunction may be more prone to develop. Short-acting ACE inhibitors (i.e., captopril or enalapril) may be reasonable for initial therapy because BP can rebound relatively quickly following discontinuation of these agents. Thereafter, once-daily ACE inhibitors should be used indefinitely to increase adherence. ARBs can be substituted in patients unable to tolerate an ACE inhibitor and outcomes trials in patients with AMI, LV systolic dysfunction, or otherwise at high cardiovascular risk, support comparable efficacy of these agents.[65,84]

Aldosterone antagonists, which decrease ventricular remodeling and myocardial fibrosis, are appropriate in patients with AMI complicated by LF systolic dysfunction or HF. In the Eplerenone Postacute Myocardial Infarction Heart Failure Efficacy and Survival (EPHESUS) study, eplerenone, as compared with placebo, reduced the risk of all-cause death by 15% and sudden cardiac death by 21%, among patients with AMI and HF and LV systolic dysfunction.[18] Importantly, these results were obtained in patients taking background therapy consisting of an ACE inhibitor or ARB (~86%), beta-blockers (75%), diuretics (~60%), aspirin (~88%), and statins (47%). Spironolactone has not been explicitly studied in patients with ACS, although data from the Randomized Aldactone Evaluation Study (RALES)[15] suggest that this drug is a reasonable (and less expensive) alternative in patients meeting EPHESUS eligibility criteria. Both agents should be avoided in patients with elevated serum creatinine and in those at risk for significant hyperkalemia. Thiazide diuretics are appropriate in patients needing additional BP control or in patients with evidence of increased filling pressures, pulmonary congestion or HF. Patients taking an ACE inhibitor, thiazide diuretic, and an aldosterone antagonist should have frequent measurements of serum potassium, especially during dose titrations.

MANAGEMENT OF HYPERTENSION IN PATIENTS WITH PERIPHERAL ARTERIAL DISEASE

Peripheral arterial disease (PAD) is the third leading cause of death from atherosclerotic disease, ranking behind only CHD and stroke. Because PAD is primarily caused by arteriosclerotic disease, it shares many of the same risk factors as CAD, including hypertension. Large population based studies have found that each 20-mm Hg increase in SBP imparts a 35 to 63% increase in the risk for developing PAD, such that those patients with SBP 180 or higher mm Hg (compared with 115 mm Hg) are at a nearly five-fold increased risk.[85,86] Patients with PAD are at a substantially increased risk for vascular events, including around a 70% increased risk of developing IHD,[86] and an approximately 2.5-fold increased risk of all-cause death.[87] Moreover, the presence of comorbid hypertension and PAD substantially increases the risk of cardiovascular events and death compared with either condition alone.

The goals of therapy in the management of hypertension in PAD include primarily controlling BP and reducing the risk of MI, stroke, HF, and cardiovascular death. In the absence of prospective trials assessing specific BP targets, the most recent guidelines recommend a goal BP less than 140/90 mm Hg in patients with hypertension and PAD and less than 130/80 mm Hg in those who also have DM or CKD.[88,89] However, observational data from the UKPDS study suggest that, at least among patients with type 2 diabetes, on-treatment SBP 130 or higher mm Hg, compared with less than 130 mm Hg is associated with a higher risk of lower extremity amputation or death from peripheral vascular disease and that the risk increases with higher on-treatment BP.[90] In contrast, a post hoc analysis of INVEST data found that the lowest risk of nonfatal MI, nonfatal stroke, or all-cause death occurred at an SBP between 135 and 145 mm Hg and DBP between 60 and 90 mm Hg.[91]

The choice of antihypertensive therapy probably matters less than achieving BP control and otherwise reducing cardiovascular risk. However, very few trials have examined outcomes in patients with PAD and most of these have methodologic or other limitations, making it difficult to draw conclusions on specific agents or classes. No large outcomes trials have been performed specifically in patients with hypertension and PAD. The most commonly used agents generally include ACE inhibitors (or ARBs), which have the most compelling evidence, as well as beta-blockers, diuretics, and CCBs.

Among 4051 patients with PAD in the HOPE trial, treatment with an ACE inhibitor, compared with placebo, reduced the risk of the primary outcome (MI, stroke, or death from cardiovascular causes) by more than 20%, probably reflecting the benefits of BP-lowering rather than a class-specific effect.[34] Nevertheless, on the basis of this trial, ACE inhibitors are a reasonable first-line option for patients with PAD. However, caution is warranted with these agents given the relatively high frequency of renal artery stenosis in patients with PAD. Beta-blockers do not increase the risk of claudication and can be used in patients with PAD, particularly those with other indications for therapy (i.e., stable angina or post-MI).

CONCLUSION

In primary and secondary prevention of CAD and in PAD in patients with arterial hypertension, BP lowering to at least less than 140/90 mm Hg is critical. Care should be exercised in lowering the DBP too low too quickly in patients with significant occlusive CAD. Recent meta-analyses suggest that all major BP-lowering classes have a similar effect in primary prevention of CHD events and stroke, and that the critical issue is BP lowering, independent of drug class. Nevertheless, it seems reasonable to recommend the use of an ACE inhibitor, usually with a thiazide diuretic, or an ACE inhibitor with a CCB, as first-line drugs in the primary prevention of CAD events in patients with hypertension. Treatment choices for the patient with hypertension and established CAD are more straightforward. Beta-blockers are effective in the management of hypertension with angina. Nondihydropyridine CCBs (verapamil or diltiazem) are an appropriate alternative if beta-blockers are contraindicated or not tolerated. If both classes of drug are needed for angina or hypertension control, then a long-acting dihydropyridine CCB should be used. An ACE inhibitor should also be included in the regimen. In ACS, therapy of the hypertension should include beta-blockers with an ACE inhibitor, especially in LV dysfunction. An ARB may be used as an alternative to ACE inhibitors in all situations, although the clinical trial data for ARBs are not as robust as those for ACE inhibitors. A thiazide diuretic and/or dihydropyridine CCB can be added for BP control. Verapamil or diltiazem may be used as alternatives to beta-blockers in unstable angina, but should not be used together with beta-blockers, or if there is depressed LV function or in AMI. In patients with PAD, BP control is most important and the specific choice of antihypertensive agents often depends on the patient's comorbid conditions.

References

1. Moran AE, Forouzanfar MH, Roth GA, et al. The global burden of ischemic heart disease in 1990 and 2010: the Global Burden of Disease 2010 study. *Circulation.* 2014;129:1493-1501.
2. Murray CJ, Vos T, Lozano R, et al. Disability-adjusted life years (DALYs) for 291 diseases and injuries in 21 regions, 1990-2010: a systematic analysis for the Global Burden of Disease Study 2010. *Lancet.* 2012;380:2197-2223.
3. Kochanek KD, Murphy SL, Xu J, Arias E. Mortality in the United States, 2013. *NCHS Data Brief.* 2014;(178):1-8.
4. Centers for Medicare and Medicaid Services. *Chronic Conditions among Medicare Beneficiaries.* Baltimore: Chartbook; 2012.
5. Franklin SS, Larson MG, Khan SA, et al. Does the relation of blood pressure to coronary heart disease risk change with aging? The Framingham Heart Study. *Circulation.* 2001;103:1245-1249.
6. Lewington S, Clarke R, Qizilbash N, Peto R, Collins R. Age-specific relevance of usual blood pressure to vascular mortality: a meta-analysis of individual data for one million adults in 61 prospective studies. *Lancet.* 2002;360:1903-1913.
7. Mitchell GF. Arterial stiffness and hypertension: chicken or egg? *Hypertension.* 2014;64:210-214.
8. Hansson L, Zanchetti A, Carruthers SG, et al. Effects of intensive blood-pressure lowering and low-dose aspirin in patients with hypertension: principal results of the Hypertension Optimal Treatment (HOT) randomised trial. HOT Study Group. *Lancet.* 1998;351:1755-1762.
9. Law MR, Morris JK, Wald NJ. Use of blood pressure lowering drugs in the prevention of cardiovascular disease: meta-analysis of 147 randomised trials in the context of expectations from prospective epidemiological studies. *BMJ.* 2009;338:b1665.
10. Rosendorff C, Black HR, Cannon CP, et al. Treatment of hypertension in the prevention and management of ischemic heart disease: a scientific statement from the American Heart Association Council for High Blood Pressure Research and the Councils on Clinical Cardiology and Epidemiology and Prevention. *Circulation.* 2007;115:2761-2788.
11. Psaty BM, Lumley T, Furberg CD, et al. Health outcomes associated with various antihypertensive therapies used as first-line agents: a network meta-analysis. *JAMA.* 2003;289:2534-2544.

12. ALLHAT Officers and Coordinators for the ALLHAT Collaborative Research Group. Major outcomes in high-risk hypertensive patients randomized to angiotensin-converting enzyme inhibitor or calcium channel blocker vs diuretic: The Antihypertensive and Lipid-Lowering Treatment to Prevent Heart Attack Trial (ALLHAT). *JAMA.* 2002;288:2981-2997.

13. Dorsch MP, Gillespie BW, Erickson SR, Bleske BE, Weder AB. Chlorthalidone reduces cardiovascular events compared with hydrochlorothiazide: a retrospective cohort analysis. *Hypertension.* 2011;57:689-694.

14. Roush GC, Holford TR, Guddati AK. Chlorthalidone compared with hydrochlorothiazide in reducing cardiovascular events: systematic review and network meta-analyses. *Hypertension.* 2012;59:1110-1117.

15. Pitt B, Zannad F, Remme WJ, et al. The effect of spironolactone on morbidity and mortality in patients with severe heart failure. Randomized Aldactone Evaluation Study Investigators. *N Engl J Med.* 1999;341:709-717.

16. Batterink J, Stabler SN, Tejani AM, Fowkes CT. Spironolactone for hypertension. *Cochrane Database Syst Rev.* 2010:Cd008169.

17. Williams B, MacDonald TM, Morant S, et al. Spironolactone versus placebo, bisoprolol, and doxazosin to determine the optimal treatment for drug-resistant hypertension (PATHWAY-2): a randomised, double-blind, crossover trial. *Lancet.* 2015;356:2015-2068.

18. Pitt B, Remme W, Zannad F, et al. Eplerenone, a selective aldosterone blocker, in patients with left ventricular dysfunction after myocardial infarction. *N Engl J Med.* 2003;348:1309-1321.

19. Zannad F, McMurray JJ, Krum H, et al. Eplerenone in patients with systolic heart failure and mild symptoms. *N Engl J Med.* 2011;364:11-21.

20. Wiysonge CS, Bradley HA, Volmink J, Mayosi BM, Mbewu A, Opie LH. Beta-blockers for hypertension. *Cochrane Database Syst Rev.* 2012;11:Cd002003.

21. Ettehad D, Emdin CA, Kiran A, et al. Blood pressure lowering for prevention of cardiovascular disease and death: a systematic review and meta-analysis. *Lancet.* 2015;387:957-967.

22. Aronow WS, Fleg JL, Pepine CJ, et al. ACCF/AHA 2011 expert consensus document on hypertension in the elderly: a report of the American College of Cardiology Foundation Task Force on Clinical Expert Consensus documents developed in collaboration with the American Academy of Neurology, American Geriatrics Society, American Society for Preventive Cardiology, American Society of Hypertension, American Society of Nephrology, Association of Black Cardiologists, and European Society of Hypertension. *J Am Coll Cardiol.* 2011;57:2037-2114.

23. Staessen JA, Fagard R, Thijs L, et al. Randomised double-blind comparison of placebo and active treatment for older patients with isolated systolic hypertension. The Systolic Hypertension in Europe (Syst-Eur) Trial Investigators. *Lancet.* 1997;350:757-764.

24. Liu L, Wang JG, Gong L, Liu G, Staessen JA. Comparison of active treatment and placebo in older Chinese patients with isolated systolic hypertension. Systolic Hypertension in China (Syst-China) Collaborative Group. *J Hypertens.* 1998;16(12 Pt 1):1823-1829.

25. Pitt B, Byington RP, Furberg CD, et al. Effect of amlodipine on the progression of atherosclerosis and the occurrence of clinical events. PREVENT Investigators. *Circulation.* 2000;102:1503-1510.

26. Borhani NO, Mercuri M, Borhani PA, et al. Final outcome results of the Multicenter Isradipine Diuretic Atherosclerosis Study (MIDAS). A randomized controlled trial. *JAMA.* 1996;276:785-791.

27. Hansson L, Hedner T, Lund-Johansen P, et al. Randomised trial of effects of calcium antagonists compared with diuretics and beta-blockers on cardiovascular morbidity and mortality in hypertension: the Nordic Diltiazem (NORDIL) study. *Lancet.* 2000;356:359-365.

28. Brown MJ, Palmer CR, Castaigne A, et al. Morbidity and mortality in patients randomised to double-blind treatment with a long-acting calcium-channel blocker or diuretic in the International Nifedipine GITS study: Intervention as a Goal in Hypertension Treatment (INSIGHT). *Lancet.* 2000;356:366-372.

29. Black HR, Elliott WJ, Grandits G, et al. Principal results of the Controlled Onset Verapamil Investigation of Cardiovascular End Points (CONVINCE) trial. *JAMA.* 2003;289:2073-2082.

30. Turnbull F, Collaboration BPLTT. Effects of different blood-pressure-lowering regimens on major cardiovascular events: results of prospectively-designed overviews of randomised trials. *Lancet.* 2003;362:1527-1535.

31. Pepine CJ, Handberg EM, Cooper-DeHoff RM, et al. A calcium antagonist vs a non-calcium antagonist hypertension treatment strategy for patients with coronary artery disease. The International Verapamil-Trandolapril Study (INVEST): a randomized controlled trial. *JAMA.* 2003;290:2805-2816.

32. Nissen SE, Tuzcu EM, Libby P, et al. Effect of antihypertensive agents on cardiovascular events in patients with coronary disease and normal blood pressure: the CAMELOT study: a randomized controlled trial. *JAMA.* 2004;292:2217-2225.

33. Jamerson K, Weber MA, Bakris GL, et al. Benazepril plus amlodipine or hydrochlorothiazide for hypertension in high-risk patients. *N Engl J Med.* 2008;359:2417-2428.

34. Yusuf S, Sleight P, Pogue J, Bosch J, Davies R, Dagenais G. Effects of an angiotensin-converting-enzyme inhibitor, ramipril, on cardiovascular events in high-risk patients. The Heart Outcomes Prevention Evaluation Study Investigators. *N Engl J Med.* 2000;342:145-153.

35. MacMahon S, Sharpe N, Gamble G, et al. Randomized, placebo-controlled trial of the angiotensin-converting enzyme inhibitor, ramipril, in patients with coronary or other occlusive arterial disease. PART-2 Collaborative Research Group. Prevention of Atherosclerosis with Ramipril. *J Am Coll Cardiol.* 2000;36:438-443.

36. Hansson L, Lindholm LH, Niskanen L, et al. Effect of angiotensin-converting-enzyme inhibition compared with conventional therapy on cardiovascular morbidity and mortality in hypertension: the Captopril Prevention Project (CAPPP) randomised trial. *Lancet.* 1999;353:611-616.

37. UK Prospective Diabetes Study Group. Efficacy of atenolol and captopril in reducing risk of macrovascular and microvascular complications in type 2 diabetes: UKPDS 39. UK Prospective Diabetes Study Group. *BMJ.* 1998;317:713-720.

38. Estacio RO, Jeffers BW, Hiatt WR, Biggerstaff SL, Gifford N, Schrier RW. The effect of nisoldipine as compared with enalapril on cardiovascular outcomes in patients with non-insulin-dependent diabetes and hypertension. *N Engl J Med.* 1998;338:645-652.

39. Malmqvist K, Ohman KP, Lind L, Nystrom F, Kahan T. Long-term effects of irbesartan and atenolol on the renin-angiotensin-aldosterone system in human primary hypertension: the Swedish Irbesartan Left Ventricular Hypertrophy Investigation versus Atenolol (SILVHIA). *J Cardiovasc Pharmacol.* 2003;42:719-726.

40. Dahlof B, Devereux RB, Kjeldsen SE, et al. Cardiovascular morbidity and mortality in the Losartan Intervention For Endpoint reduction in hypertension study (LIFE): a randomised trial against atenolol. *Lancet.* 2002;359:995-1003.

41. Julius S, Kjeldsen SE, Weber M, et al. Outcomes in hypertensive patients at high cardiovascular risk treated with regimens based on valsartan or amlodipine: the VALUE randomised trial. *Lancet.* 2004;363:2022-2031.

42. Yusuf S, Teo K, Anderson C, et al. Effects of the angiotensin-receptor blocker telmisartan on cardiovascular events in high-risk patients intolerant to angiotensin-converting enzyme inhibitors: a randomised controlled trial. *Lancet.* 2008;372:1174-1183.

43. Bloch MJ, Basile JN. In angiotensin-converting enzyme inhibitor-intolerant individuals, the angiotensin receptor blocker telmisartan does not reduce the incidence of major cardiovascular events in high-risk patients: lessons learned from the Telmisartan Randomized Assessment Study in ACE-Intolerant Subjects with Cardiovascular Disease (TRANSCEND). *J Clin Hypertens (Greenwich).* 2008;10:876-880.

44. Kannel WB, Wilson PW, Nam BH, D'Agostino RB, Li J. A likely explanation for the J-curve of blood pressure cardiovascular risk. *Am J Cardiol.* 2004;94:380-384.

45. Boutitie F, Gueyffier F, Pocock S, Fagard R, Boissel JP. J-shaped relationship between blood pressure and mortality in hypertensive patients: new insights from a meta-analysis of individual-patient data. *Ann Intern Med.* 2002;136:438-448.

46. Cushman WC, Evans GW, Byington RP, et al. Effects of intensive blood-pressure control in type 2 diabetes mellitus. *N Engl J Med.* 2010;362:1575-1585.

47. Margolis KL, O'Connor PJ, Morgan TM, et al. Outcomes of combined cardiovascular risk factor management strategies in type 2 diabetes: the ACCORD randomized trial. *Diabetes Care.* 2014;37:1721-1728.

48. Wright JT, Jr., Williamson JD, Whelton PK, et al. A Randomized Trial of Intensive versus Standard Blood-Pressure Control. *N Engl J Med.* 2015;373:2103-2116.

49. Rosendorff C, Lackland DT, Allison M, et al. Treatment of hypertension in patients with coronary artery disease: A scientific statement from the American Heart Association, American College of Cardiology, and American Society of Hypertension. *J Am Coll Cardiol.* 2015;65:1998-2038.

50. Cruickshank JM. Antihypertensive treatment and the J-curve. *Cardiovasc Drugs Ther.* 2000;14:373-379.

51. Messerli FH, Mancia G, Conti CR, et al. Dogma disputed: can aggressively lowering blood pressure in hypertensive patients with coronary artery disease be dangerous? *Ann Intern Med.* 2006;144:884-893.

52. Bangalore S, Messerli FH, Wun CC, et al. J-curve revisited: An analysis of blood pressure and cardiovascular events in the Treating to New Targets (TNT) Trial. *Eur Heart J.* 2010;31:2897-2908.

53. Dorresteijn JA, van der Graaf Y, Spiering W, Grobbee DE, Bots ML, Visseren FL. Relation between blood pressure and vascular events and mortality in patients with manifest vascular disease: J-curve revisited. *Hypertension.* 2012;59:14-21.

54. Bangalore S, Gong Y, Cooper-DeHoff RM, Pepine CJ, Messerli FH. 2014 Eighth Joint National Committee panel recommendation for blood pressure targets revisited: results from the INVEST study. *J Am Coll Cardiol.* 2014;64:784-793.

55. Winchester DE, Pepine CJ. Usefulness of Beta blockade in contemporary management of patients with stable coronary heart disease. *Am J Cardiol.* 2014;114:1607-1612.

56. Bangalore S, Makani H, Radford M, et al. Clinical outcomes with beta-blockers for myocardial infarction: a meta-analysis of randomized trials. *Am J Med.* 2014;127:939-953.

57. Bangalore S, Steg G, Deedwania P, et al. β-Blocker use and clinical outcomes in stable outpatients with and without coronary artery disease. *JAMA.* 2012;308:1340-1349.

58. Shu de F, Dong BR, Lin XF, Wu TX, Liu GJ. Long-term beta blockers for stable angina: systematic review and meta-analysis. *Eur J Prev Cardiol.* 2012;19:330-341.

59. Dargie HJ, Ford I, Fox KM. Total Ischaemic Burden European Trial (TIBET). Effects of ischaemia and treatment with atenolol, nifedipine SR and their combination on outcome in patients with chronic stable angina. The TIBET Study Group. *Eur Heart J.* 1996;17:104-112.

60. Rehnqvist N, Hjemdahl P, Billing E, et al. Effects of metoprolol vs verapamil in patients with stable angina pectoris. The Angina Prognosis Study in Stockholm (APSIS). *Eur Heart J.* 1996;17:76-81.

61. Heidenreich PA, McDonald KM, Hastie T, et al. Meta-analysis of trials comparing beta-blockers, calcium antagonists, and nitrates for stable angina. *JAMA.* 1999;281:1927-1936.

62. Bangalore S, Parkar S, Messerli FH. Long-acting calcium antagonists in patients with coronary artery disease: a meta-analysis. *Am J Med.* 2009;122:356-365.

63. Bertrand ME, Ferrari R, Remme WJ, Simoons ML, Fox KM. Perindopril and beta-blocker for the prevention of cardiac events and mortality in stable coronary artery disease patients: A European trial on Reduction of cardiac events with Perindopril in stable coronary Artery disease (EUROPA) subanalysis. *Am Heart J.* 2015;170:1092-1098.

64. Pfeffer MA, Braunwald E, Moye LA, et al. Effect of captopril on mortality and morbidity in patients with left ventricular dysfunction after myocardial infarction. Results of the survival and ventricular enlargement trial. The SAVE Investigators. *N Engl J Med.* 1992;327:669-677.

65. Pfeffer MA, McMurray JJ, Velazquez EJ, et al. Valsartan, captopril, or both in myocardial infarction complicated by heart failure, left ventricular dysfunction, or both. *N Engl J Med.* 2003;349:1893-1906.

66. Diercks DB, Owen KP, Kontos MC, et al. Gender differences in time to presentation for myocardial infarction before and after a national women's cardiovascular awareness campaign: a temporal analysis from the Can Rapid Risk Stratification of Unstable Angina Patients Suppress ADverse Outcomes with Early Implementation (CRUSADE) and the National Cardiovascular Data Registry Acute Coronary Treatment and Intervention Outcomes Network-Get with the Guidelines (NCDR ACTION Registry-GWTG). *Am Heart J.* 2010;160:80-87.e3.

67. Newby LK, Bhapkar MV, White HD, et al. Predictors of 90-day outcome in patients stabilized after acute coronary syndromes. *Eur Heart J.* 2003;24:172-181.

68. Antman EM, Cohen M, Bernink PJ, et al. The TIMI risk score for unstable angina/non-ST elevation MI: A method for prognostication and therapeutic decision making. *JAMA.* 2000;284:835-842.

69. Shlomai G, Kopel E, Goldenberg I, Grossman E. The association between elevated admission systolic blood pressure in patients with acute coronary syndrome and favorable early and late outcomes. *J Am Soc Hypertens.* 2015;9:97-103.

70. Chin CT, Chen AY, Wang TY, et al. Risk adjustment for in-hospital mortality of contemporary patients with acute myocardial infarction: the acute coronary treatment and intervention outcomes network (ACTION) registry-get with the guidelines (GWTG) acute myocardial infarction mortality model and risk score. *Am Heart J.* 2011;161:113-122.e112.

71. Mathews R, Peterson ED, Chen AY, et al. In-hospital major bleeding during ST-elevation and non-ST-elevation myocardial infarction care: derivation and validation of a model from the ACTION Registry(R)-GWTG. *Am J Cardiol.* 2011;107:1136-1143.

72. Subherwal S, Bach RG, Chen AY, et al. Baseline risk of major bleeding in non-ST-segment-elevation myocardial infarction: the CRUSADE (Can Rapid risk stratification of Unstable angina patients Suppress ADverse outcomes with Early implementation of the ACC/AHA Guidelines) Bleeding Score. *Circulation.* 2009;119:1873-1882.

73. Granger CB, Goldberg RJ, Dabbous O, et al. Predictors of hospital mortality in the global registry of acute coronary events. *Arch Intern Med.* 2003;163:2345-2353.

74. Lee D, Goodman SG, Fox KA, et al. Prognostic significance of presenting blood pressure in non-ST-segment elevation acute coronary syndrome in relation to prior history of hypertension. *Am Heart J.* 2013;166:716-722.

75. Amsterdam EA, Wenger NK, Brindis RG, et al. 2014 AHA/ACC guideline for the management of patients with non-ST-elevation acute coronary syndromes: a report of the American College of Cardiology/American Heart Association Task Force on Practice Guidelines. *Circulation.* 2014;130:e344-e426.

76. Pepine CJ, Faich G, Makuch R. Verapamil use in patients with cardiovascular disease: an overview of randomized trials. *Clin Cardiol*. 1998;21:633-641.
77. Gibson RS, Boden WE, Theroux P, et al. Diltiazem and reinfarction in patients with non-Q-wave myocardial infarction. Results of a double-blind, randomized, multicenter trial. *N Engl J Med*. 1986;315:423-429.
78. Smith NL, Reiber GE, Psaty BM, et al. Health outcomes associated with beta-blocker and diltiazem treatment of unstable angina. *J Am Coll Cardiol*. 1998;32:1305-1311.
79. Multicenter Diltiazem Postinfarction Trial Research Group. The effect of diltiazem on mortality and reinfarction after myocardial infarction. *N Engl J Med*. 1988;319:385-392.
80. Danish Study Group on Verapamil in Myocardial Infarction. Effect of verapamil on mortality and major events after acute myocardial infarction (the Danish Verapamil Infarction Trial II–DAVIT II). *Am J Cardiol*. 1990;66:779-785.
81. Holland Interuniversity Nifedipine/Metoprolol Trial (HINT) Research Group. Early treatment of unstable angina in the coronary care unit: a randomised, double blind, placebo controlled comparison of recurrent ischaemia in patients treated with nifedipine or metoprolol or both. Report of The Holland Interuniversity Nifedipine/Metoprolol Trial (HINT) Research Group. *Br Heart J*. 1986;56:400-413.
82. ACE Inhibitor Myocardial Infarction Collaborative Group. Indications for ACE inhibitors in the early treatment of acute myocardial infarction: systematic overview of individual data from 100,000 patients in randomized trials. *Circulation*. 1998;97:2202-2212.
83. Flather MD, Yusuf S, Kober L, et al. Long-term ACE-inhibitor therapy in patients with heart failure or left-ventricular dysfunction: a systematic overview of data from individual patients. ACE-Inhibitor Myocardial Infarction Collaborative Group. *Lancet*. 2000;355:1575-1581.
84. Yusuf S, Teo KK, Pogue J, et al. Telmisartan, ramipril, or both in patients at high risk for vascular events. *N Engl J Med*. 2008;358:1547-1559.
85. Rapsomaniki E, Timmis A, George J, et al. Blood pressure and incidence of twelve cardiovascular diseases: lifetime risks, healthy life-years lost, and age-specific associations in 1.25 million people. *Lancet*. 2014;383:1899-1911.
86. Emdin CA, Anderson SG, Callender T, et al. Usual blood pressure, peripheral arterial disease, and vascular risk: cohort study of 4.2 million adults. *BMJ*. 2015;351:h4865.
87. Pande RL, Perlstein TS, Beckman JA, Creager MA. Secondary prevention and mortality in peripheral artery disease: National Health and Nutrition Examination Study, 1999 to 2004. *Circulation*. 2011;124:17-23.
88. Hirsch AT, Haskal ZJ, Hertzer NR, et al. ACC/AHA 2005 Practice Guidelines for the management of patients with peripheral arterial disease (lower extremity, renal, mesenteric, and abdominal aortic): a collaborative report from the American Association for Vascular Surgery/Society for Vascular Surgery, Society for Cardiovascular Angiography and Interventions, Society for Vascular Medicine and Biology, Society of Interventional Radiology, and the ACC/AHA Task Force on Practice Guidelines (Writing Committee to Develop Guidelines for the Management of Patients With Peripheral Arterial Disease): endorsed by the American Association of Cardiovascular and Pulmonary Rehabilitation; National Heart, Lung, and Blood Institute; Society for Vascular Nursing; TransAtlantic Inter-Society Consensus; and Vascular Disease Foundation. *Circulation*. 2006;113:e463-e654.
89. Norgren L, Hiatt WR, Dormandy JA, Nehler MR, Harris KA, Fowkes FG. Inter-Society Consensus for the Management of Peripheral Arterial Disease (TASC II). *J Vasc Surg*. 2007;45(Suppl S):S5-S67.
90. Adler AI, Stratton IM, Neil HA, et al. Association of systolic blood pressure with macrovascular and microvascular complications of type 2 diabetes (UKPDS 36): prospective observational study. *BMJ*. 2000;321:412-419.
91. Bavry AA, Anderson RD, Gong Y, et al. Outcomes Among hypertensive patients with concomitant peripheral and coronary artery disease: findings from the INternational VErapamil-SR/Trandolapril STudy. *Hypertension*. 2010;55:48-53.

32 Heart Failure

Kunal N. Karmali and Clyde W. Yancy

The burden of heart failure remains ever present with a long-standing, inexorable association with hypertension. Though advances in evidence-based medical therapy for reduced ejection fraction heart failure have led to impressive reductions in morbidity and mortality, the residual burden of disease remains significant.

Heart failure is recognized as any condition characterized by a mismatched relationship between metabolic, exercise, and/or cognitive needs and cardiac performance.[1] Several important phenotypes have been clearly identified: heart failure with reduced ejection fraction (HFrEF); heart failure with preserved ejection fraction (HFpEF); and heart failure with either "improved" or "borderline" ejection fraction.[2] Especially for HFrEF, a cogent pathophysiology has been well established. Neurohormonal activation, likely initiated by ventricular deformation from acute or chronic ventricular injury, causes a cascade of maladaptive biologic responses typically characterized by renin-angiotensin-aldosterone and sympathetic nervous system activation. These perturbed systems (and other neurohormonal circuits) perpetuate left ventricular dysfunction through progressive remodeling, that is, changes in both shape and size, followed by a deterioration of systolic performance.[1] Disease severity varies from the complete absence of any symptoms of heart failure (New York Heart Association, or NYHA, class I) through progressive degrees of limitation including symptoms at rest (NYHA class II to IV).[2]

The causes of heart failure are protean. Traditional putative etiologies of left ventricular dysfunction, systolic or diastolic, include coronary artery disease, valvular heart disease, various specific cardiomyopathies, and concomitant arrhythmias leading to tachycardia-induced left ventricular dysfunction. Less frequent but still important causes include metabolic disturbances, such as diabetes and thyroid disease; myocarditis; toxic conditions mostly attributed to chemotherapeutic agents, alcohol, and illicit drugs; and human immunodeficiency virus (HIV). There are many other notable conditions leading to heart failure and like all of the foregoing considerations, there is reasonable evidence of a true causal effect.

Hypertension has traditionally been associated with heart failure, and it has been relatively easy to infer empirically a cause and effect relationship. However, although the evidence is irrefutable that hypertension is a *risk factor* for heart failure it has been less clear that hypertension is a *causal factor* for heart failure. Further, it is important to recognize the unique contribution of hypertension to HFpEF, a phenotype of heart failure which is now the predominant clinical syndrome recognized in hospital settings and responsible for more than 50% of all acute heart failure admissions.[3] Unlike HFrEF where clarity of the pathophysiology exists, the cellular and molecular aspects of the pathophysiology of HFpEF remain elusive. Prevailing considerations implicate fibrosis, ventricular noncompliance, hypertrophy, and ischemia; all of which can be impacted by hypertension.[2] Likely, there is no overarching maladaptive pathway that is the root cause of this important condition, but hypertension when aligned with coronary artery disease, obesity, diabetes and atrial fibrillation, explains the majority of concomitant comorbidities associated with clinical HFpEF.

Therapeutic considerations are clear for HFrEF, but less certain for HFpEF. Management of HFpEF is hindered by the absence of a clear mechanism of left ventricular dysfunction and by the heterogeneity of persons with HFpEF. There are reasonable but not definitive data suggesting a potential benefit of mineralocorticoid receptor antagonists (MCRAs)[4] and early signals that neprilysin inhibition in combination with renin-angiotensin-aldosterone blockade may be helpful.[5] The best guidance continues to prompt a unique focus on concomitant comorbidities, including hypertension, for which evidence-based clinical practice guidelines exist.

For HFrEF, defined treatment algorithms are available and are populated with evidence-based therapies proven to improve outcomes. Recent American College of Cardiology (ACC)/American Heart Association (AHA)/Heart Failure Society of America (HFSA) clinical practice guidelines make clear the importance of both prevailing standard bearers of therapy: angiotensin-converting enzyme (ACE) inhibitors, angiotensin receptor II blocker (ARBs), evidence-based beta-blockers, mineralocorticoid receptor antagonists (MCRAs), hydralazine and isosorbide dinitrate (ISDN), and implantable cardioverter defibrillator/cardiac resynchronization therapy (ICD/CRT); and newer therapies: valsartan/sacubitril and ivabradine.[6] The expected outcomes of optimal therapy for HFrEF are now substantially better than historical expectations. Yet, whether the condition of heart failure is HFrEF, HFpEF or even HF with improved or borderline ejection fraction, it remains clear that prevention is the more preferable intervention.

The American College of Cardiology Foundation (ACCF)/ (AHA) guideline for the management of heart failure has adopted a stepwise progression to characterize the natural history of heart failure.[2] This framework organizes treatment strategies for preventing and controlling risk factors like hypertension (stage A), treating subclinical structural and functional changes like LV hypertrophy and mechanical dysfunction (stage B), and reducing morbidity and mortality in symptomatic heart failure (stages C and D) (Fig. 32.1). This framework emphasizes the importance of intervening early in the progression of heart failure during stages A and B before development of symptoms.

Of all potential strategies that might reduce the incidence of heart failure, none appears to have higher yield than the treatment of hypertension. Thus, a greater exploration of the association of hypertension and heart failure is warranted. In this chapter, we report on: epidemiologic analyses that establish the strong association between hypertension and heart failure; longitudinal and experimental studies that elucidate mechanisms by which hypertension leads to clinical heart failure; and landmark trials in patients with and without

At Risk for Heart Failure — **Heart Failure**

Stage A	Stage B	Stage C	Stage D
High risk for HF but no structural heart disease or symptoms	**Structural heart disease but no symptoms of HF**	**Structural heart disease with prior or current symptoms of HF**	**Refractory HF requiring special intervention**
• Hypertension • Atherosclerotic disease • Diabetes mellitus • Obesity • Metabolic syndrome • Using cardiotoxins • Family history of cardiomyopathy	• Previous myocardial infarction • LV remodeling – LV hypertrophy and low EF • Asymptomatic valvular disease	• Known structural heart disease • Symptoms	• Marked HF symptoms at rest • Recurrent hospitalizations despite guideline-directed medical therapy

FIG. 32.1 Stages in the development of heart failure according to the American College of Cardiology/American Heart Association. *(Adapted from Yancy CW, Jessup M, Bozkurt B, et al. 2013 ACCF/AHA guideline for the management of heart failure: a report of the American College of Cardiology Foundation/American Heart Association Task Force on practice guidelines. Circulation. 2013;128(16):e240-327.)*

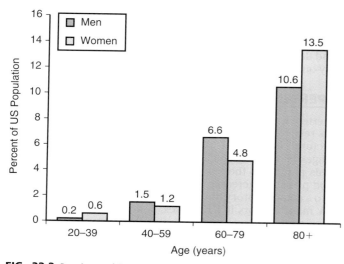

FIG. 32.2 Prevalence of heart failure among men and women aged 20 years and over in the United States from the National Health and Nutrition Examination Survey (2009-2012). Prevalence of heart failure in the United States increases with age. *(Data from Mozaffarian D, Benjamin EJ, Go AS, et al. Heart Disease and Stroke Statistics-2016 Update: A Report from the American Heart Association. Circulation. 2016;133(4):e38-60.)*

clinical heart failure that demonstrate the potent effect of antihypertensive therapy on the prevention of heart failure events in individuals with or at risk for heart failure.

THE HEART FAILURE EPIDEMIC

Worldwide there are 37 million people living with heart failure.[7] In the United States, approximately 5.7 million Americans live with heart failure and prevalence increases with older age (Fig. 32.2). Moreover, each year more than 650,000 new heart failure cases are diagnosed.[8] Although advances in heart failure treatment have improved survival, approximately 50% of people diagnosed with heart failure will die within 5 years.[8] The economic consequences of heart failure are also staggering. Heart failure accounts for more than 1 million hospitalizations each year, and many of the patients with heart failure are at high risk for repeat hospitalization with 30-day readmission rates of 25%.[9] In 2012, total costs for heart failure was estimated to be $30.7 billion. If current trends continue, projections forecast that by 2030, prevalence will increase to more than 8 million individuals, and total costs will increase to $70 billion.[10]

HYPERTENSION IN THE DEVELOPMENT OF HEART FAILURE

Population-based cohorts have played a fundamental role in establishing hypertension as the dominant, modifiable risk factor for heart failure in the general population. The Framingham Heart Study was the first study to describe the association between hypertension and heart failure. During the first 16 years of follow-up in the original Framingham cohort, antecedent hypertension was reported in 75% of the 142 individuals with a new case of heart failure.[11] Subsequent analyses in Framingham reported a two-fold greater hazard for developing heart failure in men with hypertension compared with those without hypertension (hazard ratio [HR] 2.07, 95% confidence interval [CI] 1.34 to 3.20) and a three-fold greater hazard in women (HR 3.35, 95% CI 1.67 to 6.73) (Table 32.1).[12] When coupled with the high prevalence of hypertension in the population, hypertension explained 39% of the population attributable fraction of heart failure in men and 59% in women. Longer-term analyses by Lloyd-Jones et al also highlighted the contribution of hypertension to the lifetime risk of heart failure.[13] Among men and women in Framingham, the lifetime risk of heart failure was approximately 1 in 5 but was twice as great in individuals with blood pressures 160/100 or more mm Hg compared with those with blood pressures less than 140/90 mm Hg (Fig. 32.3).

Cohort analyses have also demonstrated the unique contribution of hypertension to heart failure risk in women. In Lloyd-Jones and colleagues' lifetime risk analysis, the risk of heart failure in men was markedly lower for those without antecedent myocardial infarction. However, lifetime risk of heart failure in women was similar regardless of the history of myocardial infarction. Importantly this observation emphasizes the nonatherosclerotic mechanisms through which heart failure likely occurs in women.[13] Analyses comparing risk factors for HFpEF with HFrEF support these observations by revealing that female sex and systolic blood pressure are both associated with increased odds of HFpEF over HFrEF (odds ratio [OR] 2.29, 95% CI 1.35 to 3.90 and OR 1.13 per 10 mm Hg, 95% CI 1.04 to 1.22, respectively).[14]

In African Americans, hypertension has been implicated as a key risk factor in the racial disparities seen with heart failure.[2] In both the Atherosclerosis Risk in Communities (ARIC) study and the Multi-Ethnic Study of Atherosclerosis (MESA), heart failure incidence was higher in African Americans compared with other race/ethnic groups but differences were attenuated, yet not eliminated, after adjustment for the higher prevalence

TABLE 32.1 Hazard Ratios and Population-Attributable Risk of Multiple Heart Failure Risk Factors in Men and Women From the Framingham Heart Study 1970-1996

RISK FACTOR	MEN		WOMEN	
	Adjusted Hazard Ratio (95% CI)	Population-Attributable Risk, %	Adjusted Hazard Ratio (95% CI)	Population-Attributable Risk, %
Hypertension	2.07 (1.34-3.20)	39	3.35 (1.67-6.73)	59
Myocardial infarction	6.34 (4.61-8.72)	34	6.01 (4.37-8.28)	13
Angina pectoris	1.43 (1.03-1.98)	5	1.68 (1.23-2.30)	5
Diabetes mellitus	1.82 (1.28-2.58)	6	3.73 (2.71-5.15)	12
Left ventricular hypertrophy	2.19 (1.49-3.21)	4	2.85 (1.97-4.12)	5
Valvular heart disease	2.47 (1.70-3.60)	7	2.13 (1.54-2.94)	8

Population-attributable risk was defined as (prevalence × [hazard ratio-1])/(1+ prevalence × [hazard ratio-1]). Hazard ratio is adjusted for angina pectoris, myocardial infarction, diabetes mellitus, left ventricular hypertrophy, and valvular heart disease.
(Adapted from Levy D, Larson MG, Vasan RS, Kannel WB, Ho KK. The progression from hypertension to congestive heart failure. JAMA. 1996;275:1557-1562.)
CI, Confidence interval.

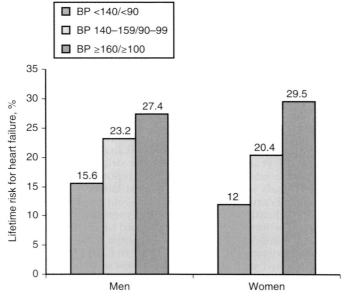

FIG. 32.3 Lifetime risk for heart failure at age 40 years through age 85 years in men and women from the Framingham Heart Study by baseline blood pressure category. Lifetime risk for heart failure is twice as great in individuals with blood pressures ≥160/≥100 mm Hg compared with individuals with blood pressures < 140/<90 mm Hg. *(Data from Lloyd-Jones DM, Larson MG, Leip EP, et al. Lifetime risk for developing congestive heart failure: the Framingham Heart Study. Circulation. 2002;106(24):3068-3072.)*

and poorer treatment of traditional risk factors like hypertension (Table 32.2).[15,16] These findings meet the definition of a true health care disparity in African Americans with hypertension.[17] Baseline characteristics from some of the earliest heart failure trials such as the Veterans Administration Vasodilator Heart Failure Trials (V-HeFT I and II) and the Studies on the Left Ventricular Dysfunction (SOLVD) also highlight the comparatively stronger association of hypertension and weaker association of myocardial infarction with systolic dysfunction in African Americans compared with whites.[18] An even more definitive set of observations emerged from the African American Heart Failure Trial (A-HeFT).[19] In this study of NYHA class II-IV heart failure completed in 1050 African Americans, approximately 50% of participants provided an antecedent history of hypertension whereas fewer than 25% had an overt history of ischemic heart disease as a cause of left ventricular systolic dysfunction.

Data from the Coronary Artery Risk Development in Young Adults study (CARDIA), a population-based cohort of young adults, further underscore how earlier onset and poorer control of hypertension contribute to early heart failure risk in African Americans.[20] Among the 5115 African American and white adults age 18 to 30 years in CARDIA, 26 out of the 27 incident heart failure events at 20 years of follow-up occurred in African Americans. As an additional observation, for every 10 mm Hg higher diastolic blood pressure there was an associated doubling in the hazard for early-onset of heart failure in African Americans (HR 2.1, 95% CI 1.4 to 3.1).[20] These profound data solidify the unique contribution of hypertension to early-onset heart failure in African Americans.

HYPERTENSIVE HEART DISEASE

Hypertensive heart disease describes a spectrum of conditions related to hypertension that progresses from subclinical structural, mechanical, cellular, and extracellular myocardial changes all the way to clinical symptoms of heart failure.[21,22] In this paradigm, the hemodynamic load caused by elevated blood pressure increases left ventricular (LV) wall stress leading to a compensatory thickening of the LV wall and an increase in LV mass. Factors like race, sex, neurohormones, cytokines, and growth factors modulate this hypertrophic response, resulting in fibrosis, myocardial stiffness, mechanical dysfunction, and eventually heart failure (Fig. 32.4).[21]

Left Ventricular Hypertrophy and Remodeling

Although LV hypertrophy can precede hypertension, it is generally considered to be the first step in the development of hypertensive heart disease.[22] Data from the Framingham Heart Study first demonstrated the association between electrocardiogram (ECG)-defined LV hypertrophy and subsequent cardiovascular events.[23] As imaging modalities improved, direct measurement of LV wall thickness and mass with echocardiogram and magnetic resonance imaging (MRI) confirmed the direct and linear association between blood pressure and LV mass, an association that was even stronger using longer-term ambulatory blood pressure monitoring.[24] Epidemiologic studies then demonstrated the association between LV mass and incident cardiovascular disease.[25-27] For example, in the Cardiovascular Health Study (CHS), higher LV mass index on echocardiogram was associated with systolic and diastolic dysfunction and future heart failure risk, independent of the prevalence of incident myocardial infarction.[26] In MESA, Bluemke et al used cardiac MRI to demonstrate the association between higher levels of LV mass and incident heart failure (HR 1.4 per 10% increment, 95% CI 1.2 to 1.5), a risk that primarily occurred in individuals with LV hypertrophy.[27]

Although the stages of hypertensive heart disease suggests a unidirectional progression, randomized trials like the Losartan Intervention for Endpoint Reduction in Hypertension (LIFE) trial have demonstrated that

TABLE 32.2 Heart Failure Incidence Rates per 1000 Person-Years by Race and Gender in the Atherosclerosis Risk in Communities Study, 1987 to 2002

	INCIDENCE RATES PER 1000 PERSON-YEARS OF FOLLOW-UP		UNADJUSTED HAZARD RATIO FOR HEART FAILURE (95% CI)	ADJUSTED HAZARD RATIO FOR HEART FAILURE (95% CI)
	African Americans	Whites		
Men	9.1	6.0	1.38 (1.16-1.63)	0.86 (0.70-1.06)
Women	8.1	3.4	1.96 (1.04-3.67)	0.93 (0.46-1.90)

Hazard ratio is for risk of heart failure in African Americans to whites. After adjustments for traditional risk factors, the higher hazard for African Americans is attenuated. Adjusted hazard ratio is adjusted for age, low-density cholesterol, smoking status, education level, body mass index, serum creatinine, left ventricular hypertrophy by electrocardiography, alcohol use, and time-varying covariates that included diabetes, hypertension, and coronary heart disease.
(Adapted from Loehr LR, Rosamond WD, Chang PP, Folsom AR, Chambless LE. Heart failure incidence and survival [from the Atherosclerosis Risk in Communities study]. Am J Cardiol. 2008;101:1016-1022.)
CI, Confidence interval.

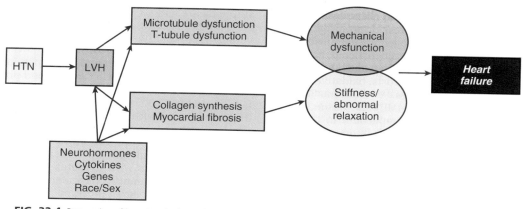

FIG. 32.4 Progression of hypertensive heart disease to heart failure. *HTN,* Hypertension; *LVH,* left ventricular hypertrophy.

antihypertensive agents can reduce LV mass, a finding that is also associated with improved outcomes in post hoc analyses.[28,29] In a meta-analysis of 80 trials comparing the efficacy of different antihypertensive drug classes for reversing LV hypertrophy in hypertensive patients, Klingbiel et al identified that LV mass index decreased by 13% reduction with ARBs, 11% with calcium channel blockers, and 10% with ACE inhibitors.[30]

Systolic and Diastolic Dysfunction

Echocardiography has also played an essential role in elucidating the effects of high blood pressure on cardiac mechanical function leading to clinical heart failure. Although the direct link between hypertension and systolic dysfunction is often complicated by concomitant cardiovascular disease, analyses like those from CHS have demonstrated the direct and stepwise relationship between LV mass and systolic dysfunction, independent of the prevalence of incident myocardial infarction.[31]

Diastolic dysfunction, referring to abnormalities in LV relaxation and filling, is a hallmark of hypertensive heart disease. Because the LV remodels in response to hypertension, cardiac myocytes hypertrophy, and fibrotic changes occur that increase LV stiffness and alter cardiac mechanical properties. In a cross-sectional survey of residents from Australia, diastolic dysfunction was prevalent in 34.7% of adults aged 60 to 86 years and was independently associated with a diagnosis of hypertension (OR 1.5, 95% CI 1.2 to 2.0),[32] an observation that has also been reported in residents from Olmsted County, Minnesota.[33] More recently, Santos et al analyzed data from 4871 participants in ARIC to demonstrate that abnormalities in LV thickness and diastolic parameters even occur in participants with prehypertension (blood pressure of 120 to 139 mm Hg systolic and/or 80 to 89 mm Hg diastolic).[34] In these analyses, prehypertensive participants had higher LV mass indices

and higher rates of mild, moderate, and severe diastolic dysfunction compared with those with optimal blood pressures (blood pressure < 120/80 mm Hg).[34]

In recent years, speckle-tracking echocardiography, which uses computer algorithms to track pixels of imaging data, has emerged as a novel technique to directly measure and quantify myocardial displacement, velocity, and deformation (stretch or contraction).[35] Abnormalities in these measures of cardiac mechanicals have been shown to be precursors of heart failure.[36,37] Choi et al demonstrated in MESA that circumferential strain was associated with future heart failure risk in asymptomatic individuals, even after adjusting for age, diabetes, hypertension, myocardial infarction, LV mass, and LV ejection fraction (HR 1.15 per 1%, 95% CI 1.01 to 1.31).[36] Blood pressure can adversely affect myocardial strain. In CARDIA, Kishi et al demonstrated that cumulative exposure to nonoptimal systolic and diastolic blood pressure in young adulthood was associated with lower longitudinal strain rate and lower early diastolic longitudinal peak strain rate, two preclinical signs of heart failure, at 25 years of follow-up.[38] Few participants in these analyses had blood pressures exceeding conventional treatment thresholds at any point during follow-up, highlighting the implications of blood pressure exposure during the lifespan and the importance of primordial prevention, that is, the prevention of hypertension per se as a means to prevent more overt cardiovascular disease including heart failure.

Cellular and Extracellular Changes

In addition to structural and mechanical changes from hypertension, multiple studies have revealed cellular changes that develop in the setting of hypertension and LV hypertrophy. In animal models of pressure-hypertrophied myocardium, stress loading increased microtubule density leading to abnormalities in cell microarchitecture that impaired myocyte contractile function.[39,40] Transverse (t)-tubules, cell structures that regulate calcium cycling for normal myocyte contractions, have also been linked to hypertensive heart disease.[41] In one study, Wei et al demonstrated that thoracic aortic banding led to t-tubule remodeling early in the development of hypertrophy.[41] This remodeling was present before echocardiographic evidence of LV dysfunction and worsened as heart failure progressed (Fig. 32.5). These findings were also confirmed by Shah et al in hearts from spontaneously hypertensive rats.[42] In response to chronic exposure to elevated blood pressures, t-tubules became disorganized, leading to impairments in intracellular calcium cycling and abnormal myocardial strain before overt evidence of LV dysfunction on echocardiogram.[42] These studies provide a biologic underpinning for ultrastructural cellular changes that lead to abnormal myocardial mechanicals and eventually precede clinical heart failure.

Changes in the extracellular matrix have also been shown to play an important role in the progression from hypertensive heart disease to heart failure. Exogenous administration of deoxycorticosterone acetate, a mineralocorticoid, has been shown in animal models of hypertension and LV-pressure hypertrophy to increase myocardial fibrosis, oxidative stress, diastolic stiffness, and filling pressures.[43,44] Abnormalities in levels of matrix metalloproteinases (MMP) and tissue inhibitors of MMP (TIMP) have also been implicated in the progression of hypertensive heart disease.[45,46] In one study that compared patients with LV hypertrophy to controls, those with hypertension and normal LV structure had normal MMP levels, whereas those with hypertension and LV hypertrophy had an MMP/TIMP profile that favored extracellular matrix degradation and collagen accumulation (low MMP-2 and MMP-13 levels, high MMP-9 levels, and high TIMP-1 levels).[45] Endomyocardial biopsies have confirmed the association between adverse MMP/TIMP levels and cardiac fibrosis and LV dilatation.[46]

Genetic

Given the substantial individual and race/ethnic variability in hypertensive heart disease, there is burgeoning interest in identifying genetic determinants of LV hypertrophy. In both the Hypertension Genetic Epidemiology Network study (HyperGEN) and the Dallas Heart Study, African-American adults with and without hypertension had a two-fold to three-fold greater odds of LV hypertrophy, even after adjusting for cardiovascular risk factors and body mass.[47,48] Although heritability analyses from family-based cohorts such as Framingham and HyperGEN have confirmed heritability of LV mass in both whites and African Americans, the correlations are modest and explain only a small portion of the variance in LV mass.[49,50] Candidate gene-based studies have identified genes that encode proteins involved in LV performance as well as proteins that modify cell signaling, myocyte growth, calcium metabolism, and blood pressure.[51] However, many of these studies are small and include subjects with vastly different ethnicities, limiting reproducibility.[51] Recently, large genome-wide association studies have been used to identify genetic loci associated with LV mass, LV wall thickness, and ECG-evidence of LV hypertrophy.[52,53] Although these genetic investigations offer much hope for targeted, molecular interventions to treat and prevent hypertensive heart disease, much remains to be discovered about the causal variants at or near candidate loci and their functional significance. These epidemiologic, imaging, and mechanistic studies provide a compelling rationale for identifying hypertension as a key risk factor in the progression of heart failure. However, it is the potent and consistent improvement in heart failure outcomes seen in clinical trials with blood pressure-lowering agents that singles out hypertension treatment as a fundamental target of any heart failure prevention strategy.

LANDMARK HYPERTENSION TRIALS TO PREVENT SYMPTOMATIC HEART FAILURE

There are significant data to suggest that the incidence of heart failure may be favorably modified through optimal management of hypertension, especially in those with a higher burden of cardiovascular risk (Table 32.3).[2] The earliest clinical trials testing antihypertensive drugs from the Veterans Administration Cooperative Study Groups reported reductions in heart failure events, but sample size was small and events were few.[54,55] The Systolic Hypertension in Elderly Program (SHEP) was one of the first hypertension trials to include a prespecified endpoint examining the efficacy of antihypertensive therapy (chlorthalidone 12.5 to 25 mg plus atenolol 25 to 50 mg, if needed) in prevention of heart failure.[56] Participants randomized to diuretic-based stepped care had a 49% reduction in fatal and nonfatal heart failure events during an average follow-up of 4.5 years (2.3% versus 4.4%; relative risk [RR] 0.51, 95% CI 0.37 to 0.71).[56] Similarly, in the Hypertension in the Very Elderly Trial (HYVET), randomization to the indapamide plus perindopril (as needed to achieve a target blood pressure of 150/80 mm Hg) group was associated with a 64% reduction in heart failure events (5.3% versus 14.8%; RR 0.36, 95% CI 0.22 to 0.58) compared with placebo at 2 years.[57] Trials such as the Heart Outcomes Prevention Evaluation (HOPE) study demonstrated that ACE inhibitors could also reduce heart failure events in high-risk participants.[58] In the HOPE study, among participants with diabetes mellitus or established vascular disease, ramipril treatment was associated with a 23% reduction in heart failure events (9.0% versus 11.5%, RR 0.77, 95% CI 0.67 to 0.87) after a mean of 4.5 years of follow-up.[58]

The Antihypertensive and Lipid-Lowering Treatment to Prevent Heart Attack Trial (ALLHAT) was one of the largest clinical trials in hypertension management that tested the efficacy of chlorthalidone compared with lisinopril, amlodipine, and doxazosin in 42,418 participants with hypertension and at least one other cardiovascular risk factor.[59] At 3.3 years, the doxazosin comparison was terminated early because of harm.[60] Among the other comparisons, chlorthalidone was associated with a 38% reduction in heart failure (7.7% versus 10.2%; RR 0.62, 95% CI 0.48 to 0.75) compared with amlodipine and was associated with a 19% reduction in heart failure (7.7% versus 8.7%; RR 0.81, 95% CI 0.69 to 0.93) compared with lisinopril at a mean follow-up of 4.9 years. It is notable that ALLHAT included a significant proportion of African-American subjects in whom reduced responsiveness to ACE inhibitor therapy was observed.[59] Sciarreta et al recently confirmed the relative efficacy of thiazide diuretics, especially chlorthalidone, compared with other antihypertensive drug classes for heart failure prevention in a network meta-analysis.[61] In the 26 trials identified, the three most effective antihypertensive drug classes for reducing heart failure were thiazide diuretics, ACE inhibitors, and ARBs (OR 0.59, 95% CI 0.47 to 0.73; OR 0.71, 95% CI 0.59 to 0.85; OR 0.76, 95% CI 0.62 to 0.90; respectively).[61] In direct and indirect comparisons, thiazide diuretics were marginally superior to ACE inhibitors and ARBs; calcium channel blockers, beta-blockers, and alpha blockers were the least effective agents for heart failure prevention.

Other meta-analyses have also focused on the magnitude of blood pressure-lowering as a key driver of heart failure prevention. In a recent high-quality meta-analysis of 123 blood pressure-lowering trials including 613,815 total participants, meta-regression demonstrated that for every 10 mm Hg reduction in systolic blood pressure the risk of heart failure was reduced by 27% (RR 0.72, 95% CI 0.67 to 0.78).[62] However, in this meta-analysis as well, investigators noted the *greater efficacy of thiazide diuretics* and *inferiority of calcium channel*

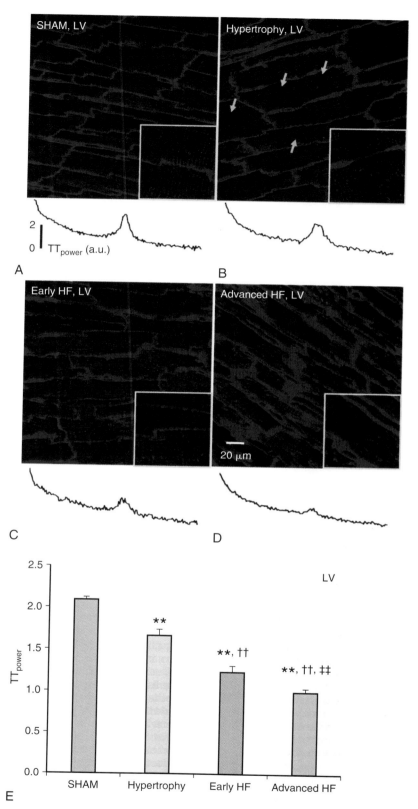

FIG. 32.5 Progressive t-tubule remodeling in rat cardiomyocytes after exposure to thoracic aortic banding pressure-load. The images display representative t-tubule images from the left ventricles of age-matched sham-operated (A), hypertrophic (B), early heart failure (C), and advanced heart failure (D) hearts. In hypertrophic hearts (B) there is loss of t-tubules *(green arrows)* that are more widespread with early and advanced heart failure. The yellow-framed inset is a zoom-in view of an area 40×40 μm from the associated images. Cumulative data for myocyte t-tubule power (TTpower), a measure of t-tubule density, at each stage is summarized (E). *(From Wei S, Guo A, Chen B, et al. T-tubule remodeling during transition from hypertrophy to heart failure. Circ Res. 2010;107(4):520-531.)*

TABLE 32.3 Treatment Effects of Blood Pressure Lowering on Heart Failure Outcomes in Landmark Hypertension Trials

STUDY	NUMBER OF PARTICIPANTS	INCLUSION CRITERIA	INTERVENTION	DURATION (YEARS)	MEAN BP DIFFERENCE BETWEEN GROUPS (mm Hg)	ABSOLUTE RATES OF HEART FAILURE (INTERVENTION VERSUS COMPARATOR)	RELATIVE RISK OF HEART FAILURE (95% CI)
SHEP 1997	4736	Age ≥ 60 years; SBP ≥ 160 mm Hg	Chlorthalidone ± atenolol	4.5	−26.0/−8.9	2.3% versus 4.4%	RR 0.51 (0.37-0.71)
HYVET 2008	3845	Age ≥ 80 years; SBP ≥ 160 mm Hg	Indapamide ± perindopril	2.1	−15.0/−6.1	5.3% versus 14.8%	RR 0.36 (0.22-0.58)
HOPE 2000	9297	Age ≥ 55 years; vascular disease or DM + 1 CV risk factor	Ramipril	4.5	−3/−2	9.0% versus 11.5%	RR 0.77 (0.67-0.87)
ALLHAT 2000, 2002	33,357	Age ≥ 55 years; HTN + 1 CV risk factor	Chlorthalidone versus amlodipine; Chlorthalidone versus lisinopril	4.9	−0.8/+0.8; −2.0/0	7.7% versus 10.2%; 7.7% versus 8.7%	RR 0.62 (0.48-0.75); RR 0.81 (0.69-0.93)
SPRINT 2015	9361	Age ≥ 50 years; SBP ≥ 130 mm Hg; high CVD risk without DM	SBP target <120 mm Hg versus SBP target <140 mm Hg	3.3	−18.2/−9.4	1.3%/years versus 2.1%/years	HR 0.62 (0.45-0.84)

In ALLHAT, data for the chlorthalidone vs. doxazosin comparison is not presented because this arm was terminated early as a result of harm from doxazosin. Data from Systolic Hypertension in the Elderly Project, SHEP[56]; Hypertension in the Very Elderly Trial, HYVET[57]; Antihypertensive and Lipid-Lowering Treatment to Prevent Heart Attack Trial, ALLHAT[59,60]; Heart Outcomes Prevention Evaluation, HOPE[58]; and Systolic Blood Pressure Intervention Trial, SPRINT.[105]
BP, Blood pressure; CI, confidence interval; CV, cardiovascular; CVD, cardiovascular disease; DM, diabetes mellitus; HR, hazard ratio; HTN, hypertension; RR, relative risk; SBP, systolic blood pressure.

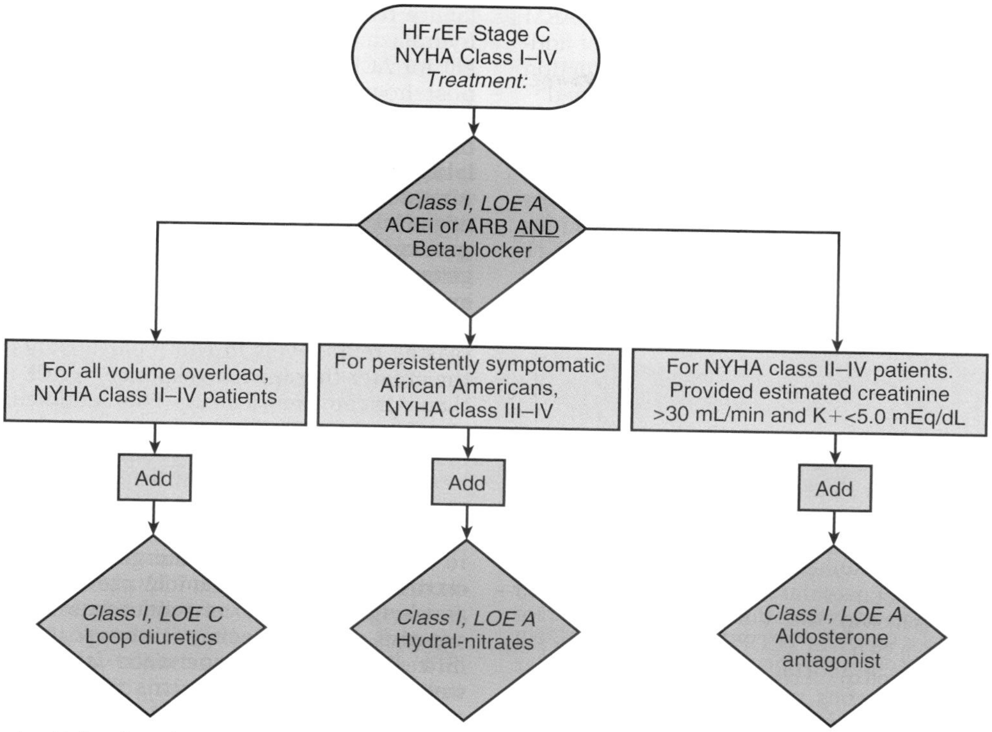

FIG. 32.6 Evidence-based, guideline-directed medical therapy for heart failure with reduced ejection fraction (HFrEF) in the American College of Cardiology/American Heart Association Heart Failure Guidelines 2013. *ACEi,* Angiotensin-converting enzyme inhibitor; *ARB,* angiotensin II receptor blocker; *hydral-nitrates,* hydralazine and isosorbide dinitrate; *LOE,* level of evidence; *NYHA,* New York Heart Association. *(From Yancy CW, Jessup M, Bozkurt B, et al. 2013 ACCF/AHA guideline for the management of heart failure: a report of the American College of Cardiology Foundation/American Heart Association Task Force on practice guidelines. Circulation. 2013;128(16):e240-327.)*

blockers for heart failure prevention. In summary, hypertension treatment and control with thiazide diuretics plus ACE inhibitors or ARBs is an essential part of a heart failure prevention strategy.

HYPERTENSION TREATMENT IN HEART FAILURE WITH REDUCED EJECTION FRACTION

In HFrEF, guideline-directed medical therapy with ACE inhibitors, ARBs, beta-blockers, and MCRAs are geared toward interruption of maladaptive neurohormonal pathways that worsen heart failure (Fig. 32.6). These agents have been shown in multiple clinical trials to improve clinical status, functional capacity, quality of life, hospitalizations, and mortality in systolic heart failure.[2] Nevertheless, elevated blood pressure in systolic heart failure can also pose a significant hemodynamic load to an already weak LV, and these agents can contribute to improved clinical status by also lowering blood pressure.

Angiotensin-Converting Enzyme Inhibitors

ACE inhibitors are one of the mainstays of heart failure therapy and have been shown in multiple trials to improve heart failure outcomes and mortality regardless of severity of heart failure.[63-67] SOLVD, which consisted of a treatment trial in symptomatic individuals and a prevention trial in asymptomatic individuals, were critical in demonstrating the efficacy of ACE inhibitor therapy in patients with HFrEF.[63,64] Other landmark ACE inhibitor trials like the Veterans Heart Failure Trial II (V-HeFT II) and the Cooperative North Scandinavian Enalapril Survival Study (CONSENSUS) established the efficacy of ACE inhibitor therapy in moderate and severe HFrEF.[65,66] In 2000, Flather et al completed a meta-analysis from five ACE inhibitor trials with individual participant data from 12,763 participants to demonstrate that ACE inhibitors lowered mortality by 20% (OR 0.80, 95% CI 0.74 to 0.87) and heart failure readmissions

by 33% (OR 0.67, 95% CI 0.61 to 0.74), supporting the widespread use of ACE inhibitors in HFrEF.[68]

Angiotensin II Receptor Blockers

ARBs also play an important role in HFrEF management and have been primarily studied as a treatment option for patients intolerant of ACE inhibitors and as an add-on therapy to background ACE inhibitor therapy. One of the largest trials testing the efficacy of ARBs in patients intolerant of ACE inhibitors was the Candesartan in Heart Failure: Assessment of Reduction in Mortality and Morbidity (CHARM)-Alternative trial.[69] In CHARM-Alternative, patients with symptomatic heart failure, LV ejection fraction 40% or less, and intolerance to ACE inhibitors were randomized to candesartan or placebo. After a median follow-up of 33.7 months, candesartan reduced the composite outcome of cardiovascular death or heart failure hospitalization by 30% compared with placebo (33% versus 40%; adjusted HR 0.70, 95% CI 0.60 to 0.81).[69] In the HEAAL study, high-dose (150 mg) versus low-dose (50 mg) losartan was compared in 3846 participants with symptomatic heart failure and LV dysfuntion.[70] Treatment with high-dose losartan compared with low-dose losartan was associated with a 10% reduction in the combined primary endpoint of death and heart failure hospitalization (43% versus 46%; HR 0.90, 95% CI 0.82 to 0.99).

The Valsartan Heart Failure Trial (Val-HeFT) was the first large trial to evaluate the effect of ARBs as an add-on to background heart failure therapy.[71] In the Val-HeFT, treatment with valsartan did not improve mortality but did reduce the coprimary composite outcome of death and cardiovascular morbidity.[71] In those patients in Val-HeFT who were unable to tolerate an ACE inhibitor, the ARB alone did improve outcomes further endorsing the outcome seen in CHARM-Alternative. However, in a post hoc subgroup analysis, participants receiving valsartan along with an ACE inhibitor and beta-blocker had increased adverse effects, raising concerns about the safety of such a treatment strategy. A follow-up study from the CHARM investigators, CHARM-Added, confirmed the benefits of add-on candesartan therapy with ACE inhibitors for reduction of cardiovascular morbidity but safety concerns remained.[72] In a Cochrane systematic review by Heran et al withdrawals because of adverse events were 34% higher in patients receiving combination ACE inhibitor and ARB therapy (absolute risk increase 3.7%; RR 1.34, 95% CI 1.19 to 1.51).[73] Because of safety concerns, the ACCF/AHA heart failure guidelines provide only a class IIb recommendation for consideration of an ARB as adjunctive therapy in persistently symptomatic patients and a class III recommendation against routine ARB, ACE inhibitor, and MCRA combination therapy.[2]

Beta-Blockers

Beta-blocker therapy is a cornerstone of HFrEF management. The first trial to demonstrate a mortality benefit with beta-blocker therapy was the U.S. Carvedilol Heart Failure Study Group trial.[74] Subsequent trials such as the Metoprolol CR/XL Randomized Intervention Trial in Congestive Heart Failure (MERIT-HF), the Cardiac Insufficiency Bisoprolol Study I (CIBIS-I), the Carvedilol Post-Infarct Survival Controlled Evaluation (CAPRICORN), and the Carvedilol Prospective Randomized Cumulative Survival (COPERNICUS) study all demonstrated reductions in mortality and cardiovascular morbidity.[75-78] A recent network meta-analysis of 21 trials comparing beta-blockers with other beta-blockers or other treatments in patients with HFrEF confirmed that beta-blocker therapy reduced mortality by 31% (OR 0.69, 95% CI 0.56 to 0.80).[79] Through indirect comparisons between different beta-blocker types, there was insufficient evidence to demonstrate a difference between types of beta-blocker. In the 2013 ACCF/AHA guidelines, carvedilol, metoprolol succinate and bisoprolol are the only recommended therapies for a patient with LV systolic dysfunction given their proven efficacy in randomized clinical trials.[2]

Mineralocorticoid Receptor Antagonists

MCRAs have recently emerged as a mainstay of therapy in patients with HFrEF who are already treated with ACE inhibitors (or ARBs) and beta-blockers. The Randomized Aldactone Evaluation Study (RALES) was the first study to demonstrate the efficacy of spironolactone in HFrEF.[80] In RALES, patients with severe symptoms (NYHA-III/IV) of heart failure and LV ejection fraction 35% or less were randomized to spironolactone or placebo. After a mean follow-up of 24 months, spironolactone was associated with a 30% reduction in all-cause mortality (35% versus 46%; RR 0.70, 95% CI 0.60 to 0.82) as well as reductions in cardiovascular death and heart failure hospitalizations.[80] The benefits of MCRAs were also demonstrated in the Eplerenone Post-Acute Myocardial Infarction Heart Failure Efficacy and Survival Study (EPHESUS)[81] and the Eplerenone in Mild Patients Hospitalizations and Survival Study in Heart Failure (EMPHASIS-HF).[82] In EMPHASIS-HF, eplerenone reduced the composite endpoint of cardiovascular death or heart failure hospitalization by 34% (18.3% versus 25.9%; HR 0.63, 95% CI 0.54 to 0.74) at a median follow-up of 21 months in patients with LV dysfunction and mild (NYHA-II) symptoms.[82] The EMPHASIS-HF trial was particularly noteworthy because it demonstrated that MCRA therapy was beneficial in all patients with symptomatic HFrEF, even those with mild symptoms.

Hydralazine/Isosorbide Dinitrate

The combination of hydralazine and isosorbide dinitrate (hydralazine/ISDN) is also an important component of heart failure treatment in patients with HFrEF. Although early heart failure trials like V-HeFT I suggested a mortality benefit for hydralazine/ISDN,[83] V-HeFT II demonstrated a survival benefit for ACE inhibitors over hydralazine/ISDN.[66] Remarkably, post hoc analyses by Carson et al suggested potentially important racial differences in response to therapy with hydralazine/ISDN.[84] In V-HeFT I, treatment with hydralazine/ISDN led to a 47% survival benefit (RR reduction) among African Americans. In V-HeFT II, the mortality benefit of enalapril over hydralazine/ISDN was only seen in white participants but African Americans responded similarly to both drugs with no evidence of a difference. Biochemical analyses demonstrated that racial differences in neurohormonal activation (higher plasma norepinephrine levels and plasma renin levels in white participants) explained in part the greater therapeutic response to ACE inhibitors in whites than African Americans.[84] This, coupled with data demonstrating diminished nitric oxide activity and increased oxidative stress in the endothelium of African Americans,[85] led to the hypothesis of the African-American Heart Failure Trial (A-HeFT), which tested whether or not hydralazine/ISDN improved survival in self-identified African Americans with HFrEF.[19] In A-HeFT, self-identified African Americans with NYHA-III/IV symptoms and LV dysfunction on ACE inhibitors and beta-blockers were randomized to hydralazine/ISDN or placebo. After a median follow-up 10 months, hydralazine/ISDN therapy was associated with a 43% reduction in all-cause mortality (6.2% versus 10.2%; HR 0.57, p = 0.01) and a 33% reduction in first heart failure hospitalization (16.4% versus 22.4%; p = 0.001).[19]

Loop Diuretics

Unlike ACE inhibitors, ARBs, beta-blockers, and MCRAs, the effects of diuretics on mortality and morbidity have not been studied in patients with HFrEF. In the ACCF/AHA heart failure guidelines, diuretics are recommended to relieve congestive symptoms of dyspnea and edema.[2] A recent Cochrane systematic review identified 14 trials with 525 participants that tested the efficacy of diuretics in heart failure.[86] In their review, loop diuretic therapy reduced mortality and heart failure hospitalization, but these outcomes were reported in only three trials (202 participants) and two trials (169 participants), respectively. Moreover, pooled treatment effects had wide confidence intervals, reducing the precision of the estimates.[86]

Newer Therapies for Heart Failure

Potential breakthrough therapies for heart failure have recently emerged. In the PARADIGM-HF trial, the combination of valsartan/sacubitril, an ARB with a neprilysin inhibitor, or ARNI, in the setting of background evidence-based medical and device therapy, reduced the primary outcome of composite of cardiovascular death and heart failure by 20% compared with ACE inhibition (21.8% versus 26.5%; HR 0.80, 95% CI 0.73 to 0.87).[87] Thus, the ARNI compound proved superior to ACE inhibitor therapy for HFrEF in the setting of otherwise indicated evidence-based medical and device therapy. As treatment for hypertension there are very few data with this new combination but an earlier iteration of an ACE inhibitor with a neprilysin inhibitor yielded quite good blood pressure-lowering efficacy but with unacceptably high rates of angioedema.[88,89] Current trials have demonstrated minimal evidence of angioedema and the events noted to date have been of lesser severity. Ivabradine, the only f-channel inhibitor of the SA node, with the singular property of heart rate slowing, has recently been demonstrated to reduce morbidity because of heart failure when added to standard evidence-based medical therapy with a persistent heart rate higher than 70 beats per minute.[90] There are no data addressing ivabradine and hypertension.

HYPERTENSION TREATMENT IN HEART FAILURE WITH PRESERVED EJECTION FRACTION

Because many of the same neurohormonal abnormalities that lead to HFrEF have been implicated in the pathogenesis of HFpEF, therapeutic trials for HFpEF have tested similar agents.[91,92] However, unlike with HFrEF, clinical trials testing beta-blockers, nitrates, ACE inhibitors, and especially ARBs and MCRAs have had largely disappointing results.

The role of ARBs in HFpEF has been studied in the Candesartan in Heart Failure: Assessment of Reduction in Mortality and Morbidity (CHARM)-Preserved and Irbesartan in Heart Failure with Preserved Ejection Fraction Study (I-PRESERVE).[93,94] Both trials failed to meet their primary outcome that included composite endpoints consisting of all-cause mortality, cardiovascular death, heart failure hospitalization, and/or hospitalization for a cardiovascular cause. Although candesartan therapy reduced heart failure hospitalizations in CHARM-Preserved in secondary analyses, this signal was not seen for I-PRESERVE.[93,94]

The Randomized Aldosterone Antagonism in Heart Failure with Preserved Ejection Fraction (RAAM-PEF) study and the Aldosterone Receptor Blockade in Diastolic Heart Failure (Aldo-DHF) both tested the effects of MCRAs in patients with HFpEF.[95,96] Both trials demonstrated improvements in diastolic function in patients treated with MCRAs but this did not translate to improvements in exercise capacity. The Treatment of Preserved Cardiac Function Heart Failure with an Aldosterone Antagonist (TOPCAT) was the largest trial to test the effects of MCRAs in patients with HFpEF.[97] After a mean follow-up of 3.3 years, spironolactone did not reduce the primary outcome of composite cardiovascular events, but it did reduce heart failure hospitalizations by 17% (12.0% versus 14.2%; HR 0.83, 95% CI 0.69 to 0.99).[97] Subsequent secondary and post hoc analyses suggested that clinical benefits primarily occurred in patients with higher B-type natriuretic peptide and those enrolled in the Americas.[97,98] In a recent review, Chen et al summarized the current state of evidence for MCRAs in HFpEF.[99] In the 14 trials identified, MCRAs reduced the risk of heart failure hospitalization by 17% (RR 0.83, 95% CI 0.70 to 0.98), improved quality of life (weighted mean difference −5.16, 95% CI −8.03 to −2.30), and improved multiple diastolic parameters on echocardiogram. However, there was no observed effect on all-cause mortality (RR 0.90, 95% CI 0.78 to 1.04).[99]

ACCF/AHA guidelines reflect the uncertainty from HFpEF trials by not recommending any specific agents with class I indications for HFpEF. Instead, guidelines recommend following hypertension guidelines for blood pressure management and treating with diuretics for volume control.[2] Post hoc analyses from ALLHAT support this approach by demonstrating the efficacy of chlorthalidone in preventing HFpEF.[100] Among the 910 ALLHAT participants hospitalized with heart failure and with ejection fraction assessment, chlorthalidone markedly reduced the risk of HFpEF (defined as LV ejection ≥ 50%) compared with amlodipine, lisinopril, and doxazosin (HR 0.69, 95% CI 0.53 to 0.91; HR 0.74, 95% CI 0.56 to 0.97; and HR 0.53, 95% CI 0.38 to 0.73; respectively).[100]

A STRATEGY FOR GUIDING HYPERTENSION TREATMENT TO PREVENT HEART FAILURE

Prevention, treatment, and control of predisposing conditions like hypertension are critical to prevent heart failure and improve cardiovascular health.

The current paradigm for primary prevention of cardiovascular diseases emphasizes the importance of absolute cardiovascular disease risk to guide the intensity of prevention efforts. This is the driving principle behind cholesterol treatment guidelines both in the United States, United Kingdom, and Europe.[101-103] In the United States, the ACC/AHA cholesterol guidelines use cardiovascular risk thresholds to guide statin initiation and intensity of treatment.[101] Although cardiovascular risk assessment is embedded in some hypertension guidelines,[103] treatment thresholds and goals have generally been the same for high and low cardiovascular risk.

Recently, Sundström et al led a meta-analysis using individual participant data from 51,917 participants included in 11 trials from the Blood Pressure Lowering Treatment Trialists' Collaboration, which provides empiric support for using risk assessment to guide blood pressure-lowering treatment decisions.[104] These analyses demonstrated that the relative risk reduction for major cardiovascular events from active or more intensive blood pressure-lowering therapy was similar across four risk strata; and consequently, absolute benefits from blood pressure-lowering therapy were progressively greater as baseline risk increased. Importantly, these findings were consistent for all cause-specific cardiovascular outcomes but were qualitatively greatest for heart failure endpoints (Fig. 32.7).

These findings are even more relevant in the context of the recently published Systolic Blood Pressure Intervention Trial (SPRINT) where participants at high risk for cardiovascular disease (e.g., 10-year cardiovascular disease [CVD] risk ≥ 15%, age ≥ 75 years, chronic kidney disease or established vascular disease) were randomized to standard blood pressure lowering (target systolic blood pressure < 140 mm Hg) versus intensive blood pressure lowering (target systolic blood pressure < 120 mm Hg).[105] After a median follow-up of 3.3 years, intensive treatment was associated with a 25% reduction in major cardiovascular events, inclusive of heart failure, compared with standard treatment (1.65% per year versus 2.19% per year; HR 0.75, 95% CI 0.64 to 0.89) (see Table 32.3). However, the beneficial effect was primarily driven by a 38% reduction in heart failure (0.41% per year versus 0.67% per year; HR 0.62, 95% CI 0.45 to 0.84) and a 43% reduction in cardiovascular death (0.25% per year versus 0.43% per year; HR 0.57, 95% CI 0.38 to 0.85). These studies establish the imperative to treat blood pressure intensively in high-risk individuals to prevent heart failure.

SUMMARY

- Heart failure is associated with substantial morbidity/mortality and is inexorably linked to hypertension.
- Hypertension is a known risk factor for heart failure, both reduced ejection fraction and preserved ejection fraction. In those with hypertension, there is a several-fold increase in the incidence of heart failure, worse in African Americans.
- Reasonable evidence strongly suggests that hypertension is a *causative factor* for heart failure.
- Ultrastructural changes, alterations in strain and pathologic left ventricular hypertrophy predispose to left ventricular dysfunction and probable heart failure.
- Evidence-based therapies for reduced ejection fraction heart failure reduce morbidity and mortality attributable to heart failure, whereas targeting concomitant comorbidities reflects current best care strategies for heart failure with preserved ejection fraction.
- Treatment of hypertension is associated with a reduction in the development of heart failure and especially so in those at highest global risk for cardiovascular disease.

CURRENT EVIDENCE GAPS

1. Parallel themes of prevention now focus on treatment of known risk factors, especially hypertension and diabetes, and the use of biomarkers to screen for subclinical evidence of ventricular dysfunction. Whether focusing on hypertension in those with increased cardiovascular risk *and* elevated biomarker profiles would further increase the benefit of definitive treatment of hypertension is unknown.

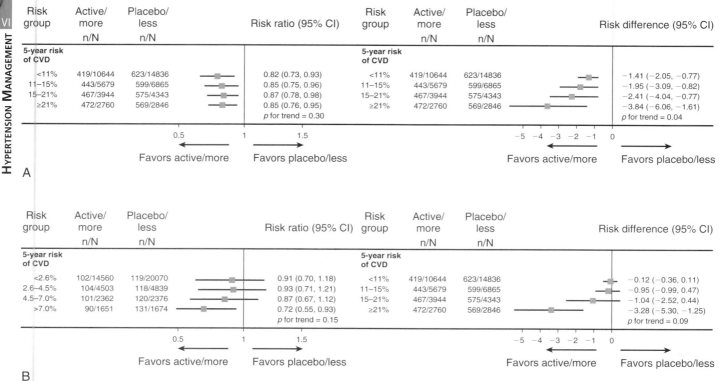

FIG. 32.7 Effects of blood pressure reduction on relative and absolute risks of cardiovascular disease (CVD) events (defined as coronary heart disease, stroke, heart failure, and cardiovascular death) (A) and heart failure (B) from 11 trials included in the Blood Pressure Lowering Treatment Trialists' Collaboration. Groups are defined by different levels of cardiovascular risk at baseline, and risk thresholds were selected to have similar event rates in each group. *(Modified from Sundström J, Arima H, Woodward M, et al. Blood pressure-lowering treatment based on cardiovascular risk: a meta-analysis of individual patient data. Lancet. 2014;384(9943):591-598.)*

2. Although it is now an evident truth that lowering systolic blood pressure to 120 mm Hg prevents heart failure in at-risk individuals, it is not known if a differential effect is seen as a function of the drug class used to treat hypertension or whether this is solely a blood pressure lowering effect.

3. The available data address the prevention of heart failure in adults with hypertension. It is not known whether earlier intervention in young adults and/or adolescents at risk for hypertension (primordial prevention) will prevent the eventual development of heart failure nor is it clear that a sufficient surrogate is available to prospectively test this hypothesis without a multiyear, even decades-long study.

4. It is plausible that newer agents, like valsartan/sacubitril, now indicated for heart failure, may represent potent therapies to reduce the progression from hypertension to heart failure if deployed in stages A or B. Testing the utility of valsartan/sacubitril in this setting is a reasonable future step in the development of specific therapies to prevent heart failure.

CONCLUSION

Heart failure is a public health burden with substantial consequences for the future of health care and the health of the population. Guidelines for the management of heart failure emphasize the progressive and gradual development of heart failure, focusing on the key role of upstream prevention to prevent downstream heart failure events. Prevention, treatment, and control of hypertension is a crucial target for prevention efforts at all stages of heart failure given the significant role of hypertension in the structural and mechanical changes that lead to heart failure. Through screening, followed by early and intensive blood pressure reduction in high-risk individuals before clinical heart failure, it is quite probable that we mitigate the burden of heart failure.

References

1. Hasenfuss G, Mann DL. Pathophysiology of Heart Failure. In: Mann DL, Zipes DP, Libby P, Bonow RO, Braunwald E, eds. *Braunwald's Heart Disease: A Textbook of Cardiovascular Medicine, 10th Edition.* Philadelphia: Elsevier, Inc.; 2015:454-472.
2. Yancy CW, Jessup M, Bozkurt B, et al. 2013 ACCF/AHA guideline for the management of heart failure: a report of the American College of Cardiology Foundation/American Heart Association Task Force on practice guidelines. *Circulation.* 2013;128:e240-327.
3. Gerber Y, Weston SA, Redfield MM, et al. A contemporary appraisal of the heart failure epidemic in Olmsted County, Minnesota, 2000 to 2010. *JAMA Int Med.* 2015;175:996-1004.
4. Pfeffer MA, Braunwald E. Treatment of heart failure with preserved ejection fraction: reflections on its treatment with an aldosterone antagonist. *JAMA Cardiol.* 2016;1:7-8.
5. Solomon SD, Zile M, Pieske B, et al. The angiotensin receptor neprilysin inhibitor LCZ696 in heart failure with preserved ejection fraction: a phase 2 double-blind randomised controlled trial. *Lancet.* 2012;380:1387-1395.
6. Yancy CW, Jessup M, Bozkurt B, et al. 2016 ACC/AHA/HFSA Focused Update on New Pharmacological Therapy for Heart Failure: An update of the 2013 ACCF/AHA guideline for the management of heart failure: a report of the American College of Cardiology/American Heart Association Task Force on clinical practice guidelines and the Heart Failure Society of America. *Circulation.* 2016;134:e282-e293.
7. Global Burden of Disease Study 2013 Collaborators. Global, regional, and national incidence, prevalence, and years lived with disability for 301 acute and chronic diseases and injuries in 188 countries, 1990-2013: a systematic analysis for the Global Burden of Disease Study 2013. *Lancet.* 2015;386:743-800.
8. Mozaffarian D, Benjamin EJ, Go AS, et al. Heart Disease and Stroke Statistics-2016 Update: A Report from the American Heart Association. *Circulation.* 2016;133:e38-60.
9. Dharmarajan K, Hsieh AF, Lin Z, et al. Diagnoses and timing of 30-day readmissions after hospitalization for heart failure, acute myocardial infarction, or pneumonia. *JAMA.* 2013;309:355-363.
10. Heidenreich PA, Albert NM, Allen LA, et al. Forecasting the impact of heart failure in the United States: a policy statement from the American Heart Association. *Circ Heart Fail.* 2013;6:606-619.
11. Kannel WB, Castelli WP, McNamara PM, McKee PA, Feinleib M. Role of blood pressure in the development of congestive heart failure. The Framingham study. *N Engl J Med.* 1972;287:781-787.
12. Levy D, Larson MG, Vasan RS, Kannel WB, Ho KK. The progression from hypertension to congestive heart failure. *JAMA.* 1996;275:1557-1562.
13. Lloyd-Jones DM, Larson MG, Leip EP, et al. Lifetime risk for developing congestive heart failure: the Framingham Heart Study. *Circulation.* 2002;106:3068-3072.
14. Lee DS, Gona P, Vasan RS, et al. Relation of disease pathogenesis and risk factors to heart failure with preserved or reduced ejection fraction: insights from the Framingham Heart Study of the National Heart, Lung, and Blood Institute. *Circulation.* 2009;119:3070-3077.
15. Loehr LR, Rosamond WD, Chang PP, Folsom AR, Chambless LE. Heart failure incidence and survival (from the Atherosclerosis Risk in Communities study). *Am J Cardiol.* 2008;101:1016-1022.
16. Bahrami H, Kronmal R, Bluemke DA, et al. Differences in the incidence of congestive heart failure by ethnicity: the Multi-Ethnic Study of Atherosclerosis. *Arch Intern Med.* 2008;168:2138-2145.

17. Institute of Medicine. *How Far Have We Come in Reducing Health Disparities? Progress Since 2000: Workshop Summary*. Washington (DC): National Academies Press (US) National Academy of Sciences; 2012.
18. Yancy CW. Heart failure in African Americans. *Am J Cardiol*. 2005;96:3i-12i.
19. Taylor AL, Ziesche S, Yancy C, et al. Combination of isosorbide dinitrate and hydralazine in blacks with heart failure. *N Engl J Med*. 2004;351:2049-2057.
20. Bibbins-Domingo K, Pletcher MJ, Lin F, et al. Racial differences in incident heart failure among young adults. *N Engl J Med*. 2009;360:1179-1190.
21. Drazner MH. The progression of hypertensive heart disease. *Circulation*. 2011;123:327-334.
22. Vasan RS, Levy D. The role of hypertension in the pathogenesis of heart failure. A clinical mechanistic overview. *Arch Intern Med*. 1996;156:1789-1796.
23. Kannel WB, Gordon T, Castelli WP, Margolis JR. Electrocardiographic left ventricular hypertrophy and risk of coronary heart disease. The Framingham study. *Ann Intern Med*. 1970;72:813-822.
24. Parati G, Pomidossi G, Albini F, Malaspina D, Mancia G. Relationship of 24-hour blood pressure mean and variability to severity of target-organ damage in hypertension. *J Hypertens*. 1987;5:93-98.
25. Levy D, Garrison RJ, Savage DD, Kannel WB, Castelli WP. Prognostic implications of echocardiographically determined left ventricular mass in the Framingham Heart Study. *N Engl J Med*. 1990;322:1561-1566.
26. de Simone G, Gottdiener JS, Chinali M, Maurer MS. Left ventricular mass predicts heart failure not related to previous myocardial infarction: the Cardiovascular Health Study. *Eur Heart J*. 2008;29:741-747.
27. Bluemke DA, Kronmal RA, Lima JA, et al. The relationship of left ventricular mass and geometry to incident cardiovascular events: the MESA (Multi-Ethnic Study of Atherosclerosis) study. *J Am Coll Cardiol*. 2008;52:2148-2155.
28. Devereux RB, Dahlof B, Gerdts E, et al. Regression of hypertensive left ventricular hypertrophy by losartan compared with atenolol: the Losartan Intervention for Endpoint Reduction in Hypertension (LIFE) trial. *Circulation*. 2004;110:1456-1462.
29. Devereux RB, Wachtell K, Gerdts E, et al. Prognostic significance of left ventricular mass change during treatment of hypertension. *JAMA*. 2004;292:2350-2356.
30. Klingbeil AU, Schneider M, Martus P, Messerli FH, Schmieder RE. A meta-analysis of the effects of treatment on left ventricular mass in essential hypertension. *Am J Med*. 2003;115:41-46.
31. Drazner MH, Rame JE, Marino EK, et al. Increased left ventricular mass is a risk factor for the development of a depressed left ventricular ejection fraction within five years: the Cardiovascular Health Study. *J Am Coll Cardiol*. 2004;43:2207-2215.
32. Abhayaratna WP, Marwick TH, Smith WT, Becker NG. Characteristics of left ventricular diastolic dysfunction in the community: an echocardiographic survey. *Heart*. 2006;92:1259-1264.
33. Redfield MM, Jacobsen SJ, Burnett JC, Jr., Mahoney DW, Bailey KR, Rodeheffer RJ. Burden of systolic and diastolic ventricular dysfunction in the community: appreciating the scope of the heart failure epidemic. *JAMA*. 2003;289:194-202.
34. Santos AB, Gupta DK, Bello NA, et al. Prehypertension is associated with abnormalities of cardiac structure and function in the Atherosclerosis Risk in Communities study. *Am J Hypertens*. 2016;29:568-574.
35. Voigt JU, Pedrizzetti G, Lysyansky P, et al. Definitions for a common standard for 2D speckle tracking echocardiography: consensus document of the EACVI/ASE/Industry Task Force to standardize deformation imaging. *J Am Soc Echocardiogr*. 2015;28:183-193.
36. Choi EY, Rosen BD, Fernandes VR, et al. Prognostic value of myocardial circumferential strain for incident heart failure and cardiovascular events in asymptomatic individuals: the Multi-Ethnic Study of Atherosclerosis. *Eur Heart J*. 2013;34:2354-2361.
37. Ersböll M, Valeur N, Mogensen UM, et al. Prediction of all-cause mortality and heart failure admissions from global left ventricular longitudinal strain in patients with acute myocardial infarction and preserved left ventricular ejection fraction. *J Am Coll Cardiol*. 2013;61:2365-2373.
38. Kishi S, Teixido-Tura G, Ning H, et al. Cumulative blood pressure in early adulthood and cardiac dysfunction in middle age: the CARDIA study. *J Am Coll Cardiol*. 2015;65:2679-2687.
39. Tsutsui H, Tagawa H, Kent RL, et al. Role of microtubules in contractile dysfunction of hypertrophied cardiocytes. *Circulation*. 1994;90:533-555.
40. Tagawa H, Rozich JD, Tsutsui H, et al. Basis for increased microtubules in pressure-hypertrophied cardiocytes. *Circulation*. 1996;93:1230-1243.
41. Wei S, Guo A, Chen B, et al. T-tubule remodeling during transition from hypertrophy to heart failure. *Circ Res*. 2010;107:520-531.
42. Shah SJ, Aistrup GL, Gupta DK, et al. Ultrastructural and cellular basis for the development of abnormal myocardial mechanics during the transition from hypertension to heart failure. *Am J Physiol Heart Circ Physiol*. 2014;306:H88-100.
43. Shapiro BP, Owan TE, Mohammed S, et al. Mineralocorticoid signaling in transition to heart failure with normal ejection fraction. *Hypertension*. 2008;51:289-295.
44. Mohammed SF, Ohtani T, Korinek J, et al. Mineralocorticoid accelerates transition to heart failure with preserved ejection fraction via "nongenomic effects". *Circulation*. 2010;122:370-378.
45. Ahmed SH, Clark LL, Pennington WR, et al. Matrix metalloproteinases/tissue inhibitors of metalloproteinases: relationship between changes in proteolytic determinants of matrix composition and structural, functional, and clinical manifestations of hypertensive heart disease. *Circulation*. 2006;113:2089-2096.
46. Lopez B, Gonzalez A, Querejeta R, Larman M, Diez J. Alterations in the pattern of collagen deposition may contribute to the deterioration of systolic function in hypertensive patients with heart failure. *J Am Coll Cardiol*. 2006;48:89-96.
47. Kizer JR, Arnett DK, Bella JN, et al. Differences in left ventricular structure between black and white hypertensive adults: the Hypertension Genetic Epidemiology Network study. *Hypertension*. 2004;43:1182-1188.
48. Drazner MH, Dries DL, Peshock RM, et al. Left ventricular hypertrophy is more prevalent in blacks than whites in the general population: the Dallas Heart Study. *Hypertension*. 2005;46:124-129.
49. Post WS, Larson MG, Myers RH, Galderisi M, Levy D. Heritability of left ventricular mass: the Framingham Heart Study. *Hypertension*. 1997;30:1025-1028.
50. Arnett DK, Hong Y, Bella JN, et al. Sibling correlation of left ventricular mass and geometry in hypertensive African Americans and whites: the HyperGEN study. Hypertension Genetic Epidemiology Network. *Am J Hypertens*. 2001;14:1226-1230.
51. Bella JN, Goring HH. Genetic epidemiology of left ventricular hypertrophy. *Am J Cardiovasc Dis*. 2012;2:267-278.
52. Vasan RS, Glazer NL, Felix JF, et al. Genetic variants associated with cardiac structure and function: a meta-analysis and replication of genome-wide association data. *JAMA*. 2009;302:168-178.
53. Shah S, Nelson CP, Gaunt TR, et al. Four genetic loci influencing electrocardiographic indices of left ventricular hypertrophy. *Circulation. Cardiovascular genetics*. 2011;4:626-635.
54. Veterans Administration Cooperative Study of Antihypertensive Agents. Effects of treatment on morbidity in hypertension. Results in patients with diastolic blood pressures averaging 115 through 129 mm Hg. *JAMA*. 1967;202:1028-1034.
55. Veterans Administration Cooperative Study of Antihypertensive Agents. Effects of treatment on morbidity in hypertension. II. Results in patients with diastolic blood pressure averaging 90 through 114 mm Hg. *JAMA*. 1970;213:1143-1152.
56. Kostis JB, Davis BR, Cutler J, et al. Prevention of heart failure by antihypertensive drug treatment in older persons with isolated systolic hypertension. SHEP Cooperative Research Group. *JAMA*. 1997;278:212-216.
57. Beckett NS, Peters R, Fletcher AE, et al. Treatment of hypertension in patients 80 years of age or older. *N Engl J Med*. 2008;358:1887-1898.
58. Yusuf S, Sleight P, Pogue J, Bosch J, Davies R, Dagenais G. Effects of an angiotensin-converting-enzyme inhibitor, ramipril, on cardiovascular events in high-risk patients. The Heart Outcomes Prevention Evaluation Study Investigators. *N Engl J Med*. 2000;342:145-153.
59. ALLHAT Collaborative Research Group. Major outcomes in high-risk hypertensive patients randomized to angiotensin-converting enzyme inhibitor or calcium channel blocker vs diuretic: The Antihypertensive and Lipid-Lowering Treatment to Prevent Heart Attack Trial (ALLHAT). *JAMA*. 2002;288:2981-2997.
60. ALLHAT Collaborative Research Group. Major cardiovascular events in hypertensive patients randomized to doxazosin vs chlorthalidone: the antihypertensive and lipid-lowering treatment to prevent heart attack trial (ALLHAT). *JAMA*. 2000;283:1967-1975.
61. Sciarretta S, Palano F, Tocci G, Baldini R, Volpe M. Antihypertensive treatment and development of heart failure in hypertension: a Bayesian network meta-analysis of studies in patients with hypertension and high cardiovascular risk. *Arch Intern Med*. 2011;171:384-394.
62. Ettehad D, Emdin CA, Kiran A, et al. Blood pressure lowering for prevention of cardiovascular disease and death: a systematic review and meta-analysis. *Lancet*. 2016;387:957-967.
63. The SOLVD Investigators. Effect of enalapril on mortality and the development of heart failure in asymptomatic patients with reduced left ventricular ejection fractions. *N Engl J Med*. 1992;327:685-691.
64. The SOLVD Investigators. Effect of enalapril on survival in patients with reduced left ventricular ejection fractions and congestive heart failure. *N Engl J Med*. 1991;325:293-302.
65. The CONSENSUS Trial Study Group. Effects of enalapril on mortality in severe congestive heart failure. Results of the Cooperative North Scandinavian Enalapril Survival Study (CONSENSUS). *N Engl J Med*. 1987;316:1429-1435.
66. Cohn JN, Johnson G, Ziesche S, et al. A comparison of enalapril with hydralazine-isosorbide dinitrate in the treatment of chronic congestive heart failure. *N Engl J Med*. 1991;325:303-310.
67. Pfeffer MA, Braunwald E, Moye LA, et al. Effect of captopril on mortality and morbidity in patients with left ventricular dysfunction after myocardial infarction. Results of the survival and ventricular enlargement trial. The SAVE Investigators. *N Engl J Med*. 1992;327:669-677.
68. Flather MD, Yusuf S, Kober L, et al. Long-term ACE-inhibitor therapy in patients with heart failure or left-ventricular dysfunction: a systematic overview of data from individual patients. ACE-Inhibitor Myocardial Infarction Collaborative Group. *Lancet*. 2000;355:1575-1581.
69. Granger CB, McMurray JJ, Yusuf S, et al. Effects of candesartan in patients with chronic heart failure and reduced left-ventricular systolic function intolerant to angiotensin-converting-enzyme inhibitors: the CHARM-Alternative trial. *Lancet*. 2003;362:772-776.
70. Konstam MA, Neaton JD, Dickstein K, et al. Effects of high-dose versus low-dose losartan on clinical outcomes in patients with heart failure (HEAAL study): a randomised, double-blind trial. *Lancet*. 2009;374:1840-1848.
71. Cohn JN, Tognoni G. A randomized trial of the angiotensin-receptor blocker valsartan in chronic heart failure. *N Engl J Med*. 2001;345:1667-1675.
72. McMurray JJ, Ostergren J, Swedberg K, et al. Effects of candesartan in patients with chronic heart failure and reduced left-ventricular systolic function taking angiotensin-converting-enzyme inhibitors: the CHARM-Added trial. *Lancet*. 2003;362:767-771.
73. Heran BS, Musini VM, Bassett K, Taylor RS, Wright JM. Angiotensin receptor blockers for heart failure. *Cochrane Database Syst Rev*. 2012(4):CD003040.
74. Packer M, Bristow MR, Cohn JN, et al. The effect of carvedilol on morbidity and mortality in patients with chronic heart failure. U.S. Carvedilol Heart Failure Study Group. *N Engl J Med*. 1996;334:1349-1355.
75. MERIT-HF Study Group. Effect of metoprolol CR/XL in chronic heart failure: Metoprolol CR/XL Randomised Intervention Trial in Congestive Heart Failure (MERIT-HF). *Lancet*. 1999;353:2001-2007.
76. CIBIS-II Investigators and Committees. The Cardiac Insufficiency Bisoprolol Study II (CIBIS-II): a randomised trial. *Lancet*. 1999;353:9-13.
77. Dargie HJ, the CAPRICORN Investigators. Effect of carvedilol on outcome after myocardial infarction in patients with left-ventricular dysfunction: the CAPRICORN randomised trial. *Lancet*. 2001;357:1385-1390.
78. Packer M, Coats AJ, Fowler MB, et al. Effect of carvedilol on survival in severe chronic heart failure. *N Engl J Med*. 2001;344:1651-1658.
79. Chatterjee S, Biondi-Zoccai G, Abbate A, et al. Benefits of beta blockers in patients with heart failure and reduced ejection fraction: network meta-analysis. *BMJ*. 2013;346:f55.
80. Pitt B, Zannad F, Remme WJ, et al. The effect of spironolactone on morbidity and mortality in patients with severe heart failure. Randomized Aldactone Evaluation Study Investigators. *N Engl J Med*. 1999;341:709-717.
81. Pitt B, Remme W, Zannad F, et al. Eplerenone, a selective aldosterone blocker, in patients with left ventricular dysfunction after myocardial infarction. *N Engl J Med*. 2003;348:1309-1321.
82. Zannad F, McMurray JJ, Krum H, et al. Eplerenone in patients with systolic heart failure and mild symptoms. *N Engl J Med*. 2011;364:11-21.
83. Cohn JN, Archibald DG, Ziesche S, et al. Effect of vasodilator therapy on mortality in chronic congestive heart failure. Results of a Veterans Administration Cooperative Study. *N Engl J Med*. 1986;314:1547-1552.
84. Carson P, Ziesche S, Johnson G, Cohn JN. Racial differences in response to therapy for heart failure: analysis of the vasodilator-heart failure trials. Vasodilator-Heart Failure Trial Study Group. *J Card Fail*. 1999;5:178-187.
85. Kalinowski L, Dobrucki IT, Malinski T. Race-specific differences in endothelial function: predisposition of African Americans to vascular diseases. *Circulation*. 2004;109:2511-2517.
86. Faris RF, Flather M, Purcell H, Poole-Wilson PA, Coats AJ. Diuretics for heart failure. *Cochrane Database Syst Rev*. 2012(2):CD003838.
87. McMurray JJ, Packer M, Desai AS, et al. Angiotensin-neprilysin inhibition versus enalapril in heart failure. *N Engl J Med*. 2014;371:993-1004.
88. Kostis JB, Packer M, Black HR, Schmieder R, Henry D, Levy E. Omapatrilat and enalapril in patients with hypertension: the Omapatrilat Cardiovascular Treatment vs. Enalapril (OCTAVE) trial. *Am J Hypertens*. 2004;17:103-111.
89. Packer M, Califf RM, Konstam MA, et al. Comparison of omapatrilat and enalapril in patients with chronic heart failure: the Omapatrilat Versus Enalapril Randomized Trial of Utility in Reducing Events (OVERTURE). *Circulation*. 2002;106:920-926.
90. Swedberg K, Komajda M, Bohm M, et al. Ivabradine and outcomes in chronic heart failure (SHIFT): a randomised placebo-controlled study. *Lancet*. 2010;376:875-885.

91. Edelmann F, Tomaschitz A, Wachter R, et al. Serum aldosterone and its relationship to left ventricular structure and geometry in patients with preserved left ventricular ejection fraction. *Eur Heart J*. 2012;33:203-212.

92. Hogg K, McMurray J. Neurohumoral pathways in heart failure with preserved systolic function. *Prog Cardiovasc Dis*. 2005;47:357-366.

93. Yusuf S, Pfeffer MA, Swedberg K, et al. Effects of candesartan in patients with chronic heart failure and preserved left-ventricular ejection fraction: the CHARM-Preserved Trial. *Lancet*. 2003;362:777-781.

94. Massie BM, Carson PE, McMurray JJ, et al. Irbesartan in patients with heart failure and preserved ejection fraction. *N Engl J Med*. 2008;359:2456-2467.

95. Deswal A, Richardson P, Bozkurt B, Mann DL. Results of the Randomized Aldosterone Antagonism in Heart Failure with Preserved Ejection Fraction trial (RAAM-PEF). *J Card Fail*. 2011;17:634-642.

96. Edelmann F, Wachter R, Schmidt AG, et al. Effect of spironolactone on diastolic function and exercise capacity in patients with heart failure with preserved ejection fraction: the Aldo-DHF randomized controlled trial. *JAMA*. 2013;309:781-791.

97. Pitt B, Pfeffer MA, Assmann SF, et al. Spironolactone for heart failure with preserved ejection fraction. *N Engl J Med*. 2014;370:1383-1392.

98. Pfeffer MA, Claggett B, Assmann SF, et al. Regional variation in patients and outcomes in the Treatment of Preserved Cardiac Function Heart Failure with an Aldosterone Antagonist (TOPCAT) trial. *Circulation*. 2015;131:34-42.

99. Chen Y, Wang H, Lu Y, Huang X, Liao Y, Bin J. Effects of mineralocorticoid receptor antagonists in patients with preserved ejection fraction: a meta-analysis of randomized clinical trials. *BMC Med*. 2015;13:10.

100. Davis BR, Kostis JB, Simpson LM, et al. Heart failure with preserved and reduced left ventricular ejection fraction in the antihypertensive and lipid-lowering treatment to prevent heart attack trial. *Circulation*. 2008;118:2259-2267.

101. Stone NJ, Robinson JG, Lichtenstein AH, et al. 2013 ACC/AHA guideline on the treatment of blood cholesterol to reduce atherosclerotic cardiovascular risk in adults: a report of the American College of Cardiology/American Heart Association Task Force on Practice Guidelines. *Circulation*. 2014;129(25 Suppl 2):S1-45.

102. National Institute for Health and Care Excellence (NICE) Clinical Guideline CG181: Cardiovascular disease: risk assessment and reduction in lipid modification, July 2014. http://nice.org.uk/guidance/cg181.

103. Perk J, De Backer G, Gohlke H, et al. European Guidelines on cardiovascular disease prevention in clinical practice (version 2012). The Fifth Joint Task Force of the European Society of Cardiology and Other Societies on Cardiovascular Disease Prevention in Clinical Practice (constituted by representatives of nine societies and by invited experts). *Eur Heart J*. 2012;33:1635-1701.

104. Sundström J, Arima H, Woodward M, et al. Blood pressure-lowering treatment based on cardiovascular risk: a meta-analysis of individual patient data. *Lancet*. 2014;384:591-598.

105. Wright JT, Jr., Williamson JD, Whelton PK, et al. A randomized trial of intensive versus standard blood-pressure control. *N Engl J Med*. 2015;373:2103-2116.

33 Hypertension and Chronic Kidney Disease

Hillel Sternlicht and George L. Bakris

Chronic kidney disease (CKD) is defined by laboratory findings of a decreased estimated glomerular filtration rate (eGFR) to less than 60 mL per minute per 1.73 m^2 or evidence of renal parenchymal injury (i.e., albuminuria > 300 mg/day) present for 3 months or more. Both the Kidney Disease Outcomes Quality Initiative (KDOQI) and Kidney Disease Improving Global Outcomes (KDIGO) classify CKD into five stages based on the degree of remaining renal function (Fig. 33.1). The stages range from histologic and/or laboratory evidence of parenchymal injury (very high albuminuria) with preserved eGFR to end-stage renal disease (ESRD) and need for renal replacement therapy.[1]

CKD is a worldwide public health problem with an increasing international prevalence, primarily related to diabetes and hypertension.[2] According to the 2012 National Health and Nutrition Examination Survey (NHANES) data, approximately 29% of the population of the United States suffers from hypertension. In contrast, hypertension affects one-third of those with stage 1 CKD, and 85% of those with stage 5 CKD.[3]

The prevalence of hypertension among hemodialysis patients is less clear, owing to variations in the threshold value for diagnosis and the timing of measurement (i.e., preceding, during, or following dialysis). In one report, 85% of the 2000 dialysis patients recruited into an iron supplementation trial possessed a predialysis blood pressure in excess of 150/85 mm Hg despite having started dialysis four years prior, a rate slightly higher than a prevalence rate of 75% observed in other studies.[4,5]

PATHOPHYSIOLOGY OF HYPERTENSION IN KIDNEY DISEASE

The key components of hypertension in patients with kidney disease include excess activation of the renin-angiotensin-aldosterone system (RAAS), inappropriately elevated sympathetic nervous activity, impaired renal salt and water excretion, increased arterial stiffness, and reduced nitric oxide release. Sympathetic overactivity results in additional efferent arteriolar vasoconstriction with increases in intraglomerular pressure and a greater plasma filtration fraction. Enhanced filtration leads to elevated oncotic pressures, further increasing intravascular volume.[6] Sympathetic activity also up-regulates the renin-angiotensin-aldosterone cascade, ultimately increasing angiotensin II. Angiotensin II promotes efferent arteriolar vasoconstriction, giving rise to hyperfiltration (increased glomerular filtration). In healthy individuals, increased sodium intake raises blood pressure and GFR, which in turn promotes sodium loss. However, in those with a GFR less than 60 mL per min, the pressure-natriuresis curve is shifted to the left such that sodium balance is only achieved at the expense of a higher blood pressure.[7] High salt loads are also poorly tolerated in such populations because of reductions in nitric oxide release, thereby blunting the vasodilatory response to increases in volume (Fig. 33.2).[8]

The pathogenesis of hypertension among dialysis patients, although related to the aforementioned mechanisms in CKD patients, is primarily related to volume overload. Among dialysis patients there is an inability to excrete sodium and water; hence, volume expansion is the driving force for hypertension. Bioelectrical impedance assessment of volume status and the reduction in blood pressure realized after volume removal confirm this precept.[9] Derangements in the sympathetic nervous system are also implicated as both the rates of sympathetic discharge and vascular resistance are more than two-fold higher among dialysis patients when compared with normotensive individuals.[10] This elevation in vascular resistance is, in part, mediated by dysfunction of the endothelial-derived compounds nitric oxide and endothelin.

Nitric oxide, a potent vasodilator, is inhibited by the endogenously produced molecule asymmetric dimethyl arginine (ADMA). Because ADMA is excreted in the urine, levels in anuric individuals are elevated and would be associated with depressed nitric oxide levels and, in experimental models, arterial constriction.[11] However, studies in dialysis patients failed to correlate ADMA concentrations with mean arterial pressure, indicating an incomplete understanding of its causal role.[12] Among endothelin subtypes, animal data demonstrate that increased levels of endothelin-1 results in elevations in systemic blood pressure. Moreover, hypertensive hemodialysis patients demonstrate elevations in endothelin-1 compared with normotensive dialysis-dependent individuals.[13]

Another contributor to persistent elevation of BP among dialysis patients includes erythropoietin-stimulating agents (EPO), provoking elevations in blood pressure in both normotensive and hypertensive individuals.[14] Although the effect is both dose and hemoglobin-target dependent, it cannot be simply explained by elevated blood volume because increases in red blood cell volume trigger compensatory reductions in plasma cell volume such that total blood volume remains unchanged.[15] Putative pathways include endothelin-1 and enhanced adrenergic sensitivity.[16]

BLOOD PRESSURE GOALS IN CHRONIC KIDNEY DISEASE

Treatment of hypertension in CKD is directed at two goals: prevention or slowing of CKD-progression and reducing the elevated cardiovascular morbidity and mortality seen among CKD patients. The target blood pressure for individuals with CKD has been established by KDIGO and the Expert Panel Report (also known as Joint National Committee Report [JNC 8]); in those with albuminuric CKD, goal blood pressure is 140/90 or lower mm Hg, and 130/80 or lower mm Hg in those with 300 mg per day or higher of albuminuria.[17,18] Despite these recommendations, the efficacy of the tighter blood pressure target has failed to show additional slowing of CKD progression (at least in nondiabetic patients with advanced CKD). Conversely, post hoc analyses of all randomized trials have demonstrated a further reduction in cardiovascular mortality including heart failure, stroke, and coronary heart events in advanced CKD patients with blood pressure levels below 130/80 mm Hg in both those with and without diabetes.[19-22]

Among dialysis patients, evidence for specific BP goals remain unclear given the paucity of randomized trials. As such, recommendations have been extrapolated from observational studies among dialysis patients and the larger hypertension literature. The most recent (2005) KDOQI guidelines for dialysis patients recommend a predialysis and postdialysis blood pressure of less than 140/90 mm Hg and 130/80 mm Hg, respectively, acknowledging a weak level of evidence and a recommendation based on expert opinion.[23] More recent evidence suggests that blood pressure measurements obtained on the morning after dialysis are the most prognostic and reproducible.[24]

Hypertension and Risk for Chronic Kidney Disease

Blood pressure has long been recognized as a manifestation and mediator of chronic kidney disease. Multiple retrospective studies have found that uncontrolled blood pressure is an independent predictor of CKD progression and the development of ESRD.[25] The Multiple Risk Factor Intervention Trial (MRFIT) of over 12,000 men prospectively studied the effects of various interventions on the incidence of coronary artery disease, and by post hoc analysis, on progression to ESRD.[26] Individuals developing ESRD had higher baseline mean systolic blood pressure (SBP) and diastolic blood pressure (DBP) than individuals without ESRD (SBP 142 versus 135 mm Hg; DBP 93 mm Hg versus 91 mm Hg, both $p < 0.001$). For every increase in systolic blood pressure of 10 mm Hg, the hazard ratio of developing ESRD increased by a factor of 1.3. These results are even more remarkable considering those individuals with baseline diastolic blood pressure in excess of 115 mm Hg were excluded.

Studies in cohorts with CKD of any etiology confirm the above association. Among more than 200 patients from the Veterans Affairs hospital population, a systolic blood pressure of 150 or greater mm Hg carried a hazard ratio of 9.1 for progression to a renal endpoint. Furthermore, rates of progression to ESRD were a function of blood pressure control with incidence rates of 7.2%, 27.7%, and 71.4% among those with systolic pressures of less than 130 mm Hg, less than 150 mm Hg, and more than 150 mm Hg, respectively.[27] Although the aforementioned studies focused on those with GFRs greater than 60 mL per minute (stages 1 to 3), studies of those with more advanced CKD show a similar association. An analysis of 4000 Canadian patients found participants' GFR declined at a rate of more than 5.0 mL per minute over the study period in those with a mean blood pressure of 145/80 mm Hg compared with reductions in GFR of less than 2.2 mL per minute in those with pressures of 137/74 mm Hg.[28]

CKD progression is even more rapid among those with diabetes and uncontrolled blood pressures (Fig. 33.3). The reduction of endpoints in noninsulin-dependent diabetes mellitus with the angiotensin II antagonist losartan (RENAAL) trial examined the effects of losartan on renal outcomes among those with diabetic nephropathy (albuminuria ≥ 300 mg/g;

Composite ranking for relative risks by GFR and albuminuria (KDIGO 2009)			Albuminuria stages, description and range (mg/g)		
			A1	A2	A3
			Optimal and high-normal	High	Very high and nephrotic
			<10	10–29	30–299	300–1999	≥2000
GFR stages, description and range (mL/min per 1.73 m²)	G1	High and optimal	>105				
			90–104				
	G2	Mild	75–89				
			60–74				
	G3a	Mild-moderate	45–59				
	G3b	Moderate-severe	30–44				
	G4	Severe	15–29				
	G5	Kidney failure	<15				

FIG. 33.1 Classification of chronic kidney disease by glomerular filtration rate and albuminuria. *(From Kidney Disease: Improving Global Outcomes (KDIGO) CKD Work Group. KDIGO clinical practice guideline for the evaluation and management of chronic kidney disease. Kidney Int Suppl. 2013; 3:1-150.)*

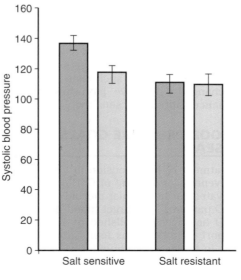

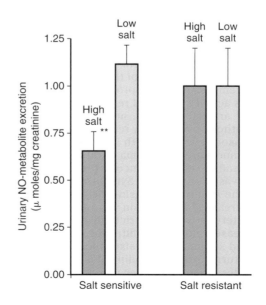

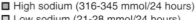

☐ High sodium (316-345 mmol/24 hours)
☐ Low sodium (21-28 mmol/24 hours)

FIG. 33.2 Urinary excretion of nitric oxide metabolites in salt-resistant and salt-sensitive individuals during high and low salt intake. Proposed pathogenesis of salt-sensitive hypertension in the setting of subtle renal parenchymal injury. *(From Cubeddu LX, Alfieri AB, Hoffmann IS, et al. Nitric oxide and salt sensitivity. Am J Hypertens. 13 (9):973-979, 2000.)*

serum creatinine 1.3 to 3.0 mg/dL). Baseline systolic blood pressure in excess of 160 mm Hg and pulse pressure greater than 70 mm Hg were both independently associated with progression to a doubling of serum creatinine, ESRD, or death. Additionally, the lower the blood pressure achieved the slower the progression of CKD (Fig. 33.4A) and to ESRD (Fig. 33.4B). There was no association between diastolic hypertension and renal outcome.[29] Among the more than 1600 hypertensive patients with diabetic nephropathy enrolled in the Irbesartan Diabetic Nephropathy Trial (IDNT), the achieved systolic BP at study completion (average follow-up: 2.6 years) was the strongest predictor of renal outcomes.[30] Those with a systolic blood pressure of more than 149 mm Hg saw a 2.2-fold increase in the risk of a doubling of serum creatinine or ESRD when compared with those with a systolic pressure of less than 134 mm Hg. Furthermore, progressive

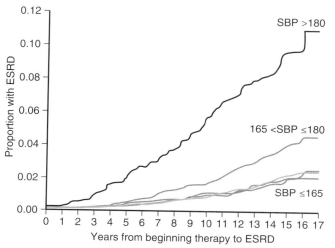

FIG. 33.3 Kaplan-Meier estimates of rates of end-stage renal disease (ESRD) by pretreatment average systolic blood pressure. *(From Perry HM, Miller JP, Fornoff JR, et al. Early predictors of 15-year end-stage renal disease in hypertensive patients.* Hypertension. *1995;25[4 Pt 1]: 587-594).*

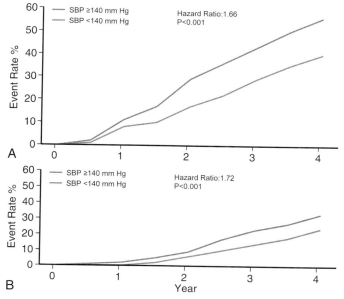

FIG. 33.4 Event rate for the primary composite endpoint (A) and end-stage renal disease (ESRD) alone (B) by systolic blood pressure level: RENAAL (reduction of endpoints in noninsulin-dependent diabetes mellitus with the angiotensin II antagonist losartan.). *(From Bakris GL, Weir MR, Shanifar S, et al. Effects of blood pressure level on progression of diabetic nephropathy: results from the RENAAL study.* Arch Intern Med. *2003;163:1555-1565.)*

lowering of systolic BP to 120 mm Hg was associated with improved renal and patient survival, an effect independent of baseline renal function. Similar to data from the RENAAL trial, there was no correlation between diastolic BP and renal outcomes.[30]

Magnitude of Blood Pressure Lowering and Chronic Kidney Disease Progression

Although the role of hypertension in the development and progression of CKD is well documented, tight control of high blood pressures has yet to be unequivocally linked to slowing the progression of CKD in either the diabetic or nondiabetic population. In the modification of diet in renal disease (MDRD) study, individuals with nondiabetic CKD (mean GFR 39 mL/min; mean proteinuria 1.1 g/d) were randomized to tight or usual mean arterial pressure (MAP) with achieved MAP of 91 mm Hg (125/75 mm Hg) or 96 mm Hg (130/80 mm Hg), respectively. After three years, the rate of GFR decline was identical in both arms at 11.5 mL per minute. However, among those with greater than 3 grams per day of proteinuria, GFR decline was 10.2 mL per minute in the usual blood pressure group but 6.7 mL per minute in those treated to the lower target.[31] Upon an additional 6 years of passive follow-up, during which no blood pressure goal was specified and blood pressures were not measured, those randomized to the intensive arm were 33% less likely to require dialysis. However, this benefit was driven exclusively by lower rates of ESRD in those with at least 1 gram per day of proteinuria.[32]

The African American Study of Kidney Disease (AASK), a trial that excluded those with diabetes, also evaluated the effects of intensive blood pressure control on CKD progression. Almost 1100 African Americans with a mean GFR of 46 mL per minute and 600 mg of proteinuria achieved a blood pressure goal of either 128/78 mm Hg (intensive therapy) or 141/85 mm Hg (usual care) with metoprolol, ramipril, or amlodipine. Over four years of follow-up, the rate of GFR decline was nearly identical in both groups at 2.1 mL per minute per year; there was no difference when stratified by antihypertensive agent.[33] The ramipril efficacy in nephropathy-2 (REIN-2) tested a similar premise with ramipril in patients with immunoglobulin a nephropathy (mean GFR 35 mL/min; mean proteinuria 2.9 g/d). Achieved blood pressures were 130/80 mm Hg (intensive group) and 134/82 (usual care). Intensive blood pressure control failed to result in further slowing of GFR decline (mean decline 2.6 mL/min in both groups) over 18 months of follow-up, an outcome noted irrespective of degree of pretreatment proteinuria.[34] In aggregate, the results of these studies indicate that control of blood pressure to less than 130/80 fails to further slow progression of nondiabetic CKD; however, there may be a modest benefit among those with proteinuria in excess of 2 to 3 grams per day. Moreover, unlike glycemic control there is no legacy effect of BP reduction on CVD outcomes.[35]

The lack of prospective trials evaluating the effects of lower blood pressure targets on the progression of diabetic nephropathy has resulted in a limited understanding of optimal blood pressure goals. One trial evaluating patients with type I diabetes with nephropathy (mean creatinine 1.2 mg/dL; mean proteinuria 1.2 mg/dL) found that both those randomized to intensive (MAP: 92 mm Hg) or usual (MAP: 100 to 107 mm Hg) blood pressure experienced a yearly decline of 10% in GFR.[36]

The appropriate blood pressure control (ABCD) trial has been the only attempt at prevention of CKD progression in type 2 diabetic patients. The study evaluated the effects of achieved blood pressure goals of 128/75 mm Hg (intensive) versus 137/81 mm Hg (usual care) among 500 normotensive individuals with type 2 diabetes, one-third of whom had diabetic nephropathy. After five years of follow up, no change in the rate of GFR decline was noted between groups.[37] Moreover, the study was extended by 2.5 years and still no difference was noted, albeit both groups had very slow decline in glomerular filtration rate.[37]

Reduction in Albuminuria

Despite the apparent lack of benefit of intensive BP lowering on CKD progression, there is consensus as to the salutary effects of albuminuria reduction associated with renal outcomes. Of note, there is considerable debate as to whether or not high albuminuria (formerly microalbuminuria; defined as 30 to 300 mg/day of urinary albumin excretion) indicates the presence of nephropathy (Fig. 33.5).[38] This is consistent with the Renin-Angiotensin System Study (RASS). It found that among normotensive normo-albuminuric patients with type I diabetes, angiotensin-converting enzyme inhibitor (ACEi) therapy suppressed albuminuria but angiotensin II receptor blocker (ARB) therapy increased it. However, neither therapy failed to alter morphologic progression of diabetic nephropathy, as documented by serial renal biopsy.[39]

The Avoiding Cardiovascular Events through Combination Therapy in Patients Living with Systolic Hypertension (ACCOMPLISH) study further highlighted the limitations of microalbuminuria as a surrogate for kidney disease. Although the primary outcome was the rate of cardiovascular events in those randomized to benazepril/hydrochlorothiazide compared with benazepril/amlodipine, the prespecified secondary endpoint of progression to ESRD was less common in benazepril/amlodipine-treated patients, despite higher rates of albuminuria.[40]

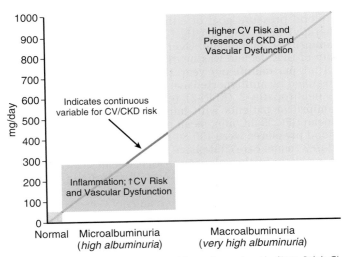

FIG. 33.5 Spectrum of albuminuria and its cardiovascular risk. *(From Bakris GL, Molitch M. Microalbuminuria as a risk predictor in diabetes: the continuing saga.* Diabetes Care. 2014;37:867-875.)

In contrast, very high albuminuria, that is more than 300 mg per day, is an unequivocal sign of renal parenchymal injury, a risk factor for CKD progression and a heightened rate of cardiovascular events.[28,41] In a post hoc analysis of the aforementioned AASK trial, every two-fold increase in baseline proteinuria was associated with an 80% increase in the risk of progression to ESRD.[42,43] Moreover, a strong association between the degree of proteinuria reduction during the first six months, and the progression to dialysis, was noted. Compared with patients who failed to achieve a reduction in proteinuria, those who achieved a 50% reduction had a slowing of progression to ESRD (Table 33.1).[42] Results from the MDRD study further reinforce this precept as only those with heavy proteinuria treated to an aggressive BP goal had a slowing of GFR decline.

Cardiovascular Risk Modification

Chronic kidney disease is as an independent risk factor for cardiovascular mortality with the risk proportionate to disease severity.[44] As such, for risk stratification purposes, the KDOQI guidelines state that those with depressed GFRs should be considered high risk for cardiovascular events. The Systolic Blood Pressure Intervention Trial (SPRINT) was an open-label randomized control trial that evaluated the effects of intensive versus usual blood pressure control among 9300 patients at an increased risk of cardiovascular events (those with a history of stroke, coronary artery disease, or CKD) without diabetes. Those in the active arm achieved a systolic blood pressure of 121 mm Hg, and those in the standard treatment arm an SBP of 135 mm Hg. 75% and 55% of patients, respectively, were on RAAS blockade. Among the 28% of patients with CKD (mean GFR 48 mL/min per m²), there was no difference between groups with respect to the prespecified outcomes of doubling of serum creatinine, progression to ESRD, or reduction in proteinuria over a follow-up of 3.3 years. There was also no reduction in cardiovascular events such as myocardial infarction, stroke, or death from a cardiovascular cause among this subgroup. Those treated to a tighter blood pressure control also had higher rates of syncope, acute kidney injury, and hypotension. Limitations include a short duration of follow-up and a mean age of only 68 years.[20]

The excess cardiac event rates attributable to kidney disease also extend to those on dialysis with 50% of patient deaths related to cardiovascular disease, specifically, heart failure and sudden death. Despite this, the relationship between hypertension and mortality remains opaque as a result of the lack of prospective studies and inconsistent interstudy methodology.[45] Because the overwhelming majority of studies are observational in nature, the influence of confounders, notably that of different classes of antihypertensive therapy, dialysis adequacy, and the possibility that predialysis hypertension may be a surrogate for interdialytic weight gain or compliance, cannot be excluded as the cause for differences in cardiovascular mortality. Moreover, variable duration of

TABLE 33.1 Clinical Trials and Renal Outcomes Based on Proteinuria Reduction

| SLOWING OF PROGRESSION TO DIALYSIS | NO CHANGE OVER CONTROL OR FASTER PROGRESSION TO DIALYSIS | |
30%-35% Reduction in Proteinuria	No Proteinuria Reduction Monotherapy	20%-35% Greater Reduction in Proteinuria vs. RAS
Captopril Trial	DHPCCB arm-IDNT	ALTITUDE
AASK	DHPCCB arm-AASK	ONTARGET
RENAAL		ACCOMPLISH
IDNT		

AASK, African American Study of Kidney Disease; *ACCOMPLISH*, Avoiding Cardiovascular Events through Combination Therapy in Patients Living with Systolic Hypertension; *ALTITUDE*, Aliskiren Trial in Type 2 Diabetes Using Cardiorenal Endpoints; *DHPCCB*, dihydropyridine calcium channel blocker; *IDNT*, Irbesartan Diabetic Nephropathy Trial; *ONTARGET*, The Ongoing Telmisartan Alone and in Combination with Ramipril Global Endpoint Trial; *RAS*, renin angiotensin system; *RENAAL*, reduction of endpoints in noninsulin-dependent diabetes mellitus with the angiotensin ii antagonist losartan.

follow-up and a reliance on predialysis blood pressures as a measure of hypertension, render accurate interpretation of such studies challenging.[46-49]

Among the more recent and larger positive studies, Mazzuchi and colleagues found both systolic and diastolic hypertension to be associated with heightened all-cause mortality. However, the study population excluded those who had been on dialysis for less than two years, thereby introducing considerable bias.[47] By far the largest study, that of Port et al, found no relationship between predialysis blood pressure and mortality. Again, patients were included only if they had been on dialysis for one or more years.[46] In contrast to the lack of consensus regarding systolic blood pressure and mortality, low diastolic pressures, defined as less than 60 to 70 mm Hg, appear to uniformly enhance all-cause mortality, a phenomenon also observed in nondialysis dependent individuals.[46,47,49,50] Possible explanations include a high burden of comorbidities, myocardial dysfunction, and patient frailty. Finally, some data support the hypothesis that moderate levels of hypertension are cardioprotective, or, perhaps, simply a manifestation of more robust health. This paradox, that low blood pressure is associated with adverse outcomes and high blood pressure with survival, has been termed the reverse epidemiology of blood pressure among those with renal failure.[51]

An analysis of 25,000 hemodialysis patients participating in the international Dialysis Outcomes and Practice Patterns Study (DOPPS) revealed an all-cause mortality hazard ratio of 1.14 for those with a predialysis systolic blood pressure of 110 to 119 mm Hg and 1.11 for pressures of 120 to 129 mm Hg, compared with a reference pressure of 130 to 139 mm Hg. Among hypertensive individuals, those with a predialysis systolic measurement of 150 to 159 mm Hg had a lower all-cause mortality (hazard ratio: 0.90) than the reference population; moreover, no correlation was noted between mortality and pressures in excess of 160 mm Hg. Similar U-shaped curves were noted for diastolic pressures, with a hazard ratio of 1.0 for predialysis values of 60 to 99 mm Hg.[52] Other post hoc analyses have confirmed this observation, suggesting that low-normal predialysis blood pressures are a marker of a higher burden of comorbid conditions, rather than a deleterious effect from lowering pressures to these levels.[46,53] Nonetheless, in the absence of prospective trials, confounding variables and the cause-effect relationship between blood pressure and mortality remain unclear.

SELECTION OF ANTIHYPERTENSIVE AGENT

Volume Control in Chronic Kidney Disease

Given the salt-avid state characteristic of CKD, appropriately dosed diuretics remain the cornerstone of hypertension management and should be instituted irrespective of the detection of edema on physical exam. This is consistent with observational data that demonstrates an association between early expansion of extracellular fluid volume and cardiac remodeling in the predialysis CKD patient.[54] In contrast to the dosing of most medications in patients with advanced CKD, diuretics require a higher dose to be effective, given decreased tubule delivery of such agents.

Before adding an antihypertensive medication to those on dialysis, optimization of the patient's volume status is critical and results in normotension in greater than 85% of patients.[55] The dry weight, the lowest blood pressure that does not result in symptoms of hypotension (rather than the absence of edema) should be sought.[56] In the prospective randomized Dry Weight Reduction in Hypertensive Hemodialysis Patients (DRIP) study, additional ultrafiltration of 0.1 kg per 10 kg body weight per session resulted in a further 0.9-kg weight loss at one month with a decrease in blood pressure of 6.9/3.1 mm

Hg by ambulatory monitoring versus control patients (Fig. 33.6).[57] Although participants in the DRIP trial benefited from a rapid decline in blood pressure, the presence of a lag phenomenon is well documented such that up to one month may be required to see an improvement in hemodynamic parameters.[58] Although no direct evaluation of dry weight reduction on left ventricular (LV) mass has been undertaken, a study comparing six-nights per week hemodialysis versus conventional thrice-weekly sessions showed improvement in this parameter.[59]

Agents That Modify the Renin-Angiotensin-Aldosterone System

As the presence of macroalbuminuria and the reduction therein has become an important consideration when selecting an antihypertensive, class differences among agents emerge. The best-studied and most effective agents are those that block the RAAS. As detailed earlier, ACEi and ARBs are effective antialbuminuric agents in kidney disease of any etiology. The aforementioned REIN-2 study, although not demonstrating the salutary effects of aggressive blood pressure control on CKD progression over 36 months of follow-up, indicated that those on ramipril therapy had significantly lower rates of GFR decline (0.53 mL/min versus 0.88 mL/min per month). Furthermore, the ramipril group demonstrated significant reductions in albuminuria that continued to improve over time: 23% reduction at 1 month of treatment, 33% at 12 months, and 55% at 36 months. This benefit was independent of blood pressure control.[60] Similarly, the Captopril Trial evaluated the effect of an ACEi compared with placebo on progression of nephropathy among those with insulin-dependent diabetes. Patients randomized to placebo experienced a 17% decline in creatinine clearance compared with 11% in the captopril arm. Doubling of creatinine occurred in 43% of placebo-treated patients versus 25% receiving captopril over three years of follow-up. The largest benefit was seen in those with the most advanced stages of CKD.[61]

Angiotensin receptor blockers appear to carry a similar benefit. The ARB irbesartan was studied in a randomized

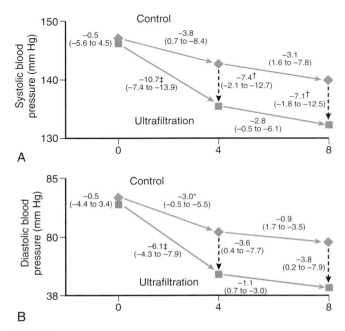

FIG. 33.6 Effect of protocol-driven dry weight reduction in hemodialysis patients on interdialytic systolic (A) and diastolic blood pressure (B). *(From Agarwal R, Alborzi P, Satyan S, Light RP. Dry-weight reduction in hypertensive hemodialysis patients [DRIP]: a randomized, controlled trial. Hypertension. 2009;53:500-507.)*

controlled trial of patients with hypertension and diabetic nephropathy. Compared with amlodipine and placebo, irbesartan reduced proteinuria to a greater degree and was associated with a 30% to 35% lower risk of doubling of serum creatinine compared with placebo or amlodipine. The risk reduction was not explained by differences in blood pressure.[62] Similarly, the previously cited RENAAL study examined the effect of losartan versus placebo in patients with type 2 diabetes and greater than 300 mg of albuminuria per day. Individuals treated with losartan achieved a 16% risk reduction of progressing to the primary endpoint of doubling of serum creatinine and an absolute, 35%, reduction of proteinuria. As in the study examining irbesartan, the benefit was not explained by differences in blood pressure.[63]

The renin inhibitor, aliskerin, was tested for both blood pressure reduction and renal outcomes in combination with the ARB, valsartan. Nearly 1150 hypertensive participants with type 2 diabetes and stage 1 or 2 CKD were randomized to receive the combination of aliskiren/valsartan 150/160 mg or valsartan 160 mg monotherapy for 2 weeks, with force-titration to 300/320 mg and 320 mg, respectively, for another 6 weeks. Changes in ambulatory blood pressure (ABP), the primary outcome, were available for 665 participants. Reductions from baseline to week 8 in 24-hour ABP were –14.1/–8.7 mm Hg with aliskiren/valsartan versus –10.2/–6.3 mm Hg among those on valsartan monotherapy. Although adverse events were noted in one-third of participants in both groups, no subject developed acute kidney injury or a serum potassium in excess of 6.0 mEq/L.[64]

In contrast, the Aliskerin Trial in Type 2 Diabetes Using Cardiorenal Endpoints (ALTITUDE) Trial evaluated the aforementioned dual therapy on cardiovascular and renal outcomes. Although there was superior proteinuria reduction among those patients on combination therapy, the trial was terminated prematurely because of significantly higher incidence of hyperkalemia, acute kidney injury, and hypotension. Moreover, there was a trend toward worse cardiovascular outcomes in those on dual therapy.[65] It is worthwhile to note that the mean eGFR in the ALTITUDE trial was below 45 mL per minute.

In addition to the ALTITUDE trial, other trials have failed to uniformly support a direct link between reduction of proteinuria and improved renal outcomes. The Gauging Albuminuria Reduction with Lotrel in Diabetic Patients with Hypertension (GUARD) study tested the combination of benazepril with either hydrochlorothiazide or amlodipine on the degree of urinary protein reduction and blood pressure decline among diabetics. Despite twice the proteinuria reduction in the diuretic arm, progression to overt nephropathy was similar between groups.[66] As a prespecified secondary analysis of the aforementioned ACCOMPLISH trial, those at high risk for a cardiovascular event were randomized to the combination of either benazepril plus amlodipine or benazepril plus hydrochlorothiazide. Ten percent of the 11,000 enrolled patients suffered from chronic kidney disease, more than half of which was attributed to diabetes. Over a 3-year period, those randomized to the ACEi with calcium channel blocker (CCB) arm achieved only half as much proteinuria reduction, yet the rate of progression to renal endpoints such as ESRD or a doubling of serum creatinine was also 50% less.[40]

Further enthusiasm for maximal proteinuria reduction has been tempered by a series of high quality trials demonstrating double RAAS blockade, while further reducing proteinuria, does so at the cost of hyperkalemia, hypotension, and increased rates of acute kidney injury. The Ongoing Telmisartan Alone or in Combination with Ramipril Global Endpoint Trial (ONTARGET) was the first large (>15,000 participants) study to compare ramipril with combination therapy with telmisartan on cardiovascular events among those

with diabetes or vascular disease. Although there was no difference in the number of cardiac endpoints reached between groups, the incidence of hyperkalemia, hypotension, and renal impairment was significantly more common in those assigned to combination therapy.[67] The Veterans Affairs Nephropathy in Diabetes (VA NEPHRON-D) trial/study specifically evaluated the effects of combination therapy with lisinopril and losartan on renal outcomes such as GFR and progression to ESRD. The trial was halted early because despite improvements in levels of proteinuria, patients randomized to ARB plus ACEi therapy experienced more hyperkalemia and acute kidney injury. Moreover, there was also a trend toward worse renal outcomes compared with placebo-treated patients.[68] In summary, the current evidence strongly supports the use of ACEi or ARB monotherapy to achieve proteinuria reduction as a means of slowing CKD progression. However, combination therapy to further reduce proteinuria, be it by double RAAS blockade or with diuretic therapy, paradoxically appears to hasten CKD progression or results in additional short-term adverse events.

Aldosterone antagonists such as spironolactone and eplerenone have grown in popularity as a means of achieving further reductions in albuminuria when used as add-on therapy among those treated with ACEi or ARB monotherapy. Physiologic grounds for their use is derived from the agents' ability to halt the aldosterone escape that occurs despite treatment with RAAS blockade.[69] This lack of suppression of the aldosterone escape pathway has been linked to persistent declines in GFR.[70] Evidence for the antiproteinuric effects of spironolactone have been demonstrated in both diabetic and nondiabetic populations. In a randomized controlled trial of 80 individuals with persistent diabetic nephropathy (mean GFR 65 mL/min; mean albuminuria 1.0 g/d) despite lisinopril (80 mg) monotherapy, either spironolactone (25 mg), losartan (100 mg), or placebo were instituted as add-on therapy. As shown in Fig. 33.7, at 2-year follow-up, only spironolactone therapy resulted in a statistically significant reduction (34%) in urinary protein excretion. Of note, nearly 50% of patients in both arms had at least one serum potassium in excess of 6.0 mEq/L.[71] Using the selective mineralocorticoid receptor blocker eplerenone, 275 diabetics with a GFR of 75 mL per min and 300 mg of albuminuria were randomly assigned to enalapril monotherapy or dual therapy with eplerenone (doses: 50 to 100 mg/day). At three months, albuminuria had decreased by 41% and 48%, respectively. However, 10% of those on low-dose and 25% on high-dose eplerenone were noted to have a serum potassium greater than 6.0 mEq/L.[72]

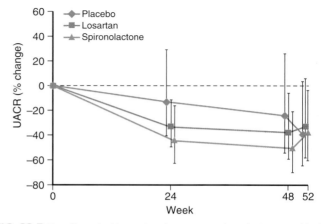

FIG. 33.7 The effect of add-on spironolactone to angiotensin II receptor blocker therapy in patients with diabetic nephropathy and persistent proteinuria on urine albumin:creatinine ratio. *(From Mehdi UF, Adams-Huet B, Raskin P, Vega GL, Toto RD. Addition of angiotensin receptor blockade or mineralocorticoid antagonism to maximal angiotensin-converting enzyme inhibition in diabetic nephropathy. J Am Soc Nephrol. 2009;20:2641-2650.)*

More recently a Phase 2b trial evaluated the nonsteroidal mineralocorticoid receptor antagonist finerenone for its ability to reduce urinary albumin excretion without attendant hyperkalemia. In the Mineralocorticoid Receptor Antagonist Tolerability Study-Diabetic Nephropathy (ARTS-DN), more than 800 participants (GFR: 65 to 70 mL/min; albuminuria: 180 mg/d) were randomized to ACEi or ARB monotherapy plus finerenone (dose 1.25 to 20 mg/d) or placebo over a 3-month period. The results revealed that at doses of 20 mg per day, a 40% reduction in albuminuria was realized. Importantly, only 5% of those with CKD stage 3 or greater suffered from a serum potassium above 5.6 mEq/L.[73] As the above trials demonstrate, the entirety of the evidence supports the efficacy of aldosterone antagonists to lower proteinuria beyond levels achieved with RAAS monotherapy, albeit at the cost of hyperkalemia. However, in the absence of trials evaluating the effects of spironolactone on clinical endpoints such as progression to ESRD or a doubling of serum creatinine, endorsement of such therapy remains limited.

The principal obstacle to the wide-spread implementation of aldosterone antagonists is the high rate of hyperkalemia among CKD patients on either ACEi or ARB therapy in spite of diuretic therapy. Such individuals have a 3.8-fold higher incidence of hyperkalemia when pretreatment serum potassium is greater than 4.5 mEq/L and GFR is less than 45 mL per minute.[74]

Until recently, apart diuretics and a low potassium diet, little has been available to manage hyperkalemia. The use of the cation exchange resin sodium polystyrene sulfonate (Kayexalate) has fallen out of favor because of unclear efficacy, poor tolerability, and an association with intestinal necrosis.[75] As of late 2015, a resin based polymer that exchanges colonic potassium for calcium, patiromer, was approved for outpatient treatment of hyperkalemia. This is distinctly different from sodium polystyrene because it uses calcium rather than sodium for exchange. A second agent with a different chemistry using sodium as the exchanger, zirconium cyclosilicate (ZS-9), is scheduled for release no earlier than 2017.[76] Both are oral, nonabsorbable agents that bind enteric potassium, thereby leading to increased fecal excretion.

The efficacy of patiromer was evaluated in the randomized open-label phase 2 trial, AMETHYST-DN. All participants had diabetes with CKD stage 3 or later, 50% of the cohort was on RAAS blockade and 40% of individuals on diuretic therapy. After the twice-daily administration of between 4.2 and 16.8 grams, reductions in serum potassium ranged from 0.35 mEq/L in those receiving the lowest dose and with potassium levels less than 5.5 mEq/L to decreases of 1.0 mEq/L among those randomized to the highest dose and with potassium levels between 5.5 mEq/L and 6.0 mEq/L. The reductions were maintained during the one-year follow-up period, with dose-dependent hypomagnesemia (7% to 13%) and constipation (5%) being the most common adverse events.[77] Based on these results, the Two-Part, Single-Blind, Phase 3 Study Evaluating the Efficacy and Safety of Patiromer for the Treatment of Hyperkalemia (OPAL-HK), was undertaken to specifically evaluate late stage 3 CKD patients on RAAS inhibitors.[78] The patient population was exclusively white with diuretic therapy in place for 50% of participants. After a four-week period during which all patients received either 4.2 g or 8.4 g twice daily, a dose-dependent reduction in serum potassium (mean decrease 1.0 mEq/L) occurred. After this 1-month period, patients were subsequently randomized to patiromer maintenance or placebo for an additional eight weeks. In contrast to a rise in potassium of 0.7 mEq/L in those transitioned to placebo (pretreatment potassium: 4.5 mEq/L), there was no rise in potassium among those continued on binder therapy. Upon trial completion, 85% of patients in the patiromer arm and 40% on placebo achieved a serum potassium of less than 5.5 mEq/L. Moreover, three times as many patients in the placebo arm required an intervention to manage recurrent hyperkalemia compared with those in the active therapy arm.

There were two double blind placebo controlled trials, to assess ZS-9 the Hyperkalemia Randomized Intervention Multidose ZS-9 Maintenance (HARMONIZE) and a larger trial by Packham et al. In these trials the selective sodium and hydrogen exchanger ZS-9 was compared with placebo at daily doses of between 1.25 g and 15 g over a 2-week to 4-week period. In both trials, those with type 2 diabetes comprised 60% of participants, 75% of participants had CKD stage 3, and 70% of patients were on concomitant RAAS therapy. Baseline potassium was between 5.3 and 5.6 mEq/L. Of note, the percentage of patients on diuretics was not reported, nearly all patients were white, and those with ESRD were excluded. Reductions in potassium were dose dependent with absolute reductions of between 0.5 and 0.8 mEq/L in the 5 g arm, 0.7 and 1.1 mEq/L in the 10-g cohort, and up to 1.2 mEq/L in those treated with 15 g.

In the HARMONIZE trial, which reported the proportion of patients achieving normokalemia, 80% to 95% were able to maintain a serum potassium of less than 5.1 mEq/L compared with only 45% of placebo-treated patients. Adverse effects between groups were similar except for edema, which occurred in 6% of patients in the 15-g arm compared with 2% in those treated with placebo.[79,80] Of note, neither trial evaluated patients with acute hyperkalemia and the trial duration was only one month.

In summary, patiromer and ZS-9, when approved, represent the first new agents in decades for the treatment of hyperkalemia that are both effective and well-tolerated. Their availability should allow for clinical trials to investigate the effects of RAAS blocking agents on CKD progression among those with advanced (i.e., GFR <30 min/min per m^2) kidney disease.

Nonrenin-Angiotensin-Aldosterone System Antihypertensive Therapy

Calcium channel blockers (CCB) are effective antihypertensive agents in those with CKD. Among cohorts with proteinuric nephropathy, there is strong evidence of an additional 30% to 40% reduction in proteinuria when a nondihydropyridine calcium channel blocker (diltiazem or verapamil) is added to a RAAS blocker.[81] Moreover, animal studies demonstrate a relative antisclerotic and antifibrotic effect of nondihydropyridine CCBs compared with amlodipine.[82]

Although no head-to-head comparison exists between CCBs, there are two long-term trials demonstrating a lack of benefit by amlodipine in the absence of a RAAS blocker on CKD progression.[62,83] There is one small long-term study demonstrating slowing of CKD progression when diltiazem was used in the absence of a RAAS blocker.[84] Likewise verapamil has been shown to reduce albuminuria compared with amlodipine in patients with diabetes in the absence of an RAAS blocker.[85] Thus, diltiazem or verapamil should be considered as an adjuvant to RAAS-blocking agents.

There is limited data regarding the effect of β-blockers in the treatment of hypertension in the setting of CKD. Those in the AASK study treated with metoprolol demonstrated rates of CKD progression similar to those in the amlodipine arm, both of which were inferior to ACEi therapy.[86] One of the few positive trials was a 45 patient study among those with Autosomal Dominant Polycystic Kidney Disease and preserved GFR. When randomized to metoprolol or ramipril, neither GFR decline nor albuminuria was slower in the ACEi arm over three years of follow-up.[87] In light of the above, β-blockers should be viewed as adjunct antihypertensive therapy, principally among those with a cardiac indication.

Diuretics, particularly those targeting the thick ascending limb of the loop of Henle ("loop" diuretics), have long been the cornerstones of management given the salt avid state characteristic of CKD. Agents acting on the distal convoluted tubule such as the thiazide-like diuretic chlorthalidone, long considered ineffective in those with a GFR less than 30 mL per min, have recently been shown to be active in those with GFRs as low as 25 mL per min.[88] A detailed review of diuretic therapy is provided in Chapter 22.

Among dialysis patients, antihypertensive agents are indicated in individuals who fail to achieve desired blood pressure goals with volume optimization alone. Among classes, there is modest evidence that certain agents provide benefits apart from their antihypertensive effects. In the open-label Hypertension in Hemodialysis Patients Treated with Atenolol or Lisinopril (HDPAL) trial, patients treated with lisinopril experienced nearly 2.5-fold more cardiovascular events than those randomized to atenolol. However, interdialytic weight gain was higher among lisinopril-treated patients as was the total number of medications required to achieve similar blood pressure levels.[89]

Despite the above evidence that lisinopril is inferior to atenolol in reducing cardiovascular events, the K/DOQI guidelines, published before the HDPAL trial, suggest ACEi or ARB therapy for those with residual renal function.[90] Moreover, although ACEi and ARB therapy both result in regression of left ventricular hypertrophy, at least one prospective trial, the Fosinopril in Dialysis Study, found no improvement in cardiovascular outcomes when ACEi therapy was compared with other classes of agents.[91] In contrast, ARB therapy may result in fewer cardiovascular events when compared with blood pressure control with other classes of agents.[92] Regardless, both ACEi and ARB therapy result in elevations of serum potassium, often by as much as 0.7 mEq/L.[93]

Angiotensin receptor blockers are not removed by hemodialysis; however, most ACE inhibitors are to some degree.[94] The strongest evidence for beta-blocker therapy comes from the aforementioned HDPAL trial showing reduced cardiovascular events when compared with lisinopril.[89] Among ESRD patients with dilated cardiomyopathy, one trial showed that carvedilol therapy resulted in nearly a two-thirds risk reduction in all-cause mortality when compared with placebo.[95] Most beta-blockers except carvedilol are removed by hemodialysis such that a supplement is needed postdialysis if taken for arrhythmia. Calcium channel blocker therapy is efficacious in lowering blood pressure but when compared with placebo, amlodipine therapy failed to decrease all-cause mortality.[96] Calcium channel blockers are not removed by dialysis. Little evidence exists regarding the benefits of aldosterone antagonists or central sympathetic agonists; however, neither are removed by hemodialysis.[94]

Although uncommon, some patients experience worsening hypertension in the final hours of a given dialysis treatment. Although the phenomenon is poorly understood, it appears to be mediated by reflex sympathetic activation in response to ultrafiltration induced volume removal. In a small study comparing thirty patients who experienced intradialytic hypertension (defined as an increase in MAP of greater than 15 mm Hg), peripheral vascular resistance increased by nearly 60% by the end of dialysis compared with less than a 20% increase in control hemodialysis patients. Moreover, endothelin-1 rose compared with control. However, neither nitric oxide, epinephrine, and renin levels were similar before and after dialysis and between groups.[97] Even less literature exists regarding treatment in such cases with anecdotal experience suggesting low-sodium dialysate, central acting sympathetic agents, and beta-blockers as potential therapies.[98]

OUT-OF-OFFICE-BLOOD PRESSURE MONITORING

Much of the existing literature on hypertension and CKD has focused on measurement and modification of blood pressure while patients are in a specific health care setting (e.g.,

in-office, in-hospital). Recently, there has been increasing recognition of the importance of out-of-office blood pressure monitoring. Specifically, continuous ambulatory blood pressure monitoring and home blood pressure monitoring have helped identify and convey the importance of white-coat hypertension, masked hypertension, and the normal diurnal variation of blood pressure. Moreover, home blood pressure measurements, if done with appropriate frequency and timing, can guide management in a fashion similar to continuous monitoring technologies.[99,100]

White-coat hypertension, defined as elevated office blood pressure readings (>140/90 mm Hg) with normal (<130/80 mm Hg) 24-hour mean readings, and masked hypertension, characterized by normal office pressures with high ambulatory pressures, have recently been implicated as risk factors for increased cardiovascular morbidity and mortality.[101,102] Continuous blood pressure monitoring also allows for the identification of individuals that fail to follow the normal diurnal variation in blood pressure characterized by a decline in the overnight hours (dipping). Individuals with CKD that do not experience nocturnal dipping may have a higher risk of cardiovascular disease and more severe renal parenchymal injury. When the relationship between blood pressure variation, GFR, and proteinuria were studied, those with CKD were more likely to be nondippers. Furthermore, severity of proteinuria was a stronger predictor of the absence of blood pressure variation than CKD stage.[103]

Data on whether or not nondipping status confers an increased cardiovascular risk among those with CKD is conflicting. In an evaluation of 80 individuals with advanced CKD, nondipping status was not an independent predictor of CKD progression or cardiovascular events.[104] However, two further studies of out-of-office blood pressure monitoring in the CKD population reveal nondipping status to be associated with an increased risk of progression to ESRD and all-cause mortality.[105] Nevertheless, the American Heart Association recommends out-of-office blood pressure monitoring as part of the routine care of hypertensive individuals.

CONCLUSION

Hypertension is found in one-third of those with early stage CKD and in the vast majority of those starting dialysis. Although the goals of therapy (prevention of CKD progression, minimization of cardiovascular complications) remain clear, the blood pressure goal to do so remains uncertain. The plurality of the evidence suggests that those with nonproteinuric CKD do not yield additional benefit below 135/85 mm Hg; those with proteinuria do so, but to a limited extent. Among those on dialysis, the lack of high quality trials precludes strong recommendations; however, observation data suggests blood pressure as high as 150 to 160/90 mm Hg do not have untoward cardiovascular effects. To achieve such blood pressure targets, diuretics for volume control and agents that modify the renin-angiotensin-aldosterone axis for proteinuria reduction should be considered first-line therapy in those with CKD. Among ESRD patients, aggressive volume control with dialysis and perhaps beta-blockers affords additional cardiovascular benefit.

References

1. (K/DOQI) KDOQI. K/DOQI clinical practice guidelines on hypertension and antihypertensive agents in chronic kidney disease. *Am J Kidney Dis.* 2004;43(5 Suppl 1):S1-290.
2. Bello AK, Nwankwo E, El Nahas AM. Prevention of chronic kidney disease: a global challenge. *Kidney Int Suppl.* 2005;98:S11-17.
3. US Renal Data System, USRDS 2009 Annual Data Report: Atlas of Chronic Kidney Disease and End Stage Renal Disease in the United States. Bethesda, MD. National Institute of Health, National Institute of Diabetes and Digestive and Kidney Diseases; 2009.
4. Agarwal R, Nissenson AR, Batlle D, Coyne DW, Trout JR, Warnock DG. Prevalence, treatment, and control of hypertension in chronic hemodialysis patients in the United States. *Am J Med.* 2003;115:291-297.
5. Salem MM. Hypertension in the hemodialysis population: a survey of 649 patients. *Am J Kidney Dis.* 1995;26:461-468.

6. Joles JA, Koomans HA. Causes and consequences of increased sympathetic activity in renal disease. *Hypertension*. 2004;43:699-706.

7. Johnson RJ, Herrera-Acosta J, Schreiner GF, Rodriguez-Iturbe B. Subtle acquired renal injury as a mechanism of salt-sensitive hypertension. *N Engl J Med*. 2002;346:913-923.

8. Cubeddu LX, Alfieri AB, Hoffmann IS, et al. Nitric oxide and salt sensitivity. *Am J Hypertens*. 2000;13:973-979.

9. Nongnuch A, Campbell N, Stern E, El-Kateb S, Fuentes L, Davenport A. Increased postdialysis systolic blood pressure is associated with extracellular overhydration in hemodialysis outpatients. *Kidney Int*. 2015;87:452-457.

10. Converse RL, Jacobsen TN, Toto RD, et al. Sympathetic overactivity in patients with chronic renal failure. *N Engl J Med*. 1992;327:1912-1918.

11. Vallance P, Leone A, Calver A, Collier J, Moncada S. Accumulation of an endogenous inhibitor of nitric oxide synthesis in chronic renal failure. *Lancet*. 1992;339:572-575.

12. Anderstam B, Katzarski K, Bergström J. Serum levels of NG, NG-dimethyl-L-arginine, a potential endogenous nitric oxide inhibitor in dialysis patients. *J Am Soc Nephrol*. 1997;8:1437-1442.

13. Shichiri M, Hirata Y, Ando K, et al. Plasma endothelin levels in hypertension and chronic renal failure. *Hypertension*. 1990;15:493-496.

14. Eschbach JW, Abdulhadi MH, Browne JK, et al. Recombinant human erythropoietin in anemic patients with end-stage renal disease. Results of a phase III multicenter clinical trial. *Ann Intern Med*. 1989;111:992-1000.

15. Krapf R, Hulter HN. Arterial hypertension induced by erythropoietin and erythropoiesis-stimulating agents (ESA). *Clin J Am Soc Nephrol*. 2009;4:470-480.

16. Kang DH, Yoon KI, Han DS. Acute effects of recombinant human erythropoietin on plasma levels of proendothelin-1 and endothelin-1 in haemodialysis patients. *Nephrol Dial Transplant*. 1998;13:2877-2883.

17. Taler SJ, Agarwal R, Bakris GL, et al. KDOQI US commentary on the 2012 KDIGO clinical practice guideline for management of blood pressure in CKD. *Am J Kidney Dis*. 2013;62:201-213.

18. James PA, Oparil S, Carter BL, et al. 2014 evidence-based guideline for the management of high blood pressure in adults: report from the panel members appointed to the Eighth Joint National Committee (JNC 8). *JAMA*. 2014;311:507-520.

19. Perkovic V, Rodgers A. Redefining Blood-Pressure Targets—SPRINT Starts the Marathon. *N Engl J Med*. 2015;373:2175-2178.

20. Wright JT, Williamson JD, Whelton PK, et al. A Randomized Trial of Intensive versus Standard Blood-Pressure Control. *N Engl J Med*. 2015;373:2103-116.

21. Margolis KL, O'Connor PJ, Morgan TM, et al. Outcomes of combined cardiovascular risk factor management strategies in type 2 diabetes: the ACCORD randomized trial. *Diabetes Care*. 2014;37:1721-1728.

22. Emdin CA, Rahimi K, Neal B, Callender T, Perkovic V, Patel A. Blood pressure lowering in type 2 diabetes: a systematic review and meta-analysis. *JAMA*. 2015;313:603-615.

23. Workgroup KD. K/DOQI clinical practice guidelines for cardiovascular disease in dialysis patients. *Am J Kidney Dis*. 2005;45(4 Suppl 3):S1-153.

24. Agarwal R. Home and ambulatory blood pressure monitoring in chronic kidney disease. *Curr Opin Nephrol Hypertens*. 2009;18:507-512.

25. Xie X, Atkins E, Lv J, et al. Effects of intensive blood pressure lowering on cardiovascular and renal outcomes: updated systematic review and meta-analysis. *Lancet*. 2016;387:435-443.

26. Ishani A, Grandits GA, Grimm RH, et al. Association of single measurements of dipstick proteinuria, estimated glomerular filtration rate, and hematocrit with 25-year incidence of end-stage renal disease in the multiple risk factor intervention trial. *J Am Soc Nephrol*. 2006;17:1444-1452.

27. Agarwal R. Blood pressure components and the risk for end-stage renal disease and death in chronic kidney disease. *Clin J Am Soc Nephrol*. 2009;4:830-837.

28. Levin A, Djurdjev O, Beaulieu M, Er L. Variability and risk factors for kidney disease progression and death following attainment of stage 4 CKD in a referred cohort. *Am J Kidney Dis*. 2008;52:661-671.

29. Bakris GL, Weir MR, Shanifar S, et al. Effects of blood pressure level on progression of diabetic nephropathy: results from the RENAAL study. *Arch Intern Med*. 2003;163:1555-1565.

30. Pohl MA, Blumenthal S, Cordonnier DJ, et al. Independent and additive impact of blood pressure control and angiotensin II receptor blockade on renal outcomes in the irbesartan diabetic nephropathy trial: clinical implications and limitations. *J Am Soc Nephrol*. 2005;16:3027-3037.

31. Klahr S, Levey AS, Beck GJ, et al. The effects of dietary protein restriction and blood-pressure control on the progression of chronic renal disease. Modification of Diet in Renal Disease Study Group. *N Engl J Med*. 1994;330:877-884.

32. Sarnak MJ, Greene T, Wang X, et al. The effect of a lower target blood pressure on the progression of kidney disease: long-term follow-up of the modification of diet in renal disease study. *Ann Intern Med*. 2005;142:342-351.

33. Appel LJ, Wright JT, Greene T, et al. Long-term effects of renin-angiotensin system-blocking therapy and a low blood pressure goal on progression of hypertensive chronic kidney disease in African Americans. *Arch Intern Med*. 2008;168:832-839.

34. Ruggenenti P, Perna A, Loriga G, et al. Blood-pressure control for renoprotection in patients with non-diabetic chronic renal disease (REIN-2): multicentre, randomised controlled trial. *Lancet*. 2005;365:939-946.

35. Holman RR, Paul SK, Bethel MA, Neil HA, Matthews DR. Long-term follow-up after tight control of blood pressure in type 2 diabetes. *N Engl J Med*. 2008;359:1565-1576.

36. Lewis JB, Berl T, Bain RP, Rohde RD, Lewis EJ. Effect of intensive blood pressure control on the course of type 1 diabetic nephropathy. Collaborative Study Group. *Am J Kidney Dis*. 1999;34:809-817.

37. Schrier RW, Estacio RO, Esler A, Mehler P. Effects of aggressive blood pressure control in normotensive type 2 diabetic patients on albuminuria, retinopathy and strokes. *Kidney Int*. 2002;61:1086-1097.

38. Bakris GL, Molitch M. Microalbuminuria as a risk predictor in diabetes: the continuing saga. *Diabetes Care*. 2014;37:867-875.

39. Mauer M, Zinman B, Gardiner R, et al. Renal and retinal effects of enalapril and losartan in type 1 diabetes. *N Engl J Med*. 2009;361:40-51.

40. Bakris GL, Sarafidis PA, Weir MR, et al. Renal outcomes with different fixed-dose combination therapies in patients with hypertension at high risk for cardiovascular events (ACCOMPLISH): a prespecified secondary analysis of a randomised controlled trial. *Lancet*. 2010;375:1173-1181.

41. Remuzzi G, Chiurchiu C, Ruggenenti P. Proteinuria predicting outcome in renal disease: nondiabetic nephropathies (REIN). *Kidney Int Suppl*. 2004;92:S90-96.

42. Lea J, Greene T, Hebert L, et al. The relationship between magnitude of proteinuria reduction and risk of end-stage renal disease: results of the African American study of kidney disease and hypertension. *Arch Intern Med*. 2005;165:947-953.

43. Norris K, Bourgoigne J, Gassman J, et al. Cardiovascular outcomes in the African American Study of Kidney Disease and Hypertension (AASK) Trial. *Am J Kidney Dis*. 2006;48:739-751.

44. Anavekar NS, McMurray JJ, Velazquez EJ, et al. Relation between renal dysfunction and cardiovascular outcomes after myocardial infarction. *N Engl J Med*. 2004;351:1285-1295.

45. Collins AJ, Foley RN, Herzog C, et al. Excerpts from the US Renal Data System 2009 Annual Data Report. *Am J Kidney Dis*. 2010;55(1 Suppl 1):S1-420. A6-7.

46. Port FK, Hulbert-Shearon TE, Wolfe RA, et al. Predialysis blood pressure and mortality risk in a national sample of maintenance hemodialysis patients. *Am J Kidney Dis*. 1999;33:507-517.

47. Mazzuchi N, Carbonell E, Fernández-Cean J. Importance of blood pressure control in hemodialysis patient survival. *Kidney Int*. 2000;58:2147-2154.

48. Salem MM. Hypertension in the haemodialysis population: any relationship to 2-years survival? *Nephrol Dial Transplant*. 1999;14:125-128.

49. Agarwal R. Hypertension and survival in chronic hemodialysis patients—past lessons and future opportunities. *Kidney Int*. 2005;67:1-13.

50. Farnett L, Mulrow CD, Linn WD, Lucey CR, Tuley MR. The J-curve phenomenon and the treatment of hypertension. Is there a point beyond which pressure reduction is dangerous? *JAMA*. 1991;265:489-495.

51. Kalantar-Zadeh K, Kilpatrick RD, McAllister CJ, Greenland S, Kopple JD. Reverse epidemiology of hypertension and cardiovascular death in the hemodialysis population: the 58th annual fall conference and scientific sessions. *Hypertension*. 2005;45:811-817.

52. Robinson BM, Tong L, Zhang J, et al. Blood pressure levels and mortality risk among hemodialysis patients in the Dialysis Outcomes and Practice Patterns Study. *Kidney Int*. 2012;82:570-580.

53. Li Z, Lacson E, Lowrie EG, et al. The epidemiology of systolic blood pressure and death risk in hemodialysis patients. *Am J Kidney Dis*. 2006;48:606-615.

54. Essig M, Escoubet B, de Zuttere D, et al. Cardiovascular remodelling and extracellular fluid excess in early stages of chronic kidney disease. *Nephrol Dial Transplant*. 2008;23:239-248.

55. Lazarus JM, Hampers C, Merrill JP. Hypertension in chronic renal failure. Treatment with hemodialysis and nephrectomy. *Arch Intern Med*. 1974;133:1059-1066.

56. Charra B, Laurent G, Chazot C, et al. Clinical assessment of dry weight. *Nephrol Dial Transplant*. 1996;11(Suppl 2):16-9.

57. Agarwal R, Alborzi P, Satyan S, Light RP. Dry-weight reduction in hypertensive hemodialysis patients (DRIP): a randomized, controlled trial. *Hypertension*. 2009;53:500-507.

58. Charra B, Bergström J, Scribner BH. Blood pressure control in dialysis patients: importance of the lag phenomenon. *Am J Kidney Dis*. 1998;32:720-724.

59. Culleton BF, Walsh M, Klarenbach SW, et al. Effect of frequent nocturnal hemodialysis vs conventional hemodialysis on left ventricular mass and quality of life: a randomized controlled trial. *JAMA*. 2007;298:1291-1299.

60. Randomised placebo-controlled trial of effect of ramipril on decline in glomerular filtration rate and risk of terminal renal failure in proteinuric, non-diabetic nephropathy. The GISEN Group (Gruppo Italiano di Studi Epidemiologici in Nefrologia). *Lancet*. 1997;349:1857-1863.

61. Lewis EJ, Hunsicker LG, Bain RP, Rohde RD. The effect of angiotensin-converting-enzyme inhibition on diabetic nephropathy. The Collaborative Study Group. *N Engl J Med*. 1993;329:1456-1462.

62. Lewis EJ, Hunsicker LG, Clarke WR, et al. Renoprotective effect of the angiotensin-receptor antagonist irbesartan in patients with nephropathy due to type 2 diabetes. *N Engl J Med*. 2001;345:851-860.

63. Brenner BM, Cooper ME, de Zeeuw D, et al. Effects of losartan on renal and cardiovascular outcomes in patients with type 2 diabetes and nephropathy. *N Engl J Med*. 2001;345:861-869.

64. Bakris GL, Oparil S, Purkayastha D, Yadao AM, Alessi T, Sowers JR. Randomized study of antihypertensive efficacy and safety of combination aliskiren/valsartan vs valsartan monotherapy in hypertensive participants with type 2 diabetes mellitus. *J Clin Hypertens (Greenwich)*. 2013;15:92-100.

65. Parving HH, Brenner BM, McMurray JJ, et al. Cardiorenal end points in a trial of aliskiren for type 2 diabetes. *N Engl J Med*. 2012;367:2204-2213.

66. Bakris GL, Toto RD, McCullough PA, et al. Effects of different ACE inhibitor combinations on albuminuria: results of the GUARD study. *Kidney Int*. 2008;73:1303-1309.

67. Yusuf S, Teo KK, Pogue J, et al. Telmisartan, ramipril, or both in patients at high risk for vascular events. *N Engl J Med*. 2008;358:1547-1559.

68. Fried LF, Emanuele N, Zhang JH, et al. Combined angiotensin inhibition for the treatment of diabetic nephropathy. *N Engl J Med*. 2013;369:1892-1903.

69. Bakris GL, Siomos M, Richardson D, et al. ACE inhibition or angiotensin receptor blockade: impact on potassium in renal failure. VAL-K Study Group. *Kidney Int*. 2000;58:2084-2092.

70. Schjoedt KJ, Andersen S, Rossing P, Tarnow L, Parving HH. Aldosterone escape during blockade of the renin-angiotensin-aldosterone system in diabetic nephropathy is associated with enhanced decline in glomerular filtration rate. *Diabetologia*. 2004;47:1936-1939.

71. Mehdi UF, Adams-Huet B, Raskin P, Vega GL, Toto RD. Addition of angiotensin receptor blockade or mineralocorticoid antagonism to maximal angiotensin-converting enzyme inhibition in diabetic nephropathy. *J Am Soc Nephrol*. 2009;20:2641-2650.

72. Epstein M, Williams GH, Weinberger M, et al. Selective aldosterone blockade with eplerenone reduces albuminuria in patients with type 2 diabetes. *Clin J Am Soc Nephrol*. 2006;1:940-951.

73. Bakris GL, Agarwal R, Chan JC, et al. Effect of Finerenone on Albuminuria in Patients With Diabetic Nephropathy: A Randomized Clinical Trial. *JAMA*. 2015;314:884-894.

74. Lazich I, Bakris GL. Prediction and management of hyperkalemia across the spectrum of chronic kidney disease. *Semin Nephrol*. 2014;34:333-339.

75. Gerstman BB, Kirkman R, Platt R. Intestinal necrosis associated with postoperative orally administered sodium polystyrene sulfonate in sorbitol. *Am J Kidney Dis*. 1992;20:159-161.

76. Pitt B, Bakris GL. New potassium binders for the treatment of hyperkalemia: current data and opportunities for the future. *Hypertension*. 2015;66:731-738.

77. Bakris GL, Pitt B, Weir MR, et al. Effect of Patiromer on Serum Potassium Level in Patients With Hyperkalemia and Diabetic Kidney Disease: The AMETHYST-DN Randomized Clinical Trial. *JAMA*. 2015;314:151-161.

78. Weir MR, Bakris GL, Bushinsky DA, et al. Patiromer in patients with kidney disease and hyperkalemia receiving RAAS inhibitors. *N Engl J Med*. 2015;372:211-221.

79. Kosiborod M, Rasmussen HS, Lavin P, et al. Effect of sodium zirconium cyclosilicate on potassium lowering for 28 days among outpatients with hyperkalemia: the HARMONIZE randomized clinical trial. *JAMA*. 2014;312:2223-2233.

80. Packham DK, Rasmussen HS, Lavin PT, et al. Sodium zirconium cyclosilicate in hyperkalemia. *N Engl J Med*. 2015;372:222-231.

81. Bakris GL, Weir MR, Secic M, Campbell B, Weis-McNulty A. Differential effects of calcium antagonist subclasses on markers of nephropathy progression. *Kidney Int*. 2004;65:1991-2002.

82. Griffin KA, Picken MM, Bakris GL, Bidani AK. Class differences in the effects of calcium channel blockers in the rat remnant kidney model. *Kidney Int*. 1999;55:1849-1860.

83. Agodoa LY, Appel L, Bakris GL, et al. Effect of ramipril vs amlodipine on renal outcomes in hypertensive nephrosclerosis: a randomized controlled trial. *JAMA*. 2001;285:2719-2728.

84. Bakris GL, Copley JB, Vicknair N, Sadler R, Leurgans S. Calcium channel blockers versus other antihypertensive therapies on progression of NIDDM associated nephropathy. *Kidney Int.* 1996;50:1641-1650.

85. Boero R, Rollino C, Massara C, et al. The verapamil versus amlodipine in nondiabetic nephropathies treated with trandolapril (VVANNTT) study. *Am J Kidney Dis.* 2003;42:67-75.

86. Wright JT, Bakris G, Greene T, et al. Effect of blood pressure lowering and antihypertensive drug class on progression of hypertensive kidney disease: results from the AASK trial. *JAMA.* 2002;288:2421-2431.

87. Zeltner R, Poliak R, Stiasny B, Schmieder RE, Schulze BD. Renal and cardiac effects of antihypertensive treatment with ramipril vs metoprolol in autosomal dominant polycystic kidney disease. *Nephrol Dial Transplant.* 2008;23:573-579.

88. Agarwal R, Sinha AD, Pappas MK, Ammous F. Chlorthalidone for poorly controlled hypertension in chronic kidney disease: an interventional pilot study. *Am J Nephrol.* 2014;39:171-182.

89. Agarwal R, Sinha AD, Pappas MK, Abraham TN, Tegegne GG. Hypertension in hemodialysis patients treated with atenolol or lisinopril: a randomized controlled trial. *Nephrol Dial Transplant.* 2014;29:672-681.

90. Group HAW. Clinical practice guidelines for hemodialysis adequacy, update 2006. *Am J Kidney Dis.* 2006;48(Suppl 1):S2-90.

91. Zannad F, Kessler M, Lehert P, et al. Prevention of cardiovascular events in end-stage renal disease: results of a randomized trial of fosinopril and implications for future studies. *Kidney Int.* 2006;70:1318-1324.

92. Suzuki H, Kanno Y, Sugahara S, et al. Effect of angiotensin receptor blockers on cardiovascular events in patients undergoing hemodialysis: an open-label randomized controlled trial. *Am J Kidney Dis.* 2008;52:501-506.

93. Hörl MP, Hörl WH. Drug therapy for hypertension in hemodialysis patients. *Semin Dial.* 2004;17:288-294.

94. Inrig JK. Antihypertensive agents in hemodialysis patients: a current perspective. *Semin Dial.* 2010;23:290-297.

95. Cice G, Ferrara L, D'Andrea A, et al. Carvedilol increases two-year survivalin dialysis patients with dilated cardiomyopathy: a prospective, placebo-controlled trial. *J Am Coll Cardiol.* 2003;41:1438-1444.

96. Tepel M, Hopfenmueller W, Scholze A, Maier A, Zidek W. Effect of amlodipine on cardiovascular events in hypertensive haemodialysis patients. *Nephrol Dial Transplant.* 2008;23:3605-3612.

97. Chou KJ, Lee PT, Chen CL, et al. Physiological changes during hemodialysis in patients with intradialysis hypertension. *Kidney Int.* 2006;69:1833-1838.

98. Inrig JK, Patel UD, Toto RD, Szczech LA. Association of blood pressure increases during hemodialysis with 2-year mortality in incident hemodialysis patients: a secondary analysis of the Dialysis Morbidity and Mortality Wave 2 Study. *Am J Kidney Dis.* 2009;54:881-890.

99. Stergiou GS, Parati G. The optimal schedule for self-monitoring of blood pressure by patients at home. *J Hypertens.* 2007;25:1992-1997.

100. Stergiou GS, Omboni S, Parati G. Home or ambulatory blood pressure monitoring for the diagnosis of hypertension? *J Hypertens.* 2015;33:1528-1530.

101. Gustavsen PH, Høegholm A, Bang LE, Kristensen KS. White coat hypertension is a cardiovascular risk factor: a 10-year follow-up study. *J Hum Hypertens.* 2003;17:811-817.

102. Bobrie G, Genès N, Vaur L, et al. Is "isolated home" hypertension as opposed to "isolated office" hypertension a sign of greater cardiovascular risk? *Arch Intern Med.* 2001;161:2205-2211.

103. Agarwal R, Light RP. GFR, proteinuria and circadian blood pressure. *Nephrol Dial Transplant.* 2009;24:2400-2406.

104. Redon J, Plancha E, Swift PA, Pons S, Muñoz J, Martinez F. Nocturnal blood pressure and progression to end-stage renal disease or death in nondiabetic chronic kidney disease stages 3 and 4. *J Hypertens.* 2010;28:602-607.

105. Agarwal R, Andersen MJ. Prognostic importance of ambulatory blood pressure recordings in patients with chronic kidney disease. *Kidney Int.* 2006;69:1175-1180.

Transplant Hypertension
Sandra J. Taler

Hypertension is a common feature after solid organ transplantation, related to preexisting disease, the vascular effects of immunosuppressive medications, and in the setting of renal transplantation, the presence of acute or chronic allograft morbidity. Transplant patients frequently carry a heavy burden of atherosclerotic disease involving multiple vascular beds and thus are at increased risk for cardiovascular events including myocardial infarction, congestive heart failure, and stroke. Hypertension may be a cause or a complication of native kidney disease or renal allograft injury. Regardless of which presents first, hypertension may accelerate further renal decline, particularly when proteinuria is present. Thus transplant recipients require meticulous attention to blood pressure (BP) control.

Hypertension following solid organ transplantation affects not only kidney recipients, but also heart, liver, and bone marrow recipients. Its presence after transplantation may be a continuation of pretransplant hypertension; a result of immunosuppressive medication effects, particularly of calcineurin inhibitors (CNIs) and corticosteroids; or a result of sodium and volume retention. The severity and persistence of this condition relate to the type of organ transplanted, primarily a result of the immunosuppression regimen used in that setting, and the level of native and/or allograft renal function. Although there are nuances for management that relate to the type of solid organ transplanted, most concepts salient to renal transplantation, which has been subject to more studies, also apply to the other posttransplant settings. The subsequent discussion will focus on renal transplant recipients.

Historically, the incidence of hypertension after renal transplant increased from between 45% and 55% to between 70% and 90% with the adoption of CNI-based (cyclosporine, then tacrolimus) immunosuppression.[1] In this setting, worsening or de novo hypertension may result from reduced renal function caused by CNI agents, rejection, chronic allograft injury, or hypoperfusion resulting from transplant renal artery stenosis (RAS). As immunosuppressive medication doses are reduced with time after transplant, hypertension severity often declines, resulting in improved control. Even so, current control rates are suboptimal,[2] and treatment can be challenging.

Concern has been raised within the transplant community regarding the flat survival rates for renal transplant recipients in recent years.[3,4] Premature death of a patient with a functioning graft, often resulting from cardiovascular (CV) disease, has become a major cause of transplant failure.[5] Nonimmunologic factors such as hypertension, are major determinants of long-term kidney graft survival.[6] Observational studies have shown hypertension to be an independent risk factor for CV disease after kidney transplantation, suggesting that transplant recipients would benefit from improved BP control.[7] Levels of BP 1 year after renal transplant predict allograft survival over subsequent years.[8] Even so, improved BP control can reduce ongoing renal allograft injury and improve long-term graft survival.[9,10] Thus it is essential that clinicians caring for transplant patients focus on hypertension control to improve CV risk, minimize renal dysfunction, and promote long-term success of the renal allograft.

PATHOGENESIS

Immunosuppressive Therapy

Posttransplant hypertension is directly related to administration of CNI agents in combination with corticosteroids. It is less common when CNIs are used without corticosteroids in the liver transplant setting,[11,12] although prevalence rates did not differ in steroid minimization trials following renal transplantation.[13,14] The rate of rise in BP and accelerated CV risk are more prominent with cyclosporine; however, prevalence rates of posttransplant hypertension with cyclosporine and tacrolimus are similar by 1 year after transplant. With the higher doses of corticosteroids used for induction, BP may be particularly elevated during the first weeks to months following transplantation. Vasoconstriction in the kidney results in decreased renal blood flow and glomerular filtration rate (GFR) within hours of CNI administration, leading to reduction in sodium excretion.[1] These changes may reverse if treatment is discontinued or the dosage is reduced. Sustained administration of CNIs results in vascular and interstitial changes that eventually become irreversible.

The primary hemodynamic consequence of CNI is an increase in systemic vascular resistance caused by widespread vasoconstriction. Calcineurin inhibitors activate the renin-angiotensin system through a direct effect on the juxtaglomerular cells and indirectly via renal vasoconstriction, with high intrarenal renin activity, yet low systemic circulating levels. Cyclosporine augments the vasoconstrictive effects of angiotensin II. CNI-induced imbalance in circulating vasoconstrictor (endothelin and thromboxane) and vasodilatory (prostacyclin and nitric oxide) compounds results in impaired vasodilation.[15] It is likely that CNIs alter function of the endothelium by shifting the relative balance of vasoconstrictive and vasodilatory pathways. Direct aggravation of hypertension by CNIs has been confirmed by the reduction in BP that occurs with later conversion to a non–CNI-based immunosuppressive regimen. This happens despite equally severe renal dysfunction in patients whose hypertension improves.

Azathioprine and mycophenolate mofetil have not been associated with hypertension. Effects of sirolimus on BP are less clear, but reports of BP-lowering with conversion from cyclosporine to sirolimus support either fewer or no hypertensive effects.[16] Belatacept-based immunosuppression is associated with higher GFR and preservation of renal function. As reported from the long-term extension of the Belatacept Evaluation of Nephroprotection and Efficacy as First-line Immunosuppression Trial (BENEFIT) Study, hypertension is still present in the majority of patients, although fewer agents were needed to achieve BP goals and reported BP levels were lower with Belatacept than for cyclosporine-treated control subjects.[17]

Glucocorticoids can cause or worsen hypertension, even in the absence of a mineralocorticoid effect, and may explain up to 15% of posttransplant hypertension. At the higher doses used early after transplantation, some activation of mineralocorticoid receptors occurs, manifested by potassium wasting, especially with high sodium intake. Glucocorticoid effects include increased cardiac output and enhanced pressor responses to epinephrine, angiotensin II, and other pressure stimuli. The role of corticosteroids in CNI-induced hypertension is complex. Although glucocorticoids alone rarely have major effects on BP in normal subjects, corticosteroids administered in immunosuppressive doses to patients with impaired renal function commonly elevate BP and aggravate hypertension. Hence, it is likely that both CNIs, corticosteroids, and their combination are major elements in the prevalence and severity of posttransplant hypertension.

Renal Allograft Factors

Blood pressure alterations may provide clues to subclinical acute rejection, hypoperfusion, or chronic allograft nephropathy. Causes of posttransplant hypertension occurring within the first 3 months after transplant generally differ from those causing late or persistent hypertension (Box 34.1). This distinction is useful when considering possible causes and choosing appropriate treatment. Transplant complications such as rejection, organ preservation injury, and transplant RAS can impair renal function and worsen hypertension. Severe hypertension during the early postoperative period is more common in those with severe hypertension before transplant, in African Americans, and in patients with delayed graft function. Primary mediators include hypervolemia, high CNI and glucocorticoid doses, withdrawal of preoperative antihypertensive medications, and postoperative pain. Beyond the first 3 months, hypertension may relate to donor variables, as donor age and donor hypertension are strongly associated with graft function. A well-functioning renal allograft frequently improves and may even normalize BP in the recipient.

Hypertension after transplantation is both a sign of kidney disease and a cause of kidney dysfunction. Renal transplant recipients with lower renal function (creatinine clearance <60 mL/min) in the first year are more likely to develop

posttransplant hypertension.[18] Alternatively, hypertension is associated with reduced renal allograft survival, independent of renal function.[5] In a retrospective series of 1600 renal transplant recipients, for each 10 mm Hg rise in systolic BP, the risk for allograft loss increased by 12% to 15%.[7] Worsening hypertension suggests acute or chronic graft pathology that may be otherwise clinically silent. Hypertension is likely to worsen with declining allograft function and may be particularly severe in those with chronic transplant glomerulopathy or focal segmental glomerulosclerosis developing late after transplant.

Transplant RAS may present as de novo or worsening hypertension, or a decline in renal function precipitated by BP treatment, particularly with use of angiotensin-converting enzyme (ACE) inhibitors or angiotensin receptor blockers (ARBs). Although it may manifest at any time, it is most commonly diagnosed between 3 months and 2 years posttransplant.[19] Anastomotic stenosis is more likely in recipients of pediatric deceased donor kidneys related to smaller donor vessels, and in recipients of living donor kidneys related to the nature of the anastomotic technique without use of a donor aortic patch. Risk factors include older recipient age, male gender, smoking, and preexisting diabetes. Stenosis of the iliac artery is likely to be as a result of atherosclerotic disease and may be associated with other symptoms of peripheral vascular disease. A critical iliac artery stenosis may present with classic features of renovascular hypertension including sudden circulatory congestion or flash pulmonary edema. Stenosis of the allograft artery may result from atherosclerotic disease of donor origin or, more often, progressive stenosis at the surgical anastomotic site.

CLINICAL FEATURES

Many features of posttransplant hypertension are similar to those of the general population with hypertension, including higher prevalence in African Americans, males, and those at higher weight or body mass index. Recipients with preexisting diabetes are more likely to be hypertensive, with primarily systolic hypertension and widened pulse pressures.[20] Studies in nontransplant populations implicate arterial stiffening as the cause for this pattern, which is associated with greater CV risk.

Hypertension developing after organ transplantation is characterized by abnormal circadian BP rhythm (Fig. 34.1), with absence or reversal of the 10% to 20% nocturnal fall commonly seen in normal subjects and those with primary hypertension. The magnitude of this fall is often blunted after transplantation, and some patients develop a paradoxical rise, with their highest pressures in the overnight hours. In the nontransplant setting, loss of nocturnal BP fall is associated with accelerated target organ damage, including left ventricular hypertrophy (LVH), lacunar stroke, and microalbuminuria. Similarly, nocturnal BP elevations may predispose transplant recipients to renal allograft injury[2,21] and accelerated atherosclerotic complications. This phenomenon is best documented using overnight ambulatory BP monitoring (ABPM). Circadian reversal has been observed following heart, liver, and kidney transplantation, most commonly in the first year. Serial studies suggest that some patients will regain more normal circadian BP patterns within the first year after transplantation. In a study of 241 renal transplant recipients at a median ABPM to transplant interval of 14 weeks, abnormal systolic diurnal variation correlated positively with age, serum creatinine, and blood cyclosporine trough level, and negatively with GFR and the time interval from transplantation.[22] In this series, 21% of patients had isolated nocturnal hypertension with normal daytime pressures. Only age and GFR were independent predictors of abnormal systolic diurnal variation.

BOX 34.1 Causes of Posttransplant Hypertension

Within the First 3 Months
- Pretransplant hypertension
- African-American race/ethnicity
- Renal allograft dysfunction
- Renal outflow obstruction
- Hypervolemia
- High-dose calcineurin inhibitors
- High-dose corticosteroids
- Postoperative pain
- Discontinuation of pretransplant antihypertensive medications

During Long-Term Care
- Donor variables
  - Increased donor age
  - African-American donor
  - Hypertensive donor
- Recipient variables
  - Older age
  - African-American race/ethnicity
  - Male gender
  - Obesity
  - Diabetes mellitus
  - Pretransplant hypertension
  - Native kidney disease
- Renal allograft dysfunction
- Recurrent primary renal disease
- Immunosuppressive medications
  - Calcineurin inhibitors
  - Corticosteroids
- Transplant renal artery stenosis

EVALUATION

The diagnosis of hypertension in transplant recipients follows criteria published in national guidelines, currently from the Joint National Committee on Prevention, Detection, Evaluation and Treatment of High Blood Pressure (JNC 7).[23] BP should be measured at every clinic visit and home self-measurement should be encouraged. Elevated office BP measurements should be verified by standardized nurse or serial device measurements, ABPM, or home self-measurement. In recent years, growing recognition of the importance of nocturnal BP levels and the presence of white coat and masked hypertension in transplant recipients has led to greater use of out-of-office measurements, particularly ABPM.

Renal function must be closely followed, as a decline in GFR may indicate rejection or hemodynamic compromise. A renal allograft biopsy often provides clinically useful information, including the presence of subclinical acute rejection, recurrent or de novo glomerulopathies, CNI toxicity, viral infections, or other pathologic changes that require modifications in treatment. Transplant RAS may be difficult to diagnose.[19] Low-pitched systolic bruits are common over the surgical anastomotic site without stenosis; even systolic-diastolic bruits may occur as a result of arteriovenous fistulas caused by allograft biopsy. Several Doppler ultrasound series report arterial stenosis prevalence rates of 9% to 12%, but the technique requires operator expertise because of variability in the angles required to visualize the transplant renal artery.[24] Magnetic resonance angiography has been reported to give a high proportion of false-positive results, although visualization is superior. Treatment by endovascular repair with angioplasty or stenting can provide recovery of blood flow with improvement or stabilization of renal function.[25] Restenosis is common and may require surgical correction of the stenotic segment.

TREATMENT

Treatment goals for posttransplant hypertension are theoretical, based on limited trial data and patterned after goals advised for the general population and particularly those designed for patients with chronic kidney disease.[26] Some transplant guidelines continue to advise BP target levels less than 130/80 mm Hg, especially for high-risk subpopulations,

including those with diabetes or proteinuric renal disease.[23,27] In the initial days after transplantation, renal perfusion is critical and blood pressure may be maintained above ideal targets to ensure optimal blood flow. During the first several weeks after transplant, rapid changes in immunosuppression, volume shifts, and changes in renal function require close monitoring of serum creatinine as a marker of renal function. Concurrent rapid changes in antihypertensive treatment may affect serum creatinine levels and implicate antihypertensive agents as the cause of renal function loss, resulting in dose reductions and inadequate control long-term. Thus, early after transplantation, BP should be lowered gradually to less than 150/90 mm Hg, with intensification of therapy later. By one month after transplant, targets should be tightened to less than 140/90 mm Hg as immunosuppression targets are reduced including corticosteroid dose for those maintained on corticosteroids long-term. Beyond the first 3 months, increasing evidence supports more aggressive efforts to achieve lower BP targets to prevent CV disease progression and kidney allograft injury. These targets are currently in evolution for the general and CKD population related to results of recent trials indicating better outcomes with targets as low as 120 mm Hg systolic.[28] Whether or not the same targets are optimal for transplant recipients are uncertain as these patients were not included in the trials. Patients should be provided with their current BP readings, along with specific BP goals.

Control of BP after transplantation can be challenging for many reasons, including polypharmacy, impaired graft function, older age, and comorbidities. Clinical inertia, defined as failure to initiate or intensify therapy when warranted, is increasingly recognized in the general population, but also occurs in the transplant setting.[29] Use of an automated device (e.g., BPTRU, Conquitlam, British Columbia, Canada, Omron Healthcare, Lake Forest, Illinois) and ABPM provide standardized, repeated measurements that more closely reflect out-of-office readings and thereby reduce measurement uncertainty for the provider and reassure the patient that changes need to be made. Use of home measurements provides essential feedback to transplant recipients, and clear targets facilitate improved and appropriate communication with providers. If there is a discrepancy between home and automated office readings, check the accuracy of the home monitor and the patient's measurement technique.

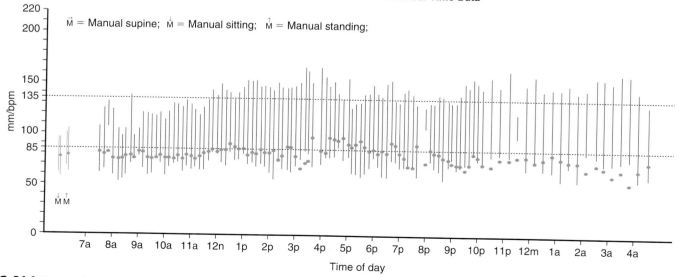

Blood Pressure and Heart Rate/Real Time Data

$\vec{M}$ = Manual supine; $\overset{\downarrow}{M}$ = Manual sitting; $\overset{\uparrow}{M}$ = Manual standing;

FIG. 34.1 Example of reversed circadian blood pressure (BP) rhythm following kidney transplantation. The magnitude of the normal nocturnal BP fall may be blunted and some patients develop a paradoxical rise in BP, with highest pressures in the overnight hours. This is sometimes associated with nocturia, headache, and disrupted sleep.

Nonpharmacologic Therapy

Although efficacy has not been demonstrated in the renal transplant population, lifestyle modification has documented value for BP-lowering in primary hypertensives, patients with chronic kidney disease (CKD), and elderly populations. These interventions are generally not harmful and may provide other health benefits; thus they should be recommended to transplant recipients as well. As in the general population, obesity is increasingly common, with most recipients gaining weight after transplantation. Weight gain is often associated with worsening hypertension, and even modest weight loss may produce measurable BP reductions.

Increased plasma volume occurs commonly as a compensatory response to antihypertensive therapy and may manifest as fluid retention (weight gain, edema) or a poor response to increased antihypertensive medications. High sodium intake and obesity contribute to increased plasma volume. Hence, sodium restriction enhances the antihypertensive efficacy of most BP medications and will minimize diuretic-induced potassium wasting. Because renal transplant recipients are more sensitive to polyuria and hypovolemia over the first several months after transplantation, extreme sodium restriction should be avoided. For chronic management, restricted sodium intake may be an effective ancillary treatment.[30] Regular exercise decreases BP primarily by facilitating weight loss. The use of the Dietary Approaches to Stop Hypertension (DASH)[31] diet may benefit transplant patients but should be introduced with caution, given that its emphasis on vegetable-based foods may worsen hyperkalemia in patients receiving CNIs.

Pharmacologic Therapy

General Concepts

Most treatment principles relevant to treating primary hypertension apply to transplant recipients as well. Treatment may require two or more antihypertensive agents to achieve recommended BP targets.

Transplant recipients are exposed to complex drug regimens with a high potential for serious drug interactions. Particular attention should be paid to selection of calcium channel blockers (CCBs) metabolized through the cytochrome P450 pathways because their effects of enhancement or blunting of CNI metabolism may induce major changes in CNI levels and trigger rejection or drug toxicity. Transplant recipients may develop unique side effects and have a higher incidence of known side effects that occur less commonly in other populations of patients with hypertension. Antihypertensive agents may affect kidney function, and agent and dose changes should be introduced gradually and require close monitoring.

Lacking prospective data testing the efficacy and safety of each agent in transplant recipients, treatment recommendations are based on clinical experience.[32] Advantages and disadvantages of specific agents and recommendations for the transplant setting are listed in Table 34.1. Several principles merit emphasis. The choice of antihypertensive agent should take into account the reduced GFR and renal vasoconstriction universally present. Uric acid levels are elevated, sometimes profoundly. Calcineurin inhibitors partially inhibit renal potassium and hydrogen ion excretion, predisposing patients

TABLE 34.1 Drug Treatment of Posttransplant Hypertension

AGENT CLASS	ADVANTAGES OR INDICATIONS FOR TRANSPLANT RECIPIENTS	DISADVANTAGES OR ADVERSE EFFECTS FOR TRANSPLANT RECIPIENTS	RECOMMENDATIONS FOR USE
Beta-blockers	Cardiac protection, myocardial infarction prophylaxis, prevent reflex tachycardia with vasodilator agents	Negative cardiac inotropic and chronotropic effects, bronchospasm, hyperglycemia, fatigue	Favored in perioperative and early posttransplant period, minimal impact on renal function. Combination alpha-blockers and beta-blocking agents preferred for their increased potency and minimal drug interactions but may cause orthostatic hypotension
Calcium channel blockers	Vasodilatory effects of dihydropyridine CCBs directly counter the vasoconstrictive effects of CNIs	*Dihydropyridines:* Edema, palpitations, headache, flushing, failure to lower proteinuria; *Nondihydropyridines:* Negative cardiac inotropic and chronotropic effects, constipation, drug interactions with CNIs	Use extended-release preparations. Dihydropyridines have minimal effects on CNI levels except nicardipine. Nondihydropyridines increase CNI levels, particularly cyclosporine.
ACE inhibitors	Slow loss of renal function especially if proteinuria is present, prevent diabetes, reduce cardiovascular risk in nontransplant settings	Cough, angioedema, anemia, hyperkalemia, azotemia	Recent prospective studies suggest lower GFR than with CCB therapy
Angiotensin receptor blockers	Slow loss of renal function especially if proteinuria is present, prevent diabetes, reduce cardiovascular risk in nontransplant settings	Anemia, hyperkalemia, azotemia	Recent prospective studies suggest lower GFR than with CCB therapy
Thiazide and thiazide-like diuretics	Potentiate effectiveness of other antihypertensive agents	Prerenal azotemia, hyponatremia, hypokalemia, hypomagnesemia, hypercalcemia, hyperglycemia, hyperuricemia	Less effective at GFR <30 mL/min
Loop diuretics	Potentiate effectiveness of other antihypertensive agents	Prerenal azotemia, hypokalemia, hypomagnesemia, hyperuricemia	Effective in azotemic patients, can be used in place of thiazide for patients with hyponatremia or hypercalcemia
Alpha-blockers	Useful as secondary agent	Orthostatic hypotension, urinary incontinence	Lack of trial data in transplant setting
Centrally acting sympathetic agents	Use for those unable to take beta-blocker	Dry mouth, sedation	Lack of trial data in transplant setting
Direct vasodilators	Potent agents	Edema, tachycardia	Lack of trial data in transplant setting

ACE, Angiotensin-converting enzyme; *CCB,* calcium channel blocker; *CNI,* calcineurin inhibitor; *GFR,* glomerular filtration rate.

to hyperkalemic metabolic acidosis. Diuretic therapy is often avoided to prevent worsening of azotemia and hyperuricemia. Aldosterone antagonists and other potassium-sparing agents must be used with caution. ACE inhibitors and ARBs, when used alone, may have limited efficacy early posttransplant and may aggravate both hyperkalemia and acidosis.

High CV risk and CV event rates in the renal failure and renal transplant populations support close attention to cardioprotection. Beta-blockers are underused in the general hypertension population and in the transplant setting. For patients with coronary artery disease, beta-blockade should be started preoperatively to reduce surgical mortality and then continued to blunt the reflex tachycardia often seen with vasodilatory or peripherally active agents (vasodilators, dihydropyridine CCBs, and/or alpha-blockers). Combination alpha-blockers and beta-blocking agents are preferred by some for their increased potency and minimal drug interactions in this setting. Fatigue, bradycardia, worsening glucose tolerance, and bronchospasm may limit use and dosage. If orthostatic hypotension becomes a problem, the alpha, beta blocker should be withdrawn and replaced by a selective B_1 blocker such as extended-release metoprolol.

Although there is theoretical evidence to support the use of ACE inhibitors or ARBs as preferred agents for long-term therapy, published trials comparing initial treatment favor calcium channel blockers. In a Cochrane analysis,[33] CCBs were noted to reduce graft loss and maintain higher GFR (by an increase of 4 mL per minute) with a suggestion of potential harm from ACE inhibitors causing anemia, hyperkalemia, and lower GFR (by a reduction of 8 mL/min). This net difference in GFR by agent class of 12 mL per minute was persistent over the time of treatment. Based on the Cochrane review, CCBs may be preferable as first-line agents for kidney transplant recipients. Compared with placebo, CCBs reduced graft loss by 25%; they avoid the anemia and hyperkalemia associated with ACE inhibitors but fail to lower proteinuria. Thus, it may be reasonable to use renin angiotensin system inhibitors for patients with hypertension and additional comorbidities such as diabetes, proteinuria, or heart failure as long as appropriate potassium and creatinine monitoring are maintained.[34]

Calcium Channel Blocking Agents

Based on the data available, CCBs are often preferred for transplant hypertension, especially in the early postoperative setting. The nondihydropyridine CCBs, verapamil and diltiazem, are less commonly used after transplantation, because of effects on gastrointestinal motility and CNI blood levels. The vasodilatory effects of dihydropyridine CCBs directly counter the vasoconstrictive effects of CNIs, but may produce significant side effects, including peripheral edema, headache, and reflex tachycardia. Edema may be severe and is a frequent cause of drug discontinuation. Nifedipine and felodipine have negligible effects on cyclosporine disposition and have been used successfully in transplant settings, whereas amlodipine has minor effects on cyclosporine levels and has been used with good results. As noted, recipients taking CCB-based treatment have higher GFRs, both immediately and at 2 years after transplantation, compared with those using other agents. Experimental studies suggest that CCBs have minor immunosuppressive properties and may blunt interstitial fibrosis. On the negative side, CCB-treated patients have higher levels of urinary protein excretion, raising concern that, as in the nontransplant setting, increased glomerular pressure caused by arterial vasodilation and increased proteinuria may accelerate renal decline.

Renin Angiotensin System Blockers

ACE inhibitors and ARBs are widely used in patients with chronic kidney disease for BP control and cardiac and renal protection, and to reduce proteinuria. Early after transplantation, patients are at risk for swings in volume status, often with volume excess where RAS inhibitors may be ineffective for BP control. In the setting of marginal renal function, ACE inhibitors and ARBs increase the risk of hyperkalemia,[35] already a risk resulting from renal insufficiency, CNI use, and common use of trimethoprim/sulfamethoxazole for infection prophylaxis. Beyond the first few months after transplant, as volume shifts become less pronounced and renal function is more clearly defined, ACE inhibitors and ARBs may be safely introduced and would be indicated for patients with proteinuria and those at risk for developing proteinuria or glomerular diseases such as diabetic nephropathy because they lower glomerular pressures and protein excretion.

A study in renal transplant recipients compared treatment with losartan to captopril and amlodipine, using prestudy and poststudy renal allograft biopsies. Treatment with losartan reduced plasma transforming growth factor beta 1 (TGF-β1) levels and 24-hour urine protein excretion.[36] Further, the rate of histologic scarring was lower in the losartan-treated group. Although unproven, ACE inhibitors may slow progression of chronic allograft nephropathy by reducing intraglomerular pressure and thus hyperfiltration. Evidence for reductions in CV events in nontransplant patients with normal renal function and those with mild renal impairment (serum creatinine 1.4 to 2.4 mg/dL) support use of these agents in the renal transplant recipient.[37] A randomized prospective trial of candesartan or placebo plus add-on therapy in 700 renal transplant recipients was stopped early (mean follow up, 19 to 21 months), as the primary event rate was lower than expected in both study arms, resulting in too few events to permit conclusions on the effects of ARB treatment.[38] Entry BP was relatively low (mean, 137/84 mm Hg) with inclusion of normotensive subjects. Of note, renal transplant recipients within 1 to 10 years of transplantation achieved better BP control with reduced protein excretion and with small increases in serum creatinine and potassium during ARB treatment. In a small trial of lisinopril versus placebo monotherapy for renal transplant recipients with persistent LVH after transplantation, greater regression in LVH was detected in the lisinopril-treated group without difference in achieved BP.[39] However, this benefit was seen only in cyclosporine-treated recipients, suggesting an interaction between lisinopril and cyclosporine rather than a hemodynamic mechanism. A large retrospective cohort study of 2031 Austrian renal transplant recipients compared patient and graft survival for patients receiving or not receiving ACE inhibitors or ARB therapy.[40] Hazard ratios for patient survival (0.57) and allograft survival (0.55) were significantly improved for ACE inhibitor/ARB users compared with nonusers. Several trials indicate that ACE inhibitors may be used safely, particularly when combined with diuretics.[41]

The benefits of ACE inhibitors and ARBs for renal and CV protection must be balanced against two major disadvantages: anemia and acute reductions in graft function. ACE inhibitors or ARBs in renal transplant recipients will cause a predictable decline in hemoglobin of 1.0 to 1.5 gm/dL. Although this side effect has been used to treat posttransplant erythrocytosis, it may require treatment with erythrocyte-stimulating agents in some patients. ACE inhibitors and ARBs may precipitate functional acute renal failure in patients with marginal arterial flow to the allograft, similar to the picture seen clinically in patients with native kidney bilateral RAS. A similar pattern may result from small vessel disease. Risk factors include higher baseline serum creatinine, higher doses or levels of CNIs, and higher plasma renin levels. ACE inhibitors or ARBs should be started at very low doses, with close monitoring of serum potassium and creatinine over the first several weeks, followed by slow dose titration.

Diuretics

Diuretics are commonly withheld after transplantation, because of concerns that they may impair renal function. Diuretics counter the sodium-retaining effects of corticosteroids, CNIs, beta-blockers, ACE inhibitors, and ARBs, allowing the kidney to maintain sodium balance at lower BP levels. Control of volume expansion improves the BP response to other agents. In the patient with renal insufficiency and sodium and volume retention, loop diuretics are often required to achieve lower BP targets. Disadvantages of diuretic therapy center on the expected rise in serum creatinine associated with their use. This is more likely in patients with compromised renal blood flow, including small vessel disease associated with allograft dysfunction, or in the setting of contracted intravascular volume. Most thiazide diuretics are ineffective at GFRs less than 30 mL/min, and in this setting, a loop diuretic such as furosemide, bumetanide, or torsemide should be considered.

Additional Treatment Choices

Although there are few data from controlled trials, other agents may be used to treat posttransplant hypertension. Peripheral alpha-blockers may be used as second-line agents. Although these agents may improve bladder outflow in men, women may develop urinary incontinence. Monitor for pronounced postural BP changes, particularly in those with autonomic dysfunction. Centrally acting sympatholytic agents are reserved for third- or fourth-line treatment because of more pronounced side effects. Clonidine is effective in patch or oral form, but its use is limited by fatigue and dry mouth. These agents magnify sodium retention and may require diuretic therapy to maintain their BP-lowering effect. Direct vasodilators are very effective, but must be used in combination with diuretics and either beta-blockers or central sympatholytic agents to counteract edema and reflex tachycardia, respectively.

Modification of Immunosuppressive Regimen

Modifications in immunosuppressive regimen may provide substantial benefits to BP control. Transitioning from cyclosporine to tacrolimus, or from a CNI to sirolimus, may effectively lower BP and simplify management. Immunologic suppression must be maintained as first priority when changes in immunosuppression are considered primarily for BP benefit. Although corticosteroid withdrawal has not been demonstrated to improve BP,[42] current trends to steroid-free immunosuppression may be of benefit for resistant patients.

Native Nephrectomy

For patients with severe hypertension before transplant, BP may remain resistant, even in the setting of a functioning allograft. Native kidney nephrectomy has been used successfully to reduce hypertension severity in select cases. Since the advent of pharmacologic renin-angiotensin system blockade, this procedure is uncommon, although interest has increased with the availability of laparoscopic nephrectomy techniques. Reports of lower BP in transplant recipients undergoing pretransplant bilateral nephrectomy support a role for native kidney disease in the maintenance of posttransplant hypertension. Particularly in the setting of a well-functioning allograft, removal of atrophic and/or infarcted native kidneys offers potential improvement in BP control and the need for fewer medications for those at low surgical risk.

SUMMARY

Hypertension occurs commonly during CNI-based immunosuppression in the transplant setting. Underlying mechanisms of altered vascular reactivity and systemic and renal vasoconstriction result in impaired glomerular filtration and sodium retention, magnified by the effects of corticosteroids. Hypertension after transplantation represents a major risk factor for CV disease and affects long-term function of the allograft. Management of this disease may be difficult and requires attention to drug-drug interactions and to the effects of antihypertensive therapy on native or renal allograft function. Therapy should include nonpharmacologic and pharmacologic modalities. Target BP levels should recognize the increased CV and renal risks of these patients. There is a need for additional randomized controlled trials to determine optimal BP treatment targets for kidney transplant recipients, the effect of reduced proteinuria on progression of CKD in kidney transplant recipients, and the long-term effects of ACE inhibitors or ARBs on patient survival and graft survival. ACE inhibitor/ARB therapy may be an important component of chronic hypertension therapy after transplant, but it has yet to be proven in a prospective trial and safety concerns remain.

References

1. Taler SJ, Textor SC, Canzanello VJ, Schwartz L. Cyclosporin-induced hypertension: incidence, pathogenesis and management. *Drug Safety*. 1999;20:437-449.
2. Paoletti E, Gherzi M, Amidone M, Massarino F, Cannella G. Association of arterial hypertension with renal target organ damage in kidney transplant recipients: the predictive role of ambulatory blood pressure monitoring. *Transplantation*. 2009;87:1864-1869.
3. Magee CC, Pascual M. Update in renal transplantation. *Arch Int Med*. 2004;164:1373-1388.
4. Hart A, Smith JM, M.A S, et al. OPTN/SRTR Annual Data Report 2014: kidney. *Am J Transplant*. 2016;16(Suppl 2):11-46.
5. Pascual M, Theruvath T, Kawai T, Tolkoff-Rubin N, Cosimi AB. Strategies to improve long-term outcomes after renal transplantation. *N Engl J Med*. 2002;346:580-590.
6. Mange KC, Feldman HI, Joffe MM, Fa K, Bloom RD. Blood pressure and the survival of renal allografts from living donors. *J Am Soc Nephrol*. 2004;15:187-193.
7. Kasiske BL, Anjum S, Shah R, et al. Hypertension after kidney transplantation. *Am J Kidney Dis*. 2004;43:1071-1081.
8. Cosio FG, Pelletier RP, Pesavento TE, et al. Elevated blood pressure predicts the risk of acute rejection in renal allograft recipients. *Kidney Int*. 2001;59:1158-1164.
9. Opelz G, Döhler B. Collaborative Transplant Study. Improved long-term outcomes after renal transplantation associated with blood pressure control. *Am J Transplant*. 2005;5:2725-2731.
10. Hillebrand U, Suwelack BM, Loley K, et al. Blood pressure, antihypertensive treatment, and graft survival in kidney transplant patients. *Transplant Int*. 2009;22:1073-1080.
11. Taler SJ, Textor SC, Canzanello VJ, et al. Role of steroid dose in hypertension early after liver transplantation with tacrolimus (FK506) and cyclosporine. *Transplantation*. 1996;62:1588-1592.
12. Textor SC, Taler SJ, Schwartz L, et al. Reduced prevalence and severity of hypertension after liver transplantation due to changes from cyclosporine to tacrolimus with steroid withdrawal. *Am J Transplant*. 2002;2(Suppl. 3):197.
13. Vincenti F, Schena FP, Paraskevas S, Hauser IA, Walker RG, Grinyo J. A randomized, multicenter study of steroid avoidance, early steroid withdrawal or standard steroid therapy in kidney transplant recipients. *Am J Transplant*. 2008;8:307-316.
14. Woodle ES, First MR, Pirsch J, Shihab F, Gaber AO, Van Veldhuisen P. A prospective, randomized, double-blind, placebo-controlled multicenter trial comparing early (7 day) corticosteroid cessation versus long-term, low-dose corticosteroid therapy. *Ann Surg*. 2008;248:564-577.
15. Textor SC, Taler SJ, Canzanello VJ, et al. Sustained urinary endothelin and suppressed prostacyclin in hypertension developing after liver transplantation. *Am J Hyper*. 1994;7:136A.
16. Johnson RW, Kreis H, Oberbauer R, Brattström C, Claesson K, Eris J. Sirolimus allows early cyclosporine withdrawal in renal transplantation resulting in improved renal function and lower blood pressure. *Transplantation*. 2001;72:777.
17. Rostaing L, Vincenti F, Grinyo J, et al. Long-term belatacept exposure maintains efficacy and safety at 5 years: results from the long-term extension of the BENEFIT study. *Am J Transplant*. 2013;13:2875-2883.
18. Fernandez-Fresnedo G, Palomar R, Escallada R, et al. Hypertension and long-term renal allograft survival: effect of early glomerular filtration rate. *Nephrol Dial Transplant*. 2001;16(Suppl 1):105-109.
19. Bruno S, Remuzzi G, Ruggenenti P. Transplant renal artery stenosis. *J Am Soc Nephrol*. 2004;15:134-141.
20. Cosio FG, Pesavento TE, Kim S, Osei K, Henry M, Ferguson RM. Patient survival after renal transplantation: IV. Impact of post-transplant diabetes. *Kidney Int*. 2002;62:1440-1446.
21. Wadei HM, Amer H, Taler SJ, et al. Diurnal blood pressure changes one year after kidney transplantation: relationship to allograft function, histology, and resistive index. *J Am Soc Nephrol*. 2007;18:1607-1615.
22. Haydar AA, Covic A, Jayawardene S, et al. Insights from ambulatory blood pressure monitoring: diagnosis of hypertension and diurnal blood presure in renal transplant recipients. *Transplantation*. 2004;77:849-853.
23. Chobanian AV, Bakris GL, Black HR, et al. The Seventh Report of the Joint National Committee on prevention, detection, evaluation, and treatment of high blood pressure: the JNC 7 report. *JAMA*. 2003;289:2560-2572.
24. Bruno S, Ferrari S, Remuzzi G, Ruggenenti P. Doppler ultrasonography in posttransplant renal artery stenosis: a reliable tool for assessing effectiveness of revascularization? *Transplantation*. 2003;76:16-17.
25. Ruggenenti P, Mosconi L, Bruno S, et al. Post-transplant renal artery stenosis: the hemodynamic response to revascularization. *Kidney Int*. 2001;60:309-318.
26. Prasad GVR, Ruzicka M, Burns KD, Tobe SW, Lebel M. Hypertension in dialysis and kidney transplant patients. *Can J Cardiol*. 2009;25:309-314.
27. Kidney Disease: Improving Global Outcomes (KDIGO) Transplant Work Group. KDIGO Clinical Practice Guideline for the Care of Kidney Transplant Recipients. *Am J Transplant*. 2009;9(Suppl 3):S1-S155.

28. Wright JT Jr., Williamson JD, Whelton PK, et al. A randomized trial of intensive versus standard blood-pressure control. *N Engl J Med.* 2015;373:2103-2116.

29. Kiberd K, Panek R, Kiberd B. Strategies to reduce clinical inertia in hypertensive kidney transplant recipients. *BMC Nephrology.* 2007;8:10.

30. Keven K, Yalçın S, Canbakan B, et al. The impact of daily sodium intake on posttransplant hypertension in kidney allograft recipients. *Transplant Proc.* 2006;38:1323-1326.

31. Sacks FM, Svetkey LP, Vollmer WM, et al. Effects on blood pressure of reduced dietary sodium and the dietary approaches to stop hypertension (DASH) diet. *N Engl J Med.* 2001;344:3-10.

32. EBPG Expert Group on Renal Transplantation. European best practice guidelines for renal transplantation: section IV: long-term management of the transplant recipient IV: 5.2. Arterial hypertension. *Nephrol Dial Transplant.* 2002;17(Suppl 4):25-26.

33. Cross NB, Webster AC, Masson P, O'Connell PJ, Craig JC. Antihypertensive treatment for kidney transplant recipients. *Cochrane Database Syst Rev.* 2009;(3):CD003598.

34. Jennings DL, Taber DJ. Use of renin-angiotensin-aldosterone system inhibitors within the first eight to twelve weeks after renal transplantation. *Ann Pharmacother.* 2008;42:116-120.

35. Formica RN Jr., Friedman Al, Lorber MI, Smith JD, Eisen T, Bia MJ. A randomized trial comparing losartan with amlodipine as initial therapy for hypertension in the early post-transplant period. *Nephrol Dial Transplant.* 2006;21:1389-1394.

36. el-Agroudy AE, Hassan NA, Foda MA, et al. Effect of angiotensin II receptor blocker on plasma levels of TGF-beta 1 and interstitial fibrosis in hypertensive kidney transplant patients. *Am J Nephrol.* 2003;23:300-306.

37. Heart Outcomes Prevention Evaluation Study Investigators: effects of an angiotensin-converting enzyme inhibitor, ramipril, on cardiovascular events in high risk patients. *N Engl J Med.* 2000;342:145-153.

38. Philipp T, Martinez F, Geiger H, et al. Candesartan improves blood pressure control and reduces proteinuria in renal transplant recipients: results from SECRET. *Nephrol Dial Transplant.* 2010;25:967-976.

39. Paoletti E, Cassottana P, Amidone M, Gherzi M, Rolla D, Cannella G. ACE inhibitors and persistent left ventricular hypertrophy after renal transplantation: a randomized clinical trial. *Am J Kidney Dis.* 2007;50:133-142.

40. Heinze G, Mitterbauer C, Regele H, et al. Angiotensin-converting enzyme inhibitor or angiotensin ii type 1 receptor antagonist therapy is associated with prolonged patient and graft survival after renal transplantation. *J Am Soc Nephrol.* 2006;17:889-899.

41. Andrés A, Morales E, Morales JM, et al. Efficacy and safety of valsartan, an angiotensin ii receptor antagonist, in hypertension after renal transplantation: a randomized multi-center study. *Transplant Proc.* 2006;38:2419-2423.

42. Pelletier RP, Akin B, Ferguson RM. Prospective, randomized trial of steroid withdrawal in kidney recipients treated with mycophenolate mofetil and cyclosporine. *Clinical Transplantation.* 2006;20:10-18.

35 Obesity
Lewis Landsberg

ASSOCIATION OF OBESITY AND HYPERTENSION

Obesity has been called the epidemic of our time with approximately 70% of the adults in the United States either overweight or obese according to the American Heart Association (AHA) and the American Physiological Society.[1,2] Estimates based on risk suggest that as much as 65% to 70% of essential hypertension occurs in association with obesity, although longitudinal population based studies indicate a somewhat lower figure.[3] It is nonetheless abundantly clear that obesity is closely associated with hypertension, with a 6.5 mm Hg increase in systolic blood pressure (SBP) for each 10% increase in body weight.[3] The importance of this association is the cardiovascular (CV) risk related to both obesity and hypertension.

Assessment of Overweight and Obesity

Calculation of body mass index (BMI) is commonly used as the basic measure of obesity. Calculated from the weight in kilograms divided by height in meters squared, the BMI gives a convenient if imperfect measure of obesity. BMI should be recorded as part of every physical examination. A BMI below 25 is considered normal, whereas overweight is indicated by a BMI of 25 to 30, and obesity by a BMI of over 30. Body fat distribution also plays a critical role in the CV risk imposed by obesity.

Body Fat Distribution

Because the upper body or abdominal form of obesity is the phenotype associated with enhanced CV risk, as compared with the lower body or gluteal form, assessment of this variable should be made for each obese or overweight individual. A convenient surrogate measurement for body fat distribution is the abdominal circumference. Over 40 inches (102 centimeters) in men and over 35 inches (88 centimeters) in women signifies the upper body form of obesity. Waist to hip ratio (W/H) has also been used to identify the upper body abdominal form of obesity but is more cumbersome and bedeviled by locating the proper places on the torso to make the measurements. W/H of over 1 in men and over 0.85 in women are indicative of the upper body phenotype. It has recently been demonstrated that even patients with a normal BMI have increased cardiovascular risk when the abdominal circumference is increased.[4] In patients with obese arms, a large BP cuff should be used to avoid the artifact resulting from the use of too small a cuff.

PATHOPHYSIOLOGY OF OBESITY-RELATED HYPERTENSION

Understanding the mechanisms associated with obesity-related hypertension provides the rationale for appropriate therapy.

Historical Milestones

Although the association of obesity with hypertension had been recognized since the measurement of blood pressures in populations in the early 1900s, the underlying mechanisms linking blood pressure (BP) and body weight were not understood until the late 1980s. The linkage of BP and obesity was reinforced by the Framingham Heart Study in the 1960s with the prospective demonstration that body weight and weight gain predicted the development of hypertension. It also became clear, by comparing obese normotensive with obese hypertensive subjects, that trivial attributions such as cuff artifact, increased salt intake, increased plasma volume, and hemodynamic factors related to cardiac output could not explain the increased peripheral resistance noted in obese hypertensives.

The pathophysiology was eventually clarified by a number of observations and studies as follows:

1. **The impact of body fat distribution:** The French clinician Jean Vague noted in the 1940s and 1950s that obesity phenotype influenced the CV and metabolic complications of obesity. These complications tracked with the upper body abdominal form of obesity, which he called "android," rather than the lower body gluteal femoral form, which he referred to as "gynoid."[5] Little noted until the 1980s, Vague's observations were strongly reinforced by large scale epidemiologic studies from Scandinavia that convincingly demonstrated that waist to hip ratio, a surrogate for the upper body phenotype, predicted CV risk (myocardial infarction, hypertension), type 2 diabetes, and overall mortality.[6-8]

2. **The role of insulin:** At the same time both epidemiological and clinical studies demonstrated that insulin resistance, hyperinsulinemia, and type 2 diabetes also tracked with the upper body phenotype.[9,10] Insulin thus emerged as a valid risk factor for CV in general and hypertension in particular.[11,12] Insulin influences BP by stimulating the sympathetic nervous system (SNS) as shown in Fig. 35.1[13,14] and by enhancing renal sodium reabsorption.

3. **Role of the SNS:** Contrary to widely held beliefs at the time, SNS activity was shown to be increased in the obese in the early 1990s[15-17] (Fig. 35.2). SNS stimulation increases cardiac output, peripheral resistance, and, importantly, renal sodium reabsorption.

4. **Role of leptin:** Leptin, the polypeptide product of the *ob/ob* gene, is synthesized in white adipose tissue; levels are higher in the obese, reflective of the fat mass of the individual. Acting at the level of the central nervous system, leptin suppresses appetite and stimulates the SNS (Fig. 35.3).[18]

5. **Role of the renin-angiotensin-aldosterone system (RAAS):** In addition to stimulation of renin release by the SNS, it has become clear that adipose tissue synthesizes all the components of the RAAS including aldosterone.[19] Obesity related hypertension is associated with increased levels of angiotensin II and aldosterone. High circulating levels of free fatty acids in obesity may also contribute to the

328

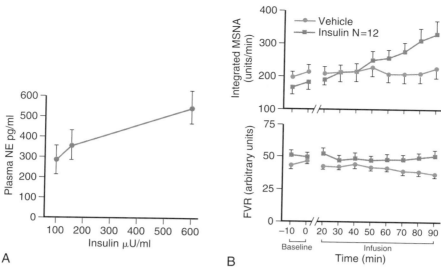

FIG. 35.1 Insulin stimulates the sympathetic nervous system (SNS). A, Plasma NE levels rise during euglycemic hyperinsulinemic clamp shown here in nine lean normotensive young men. Cardiovascular indices of SNS stimulation (pulse rate, pulse pressure, cross product, and mean arterial pressure) increased during the clamp. *(Modified from Rowe JW, Young JB, Minaker KL, Stevens AL, Pallotta JA, Landsberg L. Effect of insulin and glucose infusions on sympathetic nervous system activity in normal man. Diabetes. 1981;30:219-225.)* B, Muscle sympathetic nerve activity (MSNA) increases during euglycemic hyperinsulinemic clamp. Insulin levels were within the physiologic range. *(From Hausberg M, Mark AL, Hoffman RP, Sinkey CA, Anderson EA. Dissociation of sympathoexcitatory and vasodilator actions of modestly elevated plasma insulin levels. J Hypertens. 1995;13:1015-1021.)*

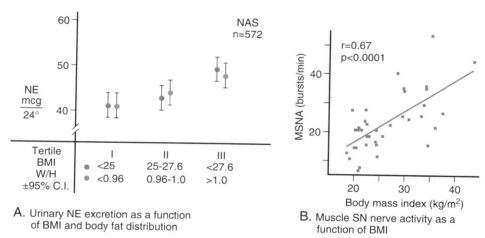

FIG. 35.2 Sympathetic activity increases with increased body weight. A, 24-hour urinary NE excretion increases as a function of body mass index and waist to hip ratio. *(Modified from Troisi RJ, Weiss ST, Parker DR, Sparrow D, Young JB, Landsberg L. Relation of obesity and diet to sympathetic nervous system activity. Hypertension. 1991;17:669-677.)* B, Muscle sympathetic nerve activity (MSNA) increases as a function of body weight. *(From Scherrer U, Randin D, Tappy L, Vollenweider P, Jéquier E, Nicod P. Body fat and sympathetic nerve activity in healthy subjects. Circulation. 1994;89:2634-2640.)*

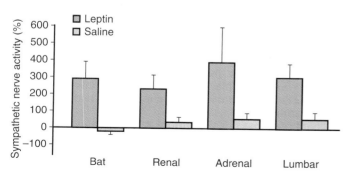

FIG. 35.3 Leptin infusion increases sympathetic nervous system activity in rats. *(From Haynes WG, Morgan DA, Walsh SA, Mark AL, Sivitz WI. Receptor-mediated regional sympathetic nerve activation by leptin. J Clin Invest. 1997;100:270-278.)*

increased secretion of aldosterone, by mechanisms that remain obscure.[20]

6. **Obstructive sleep apnea (OSA):** OSA, more common in the obese as compared with lean individuals, is recognized as a cause of both hypertension and SNS stimulation.[21] In the obese fatty infiltration of the genioglossus muscle, which pulls the base of the tongue forward in the first phase of respiration, is the likely cause.

The Pressure-Natriuresis Relationship and Salt Sensitivity

As would be anticipated from the activation of the SNS and the RAAS, the hypertension of obesity is salt sensitive.[22] The pressure-natriuresis relationship is shifted to the right by NE, insulin, and A II, all of which increase renal avidity for sodium (Fig. 35.4). The increase in BP overcomes the natriuretic handicap so volume is not expanded; the increase in BP is compensation for the increase in renal avidity for salt.

Pressure–Natriuresis Relationship

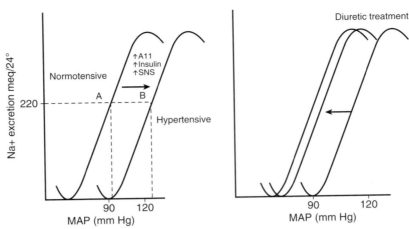

FIG. 35.4 The sympathetic nervous system, insulin, and angiotensin II (A II) shift the pressure natriuresis curve to the right. Increased renal avidity for sodium necessitates higher pressures to excrete the day's sodium load and maintain sodium balance. Diuretics shift the relationship back toward normal by helping the kidney excrete salt. *(Modified from Landsberg "On Rounds," Wolters Kluwer, 2016.)*

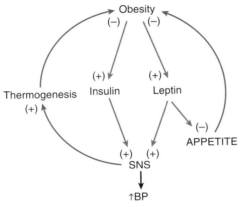

FIG. 35.5 Sympathetic nervous system stimulation in the obese, driven by insulin and leptin, increases thermogenesis tending to restore energy balance; increase in blood pressure is thus the unintended consequence of mechanisms recruited to stabilize body weight. *(From Landsberg L. Insulin-mediated sympathetic stimulation: role in the pathogenesis of obesity-related hypertension [or, how insulin affects blood pressure, and why]. J Hypertens. 2001;19[3 Pt 2]:523-528.)*

Sympathetic Stimulation and the Metabolic Economy of the Obese State

Can the linkage of obesity and hypertension, a linkage in which SNS stimulation plays a major role, be part of a metabolic adaptation to the obese state?[23] Because SNS stimulation increases energy expenditure it has been proposed that SNS activation is a mechanism recruited in the obese to restore energy balance and limit further weight gain.[24] This hypothesis (Fig. 35.5) has substantial experimental support.

THE METABOLIC SYNDROME AND CARDIOVASCULAR RISK

Since the early 1990s it has been recognized that obesity related hypertension is frequently associated with other cardiovascular risk factors (Table 35.1).

Critical Components of the Metabolic Syndrome

The four crucial components are abdominal obesity, insulin resistance (and consequent hyperinsulinemia), hypertension, and a characteristic dyslipidemia (low high-density lipoprotein [HDL]-cholesterol and high triglycerides). Considerable

TABLE 35.1 The Metabolic Syndrome

Four cardinal features	• Insulin resistance and hyperinsulinemia • Central (abdominal) obesity • Hypertension • Characteristic dyslipidemia (high triglycerides, low HDL-cholesterol)
Frequently associated	• Impaired glucose tolerance/type 2 diabetes • Microalbuminuria/impaired renal function • ↑ Plasminogen activator inhibitor-1 (PAI-1) • ↑ Small dense LDL • Hyperuricemia • ↑ Markers of inflammation

HDL, High-density lipoprotein; *LDL,* low-density lipoprotein.

debate exists as to whether this constitutes a distinct syndrome, although it seems clear that these abnormalities occur together more frequently than could be accounted for by chance alone. In addition, different diagnostic criteria have been proposed by various national and international panels[25]; the differences in criteria are, in general, small and overlapping, reflective of differences in emphasis on the four cardinal manifestations noted above. From a practical standpoint the importance of the metabolic syndrome is the recognition that these abnormalities occur together and that they convey significant CV risk. Estimates from the third National Health and Nutrition Examination Survey suggest that about 30% of adults in the U.S. have metabolic syndrome; because the incidence increases with age the figure for people over 60 years old is closer to 40%.[26]

In addition to the four critical components, other abnormalities have been noted to occur frequently in patients with metabolic syndrome,[27] including: impaired glucose tolerance and type 2 diabetes; microalbuminuria and impaired renal function; increased plasminogen activator inhibitor (PAI-1); hyperuricemia; small dense LDL-cholesterol; and markers of inflammation.

The thread that ties the various manifestations together is insulin resistance and the resultant hyperinsulinemia.

Insulin and the Metabolic Syndrome

Insulin, the major anabolic hormone of the fed state, has a myriad of biological actions but most prominent is the

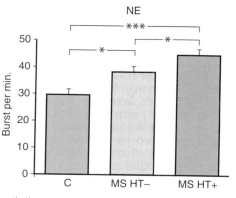

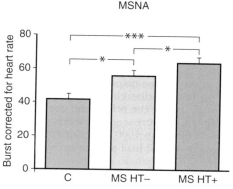

FIG. 35.6 Increased sympathetic nervous system activity in the metabolic syndrome (MS). Plasma NE and muscle sympathetic nerve activity are increased in patients with the MS; the increase is greater in hypertensive (HT) patients. *(From Grassi G, Dell'Oro R, Quarti-Trevano F, et al. Neuroadrenergic and reflex abnormalities in patients with metabolic syndrome. Diabetologia. 2005;48:1359-1365.)*

stimulation of glucose uptake in skeletal muscle. Insulin resistance, defined operationally, is an impairment in insulin-mediated glucose uptake in muscle. As a consequence of this impairment, blood glucose levels rise stimulating the release of insulin from the pancreatic beta cells. The increase in insulin compensates, partially, for the insulin resistance but results in hyperinsulinemia. When beta cell capacity to compensate for insulin resistance is exhausted impaired glucose tolerance and type 2 diabetes ensue. Patients with metabolic syndrome have increased SNS activity, as shown in Fig. 35.6.[28] The increased levels of insulin, along with leptin, stimulate the SNS contributing to the hypertension (Fig. 35.6). The increased levels of insulin are also the proximate cause of the dyslipidemia by stimulating hepatic very low-density lipoprotein synthesis.

CARDIOVASCULAR RISK OF OBESITY-RELATED HYPERTENSION

The cardiovascular risk associated with hypertension (myocardial infarction, stroke, heart failure, and renal failure) is well recognized. Although much of the CV risk associated with obesity is secondary to the comorbidity of hypertension and type 2 diabetes, evidence suggests that the long-term risk of CV disease is accentuated by obesity[29] in additive fashion with that of hypertension (Fig. 35.7). If carbohydrate intolerance develops, the risk of course is greatly accelerated.

TREATMENT OF OBESITY-RELATED HYPERTENSION

Management of Obesity-Related Hypertension by Lifestyle Changes

Management of obesity is crucial in the treatment of obesity-related hypertension. Decreasing fat burden decreases blood pressure,[30] increases responsiveness to antihypertensive medications, and beneficially affects other cardiac risk factors while preventing or delaying the development of type 2 diabetes. Weight loss and the development of a healthy lifestyle is the cornerstone in the treatment of the obese hypertensive patient. It is applicable in every case. The clinician must form a partnership with the patient, to motivate, educate, and instruct; this partnership should result in the development of a plan that takes into account the patients' health status, goals, and unique problems. Successful weight loss that is sustained will almost always require a team of professionals, including dieticians, nurses, nurse practitioners, physician assistants, and access to

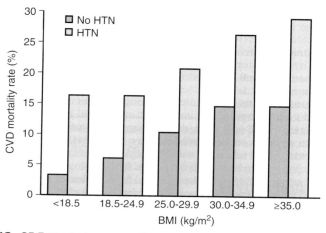

FIG. 35.7 Obesity increases cardiovascular disease (CVD) mortality with and without hypertension. *(From Landsberg L, Aronne LJ, Beilin LJ, et al. Obesity-related hypertension: pathogenesis, cardiovascular risk, and treatment: a position paper of The Obesity Society and the American Society of Hypertension. J Clin Hypertens [Greenwich]. 2013;15:14-33.)*

TABLE 35.2 Lifestyle Changes

Low energy diets	• Induce caloric deficit of 500 to 1000 kcal/day • DASH (Dietary Approaches to Stop Hypertension) diet: • High in fruits, vegetables, low fat dairy products (high in calcium, magnesium, potassium, fiber)
Sodium restriction	• 100 meq Na+/day (2.3 g sodium, 6 g salt)
Physical activity	• 30 min/day, 5 days/week (minimum) at moderate intensity (more is better)
Alcohol moderation	• Men: 2 drinks/day; Women: 1 drink/day (1 drink = 14 g ethanol: 1 oz spirits, 12 oz beer, 5 oz wine)

psychologists and exercise physiologists. An individual's weight loss plan is often best addressed by enrollment in a bona fide weight loss program headed by a physician trained in obesity management. These programs frequently stress behavioral modification techniques that have had documented success at achieving long-term weight loss.[31-33] A reasonable initial goal for weight loss is about 10% of total body weight.

The major components of lifestyle management are: low energy diets; salt restriction; increased potassium and magnesium intake; increased physical activity; and alcohol moderation (Table 35.2).

Low Energy Diets

The most important feature of therapeutic dieting is caloric restriction. Although various diets that emphasize different macronutrient content have been proposed, no one of these has been shown conclusively to be superior to the rest.[34] Nonetheless, low fat and low carbohydrate diets have their proponents and it is possible that some people, either through personal preference that favors adherence or real metabolic differences, do better with one or the other. The goal of slimming diets, in conjunction with increased physical activity, is to induce a caloric deficit of 500 to 1000 kilocalories per day. Relatively small amounts of weight loss may cause significant BP reduction.

Effect of Diet on Blood Pressure

Interestingly, diet composition does have an effect on BP independent of weight loss. The DASH (Dietary Approaches to Stop Hypertension) trial compared control (typical American diet) with a diet equal in calories and sodium but containing increased fruits and vegetables, lower saturated fats, and higher low fat dairy products.[35] After eight weeks, the DASH diet was associated with lower systolic BP (5.5 mm Hg) and diastolic BP (3.0 mm Hg) without change in weight. In patients with hypertension, the effect on BP was even greater (11.4 systolic and 5.5 mm Hg diastolic BP).[36] Inspection of the DASH diet suggests that increases in intake of potassium, magnesium, fiber, protein, and calcium, along with decreases in saturated fat intake were the important macro and micronutrient changes. The DASH type diet, along with decreased caloric intake appears to be a prudent diet for obese hypertensive patients.

Physical Activity

The energy balance equation

$$\text{Energy in} = \text{Energy out} + \text{Storage}$$

is a simple tautological expression that demonstrates the importance of energy expenditure in maintaining energy balance: increasing energy output increases the range of energy intakes over which energy balance can be maintained. An impediment to weight loss is the metabolic adaptation that occurs with a decrease in caloric intake[37]; caloric restriction is associated with a fall in resting metabolic rate that approaches 10%.[38,39] It is, therefore, no surprise that exercise has been shown to increase the effectiveness of low energy diets.[40] Because physical activity is the major currently feasible means of increasing energy expenditure, it would be expected to play an important role in the treatment of obesity (and obesity-related hypertension).

Increasing energy expenditure through exercise has been well studied in the context of weight reduction programs. Without low energy diets exercise has a small but significant effect on weight reduction[41]; in conjunction with slimming diets the effect of exercise is enhanced and appears particularly important in weight maintenance after dieting.[40,42] At least 30 minutes of exercise five days per week is generally the recommended minimum; better results are obtained with longer durations and more intense exercise. Interestingly, exercise has a beneficial effect on blood pressure independent of weight loss. The mechanism may be related to the decrease in SNS activity that occurs with training.[43,44]

Salt Restriction

In the pathophysiology of obesity-related hypertension renal avidity for sodium plays a critical role, as described above.

Obesity related-hypertension, therefore, is a salt-sensitive state[45] and sodium restriction is an important component of the lifestyle modifications that underlie the treatment of hypertension occurring in association with obesity. Salt restriction is particularly important in the obese hypertensive population because, for reasons that remain obscure, salt intake is higher in obese than in nonobese persons, an increase in salt intake of 40%, on average.[46] The effectiveness of salt restriction in obese hypertensives has been documented in many studies.[29] The reduction in blood pressure noted in the DASH diet is enhanced by accompanying sodium restriction.[36,47] Similar additive effects of weight loss and salt restriction have been noted in other studies as well.[48,49] Salt restriction is also associated with a better therapeutic response to antihypertensive drugs.

What constitutes adequate salt restriction? Guidelines generally recommend reducing salt intake to 100 meq of sodium per day from an average daily intake of about 150 to 200 meq per day. One hundred meq represents about 2.3 grams of sodium or 6 grams of salt. This is best achieved by sharply limiting the intake of processed foods which have a very high salt content.

Alcohol Moderation

Recommendations concerning alcohol ingestion are complicated by the fact that modest drinking is associated with reduced cardiovascular disease. There is no question, however, that heavy drinking contributes to hypertension, perhaps through activation of the SNS. A possible relationship of this effect to alcohol withdrawal has been suggested. Five drinks per day and beyond have an established adverse effect on BP. Recommendations are for a limit of two drinks per day for men and one for women.[36,50,51]

Long-Term Efficacy of Lifestyle Changes in Obesity Related-Hypertension

Lifestyle changes form the backbone of treatment for obese hypertensive patients because they address both the hypertension and the obesity, as well as other cardiac risk factors. The changes in blood pressure induced by lifestyle changes, particularly weight loss and salt restriction, although rarely sufficient in and of themselves to adequately treat hypertension, have demonstrated effectiveness over the long-term.[29] The lifestyle arm of the TOHMS trial (Treatment of Mild Hypertension Study), for example, showed 8 mm Hg BP reductions after four years.[52]

Blood Pressure Thresholds and Targets for Drug Treatment

Recent guidelines have generally recommended a blood pressure goal of 140/90.[53] Pressures consistently above this level after a trial of lifestyle management constitute an indication for antihypertensive medications. There remains, however, some controversy about the target of 140/90; although BP levels below this may increase the incidence of myocardial infarction, lower levels are protective against stroke. In addition the recent SPRINT (Systolic Blood Pressure Intervention Trial)[54] study indicated that more intensive treatment (target < 120 systolic) in patients at high risk for cardiovascular disease (excluding diabetes or prior stroke) had a beneficial effect on reducing cardiovascular endpoints and overall mortality as compared with those treated to the conventional target of 140 systolic. This supports previous suggestions that high-risk patients, particularly those with diabetes, should have generally lower BP targets.[53] It is too early to know how the results from SPRINT should be integrated into overall target blood pressure recommendations. For the present, a goal of 140/90 seems reasonable but a lower target for patients with diabetes or cerebrovascular disease might be considered pending further studies.

Antihypertensive Agents

Those antihypertensive agents (Box 35.1) that do not have adverse effects on weight gain or insulin resistance are preferred. RAAS inhibitors, either ACE inhibitors or angiotensin II receptor blockers are the preferred agents because of their favorable metabolic profile,[55] their nephron-protective effects, and their general tolerability. They decrease insulin resistance and diminish microalbuminuria, and delay the onset of type 2 diabetes. Calcium channel blockers are neutral with respect to metabolic effects (insulin resistance and weight gain) and are effective at lowering BP and generally well tolerated. Alpha adrenergic receptor blockers have a favorable metabolic profile but are not considered first line because the ALLHAT study suggested that they might increase heart failure.[56]

Diuretics are almost always required because of the salt sensitivity of obesity-related hypertension. This creates a bit of a problem because thiazides, the most convenient agents, have adverse effects on insulin resistance and are associated with the development of diabetes in predisposed obese patients[57,58] Low-dose thiazides in combination with RAAS inhibitors however, can be safely used. Loop diuretics and potassium sparing agents can be effectively used as well in patients that are difficult to control with low dose thiazides or thiazide-like agents.

Beta-adrenergic receptor blockers have been associated with weight gain and insulin resistance and are not therefore first-line agents for the treatment of obesity-related hypertension.[57] The newer vasodilating beta-blockers have a more favorable metabolic profile, and are appropriate in the presence of congestive heart failure. Whether or not these newer agents convey the same protective effects in the postmyocardial infarction period is not established. In the absence of a specific indication, beta-blockers should be avoided in the treatment of obesity-related hypertension.

If obstructive sleep apnea is present, weight loss and treatment with continuous positive airway pressure or a mandibular extension device is warranted and frequently effective[59] in decreasing SNS activity and BP.

Pharmacologic Treatment of Obesity

It is reasonable to assume that the effects of weight loss drugs on blood pressure are mediated through loss of weight. Several agents are now available for the treatment of obesity. Listed in Table 35.3, they should be viewed as adjuncts to the lifestyle recommendations outlined previously. Reference to the energy balance equation serves as a reminder that two major mechanisms for the pharmacologic treatment of obesity: diminishing energy intake and increasing energy expenditure. The former includes appetite suppression and interference with nutrient absorption, the latter entails increases in metabolic rate, a potential but largely unrealized mechanism. Unfortunately, because no currently approved antiobesity medications have much of an effect on metabolic rate, the expenditure side of the energy balance equation remains principally dependent on physical activity. Recent studies, however, on the activation of brown adipose tissue have raised the possibility that bioavailable agonists of the beta 3 adrenergic receptor could be developed that would safely increase energy expenditure, thereby increasing significantly the therapeutic arsenal for the treatment of obesity.

The approved medications listed in Table 35.3 impair nutrient absorption or suppress appetite and diminish food craving. The unique circumstances of the individual patient play an important role in the selection of a particular agent. Impairment in nutrient absorption with orlistat or acarbose, for example, would not be good choices for patients with gastrointestinal problems or a tendency to diarrhea. Similarly, in patients with anxiety or hypertension not under good control, phenteramine, an indirect acting sympathomimetic amine (congener of amphetamine), and a component of Qsymia, is best avoided, whereas lorcaserin, a serotonin agonist, should be used cautiously in patients on psychotropic agents. Consultation with an obesity specialist can help with the management of these agents.

Surgical Treatment of Obesity

Surgical procedures to treat obesity include the laparoscopic adjustable gastric band (lap band), which decreases the stomach volume, the roux-en-Y gastric bypass that restricts stomach volume and bypasses a portion of the small bowel, and the increasingly popular sleeve gastrectomy which removes a portion of the gastric fundus. These procedures are reserved for the morbidly obese, or those obese with significant cardiovascular

---

BOX 35.1 Antihypertensive Agents for Obesity-Related Hypertension

All agents potentiated by weight loss and salt restriction
    Target ≤ 140/90 (subject to revision downward)

Renin-Angiotensin-Aldosterone System (RAAS) Inhibition
ACE inhibitors and ARBs preferred agents: beneficial metabolic effects and neutral on weight gain

Calcium Channel Blockers
Metabolically neutral

Alpha Adrenergic Blockers
Favorable metabolic profile but not first line because of possible association with congestive heart failure

Diuretics
Important part of the regimen but thiazide should be used at low dose because of unfavorable metabolic profile (↑ insulin resistance and dyslipidemia); generally in combination with ARB or ACE inhibitors

Beta-Adrenergic Blockers
Should not be used in the treatment of hypertension unless a specific cardiac indication is present (postmyocardial infarction [MI] or congestive heart failure): ↑ insulin resistance; ↑ weight gain; ↑ new cases of diabetes; vasodilating beta-blockers do not ↑ insulin resistance but their usefulness post MI is not established

---

TABLE 35.3 Pharmacologic Treatment of Obesity

AGENT	CLASS	MECHANISM OF ACTION
Orlistat	Lipase inhibitor	Fat malabsorption
Acarbose	Glucosidase inhibitor	Carbohydrate malabsorption
Lorcaserin	Serotonin agonist (5HTc receptor)	Appetite suppressant
Liraglutide	GLP-1 agonist	Appetite suppressant
Phenteramine/ topiramate (Qysmia)	Sympathomimetic/ anticonvulsant	Appetite suppressant (↑) energy expenditure
Bupropion/naltrexone (Contrave)	Antidepressant/ opioid antagonist	Appetite suppressant (↑) energy expenditure

or metabolic complications of obesity. They prolong life, are associated with durable weight loss, and improve the associated diabetes and hypertension.[60-62] The improvement in diabetes is more profound and more long-lived than the improvement in hypertension, although the latter is not trivial. The postsurgical complications, especially following the roux-en-Y procedure, may be considerable, necessitating careful follow-up and treatment of vitamin and other nutritional deficiencies.

SUMMARY

Hypertension is one of the serious complications of obesity and obesity is the major cause of essential hypertension. Treating hypertension in the obese is predicated on treating obesity, the underlying cause of the elevated blood pressure. A therapeutic plan is required for each patient; this plan should include both lifestyle management and appropriate pharmacologic therapies. Both sides of the energy balance equation need to be addressed: dietary intake and energy expenditure. The intake side requires aggressive counseling, behavioral modification as well as appropriate appetite suppressive medications; the expenditure side, for the present is largely limited to physical activity, although safe therapeutic agents that increase metabolic rate remain a goal for the future. Increasing energy expenditure is required because decreased caloric intake is associated with conservative metabolic adaptations that diminishes the effectiveness of low energy diets.

References

1. American Heart Association, Overweight and Obesity Statistics—2009 Update. 2009; Available at: www.nanocorthx.com/Articles/HeartDiseaseStrokeStatistics.pdf.
2. Flegal KM, Carroll MD, Ogden CL, Curtin LR. Prevalence and trends in obesity among US adults, 1999-2008. *JAMA.* 2010;303:235-241.
3. Kannel WB, Brand N, Skinner JJ, Jr., Dawber TR, McNamara PM. The relation of adiposity to blood pressure and development of hypertension. The Framingham study. *Ann Intern Med.* 1967;67:48-59.
4. Sahakyan KR, Somers VK, Rodriguez-Escudero JP, et al. Normal-Weight Central Obesity: Implications for Total and Cardiovascular Mortality. *Ann Intern Med.* 2015;163:827-835.
5. Vague J. The degree of masculine differentiation of obesities: a factor determining predisposition to diabetes, atherosclerosis, gout, and uric calculous disease. *Am J Clin Nutr.* 1956;4:20-34.
6. Lapidus L, Bengtsson C, Larsson B, Pennert K, Rybo E, Sjostrom L. Distribution of adipose tissue and risk of cardiovascular disease and death: a 12 year follow up of participants in the population study of women in Gothenburg, Sweden. *Br Med J (Clin Res Ed).* 1984;289:1257-1261.
7. Larsson B, Svardsudd K, Welin L, Wilhelmsen L, Bjorntorp P, Tibblin G. Abdominal adipose tissue distribution, obesity, and risk of cardiovascular disease and death: 13 year follow up of participants in the study of men born in 1913. *Br Med J (Clin Res Ed).* 1984;288:1401-1404.
8. Cassano PA, Segal MR, Vokonas PS, Weiss ST. Body fat distribution, blood pressure, and hypertension. A prospective cohort study of men in the normative aging study. *Ann Epidemiol.* 1990;1:33-48.
9. Kissebah AH, Vydelingum N, Murray R, et al. Relation of body fat distribution to metabolic complications of obesity. *J Clin Endocrinol Metab.* 1982;54:254-260.
10. Krotkiewski M, Bjorntorp P, Sjostrom L, Smith U. Impact of obesity on metabolism in men and women. Importance of regional adipose tissue distribution. *J Clin Invest.* 1983;72:1150-1162.
11. Ferrannini E, Buzzigoli G, Bonadonna R, et al. Insulin resistance in essential hypertension. *N Engl J Med.* 1987;317:350-357.
12. Modan M, Halkin H, Almog S, et al. Hyperinsulinemia. A link between hypertension obesity and glucose intolerance. *J Clin Invest.* 1985;75:809-817.
13. Rowe JW, Young JB, Minaker KL, Stevens AL, Pallotta JA, Landsberg L. Effect of insulin and glucose infusions on sympathetic nervous system activity in normal man. *Diabetes.* 1981;30:219-225.
14. Hausberg M, Mark AL, Hoffman RP, Sinkey CA, Anderson EA. Dissociation of sympathoexcitatory and vasodilator actions of modestly elevated plasma insulin levels. *J Hypertens.* 1995;13:1015-1021.
15. Troisi RJ, Weiss ST, Parker DR, Sparrow D, Young JB, Landsberg L. Relation of obesity and diet to sympathetic nervous system activity. *Hypertension.* 1991;17:669-677.
16. Grassi G, Seravalle G, Cattaneo BM, et al. Sympathetic activation in obese normotensive subjects. *Hypertension.* 1995;25:560-563.
17. Scherrer U, Randin D, Tappy L, Vollenweider P, Jéquier E, Nicod P. Body fat and sympathetic nerve activity in healthy subjects. *Circulation.* 1994;89:2634-2640.
18. Haynes WG, Morgan DA, Walsh SA, Mark AL, Sivitz WI. Receptor-mediated regional sympathetic nerve activation by leptin. *J Clin Invest.* 1997;100:270-278.
19. Sarzani R, Salvi F, Dessi-Fulgheri P, Rappelli A. Renin-angiotensin system, natriuretic peptides, obesity, metabolic syndrome, and hypertension: an integrated view in humans. *J Hypertens.* 2008;26:831-843.
20. Goodfriend TL. Obesity, sleep apnea, aldosterone, and hypertension. *Curr Hypertens Rep.* 2008;10:222-226.
21. Narkiewicz K, Somers VK. Sympathetic nerve activity in obstructive sleep apnoea. *Acta Physiol Scand.* 2003;177:385-390.
22. Rocchini AP, Key J, Bondie D, et al. The effect of weight loss on the sensitivity of blood pressure to sodium in obese adolescents. *N Engl J Med.* 1989;321:580-585.
23. Landsberg L. Insulin-mediated sympathetic stimulation: role in the pathogenesis of obesity-related hypertension (or, how insulin affects blood pressure, and why). *J Hypertens.* 2001;19(3 Pt 2):523-528.

24. Landsberg L. Diet, obesity and hypertension: an hypothesis involving insulin, the sympathetic nervous system, and adaptive thermogenesis. *Q J Med.* 1986;61:1081-1090.
25. Reaven GM. Metabolic syndrome: To be or not to be? *The Metabolic Syndrome Epidemiology, Clinical Treatment, and Underlying Mechanisms.* Edited by Barbara Caleen Hansen and George A. Bray. 2008:11-36.
26. Ervin R. Prevalence of metabolic syndrome among adults 20 years of age and over, by sex, age, race and ethnicity, and body mass index: United States, 2003-2006. *Natl Health Stat Rep.* 2009;13:1-7.
27. Hansen BC, Bray GA. *The metabolic syndrome epidemiology, clinical treatment, and underlying mechanisms.* 2008, Humana Press.
28. Grassi G, Dell'Oro R, Quarti-Trevano F, et al. Neuroadrenergic and reflex abnormalities in patients with metabolic syndrome. *Diabetologia.* 2005;48:1359-1365.
29. Landsberg L, Aronne LJ, Beilin LJ, et al. Obesity-related hypertension: pathogenesis, cardiovascular risk, and treatment: a position paper of The Obesity Society and the American Society of Hypertension. *J Clin Hypertens (Greenwich).* 2013;15:14-33.
30. Grassi G, Seravalle G, Colombo M, et al. Body weight reduction, sympathetic nerve traffic, and arterial baroreflex in obese normotensive humans. *Circulation.* 1998;97:2037-2042.
31. Aucott L, Poobalan A, Smith WC, Avenell A, Jung R, Broom J. Effects of weight loss in overweight/obese individuals and long-term hypertension outcomes: a systematic review. *Hypertension.* 2005;45:1035-1041.
32. Aucott L, Rothnie H, McIntyre L, Thapa M, Waweru C, Gray D. Long-term weight loss from lifestyle intervention benefits blood pressure?: a systematic review. *Hypertension.* 2009;54:756-762.
33. Bray GA. Lifestyle and pharmacological approaches to weight loss: efficacy and safety. *J Clin Endocrinol Metab.* 2008;93(11 Suppl 1):S81-88.
34. Avenell A, Broom J, Brown TJ, et al. Systematic review of the long-term effects and economic consequences of treatments for obesity and implications for health improvement. *Health Technol Assess.* 2004;8:iii-iv, 1–182.
35. Appel LJ, Moore TJ, Obarzanek E, et al. A clinical trial of the effects of dietary patterns on blood pressure. DASH Collaborative Research Group. *N Engl J Med.* 1997;336:1117-1124.
36. Appel LJ. ASH position paper: Dietary approaches to lower blood pressure. *J Am Soc Hypertens.* 2009;3:321-331.
37. Landsberg L, Young JB, Leonard WR, Linsenmeier RA, Turek FW. Is obesity associated with lower body temperatures? Core temperature: a forgotten variable in energy balance. *Metabolism.* 2009;58:871-876.
38. Jung RT, Shetty PS, James WP, Barrand MA, Callingham BA. Reduced thermogenesis in obesity. *Nature.* 1979;279:322-323.
39. Shetty PS, Jung RT, James WP. Effect of catecholamine replacement with levodopa on the metabolic response to semistarvation. *Lancet.* 1979;1:77-79.
40. Cox KL, Puddey IB, Morton AR, Burke V, Beilin LJ, McAleer M. Exercise and weight control in sedentary overweight men: effects on clinic and ambulatory blood pressure. *J Hypertens.* 1996;14:779-790.
41. Thorogood A, Mottillo S, Shimony A, et al. Isolated aerobic exercise and weight loss: a systematic review and meta-analysis of randomized controlled trials. *Am J Med.* 2011;124:747-755.
42. Jakicic JM. The effect of physical activity on body weight. *Obesity (Silver Spring).* 2009; 17(Suppl 3):S34-38.
43. Jennings G, Nelson L, Nestel P, et al. The effects of changes in physical activity on major cardiovascular risk factors, hemodynamics, sympathetic function, and glucose utilization in man: a controlled study of four levels of activity. *Circulation.* 1986;73:30-40.
44. Meredith IT, Friberg P, Jennings GL, et al. Exercise training lowers resting renal but not cardiac sympathetic activity in humans. *Hypertension.* 1991;18:575-582.
45. Fujita T. Mineralocorticoid receptors, salt-sensitive hypertension, and metabolic syndrome. *Hypertension.* 2010;55:813-818.
46. Ma Y, He FJ, MacGregor GA. High salt intake: independent risk factor for obesity? *Hypertension.* 2015;66:843-849.
47. Sacks FM, Svetkey LP, Vollmer WM, et al. Effects on blood pressure of reduced dietary sodium and the dietary approaches to stop hypertension (DASH) diet. DASH-Sodium Collaborative Research Group. *N Engl J Med.* 2001;344:3-10.
48. Cook NR, Cutler JA, Obarzanek E, et al. Long term effects of dietary sodium reduction on cardiovascular disease outcomes: observational follow-up of the trials of hypertension prevention (TOHP). *BMJ.* 2007;334:885-888.
49. Appel LJ, Espeland MA, Easter L, Wilson AC, Folmar S, Lacy CR. Effects of reduced sodium intake on hypertension control in older individuals: results from the Trial of Nonpharmacologic Interventions in the Elderly (TONE). *Arch Intern Med.* 2001;161:685-693.
50. Puddey IB, Beilin LJ. Alcohol is bad for blood pressure. *Clin Exp Pharmacol Physiol.* 2006;33:847-852.
51. Puddey IB, Parker M, Beilin LJ, Vandongen R, Masarei JR. Effects of alcohol and caloric restrictions on blood pressure and serum lipids in overweight men. *Hypertension.* 1992;20:533-541.
52. Elmer PJ, Grimm R, Jr., Laing B, et al. Lifestyle intervention: results of the Treatment of Mild Hypertension Study (TOMHS). *Prev Med.* 1995;24:378-388.
53. Mancia G, De Backer G, Dominiczak A, et al. Guidelines for the management of arterial hypertension: The Task Force for the Management of Arterial Hypertension of the European Society of Hypertension (ESH) and or the European Society of Cardiology (ESC). *Eur Heart J.* 2007;28:1462-1536.
54. Group SR, Wright JT, Jr., Williamson JD, et al. A Randomized Trial of Intensive versus Standard Blood-Pressure Control. *N Engl J Med.* 2015;373:2103-2116.
55. Sharma AM, Engeli S. The role of renin-angiotensin system blockade in the management of hypertension associated with the cardiometabolic syndrome. *J Cardiometab Syndr.* 2006;1:29-35.
56. Oparil S. Antihypertensive and Lipid-Lowering Treatment to Prevent Heart Attack Trial (ALLHAT): practical implications. *Hypertension.* 2003;41:1006-1009.
57. Lindholm LH, Ibsen H, Borch-Johnsen K, et al. Risk of new-onset diabetes in the Losartan Intervention For Endpoint reduction in hypertension study. *J. Hypertens.* 2002;20:1879-1886.
58. Gupta AK, Dahlof B, Dobson J, Sever PS, Wedel H, Poulter NR. Determinants of new-onset diabetes among 19,257 hypertensive patients randomized in the Anglo-Scandinavian Cardiac Outcomes Trial—Blood Pressure Lowering Arm and the relative influence of antihypertensive medication. *Diabetes Care.* 2008;31:982-988.
59. Somers VK, Dyken ME, Clary MP, Abboud FM. Sympathetic neural mechanisms in obstructive sleep apnea. *J Clin Invest.* 1995;96:1897-1904.
60. Rubino F, R'Bibo SL, del Genio F, Mazumdar M, McGraw TE. Metabolic surgery: the role of the gastrointestinal tract in diabetes mellitus. *Nat Rev Endocrinol.* 2010;6:102-109.
61. Buchwald H, Avidor Y, Braunwald E, et al. Bariatric surgery: a systematic review and meta-analysis. *JAMA.* 2004;292:1724-1737.
62. Sjostrom L, Lindroos AK, Peltonen M, et al. Lifestyle, diabetes, and cardiovascular risk factors 10 years after bariatric surgery. *N Engl J Med.* 2004;351:2683-2693.

36 Cerebrovascular Disease

Philip B. Gorelick, Jiangyong Min, and Muhammad U. Farooq

Raised blood pressure has been referred to as the crown jewel of stroke prevention, and blood pressure lowering has been the focus of substantial study in acute stroke and recurrent stroke prevention as a means to improve outcomes. In this chapter we discuss hypertension and stroke within the context of acute and chronic stroke management. To provide a framework for subsequent discussion of acute and chronic stroke management, we begin this chapter with the definition of stroke and a brief overview of stroke epidemiology.

A NEW DEFINITION OF STROKE

Stroke has traditionally been defined based on the presence of neurological signs and symptoms and time course. The occurrence of focal neurological signs or symptoms caused by cerebrovascular disease and lasting more than 24 hours has been previously defined as stroke, whereas transient ischemic attack (TIA) has been defined as having the same clinical features as stroke but the neurological sign or symptom duration is transient lasting up to 24 hours.[1] The definitions of stroke and TIA have been criticized as being arbitrary and importantly do not take into account the underlying mechanism or etiology. In cerebrovascular disease, elucidation of stroke mechanism is the primary basis for administration of specific chronic preventative therapy and acute treatment.[2] These considerations have led to a 21st century updated definition of stroke.[3] The updated definition takes into account not only focal neurological signs or symptoms of the brain, spinal cord or retina injury, but also incorporates consideration of brain tissue status or evidence of stroke based on modern neuroimaging such as magnetic resonance imaging (MRI). In the case of TIA, it is estimated that up to 30% to 40% of persons will have evidence of correlative prior or acute cerebral ischemia on neuroimaging study. In addition, the new definition of stroke takes into account silent or unexpected strokes which may manifest as small deep infarcts, white matter disease (leukoaraiosis), and cerebral microbleeds.[3] Table 36.1 lists categories for the classification of ischemic and hemorrhagic stroke.[1,4,5]

BRIEF OVERVIEW OF STROKE EPIDEMIOLOGY

The Prospective Urban Rural Epidemiologic (PURE) cohort study was carried out among greater than 150,000 adults in 17 high-income, middle-income, and low-income countries on 5 continents. The PURE study was designed to answer questions about cardiovascular disease mortality, incidence, and risks.[6] In PURE, age-adjusted and sex-adjusted case fatality rates for stroke were highest among low-income countries followed in descending order by medium-income and high-income countries. Overall, although risk factor burden was lowest in low-income countries, rates of major cardiovascular disease and mortality were much higher in low-than high-income countries. High-income countries had a high burden of risks, but better control of these risks and more frequent administration of pharmacologic treatments and revascularization procedures may explain these disparities in outcome.[6]

In the Global Burden of Disease Study 2013 (GBD 2013) among 306 diseases and injuries in 188 countries, stroke ranked as the second leading cause of disability-adjusted life years (DALYs) behind ischemic heart disease.[7] In addition, GBD 2013 showed a greater than three times increase in burden of stroke (4.85 million stroke deaths, 91.4 million DALYs) in developing countries compared with high-income countries (1.6 million deaths, 21.5 million DALYs).[8] Overall, there were approximately 25.7 million stroke survivors (71% with ischemic stroke), 6.5 million stroke deaths (51% from ischemic stroke), 113 million DALYs attributed to stroke (58% ischemic stroke), and 10.3 million persons with new strokes (67% ischemic).[8] There was substantially greater reduction of stroke mortality rates in developed compared with developing countries.

In summary, stroke-associated rates are on the rise and are being driven by the stroke burden in low-income countries. These observations provide a potential opportunity to better prevent stroke and implement more sophisticated acute care systems in developing regions.[9] One of us (PBG) was involved in the development of a prototype Internet-based, worldwide survey of diagnostic and treatment capacitance for stroke in developing countries (Chile, Georgia, Nigeria, Qatar, India, Lithuania, Kazakhstan, Indonesia, Brazil and Bangladesh).[10] We found a significant correlation between income and access or affordability to a number of stroke diagnostics and treatments.

Hypertension and Risk for Stroke

Blood pressure is a factor associated with a continuous risk of stroke.[11,12] We no longer think of stroke risk with raised blood pressure as a threshold effect. Lawes et al. showed in cohort studies that for each 10 mm Hg lower systolic blood pressure, there was a reduction of stroke of about one-third in persons aged 60 to 79 years, and this association was continuous down to at least a blood pressure level of 115/75 mm Hg.[13] Furthermore, the relationship held according to sex, region, stroke subtype, and for fatal and nonfatal events. In randomized controlled trials, a 10 mm Hg reduction in systolic blood pressure was associated with a reduction of stroke risk by about one-third.[13] The authors emphasized that there were greater benefits of larger blood pressure lowering and maintenance of blood pressure lowering on stroke reduction, and challenged the importance of choice of initial blood pressure lowering agent.[13]

Systolic blood pressure has become the main target for stroke and cardiovascular disease prevention. Because systolic blood pressure continues to rise with age and diastolic blood pressure increases until about age 50 years and falls thereafter when stroke and other cardiovascular disease begins to substantially increase, systolic blood pressure is the major target of intervention, especially for those older

TABLE 36.1 Categories for Classification of Stroke of the Brain, Spinal Cord, and Retina

Ischemic Stroke	1. Large artery atherosclerotic extracranial or intracranial occlusive disease
	2. Embolism (cardio-aortic, artery-to-artery)
	3. Small artery occlusion (lacunar)
	4. Uncommon causes of stroke (e.g., arterial dissection, cardiac, or arterial surgery and interventions)
	5. Undetermined causes (cryptogenic): when there is suspicion of an embolism, for example, but no obvious source is identified; or incomplete evaluation
	6. Unclassified (e.g., more than one possible mechanism)
Silent or Unexpected Stroke	1. Small deep infarction
	2. White matter disease (leukoaraiosis)
	3. Cerebral microbleeds
	4. Enlarged perivascular spaces
Hemorrhagic Stroke	1. Intraparenchymal hemorrhage (hypertensive and nonhypertensive [e.g., anticoagulant or illicit drug induced])
	2. Subarachnoid hemorrhage

than 50 years.[14] Raised blood pressure is estimated to elevate stroke risk up to three-fold or four-fold compared with those without elevated blood pressure.[11] Based on a meta-analysis of individual patient data, blood pressure lowering is associated with a similar relative protection at all levels of baseline cardiovascular risk; however, there is greater absolute risk reduction as baseline risk increases.[15]

As noted above, a substantial number of observational epidemiological studies link hypertension to stroke, and numerous clinical trials show the benefit of blood pressure lowering on stroke incidence or recurrence. In addition, population attributable risk (PAR) calculations place hypertension as the most important remediable factor as it explains the highest percentage of stroke risk. The PAR for hypertension in stroke is in the 25% to almost 50% range.[12,16] In the INTERSTROKE Study, a large case-control design, there were participants from 22 countries of different geographic regions, and it was shown that 10 risk factors were associated with 90% of stroke risk.[17] The PAR for hypertension in relation to stroke was 34.6%. Overall, the relative risk or estimate of relative risk of hypertension for stroke is in the three-fold to nine-fold range.[18]

TREATMENT OF ACUTE ISCHEMIC STROKE

As previously mentioned in this chapter, the classification of stroke includes a number of major ischemic subtypes as well as the two major hemorrhagic subtypes: subarachnoid hemorrhage and intraparenchymal hemorrhage. Because the scope and depth of the topic on the management of acute stroke is so broad, we will largely limit our discussion in this chapter to management of acute ischemic stroke,[19,20] but will also review select clinical trials that address blood pressure reduction in hemorrhagic stroke. For reviews of the management of subarachnoid hemorrhage and intraparenchymal hemorrhage, the reader is referred to authoritative sources found elsewhere.[21-23]

Blood Pressure Lowering in Acute Ischemic Stroke

According to the American Heart Association(AHA)/ American Stroke Association (ASA) 2013 guidelines for the early management of acute ischemic stroke, the following evidence-based blood pressure guidance is recommended (evidence rating by Class and Level are in parenthesis).[19] (1) For patients eligible to receive intravenous tissue plasminogen activator (tPA), blood pressure should be lowered to less than 185/110 mm Hg (class I, Level of Evidence [LOE] B) and maintained before initiation of thrombolytic therapy; (2) After intravenous tPA administration, blood pressure should be maintained below 180/105 mm Hg for at least 24 hours after tPA treatment; (3) For recanalization procedures and until additional scientific study information becomes available, the recommendations just mentioned should be followed for interventional recanalization procedures including intraarterial fibrinolysis (class I, LOE C); (4) For patients with substantially raised blood pressure and who are not undergoing intravenous tPA or recanalization procedures, it is reasonable to lower blood pressure by around 15% during the first 24 hours after stroke onset. Guidance further indicates that blood pressure lowering medication should be withheld unless systolic blood pressure is greater than 220 mm Hg or diastolic is greater than 120 mm Hg (class I, LOE C), or there is a compelling indication to otherwise treat blood pressure (e.g., heart failure). Initial blood pressure lowering medications may include intravenous labetalol, nicardipine, or others[19]; (5) Administration of antihypertensive therapy within 24 hours of stroke is relatively safe. It is reasonable to restart blood pressure lowering agents 24 hours after stroke onset for persons with preexistent hypertension and who are neurologically stable (class IIa, LOE B); and (6) For patients not undergoing acute reperfusion strategies data regarding blood pressure lowering in acute ischemic stroke are inconclusive or conflicting, and the benefit of such treatment is not well established (class IIb, LOE C). It has been argued that in acute ischemic stroke too substantial blood pressure lowering could lead to extension of brain infarction in an already ischemic brain hemisphere with penumbral compromise, yet too high a blood pressure might potentiate brain edema, hemorrhagic transformation, and worsening of neurological outcome.[24,25]

Updated Trial Findings

Since the publication of the AHA/ASA 2013 guidelines for early management of acute ischemic stroke, several new major studies addressing blood pressure control have been published. The China Antihypertensive Trial in Acute Ischemic Stroke (CATIS) was a multicenter, randomized controlled study organized to test whether moderate blood pressure lowering within 48 hours of onset of acute ischemic stroke could reduce death and major disability at 14 days or at hospital discharge.[26] Patients were in their early sixties, were randomized within approximately 15 hours of stroke onset, had mild acute stroke impairment on neurological exam, and had entry blood pressures of about 167/97 mm Hg. Intravenous angiotensin-converting enzyme inhibitors were first-line treatment. Within 24 hours, blood pressure targets were met as mean systolic blood pressure (SBP) was lowered by 12.7% in the active treatment group and by 7.2% in the control group. By day 7 the corresponding group blood pressures were 137.3 mm Hg and 146.5 mm Hg, respectively. However, there was no difference in the primary (death and major disability at 14 days or discharge) or secondary (death and major disability at 3 months) outcomes between the intensive and less intensive blood pressure lowering groups. In the Efficacy of Nitric Oxide in Stroke (ENOS) trial, therapy with transdermal glyceryl trinitrate for 7 days and given within 48 hours of ischemic or hemorrhagic stroke onset was compared with control. Active blood pressure lowering therapy significantly reduced blood pressure and was safe, but it did not improve functional outcome based on the modified Rankin Scale (mRS).[27]

The above mentioned studies and others, with the exception of the Scandinavian Candesartan Acute Stroke Trial (SCAST) (there was a signal of poor outcome based on the mRS), suggest that blood pressure lowering in acute stroke is generally safe but secondary outcomes might be compromised.[28-31] Thus, there has been a call to hold blood pressure lowering therapy in acute ischemic stroke patients until they are considered to be medically and neurologically stable, and therefore have suitable oral or enteral access.[32]

Blood Pressure Variability

One of the authors (PBG) has been involved in the study of blood pressure variability after acute ischemic stroke.[33,34] Blood pressure variability after acute ischemic stroke has been associated with neurological deterioration, and thus, serves as a target for possible intervention to improve outcomes and requires further study.[32]

Blood Pressure Lowering in Acute Hemorrhagic Stroke

The AHA/ASA 2015 guidance for blood pressure management in spontaneous intracerebral hemorrhage[21] recommends: (1) Acute systolic blood pressure lowering to 140 mm Hg as a safe strategy in patients with systolic blood pressure between 150 and 220 mm Hg (class I, LOE A). In addition, this management strategy can be effective for improving functional outcome (class IIa, LOE B); and (2) For patients with systolic blood pressure higher than 220 mm Hg, aggressive reduction of blood pressure with continuous intravenous infusion therapy and frequent blood pressure monitoring may be reasonable (class IIb, LOE C).

A key consideration in the development of the above recommendations for blood pressure lowering for spontaneous intracerebral hemorrhage was the Intensive Blood Pressure Reduction in Acute Cerebral Hemorrhage Trial 2 (INTERACT2).[35] In this trial, where intensive blood pressure lowering (a target of <140 mm Hg SBP) was compared with guideline treatment (a target of <180 mm Hg systolic blood pressure), the primary outcome (death or severe disability at 90 days) was not significantly reduced with intensive treatment. However, an ordinal analysis of the mRS showed improved functional outcome with intensive blood pressure lowering.[35] Another trial of blood pressure lowering in acute cerebral hemorrhage, Antihypertensive Treatment in Acute Cerebral Hemorrhage (ATACH) II,[36] was recently halted prematurely, but the results have not been published.

2015 Guidance for Early Management of Patients With Acute Ischemic Stroke in Relation to Endovascular Treatment

Five major clinical trials of predominantly stent retrievers deployed for recanalization of large cerebral arteries in acute ischemic stroke[37-41] have led to the 2015 AHA/ASA guideline update recommendations for use of these devices in early stroke management.[20] The details of the five trials are reviewed elsewhere.[20] Key 2015 AHA/ASA guidance recommendations in relation to endovascular recanalization therapy[20] include: (1) Use of intravenous tPA as a first step for eligible patients being considered for intraarterial endovascular therapy (class I, LOE A); and (2) Endovascular therapy with a stent retriever should be deployed in patients according to the following criteria (class I, LOE A): *A.* Prestroke mRS score of 0 or 1; *B.* Administration of intravenous tPA within 4.5 hours of stroke onset; *C.* For causative occlusion of the internal carotid artery or proximal middle cerebral artery (M1); *D.* 18 years of age or older; *E.* National Institutes of Health Stroke Scale score of 6 or greater; *F.* ASPECTS (a grading scale for acute ischemic change on computed tomography [CT] head study) score of 6 or greater; and *G.* Endovascular treatment can be initiated (groin puncture) within 6 hours of stroke symptom onset. Other recommendations from this guidance statement are discussed elsewhere.[20]

TABLE 36.2 General Treatment Recommendations for Early Management of Acute Ischemic Stroke

1. Airway and ventilator support if airway compromise
2. Maintain oxygen saturation >94% (supplemental oxygen is not indicated in nonhypoxic patients)
3. Antipyretic therapy if fever occurs
4. Raised blood pressure (see text)
5. Avoid hypoglycemia and if hyperglycemic, treat to a glucose level of 140-180 mg/dL
6. Swallow evaluation to assess for aspiration potential
7. Subcutaneous anticoagulant therapy to prevent deep vein thrombosis in immobilized patients
8. Avoid indwelling bladder catheter
9. Utilize a standardized stroke order set
10. Management of acute edema or seizures (see reference 19 for details)

(From Jauch EC, Saver JL, Adams HP, et al. Guidelines for the early management of patients with acute ischemic stroke. A guideline for healthcare professionals from the American Heart Association/American Stroke Association. Stroke. 2013;44:870-947.)

General Treatment Recommendations for Early Acute Ischemic Stroke Management

Table 36.2 lists select other general treatment recommendations for the management of early acute ischemic stroke.[19]

MANAGEMENT OF CHRONIC STROKE

Persons who have experienced ischemic stroke or TIA are at high risk for recurrent stroke.[1] Of the total number of strokes occurring in the United States each year, recurrent ones make up almost 25%. It is estimated that the annual risk of a future ischemic stroke after an initial stroke or TIA is approximately 3% to 4%.[42] Given this annualized average rate of stroke recurrence over time, there is a higher risk early on (i.e., in the first year) compared with later epochs. Furthermore, as time passes, the risk of a major coronary events heightens. Thus, it is important to be aware of coronary risk in stroke patients (and vice versa).

Recurrent stroke risk will vary according to stroke subtype, age, comorbid conditions, and adherence to preventive therapy.[42] Hypertension is recognized as a risk for early and late recurrent stroke.[43] Traditionally, hypertension has not been well controlled in a number of recurrent stroke prevention trials up until more recently when it was shown that lifestyle coaching and a concerted effort to monitor and treat blood pressure is a highly efficacious strategy.[44]

It has been observed that 7-day, 30-day, and 90-day recurrent stroke rates are higher for atherosclerotic and cardiac embolic stroke subtypes compared with lacunar stroke.[45] Thus, proper definition of stroke subtype has prognostic significance and also dictates the therapeutic approach as we shall learn in the following sections.

In a single center observational study inadequate blood pressure control was linked to higher recurrence of both lobar and nonlobar intraparenchymal hemorrhage, suggesting the need for additional clinical trial study of blood pressure control in brain hemorrhage survivors.[46] Also, in a retrospective cohort study carried out at 19 German tertiary care centers among persons with oral anticoagulation-associated intraparenchymal hemorrhage, rapid reversal of an elevated international normalized ratio (INR) and SBP lowering to less than 160 mm Hg within 4 hours was associated with lower rates of hematoma enlargement.[47] Furthermore, return to oral anticoagulant therapy was linked to a lower risk of subsequent ischemic events.[47]

Management of Blood Pressure for Recurrent Stroke Prevention

The 2014 AHA/ASA guidance statement for recurrent stroke prevention recommends the following in relation to blood pressure management[42]: (1) Although initiation of blood pressure lowering therapy after stroke for persons with blood pressure less than 140/90 mm Hg is of uncertain benefit (class IIb, LOE C), blood pressure therapy may be initiated within several days after stroke for those with a blood pressure of 140 or 90 mm Hg or greater (class I, LOE B); (2) Resumption of blood pressure lowering therapy to prevent recurrent stroke and other vascular events is indicated for those with a history of hypertension (class I, LOE A); (3) It is reasonable to aim for a target blood pressure less than 140/90 mm Hg (class IIa, LOE B), and it is reasonable to target a systolic blood pressure less than 130 mm Hg in patients with recent symptomatic lacunar infarction (class IIb, LOE B); (4) Lifestyle modifications (salt restriction, weight loss, diet rich in fruits and vegetables and low-fat dairy products, regular physical exercise, and limited alcohol consumption) are a reasonable component of a blood pressure lowering therapy regimen (class IIa, LOE C); (5) The optimal drug treatment regimen remains uncertain; however, diuretics or a diuretic plus angiotensin-converting enzyme inhibitor are considered useful (class I, LOE A); and (6) Specific blood pressure lowering agents should be chosen based on pharmacologic properties, mechanism of action, and patient characteristics (e.g., presence of diabetes mellitus, heart failure, renal disease) (class IIa, LOE B).

Select Trial Data Influencing Blood Pressure Lowering Recommendations for Recurrent Ischemic Stroke Prevention

Two trials stand out as having a major influence on the above guidance for recurrent stroke prevention in relation to blood pressure management: Perindopril Protection Against Recurrent Stroke Study (PROGRESS) and Secondary Prevention of Small Subcortical Strokes (SPS3). PROGRESS featured the angiotensin-converting enzyme inhibitor, perindopril, with or without the diuretic, indapamide, versus placebo in a large trial designed to include persons with stroke or TIA in the past 5 years.[48] Active treatment reduced blood pressure by 9/4 mm Hg. Overall, there was a statistically significant 28% relative risk reduction in recurrent stroke and a 50% reduction of recurrent intracerebral hemorrhage favoring the perindopril-based treatment arm. Perindopril alone achieved a blood pressure lowering effect of 5/3 mm Hg and did not achieve statistically significant stroke reduction results. With greater blood pressure lowering (12/5 mm Hg with combination therapy), there was greater reduction of key study endpoints.

SPS3 was a randomized open-label trial of MRI brain that defined symptomatic lacunar infarcts.[49] SBP lowering treatment targets were set for two comparator groups: less than 130 mm Hg versus 130 to 149 mm Hg. The primary endpoint, similar to PROGRESS, was reduction of all-cause stroke. The higher intensity blood pressure treatment group achieved a mean systolic SBP of 127 mm Hg, whereas the less intense treatment group achieved an SBP of 138 mm Hg after 1 year. There was no statistically significant advantage of intensive blood pressure lowering on all stroke; fatal stroke; or the composite of myocardial infarction or vascular death. However, intracerebral hemorrhage was significantly reduced (63% relative reduction; $p = 0.03$). Intensive blood pressure lowering therapy was deemed to be safe. Blood pressure lowering medications were prescribed at the discretion of the study team and were provided by the local site formulary.

Meta-analysis of randomized controlled trials in recurrent stroke prevention has shown a reduction of recurrent stroke with blood pressure lowering of 29% and a reduction of cardiovascular events by 31%.[50] However, there was no advantage for reduction of myocardial infarction or all-cause mortality.[50]

TABLE 36.3 Management of Select Risks or Cerebrovascular Conditions After Ischemic Stroke or Transient Ischemic Attack

1. Lipids: statin therapy with intensive lipid lowering properties and lifestyle modification if low-density lipoprotein cholesterol 100 or more mg/dL and atherosclerotic stroke

2. Symptomatic extracranial carotid artery stenosis:
   A. Less than 50% carotid artery stenosis: medical management
   B. Between 50% and 69% carotid artery stenosis: individualize medical or medical management plus carotid endarterectomy based on patient characteristics, age, and comorbidities
   C. Between 70% and 99% carotid artery stenosis: carotid endarterectomy plus medical management
   D. Carotid artery stenting: if the carotid artery lumen is reduced by more than 70% through noninvasive imaging or more than 50% through catheter conventional cerebral angiography and direct surgical access to carotid artery is difficult (e.g., high carotid bifurcation), medical comorbidities increase risk of direct surgery, or there are local circumstances (history of neck radiation, prior carotid endarterectomy) making endarterectomy difficult

3. Large artery intracranial atherosclerosis:
   A. Extracranial to intracranial bypass is not recommended
   B. Aggressive medical management including but not limited to a high-potency statin therapy and a blood pressure target of more than 140/90 mm Hg if 50% to 99% stenosis
   C. If 70% to 99% stenosis: clopidogrel 75 mg per day plus aspirin for 90 days followed by antiplatelet monotherapy
   D. Intracranial stenting is not recommended for routine use

4. Nonvalvular atrial fibrillation:
   A. If cause of stroke uncertain, 30-day continuous cardiac rhythm monitoring
   B. Warfarin, apixaban, dabigatran or rivaroxaban (reasonable choice)[a]
   C. If oral anticoagulation is contraindicated, consider aspirin alone or aspirin plus clopidogrel

5. Antiplatelet therapy (if no indication for oral anticoagulation):
   A. Aspirin 50 to 325 mg per day or aspirin 25 mg plus extended-release dipyridamole 200 mg twice daily or clopidogrel 75 mg per day
   B. Aspirin plus clopidogrel may be considered within 24 hours of minor ischemic stroke or transient ischemic attack for 90 days followed by antiplatelet monotherapy, otherwise aspirin plus clopidogrel is not indicated unless there is some other compelling indication (e.g., coronary artery stent)

[a]Edoxaban was approved for this indication after the publication of this statement. (From Kernan WN, Ovbiagele B, Black HR, et al. Guidelines for the prevention of stroke in patients with stroke and transient ischemic attack. A guideline for healthcare professionals from the American Heart Association/American Stroke Association. Stroke. 2014;45:2160-2236.)

Management of Select Risks or Cerebrovascular Conditions After Ischemic Stroke or Transient Ischemic Attack

Management of select risks or cerebrovascular conditions for recurrent stroke prevention are listed in Table 36.3 in accordance with the AHA/ASA 2014 guidance statement.[42]

BLOOD PRESSURE MANAGEMENT FOR SELECT RECURRENT STROKE PREVENTION CONDITIONS

Preservation of Cognition and Blood Pressure

Cognitive impairment is common after stroke, and up to about one-third of these persons may have significant cognitive impairment. In addition, it has been estimated that midlife raised blood pressure may account for 5% and 8% of Alzheimer disease (AD) worldwide and in the U.S., respectively, and the relative risk of raised blood pressure on AD is about 1.6.[51] In a 2011 AHA/ASA evidence review and guidance statement it was concluded that in patients with stroke, blood pressure lowering is effective for reducing dementia after stroke (class I, LOE B); there is reasonable evidence that lowering blood pressure in middle-aged and young elderly people may prevent dementia in late life (class IIa, LOE B); and the usefulness of blood pressure lowering in persons older than 80 years for the prevention of dementia is unconfirmed (class IIb, LOE B).[52]

Uncertainty exists about the value of blood pressure lowering for preservation of cognitive function because there have been disparate study methodology, missed opportunities for study in many cardiovascular trials, a number of studies that suggest that blood pressure lowering may be useful and others that have shown no benefit, lack of long-term clinical trial data beginning in middle life or earlier, and adequate study of the phenomenon that higher blood pressure (to some degree) may be better for preservation of cognitive function in the very old.[53-55] Thus, it may turn out that blood pressure control may have different effects on cognition based on absolute age.[53] Furthermore, control of multiple cardiovascular risks including blood pressure may be needed to achieve successful cognitive preservation.[56] Currently and given the equipoise in relation to blood pressure control and maintenance of cognitive vitality, we recommend following blood pressure control parameters in the AHA/ASA 2011 guidance statement.[52]

High-Grade Occlusive Large Artery Disease

Reduction of stroke risk is highly dependent on blood pressure lowering, especially in the case of hemorrhagic stroke.[57] However, when it comes to recurrent ischemic stroke prevention there may be a "J"-shaped curve as demonstrated by Ovbiagele et al. in the Prevention Regimen for Effectively Preventing Second Strokes (PRoFESS) study, whereby systolic blood pressure levels during follow-up in the very low–normal (<120 mm Hg), high (140 to <150 mm Hg), or very high (≥150 mm Hg) range were associated with increased risk of recurrent stroke.[58] Furthermore, when there is high-grade symptomatic intracranial occlusive cerebrovascular disease, it has been shown that patients with misery perfusion based on positron emission tomography (PET) had an increased risk of ipsilateral stroke when systolic blood pressure was less than 130 mm Hg.[59] In the Carotid Occlusion Surgery Study (COSS) among a limited sample size in a nonprimary analysis, there was benefit for stroke reduction in patients who had blood pressure 130/85 or less mm Hg versus more than 130/85 mm Hg, carotid artery occlusion, and increased oxygen extraction on PET study.[60] In a nonprimary analysis of the Warfarin-Aspirin Symptomatic Intracranial Disease Study (WASID), systolic blood pressure 160 or higher mm Hg was associated with the highest ipsilateral recurrent stroke rates compared with lower blood pressure levels.[61] The above data may be interpreted to suggest a blood pressure in the range of 130 to 139/80 to 85 mm Hg as a reasonable target when there is high-grade large artery occlusive disease.

SUMMARY

Blood pressure above 140/90 mm Hg is an important and modifiable risk factor for first and recurrent stroke. Blood pressure lowering in acute ischemic stroke is generally safe but has not been shown to reduce early death or disability, and concern has been raised that such therapy may worsen functional outcomes. In relation to hemorrhagic stroke, acute intensive blood pressure lowering (i.e., a target < 140 mm Hg systolic) has not been shown to reduce death or severe disability, but may improve functional outcome. In select conditions, blood pressure lowering has not been conclusively shown to reduce risk of cognitive impairment or decline, and persons with large artery occlusion may benefit from lowering of blood pressure but too high or too low a blood pressure may lead to an increased risk of recurrent stroke. Table 36.4 lists blood pressure targets for stroke prevention and acute stroke management based on the guidance statements reviewed in this chapter and the authors' experience.

TABLE 36.4 Blood Pressure Targets for Stroke Prevention and Acute Stroke Management

The following blood pressure targets may be reasonable for stroke prevention:
1. For recurrent stroke/transient ischemic attack (TIA) prevention in general: aim for a blood pressure target less than 140/90 mm Hg (target range: 130 to 139/80 to 85 mm Hg)
2. If a lacunar infarction: consider aiming for a systolic blood pressure target less than 130 mm Hg
3. Caution must be considered when lowering blood pressure when there is symptomatic high-grade or total occlusion of large cerebral arteries such as the carotid, basilar, and middle cerebral (M1): in the absence of positron emission tomography scan guidance, it is reasonable to aim for a blood pressure target less than 140/90 mm Hg (target range: 130 to 139/80 to 85 mm Hg)
4. Although a J-shaped blood pressure lowering curve may not be a major consideration for first stroke prevention, such may exist for recurrent stroke prevention: aim for a blood pressure target less than 140/90 mm Hg (target range: 130 to 139/80 to 85 mm Hg)

The following blood pressure targets may be reasonable for acute stroke treatment:
1. For acute ischemic stroke and intravenous tissue plasminogen activator (tPA) administration or intraarterial recanalization procedures: aim for a blood pressure less than 185/110 mm Hg and maintain the blood pressure at less than 180/105 mm Hg for 24 hours after intravenous tPA therapy
2. For acute ischemic stroke without intravenous tPA administration or intraarterial recanalization procedure: unless there is a compelling indication (e.g., heart failure), blood pressure lowering may be withheld up to a systolic level of 220 mm Hg or a diastolic of 120 mm Hg
3. For acute intraparenchymal hemorrhage: aim for a systolic blood pressure of 140 mm Hg

References

1. Gorelick PB, Ruland S. Cerebrovascular disease. *Disease-a-Month.* 2010;56:33-100.
2. Gorelick PB, Farooq MU. Stroke: an emphasis on guidelines. *Lancet Neurol.* 2015;14:2-3.
3. Sacco RL, Kasner SE, Broderick JP, et al. An updated definition of stroke for the 21st century. A statement for healthcare professionals from the American Heart Association/American Stroke Association. *Stroke.* 2013;44:2064-2089.
4. Kim BJ, Kim JS. Ischemic stroke subtype classification: an Asian viewpoint. *J Stroke (Korea).* 2014;16:8-17.
5. Ay H, Benner T, Arsava M, et al. A computerized algorithm for etiologic classification of ischemic stroke. The causative classification of stroke system. *Stroke.* 2007;38:2979-2984.
6. Yusuf S, Rangarajan S, Teo K, et al. Cardiovascular risk and events in 17 low-, middle-, and high-income countries. *N Engl J Med.* 2014;371:818-827.
7. GBD 2013 DALYs and HALE Collaborators, Murray CJL, Barber RM, et al. Global, regional, and national disability-adjusted life years (DALYs) for 306 diseases and injuries and healthy life expectancy (HALE) for 188 countries, 1990-2013: quantifying the epidemiologic transition. *Lancet.* 2015;386:2145-2191.
8. Feigin VL, Krishnamurthi RV, Parmar P, et al. Update on the global burden of ischemic and hemorrhagic stroke in 1990-2013: The GBD 2013 Study. *Neuroepidemiology.* 2015;45:161-176.
9. Norrving B, Davis SM, Feigin VL, et al. Stroke prevention worldwide-what could make it work? *Neuroepidemiology.* 2015;45:215-220.
10. Aiyagari V, Pandey D, Testai FD, et al. A prototype worldwide survey of diagnostic and treatment modalities for stroke. *J Stroke Cerebral Dis.* 2015;24:2909–2296.
11. Gorelick PB. New horizons for stroke prevention; PROGRESS and HOPE. *Lancet Neurol.* 2002;1:149-156.
12. Gorelick PB. The future of stroke prevention by risk factor modification. In: Fisher M (ed): *Handbook of Clinical Neurology.* New York: Stroke Part III, Elsevier; 2009.
13. Lawes CMM, Bennett DA, Feigin VL, et al. Blood pressure and stroke. An overview of published reviews. *Stroke.* 2004;35:1024-1033.
14. Williams B, Lindholm LH, Sever P. Systolic pressure is all that matters. *Lancet.* 2008;371:2219-2221.
15. The Blood Pressure Lowering Treatment Trialists' Collaboration. Blood pressure-lowering treatment based on cardiovascular risk: a meta-analysis of individual patient data. *Lancet.* 2014;384:591-598.
16. Gorelick PB. Stroke prevention. An opportunity for efficient utilization of health care resources during the coming decade. *Stroke.* 1994;25:220-224.
17. O'Donnell MJ, Xavier D, Lui L, et al. Risk factors for ischemic and intracerebral hemorrhagic stroke in 22 countries (the INTERSTROKE study): a case-control study. *Lancet.* 2010;376:112-123.
18. Goldstein LB, Bushnell CD, Adams RJ, et al. Guidelines for the primary prevention of stroke. A guideline for healthcare professionals from the American Heart Association/American Stroke Association. *Stroke.* 2011;42:517-584.
19. Jauch EC, Saver JL, Adams HP, et al. Guidelines for the early management of patients with acute ischemic stroke. A guideline for healthcare professionals from the American Heart Association/American Stroke Association. *Stroke.* 2013;44:870-947.
20. Powers WJ, Derdeyn CP, Biller J, et al. 2015 American Heart Association/American Stroke Association focused update of the 2013 guidelines for the early management of patients with acute ischemic stroke regarding endovascular treatment. A guideline for healthcare professionals from the American Heart Association/American Stroke Association. *Stroke.* 2015;46:3020-3035.
21. Hemphill JC III, Greenberg SM, Anderson CS, et al. Guidelines for the management of spontaneous intracerebral hemorrhage. A guideline for healthcare professionals from the American Heart Association/American Stroke Association. *Stroke.* 2015;46:2032-2060.

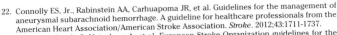

22. Connolly ES, Jr., Rabinstein AA, Carhuapoma JR, et al. Guidelines for the management of aneurysmal subarachnoid hemorrhage. A guideline for healthcare professionals from the American Heart Association/American Stroke Association. *Stroke*. 2012;43:1711-1737.

23. Steiner T, Juvela S, Unterberg A, et al. European Stroke Organization guidelines for the management of intracranial aneurysms and subarachnoid hemorrhage. *Cerebrovasc Dis*. 2013;35:93-112.

24. Gorelick PB, Aiyagari V. The management of hypertension for acute stroke: what is the blood pressure goal? *Curr Cardiol Rep*. 2013;15:366.

25. Aiyagari V, Gorelick PB. Management of blood pressure for acute and recurrent stroke. *Stroke*. 2009;40:2251-2256.

26. He J, Zhang Y, Xu T, et al. Effects of immediate blood pressure reduction on death and major disability in patients with acute ischemic stroke. The CATIS randomized clinical trial. *JAMA*. 2014;311:479-489.

27. The ENOS Trial Investigators. Efficacy of nitric oxide, with or without continuing antihypertensive treatment, for management of high blood pressure in acute stroke (ENOS): a partial-factorial randomized controlled trial. *Lancet*. 2015;385:617-628.

28. Sandset EC, Bath PMW, Boysen G, et al. on behalf of the SCAST Study Group. The angiotensin-receptor blocker candesartan for treatment of acute stroke (SCAST): a randomized, placebo-controlled, double-blind trial. *Lancet*. 2011;371:741-750.

29. Robinson TG, Potter JF, Ford GA, et al. Effects of antihypertensive treatment after acute strokein the Continue Or Stop post-Stroke Antihypertensives Collaborative Study (COSSACS): a prospective, randomized, open, blinded-endpoint trial. *Lancet Neurol*. 2010;9:767-775.

30. Potter J, Mistri A, Brodie F, et al. Controlling hypertension and hypotension immediately post stroke (CHHIPS)—a randomized controlled trial. *Health Technol Assess*. 2009;13:1-73.

31. Bath PMW, Martin RH, Palesch Y, et al. Effect of telmisartan on functional outcome, recurrence, and blood pressure in patients with acute mild ischemic stroke. A PRoFESS subgroup analysis. *Stroke*. 2009;40:3541-3546.

32. Gorelick PB. Should blood pressure be lowered in acute ischemic stroke? The CATIS Trial. *J Am Soc Hypertens*. 2015;9:331-333.

33. Kang J, Ko Y, Park JH, et al. Effect of blood pressure on 3-month functional outcome in the subacute stage of ischemic stroke. *Neurology*. 2012;79:2018-2024.

34. Chung J-W, Kim N, Kang J, et al. Blood pressure variability and the development of early neurological deterioration following acute ischemic stroke. *J Hypertension*. 2015;33:2099–2021.

35. Anderson C, Heeley E, Huang Y, et al. Rapid blood pressure lowering in patients with acute intracerebral hemorrhage. *N Engl J Med*. 2013;368:2355-2365.

36. Qureshi AI, Palesch YY. Antihypertensive Treatment in Acute Cerebral Hemorrhage (ATTACH) II: design, methods, and rationale. *Neurocrit Care*. 2011;15:559-576.

37. Berkheimer OA, Fransen PS, Beumer D, et al. A randomized trial of inta-arterial treatment for acute ischemic stroke. *N Engl J Med*. 2015;372:11-20.

38. Goyal M, Demchuk AM, Menon BK, et al. Randomized assessment of rapid endovascular treatment of ischemic stroke. *N Engl J Med*. 2015;372:1019-1030.

39. Saver JL, Goyal M, Bonafe A, et al. Stent retriever thrombectomy after intravenous t-PA vs. t-PA alone in stroke. *N Engl J Med*. 2015;372:2285-2295.

40. Campbell BC, Mitchell PJ, Kleinig TJ, et al. Endovascular therapy for ischemic stroke with perfusion imaging selection. *N Engl J Med*. 2015;372:1009-1018.

41. Jovin TG, Chamorro A, Cobo E, et al. Thrombectomy within 8 hours after symptom onset in ischemic stroke. *N Engl J Med*. 2015;372:2296-2306.

42. Kernan WN, Ovbiagele B, Black HR, et al. Guidelines for the prevention of stroke in patients with stroke and transient ischemic attack. A guideline for healthcare professionals from the American Heart Association/American Stroke Association. *Stroke*. 2014;45:2160-2236.

43. Weimar C, Diener H-C, Alberts MJ, et al. The Essen Stroke Risk Score predicts recurrent cardiovascular events. A validation within the REduction of Atherothrombosis for Continued Health (REACH) registry. *Stroke*. 2009;40:350-354.

44. Towfighi A, Markovic D, Ovbiagele B. Consistency of blood pressure control after ischemic stroke. Prevalence and prognosis. *Stroke*. 2014;45:1313-1317.

45. Lovett JK, Coull AJ, Rothwell PM. Early risk of recurrence by subtype of ischemic stroke in population-based incidence studies. *Neurology*. 2004;62:569-573.

46. Biffi A, Anderson CD, Battey TWK, et al. Association between blood pressure control and risk of recurrent intracerebral hemorrhage. *JAMA*. 2015;314:904-912.

47. Kuramatsu JB, Berner ST, Schellinger PD, et al. Anticoagulant reversal, blood pressure levels, and anticoagulant resumption in patients with anticoagulation-related intracerebral hemorrhage. *JAMA*. 2015;313:824-826.

48. PROGRESS Collaborative Group. Randomized trial of perindopril-based blood-pressure-lowering regimen among 6,105 individuals with previous stroke or transient ischemic attack. *Lancet*. 2001;358:1033-1041.

49. The SPS3 Study Group. Blood-pressure targets in patients with recent lacunar stroke: the SPS3 randomized trial. *Lancet*. 2013;382:507-515.

50. Boan AD, Lackland DT, Ovbiagele B. Lowering of blood pressure for recurrent stroke prevention. *Stroke*. 2014;45:2506-2513.

51. Gorelick PB, Nyenhuis D. ASH Position Paper. Blood pressure and treatment of persons with hypertension as it relates to cognitive outcomes including executive function. *J Am Soc Hypertens*. 2012;6:309-315.

52. Gorelick PB, Scuteri A, Black SE, et al. Vascular contributions to cognitive impairment and dementia: a statement for healthcare professionals from the American Heart Association/American Stroke Association. *Stroke*. 2011;42:2672-2713.

53. Gorelick PB. Blood pressure and the prevention of cognitive impairment. *JAMA Neurol*. 2014;71:1211-1213.

54. Williamson JD, Launer LJ, Bryan RN, et al. Cognitive function and brain structure in persons with type 2 diabetes mellitus after intensive lowering of blood pressure and lipid levels: a randomized clinical trial. *JAMA Intern Med*. 2014;174:324-333.

55. Peters R, Beckett N, Forette F, et al. Incident dementia and blood pressure lowering in the Hypertension in the Very Elderly Trial cognitive function assessment (HYVET-COG): a double-blind, placebo controlled trial. *Lancet Neurol*. 2008;7:683-689.

56. Ngandu T, Lehitsalo J, Solomon A, et al. A 2 year multidomain intervention of diet, exercise, cognitive training, and vascular risk monitoring versus control to prevent cognitive decline in at-risk elderly people (FINGER): a randomized controlled trial. *Lancet*. 2015;385:2255-2263.

57. Chrysant SG. Current status of aggressive blood pressure control. *World J Cardiol*. 2011;3:65-71.

58. Ovbiagele B, Diener H-C, Yusuf S, et al. Level of systolic blood pressure within the normal range and risk of recurrent stroke. *JAMA*. 2011;306:2137-2144.

59. Yamauchi H, Kagawa S, Kishibe Y, et al. Misery perfusion, blood pressure control, and 5-year stroke risk in symptomatic major cerebral artery disease. *Stroke*. 2015;46:265-268.

60. Powers WJ, Clarke WR, Grubb RL Jr, et al. Lower stroke risk with lower blood pressure in hemodynamic cerebral ischemia. *Neurology*. 2014;82:1027-1032.

61. Turan TN, Cotsonis G, Lynn MJ, et al. Relationship between blood pressure and stroke recurrence in patients with intracranial arterial stenosis. *Circulation*. 2007;115:2969-2975.

37 Diabetes Mellitus

Radica Z. Alicic and Katherine R. Tuttle

Diabetes mellitus ("diabetes") and hypertension, which commonly coexist, are global public health issues contributing to an enormous burden of cardiovascular disease, chronic kidney disease, and premature mortality and disability. The presence of both conditions has an amplifying effect on risk for microvascular and macrovascular complications.[1] The prevalence of diabetes is rising worldwide (Fig. 37.1). Both diabetes and hypertension disproportionately affect people in middle and low-income countries, and an estimated 70% of all cases of diabetes are found in these countries.[2,3] In the United States alone, the total costs of care for diabetes and hypertension in the years 2012 and 2011 were 245 and 46 billion dollars, respectively.[4,5] Therefore, there is a great potential for meaningful health and economic gains attached to prevention, detection, and intervention for diabetes and hypertension.

EPIDEMIOLOGY OF DIABETES, HYPERTENSION, AND DIABETIC COMPLICATIONS

The overall picture of the worldwide diabetes epidemic is sobering. In 2014, the global prevalence of diabetes was estimated to be about 9% among adults aged 18 years and older.[3] In the U.S., diabetes is present in at least 29 million people or 9.3% of people in the population with 1.4 million Americans newly diagnosed every year. About 95% (27.5 million) of the existing and new cases are type 2 diabetes, whereas about 5% (1.5 million) of U.S. children and adults have type 1 diabetes.[6] The prevalence of diabetes rises sharply in the obese population, and globally, 44% of diabetes cases are attributable to conditions of overweight and obesity. To put the worldwide scope of this risk in perspective, more than 1.9 billion adults 18 years and older were overweight and 600 million were obese.[3] Diabetes is currently the seventh leading cause of death in the U.S. with World Health Organization projections that it will be seventh leading cause of death in the world by 2030.[3,6]

Diabetes and hypertension commonly occur together. In a representative U.S. population during the years 2009 to 2012, overall 71% of adults with diabetes had hypertension defined by either blood pressure 140/90 or higher mm Hg or use of prescription medication to lower blood pressure.[7,8] Notably, hypertension is commonly present at the time of diagnosis of type 2 diabetes.[9] When prevalence of hypertension in type 2 diabetes is stratified by albuminuria status, 40% to 83% of patients with microalbuminuria and 78% to 96% of patients with macroalbuminuria are hypertensive.[10,11] In type 1 diabetes, the prevalence of hypertension is about 30% in those without kidney disease.[12] However, once diabetic kidney disease with albuminuria develops, hypertension prevalence parallels that seen in type 2 diabetes. People with diabetes have a shorter life expectancy with a high burden of comorbidities compared with those without diabetes.[11,12] They especially are at risk for developing macrovascular (cardiovascular) and microvascular complications (kidney disease, retinopathy, and neuropathy) that are worsened by hypertension.

Among adults aged 18 years and older with a diagnosis of diabetes, compared with adults without diabetes, adjusted rates of all-cause death are 1.5 times higher.[12] After adjusting for population age differences, the rates of cardiovascular death, and hospitalization rates for myocardial infarction, and stroke remain higher by 1.8, 1.7, and 1.5 times, respectively, compared with those without diabetes.[12] Overall, 10% to 12% of cardiovascular deaths are attributed to diabetes.[12-15] These risks are greatly amplified among the nearly 50% of people with diabetes who develop diabetic kidney disease. Indeed, most of the excess all-cause and cardiovascular death risk in diabetes is attributable to the presence of diabetic kidney disease.[16]

Diabetic kidney disease is also the leading cause of chronic kidney disease leading to end-stage renal disease (ESRD) and currently accounts for 44% of new cases annually.[17] Hypertension accelerates the progression of diabetic kidney disease, and kidney dysfunction further elevates blood pressure. There is an almost linear relationship between an increase in mean arterial blood pressure and yearly decrease in estimated glomerular filtration rate (eGFR).[18] The prevalence of cardiovascular disease in patients with diabetic kidney disease increases with decreasing kidney function. The 10-year mortality rate from two large population–based cohort studies of those with eGFR 15 to 60 mL/min/1.73 m², exceeds 35% in men and 20% in women.[19] Recent data demonstrate that the increased risk of cardiovascular death starts at an eGFR of about 95 mL/min/1.73 m².[20,21] The National Kidney Foundation Task Force on Cardiovascular Disease in Chronic Renal Disease has recommended that people with chronic kidney disease should be considered the "highest risk group" for cardiovascular events.[22]

In the years 2005 to 2008, 28.5% (4.2 million) of adults with diabetes aged 40 years and older had diabetic retinopathy.[4] The coexistence of hypertensive and diabetic retinopathy further magnifies the risk of blindness.[23] Diabetic peripheral neuropathy affects about 70% of patients with diabetes and is the leading cause of amputation in the U.S.[4] Manifestations of autonomic diabetic neuropathy include orthostatic hypotension, decline in vasomotor tone, and lack of normal heart rate variation, resting tachycardia, and sudden death. One of the recognized risk factors for diabetic neuropathy is hypertension.[24,25] The presence of autonomic neuropathy can be used for risk stratification for cardiovascular and diabetic kidney disease independent of other cardiovascular risk factors.[26]

PATHOGENESIS OF DIABETES, HYPERTENSION, AND DIABETIC COMPLICATIONS

Type 2 diabetes is characterized by hyperglycemia, insulin resistance, and relative impairment in insulin secretion.[27,28] Moreover, hyperglycemia itself can impair pancreatic beta-cell function ("glucose toxicity") and reduce insulin secretion.[28] Genetic predisposition for type 2 diabetes results from complex polygenic factors affecting numerous metabolic processes including pancreatic development and beta-cell function, insulin secretion and sensitivity, progression of glucose intolerance, metabolic rate, variability in body mass index and central fat distribution.[28-31]

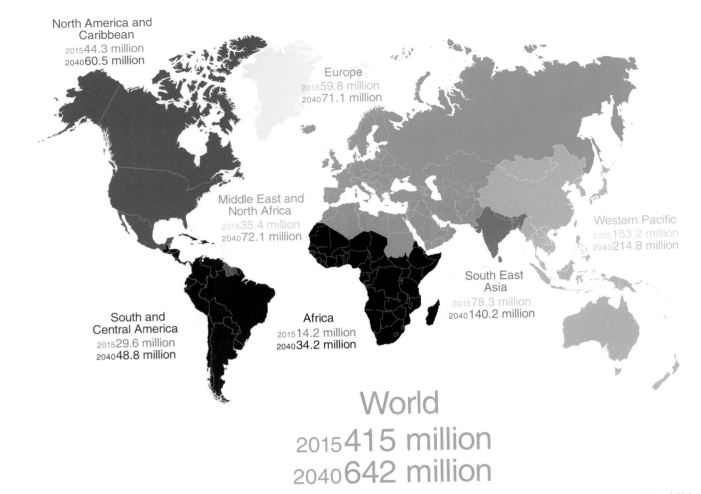

North America and
Caribbean
2015 44.3 million
2040 60.5 million

Europe
2015 59.8 million
2040 71.1 million

Middle East and
North Africa
2015 35.4 million
2040 72.1 million

Western Pacific
2015 153.2 million
2040 214.8 million

South and
Central America
2015 29.6 million
2040 48.8 million

Africa
2015 14.2 million
2040 34.2 million

South East
Asia
2015 78.3 million
2040 140.2 million

World
2015 415 million
2040 642 million

FIG. 37.1 Estimated number of people with diabetes worldwide and per region in 2015 and 2040 (20 to 79 years). *(Reused with permission from International Diabetes Federation. IDF Diabetes, 7 ed. Brussels, Belgium: International Diabetes Federation, 2015. http://www.diabetesatlas.org.)*

Obesity predisposes to insulin resistance, impaired insulin-stimulated glucose intake, and decreased sensitivity of pancreatic beta-cells to glucose.[32] Fat itself is a source of proinflammatory mediators as reflected in high circulating levels of C-reactive protein, interleukin-6, plasminogen activator inhibitor, tumor necrosis factor, and white blood cell count.[33-38] Other adipose-related factors (leptin) and increased plasma free fatty acids may promote pancreatic failure, atherosclerosis, and progressive kidney disease.[39] Moreover, deficiency of an adipocyte derived factor, adiponectin, has been inversely associated with insulin resistance and development of diabetic kidney disease.[40-41]

Diabetes, hypertension, cardiovascular, and diabetic kidney disease share common pathological mechanisms (e.g., activation of renin-angiotensin-aldosterone-system, reactive oxygen species, inflammation), which at the same time initiate and potentiate each other forming a vicious cycle of interconnected complications. Endothelial cells are essential for optimal vascular function and are at the center of diabetic complications. This cell type is especially vulnerable to injury. Endothelial dysfunction is a key initiator for atherosclerosis and thrombosis, a proximate pathway to acute events such as myocardial infarction and stroke.[42,43] Through production of both endothelium–derived relaxing factors and endothelium–derived constricting factors, the endothelium modulates function of the arterial wall. The most important endothelium produced relaxing factor is nitric oxide (NO).[42,43] A number of factors can lead to low NO production resulting in vasoconstriction including oxygen derived free radicals, angiotensin II,

lack of exercise, high salt intake, and testosterone. In addition to down-regulation of NO release, these factors may cause endothelial cell death by apoptosis. Apoptotic cells are often replaced by dysfunctional regenerated endothelial cells that are prone to inflammation and acceleration of atherosclerosis via vasoconstrictor prostanoids (endoperoxides, prostocyclines) and endothelin-1.[42,43]

In the presence of hypertension, NO production is further down-regulated by sheer stress, high salt intake, and activation of the renin-angiotensin system and aldosterone production with blunted responses to endothelium–dependent vasodilators.[42,44] Endothelin-1 contributes to high vascular tone of the glomerular afferent and efferent arterioles. Prolonged vasoconstriction of these arteries produces a decrease in renal blood flow and a reduction in glomerular filtration rate associated with enhanced filtration fraction and glomerular hypertension.[42,43,45] Endothelin-1 increases vascular reactive oxygen species (ROS) formation and is a proinflammatory and profibrotic mediator in various vascular beds.[42]

As a result of the chronic exposure to hyperglycemia, insulin resistance, and obesity, NO phosphorylation is reduced, leading to impairment of NO–mediated relaxation in arteries of diabetic and obese patients. At the same time, production of endothelium–derived vasoconstrictor prostanoids and endothelin-1 is increased in both diabetes and obesity. Both mediators instigate vasoconstriction of vascular smooth muscle cells, which magnifies endothelial dysfunction in arteries.[42,46-48] Adiponectin signaling which normally enhances NO generation and endothelium-dependent relaxations is

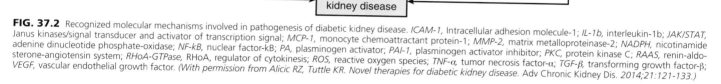

FIG. 37.2 Recognized molecular mechanisms involved in pathogenesis of diabetic kidney disease. *ICAM-1,* Intracellular adhesion molecule-1; *IL-1b,* interleukin-1b; *JAK/STAT,* Janus kinases/signal transducer and activator of transcription signal; *MCP-1,* monocyte chemoattractant protein-1; *MMP-2,* matrix metalloproteinase-2; *NADPH,* nicotinamide adenine dinucleotide phosphate-oxidase; *NF-kB,* nuclear factor-kB; *PA,* plasminogen activator; *PAI-1,* plasminogen activator inhibitor; *PKC,* protein kinase C; *RAAS,* renin-aldosterone-angiotensin system; *RHoA-GTPase,* RHoA, regulator of cytokinesis; *ROS,* reactive oxygen species; *TNF-α,* tumor necrosis factor-α; *TGF-β,* transforming growth factor-β; *VEGF,* vascular endothelial growth factor. *(With permission from Alicic RZ, Tuttle KR. Novel therapies for diabetic kidney disease.* Adv Chronic Kidney Dis. *2014;21:121-133.)*

impaired in obesity.[48] A high-fat diet per se can produce similar effects.[49]

Metabolic disturbances of diabetes initiate and sustain activation of inflammatory and injurious products and abnormal kidney hemodynamics, ultimately resulting in changes typical of diabetic kidney disease including mesangial expansion, tubulointerstitial inflammation, and kidney fibrosis[50-54] (Fig. 37.2). Early diabetes is characterized by glomerular hyperfiltration and hypertension, resulting in mechanical strain on the capillary walls. Afferent arteriolar resistance decreases along with relatively increased efferent arteriolar resistance, leading to increased glomerular capillary pressure and endothelial injury.[54] Once kidney disease develops, arterial vessels have greater prevalence and severity of atherosclerotic changes with a high degree of arterial calcifications and lower collagenous fiber content.[55-57] The frequency of advanced atherosclerotic lesions in carotid arteries increases progressively with lower eGFR.[56] Calcified lesions are commonly observed in coronary arteries of patients with diabetic kidney disease[56-58] (Fig. 37.3).

CLINICAL MANAGEMENT OF HYPERTENSION IN DIABETES

Effects of Blood Pressure Control on Diabetic Complications

The beneficial effects of blood pressure control on macrovascular and microvascular complications in diabetic patients are well recognized. The Hypertension Optimal Treatment (HOT) demonstrated improved outcomes, especially in preventing stroke, in patients assigned to lower blood pressure targets. Optimal outcomes in the HOT study were achieved in the group with a target diastolic blood pressure (DBP) of less than 80 mm Hg.[59] The United Kingdom Prospective Diabetes Study (UKPDS 38) compared a target blood pressure of less than 150/85 mm Hg and blood pressure less than 180/105 mm

Hg in newly diagnosed diabetic patients. The lower blood pressure goal demonstrated salutary effects on multiple outcomes: 24% reduced risk of predefined macrovascular and microvascular complications ($p < 0.0001$); 32% risk reduction in deaths ($p = 0.019$); 44% risk reduction in stroke ($p = 0.013$); 37% risk reduction of microvascular complications, predominantly development of albuminuria and retinopathy ($p = 0.009$).[60] In a follow-up UKPDS study, 5102 patients from the original cohort were evaluated for the relationship between systolic blood pressure over time and risk of death and macrovascular and microvascular diabetic complications.[61] The incidence of complications was significantly associated with systolic blood pressure: Each 10 mm Hg decrease in mean systolic blood pressure was associated with risk reduction of 12% ($p < 0.0001$) for any complication related to diabetes, 11% risk reduction for myocardial infarction ($p < 0.0001$), and 13% risk reduction of microvascular complications ($p < 0.0001$) with no observed threshold of risk for any end point (Fig. 37.4). Subsequent clinical trials including, The Appropriate Blood Pressure Control in Diabetes (ABCD-H, ABCD-N, ABCD-2V), Follow-up of Blood-Pressure Lowering and Glucose Control in Type 2 Diabetes (ADVANCE), Avoiding Cardiovascular Events through Combination Therapy in Patients Living with Systolic Hypertension (ACCOMPLISH) support blood pressure control to improve macrovascular and microvascular outcomes (Table 37.1).[59,62-74]

Post hoc analyses of three large clinical trials: Reduction of Endpoints in NIDDM (noninsulin-dependent diabetes mellitus) with the Angiotensin II Antagonist Losartan (RENAAL), Renoprotective Effect of the Angiotensin–Receptor Antagonist Irbesartan in Patients with Nephropathy due to Type 2 Diabetes (IDNT), and Veterans Affairs Nephropathy in Diabetes (VA NEPHRON-D) evaluated the relationship of blood pressure and kidney function.[75-77] An analysis of the RENAAL trial assessed the relationship between baseline blood pressure on individual and composite outcomes including doubling of serum creatinine, ESRD, or death. Systolic blood pressure was an

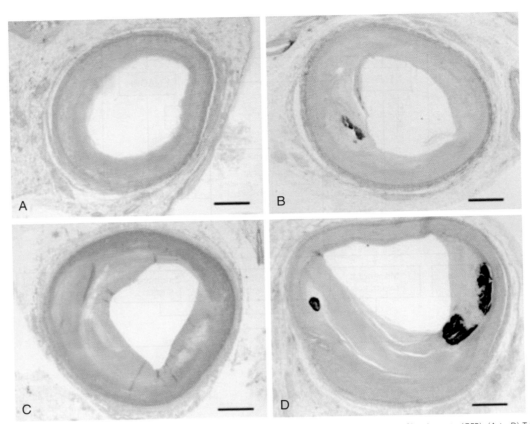

FIG. 37.3 Atherosclerosis in patients with chronic kidney disease. Typical arteries for each classification by glomerular filtration rate (GFR). (A to D) Typical light microscopic views of coronary arteries from respective cases with estimated GFR (A) 60 or over, (B) 45 to 59, (C) 30 to 44, and (D) less than 30 mL/min/1.73 m². Stenosis rates of respective arteries were (A) 36.8%, (B) 42.3%, (C) 54.2%, and (D) 58.9%. All sections were stained with hematoxylin and eosin. Scale bars = 1.0 mm. *(With permission from Nakano T, Ninomiya T, Sumiyoshi S, et al. Association of kidney function with coronary atherosclerosis and calcification in autopsy samples from Japanese elders: the Hisayama study. Am J Kidney Dis. 2010 55, 21-30.)*

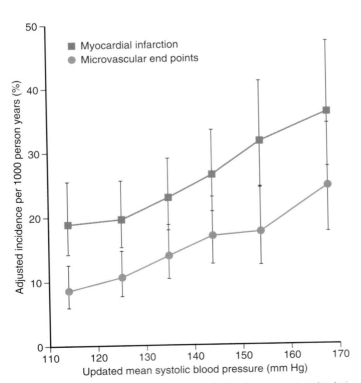

FIG. 37.4 Incidence of complications by systolic blood pressure categories. Incidence rates (95% confidence interval) of myocardial infarction, microvascular end-points by category of updated mean systolic blood pressure, adjusted for age, sex, and ethnic group expressed for white men aged 50 to 54 years at diagnosis and mean duration of diabetes of 10 years. *(From Stratton IM, Adler AI, Neil HAW, et al. Association of glycaemia with macrovascular and microvascular complications of type 2 diabetes (UKPDS 35): prospective observational study. BMJ. 2000:321: 405-412.)*

independent risk factor for ESRD and a baseline systolic blood pressure range of 140 to 159 mm Hg increased risk for ESRD or death by 38% (*p* = 0.05) compared with blood pressure less than 130 mm Hg. In multivariate analyses, every 10 mm Hg rise in baseline systolic blood pressure increased risk of ESRD or death by 6.7% (*p* = 0.007).[75] An analysis of IDNT data showed that baseline systolic blood pressure (SBP) less than 149 mm Hg was associated with 2.2-fold increase in risk for doubling serum creatinine or ESRD compared with SBP less than 134 mm Hg. Progressive lowering of SBP to 120 mm Hg was associated with improved kidney outcomes and survival, independent of baseline kidney function.[76] A VA-NEPHRON analysis evaluated association of mean on–treatment blood pressure with the decline in eGFR, ESRD, or death.[77] After multivariate adjustment, the hazard of developing the endpoint became increasingly greater with a rise of SBP from more than120 mm Hg to 150 or higher mm Hg. There was significantly higher hazard ratio for SBP 140 to 149 mm Hg versus 120 to 129 mm Hg (1.51; 95% confidence interval [CI] 1.06, 2.15; *p* = 0.02), with a monotonic relationship between systolic blood pressure and eGFR slope suggesting that lower SBP was associated with a better outcome. However, there was also a U-shaped relationship between mean DBP and eGFR with greater loss of GFR with DBP less than 60 mm Hg. The overall conclusion of this analysis was that in patients with diabetic kidney disease characterized by high-level albuminuria, mean SBP 140 or higher mm Hg and mean DBP 80 or higher mm Hg were associated with worse kidney outcomes (Fig. 37.5).

Several studies in different populations suggested that nighttime blood pressure is a strong predictor of cardiovascular events and that administration of an antihypertensive agent at bedtime resulted in lower relative risk of cardiovascular events. Another study showed that bedtime administration of antihypertensive agents resulted in significant reduction

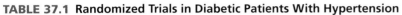
TABLE 37.1 Randomized Trials in Diabetic Patients With Hypertension

STUDY	PARTICIPANTS	FOLLOW-UP	INTERVENTION	ACHIEVED MEAN BP OR BETWEEN GROUP DIFFERENCE IN TRIAL	OUTCOMES: PRIMARY AND SECONDARY	RESULTS
HOT, 1997[59]	Subpopulation of 1501 with DM 2 and DBP 100-115 mm Hg Baseline BP 174.1/105.3 mm Hg	3.8 years (mean)	DBP ≤ 80 mm Hg vs. DBP ≤ 85 mm Hg vs. DBP ≤ 90 mm Hg	Between group difference 3.4/2.9	Major CV outcomes (fatal and nonfatal MI, all strokes, and all CV deaths)	↓CV mortality Relative risk 3.0 (CI 95%, 1.28-7.08)
UKPDS 38, 1998[60]	1148 with DM 2 and HTN (mean BP 160/94 mm Hg)	8.4 years (median)	BP < 150/85 mm Hg vs. BP < 180/105 mm Hg	144/82 mm Hg vs. 154/87 mm Hg	Fatal and nonfatal diabetes related endpoints, deaths related to diabetes and all-cause mortality, microvascular disease (albuminuria, retinopathy)	24% risk reduction in diabetes related endpoints 32% risk reduction in deaths 44% risk reduction in strokes Usual or low protein diet 37% risk reduction in microvascular endpoints (albuminuria, retinopathy)
ABCD-H, 1998[62] (hypertensive population)	470 patients with DM 2 and DBP > 90 mm Hg	5 years (mean)	Intensive (DBP 75 mm Hg) vs. moderate (DBP 80-89 mm Hg)	Intervention group DBP < 75 mm Hg Control group DBP < 90 mm Hg	Primary: change in CrCl Secondary: albumin excretion, LVH, retinopathy neuropathy	Significantly lower rate of MI in enalapril group over nisoldipine group in both intense and moderate BP control (p = 0.001)
RENAAL, 2001[63]	1513 with DM 2 and UAE >300 mg/24 hours Cr 1.3-3	3.4 years (mean)	Losartan vs. placebo	At the end of study BP 140/74 mm Hg vs. 142/74 mm Hg	Primary: composite of doubling of the baseline Cr, ESRD, or death. Secondary: composite of CV morbidity and mortality, proteinuria, progression of kidney disease	16% risk reduction of primary outcome, 28% ESRD reduction, 25% reduction of doubling of Cr, 35% proteinuria reduction in losartan group. CV mortality and morbidity similar in both groups, no difference among groups of death
IDNT, 2001[64]	1715 with DM 2 and HTN (BP > 135/85 mm Hg) Albuminuria > 900 mg/24 hours Cr 1.0-3.0 mg/dL Baseline BP 150/86.7 mm Hg	2.6 years (median)	Irbesartan vs. amlodipine vs. placebo	Target BP < 135/85 mm Hg	Primary: composite of doubling of Cr, ESRD, or death of any cause	Irbesartan group showed: ↓20% risk of primary composite endpoint ↓30% risk of doubling the creatinine 24% slower Cr concentration increase
IRMA-2, 2001[65]	590 with DM 2 and HTN (baseline BP 153/93 mm Hg) UAE 20-200 µ/min Cr < 1.5 mg/dL in men Cr < 1.1 mg/dL in women	2 years (median)	Irbesartan vs. placebo	143/83 mm Hg in 150 mg group, 141/83 mm Hg in 300 mg group, 144/83 in placebo group	Primary: developing nephropathy defined as UAE ≥ 200 µ, or UAE 30% higher than baseline. Secondary outcome: level of albuminuria, changes in CrCl, restoration of UAE < 20 µ/min	↓UEA by 24% in 150 mg/d group, ↓UEA 38% in 300 mg/d group. Nonsignificant change in creatinine decline. Nonsignificant change in nonfatal CV outcomes
BENEDICT, 2004[66]	1204 with DM 2 BP >130/85 mm Hg (baseline BP 150/86.7 mm Hg) UAE, 20 µ/min Cr, 1.5 mg/dL	3.6 years (median)	Trandolapril vs. verapamil vs. trandolapril + verapamil vs. placebo	39 ± 10/80 ± 6 mm Hg in combination group 139 ± 12/81 ± 6 mm Hg in trandolapril 141 ± 10/82 ± 6 mm Hg verapamil 142 ± 12/83 ± 6 mm Hg in placebo	Primary: onset of microalbuminuria Secondary: magnitude of treatment effect	Trandolapril + verapamil delayed albuminuria by factor 2.6. Trandalopril only delayed albuminuria by factor 2.1.

Continued

TABLE 37.1 Randomized Trials in Diabetic Patients With Hypertension—cont'd

STUDY	PARTICIPANTS	FOLLOW-UP	INTERVENTION	ACHIEVED MEAN BP OR BETWEEN GROUP DIFFERENCE IN TRIAL	OUTCOMES: PRIMARY AND SECONDARY	RESULTS
ABCD-N, 2002[67] (normotensive)	480 participants with DM 2 and BP < 140/90 mm Hg	5.3 years (mean)	Intensive (DBP < 10 mm Hg below baseline DBP) vs. moderate BP control (DBP 80-89 mm Hg)	BP128 ± 0.8/75 ± 0.3 mm Hg (intensive) vs. BP137 ± 0.7/81 ± 0.3 mm Hg (moderate)	Primary: Change in CrCl. Secondary: change in albumin excretion progression of retinopathy, neuropathy, incidence of CV disease	No difference in CrCl. Lower progression of albuminuria. Less progression of retinopathy, lower incidence of strokes in intensive group
ABCD-2V, 2006[68]	129 with DM2, BP < 140/90 mm Hg (baseline BP 126/84.7 mm Hg) UAE < 30 to 300 mg/24 hours	1.9 ± 1 year	Intensive (DBP of 75 mm Hg) vs. moderate BP control (DBP 80-90 mm Hg)	118 ± 10.9/75 ± 5.7 mm Hg vs. 124 ± 10.9/80 ± 6.5 mm Hg (p < 0.01)	Primary: change in UAE (prim). Secondary: changes in retinopathy, neuropathy, CV events	Significant reduction of UAE, no effect on progression of retinopathy, neuropathy, or incidence of CV events
ADVANCE, 2007[69]	11140 with DM2 + history of major CV disease or at least one factor for CV disease Baseline BP 145/81 mm Hg	4.3 years (mean)	Effect of routine administration of ACE inhibitor-diuretic combination on vascular events	−5.6 mm Hg SBP; −2.2 mm Hg DBP reduction in intervention group	Primary: major macrovascular and microvascular events	9% risk reduction in macrovascular and microvascular events 18% reduction of relative risk of CV death. 14% reduction of risk of death from any cause.
ACCOMPLISH, 2008[70]	11,464 (6924 with DM2) HTN	35.7 and 35.6 months (3 years)	Benazepril/amlodipine vs. benazepril/HCTZ	131.6/73.3 mm Hg (benazepril/amlodipine) 132.5/74.4 mm Hg (benazepril/HCTZ)	Primary: composite of CV death, nonfatal MI, nonfatal stroke, hospitalization for angina, coronary revascularization, resuscitation after sudden death	Absolute risk reduction of 2.2%. Relative risk reduction of 19.6% of primary outcomes in BA group
ACCORD BP, 2010[71]	4733 with DM2 34% with previous CV disease	4.7 years (mean)	SBP < 120 mm Hg (intensive) vs. SBP < 140 mm Hg (standard)		Primary: composite of nonfatal MI, nonfatal stroke of CV death	No significant difference between groups. Significant increase of SAE (eGFR, elevations of Cr, GFR < 30) in intensive group
ROADMAP, 2011[72]	4447 with DM 2 Baseline BP 136.5/80.5 mm Hg) 33% with previous CV disease	3.2 years (median)	Olmesartan vs. placebo	Mean in − treatment 3.1/1.9 mm Hg	Primary: time to onset of microalbuminuria. Secondary: composite of CV complications and CV death	Olmesartan group: Delayed onset of microalbuminuria (23% ↑time to onset) Increased fatal CV events
ALTITUDE, 2012[73]	8561 with DM 2 UACR > 20-200 mg/g eGFR > 30 ml/min, 60 mL/min 42% with previous CV disease Baseline BP 137.3/47.2 mm Hg	32.9 months 2.7 years (median)	Aliskiren 300 mg vs. placebo	Mean in treatment difference in BP 1.3/0.6 mm Hg	Primary: composite of CV death or the first occurrence of cardiac arrest, nonfatal MI, nonfatal stroke, unplanned hospitalization for CHF, ESRD, death as a result of kidney failure, doubled Cr	Primary endpoints more frequent in aliskiren group. Trial stopped for safety concerns
VA NEPHRON, 2013[74]	1448 with DM 2 UACR ≥300 mg/g eGFR 30.0-89.9 23% with CV disease Baseline BP 137/72.7 mm Hg	2.2 years (median)	Losartan vs. losartan + lisinopril	Mean in treatment difference 1.5/1 mm Hg	Primary: First occurrence of change in eGFR, ESRD or death	Combination therapy: offers no benefit with respect to mortality of CV events. Increased risk of hyperkalemia and AKI (p = 0.001) Trial stopped for safety concerns

ACE, Angiotensin-converting enzyme; *BP*, blood pressure; *CHF*, congestive heart failure; *CI*, confidence interval; *Cr*, serum creatinine in mg/dL; *CrCl*, creatinine clearance; *CV*, cardiovascular; *DBP*, diastolic blood pressure; *DM 2*, diabetes mellitus 2; *eGFR*, estimated glomerular filtration rate in mL/min/1.73m²; *ESRD*, end-stage–renal disease; *HCTZ*, hydrochlorothiazide; *HTN*, hypertension; *LVH*, left ventricular hypertrophy; *MI*, myocardial infarction; *SBP*, systolic blood pressure; *SEA*, serious adverse events; *UACR*, urine albumin-to-creatinine ratio in mg/g; *UAE*, urine albumin excretion in mg/24 hours or μg/min.

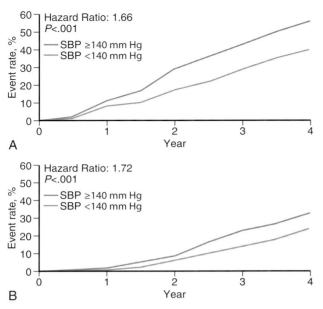

FIG. 37.5 Effects of blood pressure on progression of diabetic nephropathy. A, Event rate for the primary composite endpoint by baseline systolic blood pressure (SBP). B, Event rate for end-stage renal disease alone by baseline SBP. *(With permission from Bakris GL, Matthew RW, Shahnaz Shanifar MD. Effects of blood pressure level on progression of diabetic nephropathy: results from the RENAAL study. Arc Intern Med. 2003;163:1555-1565.)*

of the nighttime blood pressure and 24-hour blood pressure without change in daytime blood pressure.[78-80] The American Diabetes Association Standard of Medical Care in Diabetes 2016 recommend administering at least one antihypertensive agent at bedtime.[81]

What Is the Target Blood Pressure in Diabetic Patients?

The portion of the ACCORD trial testing an intensified blood pressure goal did not show reduced overall risk of major cardiovascular events or death. In this study of 4733 patients with established type 2 diabetes, intensive blood pressure lowering to a target less than 120/70 mm Hg failed to demonstrate benefits for fatal or nonfatal major cardiovascular events as compared with a target of less than 140/90 mm Hg. The only significant benefit in the group assigned to lower blood pressure was a reduction in incidence of stroke. Although the risk ratio was 0.58 (95% CI 0.39 to 0.88, $p = 0.009$), the absolute risk reduction was only 1.1%. Moreover, the lower blood pressure target was associated with a significant increase in the number of serious adverse events such as hypotension, syncope, and hypokalemia. The mean eGFR became significantly lower in the intensive-therapy group than in the standard-therapy group with significantly more instances of an eGFR less than 30 mL/min/1.73 m^2 compared with the standard-therapy group (99 versus 52 events, $p < 0.001$). Therefore, the results of this study raised major questions about recommendations of lower blood pressure targets, such as less than 120/70 mm Hg, for patients with diabetes.[82] A subsequent meta-analysis of studies designed to compare clinical outcomes in people with diabetes randomized to "lower" or to "standard" diastolic blood pressure targets (ABCD-H, ABCD-N, ABCD-2V, and subgroup of HOT trial) showed nonsignificant differences in stroke (relative risk [RR] 0.67, 95% CI 0.42 to 1.05), myocardial infarction (RR 0.95, 95% CI 0.64 to 1.40), or congestive heart failure (RR 1.06, 95% CI 0.58 to 1.92) with lower blood pressure targets. Achieved blood pressure was 128/76 mm Hg versus 135/83 mm Hg ($p < 0.0001$). Unfortunately, risk of ESRD and serious adverse events were not reported.[83] A

recent meta-analysis of 49 randomized clinical trials including 73,738 participants, most with type 2 diabetes, confirmed that antihypertensive treatment reduces risk of mortality and cardiovascular events in patients with a pretreatment blood pressure greater than 140/90 mm Hg treated to less than this level.[84] In sum, the overall evidence from randomized clinical trials to date has not supported intensified blood pressure targets of less than 140/90 mm Hg for prevention of cardiovascular complications in patients with diabetes.

The Eighth Joint National Committee (JNC-8) recently published their recommendations for blood pressure targets in patients with diabetes.[85] They recommend initiation of pharmacologic treatment at a systolic blood pressure 140 or higher mm Hg or diastolic blood pressure 90 or higher mm Hg with treatment goals less than these levels. In the general hypertensive population, including those with diabetes, initial antihypertensive treatment should include a thiazide-type diuretic, calcium channel blocker (CCB), angiotensin-converting enzyme (ACE) inhibitor, or angiotensin receptor blocker (ARB). In African-American patients with diabetes, JNC-8 recommends initial treatment with a thiazide diuretic or CCB. The same blood pressure targets are recommended for those with chronic kidney disease irrespective of diabetes status. In diabetic patients with increased levels of albuminuria or proteinuria, the medication regimen should include an ACE inhibitor or an ARB alone or in combination with medication from other drug classes (Table 37.2).

Published goals for antihypertensive treatment have been challenged by results of the Systolic Blood Pressure Intervention Trial (SPRINT) that randomized 9361 participants with hypertension and high cardiovascular risk (previous cardiovascular disease, chronic kidney disease, Framingham risk score > 15%, or age > 75 years) to either an intensive (<120 mm Hg) or standard (<140 mm Hg) SBP goal. Notably, people with diabetes were not included in SPRINT. After a mean of 3.26 years, the primary composite outcome (myocardial infarction, other acute coronary syndromes, stroke, heart failure, or death from cardiovascular causes) was reduced by 25% in the intensively treated group. All-cause mortality was similarly reduced by 27% with intensive blood pressure control. These results held across prespecified subgroups (chronic kidney disease, age over 75 years, sex, race, previous cardiovascular disease, and baseline level of SBP). However, the intensively treated group also had more frequent hypotension, syncope, acute kidney injury, hyponatremia, and hypokalemia.[91] In an accompanying editorial, a meta-analysis of SPRINT and ACCORD showed that the lower SBP goal associated with reduced risks of nonfatal myocardial infarction, stroke, heart failure, and the primary outcomes as defined in each trial. This led the editorialists to suggest that ACCORD may have been under powered to detect a cardiovascular benefit of lower SBP and that the overall results may apply to people with type 2 diabetes, too. Although compelling, this notion must be considered hypothesis-generating.[92] Until March 2016, various clinical practice guideline forming bodies have yet not altered their recommendations for hypertensive patients with or without diabetes. However, it can be reasonably expected that these groups will reevaluate their advice with an eye to shifting toward lower blood pressure goals since the release of the SPRINT trial results.

Treatment of Hyperglycemia, Blood Pressure, and Cardiovascular Outcomes

The blood pressure lowering effect of a new class of oral agents for hyperglycemia, the sodium–dependent glucose cotransporters 2 (SGLT2) inhibitors, is of great interest for reducing risks of diabetic complications. The blood pressure-lowering effect of SGLT2 inhibition appears to be a class effect and has been reported for empagliflozin,

TABLE 37.2 Current Recommendations for Hypertension Management

GUIDELINE	POPULATION	GOAL BP, MM Hg	INITIAL DRUG TREATMENT OPTIONS
2014 Hypertension guideline[85]	General ≥ 60 years	<150/90	Nonblack; thiazide-type diuretic, ACEi, ARB or CCB; black; thiazide-type diuretic or CCB
	General < 60 years	<140/90	
	Diabetes	<140-90	Thiazide-type diuretic, ACEi, ARB, or CCB
	CKD	<140/90	ACEi or ARB
ESH/ESC2013[86]	General nonelderly	<140/90	
	General elderly < 80 years	<150/90	Diuretic, β-Blocker, CCB, ACEi, or ARB
	General ≥ 80 years	<150/90	
	Diabetes	<140/90	ACEi or ARB
	CKD no proteinuria	<140/90	ACEi or ARB
	CKD + proteinuria	<130/90	
CHEP 2013[87]	General < 80 years	<140/90	Thiazide, β-Blocker (age < 60 years) ACEi (non-AA), or ARB
	General ≥ 80 years	<150/90	
	Diabetes	<130/80	ACEi or ARB with additional CVD risk ACEi, ARB, thiazide, or DHPCCB without additional CVD risk
	CKD	<140/90	ACEi or ARB
ADA 2016[81]	Diabetes	<140/80	ACEi or ARB
KDIGO 2012[88]	CKD no proteinuria	≤ 140/90	ACEi or ARB
	CKD + proteinuria	≤ 130/80	
NICE 2011[89]	General < 80 years	<140/90	<55 years: ACEi or ARB
	General ≥ 80 years	<150/90	≥55 years or AA: CCB
ISHIB 2010[90]	AA, lower risk	<135/85	Diuretic or CCB
	Target organ damage or CVD risk	<130/80	

ADA, American Diabetes Association; *CHEP,* Canadian Hypertension Education Program; *ESH/ESC,* European Society of Hypertension/European Society of Cardiology; *ISHIB,* International Society on Hypertension in Blacks; *KDiGO,* Kidney Disease: Improving Global Outcomes; *NICE,* National Institute for Health and Care Excellence.
AA, African Americans; *ACEi,* angiotensin converting enzyme inhibitor; *ARB,* angiotensin receptor blocker; *BP,* blood pressure; *β-blocker,* beta-blocker; *CCB,* calcium channel blocker; *CKD,* chronic kidney disease; *CVD,* cardiovascular disease; *DHPCCB,* dihydropyridine-type calcium channel blocker.

dapagliflozin, and canagliflozin.[93-97] The effects of dapagliflozin on blood pressure in hypertensive diabetic patients on renin–angiotensin system blockade was studied in a placebo-controlled clinical trial enrolling patients with HbA1c 7% or higher and 10.5% or lower and SBP 140 or higher mm Hg and diastolic blood pressure 85 or higher mm Hg and 105 or lower mm Hg. In addition to significant reductions in HbA1c (–0.6% vs. –0.1%, $p < 0.0001$), dapagliflozin showed significant reduction in mean seated blood pressure (–10.4 vs. –7.3 mm Hg, $p = 0.001$) and mean 24-hour ambulatory systolic blood pressure (–9.6 vs. –6.7 mm Hg, $p = 0.004$) after 12 weeks of treatment.[98] There are several proposed mechanisms for this blood pressure-lowering effect: reduction in proximal tubular sodium reabsorption and diuresis, weight loss, improved glycemic control and insulin sensitivity, decreased oxidative stress and inflammation, and improved endothelial function and vascular compliance.[99,100] Notably, the Empagliflozin, Cardiovascular Outcomes, and Mortality in Type 2 Diabetes (EMPA-REG) clinical trial recently demonstrated that empagliflozin significantly lowered rates of death from cardiovascular causes (3.7% versus 5.9%; 38% relative risk reduction), hospitalization for heart failure (2.7% versus 4.1%; 35% relative risk reduction), and death from any cause (5.7% versus 8.3%; 32% relative risk reduction) in patients with type 2 diabetes and cardiovascular disease already receiving standard-of-care for control of blood pressure and lipids.[101]

Importantly, previous large clinical trials targeting intensified glycemic control with insulin and/or various oral agents (hemoglobin A1C levels to <6 to 6.5% versus <7%) showed no to nominal effect to reduce cardiovascular risk in established 2 diabetes.[102,103] Moreover, initial findings of greater risks of cardiovascular and all-cause mortality in the intensive glucose control group in the ACCORD trial have been sustained over long term (approximately 8 years) cautioning against overly intensive glycemic control in older adults with established type 2 diabetes.[104,105]

Nonpharmacological Interventions for Diabetes and Hypertension

Delivering education and support for lifestyle modifications are effective approaches to prevention and treatment of diabetes and hypertension, as well as development and progression of diabetic complications. Studies examining influence of healthy lifestyle (physical activity, weight loss) and diet interventions in individuals with impaired glucose tolerance showed that these interventions slow down progression of impaired glucose tolerance to diabetes. Similarly, lifestyle modifications are effective strategies in prevention and control of hypertension (Table 37.3).[106-114] In a meta-analysis of 24 clinical trials with 23,858 participants, the overall pooled net effect of dietary interventions on SBP was –3.07 mm Hg (95% CI –3.85 to –2.3), and –1.81 mm Hg (95% CI, –2.24 to –1.38). The Dietary Approaches to Stop Hypertension (DASH) diet, rich in fruits, vegetables, and low-fat dairy foods had the largest net effect on SBP; 7.62 mm Hg, (95% CI, –9.95 to –5.29), and DSP –4.22 mm Hg (95% CI –5.87 to –2.57 (Fig. 37.6).[115] A posthoc analysis of The Heart Institute of Spokane-Diet Intervention and Evaluation study (THIS-DIET) showed that higher intakes of methionine and alanine, amino acids enriched in animal meat proteins, were associated with higher systolic and diastolic blood pressure. On the other hand, threonine and histidine, amino acids enriched in plant proteins were associated with lower SBP and DBP.[116]

Almost 7000 participants of the Ongoing Telmisartan Alone and Combination with Ramipril Global Endpoint Trial (ONTARGET) with type 2 diabetes and without macroalbuminuria were followed in an observational prospective study evaluating associations of diet and modifiable lifestyle and social factors on the incidence and progression of diabetic kidney disease (new micro or macroalbuminuria, eGFR decline of more than 5% per year, or progression to ESRD).[117-119] Diet was assessed using the modified Alternate Healthy Eating Index (mAHEI). Compared with participants in the least healthy

TABLE 37.3 Trials on Effect of Nonpharmacological Interventions on Incidence of Diabetes and Incidence and Control of Hypertension

STUDY	PARTICIPANTS	FOLLOW-UP	INTERVENTION	OUTCOME	RESULTS
DA Quing, 2002[106]	577 with IGT	6 years	Diet vs. exercise vs. diet + exercise	Incidence of diabetes	RR of diabetes 0.64 in diet group RR of 0.62 of diabetes in exercise group RR of 0.42 in diet + exercise group
Finnish Diabetes Prevention, 2001[107]	522 with IGT	3.2 years	Individual cancelling on WT loss, diet, physical activity	Incidence of diabetes	↓risk of diabetes by 58% (p < 0.01)
IDDP, 2006[108]	3234 with IGT	2.8 years	Metformin vs. LSM	Incidence of diabetes	↓31 % incidence of diabetes in metformin group ↓58% incidence of diabetes in LSM group
TOHP-I, 1992[109]	2182 with DBP 80-89 mm Hg, not on antihypertensive medications	1.5 years	WT loss, sodium reduction, stress management, supplements (Ca, Mg, K, fish oil)	Short term feasibility and efficacy of 7 interventions on BP	WT loss of 3.9 kg resulted in 2.3/2.9 mm Hg BP reduction −4.99% long-term absolute RR CV events −1.04% absolute RR all cause death
TOHP-II, 1997[110]	2182 with DBP 80-89 mm Hg, not on antihypertensive medications	3-4 years	WT loss vs. sodium reduction vs. WT loss + sodium reduction	Decreasing DBP, SBP, and the incidence of HTN	↓BP 3.7/2.7 mm Hg with WT loss ↓BP 2./1.6 mm Hg in sodium reduction ↓4/2.8 mm Hg in combination group
DASH, 2001[111]	412 with BP < 159/95	30 days	DASH or control diet with Na intake of 150 mmol/day vs. 100 mmol/day vs. 50 mmol/day	Effect on systolic blood pressure	DASH diet with 50 mmol/day Na intake ↓SBP by 11.5 mm Hg in participants with HTN DASH diet ↓BP at all levels of Na intake ↓BP in both diets with lower sodium intake (<100 mmol/day)
PREMIER, 2003[112]	810 with baseline BP 120-159/80-95 No antihypertensive medications	1.5 years	Behavioral intervention vs. DASH with behavioral intervention vs. advice only	BP measurement and HTN status at 6 months	↓BP by 3.7 mm Hg in behavioral intervention ↓BP by 4.3 mm Hg in DASH + behavioral intervention (at 6 months, after subtracting change in advice only group)
Hu et al, 2004[113]	17,441 men and women with no history of HTN, coronary heart disease or heart failure	11 years	Light, moderate, heavy grade physical activity	Risk of HTN	↓prevalence of HTN (in both sexes p trend < 0.001) with light activity HR 1.00 in men and women with moderate activity HR 0.63 for men, 0.82 for women with heavy activity HR 0.59 in men, 0.71 in women
Toled et al, 2013[114]	7,447 Baseline BP 148/83 At high risk of CV disease	4 years	Control group vs. Mediterranean diet with extra virgin oil vs. Mediterranean diet with extra nuts	BP effect of different diets	No difference in SBP between groups ↓DBP 1.53 mm Hg in Mediterranean diet with extra virgin oil group ↓DB 0.65 mm Hg Mediterranean diet with extra nuts group

BP, Blood pressure; *Ca,* calcium; *CV,* cardiovascular; *DASH,* dietary approaches to stop hypertension; *DBP,* diastolic blood pressure; *HR,* multivariate-adjusted hazard ratios; *HTN,* hypertension; *IGT,* impaired glucose tolerance; *K,* potassium; *LSM,* lifestyle modifications; *Mg,* magnesium; *RR,* risk reduction; *SBP,* systolic blood pressure; *WT,* weight.

tertile of mAHEI score, participants in the healthiest tertile had a lower risk of chronic kidney disease (adjusted odds ratio [OR] 0.74; 95% CI, 0.64 to 0.84), and lower risk of mortality (OR 0.61; 95% CI, 0.48 to 0.78).[118] The social network score, education, moderate alcohol intake, and regular physical activity significantly decreased risk of chronic kidney disease. The size of social network was a strong independent risk factor of chronic kidney disease and death, reducing the risk by 11% and 22% when comparing the third and first tertile of the social network score (OR of chronic kidney disease 0.89 and death 0.78). Healthy lifestyle and diet, especially increased vegetable intake, were associated with reduced risks of chronic kidney disease and mortality. Improvements in lifestyle through prevention programs can have noticeable positive impacts on reducing these risks at a population level.[117,119]

Effect of Multiple Risk Factor Intervention in Diabetes

In the Steno-2 study of multifactorial intervention in type 2 diabetes, participants had step-wise introductions of lifestyle and pharmacological interventions aimed at keeping glycated hemoglobin less than 6.5%, blood pressure less than 130/80 mm Hg, total cholesterol less than 175 mg/dL, and triglycerides less than 150 mg/dL. The lifestyle component of the intensive intervention included reduction in intake of dietary fat, regular exercise, and smoking cessation. After 7.8 years of follow-up, the differences in the group of patients receiving intensive therapy was impressive. Only 24% of participants in the intensive group had a cardiovascular event compared with 44% of participants in the conventional group, a relative risk reduction of nearly 50%. The relative risk of nephropathy, retinopathy, and autonomic neuropathy (secondary endpoints) was diminished by about 60% in the intensive group compared with the conventional treatment group.[120] Subsequently, the same participants, patients with type 2 diabetes and microalbuminuria, were followed for an additional 5.5 years (total of 13.3 years) to evaluate long-term effects of the multifactorial intervention. The importance of implementation of comprehensive, multifaceted treatment interventions is demonstrated by absolute risk reductions for death among patients who received intensive therapy: 20% for all-cause death and 13% for cardiovascular death. During the follow-up period, the rate of death among patients in the

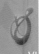
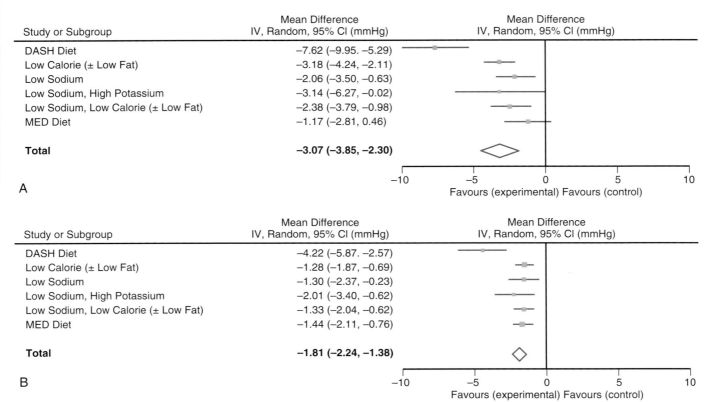

Study or Subgroup	Mean Difference IV, Random, 95% CI (mmHg)	Mean Difference IV, Random, 95% CI (mmHg)
DASH Diet	−7.62 (−9.95. −5.29)	
Low Calorie (± Low Fat)	−3.18 (−4.24, −2.11)	
Low Sodium	−2.06 (−3.50, −0.63)	
Low Sodium, High Potassium	−3.14 (−6.27, −0.02)	
Low Sodium, Low Calorie (± Low Fat)	−2.38 (−3.79, −0.98)	
MED Diet	−1.17 (−2.81, 0.46)	
Total	**−3.07 (−3.85, −2.30)**	

A   −10   −5   0   5   10   Favours (experimental) Favours (control)

Study or Subgroup	Mean Difference IV, Random, 95% CI (mmHg)	Mean Difference IV, Random, 95% CI (mmHg)
DASH Diet	−4.22 (−5.87. −2.57)	
Low Calorie (± Low Fat)	−1.28 (−1.87, −0.69)	
Low Sodium	−1.30 (−2.37, −0.23)	
Low Sodium, High Potassium	−2.01 (−3.40, −0.62)	
Low Sodium, Low Calorie (± Low Fat)	−1.33 (−2.04, −0.62)	
MED Diet	−1.44 (−2.11, −0.76)	
Total	**−1.81 (−2.24, −1.38)**	

B   −10   −5   0   5   10   Favours (experimental) Favours (control)

FIG. 37.6 Average net effect of diet on blood pressure. Average net effect for (A) systolic blood pressure and (B) diastolic blood pressure, and corresponding 95% confidence intervals summarized by diet. Average net blood pressure effect is calculated as the net incrementing change in the diet group versus control group. *(From Gay HC, Rao SG, Vaccarino V, Ali MK. Effects of different dietary interventions on blood pressure systematic review and meta-analysis of randomized controlled trials. Hypertension. 2016;67:733-739.)*

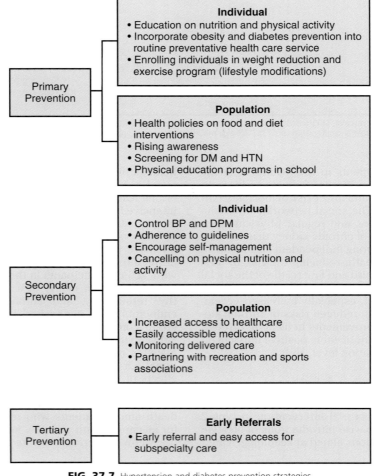

FIG. 37.7 Hypertension and diabetes prevention strategies.

conventional therapy group was 50%. One patient in the multi-factorial intervention group progressed to ESRD, as compared with six patients in the conventional-therapy group.[121]

CONCLUSION

Prevention and control of hypertension and diabetes is complex and demands multistakeholder collaboration (Fig. 37.7). In view of the enormous public health impact of diabetes and hypertension, now is the time for concerted action by engaged groups from government, professional organizations, healthcare delivery systems, pharma, the food and beverage industry, and patients. The magnitude of the problem warrants interventions on both the individual and population levels. A holistic approach to reduce the burden of diabetes and hypertension should include promotion of healthy lifestyles, identification of at-risk populations, education, programs for self-management, and implementation of evidence-based care.

References

1. American Diabetes Association. Role of cardiovascular risk factors in prevention and treatment of macrovascular disease in diabetes. *Diabetes Care*. 1989;12:573-579.
2. Long AN, Dagogo-Jack S. Comorbidities of diabetes and hypertension: mechanisms and approach to target organ protection. *J Clin Hypertens (Greenwich)*. 2011;13:244-251.
3. Global Status Report on Noncommunicable Disease. Geneva: *World Health Organization*; 2014; ISBN: 978 92 4 156485 4.
4. Centers for Disease Control and Prevention. National Diabetes Statistics Report: estimates of diabetes and its burden in the United States. Atlanta, GA: *US Department of Health and Human Services*, 2014.
5. Mozzafarian D, Benjamin EJ, Go AS, et al. Heart Disease and Stroke Statistics-2015 Update: a report from the American Heart Association. *Circulation*. 2015;131:e29-e322.
6. American Diabetes Association. *National Diabetes Statistics Report, 2014*. (released June 10, 2014) www.diabetes.org/diabetes-basics/statistics.
7. Centers for Disease Control and Prevention. National Diabetes Fact Sheet: National estimates and general information on diabetes and prediabetes in the United States. Atlanta, GA: *U.S. Department of Health and Human Services, Centers for Disease Control and Prevention*; 2011.
8. Arauz-Pacheco C, Parrott MA, Raskin P. The treatment of hypertension in adult patients with diabetes. *Diabetes Care*. 2002;25:134-147.
9. Sowers JS, Murray E, Frohlich ED. Diabetes, hypertension, and cardiovascular disease: an update. *Hypertens*. 2001;37:1053-1059.
10. National Kidney Foundation. KDOQI Clinical Practice Guidelines and Clinical Practice Recommendations for Diabetes and Chronic Kidney Disease. *Am J Kidney Dis*. 2007;49(2 Suppl 2):S1-S180.
11. American Diabetes Association. Standards of medical care in diabetes. *Diabetes Care*. 2015;38:S1-S93.
12. Task Force on diabetes, prediabetes, and cardiovascular diseases of the European Society of Cardiology (ESC); European Association for the Study of Diabetes (EASD), Rydén L, et al. ESC guidelines on diabetes, prediabetes, and cardiovascular diseases developed in collaboration with the EASD: summary. *Diab Vasc Dis Res*. 2014;11:133-173.
13. Mathers CD, Loncar D. Projections of global mortality and burden of disease from 2002 to 2003. *PLoS Med*. 2006;3:e442.
14. Centers for Disease Control and Prevention. National diabetes fact sheet: national estimates and general information on diabetes and prediabetes in the United States. Atlanta, GA: *U.S. Department of Health and Human Services, Centers for Disease Control and Prevention*; 2011.
15. Emerging Risk Factors Collaboration, Sarwar N, Gao P, et al. Diabetes mellitus, fasting blood glucose concentration, and risk of vascular disease: a collaborative meta-analysis of 102 prospective studies. *Lancet*. 2010;375:2215-2222.
16. Afkarian M, Sachs M, Kestenbaum B, et al. Kidney disease and increased mortality risk in type 2 diabetes. *J Am Soc Nephrol*. 2013;24:302-308.
17. United States Renal Data System. 2015 USRDS annual data report: Epidemiology of kidney disease in the United States. Bethesda, MD: *National Institutes of Health, National Institute of Diabetes and Digestive and Kidney Diseases*, 2015.
18. Muntner P, He J. Traditional and nontraditional risk factors predict coronary heart disease in chronic kidney disease: results from the Atherosclerosis Risk in Communities Study. *J Am Nephrol*. 2005;16:529-538.
19. Keith DS, Nichols GA. Longitudinal follow-up and outcomes among a population with chronic kidney disease in a large managed care organization. *Arch Intern Med*. 2004;164:659-663.
20. Soveri I, Arnlov J. Kidney function and discrimination of cardiovascular risk in middle-aged men. *J Intern Med*. 2009;266:406-413.
21. Foley RN, Wang C. Kidney function and risk triage in adults: threshold values and hierarchical importance. *Kidney Int*. 2011;79:99-111.
22. Sarnak MJ, Levey AS. Kidney disease as a risk factor for development of cardiovascular disease. A Statement from the American Heart Association Councils on Kidney in Cardiovascular Disease, High Blood Pressure Research, Clinical Cardiology, and Epidemiology and Prevention. *Circulation*. 2003;108:2154-2169.
23. Congdon NG, Friedman DS, Lietman T. Important causes of visual impairment in the world today. *JAMA*. 2003;290:2057-2060.
24. Tesfaye S, Chaurvedi N, Eaton SE, et al. Vascular risk factors and diabetic neuropathy. *N Eng J Med*. 2005;352:341-350.
25. Ppanas N, Ziegler D. Risk factors and comorbidities in diabetic neuropathy: an update 2015. *Rev Diabet Stud*. 2015;12:48-62.
26. Tesfaye S, Boulton AJ, Dyck PJ, et al. Diabetic neuropathies: update on definitions, diagnostic criteria, estimation of severity, and treatment. *Diabetes Care*. 2010;33:2285-2293.
27. Florez JC, Jablonski KA, Bayley N, et al. TCF7L2 polymorphisms and progression to diabetes in the Diabetes Prevention Program. *N Engl J Med*. 2006;355:241.

28. Moller DE, Flier JS. Insulin resistance-mechanisms, syndromes, and implications. *N Engl J Med*. 1991;325:938.
29. Walston J, Silver K, Bogardus C, et al. Time of onset on non-insulin-dependent diabetes mellitus and genetic variation in the beta 3-adrenergic–receptor gene. *N Engl J Med*. 1995;333-343.
30. Deeb SS, Fajas L, Nemoto M, et al. A Pro12Ala substitution in PPARgamma2 associated with decreased receptor activity, lower body mass index and improved insulin sensitivity. *Nat Genet*. 1998;20:284-287.
31. Scott LJ, Mohlke KL, Bonnycastle LL, et al. A genome-wide association study of type 2 diabetes in Finns detects multiple susceptibility variants. *Science*. 2007;316:1341-1345.
32. Boden G, Chen X. Effects of fat on glucose uptake and utilization in patients with non-insulin-dependent diabetes. *J Clin Invest*. 1995;96:1261-1268.
33. Shoelson SE, Lee J, Goldfine AB. Inflammation and insulin resistance. *J Clin Invest*. 2006;116:1793-1801.
34. Duncan BB, Schmidt MI, Pankow JS, et al. Low-grade systemic inflammation and the development of type 2 diabetes: the atherosclerosis risk in communities study. *Diabetes*. 2003;52:1799-1805.
35. Pradhan AD, Manson JE, Rifai N, et al. C-reactive protein, interleukin 6, and risk of developing type 2 diabetes mellitus. *JAMA*. 2001;286:327-334.
36. Vozarova B, Weyer C, Lindsay RS, et al. High white blood cell count is associated with a worsening of insulin sensitivity and predicts the development of type 2 diabetes. *Diabetes*. 2002;51:455-461.
37. de Rekeneire N, Peila R, Ding J, et al. Diabetes, hyperglycemia, and inflammation in older individuals: the health, aging and body composition study. *Diabetes Care*. 2006;29:1902-1908.
38. Hotamisligil GS, Shargill NS, Spiegelman BM. Adipose expression of tumor necrosis factor-alpha: direct role in obesity-linked insulin resistance. *Science*. 1993;259:87-91.
39. Morioka T, Asilmaz E, Hu J, et al. Disruption of leptin receptor expression in the pancreas directly affects beta cell growth and function in mice. *J Clin Invest*. 2007;117:2860-2868.
40. Hotamisligil GS, Johnson RS, Distel RJ, et al. Uncoupling of obesity from insulin resistance through a targeted mutation in aP2, the adipocyte fatty acid binding protein. *Science*. 1996;274:1377-1379.
41. Sharma K, Ramachandrarao S, Qui G, et al. Adiponectin regulates albuminuria and podocyte function in mice. *J Clin Invest*. 2008;118:1645-1656.
42. Vanhoutte PM, Shimokawa H, Feletou M, Tang EHC. Endothelial dysfunction and vascular disease—a 30th anniversary update. *Acta Physiol*. 2016.
43. Liu HB, Zhang J, Xin SY, et al. Mechanosensitive properties in the endothelium and their roles in the regulation of endothelial function. *J Cardiovasc Pharmacol*. 2013;61:461-470.
44. Zepeda RJ, Castillo R, Rodrigo R, et al. Effect of carvedilol and nebivolol on oxidative stress related parameters and endothelial function in patients with essential hypertension. *Basic Clin Pharmacol Toxicol*. 2012;111:309-316.
45. Laffin LJ, Bakris GL. Endothelin antagonism and hypertension: an evolving target. *Semin Nephrol*. 2015;3:168-175.
46. Wang D, Wang C, Wu X, et al. Endothelial dysfunction and enhanced contractility in microvessels from ovariectomized rats: roles of oxidative stress and perivascular adipose tissue. *Hypertens*. 2014;63:1063-1069.
47. Gollasch M. Vasodilator signals from perivascular adipose tissue. *Br J Pharmacol*. 2012;165:633-642.
48. Gu P, Xu A. Interplay between adipose tissue and blood vessels in obesity and vascular dysfunction. *Rev Endocr Metab Disord*. 2013;14:49-58.
49. Mundy AL, Haas E, Bhattacharya I, et al. Fat intake modifies vascular responsiveness and receptor expression of vasoconstrictors: implications for diet-induced obesity. *Cardiovasc Res*. 2007;73:368-375.
50. Alicic ZR, Tuttle KR. Novel therapies for diabetic kidney disease. *Adv Chronic Kidney Dis*. 2014;21:121-133.
51. Dieter BP, Alicic ZR, Meek R, et al. Novel therapies for diabetic kidney disease: stored past and forward paths. *Spectrum Diabetes*. 2015;28:167-173.
52. Sun YM, Su Y, Li J, et al. Recent advances in understanding the biochemical and molecular mechanism of diabetic nephropathy. *Biochem Biophys Res Commun*. 2013;433:359-361.
53. Thallas-Bonke V, Lindschau C, Rizkalla B, et al. Attenuation of extracellular matrix accumulation in diabetic nephropathy by the advanced glycation end product cross-link breaker ALT-711 via a protein kinase C-alpha-dependent pathway. *Diabetes*. 2004;53:2921-2930.
54. Anderberg RJ, Meek RM, Hudkins KL, et al. Serum amyloid A and inflammation in diabetic kidney disease and podocytes. *Lab Invest*. 2015;95:250-262.
55. Weiner DE, Tabatabai H. Cardiovascular outcomes and all-cause mortality: exploring the interaction between CKD and cardiovascular disease. *Am J Kidney Dis*. 2006;48:392-401.
56. Anavekar NS, McMurray JJ. Relation between renal dysfunction and cardiovascular outcomes after myocardial infarction. *N Engl J Med*. 2004;351:1285-1295.
57. Gross ML, Meyer HP. Calcification of coronary intima and media immunohistochemistry, backscatter imaging, and X-ray analysis in renal and nonrenal patients. *Clin J Am Soc Nephrol*. 2007;2:121-134.
58. Nakamura S, Ishibashi-Ueda H. Coronary calcification in patients with chronic kidney disease and coronary artery disease. *Clin J Am Soc Nephrol*. 2009;4:1892-1900.
59. Kjeldsen SE, Hedner T, Jamerson K, et al. for the HOT Study Group. Hypertension Optimal Treatment (HOT) Study. *Hypertension*. 1998;31:1014-1020.
60. Tight blood pressure control and risk of macrovascular and microvascular complications in type 2 diabetes: UKPDS 38. UK Prospective Diabetes Study Group. *BMJ*. 1998;317:703-713.
61. Adler AI, Stratton IM, Neil HA, et al. Association of systolic blood pressure with macrovascular and microvascular complications of type 2 diabetes (UKPDS 36): prospective observational study. *BMJ*. 2000;321:412-419.
62. Estacio RO, Jeffers BW, Hiatt WR, et al. The effect of nisoldipine as compared with enalapril on cardiovascular outcomes in patients with non-insulin-dependent diabetes and hypertension. *N Engl J Med*. 1998;338:645-652.
63. Brenner BM, Cooper ME, Zeeuw D, et al. for the RENAAL study investigators. Effects of losartan on renal and cardiovascular outcomes in patients with type 2 diabetes and nephropathy. *N Eng J Med*. 2001;345:861-869.
64. Lewis EJ, Hunsicker LG, Clarke WR, et al. Renoprotective effect of the angiotensin–receptor antagonist irbesartan in patients with nephropathy due to type 2 diabetes. *N Engl J Med*. 2001;345:851-860.
65. Parving HH, Lehnert H, Bröchner-Mortensen J, et al. The effect of irbesartan on the development of diabetic nephropathy in patients with type 2 diabetes. *N Engl J Med*. 2001;345:870-878.
66. Ruggenenti P, Fassi A, Ilieva AP, et al. Bergamo Nephrologic Diabetes Complications Trial (BENEDICT) Investigators. Preventing microalbuminuria in type 2 diabetes. *N Engl J Med*. 2004;351:1941-1951.
67. Schrier RW, Estacio RO, Esler A, et al. Effects of aggressive blood pressure control in normotensive type 2 diabetic patients on albuminuria, retinopathy and strokes. *Kidney Int*. 2002;61:1086-1097.

68. Estacio RO, Coll JR, Tran ZV, et al. Effect of intensive blood pressure control with valsartan on urinary albumin excretion in normotensive patients with type 2 diabetes. *Am J Hypert.* 2006;19:1241-1248.

69. Patal A, ADVANCE Collaborative group, MacMahon S, et al. Effects of a fixed combination of perindopril and indapamide on macrovascular and microvascular outcomes in patients with type 2 diabetes mellitus (the ADVANCE trial): a randomized controlled trial. *Lancet.* 2007;370:829-840.

70. Jamerson K, Weber MA, Bakris GL, et al. for the ACCOMPLISH trial investigators. Benazepril plus amlodipine or hydrochlorothiazide for hypertension in high-risk patients. *N Engl J Med.* 2008;359:2417-2428.

71. ACCORD Study Group, Cushman WC, Evans GW, et al. Effects of intensive blood-pressure control in type 2 diabetes mellitus. *N Engl J Med.* 2010;362:1575-1585.

72. Haller H, Ito S, Izzo JL, et al. Olmesartan for the delay or prevention of microalbuminuria in type 2 diabetes. *N Engl J Med.* 2011;364:907-917.

73. Parving HH, Brenner BM, McMurray JV, et al. Cardiorenal end points in a trial of aliskiren for type 2 diabetes. *N Engl J Med.* 2012;367:2204-2213.

74. Fried LF, Emanuele N, Zhang JH, et al. VA NEPHRON–D Investigators. Combined angiotensin inhibitor inhibition for the treatment of diabetic nephropathy. *N Eng J Med.* 2013;369:1892-1903.

75. Bakris GL, Weir MR, Shanifar S, et al. Effects of blood pressure level on progression of diabetic nephropathy. *Arch Intern Med.* 2003;163:1555-1565.

76. Pohl MA, Blumenthal S, Cordonnier DJ, et al. Independent and additive impact of blood pressure control and angiotensin II receptor blockade on renal outcomes in the irbesartan diabetic nephropathy trial: clinical implications and limitations. *J Am Soc Nephrol.* 2005;16(16):3027-3037.

77. Leehey DJ, Zhang JH, Emanuele NV, et al. BP and renal outcomes in diabetic kidney disease: The Veteran Affairs nephropathy in diabetes trial. *Clin J Am Soc Nephrol.* 2015;10:2159-2169.

78. Hermida RC, Ayala DE, Mojon A, et al. Influence of time of day of blood pressure lowering treatment on cardiovascular risk in hypertensive patients with type 2 diabetes. *Diabetes Care.* 2011;34:1270-1276.

79. Zhao P, Xu P, Wan C, et al. Evening versus morning dosing regimen drug therapy for hypertension. *Cochrane Database Syst Rev.* 2011;10; CD004184.

80. Rossen NB, Knudsen ST, Fleischer J, et al. Targeting nocturnal hypertension in type 2 diabetes mellitus. *Hypertens.* 2014;64:1080-1087.

81. American Diabetes Association. Risk Management Standards of Medical Care in Diabetes: Cardiovascular Disease and Risk Management. *Diabetes Care.* 2016;39(Suppl.1):S60-S71.

82. ACCORD Study Group, Cushman WC, Evans GW, et al. Effects of intensive blood-pressure control in type 2 diabetes mellitus. *N Engl J Med.* 2010;362:1575-1585.

83. Arguedas JA, Leiva V, Wright JM. Blood pressure targets for hypertension in people with diabetes mellitus. *Cochrane Database Syst Rev.* 2013;(10): CD008277.

84. Brunstro M, Carlberg B. Effect of antihypertensive treatment at different blood pressure levels in patients with diabetes mellitus: systemic review and meta-analysis. *BMJ.* 2016;352:i717.

85. James PA, Oparil S, Carter BL, et al. 2014 Evidence–based guideline for the management of high blood pressure in adults. Report from the panel members appointed to the Eight Joint National Committee (JNC8). *JAMA.* 2014;311:507-520.

86. Mancia GG, Fagard R, Narkiewicz K, et al. 2013 ESH/ESC Guidelines for the management of arterial hypertension. The Task Force for the management of arterial hypertension of the European Society of Hypertension (ESH) and of the European Society of Cardiology (ESC). *J Hypertens.* 2013;31:1281-1357.

87. Daskalopoulou SS, Rabi DM, Zarnke KB, et al. The 2015 Canadian Hypertension Education Program recommendations for blood pressure measurement, diagnosis, assessment of risk, prevention, and treatment of hypertension. *Can J Card.* 2015;31:549e-568e.

88. Kidney Disease. Improving Global Outcomes (KDIGO) CKD Work Group. KDIGO 2012 clinical practice guideline for the evaluation and management of chronic kidney disease. *Kidney Int.* 2013;3:1-150.

89. NICE guidelines [CG127] Hypertension in adults: diagnosis and management. Published date: August 2011.

90. Flack JM, Sica Domenic A, et al. Management of high blood pressure in Blacks. An update of the international society on hypertension in Black consensus statement. *Hypertens.* 2010;56:780-800.

91. Wright JT, Williamson JD, Snyder JK, et al. A randomized trial of intensive versus standard blood pressure control. *N Engl J Med.* 2015;373:2103-2116.

92. Perkovic V, Rodgers A. Redefining blood-pressure targets—Sprint starts the marathon. *N Engl J Med.* 2015;373:2175-2178.

93. Vasilakou D, Karagiannis T, Athanasiadou E, et al. Sodium-glucose cotransporter 2 inhibitors for type 2 diabetes: a systematic review and meta-analysis. *Ann Int Med.* 2013;159:262-274.

94. Baker WL, Smyth LR, Riche DM, et al. Effects of sodium-glucose cotransporter 2 inhibitors on blood pressure: a systematic review and meta-analysis. *J Am Soc Hypertens.* 2014;8:262-275.

95. Liu XY, Zhang N, Chen R, et al. Efficacy and safety of sodium-glucose cotransporter 2 inhibitors in type 2 diabetes: a meta-analysis of randomized controlled trials for 1 to 2 years. *J Diabetes Complications.* 2015;29:1295-1303.

96. Yanx XP, Lai D, Zhong XY, et al. Efficacy and safety of canagliflozin in subjects with type 2 diabetes: systematic review and meta-analysis. *Eur J Clin Pharmacol.* 2014;70:1149-1158.

97. Zhang M, Zhang L, Wu B, et al. Dapagliflozin treatment for type 2 diabetes: a systematic review and meta-analysis of randomized controlled trials. *Diabetes Metab Res Rev.* 2014;30:204-221.

98. Weber MA, Mansfield TA, Cain VA, et al. Blood pressure and glycemic effects of dapagliflozin versus placebo in patients with type 2 diabetes on combination antihypertensive therapy: a randomized, double-blind, placebo-controlled, phase 3 study. *Lancet Diabetes Endocrinol.* 2016;4:211-220.

99. Tikkanen I, Narko K, Zeller C, et al. Empagliflozin reduces blood pressure in patients with type 2 diabetes and hypertension. *Diabetes Care.* 2015;38:420-428.

100. Tikkanen I, Chilton R, Johansen OE. Potential role of sodium glucose cotransporter 2 inhibitors in the treatment of hypertension. *Curr Opin Nephrol Hypertens.* 2016;25:81-86.

101. Zinman B, Wanner C, Lachin JL, et al. Empagliflozin cardiovascular outcomes and mortality in type 2 diabetes. *N Engl J Med.* 2015;373:2117-2128.

102. ACCORD Study Group, Gerstein HC, Miller ME, et al. Effects of intensive glucose lowering in type 2 diabetes. *N Engl J Med.* 2008;358:2545-2559.

103. ADVANCE collaborative Group, Patel A, MacMahon S, et al. Intensive blood glucose control and vascular outcomes in patients with type 2 diabetes. *N Engl J Med.* 2008;12:2560-2572.

104. ACCORD Study Group. Nine-year effects of 3.7 years of intensive glycemic control on cardiovascular outcomes. *Diabetes Care.* 2016;39:701-708.

105. Zoungas S, Chalmers J, Neal B, et al. Follow-up blood-pressure lowering and glucose control in type 2 diabetes. *N Eng J Med.* 2014;371:13392-13406.

106. Li G, Hu Y, Yang W, et al. Effects of insulin resistance and insulin secretion on the efficacy of interventions to retard development of type 2 diabetes mellitus: the DA Qing IGT and Diabetes Study. *Diabetes Res Clin Pract.* 2002;58:193-200.

107. Tuomilehto J, Lindström J, Eriksson G, et al. Prevention of type 2 diabetes mellitus by changes in lifestyle among subjects with impaired glucose tolerance. *N Engl J Med.* 2001;344:1343-1350.

108. Ramachandran A, Snehalatha CS, Mary B, et al. The Indian Diabetes Prevention Programme shows that lifestyle modification and metformin prevent type 2 diabetes in Asian Indian subjects with impaired glucose tolerance (IDPP-1). *Diabetologia.* 2006;49:289-297.

109. The effects of nonpharmacologic interventions on blood pressure of persons with high normal levels. Results of the trials of hypertension prevention, phase I. *JAMA.* 1992;267:1213-1220.

110. Cutler JA. Effects of weight loss and sodium reduction intervention on blood pressure and hypertension incidence in overweight people with high-normal blood pressure: the trials of hypertension prevention, phase II. *Arch Intern Med.* 1997;157:657-667.

111. Moore TJ, Conlin PR, Ard J, et al. for the DASH Collaborative Research Group. DASH (Dietary Approaches to Stop Hypertension) Diet is effective treatment for stage 1 isolated systolic hypertension. *Hypertens.* 2001;38:155-158.

112. Appel LJ, Champagne CM, Harsha DW, et al. Effects of comprehensive lifestyle modification on blood pressure control: main results of the PREMIER clinical trial. *JAMA.* 2003;289:2083-2093.

113. Hu G, Barengo NC, Tuomilehto J, et al. Relationship of physical activity and body mass index to the risk of hypertension: a prospective study in Finland. *Hypertens.* 2004;43:25-30.

114. Toled E, Hu FB, Estruch R, et al. Effect of the Mediterranean diet on blood pressure in the PREDIMED trial: results from a randomized controlled trial. *BMC Med.* 2013;11:207.

115. Gay HC, Rao SG, Vaccarion V, Ali MK. Effects of Different Dietary Interventions on Blood Pressure: Systematic Review and Meta-Analysis of Randomized Controlled Trials. *Hypertension.* 2016;67:733-739.

116. Tuttle KR, Milton JE, Packard DP, et al. Dietary amino acids and blood pressure: a cohort study of patients with cardiovascular disease. *Am J Kidney Dis.* 2012;59:803-809.

117. Dunkler D, Kohl M, Heinze G, et al. Modifiable lifestyle and social factors affect chronic kidney disease in high-risk individuals with type 2 diabetes mellitus. *Kidney Int.* 2015;87:784-791.

118. Dunkler D, Dehghan M, Teo KK, et al. Diet and kidney disease in high-risk individuals with type 2 diabetes mellitus. *JAMA Intern Med.* 2013;173:1682-1692.

119. Dunkler D, Kohl M, Teo KK, et al. Population–Attributable fractions of modifiable lifestyle factors for CKD and mortality in individuals with type 2 diabetes: a cohort study. *Am J Kidney Dis.* 2016;68:29-40.

120. Gæde P, Vedel P, Larsen N, et al. Multifactorial intervention and cardiovascular disease in patients with type 2 diabetes. *N Engl J Med.* 2003;348:383-393.

121. Gaede P, Lund-Andersen H, Parving H, et al. Effect of a multifactorial intervention on mortality in type 2 diabetes. *N Engl J Med.* 2008;358:580-591.

38 Dyslipidemia

John W. McEvoy, Seamus P. Whelton, and Roger S. Blumenthal

EPIDEMIOLOGY OF HYPERLIPIDEMIA

Prevalence

Elevated cholesterol is a well-established and modifiable risk factor for cardiovascular disease (CVD). In 2008 there were an estimated 17.3 million CVD deaths worldwide, 2.6 million (15%) of which were caused by hyperlipidemia.[1] Data from the 2012 National Health and Nutrition Examination Survey (NHANES) indicated that nearly 31 million (13%) adults in the United States over the age of 20 years have a total cholesterol 240 mg/dL or higher and about 74 million (32%) have a low-density lipoprotein cholesterol (LDL-C) 130 mg/dL or higher and/or are taking a cholesterol lowering medication.[1] This prevalence increases with aging.

Globally, the average prevalence of hyperlipidemia, defined as a total cholesterol 240 mg/dL or higher, is estimated at 39%.[2] The global prevalence of hyperlipidemia is strongly related to socioeconomic factors, with total cholesterol levels in high income countries more than twice the levels observed in lower income countries. The highest clustering of hyperlipidemia around the world is observed in European countries with a prevalence of 54%, whereas African countries have the lowest prevalence at 23%. However, rapidly developing areas such as Southeast Asia and the Pacific region have demonstrated a mean increase in total cholesterol of approximately 3 mg/dL per decade between 1980 and 2008.[2,3]

Awareness, Treatment, and Temporal Trends

Despite widespread screening, a quarter of individuals with a high LDL-C were unaware of their diagnosis between 1999 and 2006.[4] Statin therapy is the primary medication prescribed to treat hyperlipidemia, accounting for more than 90% of prescriptions; from 2003 to 2012 and during this time the percent of U.S. adults over 40 years of age prescribed statin therapy increased from 16% to 23%.[5] Furthermore, as a result of the 2013 American College of Cardiology (ACC)/American Heart Association (AHA) cholesterol treatment guidelines, which base the decision to treat hyperlipidemia on cardiovascular risk rather than LDL-C level, the total number of U.S. adults meeting eligibility criteria for statin therapy is as high as 50%.[6] These new guidelines have an even greater impact among individuals over the age of 60 years, in whom nearly 80% would be identified to benefit from statin therapy after a clinician-patient risk discussion.

Statin therapy was approved by the United States Food and Drug Administration (FDA) in 1987 and contributed to a significant reduction in both total cholesterol (mean level from 206 to 196 mg/dL) and LDL-C (mean 129 to 116 mg/dL) among U.S. adults between 1988 and 2010.[7] In high income countries a temporal decline in total cholesterol similar to that in the U.S. has also been observed. This inverse relationship between temporal reductions in total cholesterol and per capita income, particularly among patients with prevalent vascular disease or who are at high CVD risk, is partly attributable to the higher use of cholesterol lowering medications in affluent countries.[8] Therefore, we are likely to see a continued decline in cholesterol levels among developed nations with higher per capita income as a result of an increase in cholesterol lowering medication use.

Cardiovascular Risk Factor Clustering: the Dyslipidemia and Hypertension Overlap

Among U.S. adults 50 years of age or older, less than one-third have ideal blood pressure, total cholesterol, or body mass index (BMI) and only 35% have ideal fasting blood glucose.[1] Accordingly, CVD risk factors more often occur together rather than in isolation and between 1991 and 1999, U.S. adults with hypertension had an increase in the prevalence of at least one additional CVD risk factor from 66% to 73%.[9] Similarly, more than half of hypertensive U.S. adults who do not have CVD are estimated to have one or more of the following: hyperlipidemia, diabetes, or increased BMI.[10]

High blood pressure and dyslipidemia are also closely interrelated with metabolic syndrome and in 2009 to 2010 approximately one-quarter of U.S. adults had metabolic syndrome. Adults with high blood pressure (systolic blood pressure [SBP] ≥130 and/or diastolic blood pressure [DBP] ≥ 80 mm Hg), low HDL-C (<40 mg/dL), and hypertriglyceridemia (≥150 mg/dL) meet the criteria for metabolic syndrome regardless of their other cardiovascular risk factors based on the National Heart Lung and Blood Institute (NHLBI)/AHA definition.[11] Among individuals with metabolic syndrome, 49% had high blood pressure, 85% had hypertriglyceridemia, and 60% had low HDL-C.[12]

It is no surprise, then, that between one-third to two-thirds of all U.S. adults with hypertension also have hyperlipidemia and that this coprevalence has remained unchanged over the last 20 years.[13] Among 57,573 hypertensive primary prevention patients from the Kaiser Permanente Northwest health maintenance group, 24% had concurrent hyperlipidemia (Fig. 38.1).[10,14] Similarly, in a study of 371,221 U.S. Veterans with a mean age of 58 years between 1998 and 2001, 52% had hypertension, 36% had dyslipidemia, and 31% had both hypertension and dyslipidemia.[15] There has been a significant decline in lipid levels from the early 1990s to the late 2000s and among individuals with combined hypertension and hyperlipidemia the mean total cholesterol decreased from 235 to 202 mg/dL and the mean LDL-C decreased from 154 to 120 mg/dL.[13] However, less than one-third of individuals were treated to their goal blood pressure and cholesterol goal.[13]

AMERICAN COLLEGE OF CARDIOLOGY/ AMERICAN HEART ASSOCIATION 2013 GUIDELINES FOR THE TREATMENT OF ELEVATED BLOOD CHOLESTEROL

The 2013 ACC/AHA cholesterol treatment guidelines represent a new approach to reducing atherosclerotic CVD (ASCVD).[16] There are significant changes to both the method

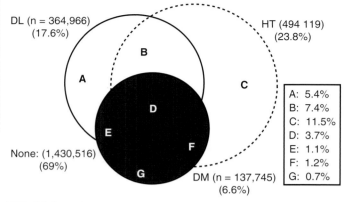

Prevalence and Co-Occurence of Hypertension (HT),
Dyslipidemia (DL) and Diabetes Mellitus (DM)
[Kaiser Permanente Members n = 2.1 million adults]

DL (n = 364,966)
(17.6%)

HT (494 119)
(23.8%)

None: (1,430,516)
(69%)

DM (n = 137,745)
(6.6%)

A: 5.4%
B: 7.4%
C: 11.5%
D: 3.7%
E: 1.1%
F: 1.2%
G: 0.7%

FIG. 38.1 Overlap between hypertension, dyslipidemia and diabetes in a contemporary managed care population. *(From Selby JV, Peng T, Karter AJ, et al. High rates of co-occurrence of hypertension, elevated low-density lipoprotein cholesterol, and diabetes mellitus in a large managed care population. Am J Manag Care. 2004;10[Part 2]:163-170.)*

of assessing which patients should be treated and in the recommended intensity of treatment. The two most important changes include: (1) the use of a new 10-year ASCVD risk estimator to identify patients who may benefit from statin therapy, and (2) the abandonment of LDL-C treatment goals. The guidelines also expand their primary treatment and prevention focus from coronary heart disease (CHD) to include ASCVD, defined as CHD, stroke, and peripheral arterial disease.

These 2013 guidelines identify four main groups who would benefit from statin therapy: (1) patients with prevalent history of ASCVD, (2) patients with an LDL-C 190 mg/dL or higher, (3) patients aged 40 to 75 years old with diabetes and an LDL-C between 70 and 189 mg/dL, and (4) nondiabetic patients aged 40 to 75 years old with an LDL-C between 70 and 189 mg/dL and an estimated 10-year ASCVD risk 7.5% or higher.

Risk Assessment

The 2013 guidelines introduced the calculation of a patient's 10-year ASCVD risk estimate based on the Pooled Cohort Risk Assessment Equations as the primary determinant to identify eligibility for lipid lowering therapy for primary prevention. However, validation analyses in modern U.S. cohorts have suggested significant overestimation of risk using the Pooled Cohort risk equation, especially for individuals in whom the estimated risk was relatively high.[17,18] Nevertheless, analyses from the Reasons for Geographic and Racial Differences in Stroke (REGARDS) study (baseline 2003 to 2007) and from the Copenhagen General Population Study (baseline 2003 to 2008) have suggested that the ASCVD equation performs better than other statin allocation approaches.[19,20]

The 7.5% cutoff for the Pooled Cohort equation dramatically increased the number of individuals who are eligible for statin therapy because it is more sensitive, but less specific than prior guideline recommendations. Accordingly, approximately one-third of all U.S. adults are now eligible for statin therapy and among these individuals, approximately two-thirds have prevalent hypertension.[6] In the context of concerns regarding overestimation, additional risk stratification information, such as a premature family history of ASCVD, a coronary artery calcium (CAC) score of more than 300 Agatston units or higher than 75th percentile for age/gender, or an elevated lifetime risk of ASCVD, are recommended by ACC/AHA as 'tiebreaker' tests for intermediate risk patients. It may also be

most reasonable to consider the use of these additional risk stratification tools (particularly CAC) in selected patients with an estimated risk that is higher than 7.5%, based on clinical judgment.[21] Furthermore, the patient-physician risk/benefit discussion is essential before the initiation of statin therapy regardless of a patient's absolute risk.[16]

Loss of Low-Density Lipoprotein Cholesterol Treatment Goals and Recommended Pharmacologic Therapy

The most controversial aspect of the 2013 lipid guidelines was the abandonment of LDL-C treatment goals. This was largely attributed to a report from the Institute of Medicine on guideline development and subsequent NHLBI Advisory Council recommendation to base guidelines on the highest-quality evidence available, specifically, randomized controlled trials.[22] Lipid lowering trials have evaluated the effect of statin therapy according to specific doses and there has not been a major lipid treatment trial with the primary outcome of evaluating treatment to a specific LDL-C goal.

Patients are now recommended for treatment with either moderate or high intensity statin therapy based on their estimated risk from the Pooled Cohort equation. High intensity statins are defined as those that lower LDL-C by 50% or more whereas moderate intensity statins are those that lower LDL-C by 30% to 50%. High intensity statin therapy is recommended for those 75 years of age or older with prevalent ASCVD, those with a LDL-C 190 mg/dL or higher, and patients with diabetes who have an estimated risk 7.5% or higher 10-year risk. Nondiabetic patients with a 7.5% or higher 10-year risk can be treated with either moderate or high intensity statin therapy. All other patients meeting statin therapy criteria are recommended to be treated with a moderate intensity statin. Low intensity statin therapy is recommended only in patients unable to tolerate moderate or high intensity statin therapy.

Despite the abandonment of LDL-C treatment goals in the ACC/AHA recommendations observational data show a consistent inverse and linear relationship between total cholesterol and CHD without an obvious lower limit of total cholesterol.[23] This relationship was also observed in an individual level meta-analysis examining the observed reductions in LDL-C among 38,153 participants enrolled in randomized controlled statin treatment trials. Participants with an achieved LDL-C less than 50 mg/dL had a 19% reduction in major CVD compared with those with an achieved LDL-C of 75 to 100 mg/dL.[24] Therefore, the majority of available evidence, inclusive of mechanistic and observational data, demonstrates that even lower LDL-C levels with proven therapy are associated with a further reduction in CVD.

Although LDL-C is expected to be reduced by 30% to 50% for moderate intensity and more than 50% for high intensity statin therapy, there is significant heterogeneity in the percent LDL-C reduction between individuals.[24] Accordingly, the 2013 Guidelines recommend to monitor a patient's individual response to statin therapy 4 to 12 weeks after statin initiation or dose adjustment and annually thereafter. Patient demographics, cigarette smoking, diet, exercise, triglyceride levels, and physical activity can contribute to differing percent LDL-C lowering between patients. However, nonadherence to statin therapy is the most frequent contributor to achieving less than anticipated reductions in LDL-C.

Interaction of Hypertension and Dyslipidemia in Estimating Atherosclerotic Cardiovascular Disease Risk

Four of the nine variables used in the Pooled Cohort equation to calculate estimated 10-year ASCVD risk incorporate blood pressure and cholesterol: (1) SBP, (2) treatment for hypertension, (3) total cholesterol, and (4) HDL-C. Observational research suggests a significant interaction between blood pressure and cholesterol on future events, although there is no formal interaction term in the ASCVD equation. Nonetheless, SBP has the largest coefficient of any variable in the ASCVD equation for African-American women and the second largest coefficient after age for African-American men. Moreover, SBP has a larger coefficient than diabetes in all gender/race versions of the equation.

In a study of U.S. Veterans, patients with combined hypertension and hyperlipidemia had a two-fold to three-fold greater prevalence of ASCVD and a three-fold to four-fold greater prevalence of myocardial infarction compared with Veterans with either hypertension or dyslipidemia alone.[15] The Multiple Risk Factor Intervention Trial (MRFIT), which included 361,662 men with an average age of 46 years, showed similar results with follow-up through 1986.[25] Participants in the lowest quintile of both SBP and total cholesterol had the lowest risk of CHD, whereas participants in the highest quintiles of SBP and total cholesterol had an approximately ten-fold increased CHD risk.

It is important to recognize the significant increase in CVD risk for patients with both hypertension and hyperlipidemia compared with patients with these risk factors in isolation. Effort should be made to ensure they are controlled in tandem to adequately reduce CVD risk. Therefore, the absence of hyperlipidemia does not equate with an absence of benefit for lipid lowering in hypertensive patients at high risk for ASCVD.

THERAPEUTIC CONSIDERATIONS SPECIFIC TO THE MANAGEMENT OF PATIENTS WITH DYSLIPIDEMIA AND HYPERTENSION

In this section, we focus on treatment options that reside in the extensive overlap between lipid abnormalities and hypertension (Fig. 38.1). Epidemiologic data demonstrate that this overlap is highly prevalent, hazardous to health, and, as embodied by the metabolic syndrome, often associated with additional CVD risk factors such as elevated fasting glucose, insulin resistance, inflammation, overweight status or frank obesity, and sedentary lifestyle.[26]

A Comprehensive Treatment Approach

A comprehensive treatment approach is required as lipid abnormalities among hypertensive adults are closely linked with other CVD risk factors.[27,28] Relying solely on the pharmacologic reduction of lipid levels represents a missed opportunity to address the underlying problems leading to a poor CVD risk factor profile. A comprehensive approach can target common modifiable factors that drive both elevated cholesterol and blood pressure levels such as unhealthy diet, low activity level, and adiposity. In addition, pharmacologic therapy should only be implemented if lifestyle modification provides inadequate results.

To this end, we recommend the simple "ABCDEF" approach (Table 38.1).[29] The ABCDEF approach is easy to use and recall by health care providers and patients, feasible in the context of clinic time constraints, and employs evidence-based recommendations. Furthermore, it is a simple tool that can translate complex and lengthy CVD prevention guidelines into a comprehensive and straightforward heuristic.[28]

It is well established that a healthy diet (one of the 'D' components of the ABCDEF tool) can improve both blood pressure and lipid parameters. This was highlighted in the Prevención con Dieta Mediterránea (PREDIMED) study that

reported a 30% reduction in myocardial infarction, stroke, or death from CVD causes among 7447 Europeans randomized to a Mediterranean diet enriched with olive oil (crude event rate 8.1 per 1000 person years, hazard ratio [HR] 0.70 [95% confidence interval {CI} 0.54 to 0.92]) or nuts (crude event rate 8.0 per 1000 person years, HR 0.72 [95% CI, 0.54 to 0.96]), with point estimates driven by reduced stroke, both compared with a control diet (11.2 per 1000 person years).[30]

A subsequent nested case-control analysis from PREDIMED demonstrated a reduction in 24 hour ambulatory blood pressure of −2.3 mm Hg (95% CI, −4.0 to −0.5) for the olive oil enriched diet and −2.6 mm Hg (95% CI, −4.3 to −0.9) for the nut enriched diet at 1 year of follow-up. Similarly, there was a reduction of changes in total cholesterol from baseline to 1 year of −11.3 mg/dL for the olive oil enriched diet and −13.6 mg/dL for the nut enriched diet.[31]

Other diets have also been shown to reduce both blood pressure (BP) and cholesterol[32,33] and therefore it is more important for patients to adhere to the overall features of a heart-healthy diet endorsed by 2013 ACC/AHA lifestyle guidelines rather than to any one rigid diet.[34] These guidelines recommend increased intake of vegetables, fruits, and whole grains and a reduced intake of sweets, sugar-sweetened beverages, and red meat. Moderate intake of low-fat dairy products, poultry, fish, legumes, nontropical vegetable oils, and nuts is also recommended. This pattern can be achieved by following plans such as the PREDIMED Mediterranean diet, DASH (dietary approaches to stop hypertension) dietary pattern, the United Department of Agriculture (USDA) food pattern, or the AHA diet. For hypertensive individuals, dietary sodium should be less than 2400 mg, and preferably closer to 1500 mg, per day. However, in the case of hypertensive individuals who have elevated cholesterol, further attention should be directed to lowering percent of calories from saturated fat (to 5% to 6% of total) and limiting *trans* fats.[34,35]

In a meta-analysis of randomized controlled trials evaluating the impact of exercise (the 'E' component of the ABCDE tool) on blood pressure control and other CVD risk factors there was an average reduction in blood pressure of −7/−5 mm Hg after exercise interventions.[36] Consistent with findings from other groups[37] there was also a reduction in triglycerides and an increase in high density lipoprotein-cholesterol (HDL-C), with nonsignificant reductions in LDL-C and total cholesterol. Mora et al reported that the 27% of the reduction in CVD outcomes as a result of exercise was accounted for by improvements in blood pressure and 19% by improvements in lipids.[38]

Finally, the effect of weight loss on lipid and blood pressure[39] control among hypertensive adults must be considered (diet and weight management is one of the 'D' components of the ABCDEF approach). Addressing diet and exercise will help most adults lose weight. However, studies assessing the durability of these interventions on sustained weight loss and long-term CVD outcomes have been mostly disappointing.[40] Although new mobile health technologies have the potential to help sustain healthy lifestyle behaviors and weight loss,[41] few data exist on the impact of these modalities on long-term lipid and blood pressure control.[42] However, bariatric surgery has proven highly effective, particularly among patients with diabetes. In the Surgical Treatment and Medications Potentially Eradicate Diabetes Efficiently (STAMPEDE) trial, which randomized 150 diabetics to one of three intervention groups (medical therapy, gastric bypass, or sleeve gastrectomy) patients with weight-loss surgery had improvements in HgbA1C, BMI, triglycerides, HDL-C, and proteinuria after 3 years of follow-up.[43] Although LDL-C and blood pressure did not differ significantly between

TABLE 38.1 The Comprehensive 'ABCDEF' Approach to the Primary Prevention of Atherosclerotic Cardiovascular Disease

	ABCDE COMPONENT	RECOMMENDATION
A	Assess Risk	Multiple Risk Calculators Available.
A	Antiplatelet Therapy	**Primary Prevention:** Aspirin 81 mg/d if >10% 10-year risk by FRS; use contraindicated if risk of bleeding outweighs benefit; no role for dual antiplatelet therapy. **Secondary Prevention:** Aspirin 81-162 mg/d indefinitely: clopidogrel, prasugrel or ticagrelor for 12 months after ACS. Clopidogrel, prasugrel or ticagrelor after PCI; duration depends on stent type; aspirin 81-325 mg/d is recommended for all patients following an ischemic stroke.
A	Atrial Fibrillation	**Primary Prevention:** Control risk factors (hypertension, obstructive sleep apnea, alcohol, obesity). **Secondary Prevention:** Warfarin or novel oral anticoagulants for CHADS$_2$ ≥ 2 or CHA$_2$DS$_2$-Vasc ≥ 2.
B	Blood Pressure	**Primary and Secondary Prevention:** Lifestyle interventions ± pharmacotherapy based on blood pressure targets. BP Goal: <150/90 mm Hg in elderly (≥60 y), <140/90 in <60 y or diabetics or history of ASCVD. Lower targets (120/80) may be reasonable given results of SPRINT trial.
C	Cholesterol	**Primary Prevention:** Only if within one of statin benefit groups. In those for whom a risk decision is uncertain, additional factors such as LDL-C ≥ 160 mg/dL, family history of premature ASCVD, high lifetime risk (these are useful in younger patients where quantitative ASCVD risk is low), and CAC score ≥ 300, ABI < 0.90, and hsCRP ≥ 2.0 mg/L (these are especially useful in older patients). **Secondary Prevention:** Lifestyle interventions ± pharmacotherapy with moderate to high intensity statins.
C	Cigarette/Tobacco Cessation	**Primary Prevention:** Education. **Secondary Prevention:** Assessment, counseling, pharmacotherapy 5As: Ask, Advise, Assess, Assist, Arrange.
D	Diet and Weight Management	**Primary and Secondary Prevention:** Goal BMI 18.5-24.9 kg/m^2; waist circumference: <40 in. (men), <35 in. (women) Lose 3% to 5% of body weight. Low calorie diet: 1200-1500 kcal/day (women); 1500-1800 kcal/day (men). Energy deficit via decreased calorie intake and increased physical activity. Comprehensive lifestyle program. Weight loss maintenance.
D	Diabetes Prevention and Treatment	**Primary Prevention:** Lifestyle interventions. Goal: Normal fasting blood glucose and hemoglobin A1c <5.7%. **Secondary Prevention:** Lifestyle interventions, metformin, oral hypoglycemic, insulin. Goal: Hemoglobin A1c<7%.
D	Discuss Risk	Ensure a Clinician-Patient Risk Discussion precedes any initiation of pharmacologic therapy, particularly statins and among patients at intermediate risk of ASCVD (e.g., 10 year risk of 5% to 15% by the Pooled Cohort estimator). Discuss patient preferences and goals of care.
E	Exercise	**Primary and Secondary Prevention:** Regular aerobic physical activity Goal: 3-4 sessions a week, lasting on average 40 minutes per session involving moderate- to vigorous-intensity physical activity; cardiac rehabilitation for patients who have had an ASCVD event.
F	Heart Failure	**Primary Prevention:** Treat HF risk factors. **Secondary Prevention:** A: Adherence to meds (ACE, ARB, BB, aldosterone antagonists, diuretics). B: Blood pressure and blood sugar control; behaviors (such as daily weights). C: Cigarette smoking cessation/cholesterol management. D: Dietary adherence, drinking limited fluids and alcohol, defibrillator. E: Exercise.

(Adapted from Kohli P, Whelton SP, Hsu S, et al. Clinician's Guide to the Updated ABCs of Cardiovascular Disease Prevention. J Am Heart Assoc. 2014;3:e001098.)
ABI, Ankle-brachial index; *ACE,* angiotensin converting enzyme; *ACS,* acute coronary syndrome; *ARB,* angiotensin II receptor blockers; *ASCVD,* atherosclerotic cardiovascular disease; *BB,* beta-blockers; *BMI,* body mass index; *CAC,* coronary artery calcium; *CHADS,* congestive heart failure, hypertension, age ≥75 years, diabetes mellitus, stroke; *FRS,* Framingham Risk Score; *HF,* heart failure; *PCI,* percutaneous coronary intervention.

the groups, this was attributed to differential medication use in the study arms over follow-up.

Evidence for Combination Treatment of Hypertension and Dyslipidemia

Although the Antihypertensive and Lipid-Lowering Treatment to Prevent Heart Attack-Lipid-Lowering Trial (ALLHAT-LLT) did not demonstrate a reduction in mortality or CHD events among 10,355 hypertensive adults with a mean baseline LDL-C of 146 mg/dL randomized to pravastatin, there was substantial crossover to statins in the control group.[44] In contrast, the Anglo-Scandinavian Cardiac Outcomes Trial-Lipid Lowering Arm (ASCOT-LLA) trial did report a reduction in nonfatal myocardial infarction, fatal CHD, and stroke over 3.3 years of follow-up for atorvastatin therapy among 19,342 hypertensive adults with a mean baseline LDL-C of 131 mg/dL.[44] Mean BP control did not differ in either the statin or control arm of both of these trials as a result of factorial randomization. However, the relative reduction in total

cholesterol of 24% in ASCOT-LLA was far higher than seen in the ALLHAT-LLT study (9.6%). Although mortality was not reduced at 3.3 years, long-term follow-up of ASCOT-LLA out to 11 years did demonstrate a significant reduction in death, despite substantial crossover to statin therapy in the control arm after trial completion.[45]

The Justification for the Use of Statins in Prevention: an Intervention Trial Evaluating Rosuvastatin (JUPITER) trial, which randomized 17,802 adults (57% had a diagnosis of hypertension) with an LDL-C less than 130 mg/dL and a high-sensitivity C-reactive protein 2 or more mg/L to rosuvastatin versus placebo also reported significant benefit for lower LDL-C.[46] Given the median SBP at the baseline visit of JUPITER was 134 mm Hg, the majority of the JUPITER population may benefit from the consideration of additional antihypertensive therapy based on results from the Systolic BP Intervention Trial (SPRINT) that showed a reduction in all-cause mortality in the group treated to a goal SBP less than 120 mm Hg.[47]

Additional evidence for aggressively reducing LDL-C in high risk hypertensive adults comes from the Improved

Reduction of Outcomes: Vytorin Efficacy International Trial (IMPROVE-IT)[48] in which 18,144 adults who were hospitalized with acute coronary syndrome with a LDL-C less than 125 mg/dL at baseline were randomized to simvastatin 40 mg (achieved LDL-C of 70 mg/dL) versus simvastatin 40 mg plus ezetimibe 10 mg (achieved LDL-C of 54 mg/dL). Over 60% of patients enrolled in this trial had hypertension and there was a 6% reduction in the primary endpoint of cardiovascular death, nonfatal myocardial infarction, unstable angina requiring rehospitalization, coronary revascularization, or nonfatal stroke ($p = 0.016$) over 7 years of follow-up. Therefore, using proven therapy, there is a linear relationship between ASCVD and the reduction of LDL-C among a wide range of hypertensive patients with a history of, or at risk for, CVD.

The Polypill

Some experts have advocated for the use of combination therapy for hyperlipidemia and hypertension in persons at elevated CVD risk: the concept of a "Polypill."[49] The motivation for a Polypill, also termed a fixed-dose combination (FDC), is to improve adherence, lower cost (particularly attractive in low-income countries where personalized medicine is more challenging as a result of limited resources), and to increase the use of preventive therapies among suitable primary prevention populations. Adherence is particularly important for hypertensive adults with elevated cholesterol because as few as one in three adults remains adherent with both hyperlipidemia and hypertension cotherapy.[50] Meta-analyses have demonstrated that, compared with placebo, FDCs resulted in meaningful reductions in SBP and DBP, and in total cholesterol and LDL-C, but that these reductions were less than what would have been expected from the component medications, based on trials of these agents taken as single medications.[51] However, it is likely that, outside of trial settings (i.e., in the real world), the Polypill would likely perform as well, if not better, than the component medications by improving adherence.

In keeping with this, the Use of a Multidrug Pill in Reducing Cardiovascular Events (UMPIRE) trial, a pragmatic study in which the control patients were not given any support with their usual care medications, reported that subjects allocated to the FDC treatment arm had improved adherence and modest reductions in SBP (2.6 mm Hg, $p < 0.001$) and LDL-C (4.2 mg/dL, $p < 0.001$) after a median follow-up of 15 months.[52] Despite these encouraging results, in the absence of evidence for reduced hard CVD outcomes, which is currently being tested in a number of outcomes trials (TIPS3 and HOPE4), it is unlikely that the Polypill will be recommended for widespread use in the near future by guideline committees.

Modifying Effects of Statins on Blood Pressure and Antihypertensive Medications on Lipid Levels

Although observational data and mechanistic trials suggest that statins may independently lower blood pressure,[53,54] posthoc exploratory blood pressure data from large outcomes trials suggest that the independent effects of statins on blood pressure lowering are likely small.[44] Nonetheless, even a 2 mm Hg reduction in blood pressure at the population level could meaningfully reduce CVD.[55]

Moreover, a number of antihypertensive medications can also alter lipid levels.[56] Thiazide diuretics can mildly increase total cholesterol levels and beta-blockers can increase triglycerides and lower HDL-C. In contrast, alpha-blockers, angiotensin-converting enzyme inhibitors, and angiotensin II receptor-blockers may have mild beneficial

effects on lipids.[56,57] However, these lipid changes are typically mild and tend to normalize within the first year of therapy.[58]

Emerging Therapies for Hyperlipidemia and Their Relationship With Blood Pressure Control

The addition of adjunctive nonstatin lipid lowering therapies to maximally tolerated statin therapy has had mixed results.[59-61] However, more recent developments have generated great enthusiasm, particularly with the approval of Proprotein convertase subtilisin/kexin type 9 (PCSK9) inhibitors, which decrease LDL-C receptor degradation and increase recirculation of the receptor to the hepatocytes cell surface, thereby lowering of serum LDL cholesterol. The classes of new lipid medication that are furthest along in development include the PCSK9 inhibitors, the cholesteryl ester transfer protein (CETP) inhibitors, mipomersen (an antisense oligonucleotide that inhibits production of apolipoprotein B-100) and loperamide (a microsomal triglyceride transfer protein inhibitor).[62,63] The latter two agents are expensive (current cost estimates are typically over $200,000 per year), associated with liver toxicities, and are only approved for use in patients with homozygous familial hypercholesterolemia and their discussion is beyond the scope of this chapter.

Although enthusiasm for the CETP inhibitors is currently waning, they are nonetheless pertinent to our discussion given their known off-target effects on blood pressure control. These agents are potent increasers of HDL-C and facilitate the exchange of cholesterol esters between HDL-C particles and apolipoprotein B-containing lipoproteins.[64] However, despite reducing LDL-C by 25% and increasing HDL-C by 72%, torcetrapib, the first agent tested, increased mortality and CVD. The excess in events has been attributed to increases in aldosterone, cortisol, endothelin-1, which resulted in an increase in SBP of about 5 mm Hg.[65] The next CETP agent tested, dalcetrapib, increased HDL-C by about 30%. Despite this, the DAL-OUTCOMES trial was stopped for futility and of note, SBP was increased by 0.6 mm Hg relative to placebo ($p < 0.001$).[66] Similarly, a large outcomes trial of evacetrapib was recently discontinued for futility. Only anacetrapib and TA-8995 remain under testing in large trials.

In contrast, the PCSK9 inhibitor class of agents has demonstrated dramatic LDL-C reductions as well as a signal for clinical benefit.[67] Alirocumab and evolocumab were recently approved for use in familial hypercholesterolemia and in persons with clinical ASCVD who would benefit from additional LDL-C lowering on top of maximally tolerated statin therapy. Thus, these agents are now available for use in a wide range of high CVD risk hypertensive patients.[68]

Both agents are given by subcutaneous injection and can cause large reductions in LDL-C levels (39% to 62% reduction for alirocumab and 47% to 56% for evolocumab) (Table 38.2).[68] Although results from definitive outcomes trials are still awaited, preliminary results point to a strong likelihood that this LDL-C reduction will translate into reduced CVD events in patients receiving these agents.[67,69] The data that have been reported on the effects of PCSK9 on blood pressure suggest that both genetic and pharmacologic inhibition of the PCSK9 pathway has no adverse impact on hypertension control.[70-72]

SUMMARY

CVD risk factors occur more often in combination than in isolation and most patients with hypertension have concurrent dyslipidemia. There is evidence that hypertension and dyslipidemia act synergistically to increase CVD risk.

TABLE 38.2 Efficacy of Novel Nonstatin Cholesterol Medications: Ezetimibe, Cholesteryl Ester Transfer Protein, and Proprotein Convertase Subtilisin/Kexin Type 9 Inhibitors

	DOSES	OTHER LIPID-LOWERING TREATMENT	% CHANGE FROM BASELINE TO END OF FOLLOW-UP BEYOND THAT WITH CONTROL[a]							CHOLESTEROL EFFLUX CAPACITY % INCREASE	OUTCOME TRIALS
			Δ Total Cholesterol	Δ LDL-C	Δ HDL-C	Δ Triglycerides	Δ APO	Δ APO-1	Δ Lipoprotein (A)		
CEPT Inhibitors											
Anacetrapib[73-75]	100 mg per day	Background statin therapy ± others	16	−36	139	−5	−18	42	−39	Increase	REVEAL in progress: results expected 2017 (>30,000 participants)
Evacetrapid[76-78]	100 mg per day	—	9.5	−26	97	−12	−16	36	—	21% to 28%[b]	ACCELERATE in progress: results expected 2016 (~12,000 participants)
TA-8995	1.0-2.5-5-10 mg per day	± Statins	−14 to 7	−28 to −69	74 to 77	−3 to −15	−21 to −51	29 to 61	−23 to −35	17% to 37%	—
PCSK-9 Inhibitors											
Allrocumab[79-81]	150 mg every 2 weeks	± Statins (± ezetimibe)	−35 to −44	−57 to −67	6 to 10	−6 to −29[c]	−44 to −58	14 (1[c])	−9 (−29[c])	—	ODYSSEE OUTCOMES expected 2018 (~18,000 participants)
Evolocumab[72,82-85]	420 mg every 4 weeks and 140mg every 2 weeks	± Statins (± ezetimibe)	−33 to −42	−50 to −66	4 to 9	−6 to −34	−42 to −56	0 to 4	−18 to −32	—	FOURIER in progress: results expected 2018 (~27,500 participants)
Cholesterol Absorption Inhibitors											
Ezetimibe[86-89]	10 mg per day	Statin	−10	−15	2	−5	−11	1	—	No significant effect	IMPROVE IT (18,144 participants) ezetimibe association with a 6.4% reduction in cardiovascular events

[a]Differences in percentage changes between active treatment and control (placebo, ezetimibe, statin/ex ezetimibe vs. statin); percentage changes are least-squares means unless otherwise specified.

[b]Pooled evacetrapib monotherapy (30, 100, and 500 mg); 28%; 100 mg evacetrapib in combination with statins: 21%.

[c]Median change.

(Adapted from Hovingh GK, Kastelein JJ, van Deventer SJ, et al. Cholesterol ester transfer protein inhibition by TA-8995 in patients with mild dyslipidaemia (TULIP): a randomised, double-blind, placebo-controlled phase 2 trial. Lancet. 2015;386:412-414.)

Based on ACC/AHA cholesterol treatment guideline recommendations, clinicians should evaluate a patient's overall ASCVD risk when considering cholesterol lowering therapy because many patients with hypertension, but without elevated LDL-C, may benefit from statin therapy. Accordingly a comprehensive approach to CVD risk factor modification, especially for hypertension and dyslipidemia, is essential to maximize the reduction in CVD. Although some CVD medications have modifying effects on blood pressure and cholesterol, these effects are generally small and overshadowed by the reductions in CVD events. Moreover, novel lipid lowering therapies like PCSK-9 inhibitors show even greater reductions in lipids without adverse changes in blood pressure, effects that may translate into further reductions in ASCVD among selected hypertensive patients with suboptimal lipid levels.

References

1. Mozaffarian D, Benjamin EJ, Go AS, et al. Heart disease and stroke statistics-2016 update: A Report From the American Heart Association. *Circulation*. 2016;133:e38-e360.
2. World Health Organization. Global Atlas CVD Prevention/Control. Geneva, Switzerland: WHO, 2011.
3. Farzadfar F, Finucane MM, Danaei G, et al. National, regional, and global trends in serum total cholesterol since 1980: systematic analysis of health examination surveys and epidemiological studies with 321 country-years and 3.0 million participants. *Lancet*. 2011;377:578-586.
4. Kuklina EV, Yoon PW, Keenan NL. Trends in high levels of low-density lipoprotein cholesterol in the United States, 1999-2006. *JAMA*. 2009;302:2104-2110.
5. Qiuping Gu, Ryne Paulose-Ram, Vicki Burt, Brian Kit. National Center for Health Statistics. Prescription cholesterol lowering medication use in adults aged 40 and over: United States, 2003-2012. December 2014. No 177.
6. Pencina MJ, Navar-Boggan AM, D'Agostino RB Sr, et al. Application of new cholesterol guidelines to a population-based sample. *N Engl J Med*. 2014;370:1422-1431.
7. Carroll MD, Kit BK, Lacher DA, Shero ST, Mussolino ME. Trends in lipids and lipoproteins in US adults, 1988-2010. *JAMA*. 2012;308:1545-1554.
8. Venkitachalam L, Wang K, Porath A, et al. Global variation in the prevalence of elevated cholesterol in outpatients with established vascular disease or 3 cardiovascular risk factors according to national indices of economic development and health system performance. *Circulation*. 2012;125:1858-1869.
9. Greenlund KJ, Zheng ZJ, Keenan NL, et al. Trends in self-reported multiple cardiovascular disease risk factors among adults in the United States, 1991-1999. *Arch Int Med*. 2004;164:181-188.
10. Weycker D, Nichols GA, O'Keeffe-Rosetti M, et al. Risk-factor clustering and cardiovascular disease risk in hypertensive patients. *Am J Hypertens*. 2007;20:599-607.
11. Grundy SM, Brewer HB Jr., Cleeman JI, Smith SC Jr, Lenfant C. Definition of metabolic syndrome: Report of the National Heart, Lung, and Blood Institute/American Heart Association conference on scientific issues related to definition. *Circulation*. 2004;109:433-438.
12. Beltran-Sanchez H, Harhay MO, Harhay MM, McElligott S. Prevalence and trends of metabolic syndrome in the adult U.S. population, 1999-2010. *J Am Coll Cardiol*. 2013;62:697-703.
13. Egan BM, Li J, Qanungo S, Wolfman TE. Blood pressure and cholesterol control in hypertensive hypercholesterolemic patients: national health and nutrition examination surveys 1988-2010. *Circulation*. 2013;128:29-41.
14. Selby JV, Peng T, Karter AJ, et al. High rates of co-occurrence of hypertension, elevated low-density lipoprotein cholesterol, and diabetes mellitus in a large managed care population. *Am J Manag Care*. 2004;10(2 Pt 2):163-170.
15. Johnson ML, Pietz K, Battleman DS, Beyth RJ. Prevalence of comorbid hypertension and dyslipidemia and associated cardiovascular disease. *Am J Manag Care*. 2004;10:926-932.
16. Stone NJ, Robinson JG, Lichtenstein AH, et al. 2013 ACC/AHA guideline on the treatment of blood cholesterol to reduce atherosclerotic cardiovascular risk in adults: a report of the American College of Cardiology/American Heart Association Task Force on Practice Guidelines. *Circulation*. 2014;129(25 Suppl 2):S1-45.
17. DeFilippis AP, Young R, Carrubba CJ, et al. An analysis of calibration and discrimination among multiple cardiovascular risk scores in a modern multiethnic cohort. *Ann Int Med*. 2015;162:266-275.
18. Ridker PM, Cook NR. Statins: new American guidelines for prevention of cardiovascular disease. *Lancet*. 2013;382:1762-1765.
19. Muntner P, Colantonio LD, Cushman M, et al. Validation of the atherosclerotic cardiovascular disease Pooled Cohort risk equations. *JAMA*. 2014;311:1406-1415.
20. Mortensen MB, Afzal S, Nordestgaard BG, Falk E. Primary prevention with statins: ACC/AHA risk-based approach versus trial-based approaches to guide statin therapy. *J Am Coll Cardiol*. 2015;66:2699-2709.
21. Blaha MJ, Cainzos-Achirica M, Greenland P, et al. Role of coronary artery calcium score of zero and other negative risk markers for cardiovascular disease: The Multi-Ethnic Study Of Atherosclerosis (MESA). *Circulation*. 2016;133:849-858.
22. Gibbons GH, Shurin SB, Mensah GA, Lauer MS. Refocusing the agenda on cardiovascular guidelines: an announcement from the National Heart, Lung, and Blood Institute. *Circulation*. 2013;128:1713-1715.
23. Lewington S, Whitlock G, Clarke R, et al. Blood cholesterol and vascular mortality by age, sex, and blood pressure: a meta-analysis of individual data from 61 prospective studies with 55,000 vascular deaths. *Lancet*. 2007;370:1829-1839.
24. Boekholdt SM, Hovingh GK, Mora S, et al. Very low levels of atherogenic lipoproteins and the risk for cardiovascular events: a meta-analysis of statin trials. *J Am Coll Cardiol*. 2014;64:485-494.
25. Neaton JD, Wentworth D. Serum cholesterol, blood pressure, cigarette smoking, and death from coronary heart disease. Overall findings and differences by age for 316,099 white men. Multiple Risk Factor Intervention Trial Research Group. *Arch Int Med*. 1992;152:56-64.
26. Grundy SM. Metabolic syndrome update. *Trends Cardiovasc Med*. 2016;16:364-373.
27. Blaha MJ, Bansal S, Rouf R, Golden SH, Blumenthal RS, Defilippis AP. A practical "ABCDE" approach to the metabolic syndrome. *Mayo Clin Proc*. 2008;83:932-941.
28. Kohli P, Whelton SP, Hsu S, et al. Clinician's guide to the updated ABCs of cardiovascular disease prevention. *J Am Heart Assoc*. 2014;3. e001098.
29. Gluckman TJ, Baranowski B, Ashen MD, et al. A practical and evidence-based approach to cardiovascular disease risk reduction. *Arch Int Med*. 2004;164:1490-1500.
30. Estruch R, Ros E, Salas-Salvado J, et al. Primary prevention of cardiovascular disease with a Mediterranean diet. *N Engl J Med*. 2013;368:1279-1290.
31. Domenech M, Roman P, Lapetra J, et al. Mediterranean diet reduces 24-hour ambulatory blood pressure, blood glucose, and lipids: one-year randomized, clinical trial. *Hypertension*. 2014;64:69-76.
32. Appel LJ, Sacks FM, Carey VJ, et al. Effects of protein, monounsaturated fat, and carbohydrate intake on blood pressure and serum lipids: results of the OmniHeart randomized trial. *JAMA*. 2005;294:2455-2464.
33. Erlinger TP, Miller ER 3rd, Charleston J, Appel LJ. Inflammation modifies the effects of a reduced-fat low-cholesterol diet on lipids: results from the DASH-sodium trial. *Circulation*. 2003;108:150-154.
34. Eckel RH, Jakicic JM, Ard JD, et al. 2013 AHA/ACC guideline on lifestyle management to reduce cardiovascular risk: a report of the American College of Cardiology/American Heart Association Task Force on Practice Guidelines. *J Am Coll Cardiol*. 2014;63(25 Pt B):2960-2984.
35. de Souza RJ, Mente A, Maroleanu A, et al. Intake of saturated and trans unsaturated fatty acids and risk of all cause mortality, cardiovascular disease, and type 2 diabetes: systematic review and meta-analysis of observational studies. *BMJ*. 2015;351:h3978.
36. Fagard RH, Cornelissen VA. Effect of exercise on blood pressure control in hypertensive patients. *Eur J Cardiovasc Prev Rehabil*. 2007;14:12-17.
37. Cox KL, Burke V, Morton AR, Gillam HF, Beilin LJ, Puddey IB. Long-term effects of exercise on blood pressure and lipids in healthy women aged 40-65 years: The Sedentary Women Exercise Adherence Trial (SWEAT). *J Hypertens*. 2001;19:1733-1743.
38. Mora S, Cook N, Buring JE, Ridker PM, Lee IM. Physical activity and reduced risk of cardiovascular events: potential mediating mechanisms. *Circulation*. 2007;116:2110-2118.
39. Crump C, Sundquist J, Winkleby MA, Sundquist K. Interactive Effects of Physical Fitness and Body Mass Index on the Risk of Hypertension. *JAMA Int Med*. 2016:1-7.
40. Look ARG, Wing RR, Bolin P, et al. Cardiovascular effects of intensive lifestyle intervention in type 2 diabetes. *N Engl J Med*. 2013;369:145-154.
41. Martin SS, Feldman DI, Blumenthal RS, et al. mActive: A Randomized Clinical Trial of an Automated mHealth Intervention for Physical Activity Promotion. *J Am Heart Assoc*. 2015;4:e002239.
42. Higgins JP. Smartphone Applications for Patients' Health and Fitness. *Am J Med*. 2016;129:11-19.
43. Schauer PR, Bhatt DL, Kirwan JP, et al. Bariatric surgery versus intensive medical therapy for diabetes—3-year outcomes. *N Engl J Med*. 2014;370:2002-2013.
44. Sever PS, Dahlof B, Poulter NR, et al. Prevention of coronary and stroke events with atorvastatin in hypertensive patients who have average or lower-than-average cholesterol concentrations, in the Anglo-Scandinavian Cardiac Outcomes Trial—Lipid Lowering Arm (ASCOT-LLA): a multicentre randomised controlled trial. *Lancet*. 2003;361:1149-1158.
45. Sever PS, Chang CL, Gupta AK, Whitehouse A, Poulter NR, Investigators A. The Anglo-Scandinavian Cardiac Outcomes Trial: 11-year mortality follow-up of the lipid-lowering arm in the U.K. *Eur Heart J*. 2011;32:2525-2532.
46. Ridker PM, Danielson E, Fonseca FA, et al. Rosuvastatin to prevent vascular events in men and women with elevated C-reactive protein. *N Engl J Med*. 2008;359:2195-2207.
47. Group SR, Wright JT Jr., Williamson JD, et al. A Randomized Trial of Intensive versus Standard Blood-Pressure Control. *N Engl J Med*. 2015;373:2103-2116.
48. Cannon CP, Blazing MA, Giugliano RP, et al. Ezetimibe added to statin therapy after acute coronary syndromes. *N Engl J Med*. 2015;372:2387-2397.
49. Wald NJ, Law MR. A strategy to reduce cardiovascular disease by more than 80%. *BMJ*. 2003;326:1419.
50. Chapman RH, Benner JS, Petrilla AA, et al. Predictors of adherence with antihypertensive and lipid-lowering therapy. *Arch Int Med*. 2005;165:1147-1152.
51. Elley CR, Gupta AK, Webster R, et al. The efficacy and tolerability of 'polypills': meta-analysis of randomised controlled trials. *PloS One*. 2012;7:e52145.
52. Thom S, Poulter N, Field J, et al. Effects of a fixed-dose combination strategy on adherence and risk factors in patients with or at high risk of CVD: the UMPIRE randomized clinical trial. *JAMA*. 2013;310:918-929.
53. Glorioso N, Troffa C, Filigheddu F, et al. Effect of the HMG-CoA reductase inhibitors on blood pressure in patients with essential hypertension and primary hypercholesterolemia. *Hypertension*. 1999;34:1281-1286.
54. Borghi C, Dormi A, Veronesi M, Sangiorgi Z, Gaddi A. Brisighella Heart Study Working P. Association between different lipid-lowering treatment strategies and blood pressure control in the Brisighella Heart Study. *Am Heart J*. 2004;148:285-292.
55. Cook NR, Cohen J, Hebert PR, Taylor JO, Hennekens CH. Implications of small reductions in diastolic blood pressure for primary prevention. *Arch Int Med*. 1995;155:701-709.
56. Kasiske BL, Ma JZ, Kalil RS, Louis TA. Effects of antihypertensive therapy on serum lipids. *Ann Int Med*. 1995;122:133-141.
57. Olsen MH, Wachtell K, Beevers G, et al. Effects of losartan compared with atenolol on lipids in patients with hypertension and left ventricular hypertrophy: the Losartan Intervention For Endpoint reduction in hypertension study. *J Hypertens*. 2009;27:567-574.
58. Lakshman MR, Reda DJ, Materson BJ, Cushman WC, Freis ED. Diuretics and beta-blockers do not have adverse effects at 1 year on plasma lipid and lipoprotein profiles in men with hypertension. Department of Veterans Affairs Cooperative study group on antihypertensive agents. *Arch Int Med*. 1999;159:551-558.
59. Keech A, Simes RJ, Barter P, et al. Effects of long-term fenofibrate therapy on cardiovascular events in 9795 people with type 2 diabetes mellitus (the FIELD study): randomised controlled trial. *Lancet*. 2005;366:1849-1861.
60. Group AS, Ginsberg HN, Elam MB, et al. Effects of combination lipid therapy in type 2 diabetes mellitus. *N Engl J Med*. 2010;362:1563-1574.
61. Group HTC, Landray MJ, Haynes R, et al. Effects of extended-release niacin with laropiprant in high-risk patients. *N Engl J Med*. 2014;371:203-212.
62. Everett BM, Smith RJ, Hiatt WR. Reducing LDL with PCSK9 inhibitors—The clinical benefit of lipid drugs. *N Engl J Med*. 2015;373(17):1588-1591.
63. Smith RJ, Hiatt WR. Two new drugs for homozygous familial hypercholesterolemia: managing benefits and risks in a rare disorder. *JAMA Int Med*. 2013;173:1491-1492.
64. Ray KK, Vallejo-Vaz AJ. The evolving role of CETP inhibition: beyond HDL cholesterol. *Lancet*. 2015;386:412-414.
65. Barter PJ, Caulfield M, Eriksson M, et al. Effects of torcetrapib in patients at high risk for coronary events. *N Engl J Med*. 2007;357:2109-2122.
66. Schwartz GG, Olsson AG, Abt M, et al. Effects of dalcetrapib in patients with a recent acute coronary syndrome. *N Engl J Med*. 2012;367:2089-2099.
67. Sabatine MS, Giugliano RP, Wiviott SD, et al. Efficacy and safety of evolocumab in reducing lipids and cardiovascular events. *N Engl J Med*. 2015;372:1500-1509.

68. Dadu RT, Ballantyne CM. Lipid lowering with PCSK9 inhibitors. *Nat Rev Cardiol.* 2014;11:563-575.

69. Robinson JG, Farnier M, Krempf M, et al. Efficacy and safety of alirocumab in reducing lipids and cardiovascular events. *N Engl J Med.* 2015;372:1489-1499.

70. Cohen JC, Boerwinkle E, Mosley TH Jr., Hobbs HH. Sequence variations in PCSK9, low LDL, and protection against coronary heart disease. *N Engl J Med.* 2006;354:1264-1272.

71. Berger JM, Vaillant N, Le May C, et al. PCSK9-deficiency does not alter blood pressure and sodium balance in mouse models of hypertension. *Atherosclerosis.* 2015;239:252-259.

72. Blom DJ, Hala T, Bolognese M, et al., DESCARTES Investigators. A 52-week placebo-controlled trial of evolocumab in hyperlipidemia. *N Engl J Med.* 2014;370(19):1809-1819.

73. Cannon CP, Shah S, Dansky HM, et al. Determining the Efficacy and Tolerability Investigators. Safety of anacetrapib in patients with or at high risk for coronary heart disease. *N Engl J Med.* 2010;363(25):2406-2415.

74. Yvan-Charvet L, Kling J, Pagler T, et al. Cholesterol efflux potential and antiinflammatory properties of high-density lipoprotein after treatment with niacin or anacetrapib. *Arterioscler Thromb Vasc Biol.* 2010;30(7):1430-1438.

75. REVEAL: Randomized EValuation of the Effects of Anacetrapib Through Lipid-modification. ClinicalTrials.gov, NCT01252953. https://clinicaltrials.gov/ct2/show/NCT01252953.

76. Nicholls SJ, Brewer HB, Kastelein JJ, et al. Effects of the CETP inhibitor evacetrapib administered as monotherapy or in combination with statins on HDL and LDL cholesterol: a randomized controlled trial. *JAMA.* 2011;306(19):2090-2109.

77. Rader DJ, Ruotolo G, Kane JP, et al. Effects of the Cholesteryl Ester Transfer Protein Inhibitor, Evacetrapib, Administered as Monotherapy or in Combination With Statins on Cholesterol Efflux and HDL Particles in Patients With Dyslipidemia. *Circulation.* 2014;130:A12252.

78. A Study of Evacetrapib in High-Risk Vascular Disease (ACCELERATE). ClinicalTrials.gov, NCT01687998. https://www.clinicaltrials.gov/ct2/show/NCT01687998.

79. Stein EA, Gipe D, Bergeron J, et al. Effect of a monoclonal antibody to PCSK9, REGN727/SAR236553, to reduce low-density lipoprotein cholesterol in patients with heterozygous familial hypercholesterolaemia on stable statin dose with or without ezetimibe therapy: a phase 2 randomised controlled trial. *Lancet.* 2012;380(9836):29-36.

80. McKenney JM, Koren MJ, Kereiakes DJ, et al. Safety and efficacy of a monoclonal antibody to proprotein convertase subtilisin/kexin type 9 serine protease, SAR236553/REGN727, in patients with primary hypercholesterolemia receiving ongoing stable atorvastatin therapy. *J Am Coll Cardiol.* 2012;59(25):2344-2353.

81. ODYSSEY Outcomes: Evaluation of Cardiovascular Outcomes After an Acute Coronary Syndrome During Treatment With Alirocumab SAR236553 (REGN727). ClinicalTrials.gov, NCT01663402. https://clinicaltrials.gov/ct2/show/NCT01663402.

82. Giugliano RP, Desai NR, Kohli P, et al. LAPLACE-TIMI 57 Investigators. Efficacy, safety, and tolerability of a monoclonal antibody to proprotein convertase subtilisin/kexin type 9 in combination with a statin in patients with hypercholesterolaemia (LAPLACE---TIMI 57): a randomised, placebo-controlled, dose-ranging, phase 2 study. *Lancet.* 2012;380(9858):2007-2017.

83. Desai NR, Kohli P, Giugliano RP, et al. AMG145, a monoclonal antibody against proprotein convertase subtilisin kexin type 9, significantly reduces lipoprotein(a) in hypercholesterolemic patients receiving statin therapy: an analysis from the LDL-C Assessment with Proprotein Convertase Subtilisin Kexin Type 9 Monoclonal Antibody Inhibition Combined with Statin Therapy (LAPLACE)-Thrombolysis in Myocardial Infarction (TIMI) 57 trial. *Circulation.* 2013;128(9):962-969.

84. Koren MJ, Lundqvist P, Bolognese M, et al. MENDEL-2 Investigators. Anti-PCSK9 monotherapy for hypercholesterolemia: the MENDEL-2 randomized, controlled phase III clinical trial of evolocumab. *J Am Coll Cardiol.* 2014;63(23):2531-2540.

85. Further Cardiovascular Outcomes Research With PCSK9 Inhibition in Subjects With Elevated Risk (FOURIER). ClinicalTrials.gov, NCT01764633. https://clinicaltrials.gov/ct2/show/NCT01764633.

86. Morrone D, Weintraub WS, Toth PP, et al. Lipid-altering efficacy of ezetimibe plus statin and statin monotherapy and identification of factors associated with treatment response: a pooled analysis of over 21,000 subjects from 27 clinical trials. *Atherosclerosis.* 2012;223(2):251-261.

87. Berthold HK, Gouni-Berthold I. Hyperlipoproteinemia(a): clinical significance and treatment options. *Atheroscler Suppl.* 2013;14(1):1-5.

88. Blazing MA, Giugliano RP, Cannon CP, et al. Evaluating cardiovascular event reduction with ezetimibe as an adjunct to simvastatin in 18,144 patients after acute coronary syndromes: final baseline characteristics of the IMPROVE-IT study population. *Am Heart J.* 2014;168(2):205-212. e1.

89. Kohno T. Report of the American Heart Association (AHA) Scientific Sessions 2014, Chicago. *Circ J.* 2015;79:34-40.

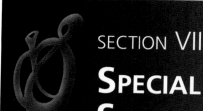

39 Hypertension in Pregnancy

Line Malha, Tiina Podymow, and Phyllis August

Hypertensive disorders are the most common medical conditions during pregnancy and are a leading cause of maternal and perinatal morbidity and mortality worldwide. Hypertension complicates 6% to 10% of pregnancies[1] and, of 4 million women giving birth in the United States each year, an estimated 240,000 are affected by hypertension.[2] Of concern, hypertension is the most important risk factor for stroke and there has been an overall rise in the incidence of pregnancy-related stroke and subsequent morbidity in the past 20 years.[3] Although maternal mortality rates are reduced considerably in developed compared with developing nations, hypertension still accounts for 15% of maternal deaths in the U.S., mostly as a result of intracerebral hemorrhage.[4]

Although the obstetrician manages most cases of hypertension during pregnancy, the internist, cardiologist, or nephrologist may be consulted if hypertension precedes conception, if end organ damage is present, or when accelerated hypertension occurs. This chapter assumes a medical perspective focusing on nonobstetrical diagnostic and therapeutic issues in the care of pregnant women with hypertension.

CLASSIFICATION AND DEFINITIONS

Hypertension in pregnancy generally refers to a blood pressure (BP) of 140/90 mm Hg or above. In most obstetric guidelines it is broken down into two categories of severity: mild-moderate (140 to 159/90 to 109 mm Hg) and severe (≥160/110 mm Hg).[5] Four major hypertensive disorders in pregnancy have been described by the American College of Obstetricians and Gynecologists (ACOG)[6]: (1) chronic hypertension; (2) preeclampsia-eclampsia; (3) chronic hypertension with superimposed preeclampsia; and (4) gestational hypertension.

Based on the 1980 to 2010 national hospital discharge survey data sets, out of 120 million births, 3.8% were complicated by preeclampsia; of these patients, 0.97% had chronic hypertension (0.24% had superimposed preeclampsia), and 2% had gestational hypertension[7] All four types may lead to maternal and perinatal complications, however, the syndrome of preeclampsia is associated with the highest maternal and fetal risks.[8]

Chronic Hypertension

Chronic hypertension is defined as blood pressure (BP) 140/90 or higher mm Hg that either predates pregnancy or develops before 20 weeks.[6] Chronic hypertension complicates 3.6% to 9.1% of pregnancies[9] and is usually (88.8%) attributed to essential hypertension.[10] Higher rates may be seen in older women, obese women, and African Americans.

Preeclampsia-Eclampsia

This syndrome occurs in 2% to 5% of pregnancies[7,11,12] and is responsible for up to 12% to 15% of maternal deaths.[8] The morbidity and mortality risks seem to be higher in women of African-American descent.[13,14]

Preeclampsia is a pregnancy-specific syndrome that develops in the latter half of pregnancy. It is characterized by a de novo onset of hypertension (BP ≥ 140/90 mm Hg) after 20 weeks of gestation and traditionally, proteinuria (>0.3 g per day). More recently, it has been recognized that nonproteinuric forms of preeclampsia exist, and guidelines[6] have updated their diagnostic criteria of preeclampsia to include additional signs/symptoms: neurological symptoms, thrombocytopenia (platelets < 100,000/μL), pulmonary edema, transaminitis (alanine aminotransferase [ALT], or aspartate aminotransferase [AST] above twice the normal range) and renal insufficiency (creatinine > 1.1 mg/dL or doubling). In the absence of proteinuria, a woman can still be diagnosed with preeclampsia if she has any of the above listed signs/symptoms assuming these findings cannot be attributed to another illness.[6]

A severe variant of preeclampsia features hemolysis, elevated liver enzymes, low platelets (HELLP) syndrome, which occurs in 1 in 1000 pregnancies. Eclampsia complicates approximately 3% of cases of preeclampsia and is the occurrence of seizures that cannot be attributed to other causes.

Chronic Hypertension With Superimposed Preeclampsia

Women with chronic hypertension are at an increased risk to develop superimposed preeclampsia, which complicates 25% of chronic hypertensive pregnancies (versus 5% of nonhypertensive pregnancies).[15] The diagnosis of superimposed preeclampsia is made in women with chronic hypertension if proteinuria or a severe feature of preeclampsia develops for the first time after 20 weeks, in association with an increase in BP.[6]

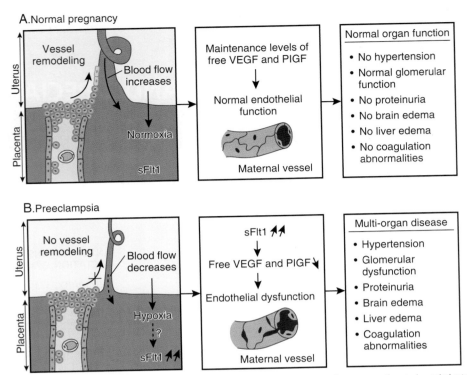

FIG. 39.1 Hypothesis on the role of soluble fms-like tyrosine kinase 1 (sFlt1) in preeclampsia. A, During normal pregnancy, the uterine spiral arteries are infiltrated and remodeled by endovascular invasive trophoblasts, thereby increasing blood flow significantly to meet the oxygen and nutrient demands of the fetus. B, In the placenta of preeclamptic women, trophoblast invasion does not occur and blood flow is reduced, resulting in placental hypoxia. In addition, increased amounts of sFlt1 are produced by the placenta and scavenge vascular endothelial growth factor (VEGF) and placental growth factor (PlGF), thereby lowering circulating levels of unbound VEGF and PlGF. This altered balance causes generalized endothelial dysfunction, resulting in multiorgan disease. It remains unknown whether hypoxia is the trigger for stimulating sFlt1 secretion in the placenta of preeclamptic mothers and whether the higher sFlt1 levels interfere with trophoblast invasion and spiral artery remodeling. *(From Luttun A, Carmeliet P. Soluble VEGF receptor Flt1: the elusive preeclampsia factor discovered? J Clin Investig. 2003;111:600-602.)*

In women with both hypertension and proteinuria before 20 weeks of gestation, superimposed preeclampsia is diagnosed (1) when there is a sudden increase in proteinuria or a sudden increase in BP in the latter half of pregnancy in a woman whose hypertension had previously been well controlled; or (2) as part of the HELLP syndrome, when there is new onset of thrombocytopenia with hemolysis and elevated levels of ALT or AST.[16]

Gestational Hypertension

Gestational hypertension, seen in 6% of pregnancies, is hypertension developing after 20 weeks not associated with the systemic features of preeclampsia (e.g., proteinuria). Some women (up to 25%) may ultimately develop signs of preeclampsia, so the final diagnosis of gestational hypertension can only be made postpartum.

CLINICAL FEATURES AND MANAGEMENT OF CHRONIC HYPERTENSION DURING PREGNANCY

Clinical Features and Diagnosis

The prevalence of hypertension in women of reproductive age (18 to 44 years old) is close to 9.3% in whites, 19.2% in African Americans, and 8.2% in Hispanics and increases with age.[17] Nearly 2% of all pregnancies are complicated by chronic hypertension.[18]

If hypertension is clearly documented before conception, the diagnosis of chronic hypertension in pregnancy is straightforward (Figs. 39.1, 39.2). Chronic hypertension is also the most likely diagnosis when hypertension is present before 20

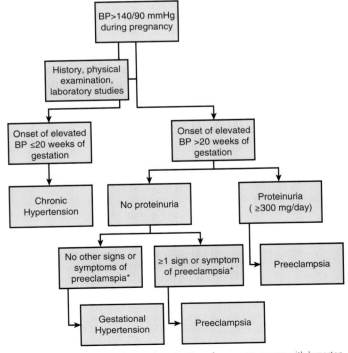

FIG. 39.2 Algorithm for diagnostic evaluation of pregnant women with hypertension. *BP*, Blood pressure. *The signs and symptoms of preeclampsia should not be attributable to any other disease and include: neurological symptoms (headaches, abnormal vision, altered mental status, etc), pulmonary edema, hepatocellular injury (serum transaminase levels ≥2 times normal), thrombocytopenia (<100,000 platelets/mm³) and renal insufficiency (creatinine>1.1 mg/dL or doubling).

weeks of gestation. Routine laboratory tests including platelets, liver function tests, blood urea nitrogen, creatinine, uric acid; and quantification of proteinuria should be performed at baseline in women with early pregnancy hypertension, to determine the clinical significance of any later changes in BP or laboratory tests.

The distinction between chronic hypertension (first noted in pregnancy) and gestational hypertension may be difficult to establish until after delivery. In some patients with undocumented chronic hypertension BPs will run normal throughout the entire pregnancy and then return to prepregnancy hypertensive levels in the postpartum period, accounting for the unusual but mysterious cases of isolated postpartum hypertension.

BP normally falls in early pregnancy; systolic blood pressure (SBP) changes little, whereas diastolic blood pressure (DBP) falls by approximately 10 mm Hg by 13 to 20 weeks, with a nadir at 24 weeks, and then rises again to prepregnancy levels in the third trimester (weeks 28 to 40). This physiologic fall may be more exaggerated in women with chronic hypertension. The BP usually rises in the third trimester to prepregnancy values and the differential in these patients includes undiagnosed chronic hypertension, gestational hypertension, or preeclampsia. In such cases, the diagnosis of preeclampsia should be ruled out by verifying the absence of proteinuria or other signs/symptoms of preeclampsia or HELLP syndrome. The patient should be asked about cerebral or visual symptoms; abdominal pain and laboratory testing for serum uric acid, liver function tests, renal function, complete blood count, and urine protein/creatinine should be done.

Although early onset hypertension (before 20 weeks gestation) is most often a result of chronic hypertension, it may, on rare occasions, be an indication of early-onset preeclampsia; such women require urine protein measurements and preeclampsia labs. They should be treated to target (see later)

and followed closely, particularly if they had no history of previous hypertension. When blood pressure increases in mid pregnancy (16 to 24 weeks), early preeclampsia should be considered because in healthy pregnancies, blood pressure usually decreases at this time.

White coat hypertension (elevated office BP with normal BP outside the medical setting) is more likely to be present in the first, rather than the second trimester, with an estimated prevalence of 32%[19] and 3% to 4%[20] respectively. White coat hypertension does not appear to predispose to preeclampsia[19] or to worsen overall pregnancy outcomes.[20] Home BP monitoring or a noninvasive 24-hour BP monitor can distinguish white coat from true hypertension in the pregnant patient.

Although most women with chronic or preexisting hypertension have essential hypertension, consider the possibility of secondary hypertension. Young women with hypertension may be somewhat more likely (compared with middle-aged women) to have secondary hypertension (e.g., intrinsic renal disease, renovascular hypertension, primary aldosteronism, Cushing syndrome, pheochromocytoma). In select patients with severely elevated BP or with attributable symptoms or laboratory abnormalities, secondary hypertension may be considered in women planning a pregnancy or even in early pregnancy, as secondary hypertension is potentially curable and some forms are associated with increased morbidity during pregnancy[6] (Fig. 39.3). For example, if proteinuria is documented in early pregnancy, then noninvasive evaluation for renal disease may be indicated, including 24-hour urinary protein excretion or creatinine clearance, renal ultrasound, and serologic testing to rule out secondary glomerulopathies.

Primary aldosteronism is the most common form of curable hypertension. The hallmarks of this disorder are an increased aldosterone production, a suppressed plasma renin activity

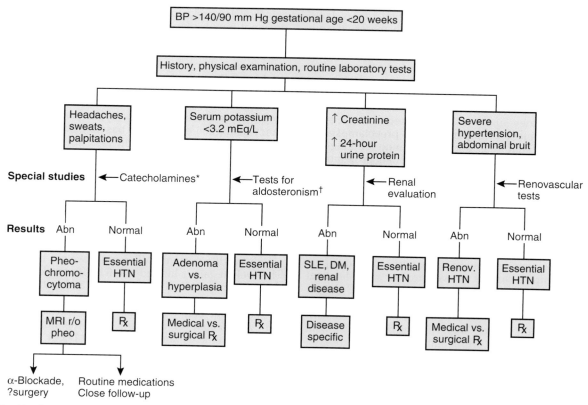

FIG. 39.3 Algorithm for diagnosis and treatment of secondary hypertension in pregnancy. Renal evaluation defined as serologic evaluation, 24-hour urine, renal ultrasound. Renovascular tests defined as renin (normally elevated in pregnancy) Doppler ultrasound of renal arteries. *Serum and urine. †Renin, urine aldosterone, urine potassium; difficult to interpret in pregnancy. *Abn,* Abnormal; *BP,* blood pressure; *DM,* diabetes mellitus; *HTN,* hypertension; *MRI,* magnetic resonance imaging; *pheo,* pheochromocytoma; *r/o,* rule out; *treatment; SLE,* systemic lupus erythematosus.

(PRA), and hypokalemia. Diagnosis in pregnancy is very difficult, as progesterone (the hormone of pregnancy) acts as an aldosterone blocker, so aldosterone levels are physiologically elevated in the normal pregnant woman; in those with secondary hyperaldosteronism who are also pregnant, they are even more so. As a result of normal volume expansion, plasma renin is physiologically increased in pregnancy; however, PRA may be lowered between 1 ng per mL per hour and 4 ng per mL per hour in primary aldosteronism. During pregnancy, the clinical manifestations of primary aldosteronism are heterogeneous and range from an improvement of hypertension/hypokalemia to difficult-to-control hypertension and hypokalemia. In cases when primary aldosteronism is quiescent during pregnancy, clinicians need to be vigilant of a rebound in hypertension and hypokalemia after delivery. If the disease is diagnosed early in pregnancy, the patient may undergo laparoscopic adrenalectomy in the late first trimester or in the second trimester.[21]

Another form of secondary hypertension that may be considered is pheochromocytoma, which, although rare, is associated with high morbidity and mortality rates during pregnancy, particularly if undiagnosed.[21] This should be considered in pregnant women with severe hypertension, especially when associated with headache, anxiety, palpitations, pallor, and sweats.

Maternal Risks

Pregnancies in women with uncomplicated chronic hypertension are usually successful although such women are more likely to undergo cesarean delivery and be hospitalized for worsening hypertension. In addition to the previously mentioned increased risk for superimposed preeclampsia, women with chronic hypertension are at a three-fold increased risk of abruptio placentae which can lead to life-threatening maternal hemorrhage.[1] Other risks include accelerated hypertension with potential target organ damage and cerebrovascular catastrophes. Both maternal and fetal morbidity and mortality are greater when superimposed preeclampsia develops[15,22,23] with an increased risk of fatal intracerebral hemorrhage, particularly if posterior reversible encephalopathy is present.[24]

Women with chronic hypertension caused by advanced chronic kidney disease (CKD) may experience irreversible deterioration in kidney function during pregnancy regardless of the development of superimposed preeclampsia. If advanced CKD is present, (e.g., serum creatinine > 1.9 mg/dL, or 168 μmol/L), maternal hypertension, worsening proteinuria, and evolution to end-stage renal disease requiring dialysis are common.[25] Fetal complications include growth restriction and preterm delivery.[26,27]

Fetal Risks

Perinatal death rates are higher in pregnancies of women with chronic hypertension than in those without, and superimposed preeclampsia confers an even greater risk. Maternal chronic hypertension is a risk factor for intrauterine growth restriction (IUGR, defined as birth weight < 10th percentile), which is seen in 5% to 13% of pregnancies of women with chronic hypertension. When superimposed preeclampsia develops, all complications are magnified; IUGR is reported in 35% of pregnancies, delivery resulting in prematurity occurs in 13% to 54%, and fetal death is the outcome in less than 1%.

Data from large surveys suggest that infants born to mothers with chronic hypertension may have as much as a 30% increased risk for congenital malformations, especially cardiac malformations.[28] This risk is not significantly altered by antihypertensive therapy.[28]

Management

Management of the pregnant woman with chronic hypertension is ideally before conception, to establish the diagnosis and to rule out secondary hypertension.

Preconception is also the appropriate time to discuss the risks of hypertension in pregnancy: a high likelihood of a favorable outcome despite risks of superimposed preeclampsia (25%) and fetal complications. Adherence to appointment keeping is essential, because frequent visits increase the likelihood of detecting preeclampsia and other complications before they become life threatening. Similarly, home BP monitoring by the patient, especially in the latter half of pregnancy, is advised. The use of medications with deleterious fetal effects, such as angiotensin-converting enzyme (ACE) inhibitors, angiotensin II receptor blockers (ARBs), and direct renin inhibitors should be addressed (see "Medications" section). Finally, in complicated conditions such as kidney transplantation or diabetes mellitus (DM) with renal disease, a multidisciplinary team consisting of obstetricians and internists familiar with the care of pregnant women can optimize the chances of a successful outcome.[29] Before conception, we also recommend the modification of certain risk factors; for example, women with obesity are at a higher risk for gestational hypertension and women who are underweight (body mass index below 18.5 kg/m^2) are at a higher risk for preterm labor.[30]

Nonpharmacologic Management

The approach to hypertension in the gravid patient represents a departure from accepted guidelines for nonpregnant hypertensive individuals. Patients are not advised to exercise vigorously because of the concern that extreme physical exertion may potentially decrease uteroplacental blood flow, and is associated with a higher rate of preeclampsia.[31] Although this has not been extensively studied, one clinical trial showed that aerobic exercise thrice weekly may reduce the risk of developing hypertension and prevent excessive weight gain[32] during pregnancy. Moderate intensity walking probably does not impair placental flow,[33] however strenuous exercise remains contraindicated in pregnancy.[34] Of note, women who work outside the home have both higher BP and an increased risk of preeclampsia compared with those who report not working.[35] Decreased work hours and more rest may theoretically increase placental blood flow and decrease BP.

Excessive weight gain (of 36 lbs or more) has been associated with an increased risk of hypertensive diseases of pregnancy in all race/ethnicity or baseline body mass index (BMI) subgroups.[36] Excessive weight loss during pregnancy is not advisable though, even in obese women because it may compromise fetal growth and increase the risk for small for gestational age infants.[37] It is therefore advisable for women to limit their weight gain during pregnancy to the 2009 Institute of Medicine (IOM) recommendation because there is currently no proven weight gain limitation strategy that would improve pregnancy outcomes.[38,39] The IOM recommends a weight gain of 1 lb per week (in the second and third trimesters) for women with a normal BMI or underweight before pregnancy. This weight gain is limited to 0.6 lb per week in women with a prepregnancy BMI 25 to 29.9 kg/m^2 and to 0.5 lb per week in those with a BMI 30 kg/m^2 or above.[40]

Significant salt restriction is not advisable during pregnancy,[6] because of concerns that the normal, physiologic plasma volume expansion would not occur. It is however reasonable for women adhering to a low-sodium diet before conception to continue their dietary habits.[41]

Blood Pressure Treatment Targets

In nonpregnant adults, BP control decreases the long-term incidence of cardiovascular (CV) disease and mortality. During the 9 months of pregnancy, however, untreated mild (stage 1) hypertension is unlikely to lead to detectable adverse outcomes and antihypertensive drugs, in this setting, are used primarily to protect the mother from acute CV or cerebrovascular events.

With regards to prevention of preeclampsia, there is unfortunately little evidence that the treatment of mild to moderate hypertension early in pregnancy reduces the incidence of superimposed preeclampsia,[42,43] preterm birth,[44] or small-for-gestational age neonates.[42,45] A major benefit of BP medication use in all hypertensive pregnancies is to decrease the incidence of severe hypertension[42,46] and possibly decrease the risk for other fetal or maternal complications.[47] In women who ultimately develop preeclampsia, the risk of cerebrovascular events increases sharply with severe hypertension.[48]

There is widespread consensus among national and international guidelines to treat any BP 160/110 or higher mm Hg.[1,6,49-53] The ACOG[6] and American Heart Association/American Stroke Association (AHA/ASA)[49] recommend initiating hypertension treatment when BP 160/105 or higher mm Hg (if either value is reached). The Society of Obstetricians and Gynaecologists of Canada[50] has the same systolic threshold in its guidelines but tolerates a DBP up to 110 mm Hg before initiation of therapy. The AHA/ASA further suggests considering pharmacologic therapy for BPs 150 to 159/100 to 109 mm Hg to prevent worsening hypertension and strokes.[49] These numbers are aligned with the targets set by the European[51] and British[52] guidelines. However, the European Society of Cardiology (ESC)[51] goes even further to recommend treatment of BP 140/90 mm Hg or above in women *with organ damage,* symptoms or superimposed gestational hypertension on chronic hypertension.

For women *without end organ damage,* current guidelines vary, with recommendations to initiate treatment for BP thresholds ranging from 140/90 to 160/110 mm Hg or higher.[50,51] Summarized recommendations in accordance with those of the National High Blood Pressure Education Program (NHBEP) Working Group on High Blood Pressure in Pregnancy in 2000[1] advising when maternal BP reaches levels 150/90 to 100 mm Hg or higher, treatment should be initiated to avoid hypertensive vascular damage. As BP normally falls in early pregnancy, even in women with chronic hypertension, if there is *no known organ damage,* clinicians can consider discontinuing antihypertensive drugs and monitoring BP in those with stage 1 hypertension. Therapy can then be restarted at a BP of 145 to 150/90 to 100 mm Hg, regardless of the type of hypertension.[53] Orally administered antihypertensive agents should be used in standard doses in pregnancy as discussed later in this chapter. Overly aggressive, acute blood pressure lowering is not advised because this may lead to reductions in uteroplacental perfusion.[45,54]

A recent large clinical trial, the Control of Hypertension In Pregnancy Study (CHIPS), has addressed treatment targets for BP in 987 pregnant women with hypertension in pregnancy.[46] The majority of participants had preexisting hypertension but the study also included women with nonproteinuric gestational hypertension. This study demonstrated that women treated to lower blood pressure targets (130 to 140/85 mm Hg) had fewer episodes of severe hypertension. Importantly, there were no adverse fetal effects in the lower blood pressure target group, challenging the previous concern that lowering blood pressure to 'normal' might be associated with reduced fetal growth.[55] The incidence of preeclampsia was similar in women treated to standard, less-tight control (target DBP, 100 mm Hg) or tight control (target DBP, 85 mm Hg).

The ACOG recommends adjusting therapy to maintain BP in the 120 to 160/80 to 105 mm Hg range during pregnancy.[6] The target range is narrower in the Canadian[50] guidelines and is further divided into 130 to 155/80 to 105 mm Hg for women with chronic hypertension without comorbidities and less than 140/90 if comorbidities are present.

Pharmacologic Management

Many women with chronic hypertension in pregnancy have stage 1 hypertension, and if, as expected, BP decreases below 130 to 140/90 mm Hg by the end of the first trimester, reduced doses or discontinuation of antihypertensive medication may be possible. When pharmacologic treatment is required to control BP, the choices for antihypertensives is limited by their safety data in pregnancy. The United States Food and Drug Administration (FDA) classification of drugs in pregnancy designates most antihypertensive drugs as category C, stating that the drug should be given only if potential benefits justify potential risks to the fetus. This category cannot be interpreted as "no risk," and it is so broad as to preclude its usefulness in clinical practice. The most recent evidence assessing risks and benefits for the drugs to treat hypertension in pregnancy is reviewed later and in Table 39.1. These medications have the longest history of safe use in pregnancy, although some are rarely used in the nonpregnant population, because of side effects or inconvenient dosing schedules. The ACOG recommends labetalol, nifedipine, or methyldopa as first-line therapy.[6]

Central Adrenergic Agonists

Methyldopa continues to be widely used for treatment of hypertension in pregnancy; it has been found to be nonteratogenic during a 40-year history of use and has no known adverse uteroplacental or fetal effects. Birth weight and development in the first year are similar in children exposed *in utero* to methyldopa compared with placebo, as is neurocognitive development up to the age of 7 years. In trials, methyldopa has compared favorably with placebo agents in decreasing the occurrence of severe hypertension, in pregnancy, as well as hospital admissions.[44,47] Recent posthoc analysis from the CHIPS trial suggests that methyldopa may be associated with less preterm delivery, severe hypertension, and perinatal loss or high-level neonatal care for more than 48 hours compared with labetalol.[56] Prior studies comparing methyldopa with labetalol failed to reveal a clear outcomes advantage to either therapy.

The adverse effects of methyldopa are primarily as a result of its action at the brainstem and include decreased mental alertness, drowsiness, impaired sleep, and decreased salivation. It can cause elevated liver enzymes in 5%, with hepatitis or hepatic necrosis rarely reported, and has been associated with Coombs positivity, with (or more commonly without) associated hemolytic anemia.

Clonidine is another alpha-2 adrenergic agonist comparable with methyldopa with respect to safety and efficacy; of some concern is a reported transient hypertension and excess of sleep disturbance in exposed infants without sequelae at 1 year of age.[57] Clonidine should be avoided in early pregnancy because of suspected embryopathy; there is little justification for its use in preference to methyldopa, given the proven safety of the latter. There is potential for rebound hypertension when clonidine is abruptly discontinued, so it is reserved for individuals who develop rash or liver dysfunction with methyldopa.

Beta-Adrenoceptor Blockers

Beta-blockers have been studied extensively in pregnancy and none have been associated with teratogenicity. Atenolol in one very small study resulted in clinically significant fetal growth restriction compared with placebo.[58] Parenteral beta-blockade has been associated with neonatal bradycardia which rarely has required intervention.[59] Reassurance is derived from a 1-year follow-up study,[60] which showed normal development of infants exposed to beta-blockers *in utero*.

Maternal outcomes improve with the use of beta-blockers, which controls maternal BP and decreases both the incidence of severe hypertension and the rate of admission to hospital

TABLE 39.1 Drugs[a] for Chronic Hypertension in Pregnancy[b]

DRUG (FDA RISK)[c]	DOSE	CONCERNS OR COMMENTS
Preferred Agent		
Methyldopa (B)	0.5-3 g/day in 2-3 divided doses	Drug of choice according to NHBEP working group; safety after first trimester well documented, including 7-year follow-up of offspring.
Second-Line Agents[d]		
Labetalol (C)	200-1200 mg/day in 2-3 divided doses	May be associated with fetal growth restriction and neonatal bradycardia.
Nifedipine (C)	30-90 mg/day of a slow-release preparation	
Hydralazine (C)	50-300 mg/day in 2-4 divided doses	Few controlled trials, but long experience with few adverse events documented; useful only in combination with sympatholytic agent. May cause neonatal thrombocytopenia.
β-Receptor blockers (C)	Depends on specific agent	May cause fetal bradycardia; this effect may be less for agents with partial agonist activity. May impair fetal response to hypoxic stress; possible risk for lower birth weight when started in first or second trimester (especially atenolol).
Hydrochlorothiazide (C)	25 mg/day	May cause volume depletion and electrolyte disorders. May be useful in combination with methyldopa and vasodilator to mitigate compensatory fluid retention.
Contraindicated		
ACE inhibitors and AT1 receptor antagonists (D)[e]		Leads to fetal loss in animals; human use in second and third trimester associated with fetopathy, oligohydramnios, growth restriction, and neonatal anuric renal failure, which may be fatal.

[a]No antihypertensive has been proven safe for use during the first trimester.
[b]Drug therapy indicated for uncomplicated chronic hypertension when diastolic blood pressure ≥100 mm Hg (using Korotkoff V phase for diastolic measurement). Treatment at lower levels may be indicated for patients with diabetes mellitus, renal disease, or target organ damage.
[c]United States Food and Drug Administration classification.
[d]Some agents are omitted (e.g., clonidine, alpha blockers) as a result of limited data on use for chronic hypertension in pregnancy.
[e]Authors would classify in category X during second and third trimeesters.
ACE, Angiotensin-converting enzyme; *AT1*, angiotensin I; *FDA*, United States Food and Drug Administration; *NHBEP*, National High Blood Pressure Education Program.

before delivery. Beta-blockers have been compared with, and found equivalent to, methyldopa in 13 trials.[61] Adverse effects resulting from beta-blockade include fatigue, lethargy, exercise intolerance, sleep disturbance, and bronchoconstriction.

Labetalol, a nonselective beta-blocker with vascular alpha₁-receptor–blocking properties has gained wide acceptance in pregnancy, and is as safe and effective as methyldopa.[61] Labetalol does not decrease uterine blood flow[62] but has been associated with fetal growth restriction in one placebo-controlled study.[63] It is used parenterally to treat severe hypertension and has been associated with a lower incidence of maternal hypotension and other side effects compared with hydralazine.[64] Prescribers should be aware of the rare, but potentially dangerous, association with hepatic injury.[65]

Alpha-Adrenergic Blockers

Alpha-adrenergic blockers are indicated during pregnancy in the management of pheochromocytoma.[21] Both prazosin and phenoxybenzamine have been used, along with β-blockers as adjunctive agents only if sufficient alpha blockade has been achieved. There is limited experience with these agents in pregnancy.

Calcium Channel Blockers

Calcium channel blockers (CCBs) have been used to treat chronic hypertension, mild preeclampsia presenting late in gestation, and severe hypertension associated with preeclampsia. Orally administered nifedipine and verapamil do not appear to pose teratogenic risk to fetuses exposed in the first trimester. Although the numbers of treated patients are small, these data are reassuring, as women with hypertension associated with kidney disease or transplantation may be difficult to manage during pregnancy without CCBs. Maternal side effects include tachycardia, palpitations, peripheral edema, and headaches (which tend to resolve after a few doses).[66]

Long-acting nifedipine is commonly used in pregnancy without causing a detectable decrease in uterine blood flow,[67] and is considered to be a safe first-line agent in the treatment of severe hypertension.[5] *Short-acting nifedipine* has been withdrawn from the market in several countries and is not recommended in older patients because of its association with an increased incidence of myocardial infarction and death in hypertensive (nonpregnant) patients with coronary artery disease. In pregnancy, short acting nifedipine continues to be used by some,[68,69] although it has been associated with maternal hypotension[70] and fetal distress.[71] Our preference is to use long-acting preparations; onset of action is similar to the short-acting preparations.

There are several reports documenting the safety of other calcium channel blockers[72] including: amlodipine,[73,74] nicardipine,[75,76] isradipine,[77-79] felodipine,[80] diltiazem,[81,82] and verapamil.[83]

Diuretics

Although diuretics are widely used in the treatment of nonpregnant hypertensives, there is reluctance on the part of obstetricians to use diuretics because of the concern that they will interfere with the physiologic volume expansion of normal pregnancy. Of interest, a 1985 meta-analysis of trials involving more than 7000 subjects suggested that diuretics prevented preeclampsia, and were not associated with adverse effects.[84] Although volume contraction might be expected to limit fetal growth, outcome data do not support these concerns. Diuretics are commonly prescribed in essential hypertension before conception and, given their apparent safety, NHBEP concluded that they may be continued through gestation or used in combination with other agents.[85] The use of the loop diuretic *furosemide* in the postpartum period in women with preeclampsia has been reported to be beneficial for blood pressure control while in the hospital[86] and potentially even after discharge.[87] More studies are required and in progress[88] to determine the role for loop diuretics in the treatment of postpartum hypertension in women with preeclampsia.

Hydrochlorothiazide can be used throughout pregnancy in low doses (12.5 to 25 mg/day), to minimize the side effects of impaired glucose tolerance and hypokalemia.[59] *Triamterene and amiloride* are not teratogenic, based on small numbers of case reports.[59] *Spironolactone* is not recommended because of antiandrogenic effects during fetal development in animal models, but does not seem to cause adverse outcomes in small human cohorts.[89] We do not recommend its use during pregnancy, and based on limited data, if a potassium-sparing diuretic is needed amiloride is recommended.

Direct Vasodilators

Hydralazine is effective orally, intramuscularly, or intravenously (IV). Adverse effects are mostly those associated with vasodilation and sympathetic nervous system activation and include headache, nausea, flushing, and palpitations. In rare cases, chronic use can lead to a polyneuropathy or to a drug-induced lupus syndrome (typically with high doses). Hydralazine has been used in all trimesters of pregnancy and has not been associated with teratogenicity, although neonatal thrombocytopenia and lupus have been reported. Other adverse effects associated with hydralazine include a decrease in uterine blood flow[62] and an increased risk for prolonged severe hypotension.[90] In acute severe hypertension during pregnancy, IV hydralazine is useful for rapid BP control, but has been associated with more adverse events compared with IV labetalol or oral nifedipine,[64] including maternal hypotension, cesarean section, placental abruption, Apgar scores lower than 7, and oliguria. Furthermore, side effects of hydralazine (headache, nausea, and vomiting) mimic the symptoms of deteriorating preeclampsia.

Oral hydralazine has been used for chronic hypertension in the second and third trimesters but has been largely supplanted by medications with more favorable side effect profiles.[66]

Nitroprusside is seldom used in pregnancy; its use is limited to cases of life-threatening refractory hypertension associated with heart failure. Adverse effects include vasodilation and syncope in volume-depleted preeclamptic women. The risk of fetal cyanide intoxication is unknown but is a concern. Given the availability of safer medications, this drug is considered a last resort.

Isosorbide dinitrate has been investigated in two small studies in women with gestational hypertension and preeclampsia.[91,92] It was found to lower BP while maintaining cerebral perfusion, thus decreasing the risk for ischemia and infarction.

Serotonin₂-Receptor Blockers

Although not approved by the FDA in the United States, *Ketanserin* is a selective serotonin₂-receptor–blocking drug that decreases systolic and diastolic BP in nonpregnant patients with acute or chronic hypertension. Ketanserin has been found to be nonteratogenic in animals and humans and has been studied primarily in Australia and South Africa in small trials of pregnant women. These studies suggest it may be safe and useful in treatment of chronic hypertension in pregnancy, preeclampsia, and HELLP syndrome.[93] However Ketanserin does not control BP as well as hydralazine in women with severe hypertension in pregnancy and is not considered a drug of choice in this clinical context.[94]

Angiotensin-Converting Enzyme Inhibitors and Angiotensin Receptor Blockers

ACE inhibitors and ARBs are contraindicated in the second or third trimesters because of toxicity associated with reduced perfusion to the fetal kidneys; their use is associated with a fetopathy similar to that observed in Potter syndrome (i.e., bilateral renal agenesis) including renal dysgenesis, oligohydramnios as a result of fetal oliguria, calvarial and pulmonary hypoplasia, IUGR, and neonatal anuric renal failure, leading to death of the fetus. ARB use in pregnancy has also been associated with fetal demise.

ACE inhibitor use and exposure in the first trimester is controversial for many physicians and requires counselling prepregnancy regarding the risks and benefits of this treatment

up to the first trimester, as well as the need for vigilance in stopping ACE inhibitors before the second trimester.

In 2006, a report linked first trimester exposure to ACE inhibitors with a greater incidence of malformations of the CV and central nervous systems.[95] Since this time, other reports, including a meta-analysis, have emerged describing an increase in cardiac malformations in fetuses exposed to *all* classes of antihypertensive drugs.[96-98] As such, current evidence does not suggest that ACE inhibitors in the first trimester are associated with a greater risk of fetal malformations than any other antihypertensives, and women in whom ACE inhibitors are of distinct benefit (e.g., diabetic nephropathy) should be counselled prepregnancy regarding the risks and benefits of this treatment up to the first trimester, as well as the need for vigilance in stopping ACE inhibitors before the second trimester. However, given the controversy and potential for risk, ACE inhibitor exposure in first trimester must be counselled and managed carefully, and in some cases where adherence to advice may be unreliable, switching to alternate agents before conception may be advisable.[99]

CLINICAL FEATURES AND MANAGEMENT OF PREECLAMPSIA

Preeclampsia is characterized by the development of hypertension in association with new-onset proteinuria, after 20 weeks gestation. It is recognized that not all women with preeclampsia will have proteinuria; therefore, additional signs and symptoms of organ dysfunction are sufficient to make the diagnosis. These newly recognized diagnostic criteria include: neurological symptoms (headaches, abnormal vision, altered mental status, etc), pulmonary edema, hepatocellular injury (serum transaminase levels ≥ 2 times normal), thrombocytopenia (<100,000 platelets/mm³), and renal insufficiency (creatinine > 1.1mg/dL or doubling). Edema has been abandoned as a marker of preeclampsia, because it is present in many normal pregnant women and lacks specificity. Nonproteinuric preeclampsia is associated with better outcomes than proteinuric preeclampsia but worse outcomes than gestational hypertension.[100]

The most recent ACOG guidelines[6] and the International Society for the study of Hypertension in Pregnancy (ISSHP)[101] guidelines have set 300 mg of urinary protein in a 24-hour collection or a urine protein/creatinine ratio of 0.3 in a spot sample as a cutoff value to diagnose proteinuria. Although protein to creatinine ratios determined on spot urines are considered to be adequate for quantification of proteinuria,[102,103] some obstetricians remain reluctant to abandon 24-hour urine collections. Proteinuria should be quantified in all patients suspected of having preeclampsia. If quantitative assays are not available, then at least 1+ proteinuria on dipstick testing is considered sufficient for a diagnosis.

The recent ACOG has recommended that the term "mild" preeclampsia be abandoned because preeclampsia can always lead to a rapidly deteriorating clinical status. All women with preeclampsia should be continuously evaluated for signs of severe features of preeclampsia. These severe features include the signs/symptoms listed above in addition to BP 160/110 or higher mm Hg (measured at least twice within 4 hours).[6] The HELLP syndrome is considered to be a manifestation of severe preeclampsia.[6,104] The magnitude of proteinuria has not been shown to correlate with adverse maternal or perinatal outcomes, and thus, is probably not a reliable indicator of the severity of preeclampsia.[105]

Risk Factors for Preeclampsia

Women at an increased risk for preeclampsia include those with chronic hypertension especially secondary forms of hypertension (renovascular hypertension, pheochromocytoma,

---

BOX 39.1 Risk Factors for Preeclampsia

- Nulliparity
- Multiple gestation
- Family history of preeclampsia
- Chronic hypertension
- Diabetes
- Renal disease
- History of preeclampsia, especially if early (before 34 weeks) in a previous pregnancy
- History of HELLP syndrome in previous pregnancy
- Obesity
- Hydatidiform mole

HELLP, Hemolysis, elevated liver enzymes, low platelets.

---

primary aldosteronism), early preeclampsia (before 34 weeks gestation) in a previous pregnancy, diabetes mellitus (DM), obesity, collagen-vascular disease, chronic kidney disease, a multifetal pregnancy, and women who themselves are the product of a pregnancy complicated by preeclampsia (Box 39.1). Recommended tests to discriminate preeclampsia from chronic or gestational hypertension later in pregnancy include hematocrit/hemoglobin, platelet count, serum creatinine and uric acid, and liver function tests. If qualitative dipstick proteinuria is documented, then protein quantification should be performed. We recommend obtaining baseline laboratory evaluation early in gestation in women with any of these risk factors.

Prediction of Preeclampsia

There is extensive literature evaluating various clinical signs or laboratory tests to predict preeclampsia[106,107]; none are considered sensitive or specific enough yet to warrant widespread clinical application. Dysregulation of angiogenic factors has been reported in pregnancies affected by preeclampsia, often before clinical signs and symptoms are apparent. There is compelling evidence that they are involved in the pathogenesis of the disease, particularly renal manifestations.[108,109] The factors that have been reported include elevated soluble fms-like tyrosine kinase-1 (sFlt-1), which is a circulating form of a receptor for vascular endothelial growth factor (VEGF),[110] decreased placental growth factor (PlGF),[110] increased endoglin,[111-113] and increased hypoxia-induced factor-1 (HIF-1).[114,115] Measurement of the ratio of sFlt-1/PlGF holds considerable promise for distinguishing preeclampsia from other hypertensive disorders, and for predicting adverse maternal and fetal outcomes in women who are being evaluated for preeclampsia.[112,116-119] Although promising, these lab tests are not readily available in most hospitals at this time, and with regards to clinically predicting the likelihood of preeclampsia, their use is a theoretical one.

Pathophysiology of Preeclampsia

The pathophysiology of preeclampsia has been divided into two stages: alterations in placental perfusion, and the later manifestations of the maternal syndrome. Abnormalities begin in the developing placenta, with impaired uteroplacental blood flow[120] leading to immune dysregulation, ischemia, and to the generation and release of substances such as angiogenic factors (e.g., sFlt-1, endoglin), syncytiotrophoblast microparticles, and others,[108] which upon reaching the maternal circulation produce endothelial dysfunction and the maternal clinical syndrome.[108]

Studies of placental tissue from women who later developed preeclampsia demonstrate impaired uterine artery remodeling and failure of the trophoblasts to invade the myometrial portion of the spiral arteries.[120] Placental blood flow is diminished, and ensuing placental ischemia early in the second trimester is thought to trigger the release of placenta-derived factors causing the multisystem maternal disorder. There is an increased incidence of preeclampsia in women with medical conditions associated with microvascular disease, such as hypertension, DM, and collagen-vascular disease, and impaired placental perfusion may be the common starting point of this disease.

Immune Dysregulation

Immune dysregulation is believed to play a role in the pathogenesis of preeclampsia. Compared with healthy pregnancies, preeclampsia is associated with decreased circulating regulatory (Foxp3 positive) CD4+ T cells, increased immune activating (Il-17 producing) CD4+ T cells,[121] and increased placental bed natural killer cells.[122] Overactivity of the complement system related to mutations in complement regulatory genes has been reported in preeclampsia.[123,124]

Additionally, angiotensin 1 receptor autoantibodies have been detected in patients with preeclampsia and placental syndromes.[125] The role of these antibodies in the pathophysiology of preeclampsia has yet to be clearly defined. Attempts to induce preeclampsia in animal models have had mixed success, and these antibodies have not been detected in all human cases.

Blood Pressure in Preeclampsia

Blood pressure in preeclampsia is often labile and elevated owing to a reversal of the vasodilation of normal pregnancy and increased peripheral vascular resistance.[126] There is reversal of the normal circadian rhythm, with BPs often being higher at night. This is mediated, at least in part, by an increase in sympathetic vasoconstrictor activity, which reverts to normal after delivery, usually within days to weeks. Investigations of gravid dogs, rats, and primates have demonstrated that acute reduction of uterine perfusion results in maternal hypertension. As mentioned, compromised uteroplacental perfusion is believed to be of pathophysiologic significance in the preeclampsia syndrome.

Metabolic Disturbances in Preeclampsia

Obesity remains an important risk factor for preeclampsia, with a strong positive association between maternal prepregnancy body mass index and the risk of preeclampsia.[127,128] Early pregnancy dyslipidemia and gestational DM are also associated with a two to three-fold increased risk of preeclampsia. These conditions may be markers of endothelial dysfunction or may cause increased oxidative stress in preeclampsia.

Renal Changes in Preeclampsia

In preeclampsia, there is a modest decrease in glomerular filtration, and filtration fraction (about 25%). Because glomerular filtration rate normally rises 35% to 50% during pregnancy, serum creatinine levels are usually still below the upper limits of normal. Fractional uric acid clearance decreases, often before overt disease is apparent, and a serum uric acid greater than 5.5 mg per dL (327 μmol/L) is a marker of preeclampsia, presumably because of decreased renal clearance and glomerular filtration. Urinary calcium excretion decreases and increased parathyroid hormone and decreased 1,25 dihydroxy vitamin D have been reported[129,130] in contrast to normal pregnancy, where vitamin D levels are usually increased as a result of placental conversion to active forms.[131] Proteinuria more than 0.3 g, but less than 3 g per day (but in some cases in the nephrotic range of >3 g/day) is a hallmark of proteinuric preeclampsia. Rarely, acute kidney injury may develop as a result of acute tubular or, rarely, cortical necrosis attributed to hypotension-associated obstetric hemorrhage.

Cardiac Function in Preeclampsia

Pulmonary artery catheterization studies of nulliparous gravidas with preeclampsia in the third trimester show decreased cardiac output (CO) in women with preeclampsia compared with controls.[132-134] The decrease in CO seems to occur after an initial increase in cardiac output[135] which has been repeatedly reported in the literature.[136-138] Peripheral vascular resistance is typically increased, and pulmonary capillary wedge pressure is in the low normal range in preeclampsia. There is impaired diastolic function[139,140] with a markedly increased afterload, also caused by increased vasoconstriction and peripheral vascular resistance. Peripartum heart failure can occur in this setting, although it is usually a complication of preexisting heart disease.

Plasma volume is increased in normal pregnancy; in preeclampsia, however, plasma volume is decreased and the renin-angiotensin system is suppressed. Thus the decreased plasma volume is as a result of vasoconstriction and a "smaller" intravascular compartment.

Central Nervous System

Eclampsia, defined as seizures in preeclampsia that cannot be attributed to another cause, is a serious central nervous system complication of pregnancy and is responsible for most maternal deaths. Seizures may occur when the BP is only modestly elevated. These are often preceded by headache (60% to 90%) and visual changes (in about 32%) including blurred vision, scotomas, and reversible cortical blindness (resulting from reversible posterior leukoencephalopathy).[141] In these cases, computed tomographic (CT) and magnetic resonance (MRI) scans show extensive bilateral white-matter abnormalities suggestive of vasogenic edema, without infarction, in the occipital and posterior parietal lobes of the cerebral hemispheres. Posterior reversible encephalopathy syndrome (PRES) is a frequent finding on neuroimaging in eclampsia.[142,143] The symptoms of PRES include headaches, altered mental status, severe hypertension, visual disturbances, and nausea/vomiting.[142] It is also more commonly seen in patients who are younger, thrombocytopenic, or proteinuric.[143]

Preeclampsia is associated with impaired cerebral blood flow auto regulation at all levels of blood pressure[144] even after lowering SBP below 140 mm Hg with medication.[145] Because of impaired auto regulation, the risk of stroke is elevated as soon as the SBP reaches 155 to 160 mm Hg.[48] DBP on the other hand has not been clearly associated with strokes in women with preeclampsia.[48] Intravenous magnesium sulfate is indicated for seizure prophylaxis in women with eclampsia, severe preeclampsia, and preeclampsia requiring C-section; it is not recommended for blood pressure treatment.[6]

Prevention of Preeclampsia

Strategies that have been studied but found not to be of benefit include sodium restriction, high-protein diets, vitamins C and E, fish oil, magnesium, and antihypertensive medication.

Aspirin has been investigated extensively for prevention of preeclampsia and as per the PARIS collaboration, has a protective effect reducing preeclampsia by 10% for those at risk, particularly if initiated early in pregnancy.[146-148] Some national[149] and international[150] guidelines, consider aspirin therapy beginning after the first trimester in any pregnant woman at a high risk for preeclampsia (see "Risk factors for preeclampsia" section). Aspirin appears most effective if taken at bedtime.[151]

Calcium supplementation in excess of the recommended dietary allowance has not been shown to reduce the incidence of superimposed preeclampsia in all populations. There is evidence from the developing world that in women with low dietary calcium intake, calcium supplementation of 1 gram daily or more may safely reduce the incidence of preeclampsia.[152]

Treatment with low molecular weight heparin (LMWH) has been investigated for the prevention of preeclampsia in high-risk groups. Clinical trials evaluating the benefits of anticoagulation have included heterogeneous study populations (e.g., patients with a history of miscarriage, thrombophilia, preeclampsia, small-for-gestational age deliveries) and have used composite endpoints to evaluate efficacy, therefore the results have been inconclusive although subgroup analysis suggests that in women with a prior history of severe or preterm preeclampsia, treatment with LMWH and low dose aspirin is associated with a lower risk of preeclampsia in a subsequent pregnancy.[153,154] Women with genetic or acquired thrombophilias such as the factor V Leiden variant, the prothrombin gene G20210A mutation, and elevated titers of the lupus anticoagulant may also benefit from LMWH.[155,156] In 2014, a Cochrane review[157] evaluated a pooled sample of 1228 women with a prior history of recurrent miscarriage with or without thrombophilia. LMWH (with enoxaparin or nadroparin) did not increase the incidence of live birth nor decrease the incidence of preeclampsia compared with aspirin or even to no treatment. Importantly, treatment with aspirin and LMWH was safe and not associated with an increase in major bleeding events. At this time, although the clinical trial evidence is inconclusive, there are encouraging results from case series and observational studies for a potential benefit of this therapy and we believe that more data from larger randomized clinical trials are needed.[158]

Treatment of Preeclampsia

Delivery

One of the most difficult management issues in preeclampsia is the timing of delivery in cases when fetal maturity is questionable. If preeclampsia presents remote from term (23 to 34 weeks gestation), bed rest, blood pressure management, and close monitoring of the maternal and fetal conditions may enable prolongation of pregnancy and improve maternal and fetal outcomes. Delivery should not be delayed if there are signs of fetal distress, or serious maternal disease (headache, abdominal pain, signs of HELLP syndrome)[159] or in cases of severe uncontrollable hypertension. Most cases of preeclampsia present close to term and can be managed with antihypertensive medication, bed rest with or without hospitalization, and delivery at 37 weeks or greater.[160] Expectant monitoring is usually preferred to delivery between 34 and 37 weeks of gestation[161] in women who do not have severe features of preeclampsia. Delivery is indicated in all women with preeclampsia when the gestational age is greater than 38 weeks.

Signs of severe maternal disease (see "Clinical features" section) are an indication for delivery when the gestational age is greater than 34 weeks. Fetal factors that may prompt delivery include fetal growth restriction, nonreassuring fetal testing results, and oligohydramnios.

The HELLP syndrome is associated with a poor prognosis and is usually an indication for urgent delivery. Women with liver involvement may develop epigastric or right upper quadrant pain from hepatocellular necrosis, ischemia, and/or edema that stretches the Glisson capsule. Elevations in liver enzymes are present. Hepatic rupture is a rare but fatal complication if not recognized early and treated aggressively with supportive therapy and surgery. The consultant should be aware of the potential severity of the development of epigastric, chest, or abdominal pain in a woman with preeclampsia.

Blood Pressure Control in Preeclampsia

The primary role of the internal medicine consultant in the care of women with preeclampsia is to participate in decisions regarding antihypertensive therapy. Lowering BP does not cure preeclampsia but may permit prolongation of pregnancy because uncontrolled hypertension is frequently an indication for delivery. In the latter half of pregnancy, if hypertension and other features of preeclampsia are detected, hospitalization should be considered to permit close monitoring of the patient.

In the days preceding and following delivery, BP can remain labile and dangerously high thereby increasing the risk for adverse maternal outcomes.[162] Oral agents are normally prescribed in this period. The main reason to lower BP in a woman with preeclampsia is to prevent maternal cerebrovascular and cardiovascular complications associated with elevated BP.[5,48] BP higher than 160/110 mm Hg requires treatment to reduce the risk of intracerebral hemorrhage and maternal death.[1] We usually initiate treatment before BP reaches 150/95 mm Hg to prevent the development of severe hypertension. If delivery is not anticipated immediately (within 24 to 48 hours), antihypertensive therapy should be considered when DBP reaches 95 to 100 mm Hg.

Women with hypertensive encephalopathy, brain hemorrhage, or eclampsia (seizures) require treatment with parenteral agents to lower mean arterial pressure (two-thirds diastolic + one-third systolic BP) by 10% to 25% over minutes to hours, and then to 160/100 mm Hg or less over subsequent hours[1] with a target of 140 to 150/90 to 100 mm Hg.[5] For blood pressure control when delivery is imminent, the three first-line agents of choice are: intravenous labetalol, intravenous hydralazine, and oral nifedipine[5] (Table 39.2). If these medications fail to control BP, the ACOG encourages consultation from a specialist and the use of continuous infusions of labetalol or nicardipine as second-line agents.[5]

Intravenous Fluid

Renal function in preeclampsia is usually well preserved, and oliguria is usually a manifestation of renal vasoconstriction rather than impaired glomerular filtration rate. It is not advisable to "push fluids" to increase urine output as aggressive hydration of women with preeclampsia may result in fluid overload and acute pulmonary edema, and if this happens, furosemide may be safely given. In women who have no oral intake before delivery, hydration should be maintained (100 to 150 mL/hour).

GESTATIONAL HYPERTENSION

This term refers to women in whom elevated blood pressure is detected for the first time during pregnancy, and no laboratory or clinical features of preeclampsia are noted. Older guidelines and texts referred to this as 'transient hypertension.' Women with gestational hypertension are at increased risk (as high as 25%) for developing preeclampsia, and should be followed closely. Treatment of hypertension is similar to women with preeclampsia or chronic hypertension. The differential diagnosis of gestational hypertension includes undiagnosed chronic hypertension where physiologic vasodilation has occurred with resultant lower BPs in the first half of pregnancy. Gestational hypertension can then only be diagnosed with certainty if blood pressure fails to normalize within 3 months postpartum.

POSTPARTUM MANAGEMENT OF HYPERTENSION

In the postpartum period, edema may worsen because of administration of intravenous fluids during delivery. Normal physiologic volume expansion and edema of pregnancy also begins to resolve, returning volume to the intravascular space. Hypertension is often worse in the first days postpartum, peaking by the fifth day, and finally resolving in the weeks postpartum.[163] Occasionally, hypertension develops for the first time in the postpartum period[164] as a result of a combination of volume expansion after cesarean section and administration of fluids, and the widespread use of high dose nonsteroidal antiinflammatory drugs for postpartum analgesia. On occasion, it may be necessary to administer small doses of diuretics if edema is debilitating.[87] Antihypertensive therapy should be used if blood pressures are consistently greater than 140/90 mm Hg. IV magnesium sulfate is routinely prescribed for 24 hours postpartum in women with preeclampsia. Although this medication may lower blood pressure, it is often necessary to use traditional antihypertensive medications for persistent hypertension. Antihypertensives prescribed antepartum should be continued in the postpartum period at the same doses; titration upward may be necessary. These medications are all safe in breastfeeding, and if ACE inhibitors are required, enalapril is considered safe in breastfeeding by the American Pediatrics Association.

If BP was normal before conception, then normalization is likely after 2 to 8 weeks postpartum. Hypertension that persists beyond 12 weeks postpartum may represent previously undiagnosed chronic hypertension or secondary

TABLE 39.2 Drugs for Urgent Control of Severe Hypertension in Pregnancy[a]

DRUG (FDA RISK)[b]	DOSE AND ROUTE	CONCERNS OR COMMENTS[c]
Labetalol (C)	20 mg IV, then 80 mg every 20-30 min, up to maximum of 300 mg; or constant infusion of 1-2 mg/min	Less risk of tachycardia and arrhythmia than with other vasodilators.
Hydralazine (C)	5 mg, IV or IM, then 5-10 mg every 20-40 min; or constant infusion of 0.5-10 mg/hour	Long experience of safety and efficacy.
Nifedipine (C)	Tablets recommended only: 10-30 mg PO	Safe to use in labor (once thought to interact with $MgSO_4$).
Relatively Contraindicated		
Nitroprusside (C)[d]	Constant infusion of 0.5-10 mcg/kg/min	Possible cyanide toxicity; agent of last resort.

[a]Indicated for acute elevation of diastolic blood pressure ≥105 mm Hg; goal is gradual reduction to 90 to 100 mm Hg.
[b]United States Food and Drug Administration classification, C, indicates that either studies in animals have revealed adverse effects on the fetus (teratogenic, embryocidal, or other) and/or there are no controlled studies in women, or studies in women and animals are not available. Drugs should only be given if the potential benefits justify the potential risk to the fetus.
[c]Adverse effects for all agents, except as noted, may include headache flushing, nausea, and tachycardia (primarily resulting from precipitous hypotension and reflex sympathetic activation).
[d]We would classify in category D: There is positive evidence of human fetal risk, but the benefits of use in pregnant women may be acceptable despite the risk (e.g., if the drug is needed in a life-threatening situation or for a serious disease for which safer drugs cannot be used or are ineffective).
IM, Intramuscular; *IV,* intravenous; *$MgSO_4$,* magnesium sulfate; *PO,* orally.

hypertension, which should be evaluated, followed, and treated (as appropriate).[163]

Evaluation should also be considered postpartum for patients with preeclampsia who developed the condition early (<34 weeks gestation), had severe or recurrent preeclampsia, or who have persistent proteinuria. In these cases, renal disease, secondary hypertension, and thrombophilias (e.g., antiphospholipid antibody syndrome) may be considered. Of note, laboratory testing for thrombophilias is usually delayed to 3 months postpartum if indicated.

Counseling for future pregnancies requires consideration of different recurrence rates for preeclampsia, depending on the pathogenesis and population characteristics. The earlier in gestation that preeclampsia develops, the higher the risk of recurrence; before week 30, recurrence rates may be as high as 40%. If preeclampsia has developed in a nulliparous woman close to term (i.e., after 36 weeks), the risk of recurrence is thought to be about 10%. Women who have had preeclampsia are also at increased risk for hypertension in future pregnancies. Patients who had HELLP syndrome have a high risk of subsequent obstetric complications, with preeclampsia occurring in 55%, although the rate of recurrent HELLP appears to be low, at only 6%.[159]

Hypertensive diseases of pregnancy have been associated with an elevated risk of hypertension, diabetes, cardiovascular disease, thromboembolism, and stroke later in life.[165] In one study, gestational hypertension was associated with a relative risk (RR) of 3.72 for subsequent hypertension, and preeclampsia with an RR of 3.98 for subsequent hypertension and 3.59 for stroke.[166] Preeclampsia is also a risk factor for coronary disease when studied retrospectively.[167] These associations may serve to inform patients of their potential risk, and to increase awareness of the need to monitor for future hypertensive and CV disorders in the decades to come. There are no evidence-based guidelines to determine a reasonable schedule for follow-up and screening. It may be of benefit to perform cardiovascular risk factor screening (blood pressure measurement, fasting glucose, weight, lipid profile) in the year following pregnancy as abnormalities may start to be detectable even this early.[168]

ANTIHYPERTENSIVE MEDICATIONS AND LACTATION

In general, drugs that are bound to plasma proteins are not transferred to breast milk. Lipid-soluble drugs may achieve higher concentrations than water-soluble drugs. Neonatal exposure to methyldopa, diltiazem, propranolol, enalapril, captopril, and nifedipine via nursing are low, and these medications are considered safe during breastfeeding.[169] Atenolol and metoprolol are concentrated in breast milk, possibly to levels that could affect the infant, and are not recommended. Labetalol can be detected in breast milk but has not been associated with adverse events in the infant.[169] Finally, although the concentration of diuretics in breast milk is low, these agents may reduce milk production as a result of mild volume contraction and may interfere with the ability to successfully breastfeed.

SUMMARY

Hypertensive disorders in pregnancy are associated with increased maternal and perinatal risks, with preeclampsia-eclampsia (regardless of BP level) and severe hypertension (regardless of type) associated with the greatest risks. It is clear that patients with a BP higher than 160/110 mm Hg must be treated to avoid cerebrovascular catastrophes in the mother. The benefits and risks of treating lower levels of BP are less clearly supported but seem to be safer than previously anticipated. There is no evidence that maintaining

lower blood pressure during pregnancy (i.e., 120/80 mm Hg) prevents preeclampsia in women with preexisting hypertension, although lower targets do appear safe for the fetus and may prevent BP spikes and hospitalization for the mother. We recommend treatment when BP levels 140 to 150/90 or higher mm Hg with oral labetalol, nifedipine, or methyldopa as first-line agents. Severe hypertension exceeding 160/110 mm Hg may result in maternal stroke or eclampsia. When delivery is imminent, parenteral therapy with intravenous labetalol, hydralazine, and/or oral nifedipine are used. Women at a high risk of preeclampsia can be treated with low dose aspirin therapy early in pregnancy. Women may remain hypertensive postpartum and require monitoring and often treatment for 2 to 8 weeks, and gestational hypertension and preeclampsia are now recognized by the American Heart Association as risk factors for future CV disease.

References

1. Report of the National High Blood Pressure Education Program Working Group on high blood pressure in pregnancy. *Am J Obstet Gynecol.* 2000;183:S1-S22.
2. Sibai BM. Antihypertensive drugs during pregnancy. *Semin Perinatol.* 2001;25:159-164.
3. Leffert LR, Clancy CR, Bateman BT, Bryant AS, Kuklina EV. Hypertensive disorders and pregnancy-related stroke: frequency, trends, risk factors, and outcomes. *Obstet Gynecol.* 2015;125:124-131.
4. Chang J, Elam-Evans LD, Berg CJ, et al. Pregnancy-related mortality surveillance—United States, 1991–1999. *MMWR Surveill Summ.* 2003;52:1-8.
5. American College of Obstetricians and Gynecologists (ACOG). Committee Opinion No 652: magnesium sulfate use in obstetrics. *Obstet Gynecol.* 2016;127:e52-e53.
6. Hypertension in pregnancy. Report of the American College of Obstetricians and Gynecologists' (ACOG) Task Force on Hypertension in Pregnancy. *Obstet Gynecol.* 2013;122:1122-1131.
7. Ananth CV, Keyes KM, Wapner RJ. Pre-eclampsia rates in the United States, 1980-2010: age-period-cohort analysis. *BMJ.* 2013;347:f6564.
8. Ghulmiyyah L, Sibai B. Maternal mortality from preeclampsia/eclampsia. *Semin Perinatol.* 2012;36:56-59.
9. Roberts CL, Ford JB, Algert CS, et al. Population-based trends in pregnancy hypertension and pre-eclampsia: an international comparative study. *BMJ Open.* 2011;1:e000101.
10. Bateman BT, Bansil P, Hernandez-Diaz S, Mhyre JM, Callaghan WM, Kuklina EV. Prevalence, trends, and outcomes of chronic hypertension: a nationwide sample of delivery admissions. *Am J Obstet Gynecol.* 2012;206:134.e131-e138.
11. Hernandez-Diaz S, Toh S, Cnattingius S. Risk of pre-eclampsia in first and subsequent pregnancies: prospective cohort study. *BMJ.* 2009;338:b2255.
12. Duley L. The global impact of pre-eclampsia and eclampsia. *Semin Perinatol.* 2009;33:130-137.
13. MacKay AP, Berg CJ, Atrash HK. Pregnancy-related mortality from preeclampsia and eclampsia. *Obstet Gynecol.* 2001;97:533-538.
14. Zhang J, Meikle S, Trumble A. Severe maternal morbidity associated with hypertensive disorders in pregnancy in the United States. *Hypertens Pregnancy.* 2003;22:203-212.
15. Sibai BM, Lindheimer M, Hauth J, et al. Risk factors for preeclampsia, abruptio placentae, and adverse neonatal outcomes among women with chronic hypertension. National Institute of Child Health and Human Development Network of Maternal-Fetal Medicine Units. *N Engl J Med.* 1998;339:667-671.
16. Sibai BM. Diagnosis, controversies, and management of the syndrome of hemolysis, elevated liver enzymes, and low platelet count. *Obstet Gynecol.* 2004;103:981-991.
17. Robbins CL, Zapata LB, Farr SL, et al. Core state preconception health indicators—pregnancy risk assessment monitoring system and behavioral risk factor surveillance system, 2009. *MMWR Surveill Summ.* 2014;63:1-62.
18. Bateman BT, Bansil P, Hernandez-Diaz S, Mhyre JM, Callaghan WM, Kuklina EV. Prevalence, trends, and outcomes of chronic hypertension: a nationwide sample of delivery admissions. *Am J Obstet Gynecol.* 2012;206:134.e131-e138.
19. Brown MA, Mangos G, Davis G, Homer C. The natural history of white coat hypertension during pregnancy. *BJOG.* 2005;112:601-606.
20. Brown MA, Robinson A, Jones M. The white coat effect in hypertensive pregnancy: much ado about nothing? *Br J Obstet Gynaecol.* 1999;106:474-480.
21. Malha L, August P. Secondary Hypertension in Pregnancy. *Curr Hypertens Rep.* 2015;17:53.
22. Vanek M, Sheiner E, Levy A, Mazor M. Chronic hypertension and the risk for adverse pregnancy outcome after superimposed pre-eclampsia. *Int J Gynaecol Obstet.* 2004;86:7-11.
23. Zetterstrom K, Lindeberg SN, Haglund B, Hanson U. Maternal complications in women with chronic hypertension: a population-based cohort study. *Acta Obstet Gynecol Scand.* 2005;84:419-424.
24. Dai X, Diamond JA. Intracerebral hemorrhage: a life-threatening complication of hypertension during pregnancy. *J Clin Hypertens (Greenwich, Conn.).* 2007;9:897-900.
25. Jones DC, Hayslett JP. Outcome of pregnancy in women with moderate or severe renal insufficiency. *N Engl J Med.* 1996;335:226-232.
26. Kendrick J, Sharma S, Holmen J, Palit S, Nuccio E, Chonchol M. Kidney disease and maternal and fetal outcomes in pregnancy. *Am J Kidney Dis.* 2015;66:55-59.
27. Maynard SE, Thadhani R. Pregnancy and the kidney. *JASN.* 2009;20:14-22.
28. Bateman BT, Huybrechts KF, Fischer MA, et al. Chronic hypertension in pregnancy and the risk of congenital malformations: a cohort study. *Am J Obstet Gynecol.* 2015;212:337.e331-e314.
29. Podymow T, August P. Pregnancy and gender issues in the renal transplant recipient. In: M W, ed. *Medical Management of Kidney Transplantation.* Philadelphia: Lippincott Williams & Wilkins; 2005:238-243.
30. Shin D, Song WO. Prepregnancy body mass index is an independent risk factor for gestational hypertension, gestational diabetes, preterm labor, and small- and large-for-gestational-age infants. *J Matern Fetal Neonatal Med.* 2015;28:1679-1686.
31. Haelterman E, Marcoux S, Croteau A, Dramaix M. Population-based study on occupational risk factors for preeclampsia and gestational hypertension. *Scan J Work Environ Health.* 2007;33:304-317.
32. Barakat R, Pelaez M, Cordero Y, et al. Exercise during pregnancy protects against hypertension and macrosomia. randomized clinical trial. *Am J Obstet Gynecol.* 2016;214:649.e1-e8.

33. de Oliveria Melo AS, Silva JL, Tavares JS, Barros VO, Leite DF, Amorim MM. Effect of a physical exercise program during pregnancy on uteroplacental and fetal blood flow and fetal growth: a randomized controlled trial. *Obstet Gynecol.* 2012;120:302-310.
34. Szymanski LM, Satin AJ. Strenuous exercise during pregnancy: is there a limit? *Am J Obstet Gynecol.* 2012;207:179.e171-e176.
35. Higgins JR, Walshe JJ, Conroy RM, Darling MR. The relation between maternal work, ambulatory blood pressure, and pregnancy hypertension. *J Epidemiol Comm Health.* 2002;56:389-393.
36. Masho SW, Urban P, Cha S, Ramus R. Body mass index, weight gain, and hypertensive disorders in pregnancy. *Am J Hypertens.* 2016;29:763-771.
37. Cox Bauer CM, Bernhard KA, Greer DM, Merrill DC. Maternal and neonatal outcomes in obese women who lose weight during pregnancy. *J Perinatol.* 2016;36:278-283.
38. Nicklas JM, Barbour LA. Optimizing weight for maternal and infant health—tenable, or too late? *Expert Rev Endocrinol Metab.* 2015;10:227-242.
39. Kapadia MZ, Park CK, Beyene J, Giglia L, Maxwell C, McDonald SD. Can we safely recommend gestational weight gain below the 2009 guidelines in obese women? A systematic review and meta-analysis. *Obes Rev.* 2015;16:189-206.
40. Determining Optimal Weight Gain. In: Rasmussen KM, Yaktine AL, eds. *Weight Gain During Pregnancy: Reexamining the Guidelines.* Washington DC: National Academy of Sciences.; 2009:241-262.
41. Duley L, Henderson-Smart D. Reduced salt intake compared to normal dietary salt, or high intake, in pregnancy. *Cochrane Database Syst Rev.* 2000;(2):CD001687.
42. Abalos E, Duley L, Steyn DW. Antihypertensive drug therapy for mild to moderate hypertension during pregnancy. *Cochrane Database Syst Rev.* 2014;(2):CD002252.
43. von Dadelszen P, Magee LA. Antihypertensive medications in management of gestational hypertension-preeclampsia. *Clin Obstet Gynecol.* 2005;48:441-459.
44. Sibai BM, Mabie WC, Shamsa F, Villar MA, Anderson GD. A comparison of no medication versus methyldopa or labetalol in chronic hypertension during pregnancy. *Am J Obstet Gynecol.* 1990;162:960-966. discussion 966-967.
45. Nakhai-Pour HR, Rey E, Berard A. Discontinuation of antihypertensive drug use during the first trimester of pregnancy and the risk of preeclampsia and eclampsia among women with chronic hypertension. *Am J Obstet Gynecol.* 2009;201:180: e181-e188.
46. Magee LA, von Dadelszen P, Rey E, et al. Less-tight versus tight control of hypertension in pregnancy. *N Engl J Med.* 2015;372:407-417.
47. Molvi SN, Mir S, Rana VS, Jabeen F, Malik AR. Role of antihypertensive therapy in mild to moderate pregnancy-induced hypertension: a prospective randomized study comparing labetalol with alpha methyldopa. *Arch Gynecol Obstet.* 2012;285:1553-1562.
48. Martin JN, Jr., Thigpen BD, Moore RC, Rose CH, Cushman J, May W. Stroke and severe preeclampsia and eclampsia: a paradigm shift focusing on systolic blood pressure. *Obstet Gynecol.* 2005;105:246-254.
49. Bushnell C, McCullough LD, Awad IA, et al. Guidelines for the prevention of stroke in women: a statement for healthcare professionals from the American Heart Association/American Stroke Association. *Stroke.* 2014;45:1545-1588.
50. Magee LA, Pels A, Helewa M, Rey E, von Dadelszen P. Diagnosis, evaluation, and management of the hypertensive disorders of pregnancy: executive summary. *JOGC.* 2014;36:416-441.
51. Regitz-Zagrosek V, Blomstrom Lundqvist C, Borghi C, et al. ESC Guidelines on the management of cardiovascular diseases during pregnancy: the Task Force on the Management of Cardiovascular Diseases during Pregnancy of the European Society of Cardiology (ESC). *Eur Heart J.* 2011;32:3147-3197.
52. Health NCCfWsaCs. *Hypertension in Pregnancy: The Management of Hypertensive Disorders During Pregnancy.* London: Royal College of Obstetricians and Gynaecologists; 2010.
53. Magee LA. Drugs in pregnancy. Antihypertensives. *Best Pract Res Clin Obstet Gynaecol.* 2001;15:827-845.
54. von Dadelszen P, Magee LA. Fall in mean arterial pressure and fetal growth restriction in pregnancy hypertension: an updated metaregression analysis. *JOGC.* 2002;24:941-945.
55. August P. Lowering diastolic blood pressure in non-proteinuric hypertension in pregnancy is not harmful to the fetus and is associated with reduced frequency of severe maternal hypertension. *Evid Based Med.* 2015;20:141.
56. Magee LA, von Dadelszen P, Singer J, et al. Do labetalol and methyldopa have different effects on pregnancy outcome? Analysis of data from the Control of Hypertension In Pregnancy Study (CHIPS) trial. *BJOG.* 2016;123:1143-1151.
57. Boutroy MJ, Gisonna CR, Legagneur M. Clonidine: placental transfer and neonatal adaption. *Early Hum Dev.* 1988;17:275-286.
58. Butters L, Kennedy S, Rubin PC. Atenolol in essential hypertension during pregnancy. *BMJ.* 1990;301:587-589.
59. Magee LA, Elran E, Bull SB, Logan A, Koren G. Risks and benefits of beta-receptor blockers for pregnancy hypertension: overview of the randomized trials. *Eur J Obstet Gynecol Reprod Biol.* 2000;88:15-26.
60. Reynolds B, Butters L, Evans J, Adams T, Rubin PC. First year of life after the use of atenolol in pregnancy associated hypertension. *Arch Dis Child.* 1984;59:1061-1063.
61. Magee LA, Duley L. Oral beta-blockers for mild to moderate hypertension during pregnancy. *Cochrane Database Syst Rev.* 2003.CD002863.
62. Baggio MR, Martins WP, Calderon AC, et al. Changes in fetal and maternal Doppler parameters observed during acute severe hypertension treatment with hydralazine or labetalol: a randomized controlled trial. *Ultrasound Med Biol.* 2011;37:53-58.
63. Sibai BM, Gonzalez AR, Mabie WC, Moretti M. A comparison of labetalol plus hospitalization versus hospitalization alone in the management of preeclampsia remote from term. *Obstet Gynecol.* 1987;70:323-327.
64. Magee LA, Cham C, Waterman EJ, Ohlsson A, von Dadelszen P. Hydralazine for treatment of severe hypertension in pregnancy: meta-analysis. *BMJ.* 2003;327:955-960.
65. Clark JA, Zimmerman HJ, Tanner LA. Labetalol hepatotoxicity. *Ann Intern Med.* 1990;113:210-213.
66. Magee LA, Miremadi S, Li J, et al. Therapy with both magnesium sulfate and nifedipine does not increase the risk of serious magnesium-related maternal side effects in women with preeclampsia. *Am J Obstet Gynecol.* 2005;193:153-163.
67. Moretti MM, Fairlie FM, Akl S, Khoury AD, Sibai BM. The effect of nifedipine therapy on fetal and placental Doppler waveforms in preeclampsia remote from term. *Am J Obstet Gynecol.* 1990;163:1844-1848.
68. Firoz T, Magee LA, MacDonell K, et al. Oral antihypertensive therapy for severe hypertension in pregnancy and postpartum: a systematic review. *BJOG.* 2014;121:1210-1218; discussion 1220.
69. Firoz T, Magee LA, Lalani S, et al. PP088. Oral antihypertensive therapy for severe hypertension in pregnancy. *Preg Hypertens.* 2012;2:288.
70. Brown MA, Buddle ML, Farrell T, Davis GK. Efficacy and safety of nifedipine tablets for the acute treatment of severe hypertension in pregnancy. *Am J Obstet Gynecol.* 2002;187:1046-1050.
71. Impey L. Severe hypotension and fetal distress following sublingual administration of nifedipine to a patient with severe pregnancy induced hypertension at 33 weeks. *Br J Obstet Gynaecol.* 1993;100:959-961.
72. Weber-Schoendorfer C, Hannemann D, Meister R, et al. The safety of calcium channel blockers during pregnancy: a prospective, multicenter, observational study. *Reproduct Toxicol (Elmsford, N.Y.).* 2008;26:24-30.
73. Vigil-De Gracia P, Dominguez L, Solis A. Management of chronic hypertension during pregnancy with furosemide, amlodipine or aspirin: a pilot clinical trial. *J Matern Fetal Neonatal Med.* 2014;27:1291-1294.
74. Ahn HK, Nava-Ocampo AA, Han JY, et al. Exposure to amlodipine in the first trimester of pregnancy and during breastfeeding. *Hypertens Preg.* 2007;26:179-187.
75. Nij Bijvank SW, Duvekot JJ. Nicardipine for the treatment of severe hypertension in pregnancy: a review of the literature. *Obstet Gynecol Surv.* 2010;65:341-347.
76. Bartels PA, Hanff LM, Mathot RA, Steegers EA, Vulto AG, Visser W. Nicardipine in pre-eclamptic patients: placental transfer and disposition in breast milk. *BJOG.* 2007;114:230-233.
77. Fletcher H, Roberts G, Mullings A, Forrester T. An open trial comparing isradipine with hydralazine and methyl dopa in the treatment of patients with severe pre-eclampsia. *J Obstet Gynaecol.* 1999;19:235-238.
78. Montan S, Anandakumar C, Arulkumaran S, Ingemarsson I, Ratnam S. Randomised controlled trial of methyldopa and isradipine in preeclampsia—effects on uteroplacental and fetal hemodynamics. *J Perinat Med.* 1996;24:177-184.
79. Wide-Swensson DH, Ingemarsson I, Lunell NO, et al. Calcium channel blockade (isradipine) in treatment of hypertension in pregnancy: a randomized placebo-controlled study. *Am J Obstet Gynecol.* 1995;173:872-878.
80. Casele HL, Windley KC, Prieto JA, Gratton R, Laifer SA. Felodipine use in pregnancy. Report of three cases. *J Reprod Med.* 1997;42:378-381.
81. Lubbe WF. Use of diltiazem during pregnancy. *NZ Med J.* 1987;100:121.
82. Khandelwal M, Kumanova M, Gaughan JP, Reece EA. Role of diltiazem in pregnant women with chronic renal disease. *J Matern Fetal Neonatal Med.* 2002;12:408-412.
83. Belfort MA, Anthony J, Buccimazza A, Davey DA. Hemodynamic changes associated with intravenous infusion of the calcium antagonist verapamil in the treatment of severe gestational proteinuric hypertension. *Obstet Gynecol.* 1990;75:970-974.
84. Collins R, Yusuf S, Peto R. Overview of randomised trials of diuretics in pregnancy. *BMJ (Clinical research ed.).* 1985;290:17-23.
85. Lenfant C. Working group report on high blood pressure in pregnancy. *J Clin Hypertens (Greenwich, Conn.).* 2001;3:75-88.
86. Magee L, von Dadelszen P. Prevention and treatment of postpartum hypertension. *Cochrane Database System Rev.* 2013;4. CD004351.
87. Ascarelli MH, Johnson V, McCreary H, Cushman J, May WL, Martin JN, Jr. Postpartum preeclampsia management with furosemide: a randomized clinical trial. *Obstet Gynecol.* 2005;105:29-33.
88. Cursino T, Katz L, Coutinho I, Amorim M. Diuretics vs. placebo for postpartum blood pressure control in preeclampsia (DIUPRE): a randomized clinical trial. *Reprod Health.* 2015;12:66.
89. Riester A, Reincke M. Progress in primary aldosteronism: mineralocorticoid receptor antagonists and management of primary aldosteronism in pregnancy. *Eur J Endocrinol/Eur Fed Endocrine Soc.* 2015;172:R23-30.
90. Duley L, Meher S, Jones L. Drugs for treatment of very high blood pressure during pregnancy. *Cochrane Database System Rev.* 2013;7:CD001449.
91. Thaler I, Amit A, Kamil D, Itskovitz-Eldor J. The effect of isosorbide dinitrate on placental blood flow and maternal blood pressure in women with pregnancy induced hypertension. *Am J Hypertens.* 1999;12:341-347.
92. Martinez-Abundis E, Gonzalez-Ortiz M, Hernandez-Salazar F, Huerta JLMT. Sublingual isosorbide dinitrate in the acute control of hypertension in patients with severe preeclampsia. *Gynecol Obstet Invest.* 2000;50:39-42.
93. Bolte AC, van Geijn HP, Dekker GA. Pharmacological treatment of severe hypertension in pregnancy and the role of serotonin(2)-receptor blockers. *Eur J Obstet Gynecol Reprod Biol.* 2001;95:22-36.
94. Bijvank SW, Visser W, Duvekot JJ, et al. Ketanserin versus dihydralazine for the treatment of severe hypertension in early-onset preeclampsia: a double blind randomized controlled trial. *Eur J Obstet Gynecol Reprod Biol.* 2015;189:106-111.
95. Cooper WO, Hernandez-Diaz S, Arbogast PG, et al. Major congenital malformations after first-trimester exposure to ACE inhibitors. *N Engl J Med.* 2006;354:2443-2451.
96. Lennestal R, Otterblad Olausson P, Kallen B. Maternal use of antihypertensive drugs in early pregnancy and delivery outcome, notably the presence of congenital heart defects in the infants. *Eur J Clin Pharmacol.* 2009;65:615-625.
97. Walfisch A, Al-maawali A, Moretti ME, Nickel C, Koren G. Teratogenicity of angiotensin converting enzyme inhibitors or receptor blockers. *J Obstet Gynaecol.* 2011;31:465-472.
98. Li DK, Yang C, Andrade S, Tavares V, Ferber JR. Maternal exposure to angiotensin converting enzyme inhibitors in the first trimester and risk of malformations in offspring: a retrospective cohort study. *BMJ.* 2011;343:d5931.
99. Podymow T, Joseph G. Preconception and pregnancy management of women with diabetic nephropathy on angiotensin converting enzyme inhibitors. *Clin Nephrol.* 2015;83:73-79.
100. Homer CS, Brown MA, Mangos G, Davis GK. Non-proteinuric pre-eclampsia: a novel risk indicator in women with gestational hypertension. *J Hypertens.* 2008;26:295-302.
101. Tranquilli AL, Dekker G, Magee L, et al. The classification, diagnosis and management of the hypertensive disorders of pregnancy: A revised statement from the ISSHP. *Preg Hypertens.* 2014;4:97-104.
102. Cote AM, Brown MA, Lam E, et al. Diagnostic accuracy of urinary spot protein:creatinine ratio for proteinuria in hypertensive pregnant women: systematic review. *BMJ.* 2008;336:1003-1006.
103. Brown MA. Pre-eclampsia: proteinuria in pre-eclampsia-does it matter any more? *Nat Rev Nephrol.* 2012;8:563-565.
104. Tranquilli AL, Brown MA, Zeeman GG, Dekker G, Sibai BM. The definition of severe and early-onset preeclampsia. Statements from the International Society for the Study of Hypertension in Pregnancy (ISSHP). *Preg Hypertens.* 2013;3:44-47.
105. Payne B, Magee LA, Cote AM, et al. PIERS proteinuria: relationship with adverse maternal and perinatal outcome. *JOGC.* 2011;33:588-597.
106. August P, Helseth G, Cook EF, Sison C. A prediction model for superimposed preeclampsia in women with chronic hypertension during pregnancy. *Am J Obstet Gynecol.* 2004;191:1666-1672.
107. Than NG, Romero R, Hillermann R, Cozzi V, Nie G, Huppertz B. Prediction of preeclampsia—a workshop report. *Placenta.* 2008;29(Suppl A):S83-85.
108. Steegers EA, von Dadelszen P, Duvekot JJ, Pijnenborg R. Pre-eclampsia. *Lancet.* 2010;376:631-644.
109. Rana S, Karumanchi SA, Lindheimer MD. Angiogenic factors in diagnosis, management, and research in preeclampsia. *Hypertension.* 2014;63:198-202.
110. Maynard SE, Min JY, Merchan J, et al. Excess placental soluble fms-like tyrosine kinase 1 (sFlt1) may contribute to endothelial dysfunction, hypertension, and proteinuria in preeclampsia. *J Clin Invest.* 2003;111:649-658.

111. Venkatesha S, Toporsian M, Lam C, et al. Soluble endoglin contributes to the pathogenesis of preeclampsia. *Nat Med.* 2006;12:642-649.
112. Rana S, Cerdeira AS, Wenger J, et al. Plasma concentrations of soluble endoglin versus standard evaluation in patients with suspected preeclampsia. *PloS One.* 2012;7:e48259.
113. Levine RJ, Lam C, Qian C, et al. Soluble endoglin and other circulating antiangiogenic factors in preeclampsia. *N Engl J Med.* 2006;355:992-1005.
114. Rath G, Aggarwal R, Jawanjal P, Tripathi R, Batra A. HIF-1 alpha and placental growth factor in pregnancies complicated with preeclampsia: a qualitative and quantitative analysis. *J Clin Lab Anal.* 2016;30:75-83.
115. Iriyama T, Wang W, Parchim NF, et al. Hypoxia-independent upregulation of placental hypoxia inducible factor-1alpha gene expression contributes to the pathogenesis of preeclampsia. *Hypertension.* 2015;65:1307-1315.
116. Stubert J, Ullmann S, Bolz M, et al. Prediction of preeclampsia and induced delivery at <34 weeks gestation by sFLT-1 and PlGF in patients with abnormal midtrimester uterine Doppler velocimetry: a prospective cohort analysis. *BMC Pregnancy Childbirth.* 2014;14:292.
117. Liu Y, Zhao Y, Yu A, Zhao B, Gao Y, Niu H. Diagnostic accuracy of the soluble Fms-like tyrosine kinase-1/placental growth factor ratio for preeclampsia: a meta-analysis based on 20 studies. *Arch Gynecol Obstet.* 2015;292:507-518.
118. Zeisler H, Llurba E, Chantraine F, et al. Predictive value of the sFlt-1:PlGF ratio in women with suspected preeclampsia. *N Engl J Med.* 2016;374:13-22.
119. Gomez-Arriaga PI, Herraiz I, Lopez-Jimenez EA, Escribano D, Denk B, Galindo A. Uterine artery Doppler and sFlt-1/PlGF ratio: prognostic value in early-onset pre-eclampsia. *Ultrasound Obstet Gynecol.* 2014;43:525-532.
120. Fisher SJ. Why is placentation abnormal in preeclampsia? *Am J Obstet Gynecol.* 2015;213:S115-122.
121. Santner-Nanan B, Peek MJ, Khanam R, et al. Systemic increase in the ratio between Foxp3+ and IL-17-producing CD4+ T cells in healthy pregnancy but not in preeclampsia. *J Immunol.* 2009;183:7023-7030.
122. Redman CW, Sargent IL. Immunology of pre-eclampsia. *Am J Reprod Immunol.* 2010;63:534-543.
123. Lynch AM, Salmon JE. Dysregulated complement activation as a common pathway of injury in preeclampsia and other pregnancy complications. *Placenta.* 2010;31:561-567.
124. Salmon JE, Heuser C, Triebwasser M, et al. Mutations in complement regulatory proteins predispose to preeclampsia: a genetic analysis of the PROMISSE cohort. *PLoS Med.* 2011;8:e1001013.
125. Wallukat G, Homuth V, Fischer T, et al. Patients with preeclampsia develop agonistic autoantibodies against the angiotensin AT1 receptor. *J Clin Invest.* 1999;103:945-952.
126. Ganzevoort W, Rep A, Bonsel GJ, de Vries JI, Wolf H. Plasma volume and blood pressure regulation in hypertensive pregnancy. *J Hypertens.* 2004;22:1235-1242.
127. Doherty DA, Magann EF, Francis J, Morrison JC, Newnham JP. Pre-pregnancy body mass index and pregnancy outcomes. *Int J Gynaecol Obstet.* 2006;95:242-247.
128. Bhattacharya S, Campbell DM, Liston WA, Bhattacharya S. Effect of Body Mass Index on pregnancy outcomes in nulliparous women delivering singleton babies. *BMC Public Health.* 2007;7:168.
129. Taufield PA, Ales KL, Resnick LM, Druzin ML, Gertner JM, Laragh JH. Hypocalciuria in preeclampsia. *N Engl J Med.* 1987;316:715-718.
130. August P, Marcaccio B, Gertner JM, Druzin ML, Resnick LM, Laragh JH. Abnormal 1,25-dihydroxyvitamin D metabolism in preeclampsia. *Am J Obstet Gynecol.* 1992;166:1295-1299.
131. Delvin EE, Arabian A, Glorieux FH, Mamer OA. In vitro metabolism of 25-hydroxycholecalciferol by isolated cells from human decidua. *J Clin Endocrinol Metabol.* 1985;60:880-885.
132. Benedetti TJ, Cotton DB, Read JC, Miller FC. Hemodynamic observations in severe pre-eclampsia with a flow-directed pulmonary artery catheter. *Am J Obstet Gynecol.* 1980;136:465-470.
133. Visser W, Wallenburg HC. Central hemodynamic observations in untreated preeclamptic patients. *Hypertension.* 1991;17:1072-1077.
134. Groenendijk R, Trimbos JB, Wallenburg HC. Hemodynamic measurements in preeclampsia: preliminary observations. *Am J Obstet Gynecol.* 1984;150:232-236.
135. Bosio PM, McKenna PJ, Conroy R, O'Herlihy C. Maternal central hemodynamics in hypertensive disorders of pregnancy. *Obstet Gynecol.* 1999;94:978-984.
136. Easterling TR, Benedetti TJ, Schmucker BC, Millard SP. Maternal hemodynamics in normal and preeclamptic pregnancies: a longitudinal study. *Obstet Gynecol.* 1990;76:1061-1069.
137. Hjertberg R, Belfrage P, Hagnevik K. Hemodynamic measurements with Swan-Ganz catheter in women with severe proteinuric gestational hypertension (pre-eclampsia). *Acta Obstet Gynecolog Scan.* 1991;70:193-198.
138. Mabie WC, Ratts TE, Sibai BM. The central hemodynamics of severe preeclampsia. *Am J Obstet Gynecol.* 1989;161:1443-1448.
139. Melchiorre K, Sutherland GR, Baltabaeva A, Liberati M, Thilaganathan B. Maternal cardiac dysfunction and remodeling in women with preeclampsia at term. *Hypertension.* 2011;57:85-93.
140. Solanki R, Maitra N. Echocardiographic assessment of cardiovascular hemodynamics in preeclampsia. *J Obstet Gynaecol India.* 2011;61:519-522.
141. Katz VL, Farmer R, Kuller JA. Preeclampsia into eclampsia: toward a new paradigm. *Am J Obstet Gynecol.* 2000;182:1389-1396.
142. Brewer J, Owens MY, Wallace K, et al. Posterior reversible encephalopathy syndrome in 46 of 47 patients with eclampsia. *Am J Obstet Gynecol.* 2013;208:468.e461-e466.
143. Fisher N, Saraf S, Egbert N, Homel P, Stein EG, Minkoff H. Clinical Correlates of Posterior Reversible Encephalopathy Syndrome in Pregnancy. *J Clin Hypertens (Greenwich).* 2016;18:522-527.
144. van Veen TR, Panerai RB, Haeri S, Griffioen AC, Zeeman GG, Belfort MA. Cerebral autoregulation in normal pregnancy and preeclampsia. *Obstet Gynecol.* 2013;122:1064-1069.
145. Sonneveld MJ, Brusse IA, Duvekot JJ, Steegers EA, Grune F, Visser GH. Cerebral perfusion pressure in women with preeclampsia is elevated even after treatment of elevated blood pressure. *Acta Obstet Gynecol Scand.* 2014;93:508-511.
146. Duley L, Henderson-Smart DJ, Meher S, King JF. Antiplatelet agents for preventing pre-eclampsia and its complications. *Cochrane Database System Rev.* 2007:CD004659.
147. Askie LM, Duley L, Henderson-Smart DJ, Stewart LA. Antiplatelet agents for prevention of pre-eclampsia: a meta-analysis of individual patient data. *Lancet.* 2007;369:1791-1798.
148. Bujold E, Roberge S, Lacasse Y, et al. Prevention of preeclampsia and intrauterine growth restriction with aspirin started in early pregnancy: a meta-analysis. *Obstet Gynecol.* 2010;116:402-414.
149. Henderson JT, Whitlock EP, O'Conner E, Senger CA, Thompson JH, Rowland MG, U.S. Preventive Services Task Force Evidence Syntheses, formerly Systematic Evidence Reviews. *Low-Dose Aspirin for the Prevention of Morbidity and Mortality From Preeclampsia: A Systematic Evidence Review for the U.S. Preventive Services Task Force.* Rockville (MD): Agency for Healthcare Research and Quality (US); 2014.
150. WHO Guidelines Approved by the Guidelines Review Committee. *WHO Recommendations for Prevention and Treatment of Pre-Eclampsia and Eclampsia.* Geneva: World Health Organization; 2011.
151. Hermida RC, Ayala DE, Fernandez JR, et al. Administration time-dependent effects of aspirin in women at differing risk for preeclampsia. *Hypertension.* 1999;34:1016-1023.
152. Hofmeyr GJ, Lawrie TA, Atallah AN, Duley L, Torloni MR. Calcium supplementation during pregnancy for preventing hypertensive disorders and related problems. *Cochrane Database System Rev.* 2014;6. CD001059.
153. de Vries JI, van Pampus MG, Hague WM, Bezemer PD, Joosten JH. Low-molecular-weight heparin added to aspirin in the prevention of recurrent early-onset pre-eclampsia in women with inheritable thrombophilia: the FRUIT-RCT. *J Thromb Haemost.* 2012;10:64-72.
154. Gris JC, Chauleur C, Molinari N, et al. Addition of enoxaparin to aspirin for the secondary prevention of placental vascular complications in women with severe pre-eclampsia. The pilot randomised controlled NOH-PE trial. *Thromb Haemost.* 2011;106:1053-1061.
155. Bouvier S, Cochery-Nouvellon E, Lavigne-Lissalde G, et al. Comparative incidence of pregnancy outcomes in thrombophilia-positive women from the NOH-APS observational study. *Blood.* 2014;123:414-421.
156. Robertson L, Wu O, Langhorne P, et al. Thrombophilia in pregnancy: a systematic review. *Br J Haematol.* 2006;132:171-196.
157. de Jong PG, Kaandorp S, Di Nisio M, Goddijn M, Middeldorp S. Aspirin and/or heparin for women with unexplained recurrent miscarriage with or without inherited thrombophilia. *Cochrane Database System Rev.* 2014;7:CD004734.
158. Roberge S, Demers S, Nicolaides KH, Bureau M, Cote S, Bujold E. Prevention of pre-eclampsia by low-molecular weight heparin in addition to aspirin: a meta-analysis. *Ultrasound Obstet Gynecol.* 2016;47:548-553.
159. Chames MC, Haddad B, Barton JR, Livingston JC, Sibai BM. Subsequent pregnancy outcome in women with a history of HELLP syndrome at < or = 28 weeks of gestation. *Am J Obstet Gynecol.* 2003;188:1504-1507; discussion 1507–1508.
160. Koopmans CM, Bijlenga D, Groen H, et al. Induction of labour versus expectant monitoring for gestational hypertension or mild pre-eclampsia after 36 weeks' gestation (HYPITAT): a multicentre, open-label randomised controlled trial. *Lancet.* 2009;374:979-988.
161. Broekhuijsen K, van Baaren GJ, van Pampus MG, et al. Immediate delivery versus expectant monitoring for hypertensive disorders of pregnancy between 34 and 37 weeks of gestation (HYPITAT-II): an open-label, randomised controlled trial. *Lancet.* 2015;385:2492-2501.
162. August P, Malha L. Postpartum Hypertension: "It Ain't Over 'til It's Over". *Circulation.* 2015;132:1690-1692.
163. Podymow T, August P. Postpartum course of gestational hypertension and preeclampsia. *Hypertens Preg.* 2010;29:294-300.
164. Goel A, Maski MR, Bajracharya S, et al. Epidemiology and mechanisms of de novo and persistent hypertension in the postpartum period. *Circulation.* 2015;132:1726-1733.
165. Lykke JA, Langhoff-Roos J, Sibai BM, Funai EF, Triche EW, Paidas MJ. Hypertensive pregnancy disorders and subsequent cardiovascular morbidity and type 2 diabetes mellitus in the mother. *Hypertension.* 2009;53:944-951.
166. Wilson BJ, Watson MS, Prescott GJ, et al. Hypertensive diseases of pregnancy and risk of hypertension and stroke in later life: results from cohort study. *BMJ.* 2003;326:845.
167. Haukkamaa L, Salminen M, Laivuori H, Leinonen H, Hiilesmaa V, Kaaja R. Risk for subsequent coronary artery disease after preeclampsia. *Am J Cardiol.* 2004;93:805-808.
168. Veerbeek JH, Hermes W, Breimer AY, et al. Cardiovascular disease risk factors after early-onset preeclampsia, late-onset preeclampsia, and pregnancy-induced hypertension. *Hypertension.* 2015;65:600-606.
169. Beardmore KS, Morris JM, Gallery ED. Excretion of antihypertensive medication into human breast milk: a systematic review. *Hypertens Preg.* 2002;21:85-95.

40 Hypertension in Older People

Athanase Benetos

Older patients represent the most rapidly increasing segment of the United States population and account for the largest health care expenditures. Age is a major risk factor for the development of hypertension, and in particular, systolic hypertension. From 1999 to 2000, approximately 10 million men over the age of 65 and at least 17 million women over the same age had hypertension.[1] From 2003 to 2006, 65.4% of men and 70.8% of women aged 65 to 74 had hypertension, whereas for ages 75 and above, the prevalence was 64.6% for men and 77.3% for women.[2] Within the hypertensive population, African Americans and Latino Americans of all ages, including older patients, exhibit higher rates of hypertension.[3]

The increased prevalence of hypertension is mainly the result of the aging of the population, in particular the very old (≥80 years of age). Over the last 40 years, this population group has expanded exponentially.[4] Currently, life expectancy for these individuals living in the Organization for Economic Cooperation and Development (OECD) group of countries is approximately 9 years compared with about 6 years in the 1970s, representing an increase of 50%.[5] The number of people in the U.S. over 85 years of age is expected to increase to 16 million[6] compared with 5.7 million in 2010. In terms of incidence of hypertension, there has been little change in the percentage of patients over the age of 60 years who have hypertension.[7] However, as more people survive into their later years, the absolute number of individuals with hypertension constantly increases. Observational data from the Framingham Heart Study suggest that the lifetime risk of developing hypertension is greater than 90% for an American 55 to 65 years of age.[8] However, the continuously increasing number of older people, especially in the over-80 age group, also leads to a growing population with high blood pressure and at the same time more prone to multimorbidity, frailty, cognitive decline, polypharmacy, and partial or complete loss of autonomy.[9,10]

High blood pressure (BP), in particular systolic hypertension, is a clinical expression of arterial stiffness[11,12] developing during the aging process. In the past, the increase in systolic blood pressure (SBP) and pulse pressure (PP) was considered part of the normal aging process and was therefore deemed not to require therapeutic intervention. However, older subjects with higher SBP and PP levels not only have higher cardiovascular morbidity and mortality[11-13] but also exhibit a higher prevalence of other age-related diseases,[14,15] loss of autonomy, and shorter life expectancy.[16,17] Importantly, several studies have also shown that the risk of neurocognitive disorders, both Alzheimer and vascular types, may be associated with elevated BP.[15] As described in the Seventh Report of the Joint National Committee on Prevention, Detection, Evaluation and Treatment of High Blood Pressure (JNC 7),[18] the association between cardiovascular (CV) events and hypertension is linear, graded, and continuous: the higher the BP, the higher the CV risk.

This dogma, that is, the association between SBP and morbidity and mortality, may not be valid however in very old frail individuals with several comorbidities. In these subjects, low SBP levels may ultimately not signify a sign of so-called "good arterial health" but more often of malnutrition and of comorbidities such as heart failure, neurological disorders, and so on, as well as other concomitant conditions associated with poor prognosis. Therefore, information provided by SBP measurements in predicting cardiovascular risk may be misleading. Currently, the majority of evidence regarding the risks of high BP as well as the benefits from its correction are derived from a simple extrapolation of data obtained in younger populations[19] and in well-selected robust older individuals.[20]

These findings show that the general term "hypertension in the elderly" is not sufficiently accurate because it amalgamates "younger" old patients (60 to 70 years of age) with the oldest old and that the management of hypertension in individuals aged 80 years and older should be specifically and separately addressed. Although this age-threshold is arbitrary, there are two major differences between these two age groups: (1) the incidence and prevalence of comorbidities, frailty, and loss of autonomy greatly increases after the age of 80 years[21]; and (2) in the "younger" old patients, there is solid evidence regarding the management of hypertension and the benefits of reducing blood pressure, whereas there is limited evidence in patients over 80 years especially in those with frailty, cognitive impairment, and loss of autonomy.[22]

Therefore, the management of older patients with high blood pressure must take into account two major differences compared with younger hypertensive subjects:
1. Presence of isolated or predominant systolic hypertension as a result of arterial aging
2. Presence of frailty, multimorbidity, polymedication, and loss of autonomy

INCREASE IN SYSTOLIC BLOOD PRESSURE IN OLDER ADULTS: A CONSEQUENCE OF THE ARTERIAL AGING

Whereas both SBP and diastolic blood pressure (DBP) are independently predictive of cardiovascular disease (CVD) risk in individuals younger than 50 years of age, epidemiological data demonstrate that SBP is a stronger predictor of risk and that DBP is inversely associated with risk for those aged 50 years and older.[12] Although this observation was originally made almost 4 decades ago, it was not included in U.S. guidelines until 1993, when the Fifth Report of the Joint National Committee on Detection, Evaluation, and Treatment of High Blood Pressure (JNC V) recognized isolated systolic hypertension (ISH) as an important marker of CVD risk.[23,24] The staging of hypertension in older individuals is usually closely related to SBP. Upon analysis of the Framingham Heart Study, knowledge of only SBP correctly classified the stage of hypertension in 99% of patients over 60 years of age.[25]

The Reasons for the Increase in Pulse Pressure With Age

Until the age of 50 to 60 years, both SBP and DBP increase as individual get older. Thereafter, in the majority of cases, SBP increases with age disproportionally to DBP. The most common cause for the disruption of the correlation between SBP and DBP (leading to an excessive increase in SBP and PP) is the progressive stiffening of the arterial wall.[26,27] Indeed, arterial stiffness develops as a consequence of several structural and functional changes in large arteries. Wall hypertrophy, calcium deposits, and changes in the extracellular matrix, including an increase in collagen and fibronectin, fragmentation and disorganization of the elastin network, nonenzymatic crosslinks, and cell-matrix interactions, are the predominant structural determinants of the decrease in elastic properties and the development of large artery stiffness.[28]

It is important to point out at this juncture that SBP is dependent on left ventricular performance and on the stiffness of the aorta and other large arteries.[26] Thus, peak systolic pressure will be greater if the arterial wall is more rigid. On the other hand, after closure of the aortic valves, arterial pressure gradually falls as blood is drained toward the peripheral vascular networks. Minimum DBP is determined by the duration of the diastolic interval and the rate at which pressure falls. The rate of drop in pressure is influenced by the rate of outflow, that is, peripheral resistance, and by viscoelastic arterial properties. Hence, at a given vascular resistance, the drop in diastolic pressure will be greater if the rigidity of large arteries is increased. The viscoelastic properties of arterial walls are also a determinant of the speed of propagation of the arterial pressure wave (pulse wave velocity-PWV) and of the timing of wave reflections. Stiffening of the arteries increases PWV and may be responsible for an earlier return of the reflected waves, which overlap the incident pressure wave, thus further contributing to the increase in SBP and PP.[26,27] Several cross-sectional and longitudinal clinical studies have shown that the increase in arterial stiffness with age is not linear, being more pronounced after the age of 55 to 60 years,[29,30] which may in turn explain the more pronounced increase in PP after this age.[31] In addition to age, any disease and/or condition that induces an accelerated increase in arterial stiffness will be clinically expressed by an increase in SBP and PP. Diabetes is a typical example of accelerated arterial aging leading to a more noticeable increase in PP with age as compared with nondiabetic patients because of a more pronounced increase in arterial stiffness.[32-34] In accordance with this concept, increased PP with age is more pronounced in diabetics with initial microalbuminuria or macroalbuminuria and retinopathy, suggesting that the progression in arterial aging is more prominent in the presence of target organ damage.[34]

The Increasing Impact of Systolic/Pulse Pressure in Older Adults

The above considerations offer a better explanation as to why SBP and PP better reflect CVD risk in older subjects, whereas DBP better reflects the risk in younger subjects.[12,35] Indeed, DBP in young patients is predominantly dependent on peripheral resistance and therefore low DBP reflects low peripheral resistance. In addition, in younger subjects with hyperkinetic circulation, DBP is less variable than SBP, thus better reflecting cardiovascular risk. In older subjects, a low DBP may reflect high arterial stiffness, which is a major manifestation of arterial aging rather than low peripheral resistance.[26,27] In this instance, low DBP is associated with high SBP and high PP as well as increased cardiovascular risk.

Furthermore, in 2003, the European guidelines on the management of hypertension[36] suggested for the first time that PP may represent an independent risk factor, and that therapeutic studies should henceforth be conducted to assess the benefits of reducing PP in terms of cardiovascular morbidity and mortality, especially amongst those over 60 years of age.[12] Indeed, since the first study conducted in 1989 which demonstrated a positive association between PP and target organ damage,[37] a large number of clinical studies, particularly over

the past 10 years, have notably shown that increased PP is a strong predictor of coronary disease, incidence of heart failure and cardiovascular morbidity and mortality, independently of mean BP levels.[31,38-43] Such observations have been made in a number of varied populations although they appear to be more pronounced in diabetics and older subjects. Threshold PP risk values have since been proposed, notably a value of approximately 65 mm Hg.[44,45] This association between PP and CV mortality has essentially been observed in older patients enrolled in large clinical trials, as shown in a meta-analysis published in 2002[46] during which seven clinical trials in older adults were analyzed (EWPHE, HEP, MRC1, MRC2, SHEP, STOP, Syst-Eur). The subjects enrolled in these trials were older patients with systolic-diastolic hypertension or isolated systolic hypertension.

FRAILTY, MULTIMORBIDITY, POLYPHARMACY, AND LOSS OF AUTONOMY

Frailty is a "biological syndrome of decreased reserve and resistance to stressors, resulting from cumulative declines across multiple physiologic systems and causing vulnerability to adverse outcomes."[9] Frailty dramatically increases after the age of 80 years; however chronological age is only one of the factors predicting frailty. Susceptibility to stressors is also influenced by biological, behavioral, environmental, and social risk factors, consequently resulting in an increased risk of multiple adverse health outcomes, including disability, morbidity, falls, hospitalization, institutionalization, and death. A standardized frailty phenotype was articulated in 2001 by Linda Fried and colleagues,[9] suggesting that with very simple tests and questions, one could identify frail individuals by the presence of three or more of the following criteria: unintended weight loss, self-reported exhaustion, weakness, slow walking speed, and low physical activity. In 2008, Bergman[47] extended the Fried definition using a life-course approach, which incorporates biological, social, clinical, psychological, and environmental determinants. Bergman's definition thus identified seven markers of frailty: nutrition, mobility, activity, strength, endurance, cognition, and mood.

Of particular note, recent clinical studies have shown a substantial influence of frailty status on the relationship between BP and outcomes, especially in old treated hypertensive individuals[48-51]: thus in the absence of major frailty assessed by various means (low walking speed, altered cognition, loss of autonomy), the higher the SBP, the higher the risk of mortality whereas in those with major signs of frailty, SBP was negatively associated with risk of death. Recent studies have shown that the increased morbidity and mortality in very old frail subjects were mainly observed in treated hypertensives and not in normotensive individuals[52] especially in those receiving several antihypertensive drugs.[53] These findings are mainly attributed to the fact that in older individuals, low BP levels are often associated with several comorbidities, which predispose to a decreased perfusion of target organs and higher mortality risk.[54]

Also, polypharmacy (generally defined as taking more than four drugs) and drug-related adverse effects are major issues in this population and may additionally contribute to morbidity, higher rates of hospitalizations, and mortality. Polypharmacy is common among frail older adults, with the age group between 75 and 84 years recording the highest intake, that is, between five and nine drugs per day in more than 50% of patients.[55,56] Polypharmacy increases the risk of drug-drug interactions, adverse drug events, and the possibility of a prescribing cascade. The risk of adverse drug-drug interactions is strongly related to the number of drugs taken, varying from less than 15% in those taking two or less drugs to more than 80% in those taking seven or more drugs per day.[57] Changes in pharmacokinetics and pharmacodynamics during the aging process, and in particular reduced renal clearance, reduced hepatic metabolism, a decline in cardiac output as well as a decrease in lean mass and total body water, can modify drug pharmacokinetics and contribute to the increased risk of adverse drug reactions.[58,59] Moreover, a decline in serum albumin attributed to acute illness or malnutrition may additionally result in transformed free-drug accumulation.[60] Likewise, reduced homeostatic mechanisms render older persons more vulnerable to adverse effects (e.g., orthostatic hypotension is more likely to occur at a 'usual dose' of a vasodilating drug in an older person, based on a slow baroreceptor response).[60]

Antihypertensive medications are often involved in adverse drug events and related hospitalizations.[60] Several methods and tools have been developed to assess medication appropriateness.[61-63] Explicit instruments, in particular the Beers list in the U.S. and the STOPP/START criteria in Europe, are increasingly used, either as a tool applied by various multidisciplinary geriatric teams or within a comprehensive geriatric assessment.[64-66] These instruments are primarily useful to identify risks that might require further intervention, although they can never substitute for global clinical judgment of each older patient.

CLINICAL EVALUATION

In old subjects with suspected hypertension, a thorough history, physical examination, and selected laboratory and complementary exams should be performed to answer four main questions:

1. Is there a permanent elevation in BP levels?
2. Is it an essential (primary) or secondary (potentially curable) hypertension?
3. What is the overall CV risk of the patient?
4. What is the global state of the subject in terms of comorbidities, comedications, frailty, and autonomy?

1. A diagnosis of hypertension should be based on at least three different BP measurements, taken on two separate office visits. At least two measurements should be obtained once the patient is seated comfortably for at least 5 minutes with the back supported, feet on the floor, arm supported in the horizontal position, and the BP cuff of adequate size at heart level. Self-assessment of BP at home and if necessary 24-hour ambulatory BP measurements can contribute to detect white coat hypertension and better identify the CV risk related to high blood pressure levels. In addition, white coat hypertension and/or an exaggerated alerting response to BP measurement in the office appear to be common in older subjects, probably more so than in younger patients. Both the American Society of Hypertension and the American Heart Association (AHA) have issued guidelines promoting the more frequent use of out-of-office BP measurements.[67]

2. Secondary (potentially curable) hypertension is uncommon in the general population; therefore it is neither cost-effective nor useful to perform an extensive work up for every old patient with hypertension. In addition, symptoms associated with high BP, especially certain typical symptoms for secondary hypertension present in younger hypertensive subjects, are much less frequent and less specific in older individuals, especially in those with multiple comorbidities. However, when an older patient presents with rapidly occurring new-onset or severe hypertension, a sudden deterioration of what was previously well-controlled hypertension, resistant hypertension, or clinical clues suggestive of a particular form of secondary hypertension, then reversible causes should be suspected and investigated. The assessment and management of secondary hypertension is often more complicated in older patients. For example, although it is not uncommon to find evidence of atherosclerotic renal artery stenosis in older patients, it is often difficult to determine whether an identified atherosclerotic lesion in the renal artery is an incidental finding or is responsible for the elevation in BP. Percutaneous or surgical intervention for renovascular hypertension may be less efficacious, and may be more risky in older individuals. Sleep apnea is an often unrecognized but relatively common cause of increased BP in older age. It should be considered in overweight individuals and those who complain of daytime hypersomnolence or are noted to have excessive snoring or irregular breathing during sleep. Chronic renal insufficiency, obstructive uropathy, and thyroid disease are other potential secondary causes of hypertension in older individuals. Assessment of serum creatinine alone may overestimate renal function in older patients. Alternatively, available formulas estimating the glomerular filtration rate (eGFR) should be used.[68] Among other causes of secondary hypertension, medication-related BP elevation should always be investigated. Older individuals are often on multiple medications, many of which can increase BP. Patients should specifically be queried regarding use of nonsteroidal antiinflammatory drugs (NSAIDs), decongestants, corticosteroids, hormone replacement therapy (HRT), ephedrine-containing supplements, and other over-the-counter preparations, which many patients do not view as "drugs" and will not mention their use unless specifically asked.

3. To determine the overall risk of CVD, cardiovascular risk factors and target organ damage should be assessed. Physical examination should include a careful funduscopic examination, auscultation of abdominal bruits, examination of pedal pulses, and abdominal palpation investigating for a widened abdominal aortic pulsation that could suggest abdominal aortic aneurysm. BP at supine position should systematically be measured in older hypertensives independently of the presence of symptoms of orthostatic hypotension. An electrocardiogram investigating for left ventricular (LV) hypertrophy, ischemic heart disease, and rhythm and conduction abnormalities as well as a urinalysis for determining albumin concentration should be performed. The assessment of subclinical organ damage, in particular systolic and diastolic dysfunction as well as arterial stiffness, can be of some help in older patients. However the question arises as to the prognostic significance of these parameters in very old hypertensive patients, and whether their improvement would actually lead to an improvement in mortality in the these subjects.[69]

4. The general term "hypertension in the elderly" is not sufficiently accurate because it amalgamates "younger" old patients (60 to 70 years) with the oldest old. Therefore the management of hypertension in individuals aged 80 years and older should be specifically addressed. Although this age threshold is arbitrary, our belief is based on several considerations: owing to a greater life expectancy, the 80-and-over population is expanding faster than any other age group[70,71]; furthermore, the incidence and prevalence of comorbidities, frailty, and loss of autonomy greatly increases after the age of 80 years[21]; finally, although there is limited evidence regarding the management of hypertension in this age group, the latest clinical studies indicate that, in these patients, treatment may not be the same as in patients in the lower age strata.
Drugs, although proven to be effective in clinical trials[20] and indicated by clinical guidelines for chronic conditions including in patients 80 years and older, should be used judiciously in older individuals with frailty and other complex conditions. A number of reasons justify a cautious prescription, including: (1) their potential to interact with coexisting diseases or geriatric syndromes; (2) the potential for incorrect use related to cognitive deficits or

disability; or (3) the limited life expectancy of the patient that might be insufficient to allow a beneficial effect of the drug to occur.[72,73] In these situations, the risk of iatrogenic illness is increased and may exceed the potential benefit observed from a given pharmacological treatment. In this sense, it seems clear that a global assessment of the patient's characteristics, frailty status, and functional capacities, including the aforementioned factors, is recommended to fully appraise iatrogenic illness and to improve the quality of prescribing.

Comprehensive geriatric assessment (CGA) has been proposed as a methodology to provide a global approach to complex older adults and their problems, allowing a specific and tailored care plan to be implemented for each patient.[74] CGA is a simultaneous assessment of various domains by a multidisciplinary team to ensure that problems are identified, quantified, and managed appropriately. In practice, medical, cognitive, psychological, functional, and social domains are assessed after which a management plan can be established. CGA allows for a complete assessment of drugs, with the goals of recognizing and preventing potential drug-related problems and improving the quality of prescribing. Several studies to date have assessed the effect of CGA and management on drug prescribing and drug-related illness, showing a substantial improvement in quality of prescription.[75,76] A global evaluation of the problems and needs of complex older adults, obtained by CGA, may be extremely helpful in simplifying drug prescription and prioritizing pharmacological and health care needs. As a result, the quality of prescribing improves whereas the risk of adverse drug events decreases.

There is growing general consensus that reducing or stopping drugs in complex older very frail patients is justified in certain situations, where "de-prescribing" rather than prescribing may in fact be beneficial.

ANTIHYPERTENSIVE THERAPY

BP control, defined as achieving goal BP, remains far from optimal in older patients. From 2007 to 2008, among patients over 60 years of age, only about 45% of all hypertensives and slightly over 50% of those on treatment were at their goal BP.[7] Although this represents substantial improvement from earlier data, BP control rates in older patients remain suboptimal. In older patients, it is virtually always SBP rather than DBP that is not at goal BP.

Benefits of Lifestyle Modifications

Lifestyle changes are beneficial in treating hypertension and should be an integral element of therapy for all older patients. A number of different lifestyle changes have been recommended.[77] In overweight or obese individuals, weight reduction is likely the most effective lifestyle intervention for lowering BP. Older patients are more likely to have salt-sensitive hypertension; thus sodium restriction is more likely to reduce BP in older than in younger individuals. The Trial of Nonpharmacologic interventions in the Elderly (TONE)[78] found that restricting dietary sodium to, at most, 80 mmol (~2 g) per day reduced SBP by 4.3 mm Hg and DBP by 2 mm Hg after 30 months of follow-up. When used together, the combination of weight loss and sodium restriction enabled almost half of the older participants to remain off antihypertensive drug therapy for the duration of the trial. Additional lifestyle changes, which have not been specifically studied in older individuals but likely to improve BP control in this population, include adopting the Dietary Approaches to Stop Hypertension (DASH) eating program,[79] reducing alcohol intake, and increasing physical activity.

Although lifestyle interventions have been shown to reduce BP, it should be noted that no clinical trial has been performed in older individuals to determine whether they actually lead to a subsequent decrease in CVD events. In addition, in old frail individuals, some of these lifestyle modifications may not be appropriate or relevant, or may even be detrimental. Accordingly, a significant weight reduction alone without exercise[80,81] could induce loss of muscle mass and even cause cachexia. Excessive salt reduction may induce hyponatremia and loss of appetite, which can lead to malnutrition, orthostatic hypotension, with increased risk of falls. Physical activity adapted to the respective capacities and sociocultural profile of the patient is of major interest, even if not meeting the level recommended by current guidelines, which is similar for older and younger adult patients.[82] Excessive alcohol intake is often underestimated in old individuals and should be discouraged, not only because of its pressor effect, but also because of increased risk of falls and confusion.

Benefits of Pharmacological Treatment

The Report from the Expert Panel Report[83] provided the following recommendation for the management of hypertension in older individuals: In the general population aged 60 years or older, initiate pharmacologic treatment to lower BP at SBP of 150 mm Hg or higher or DBP of 90 mm Hg or higher and treat to a goal SBP lower than 150 mm Hg and goal DBP lower than 90 mm Hg. Strong Recommendation: Grade A.

These guidelines are mainly the result of several well-designed prospective clinical trials comparing active treatment with placebo, which demonstrated the benefits of treating patients 60 years old and over with either systolic-diastolic hypertension[84-86] or with isolated systolic hypertension[20,87,88] (Table 40.1).

A meta-analysis of clinical trials revealed that antihypertensive treatment in adults over 65 years of age produces similar proportional reductions in the risk for total major cardiovascular events as that observed in younger adults,[19] but the absolute benefits of treatment were more pronounced in older subjects because of a higher average risk. Although evidence regarding treatment benefits in the 65 to 80 age range is based on a large number of controlled clinical trials, these benefits in the very old are thus far based on only one randomized clinical trial. Actually, only the Hypertension in the Very Elderly Trial (HYVET)[20] study has addressed this important issue. The HYVET study was an international, prospective clinical endpoint study that randomized patients at least 80 years of age with SBP 160 to 199 mm Hg and DBP less than 110 mm Hg (originally 90 to 109 mm Hg, however the inclusion criteria were amended in 2003) to placebo or a thiazide-like diuretic (indapamide) with the potential addition of an angiotensin-converting-enzyme (ACE) inhibitor (perindopril) added to reach a target BP of less than 150/80 mm Hg. The prespecified primary endpoint for HYVET was fatal and nonfatal stroke. After 2 years, the mean BP while in the sitting position was 15.0/6.1 mm Hg lower in the active treatment group than in the placebo group. On the basis of the independent Data and Safety Monitoring Committee's recommendation, the trial was terminated early after a mean of only 1.8 years of follow-up because of an apparent 21% reduction in total mortality and a 30% reduction in the primary endpoint rate. There was also a 64% reduction in the rate of incident HF. In general, the rate of serious adverse events was low and less frequent with active treatment than with placebo. Although these findings are highly relevant for a large proportion of older individuals, the benefits of antihypertensive treatment cannot be extrapolated to all patients aged 80 years and older. Moreover, the HYVET study was conducted in relatively robust ambulatory older patients with little comorbidity. Significant cognitive impairment, loss of autonomy, cardiovascular comorbidities,

TABLE 40.1 Design and Main Results of Placebo-Controlled Trials Designed to Evaluate the Benefits of Treatment in Individuals 60 Years and Older With Systolic-Diastolic Hypertension or Isolated Systolic Hypertension

	EWPHE[84]	MRC[85]	STOP[86]	SHEP[87]	SYSTEUR[88]	HYVET[20]
Number of subjects and age at enrollment	n = 840 Age > 60	n = 4396 Age = 65 to 74	n = 1627 Age = 70 to 84	n = 4736 Age > 60	n = 4695 Age > 60	n = 3845 Age > 80
Inclusion BP criteria (mm Hg)	SBP:160-239 and DBP:100-119	SBP 160-209 and DBP < 115	SBP180-230 DBP > 90 or DBP > 105-120	160-219/<90	160-219/<95	160-199/<110
Active treatment medication	HCTZ + triamterene	Atenolol or HCTZ + amiloride	Beta-blockers or diuretics	Chlorthalidone ± atenolol	Nitrendipine ± enalapril	Indapamide ± perindopril
Goal SBP levels (mm Hg)		SBP < 150 or SBP < 160	<160/95	>20 from BL or SBP < 160	>20 from BL or SBP < 150	<150/80
BP reduction (mm Hg) with active tt compared with BL	30/15	33/15	28/15	27/9	23/7	29.5/12.9
BP reduction (mm Hg) (Active tt vs. Placebo)	20/9	13/10	19.5/8.1	12/4	10/5	15.0/6.1
Achieved BP (mm Hg) with active treatment	150/85	152/76	167/87	143/64	151/79	144/78
Mean follow-up (years)	4.3	5.8	2.1	4.5	2.0	1.8
Percent Reduction in Events						
Stroke	36	25[a]	47[a]	33	42[a]	30
CAD	20	19	13[b]	27	30	28
CHF	22	—	51[a]	55[a]	29	64[a]
All CVD	29[a]	17[a]	40[a]	32[a]	31[a]	34[a]

[a]Statistically significant.
[b]Myocardial infarction only.
BL, Baseline; *BP*, blood pressure; *CAD*, coronary artery disease; *CHF*, congestive heart failure; *CVD*, cardiovascular disease; *EWPHE*, European Working Party on Hypertension in the Elderly; *HCTZ*, hydrochlorothiazide; *MRC*, Medical Research Council; *SBP*, systolic blood pressure; *STOP*, Swedish Trial in Old Patients; *tt*, treatment.

and major frailty were in fact exclusion criteria for this study. Therefore, its findings cannot be extended to frail older patients with important comorbidity and who are on multiple medications. Clinical trials enrolling very old frail hypertensive subjects are needed to assess the effects of more or less aggressive treatment in these patients.

Target Blood Pressure Levels of the Pharmacological Treatment

The Expert Panel Report[83] states there is some evidence that setting an SBP goal lower than 140 mm Hg in patients over 60 years provides no additional benefit compared with a higher goal SBP of 140 to 160 mm Hg or 140 to 149 mm Hg.

In a similar approach, the European 2013 guidelines stated that in elderly hypertensives with SBP higher than 160 mm Hg, there is solid evidence to recommend reducing SBP between 150 and 140 mm Hg.[13]

These recommendations are now challenged by the recently published Systolic Blood Pressure Intervention Trial (SPRINT).[89] This trial, conducted in patients at high cardiovascular risk and already using antihypertensive drugs, showed that targeting an SBP of 120 mm Hg resulted in lower cardiovascular events and total mortality as compared with patients targeting an SBP of 140 mm Hg; this result was also observed in the subgroup (75 years and older even in those with some degree of frailty).[89a]

However, in the SPRINT study, very old patients with advanced frailty, cognitive decline, loss of autonomy, and living in nursing home were excluded. In addition, patients with decompensated heart failure, history of stroke, and diabetes were also excluded from this study. It should furthermore be pointed out that the "120 target" group showed a significant increase in hypotension, syncope, electrolyte abnormalities, and renal failure, in other words, adverse reactions that are likely to be magnified in very old patients, and even more so if frail. Thus, although the SPRINT study may have an important impact in the management of hypertension even in aging patients, it is difficult to extrapolate the conclusions of this study to very old frail and polymorbid individuals.

Recently, an expert group on Hypertension and Geriatric Medicine proposed some general rules for the management of hypertension in very old persons with partial or total loss of autonomy[89b]: This group suggests that therapeutic decisions should be preceded by:

- Accurate information on functional capacity and cognitive status;
- Attention to multiple drug administration so common in this age stratum;
- Stratification of the frailty status by one of the available rapid methods.

In addition the group proposed "While keeping <150 mm Hg systolic BP as the evidence-based target, for safety reasons antihypertensive drugs should be reduced or even stopped if systolic BP is lowered to <130 mm Hg, thus keeping the 150 to 130 mm Hg on-treatment systolic BP values as a safety range".

Are There Specific Drugs for the Older Hypertensive Patients?

In 2003, the JNC 7 report[18] recommended five drug classes (thiazide and thiazide-type diuretics, ACE inhibitors, calcium channel blockers [CCBs], or angiotensin II receptor blockers [ARBs]) to be considered as initial therapy although recommended thiazide-type diuretics as initial therapy for most patients without compelling indication for another class. In 2014, the JNC 8 report[83] recommended selection among four specific drug classes: (ACE inhibitors, ARBs, CCBs, diuretics). In addition, the JNC 8 report recommended specific drug classes based on evidence review for racial, chronic kidney disease, and diabetic subgroups. Thus, the major change, between JNC 7 and JNC 8 reports, is the noninclusion of beta-blockers in the list of first-line treatment in the JNC 8 report with the exception of the presence of associated compelling indications such as a history of myocardial infarction, chronic angina, or heart failure. It has actually been suggested that beta-blockers may not be as effective as other drug classes in reducing stroke, particularly in elderly patients.[90]

The majority of older patients with hypertension will require two or more medications to control BP. However, it is preferable to start with a monotherapy.[89b] Thus, although current guidelines suggest considering initial combination therapy in selected patients with hypertension, particularly those who are at least 20 mm Hg above SBP goal, this is a largely untested strategy in older patients who have never taken antihypertensive therapy.

Combination therapy, particularly among the very old and those with important comorbidities, may be associated with an increased risk of adverse effects. Careful uptitration and addition of medications is prudent, especially in the setting of advanced age, renal failure, or among those who are at risk for symptomatic hypotension or falls. The French guidelines propose not to exceed three antihypertensive drugs in very old patients.[91]

Concerning the type of the combination therapy the current evidence is very weak. The Avoiding Cardiovascular Events through Combination Therapy in Patients Living with Systolic Hypertension (ACCOMPLISH) trial[92] was designed to test the hypothesis that treatment with an ACE inhibitor (benazepril) combined with a CCB (amlodipine) would result in better outcomes than the same ACE inhibitor combined with a thiazide diuretic (hydrochlorothiazide) among 11,506 patients with systolic hypertension and other high-risk characteristics. Although this was not technically a study of the older people, 66% of all randomized patients were at least 65 years of age at baseline, and 41% were at least 70 years old. In those over 65 and 70 years of age, the ACE inhibitor + CCB group was associated with approximately 20% fewer CV events.

The COLM Investigators' study using a PROBE (prospective randomized open blinded end-point) design compared ARBs with a CCB with ARB with a diuretic in Japanese patients with hypertension aged 65 to 85 years.[93,94] In this trial no difference in cardiovascular events was found between the examined groups.[93] Prespecified secondary analysis of age effects, showed lower stroke risk in the older (75 to 84 years) hypertensive patients receiving the ARB + CCB combination than those receiving the ARB + diuretic combination, for a similar BP reduction.[94]

OTHER IMPORTANT ISSUES IN OLDER HYPERTENSIVE PATIENTS

Postural Hypotension and Nocturnal Dipping

Older individuals are especially prone to orthostatic hypotension. Orthostatic hypotension, which is frequent with advancing age, has been related to increased risk of mortality, cardiovascular events, and falls.[95-98] Since 1994, the National High Blood Pressure Education Working Group[99] suggested that standing BP should also be measured and used to evaluate treatment goals in older patients such that this recommendation is now included in all subsequent recommendations.

Given the risk for potential symptomatic postural hypotension, syncope, and falls in older patients, antihypertensive therapy should often be initiated with lower doses than those used in younger patients. In older patients, drug doses should be uptitrated and medications added cautiously, particularly in those with accompanying frailty and significant comorbidities. Symptomatic postural hypotension may limit the ability to reach sitting BP goal in some patients. In this instance, it is important to carefully weigh the risks and benefits of intensified antihypertensive therapy. Whether or not certain agents or combinations of agents lead to a greater risk of postural hypotension in older patients remains unclear, but it should be borne in mind that in the ACCOMPLISH trial, treatment was

titrated every 2 weeks at the start of the study, without untoward events.[92] Noteworthy, recent studies have shown that in an old frail population, not only orthostatic hypotension but also an increase in SBP in upright position is associated with higher cardiovascular morbidity and mortality independently of sitting blood pressure levels and major comorbidities.[100] Of note, orthostatic hypertension occurs frequently in these very old frail patients and therefore health professionals should take into account not only the decrease but also the increase in blood pressure when standing up.[100]

BP is routinely measured during waking hours; thus there is concern that some older patients on antihypertensive therapy may have an exaggerated nocturnal "dipping" of BP, leading to cerebral hypoperfusion. These patients are often referred to as "excessive dippers" and have a higher risk of CV events in some studies. In an ambulatory BP monitoring substudy of Syst-Eur, the benefit for stroke risk reduction in the active treatment group was confined to those patients who maintained an average nighttime SBP 130 or higher mm Hg.[101] In another ambulatory BP monitoring study performed in Japan, old hypertensive patients with chronic ischemic cerebrovascular disease who exhibited a more pronounced nocturnal BP "dip" on therapy were more likely to have stroke recurrence and new silent ischemic lesions on cerebral imaging, compared with those who did not "dip" at night.[102] Future clinical trials using 24-hour ambulatory BP monitoring are required to further clarify this issue.

Cognitive Impairment

Multiple observational studies have found an association between elevated BP in middle age and the risk of cognitive impairment. In the Framingham study, a high BP detected 20 years previously was inversely related with cognitive performance among untreated hypertensive subjects.[103] Since this initial observation, most epidemiological studies have confirmed this relationship between hypertension and cognitive decline. Hence, the Honolulu-Asia Aging Study which followed 3735 subjects for over 30 years showed that the risk of cognitive decline at age 78 increased with the level of SBP measured 25 years earlier.[15] In a seminal study in the field, Skoog et al,[104] showed that patients with hypertension developed more frequently dementia, 10 to 15 years later than normotensive subjects. On an even shorter follow-up period of 4 years, the EVA study (Epidemiology of Vascular Aging) found the risk of cognitive decline greater among patients with untreated chronic hypertension (odds ratio = 6) compared with a normotensive group.[105] However, such relationship between BP levels and cognitive decline in older populations was not observed in other clinical studies.[106,107] Hypertension duration, BP levels, cognitive profile, and testing, as well as differences in the tested population may all contribute in explaining the discrepancy regarding the relationship between hypertension and cognitive decline. In addition, the relationship between hypertension and cognitive function is probably more complex than a simple linear relationship leading to suggest that midlife BP level is more important as a risk factor for late-life cognitive impairment and dementia than the BP levels assessed in late life. Moreover, the hypothesis of a vascular involvement, independent of blood pressure level, has been raised. Although BP levels can be decreased by antihypertensive therapy, vascular alterations (caused in part by hypertension) in a protracted, decade-long process are less sensitive to antihypertensive therapy in late life because of their already advanced stage before such intervention. Some studies have shown that markers of arterial aging may identify subjects at higher risk of cognitive decline, whereas blood pressure alone does not appear to have a significant predictive value.[108-112]

Cognitive impairment has been included as a prespecified outcome in several trials of antihypertensive treatment in older adults. Several of these studies have shown the absence of any difference between active treatment and placebo[113-115] in the evolution of the cognitive decline and the prevention of neurodegenerative diseases. For the first time a beneficial effect was found in the Vascular Dementia Project, a substudy nested within Syst-Eur.[116] Active treatment (with a dihydropyridine CCB plus add-on ACE inhibitor and/or diuretic as needed) reduced the incidence of dementia by 50% compared with placebo. Identified cases of dementia were further evaluated with cerebral imaging, and it appeared that the incidence of both Alzheimer disease and vascular dementia was reduced with active therapy. In an open-label follow-up to Syst-Eur that extended the observation period by approximately 4 years, the incidence of dementia was reduced by 55% with active treatment.[117] A beneficial effect of active treatment has also been observed in the SCOPE study using an ARB as compared with the placebo group.[118] In the Hypertension in the Very Elderly Trial (HYVET), antihypertensive treatment did not significantly reduce the incidence of dementia.[20] In the secondary analysis of HYVET, a dynamic model of cognition allowing all outcomes to be categorized (cognitive worsening, stability improvement, or death) enabled to simultaneously detect small but consistent differences between treatment and control groups (in favor of treatment) amongst very old people treated for hypertension.[119]

Recent meta-analyses tried to evaluate the effect of antihypertensive treatment but also the potential difference among different antihypertensive medications in the cognitive decline and the prevention of dementia. In a meta-analysis published in 2011,[120] Staessen and colleagues analyzed the results of eight placebo-controlled trials, which reported results on the prevention of dementia by antihypertensive drugs. When regrouping all trials, antihypertensive treatment did not reduce the risk. The authors of this meta-analysis observed, however, a beneficial effect for trials using active treatment with a diuretic or a calcium channel blocker (–18%; $p = 0.022$), but no effect when an ACE inhibitor or an ARB was used (+1%; $p = 0.91$). A more recent systematic review assessed the effects of antihypertensive treatment on cognition (19 randomized trials) and on the incidence of dementia (11 studies), in hypertensive patients without prior cerebrovascular disorders.[121] In addition a network meta-analysis was used for the comparisons among antihypertensive classes. This analysis found benefits of antihypertensive therapy on cognition and prevention of dementia in observational studies but the effect on prevention of dementia was not significant when only the randomized trials were analyzed. Interestingly, this meta-analysis found that ARBs were more effective in preventing dementia and cognitive decline than beta-blockers, diuretics, and angiotensin-converting enzyme inhibitors despite similar mean change in blood pressure. Taken together these results show that the protective effects against cognitive decline and dementia of antihypertensive drugs remains unsettled. None of the present trials, while well designed, have sufficient statistical power to examine the long-term effects of antihypertensives. This type of clinical trial should be considered of major importance in terms of public health because of the dramatic increase of the older population and therefore the incidence of neurodegenerative and cerebrovascular diseases.

SUMMARY

Hypertension is very common in older persons and is associated with considerable morbidity and mortality. Because aging is associated with decreased arterial elastic properties, hypertension in older patients is characterized by elevated systolic and pulse pressure with low DBP. Elevation in SBP in older patients is often not optimally controlled. However, in very old frail individuals, low BP is also associated with higher mortality particularly those with multiple drug regimens.

Management of older individuals with hypertension should mainly include physical activities adapted to the patient's general status and cultural context, and avoidance of excessive alcohol consumption. Sodium restriction and weight loss could have negative effects in the very old and should be proposed with great caution. There is substantial evidence to support the value of using antihypertensive drugs in most old patients with hypertension, particularly in those with baseline SBP higher than 160 mm Hg. Further data are needed in patients with moderate SBP elevation (140 to 159 mm Hg) and in very old frail people who have systematically been excluded from clinical trials. Unlike in younger patients, antihypertensive medications in the older adults should be initiated at lower doses and as monotherapy, and uptitrated more gradually, with careful monitoring for postural hypotension and other potential adverse events. Whether therapy initiation with a particular class of antihypertensive medication offers superior results remains unclear because trials demonstrating a reduction in events in older patients with hypertension have primarily used thiazide-type diuretics, ACE inhibitors, ARBs, and CCBs as first-line therapy. Optimal BP goals in older patients remain unclear. Current data would suggest that the risk to benefit ratio for antihypertensive therapy is generally favorable with treatment to an SBP less than 150 mm Hg. The recent SPRINT study suggests that a lower SBP target could provide beneficial effects even in subjects over 75 years of age. However, in this latter study, the more frail individuals were excluded. Furthermore, in the older patient population, it is imperative that planned future trials focus not only on relative, but also on absolute risk reduction, including the number needed to treat.

Given the high prevalence of hypertension in older patients with their greater likelihood of CVD events, identification and treatment of high BP in older adults remains a major health priority, especially because the absolute benefit of lowering BP in this patient population likely exceeds that of any other age group. Finally, it should be noted that hypertension has to be managed from a life-course perspective. This points out the necessity for timely diagnostics and appropriate treatment of high BP in younger age, which would have a potential to positively affect functional status and quality of life in old age.[122]

References

1. Fields LE, Burt VL, Cutler JA, et al. The burden of adult hypertension in the United States 1999-2000. *Hypertension*. 2004;44:398-404.
2. Lloyd-Jones DM, Adams RJ, Brown TM, et al. Heart disease and stroke statistics—2010 update. A Report from the American Heart Association. *Circulation*. 2010;121:e46-e215.
3. Mozaffarian D, Benjamin E, Go AS, et al. Heart Disease and Stroke Statistics-2015 update. A report from the American Heart Association. *Circulation*. 2015;131:e29-e322.
4. National Institute on Aging. National Institutes of Health. Global Health and Aging. NIH Publication no. 11-7737. Washington DC: World Health Organization, 2011.
5. Health at a glance 2009-OECD indicators. www.oecd.org/health/health-systems/health-at-a-glance-19991312.htm. Last accessed on January 2016.
6. Heart and Stroke Statistical Update, 2005. Dallas, TX: American Heart Association; 2004.
7. Egan BM, Zhao Y, Axon RN. US trends in prevalence, awareness, treatment and control of hypertension, 1988-2008. *JAMA*. 2010;303:2043-2050.
8. Vasan R, Beiser A, Seshadri S, et al. Residual lifetime risk for developing hypertension in middle-aged women and men: the Framingham Heart Study. *JAMA*. 2002;287:1003-1010.
9. Fried LP, Tangen CM, Walston J, et al. Frailty in older adults: evidence for a phenotype. *J Gerontol A Biol Sci Med Sci*. 2001;56:146-156.
10. Abellan van Kan G, Rolland Y, Bergman H, et al. The I.A.N.A Task Force on frailty assessment of older people in clinical practice. *J Nutr Health Aging*. 2008;12:29-37.
11. Safar ME, Levy BI, Struijker-Boudier. Current perspectives on arterial stiffness and pulse pressure in hypertension and cardiovascular disease. *Circulation*. 2003;107:2864-2869.
12. Franklin SS, Larson MG, Khan SA, et al. Does the relation of blood pressure to coronary heart disease risk change with aging? The Framingham Heart Study. *Circulation*. 2001;103:1245-1249.
13. Authors/Task Force M, Mancia G, Fagard R, et al. 2013 ESH/ESC Guidelines for the management of arterial hypertension: the Task Force for the management of arterial hypertension of the European Society of Hypertension (ESH) and of the European Society of Cardiology (ESC). *Eur Heart J*. 2013;34:2159-2219.
14. Alagiakrishnan K, Juby A, Hanley D, Tymchak W, Sclater A. Role of vascular factors in osteoporosis. *J Gerontol*. 2003;58:362-366.
15. Launer L, Ross GW, Petrovitch H, et al. Midlife blood pressure and dementia: the Honolulu-Asia aging study. *Neurobiol Aging*. 2000;21:49-55.
16. Franco OH, Peeters A, Bonneux L, De Laet C. Blood pressure in adulthood and life expectancy with cardiovascular disease in men and women: analysis. *Hypertension*. 2005;46:280-286.

17. Benetos A, Thomas F, Bean KE, Pannier B, Guize L. Role of modifiable risk factors in life expectancy in the elderly. *J Hypertens*. 2005;23:1803-1808.
18. Chobanian AV, Bakris GL, Black HR, et al. The seventh report of the Joint National Committee on Prevention, Detection, Evaluation, and Treatment of High Blood Pressure: the JNC 7 report. *JAMA*. 2003;289:2560-2572.
19. Blood Pressure Lowering Treatment Trialists' Collaboration, Turnbull F, Neal B, et al. Effects of different regimens to lower blood pressure on major cardiovascular events in older and younger adults: meta-analysis of randomised trials. *BMJ*. 2008;336:1121-1123.
20. Beckett NS, Peters R, Fletcher AE, et al. Treatment of hypertension in patients 80 years of age or older. *N Engl J Med*. 2008;358:1887-1898.
21. Berrut G, Andrieu S, Araujo De Carvalho I, et al. Promoting access to innovation for frail old persons. IAGG (International Association of Gerontology and Geriatrics), WHO (World Health Organization) and SFGG (Societe Francaise de Geriatrie et de Gerontologie) Workshop—Athens January 20–21, 2012. *J Nutr Health Aging*. 2013;17:688-693.
22. Benetos A, Rossignol P, Cherubini A, Joly L, Grodzicki T, Rajkumar C, Strandberg TE, Petrovic M. Polypharmacy in the Aging Patient: Management of Hypertension in Octogenarians. *JAMA*. 2015;314:170-180.
23. Kannel WB, Schwartz MJ, McNamara PM. Blood pressure and risk of coronary heart disease: the Framingham Study. *Dis Chest*. 1969;56:43-62.
24. Fifth Report of the Joint National Committee on Detection. Evaluation, and Treatment of High Blood Pressure (JNC-V). *Arch Intern Med*. 1993;153:154-183.
25. Lloyd-Jones DM, Evans JC, Larson MG, et al. Differential impact of systolic and diastolic blood pressure level on JNC-VI staging. *Hypertension*. 1999;34:381-385.
26. Safar ME, Levy BI. Struijker-Boudier. Current perspectives on arterial stiffness and pulse pressure in hypertension and cardiovascular disease. *Circulation*. 2003;107:2864-2869.
27. O'Rourke MF, Frolich ED. Pulse pressure: is this a clinically useful risk factor? *Hypertension*. 1999;34:372-374.
28. Lakatta E. Arterial and cardiac aging: major shareholders in cardiovascular disease enterprises: part III: cellular and molecular clues to heart and arterial aging. *Circulation*. 2003;107:490-497.
29. Benetos A, Adamopoulos C, Bureau JM, et al. Determinants of accelerated progression of arterial stiffness in normotensive subjects and in treated hypertensive subjects over a 6-year period. *Circulation*. 2002;105:1202-1207.
30. Benetos A, Buatois S, Salvi P, et al. Blood pressure and pulse wave velocity values in the institutionalized elderly aged 80 and over: baseline of the PARTAGE Study. *J Hypertens*. 2010;28:41-50.
31. Franklin SS, Khan SA, Wong ND, Larson MG, Levy D. Is pulse pressure useful in predicting risk for coronary heart disease? *Circulation*. 1999;100:354-360.
32. Ronnback M, Fagerudd J, Forsblom C, et al. Altered age-related blood pressure pattern in type 1 diabetes. *Circulation*. 2004;110:1076-1082.
33. Salomaa V, Riley W, Kark JD, Nardo C, Folsom AR. Non-insulindependent diabetes mellitus and fasting glucose and insulin concentrations are associated with arterial stiffness indexes. The ARIC Study. *Circulation*. 1995;91:1432-1443.
34. Schram MT, Kostense PJ, Van Dijk RA, et al. Diabetes, pulse pressure and cardiovascular mortality: the Hoorn Study. *J Hypertens*. 2002;20:1743-1751.
35. Khattar RS, Swales JD, Dore C, Senior R, Lahiri A. Effects of aging on the prognostic significance of ambulatory systolic, diastolic and pulse pressure in essential hypertension. *Circulation*. 2001;104:783-789.
36. 2003 European Society of Hypertension–European Society of Cardiology Guidelines Committee. Guidelines for the management of arterial hypertension. *J Hypertension*. 2003;21:1011-1053.
37. Darne B, Girerd X, Safar M, Cambien F, Guize L. Pulsatile versus steady component of blood pressure: a cross-sectional analysis and a prospective analysis on cardiovascular mortality. *Hypertension*. 1989;13:392-400.
38. Mitchell GF, Moye LA, Braunwald E, et al. Sphygmomanometric determined pulse pressure is a powerful independent predictor of recurrent events after myocardial infarction in patients with impaired left ventricular function. *Circulation*. 1997;96:4254-4260.
39. Chae CU, Pfeffer MA, Glynn RJ, Mitchell GF, Taylor JO, Hennekens CH. Increased pulse pressure and risk of heart failure in the elderly. *JAMA*. 1999;281:634-639.
40. Benetos A, Safar M, Rudnichi A, et al. Pulse pressure, a predictor of long-term cardiovascular mortality. *Hypertension*. 1997;30:1410-1415.
41. Kengne AP, Czernichow S, Huxley R, et al. Blood pressure variables and cardiovascular risk new findings from ADVANCE. *Hypertension*. 2009;54:399-404.
42. Bangalore S, Messerli FH, Franklin SS, Mancia G, Champion A, Pepine CJ. Pulse pressure and risk of cardiovascular outcomes in patients with hypertension and coronary artery disease: an INternational VErapamil SR-trandolapril Study (INVEST) analysis. *Eur Heart J*. 2009;30:1395-1401.
43. Miura K, Nakagawa H, Ohashi Y, et al. Four blood pressure indexes and the risk of stroke and myocardial infarction in Japanese men and women. A meta-analysis of 16 cohort studies. *Circulation*. 2009;119:1892-1898.
44. Benetos A, Rudnichi A, Safar M, Guize L. Pulse pressure and cardiovascular mortality in normotensive and hypertensive subjects. *Hypertension*. 1998;32:560-564.
45. de Simone G, Roman MJ, Alderman MH, Galderisi M, de Divitiis O, Devereux RB. Is high pulse pressure a marker of preclinical cardiovascular disease? *Hypertension*. 2005;45:575-579.
46. Gasowski J, Fagard RH, Staessen JA, et al. INDANA Project Collaborators. Pulsatile blood pressure component as predictor of mortality in hypertension: a meta-analysis of clinical trial control groups. *J Hypertens*. 2002;20:145-151.
47. Bergman H, Hogan D, Karunananthan S. Frailty: a clinically relevant concept? *Can J Geriatrics*. 2008;11:124-128.
48. Odden MC, Covinsky KE, Neuhaus JM, Mayeda ER, Peralta CA, Haan MN. The association of blood pressure and mortality differs by self-reported walking speed in older Latinos. *J Gerontol A Biol Sci Med Sci*. 2012;67:977-983.
49. Ogliari O, Westendorp RGJ, Muller M, et al. Blood pressure and 10-year mortality risk in the Milan Geriatrics 75+ Cohort Study. *Age Ageing*. 2015;44:932-937.
50. Benetos A, Gautier S, Labat C, et al. Mortality and cardiovascular events are best predicted by low central/peripheral pulse pressure amplification but not by high blood pressure levels in elderly nursing home subjects: the PARTAGE study. *J Am Coll Cardiol*. 2012;60:1503-1511.
51. Odden MC, Peralta CA, Haan MN, Covinsky KE. Rethinking the association of high blood pressure with mortality in elderly adults: the impact of frailty. *Arch Intern Med*. 2012;172:1162-1168.
52. Mossello E, Pieraccioli M, Nesti N, et al. Effects of low blood pressure in cognitively impaired elderly patients treated with antihypertensive drugs. *JAMA Intern Med*. 2015;175:578-585.
53. Benetos A, Labat C, Rossignol P, et al. Treatment with multiple blood pressure medicines, achieved blood pressure, and mortality in older nursing home residents. *JAMA Intern Med*. 2015;175:989-995.
54. Muller M, Smulders YM, de Leeuw PW, Stehouwer CD. Treatment of hypertension in the oldest old. *Hypertension*. 2014;63:433-441.
55. Mannucci PM, Nobili A. REPOSI Investigators: multimorbidity and polypharmacy in the elderly: lessons from REPOSI. *Intern Emerg Med*. 2014;9:723-734.
56. Onder G, Bonassi S, Abbatecola AM, et al. Geriatrics Working Group of the Italian Medicines Agency. High prevalence of poor quality drug prescribing in older individuals: a nationwide report from the Italian Medicines Agency (AIFA). *J Gerontol A Biol Sci Med Sci*. 2014;69:430-437.
57. Goldberg R, Mabee J, Chan L, et al. Drug-drug and drug disease interactions in the ED: analysis of a high-risk population. *Am J Emerg Med*. 1996;14:447-450.
58. Salvi F, Marchetti A, D'Angelo F, et al. Adverse drug events as a cause of hospitalization in older adults. *Drug Saf*. 2012;35(Suppl 1):29-45.
59. Petrovic M, van der Cammen T, Onder G. Adverse drug reactions in older people: detection and prevention. *Drugs Aging*. 2012;29:453-462.
60. Hutchison LC, O'Brien CE. Changes in pharmacokinetics and pharmacodynamics in the elderly patient. *J Pharm Prac*. 2007;20:4-12.
61. Beers MH, Ouslander JG, Rollingher I, et al. Explicit criteria for determining inappropriate medication use in nursing home residents. *Arch Intern Med*. 1991;151:1825-1832.
62. The American Geriatrics Society 2012 Beers Criteria Update Expert Panel. American Geriatrics Society Updated Beers Criteria for Potentially Inappropriate Medication Use in Older Adults. *J Am Geriatr Soc*. 2012;60:616-631.
63. Naugler CT, Brymer C, Stolee P, et al. Development and validation of an improving prescribing in the elderly tool. *Can J Clin Pharmacol*. 2000;7:103-107.
64. Gallagher P, Ryan C, Byrne S, Kennedy J, O'Mahony D. STOPP (Screening Tool of Older Person's Prescriptions) and START (Screening Tool to Alert doctors to Right Treatment). Consensus validation. *Int J Clin Pharmacol Ther*. 2008;46:72-83.
65. O'Mahony D, O'Sullivan D, Byrne S, O'Connor M, Ryan C, Gallagher P. STOPP/START criteria for potentially inappropriate prescribing in older people: version 2. *Age Ageing*. 2015;44:213-218.
66. Hanlon JT, Schmader KE, Samsa GP, et al. A method for assessing drug therapy appropriateness. *J Clin Epidemiol*. 1992;45:1045-1051.
67. Pickering TG, Hall JE, Appel LJ, et al. Recommendations for blood pressure measurement in humans and experimental animals. Part 1. Blood pressure measurement in humans: a statement for professionals from the sub-committee of professional and public education of the American Heart Association Council on High Blood Pressure Research. *Hypertension*. 2005;45:142-161.
68. Stevens LA, Levey AS. Clinical implications of estimating equations for glomerular filtration rate. *Ann Intern Med*. 2004;141:959-961.
69. Zhang Y, Agnoletti D, Xu Y, Wang JG, Blacher J, Safar ME. Carotid-femoral pulse wave velocity in the elderly. *J Hypertens*. 2014;32:1572-1576.
70. National Institute on Aging. National Institutes of Health. Global Health and Aging. NIH Publication no. 11-7737. Washington DC: World Health Organisation, 2011.
71. Health at a glance 2009-OECD indicators: www.google.com/url?sa=t&rct=j&q=&esrc=s&source=web&cd=1&ved=0CCIQFjAA&url=http%3A%2F%2Fwww.oecd.org%2Fhealth%2Fhealth-systems%2F44117530.pdf&ei=DvK7VN7SJMXkasibgrAl&usg=AFQjCNHKC9qNe87Gdi-Bli_VTS0dfWpigg&bvm=bv.83829542,d.d2s&cad=rja. Last accessed on October 2015.
72. Boyd CM, Darer J, Boult C, Fried LP, Boult L, Wu AW. Clinical practice guidelines and quality of care for older patients with multiple comorbid diseases: implications for pay for performance. *JAMA*. 2005;294:716-724.
73. Fusco D, Lattanzio F, Tosato M, et al. Development of CRIteria to assess appropriate Medication use among Elderly complex patients (CRIME) project: rationale and methodology. *Drugs Aging*. 2009;26(Suppl 1):3-13.
74. Abellan van Kan G, Rolland Y, Houles M, et al. The assessment of frailty in older adults. *Clin Geriatr Med*. 2010;26:275-286.
75. Onder G, Lattanzio F, Battaglia M, et al. The risk of adverse drug reactions in older patients: beyond drug metabolism. *Curr Drug Metab*. 2011;12:647-651.
76. Lampela P, Hartikainen S, Lavikainen P, et al. Effects of medication assessment as part of a comprehensive geriatric assessment on drug use over a 1-year period: a population-based intervention study. *Drugs Aging*. 2010;27:507-521.
77. Aronow WS, Fleg JL, Pepine CJ, et al. ACCF/AHA 2011 expert consensus document on hypertension in the elderly: a report of the American College of Cardiology Foundation Task Force on Clinical Expert Consensus Documents developed in collaboration with the American Academy of Neurology, American Geriatrics Society, American Society for Preventive Cardiology, American Society of Hypertension, American Society of Nephrology, Association of Black Cardiologists, and European Society of Hypertension. *J Am Soc Hypertens*. 2011;5:259-352.
78. Whelton PK, Appel LJ, Espeland MA, et al. Sodium restriction and weight loss in the treatment of hypertension on older persons: a randomized controlled trial of nonpharmacologic interventions in the elderly (TONE). Tone Collaborative Research Group. *JAMA*. 1998;279:839-846.
79. Appel L, Moore T, Obarzanek E, et al. The effect of dietary patterns on blood pressure: results from the Dietary Approaches to Stop Hypertension (DASH) randomized clinical trial. *N Engl J Med*. 1997;336:1117-1124.
80. Amati F, Dubé J, Shay C, Goodpaster B. Separate and combined effects of exercise training and weight loss on exercise efficiency and substrate oxidation. *J Appl Physiol*. 2008;105:825-831.
81. Thomas D. Loss of skeletal muscle mass in aging: examining the relationship of starvation, sarcopenia and cachexia. *Clinical Nutrition*. 2007;26:389-399.
82. Sparling PB, Howard BJ, Dunstan DW, Owen N. Recommendations for physical activity in older adults. *BMJ*. 2015;350:h100.
83. James PA, Oparil S, Carter BL, et al. Evidence-based guideline for the management of high blood pressure in adults: report from the panel members appointed to the Eighth Joint National Committee (JNC 8). *JAMA*. 2014;311:507-520.
84. Amery A, Birkenhäger W, Brixko P, et al. Mortality and morbidity results from the European Working Party on High Blood Pressure in the Elderly trial. *Lancet*. 1985;1:1349-1354.
85. Medical Research Council. Medical research trial of treatment of hypertension in older adults: principal results. *BMJ*. 1992;304:405-412.
86. Dahlöf B, Lindholm LH, Hansson L, et al. Morbidity and mortality in the Swedish Trial in Old Patients with Hypertension (STOP-Hypertension). *Lancet*. 1991;338:1281-1285.
87. SHEP Cooperative Research Group. Prevention of stroke by antihypertensive drug treatment in older persons with isolated systolic hypertension. *JAMA*. 1996;265:3255-3264.
88. Staessen JA, Fagard R, Thijs L, et al. Randomised double blind comparison of placebo and active treatment for older patients with isolated systolic hypertension: the systolic hypertension in Europe (Syst-Eur) trial investigators. *Lancet*. 1997;350:757-764.
89. SPRINT Research Group. A randomized trial of intensive versus standard blood-pressure control. *N Engl J Med*. 2015;373:2103-2116.
89a. Williamson JD, Supiano MA, Applegate WB, et al. Intensive vs Standard Blood Pressure Control and Cardiovascular Disease Outcomes in Adults Aged ≥75 Years. A Randomized Clinical Trial. *JAMA*. 2016;315:2673-2682.
89b. Benetos A, Bulpitt CJ, Petrovic M, et al. An Expert Opinion From the European Society of Hypertension-European Union Geriatric Medicine Society Working Group on the Management of Hypertension in Very Old, Frail Subjects. *Hypertension*. 2016;67(5):820-825.

90. Messerli FH, Grossman E, Goldbourt U. Are beta-blockers efficacious as first-line therapy for hypertension in the elderly? *JAMA*. 1998;279:1903-1907.

91. Blacher J, Halimi JM, Hanon O. Management of hypertension in adults: the 2013 French Society of Hypertension guidelines. *Fundam Clin Pharmacol*. 2014;28:1-9.

92. Jamerson K, Weber MA, Bakris GL, et al. Benazepril plus amlodipine or hydrochlorothiazide for hypertension in high risk patients. *N Engl J Med*. 2008;359:2417-2428.

93. Ogihara T, Saruta T, Rakugi H, et al. Combinations of olmesartan and a calcium channel blocker or adiuretic in elderly hypertensive patients: a randomized, controlled trial. *J Hypertens*. 2014;32:2054-2063.

94. Ogihara T, Saruta T, Rakugi H, et al. Combination therapy of hypertension in the elderly: a subgroup analysis of the Combination of OLMesartan and a calcium channel blocker or diuretic in Japanese elderly hypertensive patients trial. *Hypertens Res*. 2015;38:89-96.

95. Rose KM, Tyroler HA, Nardo CJ, et al. Orthostatic hypotension and the incidence of coronary heart disease: the Atherosclerosis Risk in Communities study. *Am J Hypertens*. 2000;13:571-578.

96. Masaki KH, Schatz IJ, Burchfiel CM, et al. Orthostatic hypotension predicts mortality in elderly men: the Honolulu Heart Program. *Circulation*. 1998;98:2290-2295.

97. Ooi WL, Hossain M, Lipsitz LA. The association between orthostatic hypotension and recurrent falls in nursing home residents. *Am J Med*. 2000;108:106-111.

98. Fedorowski A, Stavenow L, Hedblad B, Berglund G, Nilsson PM, Melander O. Orthostatic hypotension predicts all-cause mortality and coronary events in middle-aged individuals (The Malmo Preventive Project). *Eur Heart J*. 2010;31:85-91.

99. National High Blood Pressure Education Program Working Group Report on Hypertension in the Elderly. *Hypertension*. 1994;23:275-285.

100. Agnoletti D, Valbusa F, Labat C, Gautier S, Mourad JJ, Benetos A. Evidence for a Prognostic Role of Orthostatic Hypertension on Survival in a Very Old Institutionalized Population. PARTAGE study Investigators. *Hypertension*. 2016;67:191-196.

101. Staessen J, Thijs L, Fagard R, et al. Predicting cardiovascular risk using conventional vs. ambulatory blood pressure in older patients with systolic hypertension: systolic hypertension in Europe trial investigators. *JAMA*. 1999;282:539-546.

102. Nakamura K, Oita J, Yamaguchi T. Nocturnal blood pressure and silent cerebrovascular lesions in elderly Japanese. *Stroke*. 1996;26:1373-1378.

103. Elias MF, Wolf PA, D'Agostino RB, Cobb J, White LR. Untreated blood pressure level is inversely related to cognitive functioning: the Framingham Study. *Am J Epidemiol*. 1993;138:353-364.

104. Skoog I, Lernfelt B, Landahl S, et al. 15-year longitudinal study of blood pressure and dementia. *Lancet*. 1996;347:1141-1145.

105. Tzourio C, Dufouil C, Ducimetiere P, Alperovitch A. Cognitive decline in individuals with high blood pressure: a longitudinal study in the elderly. EVA Study Group. Epidemiology of Vascular Aging. *Neurology*. 1999;53:1948-1952.

106. Desmond DW, Tatemichi TK, Paik M, Stern Y. Risk factors for cerebrovascular disease as correlates of cognitive function in a stroke-free cohort. *Arch Neurol*. 1993;50:162-166.

107. Di Carlo A, Baldereschi M, Amaducci L, et al. Cognitive impairment without dementia in older people: prevalence, vascular risk factors, impact on disability. The Italian Longitudinal Study on Aging. *J Am Geriatr Soc*. 2000;48:775-782.

108. Kearney-Schwartz A, Rossignol P, Bracard S, et al. Vascular structure and function is correlated to cognitive performance and white matter hyperintensities in older hypertensive patients with subjective memory complaints. *Stroke*. 2009;40:1229-1236.

109. Singer J, Trollor JN, Baune BT, Sachdev PS, Smith E. Arterial stiffness, the brain and cognition: a systematic review. *Ageing Res Rev*. 2014;15:16-27.

110. Solomon A, Mangialasche F, Richard E, et al. Advances in the prevention of Alzheimer's disease and dementia. *J Int Med*. 2014;275:229-250.

111. Kaffashian S, Dugravot A, Elbaz A, et al. Predicting cognitive decline: a dementia risk score vs. the Framingham vascular risk scores. *Neurology*. 2013;80:1300-1306.

112. Watfa G, Benetos A, Kearney-Schwartz A, et al. PARTAGE study investigators. Do arterial hemodynamic parameters predict cognitive decline over a period of 2 years in individuals older than 80 years living in nursing homes? The PARTAGE Study. *J Am Med Dir Assoc*. 2015;16:598-602.

113. Prince MJ, Bird AS, Blizzard RA, et al. Is the cognitive function of older patients affected by antihypertensive treatment? Results from 54 months of the Medical Research Council's treatment trial of hypertension in older adults. *BMJ*. 1996;312:801-805.

114. Applegate WB, Pressel S, Wittes J, et al. Impact of the treatment of isolated systolic hypertension on behavioral variables: results from the systolic hypertension in the elderly program (SHEP). *Arch Intern Med*. 1994;154:2154-2160.

115. Tzuorio C, Anderson C, Chapman N, et al. Effects of blood pressure lowering with perindopril and indapamide therapy on dementia and cognitive decline in patients with cerebrovascular disease. *Arch Intern Med*. 2003;163:1069-1075.

116. Forette F, Seux MI, Staessen JA, et al. Prevention of dementia in randomized double blind placebo controlled systolic hypertension in Europe (Syst-Eur) trial. *Lancet*. 1998;352:1347-1351.

117. Rigaud AS, Olde-Rikkert MGM, Hanon O, et al. Antihypertensive drugs and cognitive function. *Current Hypertens Rep*. 2002;4:211-215.

118. Lithell H, Hansson L, Skoog I, et al. The study on cognition and prognosis in the elderly (SCOPE): principal results of randomized double blind intervention trial. *J Hypertens*. 2003;21:875-876.

119. Peters R, Beckett N, Beardmore R, et al. Modeling cognitive decline in the Hypertension in the Very Elderly Trial [HYVET] and proposed risk tables for population use. *PLoS One*. 2010;5:e11775.

120. Staessen JA, Thijs L, Richart T, Odili AN, Birkenhager WH. Placebo controlled trials of blood pressure-lowering therapies for primary prevention of dementia. *Hypertension*. 2011;57:e6-e7.

121. Marpillat L, Macquin-Mavier I, Tropeano AI, Bachoud-Levi AC, Maison P. Antihypertensive classes, cognitive decline and incidence of dementia: a network meta-analysis. *J Hypertens*. 2013;31:1073-1082.

122. Strandberg AY, Strandberg TE, Stenholm S, Salomaa VV, Pitkälä KH, Tilvis RS. Low midlife blood pressure, survival, comorbidity, and health-related quality of life in old age: the Helsinki Businessmen Study. *J Hypertens*. 2014;32:1797-1804.

41 Hypertension in African Americans

George A. Mensah

Worldwide, hypertension remains a powerful, independent marker of cardiovascular mortality and death from all causes. In 2013, high systolic blood pressure (BP) accounted for more than 10 million deaths globally.[1] In the United States, hypertension caused nearly 397,000 deaths in 2013; an increase of 61.8% since 2000.[2] The highest hypertension-related age-adjusted death rate was seen in African Americans in whom the rate was 44% and 42% higher than in Hispanics and non-Hispanic whites, respectively.[2,3] Thus, hypertension remains a major contributor to death from stroke, heart failure, kidney failure, and ischemic heart disease in African Americans.

This chapter discusses the epidemiology of hypertension in African Americans as well as the pathophysiological characteristics and strategies for prevention, treatment, and control of hypertension in this population. The magnitude and trends in disparities in care and clinical outcomes are explored and so are opportunities for eliminating these disparities. The role of implementation research and practice-based evidence to inform hypertension treatment and control in African Americans is also addressed. This chapter does not discuss specific forms of hypertension such as pregnancy-related hypertension, white coat hypertension, renovascular hypertension or the strategies for their detection and evaluation which are addressed in other sections of this book.

EPIDEMIOLOGY OF HYPERTENSION IN AFRICAN AMERICANS

Hypertension Risk Factors

Important risk factors that predispose to hypertension include advancing age, a strong family history of hypertension, obesity, physical inactivity, high dietary sodium intake, low dietary potassium intake, low vitamin D intake, harmful use of alcohol, psychosocial stress, low socioeconomic status, low educational attainment, and psychological traits such as anger and hostility. These factors are as important in African Americans as they are in other race-ethnic population subgroups. However, they take on additional significance when a greater prevalence of any of them in African Americans is used to explain the greater prevalence of hypertension in this population.

Hypertension Incidence

Hypertension incidence is strongly influenced by age, baseline BP level, the definition of hypertension, and duration of follow-up. It is also influenced by sex, race, ethnicity, family history, obesity, geography, and several psychosocial, environmental, and biomedical risks. Although older studies showed a higher incidence of hypertension in African Americans, more recent, carefully controlled studies of longer duration paint a more nuanced picture. For example, in younger adults who were aged 18 to 30 years when recruited in 1985 to 1986 in the community-based Coronary Artery Risk Development in Young Adults (CARDIA) cohort,[4] hypertension incidence after 20 years of follow-up was significantly higher in African Americans, especially women, even after adjustment for age, race, heart rate, body mass index, smoking, family history, education, uric acid, alcohol use, physical activity, and baseline systolic BP. For example, when the mean age was approximately 45 years, the 20-year incidence was 34.5% in black men, 37.6% in black women, 21.4% in white men, and 12.3% in white women; $p < 0.001$.[4] Hypertension incidence also varied significantly across urban areas and by race and sex, with higher rates in the southeast and in blacks, especially African-American women.[4] In the Trials of Hypertension Prevention, the incidence of hypertension (defined as BP $\geq$ 160/95 mm Hg or taking antihypertensive medications) over 7 years of follow-up in middle-aged African Americans and whites was nearly identical (25.7% in African Americans and 25.3% in whites).[5] In the Multi-Ethnic Study of Atherosclerosis, participants aged 45 to 84 years at baseline were followed for a median of 4.8 years for incident hypertension, defined as systolic BP 140 or higher mm Hg, diastolic BP 90 or higher mm Hg, or the initiation of antihypertensive medications.[6] After adjustment for age, sex, and study site, hypertension incidence was higher for African Americans aged 45 to 64 compared with whites but not for those 75 to 84 years of age.[6]

Hypertension Prevalence

Most published studies demonstrate that hypertension prevalence is significantly greater in African Americans compared with other race-ethnic groups in the United States.[7] As shown in Fig. 41.1, the age-adjusted prevalence in the most recent National Health and Nutrition Examination Survey (2011–2014) was higher in non-Hispanic African-African women (41.5%) and men (40.8%) compared with all other race-ethnic-sex groups.[8] Importantly, in both non-Hispanic African-African women and men, the age-adjusted prevalence has steadily increased in graded fashion over all three national surveys in 1988 to 1994, 1999 to 2006, and 2007 to 2012.[9] Fig. 41.2 shows the extent of the increase in hypertension prevalence in U.S. counties from 2001 to 2009 and the particularly marked increase seen in African-African men and women.[10]

Hypertension Severity

In addition to their greater prevalence of hypertension, African Americans (in comparisons with whites) develop hypertension at an earlier age[11,12]; have higher average BP levels; and higher average nondipping nocturnal BP and greater 24-hour BP variability on ambulatory monitoring.[13] Additionally, African Americans are more likely to experience accelerated conversion from prehypertension to hypertension.[14] As a result, severe hypertension is more common in African Americans compared with whites and is often more likely to be associated with a greater prevalence of target organ damage. However, there is little, if any, evidence that hypertension is a different disease or is "more severe" in African Americans.[15] Thus race, per se, does not cause more severe hypertension.

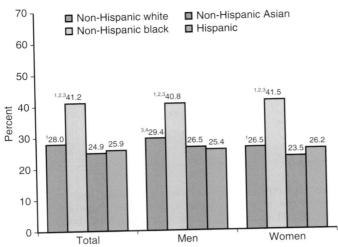

FIG. 41.1 Prevalence of hypertension among adults aged 18 years and over, by sex and race and Hispanic origin: United States, 2011 to 2014. *(Reproduced from Yoon SS, Carroll MD, Fryar CD. Hypertension prevalence and control among adults: United States, 2011-2014. NCHS Data Brief. 2015;(220):1-8.) Notations: [1]Significant difference from non-Hispanic Asian. [2]Significant difference from non-Hispanic white. [3]Significant difference from Hispanic. [4]Significant difference from women in same race and Hispanic origin group. NOTE: Estimates are age-adjusted by the direct method to the 2000 U.S. census population using age groups 18 to 39, 40 to 59, and 60 and over; see reference 9. From CDC/NCHS, National Health and Nutrition Examination Survey, 2011–2014.*

As Schmieder et al.[16] demonstrated in a matched-pair analysis of early target organ damage that also controlled for confounding factors such as age, sex, body weight, and BP level, race per se does not predict hypertension severity or extent of target organ damage.

Awareness, Treatment, and Control

Over the last three decades, awareness and treatment of hypertension in African Americans have improved significantly as it has in the general population (Fig. 41.3).[17] In fact, hypertension awareness has been higher in non-Hispanic blacks compared with the total U.S. population or in non-Hispanic whites and Hispanics in most years of the survey (Fig. 41.3).[17] In 2011 to 2012, hypertension treatment rates were similar among non-Hispanic blacks (76.5%), and non-Hispanic whites (75.8%) but lower in Mexican Americans (69.6%).[17]

Although hypertension control has also improved steadily over the last three decades, the most recent control rate in African Americans (49.4%) is lower than that in non-Hispanic whites (54.3%) and also lower than achievable in an integrated health system model that uses implementation, dissemination, and performance feedback strategies in chronic disease care.[18-20] For example, the Kaiser Permanente Southern California health care system was able to improve hypertension control in a multiethnic population from 54% to 86% in the

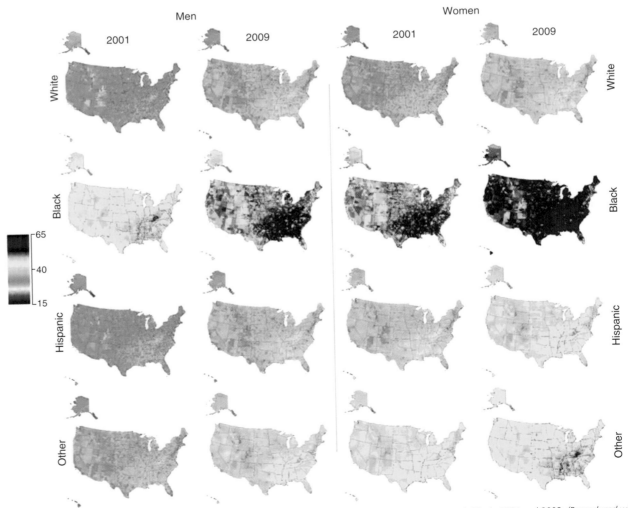

FIG. 41.2 Age-standardized prevalence of total hypertension in U.S. counties by sex and race among adults 30 years and older in 2001 and 2009. *(Reproduced with permission from Olives C, Myerson R, Mokdad AH, Murray CJ, Lim SS. Prevalence, awareness, treatment, and control of hypertension in United States counties, 2001-2009. PLoS One. 2013;8:e60308.)*

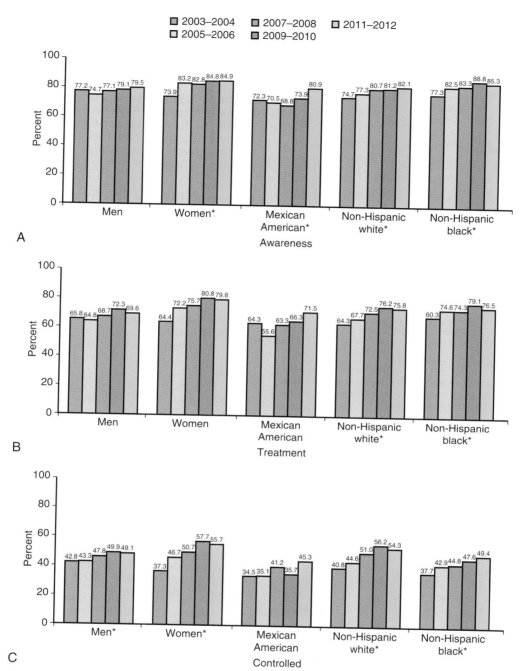

FIG. 41.3 Age-adjusted awareness, treatment, and control of hypertension among adults with hypertension by sex and race/ethnicity (other racial/ethnic groups not shown separately), 2003 to 2004 through 2011 to 2012. A, Age standardization was computed by the direct method using weights based on the subpopulation of individuals with hypertension in The National Health and Nutrition Examination Survey (NHANES) 2007 to 2008. *p-trend < 0.05. B, Age standardization was computed by the direct method using weights based on the subpopulation of individuals with hypertension in NHANES 2007 to 2008. *p-trend < 0.05. C, Age standardization was computed by the direct method using weights based on the subpopulation of individuals with hypertension in NHANES 2007 to 2008. *p-trend < 0.05. (Reproduced from Yoon SS, Gu Q, Nwankwo T, Wright JD, Hong Y, Burt V. Trends in blood pressure among adults with hypertension: United States, 2003 to 2012. Hypertension. 2015;65:54-61.)

total population and achieved a control rate of 80% or more in African Americans and other population subgroups, regardless of preferred language or type of health insurance plan.[20]

Mortality and Morbidity

The age-adjusted hypertension-related mortality rate in non-Hispanic blacks is nearly double the rate seen in non-Hispanic whites and Hispanics (Fig. 41.4).[2] The disparity is even starker when examined by sex.[9] For example, in 2013, the death rates per 100,000 population were 51.6 for non-Hispanic black males but 18.9 for non-Hispanic white males,

and 20.0 for Hispanic males.[9] The corresponding rates for women were 36.5 for non-Hispanic black females, 15.8 for non-Hispanic white females, and 15.3 for Hispanic females.[9] Hypertension is also an important contributor to stroke, myocardial infarction (MI), heart failure, kidney failure, and other morbid events and reduced quality of life in African Americans. The greater prevalence of hypertension, onset at an earlier age, and lower control rates in African Americans, compared with whites, contribute to the greater prevalence of hypertensive target organ damage in the heart, brain, kidney, and arterial vasculature with resulting chronic organ failure and reduced quality of life.[21,22]

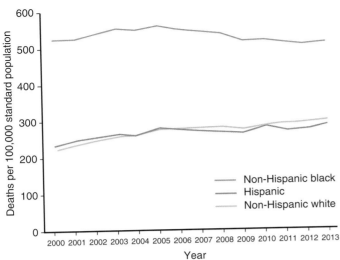

FIG. 41.4 Age-adjusted hypertension-related death rates, by race and Hispanic origin: United States, 2000 to 2013. (*Reproduced from Kung HC, Xu J. Hypertension-related Mortality in the United States, 2000-2013.* NCHS Data Brief. *2015;(193):1-8.) NOTES: Linear increases for the non-Hispanic white population from 2000 through 2013 and for the Hispanic and non-Hispanic black populations from 2000 through 2005 are statistically significant at the p < 0.05 level. Linear decreases for the non-Hispanic black population from 2005 to 2013 and for the Hispanic population from 2005 to 2009 are statistically significant at the p < 0.05 level. Hypertension-related deaths are identified using ICD–10 codes I10, I11, I12, I13, and I15 for underlying and contributing causes of death, according to the* International Classification of Diseases, 10th revision *(ICD–10). Access data table at:* www.cdc.gov/nchs/data/databriefs/db193_table.pdf#3. *(CDC/NCHS, National Vital Statistics System, Mortality.)*

PATHOPHYSIOLOGY

The pathophysiological mechanisms that initiate and maintain chronic hypertension are complex, interrelated, dynamic, and have multiple feedback loops that, to a large extent, contribute to the marked heterogeneity seen in the phenotypic expression of chronic hypertension at the population level. Among the most studied of these mechanisms are increased sympathetic nervous system (SNS) activity; alterations in the renin-angiotensin-aldosterone axis; other neurohormonal influences; alterations in the circadian control of BP; exaggerated BP responses to various stimuli; increased sodium sensitivity; excess intake of dietary sodium; impaired renal handling of sodium; endothelial dysfunction; and other chronic alterations in vascular structure and function. These mechanisms are discussed in detail in Chapter XX of this book.

In light of this complexity and the fact that African Americans are not a biologically monolithic population, a definitive pathophysiological basis for their greater prevalence of hypertension remains speculative. Most likely, all of these mechanisms play some role in the long-term maintenance of hypertension in African Americans but the literature suggests that some may play a greater role than others in contributing to the higher prevalence of hypertension in this population. In this section, the current evidence on mechanisms that likely contribute to the pathophysiological basis for hypertension in African Americans is discussed.

INCREASED SYMPATHETIC NERVOUS SYSTEM ACTIVITY

Increased SNS activity and an exaggerated adrenergic response to stress are important contributors to acute and chronic BP elevation. Increased SNS activity directly contributes to the initiation as well as chronic maintenance of hypertension through its effect on cardiac output, peripheral vascular resistance, and renal fluid and sodium retention.[23] Several studies demonstrate a greater prevalence of increased SNS activity in African Americans compared with whites.[24,25] For example, in

African American men and women in the CARDIA study, systolic blood pressure (SBP) hyper-responsivity to two laboratory-induced psychological stressors was associated with a higher SBP at 3 years of follow-up.[26] Chronic repeated exaggerated SNS responses to various stressors may be important mechanisms for the increased prevalence of hypertension and target organ damage in African Americans. In fact, it has been suggested that SNS over-reactivity in young adulthood may be an important explanations for both the high incidence of obesity-related hypertension in African-American women and the disproportionately high incidence of hypertension in lean African-American men.[27]

Increased Dietary Salt Intake and Salt Sensitivity

Increased intake of dietary salt, especially in the setting of increased salt sensitivity, has been suggested as an important contributor to the increased prevalence of hypertension in African Americans. Although widely varying methodologies and criteria have been used to diagnose or define salt sensitivity, the phenomenon is generally considered to be present when mean arterial BP increases by at least 5% in normotensive and borderline hypertensive individuals and greater than 10% in hypertensive patients in response to sodium loading.[28] Other definitions require a 10 mm Hg absolute increase or a 10% relative increase between mean arterial pressure on low-versus high-salt diets.[29]

In general, most studies show a greater prevalence of salt-sensitivity in African American hypertensive patients often associated with increased forearm vascular resistance, decreased venous compliance, suppressed plasma renin activity, and reduced circulating aldosterone concentration.[28] The myriad factors that can contribute to salt-sensitivity in African Americans include reduced dietary potassium intake, decreased urinary kallikrein excretion, upregulation of sodium channel activity, and alterations in atrial natriuretic peptide production.[29] Importantly, salt sensitivity has also been associated with increased prevalence of target organ damage and excess mortality, especially from cardiovascular and renal causes independent of the BP rise.[30-33] These findings provide a firm foundation for dietary salt reduction and the clinical use of thiazide-type diuretic antihypertensive medications as essential components of multidrug therapy for BP control in African American patients.

Impaired Renal Handling of Sodium and Expanded Extracellular Plasma Volume

Abnormalities in the renal handling of sodium excretion, expanded extracellular plasma volume, and impaired tubuloglomerular feedback have been suggested as important factors in the greater prevalence of hypertension and hypertensive renal damage in African Americans.[34,35] These abnormalities are not present in all African Americans or even the majority of African Americans; nevertheless, their greater prevalence in African Americans compared with whites may contribute to the known racial disparities in hypertension and hypertension-related renal damage. These mechanisms are likely to take on even greater importance when dietary sodium intake is increased in salt-sensitive individuals. For example, in a recent study that examined the association of dietary sodium and potassium intakes with blood pressure separately by race/ethnicity, age, and sex among 1568 participants, Bartley et al.[36] noted that African-American and Hispanic males aged 50 years and younger consumed considerably more sodium and less potassium compared with their white counterparts. Weinberger et al. demonstrated more than three decades ago, the importance of sodium in blood pressure regulation, especially in individuals predisposed to avid sodium conservation.[37]

Renin-Angiotensin-Aldosterone System Activation

Activation of the renin-angiotensin-aldosterone system (RAAS) is one of the primary pathophysiological mechanisms in acute and chronic regulation of systemic BP level as well as a major modulator of cardiovascular structure and function and hypertension-related target organ damage. Not surprisingly, some of the most powerful antihypertensive medications target this system using angiotensin-converting enzyme (ACE) inhibitors, angiotensin II receptor blockers (ARBs), renin inhibitors, and mineralocorticoid receptor blockers. African-American hypertensive patients, especially those who are salt sensitive, have a high dietary sodium intake, and therefore have suppressed circulating plasma renin activity, invoking an activated RAAS seems counterintuitive and paradoxical. However, Michel et al.[38] recently demonstrated in a community sample of African ancestry participants that in the presence of high-sodium, low-potassium diets, and suppressed renin release, RAAS system activation downstream from renin and its impact on BP are maintained in part by circulating angiotensinogen concentrations.[38] In fact, the study further demonstrated a positive relationship between angiotensinogen and serum aldosterone concentrations and SBP, independently of confounders in the setting of high dietary sodium intake.[38] It is therefore reasonable to conclude that the RAAS may play an important role in hypertension in African Americans and the greater prevalence of severe target organ damage.

Circadian Biology and Nocturnal Blood Pressure Levels

Abnormal circadian regulation of BP manifests as an absence or a blunted nocturnal "dipping" of BP, higher average sleep BP, and exaggerated morning BP surge seen during ambulatory monitoring. These derangements have been reported to be associated with increased prevalence of hypertension and hypertension-related target organ damage. Most studies suggest a greater prevalence of blunted nocturnal dipping in African Americans that may contribute to greater prevalence of hypertension and hypertension-related target organ damage.[39-44] Impaired renal handling of sodium has been suggested as a likely explanation for nocturnal nondipping of BP[45]; however, many other factors such as physical activity, salt sensitivity, dietary electrolyte intake, sex, body size, socioeconomic status, age, psychological factors, stressful life circumstances, perceived racism, and neighborhood environment all influence the pattern of ambulatory BP variation and therefore confound unadjusted racial comparisons.

Psychosocial Stress

The weight of the evidence suggests that several categories of chronic psychosocial stress including occupational stress, job strain, housing instability, social isolation, and perceived racism and hostility contribute to the onset and maintenance of chronic hypertension.[46-51] These factors occur more often in African Americans than in whites and have been considered contributory to the greater prevalence of hypertension in African Americans. Although the definitive underlying mechanisms remain incompletely understood, prominent roles have been described for the sympathetic nervous system, neuroendocrine system, renal handling of sodium, endothelial function, and gene-environment interactions.

STRATEGIES FOR HYPERTENSION TREATMENT AND CONTROL

In the African-American patient with hypertension, an effective strategy for the treatment and control of hypertension must begin with the establishment of a trusting patient-provider relationship and a commitment to follow through on an action plan. The initial clinical history and physical examination help establish a diagnosis and stage of primary hypertension at the same time as clues for secondary hypertension, masked hypertension, or white coat hypertension are explored and excluded.[52] An assessment for the presence and extent of hypertension-related target organ damage, comorbid clinical diagnoses, and determination of short-term and long-term total cardiovascular risk is essential. The initial laboratory tests will be invaluable in the calculation of cardiovascular risk. Additionally, an assessment of the patient's health literacy, educational level, social support, and self-management skills is necessary. Collectively, these initial assessments and their findings help match the intensity of hypertension treatment strategy to the stage and level of cardiovascular risk of the patient.[52]

Behavioral and Lifestyle Interventions

Behavioral and lifestyle interventions are as important in the African-American patient as they are in other patients. These include changes in diet, physical activity, sleep duration and pattern, weight management, alcohol consumption, and psychosocial stress. Although cigarette smoking does not directly contribute to long-term BP elevation, it contributes to total cardiovascular risk and it is therefore included as an important part of behavioral and lifestyle changes.

Dietary Interventions

A diet that is rich in fruits and vegetables and low in sodium is important in the management of hypertension. This dietary pattern, as used in the Dietary Approaches to Stop Hypertension (DASH) trial,[53,54] leads to BP reduction in hypertensive patients, an effect that persists as long as the recommended dietary pattern is maintained. This phenomenon has been demonstrated in many adult patient populations including African Americans. For example, in the DASH trial, a combination diet rich in fruits and vegetables and low in saturated fat, total fat, and cholesterol reduced SBP in African Americans (−6.8 mm Hg) and whites (−3.0 mm Hg) and was particularly effective in patients with hypertension, lowering systolic BP by −11.5 mm Hg. In fact, the dietary pattern's effect on BP was independent of changes in body weight and sodium intake and is considered to be of a magnitude sufficient to prevent progression from prehypertension to hypertension and serve as an important strategy in the nonpharmacologic treatment of hypertension or as a supplement in drug therapy.[55]

Physical Activity Interventions

The independent beneficial impact of regular physical exercise on BP control in hypertensive subjects has been well demonstrated. A recent narrative review of 27 randomized controlled trials of regular medium-to-high-intensity aerobic activity demonstrated mean BP reductions of 11/5 mm Hg in hypertensive persons.[56] Staffileno et al. have demonstrated that tailored interventions that incorporate lifestyle-compatible physical activity in young, hypertension-prone African-American women result in significant reductions in SBP and diastolic BP (DBP) and greater reductions in nocturnal BP load compared with women in the control "No Exercise" group.[57]

Comprehensive Multifaceted Lifestyle Interventions

Ideally, simultaneous implementation of multifaceted interventions that are considered culturally acceptable, affordable, and can be sustained long-term have the greatest potential for most benefit in hypertension control. These interventions include increased physical activity; weight loss

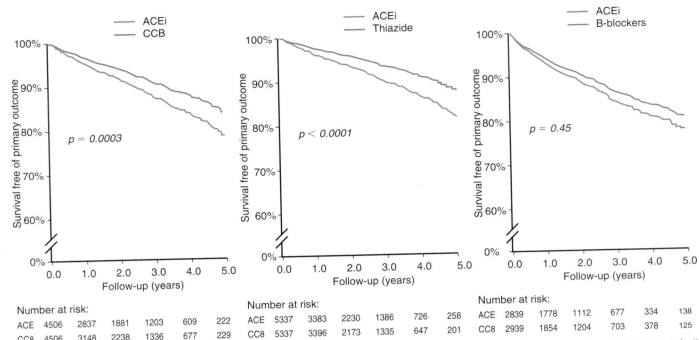

FIG. 41.5 The risk of a primary outcome (a composite of death, myocardial infarction, and stroke) in a real-world cohort of hypertensive African Americans treated with angiotensin-converting enzyme inhibitors, thiazide-type diuretic, or beta-blockers. Angiotensin-converting enzyme inhibitor treatment compared with calcium channel blocker or beta-blocker treatment. *ACEi,* Angiotensin-converting enzyme inhibitor; *CCB,* calcium channel blocker. *(Reproduced from Bangalore S, Ogedegbe G, Gyamfi J, et al. Outcomes with angiotensin-converting enzyme inhibitors vs other antihypertensive agents in hypertensive blacks. Am J Med. 2015;128:1195-203.)*

or ideal weight maintenance; reduced alcohol intake in those who drink alcohol; strategies to reduce or address psychosocial stress; dietary sodium reduction; increased fruit and vegetable intake; and other dietary approaches to lower BP. The PREMIER trial, whose participants included 34% African Americans and 62% women, was an example of such multifaceted interventions.[58] It demonstrated the feasibility of comprehensive multifaceted interventions and their beneficial effects on BP control in hypertensive patients not on medical therapy as well as in the prevention of hypertension in at-risk subjects with above-optimal BP.[58]

Sleep-Disordered Breathing and Sleep Apnea

Sleep-disordered breathing, manifesting as apneic or hypopneic episodes during sleep, together with reduced duration and quality of sleep have been associated with the development of hypertension.[59-61] African Americans, compared with whites, have a disproportionately greater risk of having poor sleep quality and duration and, thus, may be at greater risk of sleep-related hypertension.[62] For example, the CARDIA study reported that objectively measured average sleep duration was 6.7 and 6.1 hours for white women and men, respectively, but 5.9 and 5.1 hours for African-American women and men, respectively and that the race-sex differences remained significant ($p < 0.001$) after adjustment for socioeconomic, employment, household, and lifestyle factors and for apnea risk. In addition, African Americans are at greater risk of living in environments with a greater exposure to environmental factors that impair sleep duration and quality. Interventions to address adverse sleep habits and the use of continuous positive airway pressure (CPAP) to treat sleep apnea when present can be important strategies in a comprehensive approach to the treatment and control of hypertension.

Drug Treatment

The primary objective in the drug treatment of hypertension is to use safe, effective, and affordable medications to reach goal BP and reduce mortality and morbidity in patients already

using behavioral and lifestyle interventions in the long-term control of hypertension. Ideally, drug treatment should be informed by published guidelines that meet national or international standards for trustworthiness.[63,64] It is not enough for patients to be simply started on antihypertensive medications; every effort must be used to reach goal BP as safely as possible and as tolerated by the patient. Although the threshold BP for initiating drug treatment in hypertension and the goal BP to be attained remain controversial,[65] all recent major guidelines remain consistent in the selection of medications for treating African Americans. In addition, there is now compelling evidence that systemic implementation of specific strategies, such as the use of an evidence-based treatment algorithm and a multidisciplinary approach using community health workers, medical assistants, nurses, and pharmacists as key stakeholders, can result in a similar level of good BP control as seen in patients of other race and ethnicities.[18]

In African-American patients with stage 1 hypertension, including those with diabetes, there is moderate evidence to support initiating treatment with a calcium channel blocker (CCB) or thiazide-type diuretic.[66,67] There is also moderate evidence to recommend the use of an ACE inhibitor or ARB as initial or add-on drug therapy in the presence of chronic kidney disease (CKD) to improve kidney outcomes.[67] When stage 1 hypertension is complicated by the presence of chronic heart failure, coronary artery disease, or stroke, drug selection from an appropriate drug class is recommended based on the compelling indication.[68,69] However, the use of an ACE inhibitor is not recommended as monotherapy in African Americans.[66,70] This is supported by several recent guidelines and findings from recent clinical trials suggesting that hypertensive African Americans have higher risk of cardiovascular events when treated with an ACE inhibitor-based regimen compared with CCBs or thiazide diuretics.[71,72] For example, in one cohort study of patients using data from a clinical data warehouse of 434,646 patients from January 2004 to December 2009, a propensity score-matched comparisons, ACE inhibitors were associated with a higher risk of primary outcome, MI, stroke, and heart failure when compared with CCBs or thiazide-type diuretic (Fig. 41.5).[71,72]

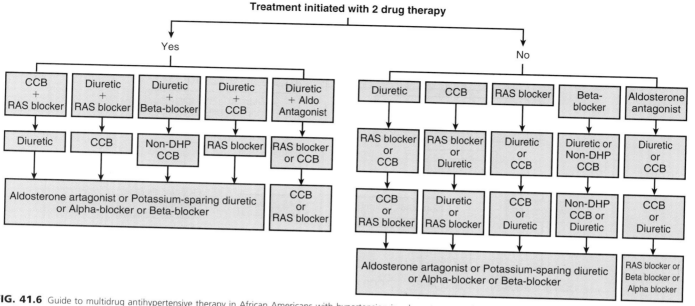

FIG. 41.6 Guide to multidrug antihypertensive therapy in African Americans with hypertension in whom treatment is initiated with one or two drugs. *Aldo,* Aldosterone; *non-DHP,* non-dihydropyridine. *(Reproduced from Flack JM, Sica DA, Bakris G, et al. Management of high blood pressure in Blacks: an update of the International Society on Hypertension in Blacks consensus statement. Hypertension. 2010;56:780-800.)*

Most African-American patients with stage 2 hypertension will require two or more drugs to achieve BP control; thus, monotherapy in this setting is not recommended.[69] Importantly, drug treatment is recommended immediately after diagnosis, ideally beginning with a two-drug combination, without first waiting to assess the effects of lifestyle and behavioral interventions.[66,69] When stage 2 hypertension is complicated by the presence of diabetes, coronary artery disease, a history of stroke, or heart failure, it is recommended that the choice of drug classes from which multidrug and/combination drug therapy is chosen be informed by the compelling indication.[68,69]

In African-American patients, as it is with all hypertensive patients, a diligent search is necessary to identify the reasons why BP remains uncontrolled during treatment with maximum or near-maximum doses of drugs from three or more recommended classes. In this setting, it is important to confirm that patients can afford the medications and have not only filled the prescriptions but are actually taking the medications as prescribed. When medication nonadherence is excluded, other factors that contribute to resistant hypertension such as plasma volume expansion, obesity, type 2 diabetes mellitus, CKD, and other physiological perturbations should be considered.[68,69]

CLINICAL PRACTICE GUIDELINES

Numerous clinical practice guidelines (CPGs) have been published[73] but few focus primarily on the management of hypertension in African Americans. A recent systematic review of CPGs for hypertension identified 375 CPGs from 6 continents, 33 countries, 4 regions, and 3 international organizations.[73] Among published CPGs and scientific statements from the United States, only a few focus specifically on the management of hypertension in African Americans[69,74-76] although several of them provide prominent discussions on the prevention, treatment, and control of BP in African Americans.[66,68]

For nearly three decades, the International Society of Hypertension in Blacks (ISHIB) has provided leadership and guidance for the management of hypertension in African Americans. The ISHIB consensus statement of 2010 updated the previous consensus statement[76] and strongly recommended the initiation of comprehensive lifestyle modification in African Americans, lowered the minimum goal BP level for the lowest-risk African Americans, emphasized effective multidrug regimens, and deemphasized hypertension monotherapy.[69] An algorithm was provided (Fig. 41.6) to guide multidrug antihypertensive therapy for African Americans with hypertension in whom treatment is initiated with one or two drugs.[69] A further refinement of this is seen in Fig. 41.7 which represents the algorithm summarizing the clinical practice guidelines for the management of hypertension in the community published by the American Society of Hypertension and the International Society of Hypertension.[66] These algorithms are likely to be further refined, especially with reference to the number of antihypertensive drugs needed and the desirable goal BP because of recent findings from the Systolic Blood Pressure Intervention Trial (SPRINT).[77] The SPRINT trial showed that among patients at high risk for cardiovascular events but without diabetes, an intensive treatment strategy targeting an SBP goal of less than 120 mm Hg reduced the primary composite outcome of MI, non–MI acute coronary syndrome, stroke, acute decompensated heart failure, and cardiovascular death by approximately 25%, and all-cause mortality by about 27%, as compared with the standard treatment SBP goal of less than 140 mm Hg.[77,78]

DISPARITIES IN CARE AND CLINICAL OUTCOMES

Although hypertension treatment and control rates in African Americans have improved substantially over the last 30 years, they remain lower than in non-Hispanic whites and important racial and ethnic disparities in clinical outcomes for hypertension-related morbidity and mortality persist. Important barriers and challenges for providers and health systems in the management of hypertension in African Americans are many and deserve to be addressed. In the interim however, there is compelling evidence that parity in the delivery of high quality care and BP control across race and ethnic groups is feasible and should be the goal of providers and health systems.[79,80] The primary drivers of such high-quality care include

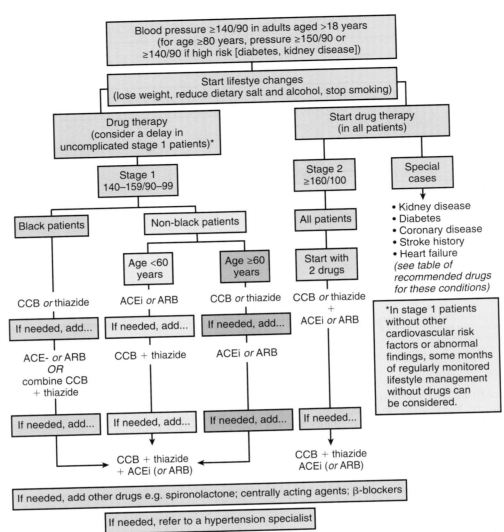

FIG. 41.7 Algorithm summarizing the clinical practice guidelines for the management of hypertension in the community published by the American Society of Hypertension and the International Society of Hypertension. *ACEi,* Angiotensin-converting enzyme inhibitor; *ARB,* angiotensin receptor blocker; *CCB,* calcium channel blocker; *thiazide,* thiazide or thiazide-like diuretics. Blood pressure values are mm Hg. *(Reproduced from Weber MA, Schiffrin EL, White WB, et al. Clinical practice guidelines for the management of hypertension in the community a statement by the American Society of Hypertension and the International Society of Hypertension. J Hypertens. 2014;32:3-15.)*

patient-centered interventions of trust building; provider- and health-systems-focused interventions in culturally responsive care; physician-led educational programs on treatment intensification, medication adherence, and consistent use of clinical practice guidelines; strong multidisciplinary care teams with clear definitions of roles in hypertension management; effective strategies to improve and expand access to care; and a commitment to embrace implementation, dissemination, and performance feedback strategies in chronic disease care.[18-20,81] Favorable results of comprehensive interventions such as the examples from Kaiser Permanente (Fig. 41.8)[18-20,81] provide the evidence and assurance that successful control of hypertension in African Americans and reduction or eventual elimination of related health disparities is feasible. What is needed now are focused dissemination and implementation research efforts to explore strategies for widespread dissemination, scale-up, and sustained implementation of effective strategies.

RESEARCH IMPLICATIONS

Research challenges in the management of hypertension in African Americans are many and include importantly, the

relative lack of objective clinical trial data on which to base decisions.[79] At the root of this challenge is the continuing underrepresentation of African Americans in clinical trials. Impediments at the level of participants, researchers, and health systems all contribute to this challenge.[82-87] Efforts to increase the participation of African Americans in clinical trials will help to address this challenge. There is compelling evidence that high rates of clinical trial participation and retention are attainable even in the high risk populations of underserved, inner-city, hypertensive young African-American men, especially when culturally acceptable strategies that employ nurse-community health worker teams in combination with usual medical care are used.[87]

Other research challenges include the need for practice-based evidence in hypertension treatment and control; further exploration of strategies for the prevention of hypertension beginning in at-risk youth; and primary drivers of increased susceptibility to hypertensive target organ damage. Additionally, renewed emphasis is needed in dissemination and implementation research to help turn fundamental discoveries and major clinical trial findings into population health impact and the elimination of hypertension-related health inequities.

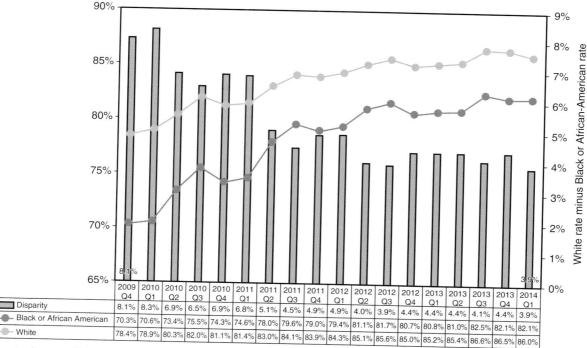

	2009 Q4	2010 Q1	2010 Q2	2010 Q3	2010 Q4	2011 Q1	2011 Q2	2011 Q3	2011 Q4	2012 Q1	2012 Q2	2012 Q3	2012 Q4	2013 Q1	2013 Q2	2013 Q3	2013 Q4	2014 Q1
Disparity	8.1%	8.3%	6.9%	6.5%	6.9%	6.8%	5.1%	4.5%	4.9%	4.9%	4.0%	3.9%	4.4%	4.4%	4.4%	4.1%	4.4%	3.9%
Black or African American	70.3%	70.6%	73.4%	75.5%	74.3%	74.6%	78.0%	79.6%	79.0%	79.4%	81.1%	81.7%	80.7%	80.8%	81.0%	82.5%	82.1%	82.1%
White	78.4%	78.9%	80.3%	82.0%	81.1%	81.4%	83.0%	84.1%	83.9%	84.3%	85.1%	85.6%	85.0%	85.2%	85.4%	86.6%	86.5%	86.0%

FIG. 41.8 Hypertension control for Kaiser Permanente program wide. *(Reproduced from Bartolome RE, Chen A, Handler J, Platt ST, Gould B. Population care management and team-based approach to reduce racial disparities among African Americans/Blacks with hypertension. Perm J. 2016;20:53-59.) Percentage of members in hypertension registry with blood pressure below 140/90 mm Hg (left x-axis) and disparity between control rates for white and black members (bars), 2009 Quarter (Q) 4 through 2014 Q1. (Reprinted from Perm J 2016;20(1):53-9. Bartolome RE, Chen A, Handler J, Platt ST, Gould B. Population Care Management and Team-Based Approach to Reduce Racial Disparities among African Americans/Blacks: 53-9. Copyright 2016, with permission from, The Permanente Press.)*

SUMMARY

Hypertension is a common chronic condition that affects one in three African Americans. It is a major and disproportionate contributor to death and disability from stroke, heart failure, kidney failure, and ischemic heart disease. Definitive pathophysiological mechanisms that explain the greater prevalence of hypertension and severe target organ damage remain elusive. However, increased SNS activity; increased dietary salt intake and salt sensitivity; impaired renal handling of sodium and expanded extracellular plasma volume; RAAS activation; alterations in the circadian control of nocturnal blood pressure; and psychosocial stress all play a role in the pathogenesis and maintenance of chronic hypertension in African Americans.

Over the last three decades, hypertension awareness, treatment, and control in African Americans have improved significantly. In fact, control rates of 80% and higher are achievable in African Americans when evidence-based strategies are used within integrated and supportive health care systems. Effective strategies begin with therapeutic lifestyle changes that emphasize individual's cultural heritage, beliefs, and behavioral norms and are instituted within the context of improved patient self-management and self-efficacy. Safe, effective, and affordable antihypertensive medications used in combination to attain goal blood pressure and overall community, health systems, and policy support are essential. Referral to a hypertension specialist is indicated when BP remains uncontrolled despite treatment with maximum doses of drugs from three or more recommended classes.

Increasing the recruitment and retention of African Americans in hypertension clinical trials remains an important research challenge. Other challenges include increasing the numbers of African American and other underrepresented racial and ethnic minority researchers with interest in hypertension research. The scope for such an endeavor appropriately includes all aspects of biomedical, behavioral, and social science research

in hypertension and hypertension-related target organ damage. Dissemination and implementation research strategies for accelerating the translation of research discoveries into sustained BP control, successful reduction in target organ damage, and elimination of related health inequities deserve emphasis.

Disclaimer

The views expressed in this chapter are those of the author and do not necessarily represent the views of the National Heart, Lung, and Blood Institute; National Institutes of Health; or the United States Department of Health and Human Services.

References

1. Forouzanfar MH, Alexander L, Anderson HR, et al. Global, regional, and national comparative risk assessment of 79 behavioural, environmental and occupational, and metabolic risks or clusters of risks in 188 countries, 1990-2013: a systematic analysis for the Global Burden of Disease Study 2013. *Lancet.* 2015;386:2287-2323.
2. Kung HC, Xu J. Hypertension-related Mortality in the United States, 2000-2013. *NCHS Data Brief.* 2015;(193):1-8.
3. Apostolides AY, Cutter G, Daugherty SA, et al. Three-year incidence of hypertension in thirteen U.S. communities. *Prev Med.* 1982;11:487.
4. Levine DA, Lewis CE, Williams OD, et al. Geographic and demographic variability in 20-year hypertension incidence: the CARDIA study. *Hypertension.* 2011;57:39-47.
5. Carson AP, Howard G, Burke GL, Shea S, Levitan EB, Muntner P. Ethnic differences in hypertension incidence among middle-aged and older adults: the multi-ethnic study of atherosclerosis. *Hypertension.* 2011;57:1101-1107.
6. He J, Klag MJ, Appel LJ, Charleston J, Whelton PK. Seven-year incidence of hypertension in a cohort of middle-aged African Americans and whites. *Hypertension.* 1998;31:1130-1135.
7. *Hypertension in Blacks: Epidemiology, Pathophysiology and Treatment.* Chicago: Year Book Medical Publishers; 1985.
8. Yoon SS, Carroll MD, Fryar CD. Hypertension Prevalence and Control Among Adults: United States, 2011-2014. *NCHS Data Brief.* 2015;(220):1-8.
9. Mozaffarian D, Benjamin EJ, Go AS, et al. Heart Disease and Stroke Statistics-2016 Update: a Report From the American Heart Association. *Circulation.* 2016;133:e38-e360.
10. Olives C, Myerson R, Mokdad AH, Murray CJ, Lim SS. Prevalence, awareness, treatment, and control of hypertension in United States counties, 2001-2009. *PLoS One.* 2013;8:e60308.
11. Voors AW, Webber LS, Berenson GS. Time course study of blood pressure in children over a three-year period. *Hypertension.* 1980;2(4 Pt 2):102-108.
12. Voors AW, Webber LS, Berenson GS. Time course studies of blood pressure in children—the Bogalusa Heart Study. *Am J Epidemiol.* 1979;109:320-334.
13. Muntner P, Lewis CE, Diaz KM, et al. Racial differences in abnormal ambulatory blood pressure monitoring measures: results from the Coronary Artery Risk Development in Young Adults (CARDIA) study. *Am J Hypertens.* 2015;28:640-648.

14. Selassie A, Wagner CS, Laken ML, Ferguson ML, Ferdinand KC, Egan BM. Progression is accelerated from prehypertension to hypertension in blacks. *Hypertension*. 2011;58:579-587.

15. Cooper RS, Liao Y, Rotimi C. Is hypertension more severe among U.S. blacks, or is severe hypertension more common? *Ann Epidemiol*. 1996;6:173-180.

16. Schmieder RE, Rockstroh JK, Luchters G, Hammerstein U, Messerli FH. Comparison of early target organ damage between blacks and whites with mild systemic arterial hypertension. *Am J Cardiol*. 1997;79:1695-1698.

17. Yoon SS, Gu Q, Nwankwo T, Wright JD, Hong Y, Burt V. Trends in blood pressure among adults with hypertension: United States, 2003 to 2012. *Hypertension*. 2015;65:54-61.

18. Sim JJ, Handler J, Jacobsen SJ, Kanter MH. Systemic implementation strategies to improve hypertension: the Kaiser Permanente Southern California experience. *Can J Cardiol*. 2014;30:544-552.

19. Jaffe MG, Lee GA, Young JD, Sidney S, Go AS. Improved blood pressure control associated with a large-scale hypertension program. *JAMA*. 2013;310:699-705.

20. Shaw KM, Handler J, Wall HK, Kanter MH. Improving blood pressure control in a large multiethnic California population through changes in health care delivery, 2004-2012. *Prev Chronic Dis*. 2014;11:E191.

21. Ogunniyi MO, Croft JB, Greenlund KJ, Giles WH, Mensah GA. Racial/ethnic differences in microalbuminuria among adults with prehypertension and hypertension: National Health and Nutrition Examination Survey (NHANES), 1999-2006. *Am J Hypertens*. 2010;23:859-864.

22. Mensah GA, Croft JB, Giles WH. The heart, kidney, and brain as target organs in hypertension. *Cardiol Clin*. 2002;20:225-247.

23. Izzo JL, Jr., Taylor AA. The sympathetic nervous system and baroreflexes in hypertension and hypotension. *Curr Hypertens Rep*. 1999;1:254-263.

24. Musante L, Treiber FA, Strong WB, Levy M. Family history of hypertension and cardiovascular reactivity to forehead cold stimulation in black male children. *J Psychosom Res*. 1990;34:111-116.

25. Anderson NB. Racial differences in stress-induced cardiovascular reactivity and hypertension: current status and substantive issues. *Psychol Bull*. 1989;105:89-105.

26. Knox SS, Hausdorff J, Markovitz JH. Reactivity as a predictor of subsequent blood pressure: racial differences in the Coronary Artery Risk Development in Young Adults (CARDIA) Study. *Hypertension*. 2002;40:914-919.

27. Nesbitt S, Victor RG. Pathogenesis of hypertension in African Americans. *Congest Heart Fail*. 2004;10:24-29.

28. Sullivan JM. Salt sensitivity. Definition, conception, methodology, and long-term issues. *Hypertension*. 1991;17(1 Suppl):I61-I68.

29. Richardson SI, Freedman BI, Ellison DH, Rodriguez CJ. Salt sensitivity: a review with a focus on non-Hispanic blacks and Hispanics. *J Am Soc Hypertens*. 2013;7:170-179.

30. Weinberger MH. Salt sensitivity is associated with an increased mortality in both normal and hypertensive humans. *J Clin Hypertens (Greenwich)*. 2002;4:274-276.

31. Basile JN. Salt sensitivity predicts mortality independently of elevated blood pressure: a 27-year follow-up study. *J Clin Hypertens (Greenwich)*. 2001;3:258-259.

32. Weinberger MH, Fineberg NS, Fineberg SE, Weinberger M. Salt sensitivity, pulse pressure, and death in normal and hypertensive humans. *Hypertension*. 2001;37(2 Pt 2):429-432.

33. Bihorac A, Tezcan H, Ozener C, Oktay A, Akoglu E. Association between salt sensitivity and target organ damage in essential hypertension. *Am J Hypertens*. 2000;13:864-872.

34. Weinberger MH. Hypertension in African Americans: the role of sodium chloride and extracellular fluid volume. *Semin Nephrol*. 1996;16:110-116.

35. Aviv A, Hollenberg NK, Weder AB. Sodium glomerulopathy: tubuloglomerular feedback and renal injury in African Americans. *Kidney Int*. 2004;65:361-368.

36. Bartley K, Jung M, Yi S. Diet and blood pressure: differences among whites, blacks and Hispanics in New York City 2010. *Ethn Dis*. 2014;24:175-181.

37. Weinberger MH, Luft FC, Bloch R, et al. The blood pressure-raising effects of high dietary sodium intake: racial differences and the role of potassium. *J Am Coll Nutr*. 1982;1:139-148.

38. Michel FS, Norton GR, Majane OH, et al. Contribution of circulating angiotensinogen concentrations to variations in aldosterone and blood pressure in a group of African ancestry depends on salt intake. *Hypertension*. 2012;59:62-69.

39. Tientcheu D, Ayers C, Das SR, et al. Target organ complications and cardiovascular events associated with masked hypertension and white-coat hypertension: analysis from the Dallas Heart Study. *J Am Coll Cardiol*. 2015;66:2159-2169.

40. Profant J, Dimsdale JE. Race and diurnal blood pressure patterns. A review and meta-analysis. *Hypertension*. 1999;33:1099-1104.

41. Hebert LA, Agarwal G, Ladson-Wofford SE, et al. Nocturnal blood pressure in treated hypertensive African Americans Compared to treated hypertensive European Americans. *J Am Soc Nephrol*. 1996;7:2130-2134.

42. Harshfield GA, Treiber FA, Wilson ME, Kapuku GK, Davis HC. A longitudinal study of ethnic differences in ambulatory blood pressure patterns in youth. *Am J Hypertens*. 2002;15:525-530.

43. Harshfield GA, Hwang C, Grim CE. Circadian variation of blood pressure in blacks: influence of age, gender and activity. *J Hum Hypertens*. 1990;4:43-47.

44. Napan S, Kwagyan J, Randall OS, Xu S, Ketete M, Maqbool AR. Nocturnal blood pressure nondipping in obese African-Americans. *Blood Press Monit*. 2011;16:111-116.

45. Burnier M, Coltamai L, Maillard M, Bochud M. Renal sodium handling and nighttime blood pressure. *Semin Nephrol*. 2007;27:565-571.

46. Cuffee Y, Ogedegbe C, Williams NJ, Ogedegbe G, Schoenthaler A. Psychosocial risk factors for hypertension: an update of the literature. *Curr Hypertens Rep*. 2014;16. 483-483.

47. Rosenthal T, Alter A. Occupational stress and hypertension. *J Am Soc Hypertens*. 2012;6:2-22.

48. Sparrenberger F, Cichelero FT, Ascoli AM, et al. Does psychosocial stress cause hypertension? A systematic review of observational studies. *J Hum Hypertens*. 2009;23:12-19.

49. Spruill TM, Gerin W, Ogedegbe G, Burg M, Schwartz JE, Pickering TG. Socioeconomic and psychosocial factors mediate race differences in nocturnal blood pressure dipping. *Am J Hypertens*. 2009;22:637-642.

50. Bosworth HB, Powers B, Grubber JM, et al. Racial differences in blood pressure control: potential explanatory factors. *J Gen Intern Med*. 2008;23:692-698.

51. Brondolo E, Rieppi R, Kelly KP, Gerin W. Perceived racism and blood pressure: a review of the literature and conceptual and methodological critique. *Ann Behav Med*. 2003;25:55-65.

52. Sampson UK, Mensah GA. Initial clinical encounter with the patient with established hypertension. *Cardiol Clin*. 2010;28:587-595.

53. Sacks FM, Svetkey LP, Vollmer WM, et al. Effects on blood pressure of reduced dietary sodium and the Dietary Approaches to Stop Hypertension (DASH) diet. DASH-Sodium Collaborative Research Group. *N Engl J Med*. 2001;344:3-10.

54. Appel LJ, Moore TJ, Obarzanek E, et al. A clinical trial of the effects of dietary patterns on blood pressure. DASH Collaborative Research Group. *N Engl J Med*. 1997;336:1117-1124.

55. Eckel RH, Jakicic JM, Ard JD, et al. 2013 AHA/ACC Guideline on lifestyle management to reduce cardiovascular risk: a report of the American College of Cardiology/American Heart Association Task Force on Practice Guidelines. *J Am Coll Cardiol*. 2014;63(25 Pt B): 2960-2984.

56. Borjesson M, Onerup A, Lundqvist S, Dahlof B. Physical activity and exercise lower blood pressure in individuals with hypertension: narrative review of 27 RCTs. *Br J Sports Med*. 2016;50:1-8.

57. Staffileno BA, Minnick A, Coke LA, Hollenberg SM. Blood pressure responses to lifestyle physical activity among young, hypertension-prone African-American women. *J Cardiovasc Nurs*. 2007;22:107-117.

58. Appel LJ, Champagne CM, Harsha DW, et al. Effects of comprehensive lifestyle modification on blood pressure control: main results of the PREMIER clinical trial. *JAMA*. 2003;289:2083-2093.

59. Akinseye OA, Williams SK, Seixas A, et al. Sleep as a mediator in the pathway linking environmental factors to hypertension: a review of the literature. *Int J Hypertens*. 2015;2015:926414.

60. Smith ML, Pacchia CF. Sleep apnoea and hypertension: role of chemoreflexes in humans. *Exp Physiol*. 2007;92:45-50.

61. Hoffstein V, Chan CK, Slutsky AS. Sleep apnea and systemic hypertension: a causal association review. *Am J Med*. 1991;91:190-196.

62. Hale L, Do DP. Racial differences in self-reports of sleep duration in a population-based study. *Sleep*. 2007;30:1096-1103.

63. Institute of Medicine. Clinical Practice Guidelines We Can Trust. *National Academy of Sciences*. 2013; www.iom.edu/Reports/2011/Clinical-Practice-Guidelines-We-Can-Trust.aspx.

64. Institute of Medicine. Finding What Works in Health Care: Standards for Systematic Reviews. *National Academy of Sciences*. 2013; www.iom.edu/Reports/2011/Finding-What-Works-in-Health-Care-Standards-for-Systematic-Reviews.aspx.

65. Weber MA. Recently published hypertension guidelines of the JNC 8 panelists, the American Society of Hypertension/International Society of Hypertension and other major organizations: introduction to a focus issue of the Journal of Clinical Hypertension. *J Clin Hypertens (Greenwich)*. 2014;16:241-245.

66. Weber MA, Schiffrin EL, White WB, et al. Clinical practice guidelines for the management of hypertension in the community a statement by the American Society of Hypertension and the International Society of Hypertension. *J Hypertens*. 2014;32:3-15.

67. James PA, Oparil S, Carter BL, et al. 2014 evidence-based guideline for the management of high blood pressure in adults: report from the panel members appointed to the Eighth Joint National Committee (JNC 8). *JAMA*. 2014;5(311):507-520.

68. Chobanian AV, Bakris GL, Black HR, et al. The Seventh Report of the Joint National Committee on prevention, detection, evaluation, and treatment of high blood pressure: the JNC 7 Report. *JAMA*. 2003;289:2560-2572.

69. Flack JM, Sica DA, Bakris G, et al. Management of high blood pressure in Blacks: an update of the International Society on Hypertension in Blacks consensus statement. *Hypertension*. 2010;56:780-800.

70. Daskalopoulou SS, Rabi DM, Zarnke KB, et al. The 2015 Canadian Hypertension Education Program recommendations for blood pressure measurement, diagnosis, assessment of risk, prevention, and treatment of hypertension. *Can J Cardiol*. 2015;31:549-568.

71. Bangalore S, Ogedegbe G, Gyamfi J, et al. Outcomes with angiotensin-converting enzyme inhibitors vs other antihypertensive agents in hypertensive blacks. *Am J Med*. 2015;128:1195-1203.

72. Ogedegbe G, Shah NR, Phillips C, et al. Comparative effectiveness of angiotensin-converting enzyme inhibitor-based treatment on cardiovascular outcomes in hypertensive blacks versus whites. *J Am Coll Cardiol*. 2015;15(66):1224-1233.

73. Chen Y, Hu S, Li Y, Yan B, Shen G, Wang L. Systematic review of hypertension clinical practice guidelines based on the burden of disease: a global perspective. *J Evid Based Med*. 2014;7:52-59.

74. Egan BM, Bland VJ, Brown AL, et al. Hypertension in african americans aged 60 to 79 years: statement from the international society of hypertension in blacks. *J Clin Hypertens (Greenwich)*. 2015;17:252-259.

75. Williams RA, Flack JM, Gavin JR, III, Schneider WR, Hennekens CH. Guidelines for management of high-risk African Americans with multiple cardiovascular risk factors: recommendations of an expert consensus panel. *Ethn Dis*. 2007;17:214-220.

76. Douglas JG, Bakris GL, Epstein M, et al. Management of high blood pressure in African Americans: consensus statement of the Hypertension in African Americans Working Group of the International Society on Hypertension in Blacks. *Arch Intern Med*. 2003;163:525-541.

77. Wright JT, Jr., Williamson JD, Whelton PK, et al. A Randomized Trial of Intensive versus Standard Blood-Pressure Control. *N Engl J Med*. 2015;373:2103-2116.

78. Cushman WC, Whelton PK, Fine LJ, et al. SPRINT Trial Results: latest news in hypertension management. *Hypertension*. 2016;67:263-265.

79. Bakris GL, Ferdinand KC, Douglas JG, Sowers JR. Optimal treatment of hypertension in African Americans. Reaching and maintaining target blood pressure goals. *Postgrad Med*. 2002;112:73-80, 83.

80. Ferdinand KC. Recommendations for the management of special populations: racial and ethnic populations. *Am J Hypertens*. 2003;16(11 Pt 2):50S-54S.

81. Bartolome RE, Chen A, Handler J, Platt ST, Gould B. Population care management and team-based approach to reduce racial disparities among African Americans/Blacks with hypertension. *Perm J*. 2016;20:53-59.

82. Branson RD, Davis K, Jr., Butler KL. African Americans' participation in clinical research: importance, barriers, and solutions. *Am J Surg*. 2007;193:32-39.

83. Park IU, Taylor AL. Race and ethnicity in trials of antihypertensive therapy to prevent cardiovascular outcomes: a systematic review. *Ann Fam Med*. 2007;5:444-452.

84. Sheikh A. Why are ethnic minorities under-represented in US research studies? *PLoS Med*. 2006;3:e49.

85. Oddone EZ, Olsen MK, Lindquist JH, et al. Enrollment in clinical trials according to patients race: experience from the VA Cooperative Studies Program (1975-2000). *Control Clin Trials*. 2004;25:378-387.

86. Freimuth VS, Quinn SC, Thomas SB, Cole G, Zook E, Duncan T. African Americans' views on research and the Tuskegee Syphilis Study. *Soc Sci Med*. 2001;52:797-808.

87. Hill MN, Bone LR, Hilton SC, Roary MC, Kelen GD, Levine DM. A clinical trial to improve high blood pressure care in young urban black men: recruitment, follow-up, and outcomes. *Am J Hypertens*. 1999;12:548-554.

42   Orthostatic Hypotension

Italo Biaggioni

Orthostatic hypotension (OH) is a significant medical problem; it occurs in about 6% of healthy elderly in the community, 18% to 54% of nursing home residents, and up to 60% in hospitalized elderly.[1] The incidence of OH increases exponentially after age 65, and its importance is likely to increase as our population ages.[2] OH is not only a cause of disability and impaired quality of life, but it is also associated with a 2.6-fold increase in the risk of falls,[3] and is an independent risk factor for increased mortality.[4] The prototypical patient with orthostatic hypotension is a frail elderly, with multiple comorbidities and on multiple medications.[5] Hypertension is the most common comorbidity among patients with OH; it is present in approximately 70% of patients.[5] Conversely, orthostatic hypotension is present in about 10% of patients referred to hypertension specialists,[6] and in community studies hypertension is strongly associated with OH.[7] Coexistence of hypertension with orthostatic hypotension represents a management challenge as the treatment of one condition can worsen the other. It is important, therefore, that physicians treating hypertensive patients be knowledgeable of the pathophysiology of orthostatic hypotension, which will ultimately guide its treatment.

PATHOPHYSIOLOGY

When a normal individual stands, up to 700 mL of blood pools in the legs and lower abdominal veins. Venous return decreases, resulting in a transient decline in cardiac output. The reduction in central blood volume and arterial pressure is sensed by cardiopulmonary volume receptors and arterial baroreceptors. Afferent signals from these receptors reach vasomotor centers in the brainstem. Efferent fibers from these centers reduce parasympathetic output and increase sympathetic outflow. Norepinephrine is released from postganglionic sympathetic nerve terminals at target organs, resulting in an increase in heart rate and cardiac contractility, partial restoration of venous return and diastolic ventricular filling by venoconstriction, and an increase in peripheral resistance by arteriolar vasoconstriction. As a net effect of these adaptive mechanisms, upright cardiac output remains reduced by 10% to 20% compared with supine, systolic blood pressure (SBP) is reduced by 5 to 10 mm Hg, diastolic blood pressure increases by 2 to 5 mm Hg, mean blood pressure remains almost unchanged, and heart rate increases by 5 to 20 beats per minute.

Impairment in these compensatory autonomic neural mechanisms results in OH. Primary neurodegenerative disorders of the autonomic nervous system are the cause of the most severe cases of OH. The common pathology of these disorders are deposits of alpha-synuclein forming Lewy bodies in peripheral noradrenergic nerves (pure autonomic failure, Parkinson disease) or glial cytoplasmic inclusions in central autonomic pathways (multiple system atrophy).[8,9] In the vast majority of patients, however, OH is the result of milder forms of autonomic impairment (often related to aging or diabetes) superimposed with other aggravating factors (often medications).

CLINICAL CONSEQUENCES OF ORTHOSTATIC HYPOTENSION

OH impairs the functional status and quality of life of patients affected by it. Furthermore, it is associated with a 2.6-fold increase in the risk of falls in the elderly, and this association remains after correcting for other risk factors.[3] Patients with OH commonly experience syncope and falls,[10,11] an association that has been documented in 24% to 31% of patients presenting to emergency department visits.[12,13] Multiple epidemiological studies have reported that OH is associated with coronary artery disease, stroke, and heart failure.[10,11] The presence of OH doubles the risk of developing chronic kidney disease,[12] and as an independent risk factor it is comparable with having coronary artery disease, smoking, hypertriglyceridemia, and other risk factors that receive more attention.[2] Importantly, during the past 2 decades, evidence from cross-sectional and longitudinal epidemiological studies has identified OH as an independent risk factor for cardiovascular morbidity and all-cause mortality.[4,13]

Orthostatic hypotension, therefore, represents a burden to the United States health care system. A recent report showed that the overall annual rate for OH-related hospitalization is 36 per 100,000 U.S. adults, and this rate increases steadily with age and can be as high as 233 per 100,000 in those age 75 or older.[5] Considering that the U.S. demographic is rapidly changing, with the elderly population representing nearly 20% of the total U.S. population in the next 20 years, the impact of OH-related hospitalizations will be a greater challenge to our health services and the medical community.

EVALUATION OF THE PATIENT WITH ORTHOSTATIC HYPOTENSION

OH is defined as a sustained reduction of SBP of at least 20 mm Hg or diastolic blood pressure (DBP) of 10 mm Hg within 3 min of standing, or head-up tilt to at least 60 degrees.[14] In hypertensive patients, a reduction in SBP of 30 mm Hg is considered a more appropriate criterion for orthostatic hypotension because the magnitude of the orthostatic blood pressure fall is dependent on the baseline blood pressure.[14] Typical symptoms of OH are lightheadedness, dizziness, fatigue, dimming of vision, and shoulder ("coat hanger") pain. Patients may be asymptomatic or may have difficulty identifying their symptoms. It is useful to consider that, as a general rule, symptoms should never start while the patient is supine, should occur mostly while standing, and should be quickly relived by seating or lying down. Symptoms tend to be worse in hot

393

environments and if patients stand still. The severity of OH is also greater in the morning, so much so that the diagnosis of OH is more likely to be made if orthostatic vitals are taken in the morning than in the afternoon.[15]

The evaluation and diagnosis of OH can be done at the bedside. Autonomic testing, often restricted to specialized units, is helpful to assess the presence and severity of autonomic impairment (neurogenic OH). It is, however, not essential. Measuring orthostatic blood pressure and heart rate is often all that is needed. A significant decrease in orthostatic blood pressure that is not associated with an appropriate increase in heart rate is indicative of neurogenic OH. Another practical alternative to specialized testing is to clinically try to improve OH by removing factors that can trigger or aggravate OH (see below under management); any significant OH that remains is likely to have an important neurogenic component.

The list of etiologies that cause neurogenic OH is long but most become apparent after a comprehensive evaluation. In principle, any disease that causes peripheral neuropathy can cause autonomic neuropathy and neurogenic OH. In practice, diabetes mellitus (DM) is the most common culprit. Tight glucose control can delay the progression of autonomic neuropathy in type 1 diabetes,[16] but the evidence for type 2 diabetes is less clear. B12 deficiency should be ruled out because its treatment can lead to improvement of OH.[17] Special attention should be given to patients that develop severe OH with a subacute onset and rapid progression, for they often have an autoimmune or paraneoplastic syndrome; in some cases neurogenic OH can be the presenting problem which leads to the diagnosis of the underlying disease.[18]

MANAGEMENT OF HYPERTENSION IN THE PATIENT WITH ORTHOSTATIC HYPOTENSION

When encountering a hypertensive patient with concomitant orthostatic hypotension, it is tempting to ease the antihypertensive treatment, in an attempt to prevent syncope and falls. Current evidence, however, suggest that such an approach is misguided. In studies of elderly living in the community, the incidence of OH increased from 2% to 5% when hypertension was present, but was greatest (19%) in those with uncontrolled hypertension.[7,19] Importantly, the presence of OH per se did not increase the risk of falls, whereas elderly with uncontrolled hypertension and OH had more than a twofold increase risk of falls.[19] This observation argues in favor of treating both OH and hypertension in these patients.

The obvious question is what antihypertensives should be used in patients with OH, and which should be avoided? There is limited evidence from randomized controlled trials on which to base recommendations. It stands to reason that antihypertensives that interfere with autonomic orthostatic compensatory mechanisms will worsen OH, and observational studies have indeed found that the use of alpha blockers,[6,7] beta-blockers,[6,7,20] and central sympatholytics[6] are associated with OH. A similar association is also found with the use of thiazide diuretics.[6,7] No significant associations were found between the presence of OH and the use of calcium channel blockers.[7,20] The presence of OH was reduced in patients receiving angiotensin receptor blockers in one study,[6] increased in patients taking angiotensin-converting enzyme (ACE) inhibitors in another,[7] and no association was observed in patients using antihypertensives targeting the renin-angiotensin system in a third study.[20]

Some patients may have isolated supine hypertension. This is most commonly observed in patients with severe primary forms of autonomic failure,[21] in whom seated blood pressure may be completely normal or only slightly elevated. There is no agreement as to whether or not isolated supine hypertension should be treated. Supine hypertension, however, is associated with left ventricular hypertrophy[22] and decreased renal

function.[23] Furthermore, severely affected patients can lose up to 2 kilograms of weight during the night.[24] This is caused by pressure diuresis and explains why patients are worse early in the morning. Treatment of supine hypertension, therefore, could theoretically improve OH. During the day, simply avoiding the supine position is the best way to treat these patients. During the night, several antihypertensives given at bedtime have been shown to reduced supine hypertension, including nitroglycerine patch (to be removed first thing in the morning),[21] nebivolol,[25] losartan,[24] and sildenafil.[26] Unfortunately none have been shown to improve next morning OH either because they do not reduce nighttime diuresis or they have residual hypotensive effects in the morning.

MANAGEMENT OF ORTHOSTATIC HYPOTENSION IN THE HYPERTENSIVE PATIENT

Goal of Treatment and Overall Strategy

The main goal of treatment of OH is to reduce symptoms and improve the patients' functional status and quality of life. This requires an increase in standing blood pressure. A recent study in patients with Parkinson disease and OH found that symptoms were absent if mean standing blood pressure (BP) was above 75 mm Hg.[27] This likely reflects the threshold BP below which cerebral autoregulation is overcome. Conversely, increasing BP above that level provides no additional therapeutic benefit. Thus, the goal should not be to "normalize" upright blood pressure, but to raise it only enough to alleviate symptoms.

The ideal therapy will selectively improve upright BP while having no effect on supine BP. Most pressor agents, however, have an opposite effect, and produce a greater increase in supine or seated BP than in standing BP. In the absence of orthostatic pressor selectivity, therapies should have a quick onset and short duration of action to avoid worsening supine hypertension. Particularly in patients with hypertension, therefore, it is preferable to use short-acting pressor agents only to prepare patients to stand up, and should be avoided when patients lie down.

We assume that reducing orthostatic hypotension will result in prevention of syncope and falls, but this has not been shown for any of the therapies currently available. Even less certain is that the treatment will prevent the increase in mortality associated with OH. It could be argued that pharmacological treatment (e.g., with fludrocortisone or pressor agents) may even have a negative impact on cardiovascular outcomes.

Current treatment recommendations are based mostly on studies in small numbers of patients with primary forms of autonomic failure and severe OH, with limited evidence of long-term efficacy in randomized controlled clinical trials.[28] No studies have been designed to include the most common forms of OH, patients with diabetes, or elderly hypertensive patients with multiple comorbidities.

Remove Offending Factors

The first step in the management of OH is to remove any potential factor that could precipitate or contribute to OH. Medications are among the common offenders. Amitriptyline, often used to treat pain in sensory neuropathies (which is often seen in patients with autonomic neuropathies), is a common culprit. In patients with hypertension and OH, certain medications should be avoided, such as diuretics and alpha-blockers but without abandoning antihypertensive treatment altogether (see previously). Physicians also need to be aware of "hidden" antiadrenergic agents. Tamsulosin, commonly used to treat benign prostatic hyperplasia, is an alpha-blocker with preferential selectivity for the α_{1A} receptor in the prostate versus the α_{1B} receptor in blood vessels. This selectivity, however, is not absolute, and tamsulosin increases the risk of orthostatic hypotension in susceptible individuals.[29] Trazodone is used as an antidepressant, but it is often overlooked that it is also a potent alpha$_1$-blocker that can worsen or trigger OH.[30] Tizanidine is marketed as a "central muscle relaxant," but pharmacologically it is an α_2 agonist very similar in chemical structure and antihypertensive properties to clonidine[31] and can also cause orthostatic hypotension. Congestive heart failure is a common comorbidity in patients with OH, and is often treated with "vasodilating" beta-blockers than have alpha-blocking properties (carvedilol, labetalol) or that promote nitric oxide (nebivolol). These agents do lower BP in autonomic failure patients,[25] and if cardioprotection is desired it would seem preferable to use nonvasodilating beta-blockers. Finally, erectile dysfunction is often an early (albeit nonspecific) sign of autonomic impairment, and phosphodiesterase inhibitors used in its treatment can produce profound decreases in BP in patients with autonomic failure.[26]

Food digestion induces pooling of blood in the splanchnic circulation with hemodynamic consequences that are similar to those that occur on standing. It is not surprising then that patients with autonomic failure can have substantial drops in BP after meals. The nadir in BP is usually seen 30 minutes after a meal, is worse with high carbohydrate foods, and can be prevented by delaying glucose absorption with 50 to 100 mg acarbose.[32] The presence of postprandial hypotension should be investigated in all patients with significant OH because its treatment can provide significant symptomatic relief without the use of pressor agents.

Nonpharmacological Countermeasures

Patients should use physical countermeasures that reduce venous pooling, thereby improving venous return and cardiac output. These include standing slowly and in stages, avoid standing motionless, and tensing the leg muscles.[33] Compression stockings can be used to decrease venous pooling on standing, but because most of the pooling occurs in the abdomen[34] waist-high stockings that produce at least 15 to 20 mm Hg pressure are required, but they are difficult to put on, limiting compliance. Many patients and physicians rely on knee-high or thigh-high stockings, but experimental data indicate that leg compression does not improve orthostatic tolerance. On the other hand selective abdominal compression is effective.[35] This provides a rationale to use abdominal binders, worn as tight as possible, as an alternative to waist-high compression stockings. We have recently found that an automated abdominal binder, servo-controlled to maintain an abdominal pressure of 40 mm Hg, is as effective as midodrine in improving orthostatic tolerance acutely. Theoretically, an abdominal binder has all the properties of an ideal treatment for OH, particularly in patients with hypertension; because it is applied only on standing, it selectively increases upright blood pressure, and its onset and offset of action are immediate (Table 42.1). However, the long-term effectiveness and tolerability of this approach has not been tested.

Pressor Agents

A bolus ingestion of 16 ounces of tap water can produce dramatic increases in BP in autonomic failure patients.[36] This is not a volume effect, because intravenous infusion of the same volume has negligible effects on BP. Recent animal studies indicate that this effect is triggered by hypotonicity at the level of the portal circulation, which then triggers a sympathetic pressor reflex.[37] Of the interventions designed to increase BP in autonomic failure, oral water bolus is arguably the closest to an ideal pressor agent; it acts quickly, the increase in BP is apparent in the first 5 to 10 minutes and peaks around 30 minutes, and it is short-lived. The increase in BP produced by oral water boluses can be dramatic in patients with autonomic failure. In normal elderly it is also present but of less magnitude,[38] and this approach has not been tested in the vast majority of patients with OH associated with milder impairments of autonomic function.

Pyridostigmine, a cholinesterase inhibitor that potentiates the actions of acetylcholine, can increase BP in autonomic failure patients by facilitating cholinergic neurotransmission at the level of autonomic ganglia. In essence, it harnesses the patient's residual sympathetic activity. Because of this mechanism of action, the increase in BP is preferentially seen on standing, when residual sympathetic tone is increased; 60 mg pyridostigmine increases upright BP and reduces symptoms in patients with OH and has the added advantage of not affecting supine BP.[39] Because it requires residual sympathetic tone, it may not be as effective in patients with severe neurogenic OH,[40] and dose escalation is limited by side effects (abdominal cramping and other gastrointestinal side effects, and urinary urgency). Nonetheless, because it does not worsens supine hypertension, it may be particularly useful to try in hypertensive patients.

Fludrocortisone is a synthetic mineralocorticoid aldosterone analog that is often used to treat OH[41] under the concept that it expands intravascular volume by increasing renal sodium reabsorption. This increase in plasma volume, however, is only transient and plasma volume returns to baseline values in about 2 weeks[42] likely as a result of mineralocorticoid escape. The long-term benefit of fludrocortisone may be related to potentiation of the pressor effect of norepinephrine and angiotensin II. Fludrocortisone should not be given in patients with congestive heart failure and is best avoided in patients with hypertension.

TABLE 42.1 Clinical Characteristics of Therapeutic Modalities for Orthostatic Hypotension

	PREFERENTIAL INCREASE IN UPRIGHT BP	TIME TO PEAK ACTION	DURATION OF ACTION	EVIDENCE FROM RCT?	SIDE EFFECTS COMMENTS
Abdominal Binder	Yes	Immediate	As required	No	Uncomfortable
Oral Water Bolus	No	~20-30 min	~1 hour	No	Diuresis Best for patients with severe autonomic failure
Pyridostigmine	Yes	~1 hour	~3-4 hours	Limited	Not very potent Best for milder patients
Fludrocortisone	No	?	?	No	Supine HTN, hypokalemia
Midodrine	No	~1 hour	~3-4 hours	Yes[a]	Supine HTN, urinary obstruction
Droxidopa	No	~3 hours	~4-6 hours	Yes	Supine HTN

[a]Midodrine was approved based on an acute increase in upright blood pressure.

BP, Blood pressure; HTN, hypertension; RTC, randomized clinical trial.

Midodrine was approved in 1996 for the treatment of symptomatic orthostatic hypotension based on studies showing an improvement in 1-minute standing systolic pressure. The United States Food and Drug Administration (FDA) granted accelerated approval using this increase in BP as a surrogate end-point for clinical efficacy. A recent postmarketing study required by the FDA demonstrated a reduction of orthostatic symptoms.[43] Even though an acute increase in BP has been repeatedly documented with midodrine in patients with autonomic failure, the improvement of symptoms has not always been significant.[44] Its relatively short half-life is particularly useful in patients with hypertension, who are instructed not to lie down for 3 to 4 hours after each dose to avoid supine hypertension. Treatment should begin with a 2.5 to 5 mg dose, which can then be increased up to 10 mg thrice daily. We routinely try to hold the last daily dose, as OH tends to improve spontaneously during the day.

Droxidopa (L-threo-3,4-dihydroxyphenylserine, L-threo-DOPS, or L-DOPS) is structurally similar to norepinephrine but has an additional carboxyl group. It is absorbed orally and is converted to norepinephrine through the enzyme dopa-decarboxylase (L-aromatic amino acid decarboxylase) that is ubiquitous in tissues. This is the same enzyme that converts levodopa to dopamine for the treatment of Parkinson disease. Multicenter, randomized, placebo-controlled studies have shown droxidopa to be effective in increasing upright BP and reducing orthostatic symptoms in patients with primary forms of neurogenic OH.[45-47] The effectiveness of droxidopa beyond the 2 weeks efficacy tested in these trials is currently being assessed. More common causes of OH (e.g., diabetic neuropathy) were not included in these studies, in keeping with the development of the drug for orphan product designation.

The dose of droxidopa needs to be individualized, from 100 to 600 mg thrice daily. The increase in BP after a single dose peaks at about 3 to 4 hours and persists for about 6 hours. Droxidopa appears to have a good safety profile, with a relatively low incidence of adverse events related to supine hypertension (4.9% versus 2.5%). We would expect a higher incidence of supine hypertension when droxidopa is prescribed outside a controlled clinical trial, especially if physicians use it on a scheduled three times daily basis, instead of thrice daily with the last dose no later than 5 hours before bedtime. It is not clear if a thrice-daily dose is needed, or with twice daily dosing would be sufficient as suggested by a European open label study.[48]

SUMMARY

Orthostatic hypotension is an important and common medical problem, particularly in the frail elderly with multiple comorbidities and polypharmacy. OH is an independent risk factor for falls and overall mortality. Hypertension is among the most common comorbidities associated with OH. Coexistence of hypertension and OH may complicate the management of patients because treatment of one can worsen the other. However, there is evidence that uncontrolled hypertension makes OH worse, so both should be managed. The limited data available suggest that angiotensin receptor blockers and calcium channel blockers are preferable antihypertensives for these patients. Patients with isolated supine hypertension can be treated by simply avoiding the supine position during the day, and with bedtime doses of short-acting antihypertensives. Treatment of OH in the hypertensive patients should focus first on conservative countermeasures and therapeutic approaches that do not worsen hypertension. Foremost, removal of drugs that can trigger or worsen OH, including ones that are easily overlooked (e.g., tamsulosin, tizanidine, sildenafil, trazodone, and vasodilating beta-blockers). OH and postprandial hypotension can be prevented with abdominal binders and acarbose, respectively, without the need to increase baseline blood pressure. Pyridostigmine can selectively improve standing BP in patients with milder forms of autonomic impairment, and oral water bolus can acutely but transiently increase blood pressure in patients with severe autonomic failure. If traditional pressor agents are needed, midodrine and droxidopa can be used. The goal is to use the lowest dose that will improve symptoms, given only when needed, which in most patients is early morning and early afternoon.

Disclaimer

The author has been a consultant for Shire PLC, is a consultant for Lundbeck, and has applied for a patent for an automated abdominal binder to treat orthostatic hypotension.

References

1. Low PA. Prevalence of orthostatic hypotension. *Clin Auton Res*. 2008;18(Suppl 1):8-13.
2. Shibao C, Biaggioni I. Orthostatic hypotension and cardiovascular risk. *Hypertension*. 2010;56:1042-1044.
3. Ooi WL, Hossain M, Lipsitz LA. The association between orthostatic hypotension and recurrent falls in nursing home residents. *Am J Med*. 2000;108:106-111.
4. Xin W, Lin Z, Mi S. Orthostatic hypotension and mortality risk: a meta-analysis of cohort studies. *Heart*. 2014;100:406-413.
5. Shibao C, Grijalva CG, Raj SR, Biaggioni I, Griffin MR. Orthostatic hypotension-related hospitalizations in the United States. *AmJ Med*. 2007;120:975-980.
6. Di Stefano C, Milazzo V, Totaro S, et al. Orthostatic hypotension in a cohort of hypertensive patients referring to a hypertension clinic. *J Hum Hypertens*. 2015;29:599-603.
7. Kamaruzzaman S, Watt H, Carson C, Ebrahim S. The association between orthostatic hypotension and medication use in the British Women's Heart and Health Study. *Age Ageing*. 2010;39:51-56.
8. Biaggioni I. Sympathetic control of the circulation in hypertension: lessons from autonomic disorders. *Curr Opin Nephrol Hypertens*. 2003;12:175-180.
9. Shannon JR, Jordan J, Diedrich A, et al. Sympathetically mediated hypertension in autonomic failure. *Circulation*. 2000;101:2710-2715.
10. Rose KM, Tyroler HA, Nardo CJ, et al. Orthostatic hypotension and the incidence of coronary heart disease: the Atherosclerosis Risk in Communities study. *Am J Hypertens*. 2000;13:571-578.
11. Luukinen H, Koski K, Laippala P, Airaksinen KE. Orthostatic hypotension and the risk of myocardial infarction in the home-dwelling elderly. *J Intern Med*. 2004;255:486-493.
12. Franceschini N, Rose KM, Astor BC, Couper D, Vupputuri S. Orthostatic hypotension and incident chronic kidney disease: the atherosclerosis risk in communities study. *Hypertension*. 2010;56:1054-1059.
13. Masaki KH, Schatz IJ, Burchfiel CM, Sharp DS, Chiu D, Foley D, Curb JD. Orthostatic hypotension predicts mortality in elderly men: the Honolulu Heart Program. *Circulation*. 1998;98:2290-2295.
14. Freeman R, Wieling W, Axelrod FB, et al. Consensus statement on the definition of orthostatic hypotension, neurally mediated syncope and the postural tachycardia syndrome. *Clin Auton Res*. 2011;21:69-72.
15. Ooi WL, Barrett S, Hossain M, Kelley-Gagnon M, Lipsitz LA. Patterns of orthostatic blood pressure change and their clinical correlates in a frail, elderly population. *J Amer Med Assoc*. 1997;277:1299-1304.
16. The effect of intensive treatment of diabetes on the development and progression of long-term complications in insulin-dependent diabetes mellitus. The Diabetes Control and Complications Trial Research Group. *N Engl J Med*. 1993;329:977-986.
17. Moore A, Ryan J, Watts M, Pillay I, Clinch D, Lyons O. Orthostatic tolerance in older patients with vitamin B12 deficiency before and after vitamin B12 replacement. *Clin Auton Res*. 2004;14:67-71.
18. Shibao C, Muppa P, Semler MW, Peltier AC, Biaggioni I. A standing dilemma: autonomic failure preceding Hodgkin's lymphoma. *Am J Med*. 2014;127:284-287.
19. Gangavati A, Hajjar I, Quach L, et al. Hypertension, orthostatic hypotension, and the risk of falls in a community-dwelling elderly population: the maintenance of balance, independent living, intellect, and zest in the elderly of Boston study. *J Am Geriatr Soc*. 2011;59:383-389.
20. Canney M, O'Connell MD, Murphy CM, et al. Single agent antihypertensive therapy and orthostatic blood pressure behaviour in older adults using beat-to-beat measurements: the Irish longitudinal study on ageing. *PLoS One*. 2016;11:e0146156.
21. Shannon J, Jordan J, Costa F, Robertson RM, Biaggioni I. The hypertension of autonomic failure and its treatment. *Hypertension*. 1997;30:1062-1067.
22. Vagaonescu TD, Saadia D, Tuhrim S, Phillips RA, Kaufmann H. Hypertensive cardiovascular damage in patients with primary autonomic failure. *Lancet*. 2000;355:725-726.
23. Garland EM, Gamboa A, Okamoto L, et al. Renal impairment of pure autonomic failure. *Hypertension*. 2009;54:1057-1061.
24. Arnold AC, Okamoto LE, Gamboa A, et al. Angiotensin II, independent of plasma renin activity, contributes to the hypertension of autonomic failure. *Hypertension*. 2013;61:701-706.
25. Okamoto LE, Gamboa A, Shibao CA, et al. Nebivolol, but not metoprolol, lowers blood pressure in nitric oxide-sensitive human hypertension. *Hypertension*. 2014;64:1241-1247.
26. Gamboa A, Shibao C, Diedrich A, et al. Excessive nitric oxide function and blood pressure regulation in patients with autonomic failure. *Hypertension*. 2008;51:1531-1536.
27. Palma JA, Gomez-Esteban JC, Norcliffe-Kaufmann L, et al. Orthostatic hypotension in Parkinson disease: how much you fall or how low you go? *Mov Disord*. 2015;30:639-645.
28. Logan IC, Witham MD. Efficacy of treatments for orthostatic hypotension: a systematic review. *Age Ageing*. 2012;41:587-594.
29. Bird ST, Delaney JA, Brophy JM, Etminan M, Skeldon SC, Hartzema AG. Tamsulosin treatment for benign prostatic hyperplasia and risk of severe hypotension in men aged 40-85 years in the United States: risk window analyses using between and within patient methodology. *BMJ*. 2013;347:f6320.
30. Poon IO, Braun U. High prevalence of orthostatic hypotension and its correlation with potentially causative medications among elderly veterans. *J Clin Pharm Ther*. 2005;30:173-178.

31. Miettinen TJ, Kanto JH, Salonen MA, Scheinin M. The sedative and sympatholytic effects of oral tizanidine in healthy volunteers. *Anesth Analg*. 1996;82:817-820.
32. Shibao C, Gamboa A, Diedrich A, et al. Acarbose, an alpha-glucosidase inhibitor, attenuates postprandial hypotension in autonomic failure. *Hypertension*. 2007;50:54-61.
33. Krediet CT, van Lieshout JJ, Bogert LW, Immink RV, Kim YS, Wieling W. Leg crossing improves orthostatic tolerance in healthy subjects: a placebo-controlled crossover study. *Am J Physiol Heart Circ Physiol*. 2006;291:H1768-H1772.
34. Diedrich A, Biaggioni I. Segmental orthostatic fluid shifts. *Clin Auton Res*. 2004;14:146-147.
35. Smit AAJ, Wieling W, Fujimura J, et al. Use of lower abdominal compression to combat orthostatic hypotension in patients with autonomic dysfunction. *Clin Auton Res*. 2004;14:167-175.
36. Jordan J, Shannon JR, Grogan E, Biaggioni I, Robertson D. A potent pressor response elicited by drinking water. *Lancet*. 1999;353:723.
37. McHugh J, Keller NR, Appalsamy M, et al. Portal osmopressor mechanism linked to transient receptor potential vanilloid 4 and blood pressure control. *Hypertension*. 2010;55:1438-1443.
38. Jordan J, Shannon JR, Black BK, et al. The pressor response to water drinking in humans: a sympathetic reflex? *Circulation*. 2000;101:504-509.
39. Singer W, Opfer-Gehrking TL, McPhee BR, Hilz MJ, Bharucha AE, Low PA. Acetylcholinesterase inhibition: a novel approach in the treatment of neurogenic orthostatic hypotension. *J Neurol Neurosurg Psychiatry*. 2003;74:1294-1298.
40. Shibao C, Okamoto LE, Gamboa A, et al. Comparative efficacy of yohimbine against pyridostigmine for the treatment of orthostatic hypotension in autonomic failure. *Hypertension*. 2010;56:847-851.
41. van Lieshout JJ, ten Harkel AD, Wieling W. Fludrocortisone and sleeping in the head-up position limit the postural decrease in cardiac output in autonomic failure. *Clin Auton Res*. 2000;10:35-42.
42. Chobanian AV, Volicer L, Tifft CP, Gavras H, Liang CS, Faxon D. Mineralocorticoid-induced hypertension in patients with orthostatic hypotension. *N Engl J Med*. 1979;301:68-73.
43. Smith W, Wan H, Much D, et al. Clinical benefit of midodrine hydrochloride in symptomatic orthostatic hypotension: a phase 4, double-blind, placebo-controlled, randomized, tilt-table study. *Clin Auton Res*. 2016;26:269-277.
44. Ramirez CE, Okamoto LE, Arnold AC, et al. Efficacy of atomoxetine versus midodrine for the treatment of orthostatic hypotension in autonomic failure. *Hypertension*. 2014;64:1235-1240.
45. Biaggioni I, Freeman R, Mathias CJ, et al. Randomized withdrawal study of patients with symptomatic neurogenic orthostatic hypotension responsive to droxidopa. *Hypertension*. 2015;65:101-107.
46. Hauser RA, Isaacson S, Lisk JP, Hewitt LA, Rowse G. Droxidopa for the short-term treatment of symptomatic neurogenic orthostatic hypotension in Parkinson's disease (nOH306B). *Mov Disord*. 2015;30:646-654.
47. Kaufmann H, Freeman R, Biaggioni I, et al. Droxidopa for neurogenic orthostatic hypotension: a randomized, placebo-controlled, phase 3 trial. *Neurology*. 2014;83:328-335.
48. Mathias CJ, Senard JM, Braune S, Watson L, Aragishi A, Keeling JE, Taylor MD. L-threo-dihydroxyphenylserine (L-threo-DOPS; droxidopa) in the management of neurogenic orthostatic hypotension: a multi-national, multi-center, dose-ranging study in multiple system atrophy and pure autonomic failure. *Clin Auton Res*. 2001;11:235-242.

43 Resistant Hypertension

Guillaume Bobrie, Laurence Amar, Anne-Laure Faucon, Anne-Marie Madjalian, and Michel Azizi

Hypertension is the most common chronic disease in developed countries, with a prevalence of approximately 25% to 30% in adults.[1] High blood pressure (BP) remains one of the leading risk factors influencing cardiovascular morbidity and mortality.[2,3] The current management of hypertension is based on knowledge accumulated over more than a half a century, the availability of multiple orally active and potent antihypertensive drugs targeting different pathophysiological pathways, the cumulative evidence from several randomized controlled trials and meta-analyses, and hundreds of pages of guidelines regularly updated by experts from around the world. Nevertheless, hypertension remains poorly controlled worldwide, and its incidence is increasing, because of the aging of the population and the obesity epidemic.[1,4] However, only some of the patients for whom the recommended BP thresholds are not reached actually have resistant hypertension (RHTN).

According to the joint European Society of Hypertension (ESH)/European Society of Cardiology (ESC) guidelines,[5] hypertension is defined as resistant to treatment "when a therapeutic strategy that includes appropriate lifestyle measures plus a diuretic and two other antihypertensive drugs belonging to different classes at adequate doses (but not necessarily including a mineralocorticoid receptor antagonist) fails to lower systolic BP (SBP) and diastolic BP (DBP) values to less than 140 and 90 mm Hg, respectively." These guidelines do not specify which classes of antihypertensive drugs other than a diuretic should be used to define RHTN. The NICE-UK (National Institute for Health and Care Excellence-United Kingdom) guidelines recommend that the three-drug regimen should include a renin angiotensin system (RAS) blocker (i.e., an angiotensin-converting enzyme [ACE] inhibitor, or angiotensin II receptor blocker [ARB], but not both), a long-acting calcium channel blocker (CCB) and a thiazide (or thiazide-like) diuretic in the absence of renal insufficiency.[6] The American Heart Association guidelines also include BP controlled by four or more drugs in the definition of RHTN[7]; this approach aims at identifying patients likely to benefit from particular (1) diagnostic procedures to screen for secondary hypertension or (2) treatment options. The BP goals generally recommended for all hypertensive patients are an SBP of less than 140 mm Hg and a DBP of less than 90 mm Hg. Some guidelines recommend lower BP targets for patients with diabetes or chronic kidney disease and higher thresholds for patients over the age of 80 years,[8-11] as shown in Table 43.1. The NICE-UK guidelines also suggest defining RHTN after confirmation by ambulatory BP monitoring in case of a mean daytime BP greater than 135/85 mm Hg despite treatment with the combination of a RAS blocker, a CCB and a diuretic.[6]

The United States guidelines provide a list of the optimal/adequate doses of a limited number of antihypertensive drugs available in the U.S. that should be used to treat hypertensive patients.[7] No such detailed list is available in other guidelines and the antihypertensive drugs used, together with their doses, vary considerably between countries. Moreover, the optimal/adequate doses of antihypertensive drugs may differ between individuals, not only in terms of efficacy, but also

in terms of tolerability. Furthermore, none of the guidelines clearly stress that preferential use should be made of long-acting drugs, which are more forgiving in case of a missed dose, or of fixed-dose triple combination therapy in a single pill, to reduce the daily pill burden, thereby favoring adherence to treatment (see later). Finally, the publication of the PATHWAY2 (Prevention And Treatment of Hypertension With Algorithm based therapY)[12] and SPRINT (Systolic blood PRessure INtervention Trial)[13] studies in 2015 may influence the definition of RHTN by (1) including the combination of a low-dose spironolactone with the above-mentioned triple therapy, and (2) favoring the use of lower BP thresholds, respectively.

PREVALENCE AND INCIDENCE OF RESISTANT HYPERTENSION

It is difficult to estimate the prevalence of true RHTN.[14-16] This prevalence is clearly lower than that of "apparent" RHTN, which may be attributed to inadequate office BP measurement, white coat hypertension, the use of nonoptimal combinations of drugs at nonadequate doses, or nonadherence to treatment. Its estimation thus depends on multiple factors, including the clinical setting (general population, tertiary referral center, clinical trial), the time frame of evaluation, the classes and optimal doses of antihypertensive treatment used, the exclusion or retention of patients not complying with treatment, and the BP threshold selected. In the 2003 to 2008 National Health and Nutrition Examination Surveys (NHANES) survey, 8.9% of the U.S. adults with hypertension included in the survey (12.8% of those treated) were classified as resistant because their office BP was 140/90 mm Hg and they reported using antihypertensive drugs from three different classes, or because they reported using antihypertensive drugs from four different classes regardless of BP.[17] The prevalence of apparent RHTN increased from 15.9% of treated patients in 1998 to 2004 to 28% of treated patients in 2005 to 2008.[18] An analysis of electronic record data from more than 200 community-based clinics in the U.S. between 2007 and 2010 showed that 31.5% of 468,877 hypertensive patients had uncontrolled BP (office BP >140/90 mm Hg), but that only 9.5% were treated with three or more antihypertensive drugs.[19] The triple-drug combination therapy was considered optimal in only 4.7% of the total study population.[19]

Unsurprisingly, the prevalence of RHTN is higher in tertiary referral centers than elsewhere. RHTN was confirmed by ambulatory BP monitoring (ABPM) in 19.3% of the 1034 patients aged 18 to 80 years hospitalized at a university hospital tertiary referral center in Paris.[20] Another way of estimating the prevalence of RHTN is to analyze the results of randomized controlled trials. A meta-analysis of 20 observational studies and randomized controlled trials estimated the prevalence of RHTN at 13.72% (95% confidence interval [CI]:11.19% –16.24%) for the observational studies and 16.32% (95% CI: 10.68% –21.95%) for the randomized controlled trials.[16] Finally, the prevalence of RHTN is highest in patients with a low glomerular filtration rate (GFR) and albuminuria (i.e., chronic kidney disease), in which it may be a

TABLE 43.1 Office Blood Pressure Goals According to Guidelines and Patient Characteristics

YEAR	GUIDELINE	POPULATION	GOAL OFFICE BP (MM HG)
2015	Canadian Hypertension Education Program recommendations[8]	Adults <80 years Adults ≥80 years Adults with diabetes Adults with CKD	<140/90 <150 <130/80 <140/90
2014	Eighth Joint National Committee (JNC 8) Hypertension Guidelines[10]	Adults <60 years Adults ≥60 years Adults with diabetes Adults with CKD	<140/90 <150/90 <140/90 <140/90
2014	American Society of Hypertension/International Society of Hypertension (ASH/ISH) Clinical practice guidelines[9]	Adults <80 years Adults ≥80 years Adults ≥80 years with CKD or diabetes Adults <80 years with CKD and albuminuria	<140/90 <150/90 <140/90 <130/80
2013	European Society of Hypertension/European Society of Cardiology (ESH/ESC) guidelines for the management of arterial hypertension[5]	Adults <80 years Adults ≥80 years Adults with diabetes Adults with CKD without proteinuria Adults with CKD with overt proteinuria Adults with CHD	<140/90 <150/90 <140/85 <140/90 <130/90 <140/90
2012	Kidney Disease: Improving Global Outcomes Chronic Kidney Disease clinical practice guideline (KDIGO)[11]	Adults with CKD and urine albumin <30 mg/24 h Adults with CKD and urine albumin ≥30 mg/24 h	<140/90 <130/80
2011	National Institute for Health and Care Excellence-United Kingdom (NICE-UK) guidance[6]	Adults <80 years Adults ≥80 years	<140/90 <150/90

BP, Blood pressure; *CKD,* chronic kidney disease; *CHD,* coronary heart disease.

high as 50%.[21,22] In a population-based cohort, the prevalence of refractory hypertension, the extreme phenotype of RHTN, defined as uncontrolled BP (≥140/90 mm Hg) on five or more antihypertensive drugs, was 3.6% in participants with RHTN (n = 2144) and 41.7% in participants taking drugs from five or more antihypertensive drug classes.[23] In all these settings, the prevalence of RHTN is probably overestimated because it is generally defined on the basis of office BP measurements. The systematic use of ABPM in a Spanish registry including more than 8000 patients with RHTN defined on the basis of an office BP of at least 140/90 mm Hg despite treatment with three antihypertensive drugs showed that 37.5% of these patients actually had pseudoresistant hypertension (HTN) because of (1) a "white coat phenomenon" causing isolated office HTN or (2) a poor method of office BP measurement.[24] These results suggest that out-of-office BP measurements (i.e., ABPM or self-BP measurement at home) should be used systematically for the definition and confirmation of RHTN, to exclude pseudoresistance.[6,7,25-27]

Data on the incidence of RTHN are scarce. A single retrospective cohort study of two integrated health plans evaluated the incidence of RHTN in a population of 205,750 patients with newly diagnosed hypertension.[28] The incidence of RHTN was 16.2% (1.9% of the initial cohort) after a median follow-up of 1.5 years among the patients taking three or more antihypertensive drugs for at least 1 month for whom follow-up office BP measurements were available (n = 24,499).[28] In a randomized controlled trial assessing the BP-lowering efficacy of single-pill, fixed-dose, triple combination therapy, 29% of the patients treated with the highest daily dose (25 mg hydrochlorothiazide/320 mg valsartan/10 mg amlodipine) for 8 weeks still had an office BP above 140/90 mm Hg.[29]

FACTORS CONTRIBUTING TO RESISTANT HYPERTENSION

Characteristics of Patients With Resistant Hypertension

RHTN is significantly associated with older age, being male, African origin, initial BP at the diagnosis of hypertension, highest BP ever reached during the patient's lifetime, frequent outpatient visits, obesity, diabetes, a Framingham 10-year coronary risk greater than 20%, chronic kidney disease, and the presence of target organ damage.[17,19,30-33] Obstructive sleep apnea (OSA) is also frequently associated with hypertension, particularly in obese patients, and is almost four times more frequent in patients with RHTN than in patients with controlled hypertension.[34] This higher prevalence may reflect the higher frequency of obesity, excess aldosterone, or sympathetic overdrive in these patients.[35,36] OSA should be suspected in obese patients with a short neck who snore and present daytime sleepiness and frequent night-time awakenings, in whom apnea is witnessed.[37] The Epworth questionnaire is used to screen for OSA, which is diagnosed by polysomnography.

RHTN is also associated with a higher prevalence of end-organ damage, including left ventricular hypertrophy (LVH) carotid intima–media thickening, microalbuminuria, and retinal lesions, than well-controlled hypertension.[38,39] The frequent association of target organ damage and the clustering of cardiovascular risk factors in patients with RHTN accounts for the higher risk of a major cardiovascular event in these patients and, thus, of a poor short-term prognosis.[28] Indeed, after a median follow-up of 3.8 years, patients with incident RHTN had a higher risk of cardiovascular events (adjusted hazard ratio [HR], 1.47; 95% CI, 1.33 to 1.62) than those with controlled hypertension.[28] The long-term risk of major adverse events, including death, is much higher in women displaying signs of myocardial ischemia and RHTN (HR, 1.77; 95% CI, 1.26 to 2.49) than in those with controlled hypertension.[40] In patients with chronic kidney disease, RHTN is also associated with a higher cardiovascular risk (HR: 1.98, 95% CI: 1.14 to 3.43) and renal events (HR: 2.66, 95% CI: 1.62 to 4.37).[41,42]

Consequently, patients with RHTN report a higher degree of concern about their high BP levels and a greater emotional burden, including a poorer perception of their overall health, than patients with uncontrolled hypertension.[43]

Lifestyle Factors

Excessive salt consumption promotes hypervolemia, which is frequently observed in patients with RHTN, and decreases the effectiveness of diuretics and RAS blockers.[44-48] The effects of excessive salt consumption are particularly marked in elderly patients, in those of African origin and in those with chronic kidney disease. Daily salt intake can be assessed by food records, questionnaires or by measuring sodium excretion over a 24-hour period.

Alcohol abuse is also a major factor underlying poor BP control[33,46] through a direct vasoconstrictive effect mediated, at least in part, by sympathetic overdrive (see later). It is also associated with being overweight and low compliance with treatment, both of which also contribute to RHTN (see later).

Finally, BP increases steadily with body mass index (BMI). Being overweight or obese is associated with significantly poorer BP control. Overweight and obesity are frequently observed in patients with RHTN.[32]

Nonadherence to Antihypertensive Treatment

Nonadherence to antihypertensive medications and life-style measures is a key factor underlying resistance to treatment and this remains a major public health challenge.[49] Nonadherence is associated with poor cardiovascular prognosis.[50-52] Several disease-related, physician-related, treatment-related, and patient-related factors, either alone or in combination, promote nonadherence to treatment and are common to all chronic diseases, including hypertension.[49,53] These factors include (1) a lack of symptoms in patients with hypertension; (2) inadequate patient education leading to a poor understanding of the BP goal to be achieved, the treatment strategy, the balance between the benefits and risk of treatment, and the need for life-long treatment; (3) cognitive impairment, particularly in elderly patients or in patients with a history of stroke or other causes of dementia; (4) the use of complex antihypertensive drug regimens, particularly if combined with treatments for diabetes, dyslipidemia, or other comorbid conditions, increasing the pill burden and the number of drug intakes per day[54]; (5) illegible prescriptions; (6) the occurrence of drug-related side effects, which can alter quality of life, particularly in patients who were previously asymptomatic (e.g., coughing with ACE inhibitors, flushing or leg edemas with CCBs, sexual dysfunction with diuretics or beta-blockers, gout with diuretics, symptomatic hypotension etc.); and (7) a poor health care provider-patient relationship including (a) too little time spent with patients, (b) a lack of explanation about hypertension and the benefits of treatment, or (c) a lack of consideration of the patient's complaints about drug-related side effects on the part of the physician.[55] Psychosocial factors, perceptions of treatment concerns, depression, excessive alcohol consumption, a lack of belief in the efficacy of the treatment, practical barriers to treatment and poor access to busy nonempathetic physicians, high drug and appointment costs, a lack of health insurance, unemployment, low income, and poor compliance with lifestyle changes have also been associated with poor compliance with drug treatment.[56-58] It is important to take the patient's viewpoint and beliefs about the causes and effects of hypertension and its treatment into account.[59] A systematic review of 53 studies from 16 countries showed that a large proportion of patients (1) felt that their hypertension was principally caused by stress and, therefore, did not believe that treatment was required once the stress had been relieved, (2) were reluctant to use antihypertensive treatment, and (3) had concerns about side effects and the risk of drug addiction.[59]

Various direct and indirect methods for assessing adherence to drug treatments have been developed.[49,53] The direct methods include the direct observation of treatment intake in a medicalized setting, such as a BP clinic, the detection of a drug or its metabolite in blood or urine, or the determination of a pharmacodynamic marker.[49,53] Indirect methods include patient questionnaires such as the eight-item Morisky questionnaire (MMAS-8),[60] self-reports, patient diaries, pill counts, prescription refill rates, the assessment of patient clinical

response, electronic drug monitoring systems, and the determination of physiological markers.[49,53] Pharmacodynamic markers of exposure to a given antihypertensive treatment include, for example, bradycardia in patients on beta-blockers, hyperuricemia or gout in patients on diuretics, increases in plasma renin concentration in patients on diuretics or RAS blockers, increases in urine N-acetyl-seryl-aspartyl-lysyl-proline (AcSDKP) concentration in patients on ACE inhibitors,[61] and drug-related side effects.

The prevalence of nonadherence to antihypertensive treatment in patients with RHTN remains high when assessed by toxicological analyses based on high-performance or ultra-high-performance liquid chromatography with tandem mass spectrometry (HP LC-MS/MS) to detect the presence of a given prescribed drug in plasma or urine samples. About 50% of patients attending specialized BP clinics for RHTN have been found not to be complying with the prescribed drug regimen on the basis of a lack of detection of one or more of the multiple antihypertensive drugs prescribed in plasma or urine.[62-65] However, the nondetection of a drug is not sufficient to conclude with certainty that the patient is not complying with antihypertensive treatment. Alterations or between-subject variability in drug pharmacokinetics (absorption, distribution, metabolism, or elimination) related to (1) associated comorbid conditions (e.g., gastrointestinal bypass, etc.), (2) genetic factors, including polymorphisms of genes encoding drug-metabolizing enzymes or transporters, (3) drug-drug interactions (involving transport proteins, the inhibition or induction of enzymes, such as cytochromes P450, especially CYP3A4, or of drug transporters, such as P-glycoprotein,[66-68] etc.), or (4) interference with food (e.g., high sodium intake,[69] grapefruit juice, herbal teas[67,68]) may strongly influence the pharmacokinetics of antihypertensive drugs, resulting in their nondetection in biological samples. Conversely, the detection of significant quantities of drugs in plasma or urine is not sufficient to confirm optimal adherence to treatment on a daily basis. Indeed, patients often display better adherence to treatment during the week before and the week immediately after medical visits.[53] This phenomenon, known as "the toothbrush effect," may be amplified if the patients are aware that regular drug monitoring is carried out at each visit.[53]

In conclusion, each method for measuring treatment adherence has advantages and disadvantages, and the method chosen depends on availability in the clinical setting.[53] Some methods are easy to use (standardized questionnaire, determination of physiological variables), whereas others, such as drug detection or the direct observation of treatment intake, are much more difficult to implement.

Multiple modes of intervention are required to improve compliance, but their long-term efficacy has yet to be clearly established.[70] These modes of intervention include improving the physician-patient relationship, empathy on the part of the physician when the patients are describing their complaints, patient education, the provision of reminders in the packaging of the drugs, frequent clinic visits, the self-monitoring of BP, patient empowerment and self-management, text messaging, the use of single-pill combination treatments, and assistance from other health care providers and families.[70-72] However, the complexity of these interventions may make them difficult to implement in everyday practice, in which physicians are subject to a number of constraints potentially limiting the time available.

Self-BP monitoring at home may improve the patient's compliance with drug treatment, but clinical trials have reported mixed benefits.[73] In 6 of 11 randomized controlled trials included in a systematic review, the use of "multimodal complex" interventions involving self-BP measurement was associated with significant improvements in adherence to treatment.[74] Treatment adherence was measured by pill counting, pharmacy refill rates, self-reporting, and electronic monitoring devices, but not by LC-MS/MS. A meta-analysis of 23 randomized controlled trials including 7037 patients showed that the teletransmission of self-BP measurements resulted in a lower BP (SBP lower by 4.7 mm Hg and DBP lower by 3.3 mm Hg) than usual care. This approach thus improved BP control, despite the absence of a significant influence on adherence to treatment.[75]

Self-BP management coupled to self-BP monitoring may improve adherence to treatment further, as shown in the TASMIN-SR randomized controlled trial.[76] This trial compared self-BP management with the self-titration of antihypertensive medication, using a precise treatment algorithm with usual care in 450 patients with a high cardiovascular risk. After 12 months, a difference in BP of 9.2/3.1 mm Hg in favor of the self-management group was reported.[76]

These studies did not specifically include patients with RHTN or monitor compliance with treatment, but it seems likely that the teletransmission of self-monitoring BP measurements and the self-titration of medication improve BP control through better compliance with treatment. However, the long-term efficacy of this approach and its external applicability to all patients remains questionable. This approach probably requires the active and motivated participation of well-educated and trained patients without cognitive deficiencies.

Support from health professionals, including pharmacists and nurses, counseling, motivational support or cognitive behavioral therapy, and additional help from the family may also increase compliance with treatment.[70] Technological interventions for education, counseling, self-monitoring, feedback, and electronic reminders are increasingly being used, but the evidence concerning their efficacy for improving compliance with treatment is inconsistent.[77]

The use of once-daily single-pill double or triple combination therapies reduces pill burden,[72] simplifies treatment regimens without increasing the incidence of side effects, and has been shown to improve compliance with treatment. All of this should, in turn, help patients to reach and maintain their target BP and to achieve the short-term and long-term treatment goal of cardiovascular risk reduction.[78,79] Finally, the use of electronic pill monitors improves BP control, probably by improving compliance with treatment,[80,81] but these devices are expensive and not readily available outside of clinical trials.

Clinical Inertia

Clinical inertia is defined as a lack of treatment intensification in a patient whose treatment goals have not been attained. This inertia is another major factor contributing to inadequate BP control and other associated risk factors. It was first assessed in 1998, in a Veterans Administration study, in which the clinical inertia rate reached 75%.[82] Clinical inertia is, unfortunately, frequent. In the nationally representative CardioMonitor 2004 survey, treatment was intensified for uncontrolled hypertension at 32% of patient visits in the U.S., and at 14% to 26% of patient visits in European countries.[83] An analysis of electronic record data for patients at 200 U.S. clinical sites showed that only 4.7% of the hypertensive patients included in the analysis were prescribed optimal triple therapy including a diuretic and at least two other BP drugs at a dose at least 50% the maximum dose recommended for hypertension.[19] This low proportion highlights deficiencies in the prescription of optimal triple therapy to hypertensive patients by health care providers, despite the need for this treatment.

There are many reasons for this clinical inertia and a systematic review identified 293 potential barriers to compliance with guidelines for physicians.[84,85] The most frequently cited reasons for an absence of antihypertensive treatment intensification related to (1) physicians being satisfied with the change in BP achieved with their prescription, despite

the persistence of systolic BP above the threshold in their patients[86]; (2) the number of associated cardiovascular risk factors and comorbid conditions to be taken into account simultaneously[87]; (3) the side effects of antihypertensive treatments reported by the patients during the visit[88]; and (4) the lack of time to find a well-tolerated drug regimen.[89]

The use of strict protocol-based treatment algorithms may overcome clinical inertia by providing health care providers with simple, accessible prescription rules, as shown in the Canadian Simplified Treatment Intervention To Control Hypertension (STITCH) cluster-randomized, controlled trial.[90] Indeed, this trial showed that a simplified antihypertensive algorithm including (1) initial low-dose fixed-dose combination therapy with a diuretic and a RAS blocker; (2) the uptitration of combination therapy; (3) the addition and uptitration of a calcium channel blocker, and (4) the addition of a non–first-line antihypertensive agent, was superior to guideline-based practice for achieving a target office BP < 140/90 mm Hg after 6 months of follow-up (64.7% versus 52.7%; respectively, $p = 0.026$).[90] Such algorithms can be incorporated into clinical support decision tools to reduce clinical inertia, but the resulting hypothetical improvement in BP control in patients with RHTN is uncertain. Indeed, in the Renal Denervation for Hypertension (DENERHTN) trial, only 18% of the patients with RHTN on standardized triple therapy randomized to the control group achieved BP control (<130/80 mm Hg on 24-hour ABPM) despite treatment according to a strict algorithm including the sequential addition of 25 mg spironolactone, 10 mg bisoprolol, 5 mg prazosin, and 1 mg rilmenidine at monthly visits, according to home BP results.[91]

Screening for Secondary Hypertension

The prevalence of secondary hypertension is much higher in patients with RHTN. The frequency of secondary hypertension has been estimated at 5% in the general population, but may be as high as 10% to 20% in patients with RHTN.[20] Up to 50% of patients with RTHN referred for renal denervation may have secondary hypertension.[91]

Patients with confirmed RHTN should thus be screened for secondary hypertension.[7,25-27,92] Additional reasons to screen for secondary hypertension are:

1. Early hypertension onset (i.e., before the age of 30 years) in patients without other risk factors (family history, obesity, etc.)
2. Grade III hypertension (>180/110 mm Hg) or hypertensive emergencies
3. Sudden increase in BP in a previously stable patient
4. Nondipping or reverse dipping during 24-hour ambulatory BP monitoring
5. Presence of target organ damage (LVH, hypertensive retinopathy, etc.)

Some etiologies of secondary hypertension are common, whereas others are much less common[7,25-27,92] as indicated in Table 43.2.

Screening for Drug-Induced Hypertension

Drug-induced RHTN is often underestimated. Several drugs prescribed for conditions other than hypertension can increase BP per se or blunt the BP-lowering effect of antihypertensive treatments (Table 43.3). Some drugs induce sodium retention associated with extracellular volume expansion. Others directly or indirectly activate the sympathetic nervous system, act directly on arterial smooth muscle tone, or have no clear mechanism of action (for review, see references 67,68,93). Finally, some drugs may directly or indirectly interfere with the pharmacokinetic and/or pharmacodynamic profile of the antihypertensive drug.[66,68] A systematic examination of the recommendations in 12 UK national clinical

TABLE 43.2 Common and Uncommon Causes of Secondary Hypertension

Common Causes	
Primary hyperaldosteronism (reported prevalence: 7% to 20%)	• Spontaneous or diuretic-induced hypokalemia, left ventricular hypertrophy, high aldosterone and low renin levels. • Screening: plasma aldosterone/renin ratio or plasma aldosterone/plasma renin activity ratio under standardized conditions (correction of hypokalemia and withdrawal of drugs affecting the RAS). Confirmatory test: saline infusion test, captopril test, fludrocortisone test, oral sodium test. • Imaging: adrenal CT or MRI, adrenal vein sampling.
Renal artery stenosis (reported prevalence: 2% to 24%)	• Generalized atherosclerotic disease (coronary or peripheral artery disease, carotid, abdominal, or femoral bruits); smoking, diabetes; history of flash pulmonary edema; young female patients (fibromuscular dysplasia); acute deterioration of renal function after ACE inhibitors or ARB, recent renal insufficiency, small unilateral kidney. • Screening: duplex ultrasound, CT angiogram or MR angiogram. • Renovascular hypertension may also be caused by other rare etiologies, including Takayasu arteritis, renal artery dissection, neurofibromatosis, tuberous sclerosis, pseudoxanthoma elasticum, vascular Ehlers-Danlos syndrome, Alagille syndrome, Williams syndrome, Turner syndrome, segmental arterial mediolysis.
Renal parenchymal disease (reported prevalence: 1% to 2%)	• Albuminuria or microscopic hematuria, renal insufficiency, leg edema. • Screening: plasma creatinine or cystatin C concentration, urine albumin concentration, blood electrolytes, blood count. • Imaging: renal ultrasound. If necessary, renal biopsy.
Uncommon (Reported Prevalence: <1%)	
Pheochromocytoma	• Paroxysmal hypertension; palpitation; sweating; pallor; headaches; family history of pheochromocytoma; associated genetic diseases (MEN 2, von Hippel Lindau, neurofibromatosis, hereditary paraganglioma). • Screening: plasma metanephrine concentration or 24-hour urinary metanephrine determination. • Imaging: Adrenal CT or MR. If abdominal imaging results are negative, scintigraphic localization with ^{123}I-labeled metaiodobenzylguanidine scanning or ^{18}F-fluorodeoxyglucose PET scan or additional whole-body MRI may be indicated. • Genetic screening for pathogenic mutations.
Thyroid diseases	• Eye signs, weight loss or gain, heat or cold intolerance, heart failure, tachycardia, bradycardia, anxiety or fatigue. • Screening: TSH, T4L, T3L. • Imaging: thyroid ultrasound; thyroid scintigraphy.
Cushing syndrome	• Easy bruising, facial plethora, proximal myopathy, trunk obesity, moon facies, abdominal striae, dorsocervical fat pad, thin skin, depression. • Screening: 24-hour urinary free cortisol concentration, late salivary cortisol concentration, 1-mg overnight dexamethasone suppression test. • Imaging: adrenal CT or MRI, brain MRI.
Other rare causes of endocrine hypertension	• Acromegaly. • Exceptional renin tumors (benign). Hypertension with hypokalemia and high plasma renin, prorenin, and aldosterone concentrations.
Urological causes	• Reflux nephropathy with cortical kidney scars, congenital renal hypoplasia, sequelae of hematoma or infections (tuberculosis), kidney cancers.
Coarctation of the thoracic or abdominal aorta	• Diminished femoral pulses, rib notching on chest x-ray. • Imaging: cardiac echocardiogram, whole-body CT- or MR-angiogram.
Intracranial tumor	• Early morning headache, family history. • Imaging: brain CT or MRI.

ACE, Angiotensin-converting enzyme; *ARB*, angiotensin II receptor blocker; *CT*, computed tomography; *MEN 2*, multiple endocrine neoplasia type 2; *MRI*, magnetic resonance imaging; *MR*, magnetic resonance; *PET*, positron emission tomography; *RAS*, renin angiotensin system.

guidelines revealed 32 potentially serious drug-disease interactions between drugs recommended for type 2 diabetes and the other 11 conditions considered: 6 for drugs recommended for depression and 10 for drugs recommended for heart failure.[94] Careful evaluation of the drugs taken by patients for conditions other than cardiovascular diseases, through the completion of a standardized questionnaire[95] or the use of drug-drug interaction-checking websites, can help to identify drug-related hypertension.

Drugs or Substances Associated With Apparent Mineralocorticoid Excess or Activation of the Renin Angiotensin System

Glucocorticoids and their derivatives, regardless of the route of administration, including eye drops and topical creams, can have mineralocorticoid effects. Glycyrrhizin acid (licorice) inhibits 11-beta-hydroxysteroid dehydrogenase type II in the kidney. This enzyme converts cortisol into inactive cortisone, and its inhibition results in the presence of excess cortisol. Cortisol binds renal mineralocorticoid receptors (MCR) with high affinity, leading to mineralocorticoid–induced

hypertension with hypokalemia, sodium and fluid retention, and a decrease in plasma renin and aldosterone levels.[96,97] At high doses, ketoconazole, an antifungal imidazole derivative, inhibits several enzymes involved in steroid synthesis, including the 11 beta-hydroxylase responsible for converting 11-deoxycortisol into cortisol. The resulting increase in adrenocorticotropic hormone (ACTH) stimulates aldosterone and 11-deoxycorticosterone synthesis, leading to apparent mineralocorticoid excess and a concomitant decrease in renin levels.[67,68,93] Itraconazole use has also been associated with RHTN.[98] The CYP17A1 inhibitor abiraterone acetate, which decreases androgen synthesis, is used to treat castration-resistant metastatic prostate cancer, but it leads to the synthesis of excessive amounts of 11-deoxycorticosterone via the counter-regulatory stimulation of ACTH release in response to a decrease in cortisol synthesis.[99] The binding of 11-deoxycorticosterone to the MCR induces hypertension with hypokalemia, sodium and fluid retention, and decreases plasma renin and aldosterone levels.[100]

The combination of synthetic estrogens and progestins in oral contraceptive pills may increase BP moderately, by

TABLE 43.3 Drug or Substances Increasing Blood Pressure

Drugs or substances associated with apparent mineralocorticoid excess or activation of the renin angiotensin system	• Glucocorticoids and their derivatives • Glycyrrhizin acid (licorice) • Ketoconazole, itraconazole • Abiraterone acetate • Synthetic estrogens combined with progestin
Drugs or substances with direct vasopressor properties	• Alcohol • Immunosuppressive agents (cyclosporine, tacrolimus, and calcineurin inhibitors) • Recombinant human erythropoietin • Drugs targeting the vascular endothelial growth factor (VEGF) pathway, including monoclonal antibodies and small-molecule receptor tyrosine kinase inhibitors
Drugs or substances activating the sympathetic nervous system	• Illicit drugs of abuse, such as cocaine and amphetamines • Epinephrine or phenylephrine derivatives present in over-the-counter oral, nasal, or ophthalmic decongestants • Ephedrine alkaloids (Ephedra or herbal ma-huang) • Antidepressants, including venlafaxine, bupropion, monoamine oxidase inhibitors, and tricyclic agents • Appetite suppressants for weight loss • Modafinil
Drugs or substances with diverse mechanisms of action	• Antiretroviral drugs (lopinavir and ritonavir) • Nonselective nonsteroidal antiinflammatory drugs (NSAIDs) and selective cyclooxygenase 2 inhibitors

increasing angiotensinogen synthesis, angiotensin II production, aldosterone secretion, and extracellular volume.[93,101] No such effect is observed with hormone replacement therapy.[67,68,93]

Drugs or Substances With Direct Vasopressor Properties

Excess alcohol consumption acutely and chronically increases BP, potentially resulting in treatment resistance. The regular consumption of three or more alcoholic drinks per day has been shown to be a risk factor for hypertension.[102] The effects of alcohol on BP are independent of age, sex, ethnicity, obesity, salt intake, cigarette smoking, coffee use, and potassium intake. Alcohol induces an increase in BP through a stimulation of sympathetic activity, activation of the RAS, and calcium-mediated vasoconstriction.[66,67,91]

Immunosuppressive agents, such as cyclosporine, tacrolimus, and calcineurin inhibitors, increase BP in a dose-dependent manner, by increasing the cytosolic calcium content of the vascular smooth muscle cells, activating the local RAS, increasing endothelin (ET)-1 production, decreasing nitric oxide (NO) availability, and increasing the response to catecholamines.[66,67,91] Dose reduction may cure hypertension. CCBs should be used with caution as they increase cyclosporine concentration in the blood. The recombinant human erythropoietin used to treat anemia in patients with chronic kidney diseases or cancers may cause a moderate increase in BP via the mechanisms described above.

Drugs targeting the vascular endothelium growth factor (VEGF) pathway for the treatment of various cancers,[103] including monoclonal antibodies and small-molecule receptor tyrosine kinase inhibitors (RTKIs), can increase BP[104] via multiple mechanisms such as decreases in NO availability, capillary rarefaction, or activation of the ET-1 pathway.[66,67,91] Hypertension has been reported in more than 20% of patients

receiving the RTKIs sorafenib or sunitinib, and about 6% of patients on these drugs develop severe hypertension.[105,106] Dose reduction may reverse the increase in BP.[107] NO donors, including nebivolol and nitrates, and RAS blockers should be preferred as antihypertensive treatments.[107] RTKIs are metabolized by CYP3A4, which inactivates verapamil and diltiazem; there is, therefore, a high risk of drug-drug interaction that may require adjustment of the doses of both RTKIs and CCBs.[107] Thiazide diuretics, which may increase serum calcium concentration in patients with bone metastasis, should be used with caution.[107] Dose reduction or the temporary or permanent discontinuation of anti-VEGF drugs should be considered in cases of severe RHTN or abundant proteinuria.[107]

Some drugs or substances have a pressor effect mediated by direct activation of the sympathetic nervous system. Illicit drugs of abuse, such as cocaine and amphetamines, have such an effect, as do the epinephrine or phenylephrine derivatives present in over-the-counter oral, nasal, and ophthalmic decongestants and plants containing ephedrine alkaloids used as stimulants for weight loss or as energy supplements (Ephedra or herbal ma-huang).[66,67,91] Several antidepressants, including venlafaxine, a serotonin and norepinephrine reuptake inhibitor, bupropion, a dopamine reuptake inhibitor, monoamine oxidase inhibitors, and tricyclic agents, appetite suppressants taken for weight loss, and modafinil, a nonamphetamine stimulant, can also increase BP via the same mechanism.[66,67,91]

Drugs or Substances With Diverse Mechanisms of Action

Some antiretroviral drugs (lopinavir and ritonavir) increase BP through a drug-related increase in body mass index.[108] Nonselective nonsteroidal antiinflammatory drugs (NSAIDs) and selective cyclooxygenase 2 inhibitors can increase BP in normotensive subjects[109] and blunt the antihypertensive efficacy of diuretics or RAS blockers in hypertensive patients, by inhibiting prostaglandin-mediated renal vasodilation and promoting sodium retention.[110,111] NSAIDs differ considerably in their effects on BP.[112]

Drugs or Substances Affecting the Pharmacokinetics or Pharmacodynamic Effects of Antihypertensive Drugs

Some antihypertensive drugs are P glycoprotein substrates (aliskiren, candesartan, verapamil), whereas others are substrates of CYP2D6 (metoprolol) or CYP3A4 (CCBs, eplerenone). Their pharmacokinetic profiles and, thus, their pharmacodynamic effects, can be strongly affected by inhibitors/inducers of these transporters or CYP450, including St. John's wort, anticonvulsants (carbamazepine, phenobarbital, phenytoin), and by some antiinfection drugs (rifampicin, rifabutin, efavirenz, nevirapine, griseofulvin).[66,67,91]

In conclusion, the factors contributing to RHTN include nonadherence to treatment and the inertia of the physician, excessive dietary sodium and alcohol intake, obesity, substance abuse, drug-drug interactions, and the presence of underlying secondary hypertension, all of which should be considered in the diagnostic procedure for RHTN.

PROPOSED TREATMENT FOR PATIENTS WITH RESISTANT HYPERTENSION

In addition to the contributory factors listed above, the pathophysiology of RHTN involves complex interplay between multiple factors involving (1) various neurohormonal pathways, including the excess aldosterone,[47] sympathetic overactivity,[113] and ET-1[114] overactivity, (2) complex counter-regulatory mechanisms upregulating sodium reabsorption in the tubules of the kidney,[115,116] and (3) target organ damage, including vascular and renal damage. These factors contribute to different extents to volume and sodium overload, increases in arterial stiffness, and renal fibrosis in the mid- and long-term.

Multidrug regimens are, therefore, usually required to achieve BP goals through interference with the different pathways implicated in the pathogenesis of RHTN. Treatment should also be personalized, to take into account patient age and ethnicity, the presence of compelling indications for certain classes of drugs, associated comorbid conditions, chronic kidney disease and proteinuria, and the risk of drug-drug interactions.[5,7,25-27]

Lifestyle Changes

Lifestyle changes should include a reduction of sodium and alcohol intake, together with regular exercise and weight loss.[5,7,25-27] A systematic review of 105 trials randomizing 6805 patients showed that a weight-reducing diet, regular exercise, and the reduction of alcohol and salt intake were associated with a decrease in SBP of 4.0 to 6.0 mm Hg in the short term.[117] However, it remains unclear whether patients remain sufficiently motivated to maintain lifestyle changes in the long term.

For those with OSA, continuous positive airway pressure (CPAP) may also be of moderate benefit, as shown in meta-analyses[118] but this remains a matter of debate for patients with RHTN.[119,120] Alternatively, mandibular advancement devices can be used in patients with OSA and have been shown to have a modest BP-lowering effect similar to that of CPAP.[121] Long-term compliance with CPAP may be problematic: in a prospective, multicenter study including 357 non-sleepy patients, only 64.4% displayed good compliance with CPAP after 4 years of follow-up.[122]

Optimization of Ongoing Triple Therapy and Intensification of Sodium Depletion

The first step is to optimize the doses of current treatment or to prescribe appropriate antihypertensive drug combinations.[5,7,25-27] By definition, patients with RHTN should receive at least three antihypertensive drugs of different classes at the maximally tolerated doses, and the combination used should preferentially include a thiazide or thiazide-like diuretic, a RAS blocker, and a CCB. One of the causes of RHTN is inappropriate refractory volume retention of multifactorial origin, as suggested by the low renin levels frequently detected in patients with RHTN.[31,47,123] International guidelines, therefore, principally recommend reducing sodium intake to below100 mmol per day and increasing the intensity of diuretic therapy. Indeed, the cornerstone of therapy is diuretic treatment to decrease volume overload, together with salt intake restriction, particularly in patients with chronic kidney disease.[5,7,11,25-27] BP control can be improved by increasing the dose of the diuretic, or by switching to a more potent thiazide-like diuretic (chlorthalidone and indapamide) if estimated GFR (eGFR) is 30 or more mL per minute.[5,7,11,25-27] Indeed, chlorthalidone or indapamide should be preferred over hydrochlorothiazide or bendroflumethiazide, on the basis of their pharmacokinetic characteristics (greater bioavailability, longer half-life) and greater efficacy for decreasing BP[124-127] and, possibly, cardiovascular events.[128] However, chlorthalidone use may be associated with a higher risk of adverse events, including hypokalemia or hyponatremia.[129] Indeed, thiazides yield a flat dose-response curve for BP and steeper dose-response curves for adverse electrolytic and metabolic effects.[130] The use of a potassium-sparing diuretic[131] or of an MCR antagonist in combination[132,133] with thiazides can prevent thiazide-induced hypokalemia whilst improving BP control (see later).

Loop diuretics should be used when eGFR is less than 30 mL per minute, as recommended by the NICE and KDIGO (Kidney Disease Improving Global Outcomes) guidelines,[6,11] although small studies have shown that thiazides retain their short-term and mid-term natriuretic and antihypertensive effects when GFR is less than 30 mL per minute.[134,135] Furosemide and bumetanide should be administered twice daily, because of their short duration of action, whereas longer-acting agents, such as torsemide, can be administered once daily.[136] The dose or intake frequency of the loop diuretic may need to be increased in patients with severe chronic kidney disease and/or albuminuria.[11,136] Careful monitoring of renal function, serum electrolyte levels, and fluid status is required to detect dehydration, hypokalemia, hyponatremia, hypovolemia or renal dysfunction.

Adding a Fourth-Line Treatment: A Mineralocorticoid Receptor Blocker

After optimizing ongoing triple therapy and sodium depletion in addition to lifestyle management, the stepwise addition of other antihypertensive drugs should be considered. There is growing evidence to suggest that the fourth-line treatment should involve a blockade of the biological effects of aldosterone through the use of MCR antagonists, such as spironolactone and eplerenone. Eplerenone is a short-acting MCR antagonist that is less potent than spironolactone[132,133,137,138] but more selective than spironolactone for the MCR.[139] Eplerenone does not interfere with progesterone or androgen receptors at the doses available commercially (50 to 100 mg). It does not, therefore, have the sexual side effects of spironolactone, such as impotence, gynecomastia, breast tenderness, and menstrual irregularities, which may limit its use in the long term.[133,139] However, eplerenone has not been approved for use to treat hypertension in many European countries.

MCR blockade is an effective way to decrease BP in patients with RHTN for multiple pathophysiological reasons,[133,139,140] as shown in randomized trials and meta-analyses. In a meta-analysis including three randomized controlled trials and 12 observational studies (1024 patients), spironolactone (12.5 to 100 mg) and eplerenone (50 to 100 mg) resulted in a 24-hour ambulatory SBP lower, by 9.32 mm Hg (6.2 to 12.44, $p < 0.00001$), than that achieved with the placebo, and nonsignificant decrease in 24-hour ambulatory DBP by 2.57 mm Hg (-0.27 to 5.4, $p = 0.08$) in patients with RHTN after follow-up for 1.4 to 10.3 months.[141] The PATHWAY2 double-blind crossover study has provided strong evidence in favor of the use of spironolactone as a fourth-line treatment added to a preexisting three-drug regimen (an ACE inhibitor, a CCB, and a low dose of bendroflumethiazide) in overweight patients with RHTN, eGFR 45 or higher mL per minute, and plasma potassium concentrations within the normal range.[12] Targeting the MCR with 25 to 50 mg spironolactone was the most effective fourth-line treatment, yielding better results than the targeting of beta 1 receptors with bisoprolol (5 to 10 mg) or the targeting of alpha receptors with doxazosin (4 to 8 mg). Indeed, after 12 weeks of treatment, BP control was achieved in 58% of patients treated with spironolactone but in only 42% of those treated with doxazosin, and 43% of those treated with bisoprolol. Moreover, there was an inverse linear relationship between plasma renin concentration on the initial triple combination therapy and BP response to spironolactone, suggesting that spironolactone is more effective in those with a low renin profile (i.e., with persistent volume and sodium overload). No such relationship was observed for bisoprolol or doxazosin.

However, the PATHWAY2 study was subject to a number of limitations:
- About 150 patients had at least one serum potassium concentration determination of 3.5 mmol/L or less on treatment with the three-drug regimen plus doxazosin, bisoprolol, or placebo. This finding suggests that an unknown proportion of patients may have had undiagnosed primary aldosteronism, a condition that was not specifically excluded, enhancing the BP-lowering efficacy of spironolactone.

- The low dose of bendroflumethiazide, a drug less effective than chlorthalidone or indapamide, in PATHWAY2 may have enhanced the BP-lowering efficacy of spironolactone.
- The mean baseline BP obtained by self-monitoring for patients on triple therapy was relatively low (148/84 mm Hg), making it easier to achieve BP control.[33]
- The short time (6 weeks) of exposure to the maximum dose of spironolactone (50 mg/d) was insufficient for an accurate assessment of the long-term tolerability of this drug. Indeed, there was an unexpectedly low rate of side effects, including gynecomastia and impotence, which are known to occur in the long term[142] and may lead to treatment being stopped at the request of the health care provider or patient.
- It is unclear whether BP-lowering efficacy would be similar in patients of African origin.
- The risk of hyperkalemia may be greater in patients with chronic kidney disease, particularly if spironolactone is added to a treatment regimen already including a RAS blocker,[143] making it necessary to monitor plasma potassium and creatinine concentrations closely.

In summary, spironolactone (25 to 50 mg/day) or eplerenone (50 to 100 mg/day) should be used in patients with RHTN but restricted to those with an eGFR 30 or higher mL per minute and a plasma potassium concentration 4.5 or lower mmol/L, particularly in cases of a compelling indication, such as heart failure, in accordance with guidelines.[5,6,11]

The efficacy of spironolactone to reverse sodium overload and, thus, to lower BP in patients with RHTN may be enhanced by using a combination of loop diuretics and thiazides at low doses or by sequential nephron blockade as shown in a French study.[144] In this prospective, randomized, open, blinded, endpoint study, 167 patients with hypertension resistant to 300 mg per day irbesartan, 12.5 mg per day hydrochlorothiazide, and 5 mg per day amlodipine were randomized to sequential nephron blockade (sequential administration of 25 mg/day spironolactone, followed by 20 and then 40 mg/day furosemide, and 5 mg/day amiloride) or sequential RAS blockade (sequential administration of 5 mg/day ramipril uptitrated to 10 mg/day ramipril, followed by 5 mg/day bisoprolol uptitrated to 10 mg/day) on the basis of home BP results. In week 12, the mean between-group difference in daytime ambulatory BP was 10/4 mm Hg in favor of sequential nephron blockade, providing strong support for the use of approaches aiming to reverse sodium overload for the treatment of patients with RHTN. However, although well-tolerated in this trial, sequential nephron blockade strategy requires the careful monitoring of renal function, serum electrolyte levels, and fluid status, for the detection of dehydration, hypokalemia, hyponatremia, hypovolemia, or renal dysfunction.

Further Addition of Antihypertensive Treatments: Seeking Specialist Advice

International guidelines suggest that specialist advice should be sought at a dedicated BP clinic if BP remains uncontrolled.[5-7] At this stage, a stepped-care approach is preferred, including sequential sympathetic nervous system blockade through the stepwise addition of a beta-blocker, an alpha-blocker, and a centrally acting alpha-agonist. Beta-blockers can be used at any step, particularly in patients with coronary artery disease, heart failure, arrhythmia, or chronic kidney disease.[5-7] Direct vasodilators, such as hydralazine or minoxidil, should be used parsimoniously, because they may cause severe fluid retention and tachycardia. This is particularly true for minoxidil, which also has other side effects (e.g., hirsutism, pericardial effusion).[5-7]

Dual RAS blockade with ACE inhibitors and ARBs or with direct renin inhibitors should no longer be used in patients with RHTN because such combinations are not sufficiently effective for lower BP[144] and are associated with a higher risk of potential harm, including hyperkalemia, hypotension, and acute renal failure.[145,146] Dual RAS blockade is discouraged by the NICE and ESH guidelines[5,6] and by the FDA and the European Medicines Agency.

The complexity of the multidrug therapeutic regimens used in patients with RHTN increases the likelihood of drug-related side effects and contributes to the lack of compliance with treatment in patients who may already be taking large numbers of other drugs for comorbid conditions. Device-based therapies are still being investigated, but could potentially be offered as an alternative to patients with severe RHTN (see Chapter 28).

New Drugs

There is a persistent need for the development of new antihypertensive drugs based on new concepts, because BP control remains unachievable in a significant proportion of patients.[147] Indeed, not all the pathophysiological mechanisms involved in RHTN may be entirely neutralized by the various classes of antihypertensive treatments currently available, and the counter-regulatory mechanisms triggered by these treatments may also partly overcome their BP-lowering effect.

Blockade of the ET1 pathway is a rational approach to the treatment of RHTN. The dual ETA/ETB antagonist darusentan was more effective than placebo for decreasing BP in patients with RHTN, but it increased the risk of fluid retention, edema, and cardiac events.[114] The dual angiotensin II receptor-neprilysin inhibitor LCZ696, which decreases the effects of vasoconstrictor and antinatriuretic peptide (angiotensin II) and strengthens the effects of vasodilatory and natriuretic peptides (ANP and bradykinin), lowers BP in hypertensive patients[148] but is marketed for heart failure.[149,150] Aldosterone synthase inhibitors[151] and the fourth-generation nonsteroidal dihydropyridine-based MCR blockers (finerenone) could also be used to target the multiple noxious effects of aldosterone in the kidney, vessels, and heart.[133,152,153] Centrally acting aminopeptidase A inhibitors block the formation of brain angiotensin III, one of the main effector peptides of the brain renin angiotensin system, are in the early phase of clinical development.[154,155]

SUMMARY

RHTN is defined as the failure to lower BP values to the target value despite appropriate treatment with optimal doses of at least three antihypertensive drugs from three different classes, including one diuretic. Pseudoresistance should be excluded by determining 24-hour ambulatory BP or through BP determination at home. RHTN management includes screening for secondary forms of hypertension and the identification of lifestyle factors, such as obesity, excessive alcohol and dietary sodium intake, volume overload, and drug-induced hypertension. Treatment combines lifestyle changes, the discontinuation of interfering substances, and the sequential addition of antihypertensive drugs to the initial triple therapy (diuretic, RAS blocker, and CCB), including MCR antagonists as a fourth-line treatment, followed by sequential sympathetic nervous system blockade (Figs. 43.1 and 43.2). New pharmacological treatments targeting new pathways and device-based approaches aiming to decrease sympathetic tone, including renal denervation and baroreceptor stimulation, are currently being developed (see Chapters 27 and 28). However, it will take a long time to evaluate the efficacy and safety of these new approaches thoroughly. In the meantime, the use of appropriate and personalized daily doses of the available drugs, efforts to decrease physician inertia, to improve compliance with treatment, and access to healthcare and to decrease treatment costs remain major objectives for reducing the incidence of RHTN and the associated target organ damage and poor prognosis.

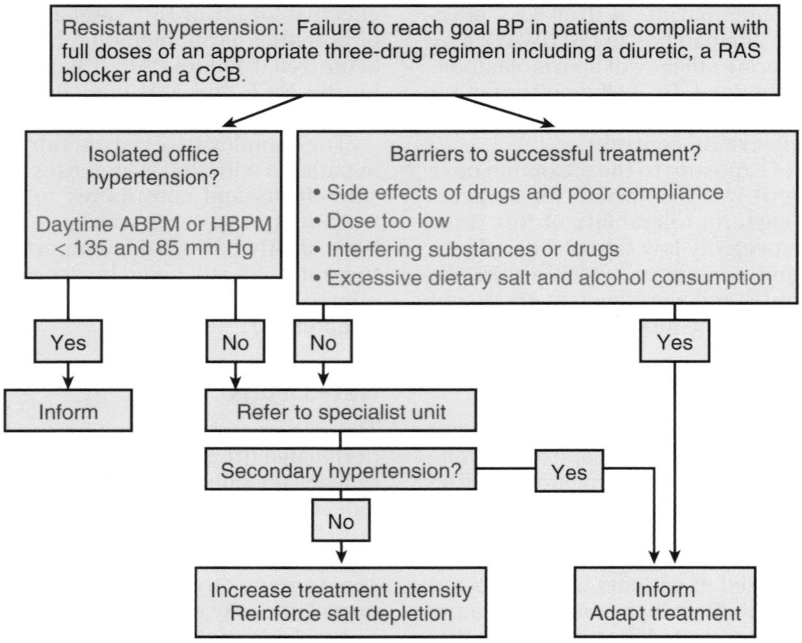

FIG. 43.1 Work up for resistant hypertension. *ABPM*, Ambulatory BP monitoring; *HBPM*, home BP monitoring.

Pharmacological treatment for resistant hypertension

General measures

- Take into account cardiovascular or other comorbid conditions, age, sex, ethnicity, the presence of chronic kidney disease, the risk of drug-drug interactions due to joint prescription, contraindications, previous side effects.
- Use fixed-dose combinations in a single pill to reduce pill burden, home BP monitoring, regular appointments, and the help of other health care professionals (nurses, pharmacists) and of the patient's family, to improve compliance with treatment.
- Regular monitoring of plasma electrolytes (K and Na) and creatinine (or cystatin C) concentrations

Reinforce sodium depletion by maximizing diuretic therapy in addition to a low Na diet

- Switch to a more potent thiazide with a longer duration of action (chlortalidone and indapamide instead of hydrochlorothiazide) when eGFR is ≥30 mL/min/1.73 m^2 or to loop diuretics when eGFR is <30 mL/min/1.73 m^2.
- Increase the diuretic dose or consider sequential nephron blockade (loop diuretic + thiazide).
- Monitor plasma electrolytes and creatinine (or cystatin C) concentrations closely.

Add a mineralocorticoid receptor antagonist at low dose

- Patients with eGFR ≥30 mL/min/1.73 m^2 and plasma K levels ≤4.5 mmol/or especially in cases of a compelling indication, such as heart failure or left ventricular dysfunction.
- Withdraw potassium supplements if part of current medication; Monitor plasma K and creatinine (or cystatin C) concentrations closely.

Consider adding other antihypertensive drugs step-by-step

- A beta-blocker. Monitor ECG
- An alpha-blocker
- A centrally acting alpha-agonist

FIG. 43.2 Pharmacological treatment for resistant hypertension.

References

1. Kearney PM, Whelton M, Reynolds K, et al. Global burden of hypertension: analysis of worldwide data. *Lancet.* 2005;365:217-223.
2. Rapsomaniki E, Timmis A, George J, et al. Blood pressure and incidence of twelve cardiovascular diseases: lifetime risks, healthy life-years lost, and age-specific associations in 1.25 million people. *Lancet.* 2014;383:1899-1911.
3. Prince MJ, Wu F, Guo Y, et al. The burden of disease in older people and implications for health policy and practice. *Lancet.* 2015;385:549-562.
4. Chobanian AV. Shattuck Lecture. The hypertension paradox—more uncontrolled disease despite improved therapy. *N Engl J Med.* 2009;361:878-887.
5. Mancia G, Fagard R, Narkiewicz K, et al. 2013 ESH/ESC Guidelines for the management of arterial hypertension: The Task Force for the management of arterial hypertension of the European Society of Hypertension (ESH) and of the European Society of Cardiology (ESC). *Eur Heart J.* 2013;34:2159-2219.
6. Krause T, Lovibond K, Caulfield M, et al. Management of hypertension: summary of NICE guidance. *BMJ.* 2011;343:d4891.
7. Calhoun DA, Jones D, Textor S, et al. Resistant hypertension: diagnosis, evaluation, and treatment. A scientific statement from the American Heart Association Professional Education Committee of the Council for High Blood Pressure Research. *Hypertension.* 2008;51:1403-1419.

8. Daskalopoulou SS, Rabi DM, Zarnke KB, et al. The 2015 Canadian Hypertension Education Program recommendations for blood pressure measurement, diagnosis, assessment of risk, prevention, and treatment of hypertension. *Can J Cardiol.* 2015;31:549-568.

9. Weber MA, Schiffrin EL, White WB, et al. Clinical practice guidelines for the management of hypertension in the community a statement by the American Society of Hypertension and the International Society of Hypertension. *J Hypertens.* 2014;32:3-15.

10. James PA, Oparil S, Carter BL, et al. 2014 evidence-based guideline for the management of high blood pressure in adults: report from the panel members appointed to the Eighth Joint National Committee (JNC 8). *JAMA.* 2014;311:507-520.

11. Kidney Disease Improving Global Outcomes (KDIGO) Blood Pressure Work Group. KDIGO clinical practice guideline for the management of blood pressure in chronic kidney disease. *Kidney Int Suppl.* 2012;2:337-414.

12. Williams B, MacDonald TM, Morant S, et al. Spironolactone versus placebo, bisoprolol, and doxazosin to determine the optimal treatment for drug-resistant hypertension (PATHWAY-2): a randomised, double-blind, crossover trial. *Lancet.* 2015;386:2059-2068.

13. Wright JT, Jr. Williamson JD, Whelton PK, et al. A randomized trial of intensive versus standard blood-pressure control. *N Engl J Med.* 2015;373:2103-2116.

14. Sarafidis PA, Bakris GL. Resistant hypertension: an overview of evaluation and treatment. *J Am Coll Cardiol.* 2008;52:1749-1757.

15. Judd E, Calhoun DA. Apparent and true resistant hypertension: definition, prevalence and outcomes. *J Hum Hypertens.* 2014;28:463-468.

16. Achelrod D, Wenzel U, Frey S. Systematic review and meta-analysis of the prevalence of resistant hypertension in treated hypertensive populations. *Am J Hypertens.* 2015;28:355-361.

17. Persell SD. Prevalence of resistant hypertension in the United States, 2003-2008. *Hypertension.* 2011;57:1076-1080.

18. Egan BM, Zhao Y, Axon RN. US trends in prevalence, awareness, treatment, and control of hypertension, 1988-2008. *JAMA.* 2010;303:2043-2050.

19. Egan BM, Zhao Y, Li J, et al. Prevalence of optimal treatment regimens in patients with apparent treatment-resistant hypertension based on office blood pressure in a community-based practice network. *Hypertension.* 2013;62:691-697.

20. Savard S, Frank M, Bobrie G, et al. Eligibility for renal denervation in patients with resistant hypertension: when enthusiasm meets reality in real-life patients. *J Am Coll Cardiol.* 2012;60:2422-2424.

21. Tanner RM, Calhoun DA, Bell EK, et al. Prevalence of apparent treatment-resistant hypertension among individuals with CKD. *Clin J Am Soc Nephrol.* 2013;8:1583-1590.

22. Muntner P, Anderson A, Charleston J, et al. Hypertension awareness, treatment, and control in adults with CKD: results from the Chronic Renal Insufficiency Cohort (CRIC) Study. *Am J Kidney Dis.* 2010;55:441-451.

23. Calhoun DA, Booth 3rd JN, Oparil S, et al. Refractory hypertension: determination of prevalence, risk factors, and comorbidities in a large, population-based cohort. *Hypertension.* 2014;63:451-458.

24. de la Sierra A, Segura J, Banegas JR, et al. Clinical features of 8295 patients with resistant hypertension classified on the basis of ambulatory blood pressure monitoring. *Hypertension.* 2011;57:898-902.

25. Myat A, Redwood SR, Qureshi AC, et al. Resistant hypertension. *BMJ.* 2012;345:e7473.

26. Vongpatanasin W. Resistant hypertension: a review of diagnosis and management. *JAMA.* 2014;311:2216-2224.

27. Rimoldi SF, Messerli FH, Bangalore S, et al. Resistant hypertension: what the cardiologist needs to know. *Eur Heart J.* 2015;36:2686-2695.

28. Daugherty SL, Powers JD, Magid DJ, et al. Incidence and prognosis of resistant hypertension in hypertensive patients. *Circulation.* 2012;125:1635-1642.

29. Calhoun DA, Lacourciere Y, Chiang YT, et al. Triple antihypertensive therapy with amlodipine, valsartan, and hydrochlorothiazide: a randomized clinical trial. *Hypertension.* 2009;54:32-39.

30. Degoulet P, Menard J, Vu HA, et al. Factors predictive of attendance at clinic and blood pressure control in hypertensive patients. *BMJ (Clin Res Ed).* 1983;287:88-93.

31. Gaddam KK, Nishizaka MK, Pratt-Ubunama MN, et al. Characterization of resistant hypertension: association between resistant hypertension, aldosterone, and persistent intravascular volume expansion. *Arch Intern Med.* 2008;168:1159-1164.

32. Martins LC, Figueiredo VN, Quinaglia T, et al. Characteristics of resistant hypertension: ageing, body mass index, hyperaldosteronism, cardiac hypertrophy and vascular stiffness. *J Hum Hypertens.* 2011;25:532-538.

33. Gupta AK, Nasothimiou EG, Chang CL, et al. Baseline predictors of resistant hypertension in the Anglo-Scandinavian Cardiac Outcome Trial (ASCOT): a risk score to identify those at high-risk. *J Hypertens.* 2011;29:2004-2013.

34. Ruttanaumpawan P, Nopmaneejumruslers C, Logan AG, et al. Association between refractory hypertension and obstructive sleep apnea. *J Hypertens.* 2009;27:1439-1445.

35. Dudenbostel T, Calhoun DA. Resistant hypertension, obstructive sleep apnoea and aldosterone. *J Hum Hypertens.* 2012;26:281-287.

36. Pimenta E, Calhoun DA, Oparil S. Sleep apnea, aldosterone, and resistant hypertension. *Prog Cardiovasc Dis.* 2009;51:371-380.

37. Pedrosa RP, Drager LF, Gonzaga CC, et al. Obstructive sleep apnea: the most common secondary cause of hypertension associated with resistant hypertension. *Hypertension.* 2011;58:811-817.

38. Cuspidi C, Macca G, Sampieri L, et al. High prevalence of cardiac and extracardiac target organ damage in refractory hypertension. *J Hypertens.* 2001;19:2063-2070.

39. Muiesan ML, Salvetti M, Rizzoni D, et al. Resistant hypertension and target organ damage. *Hypertens Res.* 2013;36:485-491.

40. Smith SM, Huo T, Delia Johnson B, et al. Cardiovascular and mortality risk of apparent resistant hypertension in women with suspected myocardial ischemia: a report from the NHLBI-sponsored WISE Study. *J Am Heart Assoc.* 2014;3:e000660.

41. De Nicola L, Gabbai FB, Agarwal R, et al. Prevalence and prognostic role of resistant hypertension in chronic kidney disease patients. *J Am Coll Cardiol.* 2013;61:2461-2467.

42. Rossignol P, Massy ZA, Azizi M, et al. The double challenge of resistant hypertension and chronic kidney disease. *Lancet.* 2015;386:1588-1598.

43. Schmieder RE, Grassi G, Kjeldsen SE. Patients with treatment-resistant hypertension report increased stress and anxiety: a worldwide study. *J Hypertens.* 2013;31:610-615. discussion 615.

44. Pimenta E, Gaddam KK, Oparil S, et al. Effects of dietary sodium reduction on blood pressure in subjects with resistant hypertension: results from a randomized trial. *Hypertension.* 2009;54:475-481.

45. Pimenta E, Gaddam KK, Pratt-Ubunama MN, et al. Relation of dietary salt and aldosterone to urinary protein excretion in subjects with resistant hypertension. *Hypertension.* 2008;51:339-344.

46. Shimbo D, Levitan EB, Booth JN 3rd, et al. The contributions of unhealthy lifestyle factors to apparent resistant hypertension: findings from the Reasons for Geographic And Racial Differences in Stroke (REGARDS) study. *J Hypertens.* 2013;31:370-376.

47. Calhoun DA. Hyperaldosteronism as a common cause of resistant hypertension. *Annu Rev Med.* 2013;64:233-247.

48. Pimenta E, Stowasser M, Gordon RD, et al. Increased dietary sodium is related to severity of obstructive sleep apnea in patients with resistant hypertension and hyperaldosteronism. *Chest.* 2013;143:978-983.

49. Osterberg L, Blaschke T. Adherence to medication. *N Engl J Med.* 2005;353:487-497.

50. Simpson SH, Eurich DT, Majumdar SR, et al. A meta-analysis of the association between adherence to drug therapy and mortality. *BMJ.* 2006;333:15.

51. Ho PM, Bryson CL, Rumsfeld JS. Medication adherence: its importance in cardiovascular outcomes. *Circulation.* 2009;119:3028-3035.

52. Mazzaglia G, Ambrosioni E, Alacqua M, et al. Adherence to antihypertensive medications and cardiovascular morbidity among newly diagnosed hypertensive patients. *Circulation.* 2009;120:1598-1605.

53. Burnier M, Wuerzner G, Struijker-Boudier H, et al. Measuring, analyzing, and managing drug adherence in resistant hypertension. *Hypertension.* 2013;62:218-225.

54. Claxton AJ, Cramer J, Pierce C. A systematic review of the associations between dose regimens and medication compliance. *Clin Ther.* 2001;23:1296-1310.

55. Knight EL, Bohn RL, Wang PS, et al. Predictors of uncontrolled hypertension in ambulatory patients. *Hypertension.* 2001;38:809-814.

56. Mancia G, Zambon A, Soranna D, et al. Factors involved in the discontinuation of antihypertensive drug therapy: an analysis from real life data. *J Hypertens.* 2014;32:1708-1715; discussion 1716.

57. Cene CW, Dennison CR, Powell Hammond W, et al. Antihypertensive medication nonadherence in black men: direct and mediating effects of depressive symptoms, psychosocial stressors, and substance use. *J Clin Hypertens (Greenwich).* 2013;15:201-209.

58. Holt E, Joyce C, Dornelles A, et al. Sex differences in barriers to antihypertensive medication adherence: findings from the cohort study of medication adherence among older adults. *J Am Geriatr Soc.* 2013;61:558-564.

59. Marshall IJ, Wolfe CD, McKevitt C. Lay perspectives on hypertension and drug adherence: systematic review of qualitative research. *BMJ.* 2012;345:e3953.

60. Morisky DE, Ang A, Krousel-Wood M, et al. Predictive validity of a medication adherence measure in an outpatient setting. *J Clin Hypertens (Greenwich).* 2008;10:348-354.

61. Azizi M, Menard J, Peyrard S, et al. Assessment of patients' and physicians' compliance to an ACE inhibitor treatment based on urinary N-acetyl Ser-Asp-Lys-Pro determination in the Noninsulin-Dependent Diabetes, Hypertension, Microalbuminuria, Proteinuria, Cardiovascular Events, and Ramipril (DIABHYCAR) study. *Diabetes Care.* 2006;29:1331-1336.

62. Jung O, Gechter JL, Wunder C, et al. Resistant hypertension? Assessment of adherence by toxicological urine analysis. *J Hypertens.* 2013;31:766-774.

63. Strauch B, Petrak O, Zelinka T, et al. Precise assessment of noncompliance with the antihypertensive therapy in patients with resistant hypertension using toxicological serum analysis. *J Hypertens.* 2013;31:2455-2461.

64. Patel P, Gupta PK, White CM, et al. Screening for non-adherence to antihypertensive treatment as a part of the diagnostic pathway to renal denervation. *J Hum Hypertens.* 2016;30:368-373.

65. Tomaszewski M, White C, Patel P, et al. High rates of non-adherence to antihypertensive treatment revealed by high-performance liquid chromatography-tandem mass spectrometry (HP LC-MS/MS) urine analysis. *Heart.* 2014;100:855-861.

66. Flockhart DA, Tanus-Santos JE. Implications of cytochrome P450 interactions when prescribing medication for hypertension. *Arch Intern Med.* 2002;162:405-412.

67. Grossman A, Messerli FH, Grossman E. Drug induced hypertension—An unappreciated cause of secondary hypertension. *Eur J Pharmacol.* 2015;763:15-22.

68. Grossman E, Messerli FH. Drug-induced hypertension: an unappreciated cause of secondary hypertension. *Am J Med.* 2012;125:14-22.

69. Azizi M, Blanchard A, Charbit B, et al. Effect of contrasted sodium diets on the pharmacokinetics and pharmacodynamic effects of renin-angiotensin system blockers. *Hypertension.* 2013;61:1239-1245.

70. Nieuwlaat R, Wilczynski N, Navarro T, et al. Interventions for enhancing medication adherence. *Cochrane Database Syst Rev.* 2014;11. CD000011.

71. Haynes RB, McDonald HP, Garg AX. Helping patients follow prescribed treatment: clinical applications. *JAMA.* 2002;288:2880-2883.

72. Schroeder K, Fahey T, Ebrahim S. How can we improve adherence to blood pressure-lowering medication in ambulatory care? Systematic review of randomized controlled trials. *Arch Intern Med.* 2004;164:722-732.

73. Ogedegbe G, Schoenthaler A. A systematic review of the effects of home blood pressure monitoring on medication adherence. *J Clin Hypertens (Greenwich).* 2006;8:174-180.

74. Parati G, Stergiou G, O'Brien E, et al. European Society of Hypertension practice guidelines for ambulatory blood pressure monitoring. *J Hypertens.* 2014;32:1359-1366.

75. Omboni S, Gazzola T, Carabelli G, et al. Clinical usefulness and cost effectiveness of home blood pressure telemonitoring: meta-analysis of randomized controlled studies. *J Hypertens.* 2013;31:455-467; discussion 467–468.

76. McManus RJ, Mant J, Haque MS, et al. Effect of self-monitoring and medication self-titration on systolic blood pressure in hypertensive patients at high risk of cardiovascular disease: the TASMIN-SR randomized clinical trial. *JAMA.* 2014;312:799-808.

77. Mistry N, Keepanasseril A, Wilczynski NL, et al. Technology-mediated interventions for enhancing medication adherence. *J Am Med Inform Assoc.* 2015;22:e177-e193.

78. Sherrill B, Halpern M, Khan S, et al. Single-pill vs free-equivalent combination therapies for hypertension: a meta-analysis of health care costs and adherence. *J Clin Hypertens (Greenwich).* 2011;13:898-909.

79. Panjabi S, Lacey M, Bancroft T, et al. Treatment adherence, clinical outcomes, and economics of triple-drug therapy in hypertensive patients. *J Am Soc Hypertens.* 2013;7:46-60.

80. Christensen A, Osterberg LG, Hansen EH. Electronic monitoring of patient adherence to oral antihypertensive medical treatment: a systematic review. *J Hypertens.* 2009;27:1540-1551.

81. Vrijens B, Vincze G, Kristanto P, et al. Adherence to prescribed antihypertensive drug treatments: longitudinal study of electronically compiled dosing histories. *BMJ.* 2008;336:1114-1117.

82. Berlowitz DR, Ash AS, Hickey EC, et al. Inadequate management of blood pressure in a hypertensive population. *N Engl J Med.* 1998;339:1957-1963.

83. Wang YR, Alexander GC, Stafford RS. Outpatient hypertension treatment, treatment intensification, and control in Western Europe and the United States. *Arch Intern Med.* 2007;167:141-147.

84. Casey Jr DE. Why don't physicians (and patients) consistently follow clinical practice guidelines? *JAMA Intern Med.* 2013;173:1581-1583.

85. Cabana MD, Rand CS, Powe NR, et al. Why don't physicians follow clinical practice guidelines? A framework for improvement. *JAMA.* 1999;282:1458-1465.

86. Oliveria SA, Lapuerta P, McCarthy BD, et al. Physician-related barriers to the effective management of uncontrolled hypertension. *Arch Intern Med.* 2002;162:413-420.

87. Turner BJ, Hollenbeak CS, Weiner M, et al. Effect of unrelated comorbid conditions on hypertension management. *Ann Intern Med.* 2008;148:578-586.

88. Kerr EA, Zikmund-Fisher BJ, Klamerus ML, et al. The role of clinical uncertainty in treatment decisions for diabetic patients with uncontrolled blood pressure. *Ann Intern Med.* 2008;148:717-727.

89. Margolis KL, Rolnick SJ, Fortman KK, et al. Self-reported hypertension treatment beliefs and practices of primary care physicians in a managed care organization. *Am J Hypertens.* 2005;18:566-571.

90. Feldman RD, Zou GY, Vandervoort MK, et al. A simplified approach to the treatment of uncomplicated hypertension: a cluster randomized, controlled trial. *Hypertension.* 2009;53:646-653.

91. Azizi M, Sapoval M, Gosse P, et al. Optimum and stepped care standardised antihypertensive treatment with or without renal denervation for resistant hypertension (DENERHTN): a multicentre, open-label, randomised controlled trial. *Lancet.* 2015;385:1957-1965.

92. Rimoldi SF, Scherrer U, Messerli FH. Secondary arterial hypertension: when, who, and how to screen? *Eur Heart J.* 2014;35:1245-1254.

93. Rossi GP, Seccia TM, Maniero C, et al. Drug-related hypertension and resistance to antihypertensive treatment: a call for action. *J Hypertens.* 2011;29:2295-2309.

94. Dumbreck S, Flynn A, Nairn M, et al. Drug-disease and drug-drug interactions: systematic examination of recommendations in 12 UK national clinical guidelines. *BMJ.* 2015;350:h949.

95. Postel-Vinay N, Bobrie G, Steichen O, et al. HY-Quest, standardized patient questionnaire to be completed at home before a first visit for hypertension: a validation study in specialized centres in France. *J Hypertens.* 2014;32:693-698.

96. Stewart PM, Wallace AM, Atherden SM, et al. Mineralocorticoid activity of carbenoxolone: contrasting effects of carbenoxolone and liquorice on 11 beta-hydroxysteroid dehydrogenase activity in man. *Clin Sci (Lond).* 1990;78:49-54.

97. Stewart PM, Wallace AM, Valentino R, et al. Mineralocorticoid activity of liquorice: 11-beta-hydroxysteroid dehydrogenase deficiency comes of age. *Lancet.* 1987;2:821-824.

98. Denolle T, Azizi M, Massart C, et al. [Itraconazole: a new drug-related cause of hypertension]. *Ann Cardiol Angeiol (Paris).* 2014;63:213-215.

99. Roviello G, Sigala S, Danesi R, et al. Incidence and relative risk of adverse events of special interest in patients with castration resistant prostate cancer treated with CYP-17 inhibitors: a meta-analysis of published trials. *Crit Rev Oncol Hematol.* 2016;101:12-20.

100. Attard G, Reid AH, Auchus RJ, et al. Clinical and biochemical consequences of CYP17A1 inhibition with abiraterone given with and without exogenous glucocorticoids in castrate men with advanced prostate cancer. *J Clin Endocrinol Metab.* 2012;97:507-516.

101. Pechere-Bertschi A, Maillard M, Stalder H, et al. Renal hemodynamic and tubular responses to salt in women using oral contraceptives. *Kidney Int.* 2003;64:1374-1380.

102. Klatsky AL, Friedman GD, Siegelaub AB, et al. Alcohol consumption and blood pressure Kaiser-Permanente Multiphasic Health Examination data. *N Engl J Med.* 1977;296:1194-1200.

103. Ranpura V, Pulipati B, Chu D, et al. Increased risk of high-grade hypertension with bevacizumab in cancer patients: a meta-analysis. *Am J Hypertens.* 2010;23:460-468.

104. Azizi M, Chedid A, Oudard S. Home blood-pressure monitoring in patients receiving sunitinib. *N Engl J Med.* 2008;358:95-97.

105. Zhu X, Stergiopoulos K, Wu S. Risk of hypertension and renal dysfunction with an angiogenesis inhibitor sunitinib: systematic review and meta-analysis. *Acta Oncol.* 2009;48:9-17.

106. Wu S, Chen JJ, Kudelka A, et al. Incidence and risk of hypertension with sorafenib in patients with cancer: a systematic review and meta-analysis. *Lancet Oncol.* 2008;9:117-123.

107. Steingart RM, Bakris GL, Chen HX, et al. Management of cardiac toxicity in patients receiving vascular endothelial growth factor signaling pathway inhibitors. *Am Heart J.* 2012;163:156-163.

108. Crane HM, Van Rompaey SE, Kitahata MM. Antiretroviral medications associated with elevated blood pressure among patients receiving highly active antiretroviral therapy. *AIDS.* 2006;20:1019-1026.

109. Wang J, Mullins CD, Mamdani M, et al. New diagnosis of hypertension among celecoxib and nonselective NSAID users: a population-based cohort study. *Ann Pharmacother.* 2007;41:937-943.

110. Aw TJ, Haas SJ, Liew D, et al. Meta-analysis of cyclooxygenase-2 inhibitors and their effects on blood pressure. *Arch Intern Med.* 2005;165:490-496.

111. Sowers JR, White WB, Pitt B, et al. The Effects of cyclooxygenase-2 inhibitors and nonsteroidal anti-inflammatory therapy on 24-hour blood pressure in patients with hypertension, osteoarthritis, and type 2 diabetes mellitus. *Arch Intern Med.* 2005;165:161-168.

112. Armstrong EP, Malone DC. The impact of nonsteroidal anti-inflammatory drugs on blood pressure, with an emphasis on newer agents. *Clin Ther.* 2003;25:1-18.

113. Esler M. Sympathetic nervous system moves toward center stage in cardiovascular medicine: from Thomas Willis to resistant hypertension. *Hypertension.* 2014;63:e25-e32.

114. Weber MA, Black H, Bakris G, et al. A selective endothelin-receptor antagonist to reduce blood pressure in patients with treatment-resistant hypertension: a randomised, doubleblind, placebo-controlled trial. *Lancet.* 2009;374:1423-1431.

115. Na KY, Oh YK, Han JS, et al. Upregulation of Na+ transporter abundances in response to chronic thiazide or loop diuretic treatment in rats. *Am J Physiol Renal Physiol.* 2003;284:F133-F143.

116. Nielsen J, Kwon TH, Masilamani S, et al. Sodium transporter abundance profiling in kidney: effect of spironolactone. *Am J Physiol Renal Physiol.* 2002;283:F923-F933.

117. Dickinson HO, Mason JM, Nicolson DJ, et al. Lifestyle interventions to reduce raised blood pressure: a systematic review of randomized controlled trials. *J Hypertens.* 2006;24:215-233.

118. Hu X, Fan J, Chen S, et al. The role of continuous positive airway pressure in blood pressure control for patients with obstructive sleep apnea and hypertension: a meta-analysis of randomized controlled trials. *J Clin Hypertens (Greenwich).* 2015;17:215-222.

119. Martinez-Garcia MA, Capote F, Campos-Rodriguez F, et al. Effect of CPAP on blood pressure in patients with obstructive sleep apnea and resistant hypertension: the HIPARCO randomized clinical trial. *JAMA.* 2013;310:2407-2715.

120. Muxfeldt ES, Margallo V, Costa LM, et al. Effects of continuous positive airway pressure treatment on clinic and ambulatory blood pressures in patients with obstructive sleep apnea and resistant hypertension: a randomized controlled trial. *Hypertension.* 2015;65:736-742.

121. Bratton DJ, Gaisl T, Wons AM, et al. CPAP vs Mandibular Advancement Devices and Blood Pressure in Patients With Obstructive Sleep Apnea: A Systematic Review and Metaanalysis. *JAMA.* 2015;314:2280-2293.

122. Campos-Rodriguez F, Martinez-Alonso M, Sanchez-de-la-Torre M, et al. Long-term adherence to continuous positive airway pressure therapy in non-sleepy sleep apnea patients. *Sleep Med.* 2016;17:1-6.

123. Eide IK, Torjesen PA, Drolsum A, et al. Low-renin status in therapy-resistant hypertension: a clue to efficient treatment. *J Hypertens.* 2004;22:2217-2226.

124. Roush GC, Ernst ME, Kostis JB, et al. Head-to-head comparisons of hydrochlorothiazide with indapamide and chlorthalidone: antihypertensive and metabolic effects. *Hypertension.* 2015;65:1041-1046.

125. Ernst ME, Carter BL, Goerdt CJ, et al. Comparative antihypertensive effects of hydrochlorothiazide and chlorthalidone on ambulatory and office blood pressure. *Hypertension.* 2006;47:352-358.

126. Pareek AK, Messerli FH, Chandurkar NB, et al. Efficacy of Low-Dose Chlorthalidone and Hydrochlorothiazide as Assessed by 24-h Ambulatory Blood Pressure Monitoring. *J Am Coll Cardiol.* 2016;67:379-389.

127. Peterzan MA, Hardy R, Chaturvedi N, et al. Meta-analysis of dose-response relationships for hydrochlorothiazide, chlorthalidone, and bendroflumethiazide on blood pressure, serum potassium, and urate. *Hypertension.* 2012;59:1104-1109.

128. Roush GC, Holford TR, Guddati AK. Chlorthalidone compared with hydrochlorothiazide in reducing cardiovascular events: systematic review and network meta-analyses. *Hypertension.* 2012;59:1110-1117.

129. Dhalla IA, Gomes T, Yao Z, et al. Chlorthalidone versus hydrochlorothiazide for the treatment of hypertension in older adults: a population-based cohort study. *Ann Intern Med.* 2013;158:447-455.

130. Tamargo J, Segura J, Ruilope LM. Diuretics in the treatment of hypertension. Part 1: thiazide and thiazide-like diuretics. *Expert Opin Pharmacother.* 2014;15:527-547.

131. Roush GC, Ernst ME, Kostis JB, et al. Dose doubling, relative potency, and dose equivalence of potassium-sparing diuretics affecting blood pressure and serum potassium: systematic review and meta-analyses. *J Hypertens.* 2016;34:11-19.

132. Jansen PM, Danser AH, Imholz BP, et al. Aldosterone-receptor antagonism in hypertension. *J Hypertens.* 2009;27:680-691.

133. Colussi G, Catena C, Sechi LA. Spironolactone, eplerenone and the new aldosterone blockers in endocrine and primary hypertension. *J Hypertens.* 2013;31:3-15.

134. Dussol B, Moussi-Frances J, Morange S, et al. A pilot study comparing furosemide and hydrochlorothiazide in patients with hypertension and stage 4 or 5 chronic kidney disease. *J Clin Hypertens (Greenwich).* 2012;14:32-37.

135. Agarwal R, Sinha AD, Pappas MK, et al. Chlorthalidone for poorly controlled hypertension in chronic kidney disease: an interventional pilot study. *Am J Nephrol.* 2014;39:171-182.

136. Tamargo J, Segura J, Ruilope LM. Diuretics in the treatment of hypertension. Part 2: loop diuretics and potassium-sparing agents. *Expert Opin Pharmacother.* 2014;15:605-621.

137. Calhoun DA, White WB. Effectiveness of the selective aldosterone blocker, eplerenone, in patients with resistant hypertension. *J Am Soc Hypertens.* 2008;2:462-468.

138. Weinberger MH, Roniker B, Krause SL, et al. Eplerenone, a selective aldosterone blocker, in mild-to-moderate hypertension. *Am J Hypertens.* 2002;15:709-716.

139. Menard J. The 45-year story of the development of an anti-aldosterone more specific than spironolactone. *Mol Cell Endocrinol.* 2004;217:45-52.

140. Epstein M, Duprez DA. Resistant hypertension and the pivotal role for mineralocorticoid receptor antagonists: a clinical update-2016. *Am J Med.* 2016;129:661-666.

141. Dahal K, Kunwar S, Rijal J, et al. The effects of aldosterone antagonists in patients with resistant hypertension: a meta-analysis of randomized and nonrandomized studies. *Am J Hypertens.* 2015;28:1376-1385.

142. Jeunemaitre X, Charru A, Chatellier G, et al. Long-term metabolic effects of spironolactone and thiazides combined with potassium-sparing agents for treatment of essential hypertension. *Am J Cardiol.* 1988;62:1072-1077.

143. Bolignano D, Palmer SC, Navaneethan SD, et al. Aldosterone antagonists for preventing the progression of chronic kidney disease. *Cochrane Database Syst Rev.* 2014;4. CD007004.

144. Bobrie G, Frank M, Azizi M, et al. Sequential nephron blockade versus sequential reninangiotensin system blockade in resistant hypertension: a prospective, randomized, open blinded endpoint study. *J Hypertens.* 2012;30:1656-1664.

145. Makani H, Bangalore S, Desouza KA, et al. Efficacy and safety of dual blockade of the renin-angiotensin system: meta-analysis of randomised trials. *BMJ.* 2013;346:f360.

146. Susantitaphong P, Sewaralthahab K, Balk EM, et al. Efficacy and safety of combined vs. single renin-angiotensin-aldosterone system blockade in chronic kidney disease: a metaanalysis. *Am J Hypertens.* 2013;26:424-441.

147. Monge M, Lorthioir A, Bobrie G, et al. New drug therapies interfering with the reninangiotensin-aldosterone system for resistant hypertension. *J Renin Angiotensin Aldosterone Syst.* 2013;14:285-289.

148. Ruilope LM, Dukat A, Bohm M, et al. Blood-pressure reduction with LCZ696, a novel dual-acting inhibitor of the angiotensin II receptor and neprilysin: a randomised, doubleblind, placebo-controlled, active comparator study. *Lancet.* 2010;375:1255-1266.

149. McMurray JJ, Packer M, Desai AS, et al. Angiotensin-neprilysin inhibition versus enalapril in heart failure. *N Engl J Med.* 2014;371:993-1004.

150. Hubers SA, Brown NJ. Combined Angiotensin Receptor Antagonism and Neprilysin Inhibition. *Circulation.* 2016;133:1115-1124.

151. Azizi M, Amar L, Menard J. Aldosterone synthase inhibition in humans. *Nephrol Dial Transplant.* 2013;28:36-43.

152. Kolkhof P, Nowack C, Eitner F. Nonsteroidal antagonists of the mineralocorticoid receptor. *Curr Opin Nephrol Hypertens.* 2015;24:417-424.

153. Bakris GL, Agarwal R, Chan JC, et al. Effect of finerenone on albuminuria in patients with diabetic nephropathy: a randomized clinical trial. *JAMA.* 2015;314:884-894.

154. Bodineau L, Frugiere A, Marc Y, et al. Orally active aminopeptidase A inhibitors reduce blood pressure: a new strategy for treating hypertension. *Hypertension.* 2008;51:1318-1325.

155. Balavoine F, Azizi M, Bergerot D, et al. Randomised, double-blind, placebo-controlled, dose-escalating phase I study of QGC001, a centrally acting aminopeptidase a inhibitor prodrug. *Clin Pharmacokinet.* 2014;53:385-395.

44 Hypertension and the Perioperative Period

Robert L. Bard and Robert D. Brook

There are few contemporary studies concerning the cardiovascular (CV) risks caused by hypertension or the benefits of its treatment during the perioperative period. Conversely, numerous trials have evaluated the potential benefits of specific antihypertensive medications, in particular beta-blockers. The 2007 American Heart Association (AHA) guidelines took a precautionary approach and considered severe high blood pressure (BP) (≥180 mm Hg systolic and/or ≥100 mm Hg diastolic) a "minor" clinical risk predictor for adverse perioperative CV events and suggested that clinicians lower BP below this threshold before elective surgery. However, the more recent AHA guidelines published in 2014 do not specifically address perioperative hypertension. The optimal management of high BP during the surgical period therefore remains uncertain. In this chapter we review the common hemodynamic alterations and surgical risks related to hypertension during the perioperative period. We summarize the findings from relevant clinical trials, the roles for specific antihypertensive agents (e.g., beta-blockers), and provide a pragmatic algorithm for the management of hypertensive patients undergoing surgery.

Hypertension affects over 1 billion people and is the leading risk factor for global morbidity and mortality.[1] Given that roughly one-third of the adult population has hypertension, it is not surprising that high BP is commonly encountered in patients preparing for surgery.[2,3] Estimates of the prevalence range from 8% to 80% depending upon the clinical scenario, with an overall average of approximately 25% of surgical patients. However, it is important to highlight that there is no universally accepted consensus definition of perioperative hypertension.[2] In addition, few studies have focused on the optimal therapeutic approach to high BP during the perioperative period.

PERIOPERATIVE BLOOD PRESSURE CHANGES

The most typical alterations in BP that occur throughout the perioperative period have been evaluated in detail.[2,3] Acute BP elevations, occasionally reaching severe levels (i.e., ≥180/110 mm Hg), can occur before surgery in response to a number of transient factors (e.g., anxiety, pain, white coat effect, medication withdrawal). Several observational studies have demonstrated that uncontrolled hypertension ranks among the most common causes for surgical or procedural postponement.[4-7] Intubation and the induction of anesthesia can also induce rapid elevations in both BP and heart rate, responses that are often exaggerated in hypertensive patients. Conversely, anesthesia (intravenous, spinal, or inhaled volatile agents) is most often a cause of hypotension during surgery itself as a result of reduced sympathetic tone, pain control, sedation, and direct hemodynamic actions. Other possible causes of low BP during surgery include blood loss, upright patient position,

mechanical ventilation, infection/anaphylaxis or intraoperative CV events (e.g., reduced cardiac output). It is also generally accepted that patients with hypertension are at increased risk for excessive BP variability during the intraoperative period. This has been defined as increases and/or decreases in mean arterial pressure by 20% or more from baseline levels and has been associated with worse perioperative CV outcomes.[2,3,8] Finally, acute elevations in BP predominate during the postoperative period.[2,9]

Perioperative high BP may occur for two general reasons. Patients may present with an acute worsening of underlying chronic hypertension or it may be a new isolated response to one or more transient factors. Anxiety, pain, drug/medication withdrawal (e.g., alpha 2-agonists, beta-blockers, and alcohol), and stress-induced sympathetic nervous system activation can acutely increase BP and heart rate. Postoperative hypertension may be further worsened or induced by hypothermia, hypoxemia, inadequate ventilation with subsequent hypercarbia, or bladder distention. Intraoperative intravenous fluid administration, especially in patients with chronic kidney disease and/or postoperative renal dysfunction, is also commonly responsible. The initial step in the management of postoperative hypertension is to identify and remedy the factor(s) responsible.[9] Treatment of persistent severe elevations in BP (≥180 mm Hg systolic and/or ≥100 mm Hg diastolic) with intravenous or oral antihypertensive agents is thereafter commonly recommended based upon expert opinions and the precautionary principle. However, there are few outcome data supporting the CV benefits of acute perioperative BP-lowering or outlining the optimal therapeutic approach (i.e., BP targets, most effective medications).[2,3,9]

CLINICAL GUIDELINES AND PERIOPERATIVE HYPERTENSION

Studies that have assessed the effect of hypertension on operative outcomes have been largely limited to patients with chronic hypertension and not those with acute BP elevations in response to transient conditions. The overall evidence supports that chronic hypertension plays a relatively minor role in the risk for CV complications in surgical candidates.[10] In previous versions of the American College of Cardiology (ACC) and the AHA guidelines published in 2007, hypertension was deemed a "minor clinical predictor" of adverse outcomes only when reaching severe levels (systolic BP ≥180 mm Hg and/or diastolic BP ≥110 mm Hg). It was recommended that acute treatment of severe hypertension and/or delay of surgery to control BP should be considered on a case-by-case basis. However, lower stages of hypertension (140 to 179/90 to 109 mm Hg) were not deemed independent predictors of CV complications by their analyses of the pooled results from observational studies.[10] Mild hypertension was therefore not considered in the calculation of global perioperative CV risk, nor was it a factor that required treatment or delay of surgery under most clinical scenarios.

The more recent ACC/AHA guidelines published in 2014 do not specifically discuss the surgical risks associated with high BP.[11] Hypertension is only listed as a single factor among many parameters to calculate global preoperative CV risk in one of the three calculators promulgated for clinical usage (National Surgical Quality Improvement Program). The simpler and likely more often used tool, the Revised Cardiac Risk Index (RCRI), does not include hypertension (Box 44.1). There is also no discussion about the consideration to treat or delay surgery to control severe hypertension (i.e., BP ≥ 180/110 mm Hg). As such, we believe it is reasonable to continue to follow the approach previously outlined in 2007 because there have been no new practice-changing studies published regarding the importance of hypertension or outcome trials challenging the validity of the prior precautionary recommendations.

Note that hypertension is frequently associated with and/or is a cause of other CV diseases (e.g., diabetes mellitus, ischemic heart disease, heart failure) that are more potent risk factors for perioperative complications.[10,11] As such, an elevated BP should cue clinicians to more thoroughly evaluate patients for other higher risk parameters (Box 44.1). The identification of hypertension during preoperative risk

---

BOX 44.1 The Revised Cardiac Risk Index for Perioperative Risk Assessment[11]

Revised Cardiac Risk Index Parameters
Chronic kidney disease (creatinine ≥ 2.0 mg/dL)
Heart failure
Insulin-dependent diabetes mellitus
High risk surgery
(Intrathoracic, intraabdominal, or suprainguinal vascular surgery)
History of stroke or transient ischemic attack
Ischemic heart disease

   Current 2014 ACC/AHA guidelines[11] recommend that a validated risk-prediction tool (e.g., RCRI) can be useful in predicting the risk of perioperative major adverse cardiovascular events (MACE) in patients undergoing noncardiac surgery (level of evidence B). For the RCRI, MACE includes myocardial infarction, pulmonary edema, ventricular fibrillation, cardiac arrest, or complete heart block.
   Online RCRI tool: www.mdcalc.com/revised-cardiac-risk-index-for-pre-operative-risk.
   Note: Neither mild nor severe hypertension (BP ≥ 180/110 mm Hg) are listed among the parameters in RCRI to calculate perioperative cardiovascular risk.
   The RCRI score is calculated as the sum of each of the 6 parameters listed. Patients with a score 2 or higher are considered "elevated risk." Stable patients without unstable conditions (i.e., ischemic heart disease or recent acute coronary syndrome within last 60 days, decompensated heart failure, high risk/uncontrolled arrhythmia, severe valve disease, or severe pulmonary hypertension) and a Revised Cardiac Risk Index score 1 or higher can procedure with surgery without further CV testing. Those with a score 2 or higher at "elevated risk" may be candidates for further evaluation including pharmacological stress testing. Patients requiring emergent or urgent surgery that cannot be delayed and those with an excellent (≥10 METS) or moderate/good (≥4 METS) estimated functional capacity should procedure with surgery without further testing. Patients with elevated risk and an unknown or poor (<4 METS) functional capacity are candidates for stress testing and subsequent intervention (i.e., revascularization and/or added beta-blockade) if appropriate.

(From Fleisher LA, Fleischmann KE, Auerbach AD, et al. 2014 ACC/AHA Guideline on perioperative cardiovascular evaluation and management of patients undergoing noncardiac surgery. J Am Coll Cardiol. 2014;64:e77-e137.)

---

assessment also offers a valuable clinical opportunity for a more complete evaluation of the patient's overall long-term CV risk. Lifestyle modifications (e.g., diet and exercise) and control of CV risk factors in addition to hypertension (e.g., hyperlipidemia) should be initiated as clinically indicated irrespective of the upcoming surgery. On the other hand, clinical trial evidence does not support performing coronary revascularizations (e.g., angioplasty/stent or bypass surgery) with the sole intention of preventing surgical complications, even among patients with significant cardiac ischemia. Rather, CV diseases (e.g., coronary heart disease, heart failure) should be managed per published guidelines with the goal of reducing life-limiting symptoms (e.g., angina) and improving long-term CV risk. Clinicians need to consider that any coronary revascularization will involve a significant delay in surgery from 1 to 12 months depending upon the procedure and subsequent duration of dual antiplatelet therapy. Guidelines recommend that the risks versus benefits of proceeding with surgery versus delaying the procedure to control hypertension or treat underlying CV diseases need to be carefully evaluated on a case-by-case basis.[11]

HYPERTENSION AND PERIOPERATIVE CARDIOVASCULAR RISK

In 1953 Smithwick and Thompson[12] reported that hypertensive patients undergoing sympathectomy had six times the rate of mortality as compared with normotensive patients.[13] Several studies have confirmed that hypertensive patients are at elevated risk for postsurgical CV complications,[13] including the Department of Veterans Affairs National Surgical Quality Improvement Program involving more than 83,000 patients.[14] However, the overall published findings during the past few decades have been mixed in regards to the risks as a result of high BP or benefits of perioperative antihypertensive medications (in particular beta-blockers).[15-25] For example, in 1977 Goldman et al[15] reported that hypertension was not a significant risk factor among 1001 patients. These observations were confirmed in 1979[21] among 676 surgical patients as preoperative BP did not correlate with adverse events. Lette et al[16] also demonstrated that numerous clinical parameters, including hypertension, did not predict adverse surgical outcomes; whereas the amount of jeopardized myocardium during stress perfusion testing successfully identified higher risk patients. On the other hand, Rose[22] studied 18,380 general surgery patients and showed that patients with postoperative hypertension had greater rates of unplanned critical care admissions (2.6% versus 0.2%) and excess mortality (1.9% versus 0.3%). It is also important to note that several studies have shown that rather than hypertension per se, the CV risks and complications related to surgery may be more strongly associated with excessive BP variability (both low and high BP outside an "optimal" range) during the perioperative period.[2,8]

The risks of hypertension in the absence of other higher risk conditions (Box 44.1), as well as the efficacy of lowering of BP on perioperative morbidity and mortality, remain unclear. This is because most published studies have evaluated the impact of hypertension in the setting of multiple other risk factors, in the presence of underlying CV disease or abnormal stress test results, and/or the assessed benefits of a specific class of antihypertensive agent (e.g., beta-blockers). To date, there are few studies that have investigated CV risk associated with mild-to-moderate hypertension (140 to 179/90 to 109 mm Hg) measured in the immediate preoperative setting. Additionally, the little published evidence does not demonstrate that CV outcomes are improved by delaying surgery to control BP among stable patients with mild or even more severe hypertension (i.e., diastolic ≥ 110 mm Hg).[4,26] The safety and efficacy of an acute treatment strategy for perioperative BP control (i.e., intravenous medications without surgical delay) versus a delayed therapeutic approach (i.e., outpatient management before surgery) among individuals presenting with severe hypertension has rarely been evaluated.[4,26] Thus far, the available published evidence does not support any clear CV benefits of the latter more cautious approach of delaying surgery to assure satisfactory preoperative BP control as an outpatient.

There are several additional methodological issues to further consider when reviewing the literature regarding hypertension and perioperative risk. Fleisher criticized the statistical design of studies, stating that the majority of studies were underpowered to appropriately evaluate the primary endpoints of myocardial infarction and death, and was particularly critical of trials that used surrogate markers.[27] For example, some studies use electrocardiographic changes to suggest ischemia as a surrogate for myocardial infarction and death, but suppressing myocardial ischemia alone does not necessarily correlate with a reduced incidence of myocardial infarction or death. The methodology of perioperative BP studies may be inherently flawed or limited because the perioperative environment that influences BP cannot be replicated during follow-up. Lastly, proper measurement of consecutive, resting, seated BPs may not have been obtained, or may have been impossible to obtain, during the preoperative evaluation.

In summary, the overall evidence as reported by several reviews,[2,3] a meta-analysis of 30 observational studies (odds ratio of 1.35 for cardiac complications),[28] and by the analysis performed in the 2007 AHA guidelines[10] is that mild-moderate hypertension (i.e., BP < 180/110 mm Hg) is not a "clinically-relevant" independent risk factor for perioperative CV complications. In the absence of other higher risk parameters, this degree of hypertension does not require clinical attention or treatment before surgery.[10,11] Conversely, the evidence that BP levels 180/110 or higher mm Hg cause perioperative CV events is mixed[10,28]; thus explaining the current clinical equipoise regarding the therapeutic approach to patients with more severe hypertension among guidelines.[10,11]

ANTIHYPERTENSIVE MEDICATIONS DURING THE PERIOPERATIVE PERIOD

Numerous intravenous and oral antihypertensive agents are capable of rapidly lowering BP. However, there have been few head-to-head trials assessing the comparative benefits of the available medications to reduce CV events during the perioperative period. The prudent clinician should therefore focus on using medications with the most predictable hemodynamic responses and that offer potential ancillary benefits (e.g., antianginal effects). Table 44.1 provides an overview of several BP-lowering medications commonly employed during the perioperative period.[2,3,9,13]

Older Medications

During the perioperative period, medications such as nitroglycerin, hydralazine, and enalapril should be considered second-line agents because of unpredictable BP responses. Intravenous nitroglycerin may be useful in low doses in combination with other BP-lowering agents, such as beta-blockers, in the presence of acute coronary syndromes or pulmonary edema. Further sequelae of nitroglycerin usage include the potential for tolerance, severe hypotension, and reflex tachycardia; thus it is not recommended for routine BP control as a sole agent.[9] Hydralazine is difficult to titrate and can cause an overly zealous and long-lasting reduction in BP. The utility of enalapril is generally limited to combination with other agents because it has a long duration of action and difficulty to rapidly titrate.

Nitroprusside has historically been considered the drug of choice during the postoperative period. It has an extremely rapid onset and offset of action and a comparatively predictable BP-lowering response. However, nitroprusside carries significant risks including cyanide and thiocyanate toxicity, particularly in the setting of renal disease. It can also unfavorably redistribute blood flow which may adversely affect renal, myocardial, or cerebral perfusion.[13] These factors, the reported association with increased mortality compared with clevidipine,[8,29] as well as the availability of newer agents should now limit its usage most often to second-line therapy.[13]

Calcium Channel Blockers

Clevidipine is an ultra-short-acting and highly selective (vasodilating) dihydropyridine calcium channel blocker (CCB).[29] It is quickly metabolized by blood esterases leading to a rapid onset and offset of action within minutes. It has a predictable and titratable dose-response curve and can be used continuously for days (i.e., 72 hours in trials) without evidence for tolerance or side effects. The results of the ECLIPSE (Evaluation of Clevidipine in the Perioperative Treatment of Hypertension Assessing Safety Events) trial[8,29] demonstrated that clevidipine was more effective in controlling BP and resulted in a lower perioperative mortality rate compared with nitroprusside. ECLIPSE randomized 1964 cardiac patients requiring treatment for perioperative hypertension to receive clevidipine or one of several other medications (nitroprusside, nitroglycerin, or nicardipine). There were no differences in the incidences of myocardial infarction, stroke, or renal dysfunction among the treatment limbs but mortality was significantly higher in patients treated with nitroprusside compared with clevidipine (1.7% versus 4.7%, p = 0.04). Furthermore, clevidipine was overall the most effective agent in maintaining BP stability within a prespecified narrow range. As excessive BP lability during surgery has been associated with worse CV outcomes, this finding along with its favorable pharmacological properties places clevidipine among the leading medication choices for perioperative BP control in the modern era.[8,29]

In 2003, a meta-analysis of all other CCBs involving 11 trials of 1007 patients in the perioperative period was published.[10,30] CCBs were associated with reductions in both ischemia and super-ventricular tachycardia and trends toward decreases in myocardial infarction and death. Most of these benefits were attributed specifically to diltiazem. The 2007 ACC/AHA guidelines[10] recognized the potential cardioprotective benefits of perioperative CCBs but stopped short of recommending their use; it was noted that further high-quality trials are required. Because no such studies have been published in the interim, this conclusion still stands.

Alpha 2 Agonists

Alpha 2 agonists, including clonidine, reduce sympathetic nervous system activity and heart rate. For this reason, it has been promoted that they could be cardioprotective during the perioperative period. A meta-analysis published in 2008 of 31 small trials composed of 4578 patients suggested that alpha 2 agonists are indeed beneficial.[10,31] However, the recent results from the large multicenter POISE-2 trial evaluating the role of perioperative clonidine challenged these older findings.[32] In over 10,000 patients, clonidine did not reduce the primary composite endpoint of death or myocardial infarction but was associated with a higher rate of adverse events including serious hypotension and cardiac arrests. A subsequent analysis also demonstrated that clonidine did not reduce the risk of perioperative acute kidney injury.[33] As such, the 2014 ACC/AHA guidelines recommended against

TABLE 44.1 Summary of the Blood Pressure Effects and Concerns Regarding Different Blood Pressure Controlling Agents During the Perioperative Period.: Short: <5 Min, Medium: 5-15 Min, Long: 15-60 Min, Extended: >60 Min

	ONSET OF ACTION	DURATION OF BP EFFECTS	PREDICTABLE BP RESPONSE	COMMENTS	RECOMMENDED
Intravenous Agents:					
Clevidipine	Short	Medium	Predictable	1. Useful for tight BP control. 2. Maintains renal blood flow. 3. Decreased mortality compared with nitroprusside or nicardipine.[8] 4. Contraindicated in patients with allergies to eggs or soybeans.	Yes
Enalaprilat	Long	Extended	Unpredictable	1. Contraindicated in renal artery stenosis. 2. Has been used in combination with shorter acting, easier to titrate medications.	No
Esmolol	Short	Medium	Predictable	1. First degree heart block. 2. Ideal postoperatively with tachycardia for fast, predictable response.	+/−
Fenoldopam	Short	Long/Extended	Predictable	1. Does not cause rebound hypertension. 2. Improves renal function. 3. Contraindicated in patients with glaucoma.	+/−
Hydralazine	Long	Extended	Unpredictable	1. Rapid onset from catecholamine surge. 2. BP effects can last up to 12 hours.	No
Labetalol	Short	Extended	Predictable	1. Cardiac output is maintained unlike pure beta-blockers.	+/−
Nicardipine	Medium	Extended	Predictable	1. No coronary steal, unlike nitroprusside. 2. Easy to titrate.	Yes
Nitroglycerin	Short	Short/Medium	Unpredictable	1. Hypotension and reflex tachycardia. 2. May develop tolerance.	+/−
Nitroprusside	Short	Short	Predictable	1. Cyanide toxicity. 2. Reduced regional blood flow. 3. Requires intensive monitoring. 4. Increased mortality compared with clevidipine.	No
Oral Agents:					
ACE Inhibitors	Long	Extended	Unpredictable	1. Risk of severe hypotension.	No
ARBs	Extended	Extended	Unpredictable	1. Risk of severe hypotension.	No
Clonidine	Long	Extended	Unpredictable	1. Based on long duration and slow onset. 2. Not well studied in postoperative hypertension. 3. Hypertension may present from clonidine withdrawal syndrome in patients who abruptly discontinue drug.	No
Labetalol	Long	Extended			+/−
Metoprolol	Long	Extended	Predictable	1. Well studied in preoperative setting, considered safe and effective.	+/−
Nifedipine	Long	Extended	Unpredictable	1. Cerebral hypoperfusion. 2. Tachycardia. 3. Myocardial ischemia.	No

Recommended: Yes = evidence from clinical trials supporting the comparative benefits of the medication;
No = evidence against usage or data is not generally supportive of its wide usage among most surgical patients;
+/− = little available outcome evidence or potentially advantageous medication in certain clinical scenarios.
ACE, Angiotensin-converting enzyme; *ARBs,* angiotensin receptor blockers; *BP,* blood pressure.

(class III) using alpha 2 agonists specifically for the prevention of CV events in patients undergoing noncardiac surgery.

Fenoldopam

Fenoldopam is a short-acting intravenous antihypertensive agent with the unique mechanism of action of dopamine 1 receptor agonism leading to peripheral and renal arteriole vasodilatation.[34-36] Many small trials have suggested that fenoldopam may provide protection against renal ischemia or injury in several scenarios while also maintaining total body fluid homeostasis by promoting diuresis. However, in a recent large scale multi-center trial of 667 patients with acute kidney injury following cardiac surgery, fenoldopam did not reduce the need for renal replacement procedures or decrease the

risk of 30-day mortality.[35] Although fenoldopam possess several favorable pharmacological and hemodynamic properties, no formal recommendations in the 2014 ACC/AHA guidelines were provided in regards to its usage.

Beta-Blockers

Perioperative beta-blockade (regardless of hypertension status) has undergone several clinical trials[19,20,23-25] and was the subject of a recent systematic review and clinical practice guideline by the ACC/AHA in 2014.[37,38] Beta-blockers have traditionally been considered a first line of therapy because they can rapidly lower BP and heart rate, prevent wide fluctuations in BP, and reduce the evidence for perioperative myocardial ischemia.[27] Studies have shown that preoperative beta-blocker administration can decrease the incidence of atrial fibrillation,[1] all-cause mortality,[19] and several CV complications[19] in both patients with and at risk for ischemic heart disease.

The ACC/AHA review[37] reported that among 12,043 patients in 17 studies (16 clinical trials) beta-blockers started within 1 day of surgery decreased nonfatal myocardial infarction (relative risk [RR]: 0.69) but increased nonfatal stroke (RR: 1.76), hypotension (RR: 1.47), and bradycardia (RR: 2.61). Note that the integrity of the trial results from a team of investigators has been seriously challenged; nonetheless, the main findings were qualitatively unchanged after excluding these data. Conversely, beta-blockers were associated with a trend toward reduced all-cause and CV mortality rates in the trials of questionable integrity but with increased rates in all other trials. The expert reviewers concluded that perioperative beta-blockade should not be routinely started within 1 day of noncardiac surgery and that there is still currently insufficient evidence to support starting beta-blockade 2 or more days preoperatively in higher risk patients.

Further recommendations regarding beta blockers were given in the full 2014 ACC/AHA guidelines.[11] Patients already taking a beta-blocker should continue it throughout the perioperative period (class I). It was also deemed reasonable to start a beta-blocker at least 2 to 7 days beforehand in individuals with evidence of intermediate or high risk ischemia on stress testing and those with a score of 3 or more in the RCRI. All other patients should not start a beta-blocker for the purpose of reducing perioperative risk. When prescribed, cardioselective agents (e.g., bisoprolol and atenolol) are favored over nonselective agents and the dosage should be titrated to achieve adequate heart rate control over a several-day period (2 to 30 days) before surgery to avoid bradycardia or hypotension.

Renin Angiotensin System Blockers

Unlike other antihypertensive medications, there has been concern that perioperative initiation or continuation of an angiotensin-converting enzyme (ACE) inhibitor or angiotensin receptor blocker (ARB) can lead to unacceptable rates of clinically significant hypotension.[39,40] This may occur because these medications block the remaining physiologically important pathway responsible for maintaining hemodynamic stability following anesthesia induction. In some cases, hypotension during general anesthesia refractory to usual therapeutic interventions has been reported (fluids, ephedrine, or phenylephrine).[2] Discontinuation of ACE inhibitors or ARB therapy at least 10 hours before anesthesia is associated with a reduced risk for immediate postinduction hypotension and patients who discontinued these agents required lower doses of ephedrine and phenylephrine.[2] Contrary to the general recommendations that patients should continue all antihypertensive medications throughout the perioperative period, it has been suggested by some experts to consider holding ACE inhibitors or ARBs the morning of surgery. Although the 2014 ACC/AHA guidelines acknowledged the potential for perioperative hypotension,[11] the authors highlighted that the overall risks versus benefits support the continuation of an ACE inhibitor or ARB even on the day of surgery. If they are held, it was also emphasized that they should be restarted as soon as clinically feasible postoperatively.

ALGORITHM FOR THE MANAGEMENT OF HYPERTENSIVE PATIENTS UNDERGOING SURGERY

As a general rule, patients with hypertension and those taking medications with BP-lowering properties (e.g., beta-blockers for ischemic heart disease) should continue to take all their antihypertensive medications throughout the perioperative period, including on the morning of surgery. The dosages of medications may be adjusted or even held (e.g., ACE inhibitor or ARB) as clinically indicated in relation to the patients' BP levels before and following surgery on a case-by-case basis. It is critical to emphasize that patients should not stop or withhold agents perioperatively that commonly provoke rebound tachycardia and/or hypertension (e.g., beta-blockers, alpha 2 agonists).

Fig. 44.1 provides a flow diagram for the perioperative management of hypertensive patients. The algorithm has been modified from the 2014 ACC/AHA guidelines to incorporate the consideration of BP levels into the management process.[11] The initial step in the preoperative evaluation of patients is to determine if they require emergent surgery (i.e., life-threatening conditions). These individuals should immediately proceed with surgery under careful cardiac and hemodynamic monitoring regardless of their BP level or CV risk status. For less time-sensitive procedures, unstable and high-risk conditions including severe cardiac valve disease (e.g., aortic stenosis), unstable angina or recent acute coronary syndrome (within the prior 60 days), decompensated heart failure, and uncontrolled arrhythmias should be appropriately addressed by standard guideline practices before surgery in most scenarios.

Among the remaining "stable" patients with or without hypertension undergoing elective surgery, the first step is to estimate global CV risk related to the surgical procedure by one of the validated risk prediction tools such as the RCRI.[11] Several web-based online calculators are available (Fig. 44.1). Patients considered to be at "elevated risk" (i.e., RCRI ≥ 2) have a perioperative major adverse CV event rate of 1% or more and their appropriate management is briefly outlined in Box 44.1. Stable low-risk patients (RCRI ≤ 1) should proceed with surgery regardless of their BP level. Severe perioperative hypertension can be treated acutely in these low-risk patients on an individual basis with intravenous and/or oral agents.

For patients deemed to be at "elevated risk" (RCRI ≥ 2), the next step is to assess cardiopulmonary functional status. Several tables and questionnaires are available to aid clinicians in the estimation of maximal attainable metabolic equivalents (METs) during daily activity or exercise.[11] Patients unable to achieve at least 4 METs as a result of poor functional status limited by symptoms (e.g., dyspnea, angina, or fatigue) or in whom exercise or functional capacity cannot be reliably evaluated (e.g., activity limitations attributed to other conditions such as arthritis; poor historians) are likely at higher operative CV risk. Further evaluation before surgery such as pharmacological stress testing should be considered and appropriate medical management of risk factors initiated or intensified (e.g., adding or increasing the dosage of beta-blockers) based upon the results (see beta-blocker section). Any intervention (e.g., coronary revascularization) should be performed based upon standard guideline practices[11] irrespective of the upcoming surgery with the main objective of symptom management (e.g., medical refractory angina). Coronary interventions are not recommended for the sole purposes of reducing perioperative risk because preoperative revascularizations have not been shown to reduce CV events.[11] It is important that clinicians understand that any intervention will lead to a delay of an elective surgery (e.g., as a result of prolonged dual antiplatelet therapy for 1 to 12 months). The risks versus potential clinical benefits of postponing surgery to perform medical or procedural interventions need to be carefully considered and weighed on a case-by-case basis.

Patients at "elevated" CV risk (RCRI ≥ 2) who are able to achieve at least 4 METs of activity without limitations or cardiopulmonary symptomatology have a functional status associated with good surgical outcomes. Those with even higher exercise capacities (>7 to 10 METs) are at even lower

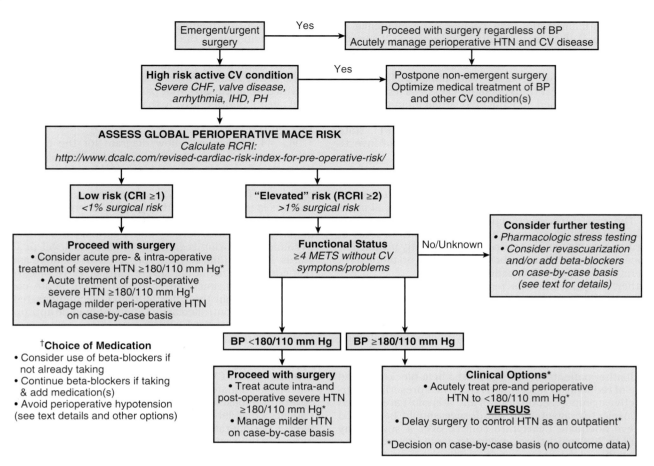

FIG. 44.1 Approach to high blood pressure during the perioperative period. *BP,* Blood pressure; *CHF,* congestive heart failure; *CV,* cardiovascular; *HTN,* hypertension; *IHD,* ischemic heart disease; *PH,* pulmonary hypertension; *RCRI,* Revised Cardiac Risk Index.

risk. We propose at this juncture that the BP level of the individual patient be taken into consideration, because it may alter subsequent management (Fig. 44.1). It should be noted that preoperative BP measurement should be performed in the least anxiety-provoking environment and using the careful methodologies detailed by guidelines.[11,41] Postponement of surgery to perform additional office, home, or ambulatory BP measurements may occasionally be necessary when transient factors (e.g., stress, pain, anxiety, or white coat hypertension) are suspected as the cause(s) of elevated BP. Based upon our opinion, the recommendations of other reviewers,[3] and the 2007 AHA guidelines,[10] clinicians should strongly consider treating severe hypertension (BP ≥ 180 mm Hg systolic and/or 110 mm Hg diastolic) before surgery in patients at "elevated" risk. The strategy to achieve adequate preoperative BP control and the specific medication(s) prescribed should be selected on a case-by-case basis (e.g., urgency of surgery, concomitant CV conditions, and other indications for specific antihypertensive agents). Unless contraindicated, the greatest evidence supports using selective beta-1 blockade as part of the regimen (see beta-blocker section). The optimal goal BP to lower perioperative CV risk has not been established; nonetheless, expert opinions suggest that a reduction to a level at least below 180/110 mm Hg should be a minimal target.

SUMMARY

Relatively few published studies have evaluated the management of hypertension during the perioperative period. Nevertheless, the evidence supports that most stable patients, regardless of their surgical risk who have only mild-to-moderate hypertension, do not require further risk assessments or BP-lowering interventions before surgery. Individuals at "elevated" CV risk who also have a BP 180/110 or higher mm Hg may be at excessive risk of a perioperative complications. Based upon precautionary principles, we suggest that these patients should have their severe hypertension addressed by an individualized treatment approach before proceeding with surgery. Additional clinical trials are needed to provide a stronger evidence-based management strategy for patients with hypertension during the perioperative period.

References

1. Bromfield S, Muntner P. High blood pressure: the leading global burden of disease risk factor and the need for worldwide prevention programs. *Curr Hypertens Rep.* 2013;15:134-136.
2. Lonjaret L, Lairez O, Minville V, et al. Optimal perioperative management of arterial blood pressure. *Integrated Blood Pressure Control.* 2014;7:49-59.
3. Lien SF, Bisognano JD. Perioperative hypertension: defining at-risk patients and their management. *Curr Hypertens Rep.* 2012;14:432-441.
4. Weksler N, Klein M, Szendro G, et al. The dilemma of immediate preoperative hypertension: to treat and operate, or to postpone surgery? *J Clin Anesth.* 2003;15:179-183.
5. Kumar R, Gandhi R. Reasons for cancellation of operation on the day of intended surgery in a multidisciplinary 500 bedded hospital. *J Anaesthesiol, Clin Pharmacol.* 2012;28:66-69.
6. Dix P, Howell S. Survey of cancellation rate of hypertensive patients undergoing anaesthesia and elective surgery. *Br J Anaesth.* 2001;86:789-793.
7. Sultan N, Rashid A, Abbas SM. Reasons for cancellation of elective cardiac surgery at Prince Sultan Cardiac Centre, Saudi Arabia. *J Saudi Heart Assoc.* 2012;24:29-34.
8. Aronson S, Dyke CM, Levy JH, et al. Does perioperative systolic blood pressure variability predict mortality after cardiac surgery? An exploratory analysis of the ECLIPSE trials. *Anesth Analg.* 2011;113:19-30.
9. Haas CE, LeBlanc JM. Acute postoperative hypertension: a review of therapeutic options. *Am J Health Syst Pharm.* 2004;61:1661-1673.
10. Fleisher LA, Beckman JA, Brown KA, et al. ACC/AHA 2007 Guidelines on Perioperative Cardiovascular Evaluation and Care for Noncardiac Surgery: a report of the American College of Cardiology/American Heart Association Task Force on Practice Guidelines (Writing Committee to Revise the 2002 Guidelines on Perioperative Cardiovascular Evaluation for Noncardiac Surgery). *Circulation.* 2007;116:e418-e500.

11. Fleisher LA, Fleischmann KE, Auerbach AD, et al. 2014 ACC/AHA Guideline on perioperative cardiovascular evaluation and management of patients undergoing noncardiac surgery. *J Am Coll Cardiol.* 2014;64:e77-e137.

12. Smithwick RH, Thompson JE. Splanchnicectomy for essential hypertension; results in 1,266 cases. *J Am Med Assoc.* 1953;152:1501-1504.

13. Marik PE, Varon J. Perioperative hypertension: a review of current and emerging therapeutic agents. *J Clin Anesth.* 2009;21:220-229.

14. Khuri SF, Daley J, Henderson W, et al. The National Veterans Administration Surgical Risk Study: risk adjustment for the comparative assessment of the quality of surgical care. *J Am Coll Surg.* 1995;180:519-531.

15. Goldman L, Caldera DL, Nussbaum SR, et al. Multifactorial index of cardiac risk in noncardiac surgical procedures. *N Engl J Med.* 1977;297:845-850.

16. Lette J, Waters D, Bernier H, et al. Preoperative and long-term cardiac risk assessment. Predictive value of 23 clinical descriptors, 7 multivariate scoring systems, and quantitative dipyridamole imaging in 360 patients. *Ann Surg.* 1992;216:192-204.

17. Raby KE, Barry J, Creager MA, Cook EF, Weisberg MC, Goldman L. Detection and significance of intraoperative and postoperative myocardial ischemia in peripheral vascular surgery. *JAMA.* 1992;268:222-227.

18. Ashton CM, Petersen NJ, Wray NP, et al. The incidence of perioperative myocardial infarction in men undergoing noncardiac surgery. *Ann Intern Med.* 1993;118:504-510.

19. Mangano DT, Layug EL, Wallace A, Tateo I. Effect of atenolol on mortality and cardiovascular morbidity after noncardiac surgery. Multicenter Study of Perioperative Ischemia Research Group. *N Engl J Med.* 1996;335:1713-1720.

20. Poldermans D, Boersma E, Bax JJ, et al. The effect of bisoprolol on perioperative mortality and myocardial infarction in high-risk patients undergoing vascular surgery. *N Engl J Med.* 1999;341:1789-1794.

21. Goldman L, Caldera DL. Risks of general anesthesia and elective operation in the hypertensive patient. *Anesthesiology.* 1979;50:285-292.

22. Rose DK, Cohen MM, DeBoer DP. Cardiovascular events in the postanesthesia care unit: contribution of risk factors. *Anesthesiology.* 1996;84:772-781.

23. Juul AB, Wetterslev J, Gluud C, et al. Effect of perioperative beta blockade in patients with diabetes undergoing major non-cardiac surgery: randomised placebo controlled, blinded multicentre trial. *BMJ.* 2006;332:1482.

24. Yang H, Raymer K, Butler R, et al. The effects of perioperative beta-blockade: results of the Metoprolol after Vascular Surgery (MaVS) study, a randomized controlled trial. *Am Heart J.* 2006;152:983-990.

25. Devereaux PJ, Yang H, Yusuf S, et al. Effects of extended-release metoprolol succinate in patients undergoing noncardiac surgery (POISE trial): a randomised controlled trial. *Lancet.* 2008;371:1839-1847.

26. Casadei B, Abuzeid H. Is there a strong rationale for deferring elective surgery in patients with poorly controlled hypertension? *J Hypertens.* 2005;23:19-22.

27. Fleisher LA. Preoperative evaluation of the patient with hypertension. *JAMA.* 2002;287:2043-2046.

28. Howell SJ, Sear JW, Foëx P. Hypertension, hypertensive heart disease, and perioperative cardiac risk. *Br J Anaesth.* 2004;92:570-583.

29. Keating GM. Clevidipine: a review of its use for managing blood pressure in perioperative and intensive care settings. *Drugs.* 2014;74:1947-1960.

30. Wijeysundera DN, Beattie WS. Calcium channel blockers for reducing cardiac morbidity after noncardiac surgery: a meta-analysis. *Anesth Analg.* 2003;97:634-641.

31. Wijeysundera DN, Bender JS, Beattie WS. Alpha-2 adrenergic agonists for the prevention of cardiac complications among patients undergoing surgery. *Cochrane Database Syst Rev.* 2009;(4):CD004126.

32. Devereaux PJ, Sessler DI, Leslie K, et al. Clonidine in patients undergoing noncardiac surgery. *N Engl J Med.* 2014;17:1504-1513.

33. Garg AX, Kurz A, Sessler DI, et al. Perioperative aspirin and clonidine and risk of acute kidney injury: a randomized clinical trial. *JAMA.* 2014;312:2254-2264.

34. Zangrillo A, Biondi-Zoccai GG, Frati E, et al. Fenoldopam and acute renal failure in cardiac surgery: a meta-analysis of randomized placebo-controlled trials. *J Cardiothorac Vasc Anesth.* 2012;26:407-413.

35. Bove T, Zangrillo A, Guarracino F, et al. Effect of fenoldopam on use of renal replacement therapy among patients with acute kidney injury after cardiac surgery: a randomized clinical trial. *JAMA.* 2014;312:2244-2253.

36. Murphy MB, Murray C, Shorten GD. Fenoldopam: a selective peripheral dopamine-receptor agonist for the treatment of severe hypertension. *N Engl J Med.* 2001;345:1548-1557.

37. Wijeysundera DN, Duncan D, Nkonde-Price C, et al. Perioperative beta blockade in noncardiac surgery: a systematic review for the 2014 ACC/AHA guideline on perioperative cardiovascular evaluation and management of patients undergoing noncardiac surgery: a report of the American College of Cardiology/American Heart Association Task Force on Practice Guidelines. *Circulation.* 2014;130:2246-2264.

38. Fleisher LA, Beckman JA, Brown KA, et al. 2009 ACCF/AHA focused update on perioperative beta blockade incorporated into the ACC/AHA 2007 guidelines on perioperative cardiovascular evaluation and care for noncardiac surgery: a report of the American College of Cardiology Foundation/American Heart Association task force on practice guidelines. *Circulation.* 2009;120:e169-e276.

39. Coriat P, Richer C, Douraki T, et al. Influence of chronic angiotensin-converting enzyme inhibition on anesthetic induction. *Anesthesiology.* 1994;81:299-307.

40. Bertrand M, Godet G, Meersschaert K, Brun L, Salcedo E, Coriat P. Should the angiotensin II antagonists be discontinued before surgery? *Anesth Analg.* 2001;92:26-30.

41. Pickering TG, and the Subcommittee of Professional and Public Education of the American Heart Association Council on High Blood Pressure Research. Recommendations for blood pressure measurement in humans and experimental animals: part 1: blood pressure measurement in humans: a statement for professionals from the Subcommittee of Professional and Public Education of the American Heart Association Council on High Blood Pressure Research. *Hypertension.* 2001;45:142-161.

45 Aorta and Peripheral Arterial Disease in Hypertension

Luke J. Laffin, Akiko Tanaka, Ross Milner, and Takeyoshi Ota

Aortic and peripheral arterial diseases may coexist in patients with hypertension. Although aortopathies and peripheral arterial disease can be seen in isolation, more often than not they present in patients with multiple cardiovascular risk factors, hypertension being chief among them. The following addresses the epidemiology and natural history of aortic and peripheral arterial disease, with a specific focus on the contribution of blood pressure to disease progression and mortality. With a vast array of pharmacological options available to treat primary hypertension, subsequently addressed is the issue of which antihypertensive agents are best suited and studied to treat patients with aortic and peripheral arterial disease.

AORTIC DISEASE IN HYPERTENSION

Aortic pathologies represent a wide spectrum of disease processes and cross multiple medical and surgical subspecialties. Aortic disease can present suddenly and catastrophically, or may be found incidentally on unrelated imaging studies. Although many infectious, inflammatory, and genetic conditions can contribute to disease processes found in the aorta, appropriate blood pressure control represents a pillar in the prevention of disease progression. The focus of the following is thoracic aortic disease with some discussion of abdominal aortic aneurysmal disease in the setting of hypertension.

Thoracic Aortic Disease

The term thoracic aortic disease (TAD) encompasses a varied range of disease processes that range from life threatening upon presentation, to incidentally discovered and asymptomatic. A comprehensive review of all aspects of TAD management is addressed in guidelines published in 2010.[1] Hypertension plays a significant role in the development of TAD in combination with multiple other risk factors including age, atherosclerosis, smoking, and underlying genetic and congenital factors.

The normal adult thoracic aorta is composed of three layers (intima, media, and adventitia) and four primary portions including the aortic root, the ascending aorta, the aortic arch, and the descending aorta (Fig. 45.1). Normal size ranges have been published based on two-dimensional echocardiographic and computed tomography data accounting for factors such as an individual's age, sex, and body size.[2] These tables aid the clinician in identifying patients with aneurysms or those at risk for aneurysm formation, but do not necessarily account for certain genetic abnormalities and tissue characteristics that place patients at risk for disease processes such as dissection. The major histopathological disease processes that affect the thoracic aorta include atherosclerosis, inflammatory disease, and vasculitides, as well as dissection and aneurysm formation.

Genetic, inflammatory, and congenital conditions are associated with TAD and increase the risk of aneurysm, dissection, and rupture. Genetic syndromes strongly associated with TAD in the form of aneurysms and dissection include Marfan, Loeys-Dietz, vascular Ehlers-Danlos, and Turner syndromes. Other cardiovascular conditions that place individuals at risk for dissection and aneurysm formation include individuals with bicuspid aortic valve and/or aortic coarctation.

Acute Aortic Syndromes (i.e., Aortic Dissection)

Disease processes classified as acute aortic syndromes (AAS) include, most commonly, aortic dissection (AoD) and the less frequently encountered intramural hematoma (IMH), and penetrating atherosclerotic ulcer (PAU). They represent interconnected emergent aortic conditions with similar clinical features and oftentimes are challenging to treat effectively. IMH and PAU may be thought of as variants or precursors to AoD and data regarding blood pressure management in these patients are similar to patients with AoD. Traumatic aortic disease (i.e., aortic disruption) may also be classified as an AAS, but is beyond the scope of this chapter.

Aortic Dissection

The incidence of AoD is difficult to define given that dissections may be rapidly fatal and are frequently missed on initial presentation. When patients die before reaching, or shortly after presenting to, a hospital, death may be mistakenly attributed to another more common cause such as myocardial infarction (MI) or sudden cardiac death. A recent prospective population-based study reveals the incidence of AoD to be 6 cases per 100,000 person years, a significant increase from prior estimates.[3] Risk of aortic dissection increases with age and male sex is a risk factor.[4]

Classification of aortic dissections is based on two major systems, Stanford and DeBakey classification schema. The Stanford system is more widely used in clinical practice. Stanford type A dissections involve the ascending aorta with or without the aortic arch or descending aorta. Type B dissections involve the descending aorta without any involvement of the ascending aorta (Fig. 45.2). Dissections involving the ascending aorta and aortic arch vessels are at highest risk for complications including stroke. These Type A dissections are best treated with emergent surgical management. A key factor in management of type B dissections is determining the presence of complications. Complications are defined as organ or limb malperfusion, progressive dissection, extra aortic blood collection (impending rupture), intractable pain, or uncontrolled hypertension. Short-term survival (3-year) appears to be unaffected by endovascular treatment in acute *uncomplicated* type B dissections compared with medical management as demonstrated by the INSTEAD trial.[5] However, the INSTEAD XL-trial demonstrated that endovascular treatment in addition to optimal medical therapy is associated with improved 5-year aorta-specific survival and delayed disease progression.[6]

On the other hand, complicated type B dissections may benefit from endovascular intervention as described in Study for the Treatment of complicated type B Aortic Dissection using Endoluminal repair (STABLE) trial, a prospective, multicenter study evaluating safety and effectiveness of a

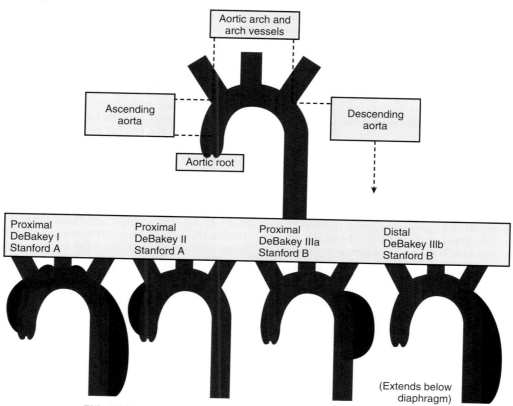

FIG. 45.1 Aortic anatomy (with Stanford versus Debakey Dissection Classification).

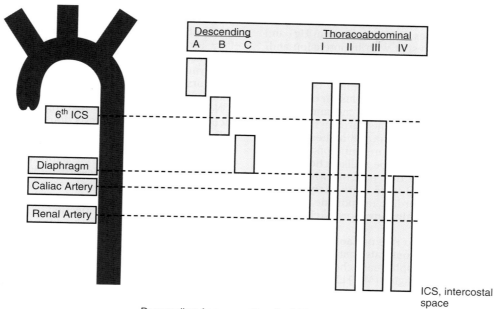

Descending Aneurysm Crawford Classification:

A involves *proximal* 3rd of the descending aorta
B involves *middle* 3rd of the descending aorta
C involves *distal* 3rd of the descending aorta

Thoracoabdominal aneurysms
according to the Crawford Classification:

Type I extends from below the subclavian artery to above the celiac/
    cupramesenteric/renal arteries
Type II extends below the subclavian artery to above the iliac bifurcation
Type III extends from the 6th ICS to above the iliac bifurcation
Type IV extends from the 12th ICS to above the iliac bifurication

FIG. 45.2 Descending aneurysm classification.

pathology-specific endovascular system (proximal stent graft and distal bare metal stent) for the treatment of complicated type B aortic dissection.[7] It demonstrates that endovascular repair of complicated type B dissections with the use of a composite construct results in early clinical outcomes and aortic remodeling. Of note, patients treated acutely may be prone to aortic growth and may require close observation. Patient follow-up is still on-going.

Timely identification of the intimal disruption, location of dissection, and the involved vessels is crucial to prognosis as well as management decisions (open-surgical, medical, and/or endovascular). Classically, aortic dissection has been temporally categorized based on time of symptom onset with acute aortic dissection defined as diagnosis less than 14 days from symptom onset, and chronic defined as diagnosis greater than 14 days from symptom onset. Given the advances in care for patients with AoD, recent work proposes more nuanced categorization (hyperacute [symptom onset to 24 hours], acute [2 to 7 days], subacute [8 to 30 days], and chronic [>30 days]) based on Kaplan-Meier survival curves developed using the International Registry of Acute Aortic Dissection (IRAD: a consortium of research centers that are evaluating the current management and outcomes of acute aortic dissection involving 30 large referral centers in 11 countries), although this has not yet been formally adopted in guidelines.[1,8]

Increased aortic wall stress and conditions that encourage aortic medial degeneration increase one's risk of dissection. The majority of patients diagnosed with AoD have hypertension and the prevalence is increasing.[9] Underlying genetic syndromes are not uncommon in patients with AoD, especially younger patients.[10] Presentation of aortic dissection and complications are varied and numerous, with rapid assessment, diagnosis, and treatment resulting in much better outcomes.

Half of all patients with aortic dissections present with elevated systolic blood pressures (SBPs) (>150 mm Hg) and alternatively, 20% of patients present with hypotension and/or shock. As outlined in comprehensive thoracic aortic disease guidelines published in 2010, accurate blood pressure (BP) measurement at the time of dissection may be complicated in the setting of dissection-related occlusion of branching arteries, resulting in incorrectly low BP measurement in affected limbs. As such, BPs should be measured in both arms and, oftentimes, both legs to determine the highest central BP.[1] Pulse pressure (PP), at the time of presentation, may also be a prognostic value in those with type A dissections. IRAD investigators recently determined that patients with type A AoD with narrow PP (<40 mm Hg) were more likely to have cardiac complications such as cardiac tamponade, whereas those with PP greater than 75 mm Hg were more likely to have abdominal aortic involvement.[11]

Diagnosis imaging modalities to rule out aortic dissection are numerous. Meta-analyses demonstrate that contrast computed tomography (CT), transesophageal echocardiography (TEE), and magnetic resonance imaging (MRI) all provide valuable diagnostic information. Given that it is the most readily available imaging modality, CT is often the imaging modality of choice in hemodynamically stable patients. Those that are unstable are better suited for TEE.

Upon diagnosis of thoracic AoD, initial management should focus on decreasing aortic wall stress, by controlling heart rate and BP, to prevent propagation of the false lumen potentially leading to subsequent complications including rupture and/or malperfusion. Simultaneous discussion for definitive management should also be undertaken with surgical colleagues (regardless of dissection location, ascending or descending). Intravenous beta-blockade (in the absence of contraindications) should be administered to target a heart rate of less than 60 beats per minute. In patients with a contraindication to beta-blockade, nondihydropyridine

calcium channel blockers should be administered with the goal of similar heart rate reduction (for example diltiazem or verapamil). Simultaneously, with heart rate control, the SBP should be addressed. If a patient's SBP remains above 110 mm Hg with medication administration as noted above, angiotensin-converting enzyme inhibitors and/or other vasodilators should be given to further reduce SBP while maintaining adequate end-organ perfusion.[12] Rapid diagnosis and initial blood pressure/heart rate management for acute type A dissection is the key for successful management transition to definitive surgical therapy. At our institution, we developed an aortic dissection flowsheet to facilitate and generalize the management (Fig. 45.3). Appropriate initial heart rate control is critical before initiating vasodilator therapy, because the reflex tachycardia induced by vasodilators can increase aortic wall stress and worsen the existing dissection. Along similar lines, cautious beta-blocker administration in those patients with aortic insufficiency is warranted given the appropriate need for a compensatory tachycardia to maintain cardiac output.

The choice of beta-blocker is not crucial, as long as the desired heart rate and blood pressure lowering is achieved. However, intravenous labetalol may be the best initial choice given that it is both an alpha-receptor and beta-receptor antagonist. Theoretically, in addition to effective heart rate lowering, it also offers more BP lowering than beta-blockers that do not have additional alpha-blocking properties, potentially eliminating the need for multiple antihypertensive vasodilators. This is not an insignificant factor given that it is oftentimes difficult to reduce BP to endorsed levels and multiple antihypertensive agents may ultimately be needed.[13] In addition to beta-blockers, other established agents for BP control during this critical time include intravenous nicardipine, nitroglycerin, fenoldopam among others whereas sodium nitroprusside should be considered a contraindication in the setting of acute type dissection as a result of an aggravating effect for spinal ischemia.[14] An additional key intervention after diagnosis of aortic dissection is appropriate pain control. Sympathetic activation in setting of uncontrolled pain may worsen a patient's tachycardia, raise BP, and will be difficult to treat.

Not surprisingly IRAD investigators demonstrated that uncomplicated type B dissections with appropriately controlled pain and hypertension have lower in-hospital mortality than those patients with uncontrolled hypertension and/or pain.[15] Interestingly, the basis for the widely accepted for intensive SBP control (less than 120 mm Hg) in acute aortic dissection is decades old case series evidence and although the recommendation is class I, it is level of evidence C. This suggests that further investigation of BP goals in acute medical treatment of aortic dissection is needed.[16]

Following initial stabilization with intravenous antihypertensives, and in certain cases surgical management (open or endovascular) based on the location and complexity of the dissection, most patients will require long-term antihypertensive treatment. This should include a beta-blocker plus additional classes of BP lowering medications as detailed later.

Long-Term Blood Pressure Management Following Repair of Type A Dissections

In-hospital mortality for type A dissections has decreased from 31% to 22% in the past 17 years in the IRAD registry.[17] Interestingly, more contemporary large single center data reflect a lower in-hospital mortality rate of closer to 10%.[18-20] As such, long-term management strategies for these patients is crucial to prevent future events and complications. Data with respect to long-term survival of patients with repaired type A dissections are not robust, although the IRAD investigators report relatively high 3-year survival among patients

SUSPICIOUS FOR AORTIC DISSECTION

SYMPTOMS
- Severe chest, back, or abdominal pain – often abrupt in onset AND/OR ripping, tearing, stabbing quality AND/OR migratory
- Severe uncontrolled hypertension
- Syncope/loss of consciousness/change of mental status
- Weakness, difficulty walking, slurred speech, or change/loss of vision
- Feeling of impending death

RISK FACTORS
- Known aortic aneurysm
- Previous cardiac surgery
- Recent aortic manipulation (surgical or catheter based)
- Family history of aortic dissection, aortic aneurysms, and/or sudden death including massive heart attack
- Marfan syndrome, Loeys-Dietz syndrome, Ehlers-Danlos syndrome, Turner syndrome, or other connective tissue disease

PHYSICAL FINDINGS
- Pulse deficit in arm or leg
- Tachycardia
- Murmur or aortic regurgitation (new)
- SBP differential >20 mm Hg in right arm/leg vs. left arm/leg
- Limb pain or loss of sensation

DIAGNOSTIC
- 12-lead EKG
- Lab work: basic metabolic panel, INR, CBC with platelets, lactate, D-dimer
- CT scan protocol: CT chest/abdomen/pelvis with and without contrast STAT Label "STAT Aortic Dissection" and send films with patient.

DIAGNOSED ACUTE AORTIC DISSECTION OR CANNOT RULE OUT AORTIC DISSECTION

FIRST LINE: BETA BLOCKERS

Immediately start IV agents to control blood pressure (target SBP <110 mm Hg)

- Labetolol: 20 mg bolus IV followed by repeated incremental bolus or 5–20 mg every 10 minutes prn; may start continuous IV at 1–2 mg/min.

OR

- Esmolol: 500 mcg/kg IV loading dose over 1 minute; followed by a continuous infusion of 25-50 mcg/kg/min; increase every 4 minutes by 25 mcg/kg/min to a maximum infustion rate of 300 mcg/kg/min

OR

- Metoprolol: 5 mg IV over 5 minutes. Repeat 2× if necessary. Titrate for HR <60

SECOND LINE, OR IF BETA BLOCKADE CONTRAINDICATED
- IV Nicardipine start infusion 5 mg/hour, increasing 2.5 mg/hour every 5 minutes to maximum of 30 mg/hour

THIRD LINE
- Nitroglycerin
- Start at 5 mcg/min continuous infusion
- Increase by 5 mcg/min every 5 min up to 20 mcg/min, then 10 mcg/min every 5 min up to maximum 200 mcg/min

FOR SHOCK OR HYPOTENSION
- IVF fluid bolus (NaCl 0.9% IV 500 mL) repeat PRN
- If hypotension still, begin intravenous vasopressor agent (e.g. norepinephrine 0.05 mcg/kg/min) and/or inotropic agent (e.g. dopamine 5 mcg/kg/min) titiating with target SBP 80–110 mm Hg

- Place on cardiac monitor
- Place 2 large bore peripheral IV
- Oxygen nasal cannula
- Pain control: morprhine sulfate 2–4 mg IV push every 10 minutes as needed

PREPARE FOR TRANSFER

TRANSFER FROM OUTSIDE CHECKLIST
- All EKGs
- Transferring physician H&P
- Lab results
- CT films on disk

TRANSFER TO:
- The operating room for emergent surgery
- Intensive care unit for medical management

FIG. 45.3 Aortic dissection immediate management algorithm.

who survived operative repair of their dissection.[21] The study of patient characteristics impacting survival primarily focuses on preoperative and intraoperative characteristics, such as a patient's comorbidities and the type of repair chosen. However, a recent retrospective review of patient characteristics impacting long-term outcomes following type A dissection repair, highlights the importance of blood pressure control and choice of antihypertensive medication, even after operative repair.

Amongst patients who survived operative repair, four main factors, male sex, Marfan syndrome, elevated SBP, and the absence of beta-blocker therapy significantly impacted the need for reoperation.[22] Further, at 10-year follow-up, of those patients that maintained an SBP less than 120 mm Hg, only 8% required reoperation, compared with 26% in patients with SBP

between 120 and 140 mm Hg, and 51% in those with SBP greater than 140 mm Hg. Similarly, patients taking beta-blockers at 10 years postrepair had an 86% freedom from reoperation, compared with 57% for those not taking beta-blockers. The IRAD investigators demonstrate similar beneficial effects of beta-blockade in survivors of type A AoDs, albeit over a shorter follow-up time (less than 5 years).[23] Although the data are retrospective and include relatively low numbers, the pathophysiologic mechanism is sound. Beta-blockers, and strict BP control, diminish stress on the already diseased aorta, with a concurrent decrease in dP/dT (impulse), resulting in less aortic damage over time. Further long-term prospective study is needed, but it is very reasonable to aim for strict BP control in this subgroup of patients, with beta-blocker therapy as a first-line agent.

Long-Term Blood Pressure Management Type B Dissections

Recently, management paradigms of type B dissections have shifted based on the use of thoracic endovascular aortic repair (TEVAR) in complicated dissections, and some suggestion that even uncomplicated low-risk patients may demonstrate long-term benefit from preemptive or early endovascular repair.[24] Irrespective of interventional management, control of BP remains a hallmark of immediate and long-term management of type B AoDs.

Similar to type A dissections, no high-level of evidence data exist regarding specific BP goals in patients with a history of type B AoD. Current guidelines recommend BP control similar to that of the general population[1]; however this may change in the wake of results from the SPRINT BP trial that demonstrated increased survival with more intensive BP goals in the general population.[25] Beta-blockers are currently recommended in all patients with type B AoD based on data in Marfan syndrome patients that beta-blockade attenuates aneurysmal expansion. A recent systematic review attempted to establish the efficacy of beta-blockers versus other antihypertensives in this patient population. Unfortunately, no randomized control trials (RCTs) compare first-line beta-blockade with other first-line antihypertensive medications in the treatment of chronic type B AoD. The authors conclude that it is unknown whether beta-blockers as first-line therapy is appropriate, and future randomized controlled trials are needed.[26]

However, there are some nonrandomized data to help guide clinical decision-making. A study of 71 patients with type B dissection that survived to hospital discharge, with approximately of 4 years of follow-up, suggests benefit of beta-blockade. Of the 50 patients treated with beta-blockers chronically, 10 required surgery for aortic dissection. This stands in contrast to 9 of 20 patients not treated with beta-blockers who required surgery for aortic dissection.[27] Contrasting that data is a study from 2008, of patients with type B AoD treated medically with an average of 2.5 years of follow-up. Multivariate analysis did not demonstrate a reduction in long-term aortic events with beta-blocker administration, but did see a benefit in those patients prescribed angiotensin-converting enzyme inhibitors. Similarly, data from the 5-year IRAD follow-up do not demonstrate long-term benefit of beta-blockade on survival in patients with type B dissections. Interestingly, this multivariate analysis found that use of calcium channel blockers was associated with improved survival.[23]

Aortic dissection is not a common end-point (primary or secondary) in large cardiovascular (CV) trials, including those looking at antihypertensive therapy. Taken as a whole, data with respect long-term BP management in type B dissections are limited at best and no specific class of antihypertensive demonstrates superiority aside from patients with Marfan syndrome.

Physical Activity and Lifestyle Recommendations Following Aortic Dissection

Lifestyle and physical activity restrictions are reasonable in patients with a history of thoracic aortic disease, even in those with repaired AoD, as a result of their effect on BP and aortic stress. Aerobic exercise should be encouraged in these patients because it is beneficial for overall cardiovascular health and wellbeing. However, sudden increases in dP/dt and blood pressure associated with certain physical stressors, particularly isometric exercise, may trigger AoD or rupture of aneurysms. Guidelines recommend advising patients to refrain from activities such as weightlifting and sports that may result in thoracic stress and trauma, or involve rotational movement while straining or breath-holding (Valsalva maneuver). Similarly, the sudden increase in aortic stress and systemic arterial pressure produced by activities such as lifting boxes and moving furniture should preclude patients with a history of TAD from the occupations.

BOX 45.1 Conditions Associated With Thoracic Aortic Aneurysms and Dissections

Inflammatory
- Takayasu arteritis
- Giant cell arteritis
- Behçet disease
- Ankylosing spondylitis (spondylarthropathies)
- Infective thoracic aortic aneurysms
- Syphilis

Congenital
- Bicuspid aortic valve
- Abberrant right/left subclavian artery
- Coarctation of the aorta
- Right aortic arch, double aortic arch

Genetic
- Marfan syndrome
- Loeys-Dietz syndrome (TGF-β Thoracic Aortic Disease Syndromes)
- Vascular Ehlers-Danlos syndrome
- Turner Syndrome
- Familial thoracic aortic aneurysm and dissection (ACTA 2, MYH11, TGFBR1, FBN1)

Trauma
- Motor vehicle accident
- Catheter procedure
- Open heart/aortic/vascular surgery

Thoracic Aortic Aneurysms

Degenerative disease results in dilatation of the aorta, leading to thoracic aortic aneurysm formation (TAA). The incidence of TAA is increasing (it is currently 10.4 cases per 100,000 persons years) and influenced by risk factors similar to those for atherosclerosis, including age, smoking, hypertension, a family history of aneurysmal disease, and hypercholesterolemia.[28] Inflammatory, genetic, and certain congenital conditions also influence and increase the risk of aneurysm formation or dissection (see Box 45.1). Oftentimes patients are asymptomatic at the time of diagnosis and the aneurysm is found due on unrelated chest imaging, such as chest x-ray or CT. However, patients may present with symptoms related to anatomic enlargement of the aneurysm, including compression of surrounding structures.

The definition of a true aneurysm is a segmental, full-thickness dilation of a blood vessel having at least a 50% increase in diameter compared with the expected normal diameter.[1] In the case of the aorta, true aneurysms involve all three layers (intima, media, and adventitia). Similar to AoD, TAAs may affect varying segments of the aorta (Fig. 45.1). The majority of aneurysms of the TAA affect the ascending aorta (60%), followed by descending, with only approximately 10% involving the aortic arch,[29] although there is a variation depending on race and regions. Descending thoracic aortic aneurysms have a unique classification system that allows for more detailed information regarding the extent of aortic involvement (Fig. 45.2).

The natural history of all aortic aneurysms is slow but progressive enlargement with increasing risk of aortic rupture or dissection as size increases. Rates of growth/expansion vary based on aneurysm location, pathogenesis, and size. Given the progressive nature of this disease process, regular surveillance and screening are recommended in certain high-risk populations, with more frequent imaging recommended as aneurysmal size increases and operative repair recommended at specific thresholds. In addition, control of risk factors for further aneurysm growth is recommended, including aggressive BP and cholesterol management, as well as smoking cessation.[1]

Multiple studies have been undertaken in an attempt to limit or halt the progression of thoracic aortic aneurysmal growth via medical therapy in patients with asymptomatic disease, who do not have an indication for surgery (i.e., aneurysm is not rapidly expanding, nor has it reached the size threshold for surgical intervention). The most significant study, which demonstrates a slowing of aortic dilation, was performed in patients with Marfan syndrome who are at very high-risk for aortic dilation and aneurysm formation. Seventy patients were randomized to propranolol, versus no beta-blockade, in an open-label study with 10 years of follow-up. The rate of aortic dilation was 73% less in the propranolol group, when compared with the control group.[30]

Similar to beta-blockade in AoD, the mechanism is thought to be a decrease in left ventricular dP/dt and shear stress. Although this beta-blockade benefit has not been specifically demonstrated in non-Marfan syndrome patients, the valid physiological basis has led to general consensus for medical therapy of TAAs to include beta-blockade as first-line therapy.

Further study of Marfan patients has addressed the role of renin-angiotensin system blockade, and attempted to determine if that could also reduce the rate of aneurysmal expansion. An initial small study of 17 adult patients demonstrated when perindopril is added to beta-blocker therapy aortic wall stiffness and aortic root stiffness are decreased.[31] Subsequently, a larger open-label randomized study of losartan versus placebo treatment in 233 adult patients with Marfan syndrome demonstrated a significantly decreased rate of aortic root dilation in those treated with losartan. Over 70% of patients enrolled in this study were also taking beta-blockers.[32] The most recent work evaluating medical therapy's role in decreasing aortic root dilation/aneurysmal progression was published in 2014. A total of 608 adult and pediatric subjects were assigned to treatment with losartan or atenolol. No significant difference in the rate of aortic-root dilatation between the two treatment groups was seen over a 3-year period. Rates of aortic-root surgery, aortic dissection, death, and a composite of these events also did not differ significantly between the two treatment groups.[33]

Again, the degree of BP lowering in patients with TAAs is not well established. It may be reasonable to aim for aggressive BP goals (<120 mm Hg), in the absence of other comorbidities such as diabetes mellitus. Using data extrapolated from patients with Marfan syndrome, the use of beta-blockers is recommended to slow TAA progression, and the use angiotensin-receptor blockers are reasonable as second-line therapy in hypertensive patients with TAA.

Abdominal Aortic Aneurysms

Abdominal aortic aneurysms (AAA) are the most common form of arterial aneurysm and accounted for 151,500 deaths in the United States in 2013.[34] In the majority of adults an abdominal aortic diameter of greater than 3.0 cm is defined as aneurysmal and occurs most frequently below the renal arteries. The natural history of AAAs includes progressive increases in size, the rate of which varies based on a variety of risk factors including increasing age, male sex, smoking, hypertension, and atherosclerosis. Interestingly, diabetes appears to lessen the likelihood of developing an AAA.[35]

Of course, with increasing aneurysmal size the risk of rupture, and subsequent mortality, increases. Independently, the rate of AAA expansion also increases the risk of rupture. A 2015 study assessed factors associated with small AAA expansion rate and determined that elevations in diastolic blood pressure were tied to increased expansion rates.[36] This is similar to a 2014 study of 1.25 million individuals aged 30 and above that were free from atherosclerotic cardiovascular disease

that were followed for a median of 5.2 years. Although AAA was very weakly associated with systolic hypertension, of all cardiovascular conditions, AAA demonstrated the strongest association with diastolic blood pressure (DBP) and mean arterial pressure. It also was the only cardiovascular condition studied that demonstrated a reverse relationship with increasing PP (i.e., less AAA development with increasing PP.) This may reflect that arterial rigidity seen with increasing PP is in fact protective against aneurysm formation.[37]

The United States Preventive Task Force (USPTF) developed guidelines for AAA screening in the general population that includes the recommendation for ultrasound screening of men with a smoking history between the ages of 65 and 75 years. "Clinically selective" screening is recommended in men ages 65 to 75 years who have never smoked but have risk factors for AAA. Women who have never smoked should not be screened, and there is insufficient evidence to recommend screening in women who have smoked according to the USPTF.[38] There are also recommendations based on randomized control trials and a recent meta-analysis favoring elective operative repair (be it open or more commonly endovascular repair) when aneurysm size reaches greater than 5.5 cm in diameter.[39] However only a small proportion of patients, when initially diagnosed with an AAA, meet criteria for aneurysm repair. Thus, before operative repair is indicated, observation and medical management are therapy mainstays.

As one would imagine, medical therapy includes overall cardiovascular risk reduction with the goal of slowing aneurysm growth and optimizing cardiovascular risk factors. Smoking cessation is the most significant modifiable risk factor when attempting to limit aneurysmal expansion.[40] Other common modifiable risk factors, such as statins and antiplatelet therapy, have been studied with respect to aneurysmal size changes and do not demonstrate a significant difference.

Antihypertensive Treatment in Setting of AAA

Of course, appropriate blood pressure control reduces an individual's overall cardiovascular risk and this benefit is seen in patients with abdominal aortic disease. Multiple studies have investigated whether antihypertensive medications decrease aneurysm expansion rates, but none demonstrates a clear impact on AAA size. Diuretics do not appear to have any effect on expansion rates. Beta-blockers are amongst the most studied and are of uncertain benefit in limiting AAA expansion. Although animal and retrospective studies suggested beta-blockers may limit AAA growth, prospective randomized control trials do not demonstrate a significant difference. A 548-subject randomized placebo controlled trial of propranolol administration to limit expansion of small AAA (mean size of 3.8 cm) demonstrated no significant difference in growth rate and demonstrated poor tolerance of beta-blockade in the active treatment group.[41] It is unknown whether a better tolerated (i.e., more selective beta-blocker) may result in better patient compliance and a beneficial effect.

Blockade of the renin-angiotensin-aldosterone system, with angiotensin receptor blockers or angiotensin converting enzyme inhibitors, has also been studied in attempts to decrease AAA growth. Data from these trials are conflicting and current studies are ongoing as noted below. A 2010 prospective cohort study suggested that treatment with angiotensin converting enzyme inhibitors may in fact lead to aneurysm growth in patients with small AAAs.[42] This stands in contrast to a 2006 population-based case control study suggesting the opposite.[43] Clearly further investigation is needed in the form of randomized control trials. A current phase 2 trial has been completed, but not yet published (ClinicalTrials.gov NCT01118520) comparing rates of AAA expansion when treated with perindopril versus amlodipine versus placebo. A stage 4 trial of telmisartan versus placebo treatment

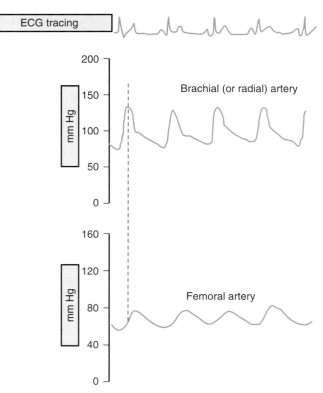

FIG. 45.4 Femoral and brachial blood pressure measurements in a patient with aortic coarctation. It demonstrates a delay in the peak systolic pressure.

(ClinicalTrials.gov NCT01683084) in AAA is also ongoing, with anticipated completion in mid-2016.

Aortic Coarctation

Coarctation of the aorta is most commonly described as a narrowing of the descending aorta located opposite the closed ductus arteriosus (ligamentum arteriosum), just distal to left subclavian artery. Anatomically, there is a ridge-like in-folding of the aorta, resulting in encroachment upon the aortic lumen. Classically an "infantile" form of aortic coarctation also exists, with narrowing proximal to a *patent* ductus arteriosum (PDA), which manifests early in childhood as cyanosis, and requires surgical and/or catheter-based interventions in the neonatal period. Taken together, coarctation of the aorta is a congenital heart defect that accounts for approximately 5% of all congenital cardiac malformations[44] and can be seen as a solitary defect, or in combination with other cardiac abnormalities such as a bicuspid aortic valve.[45] Rarely, aortic coarctation may be acquired following inflammatory disease of the aorta or severe atherosclerosis.

Coarctation of the aorta without a PDA is a commonly discussed cause of secondary hypertension and is oftentimes unrecognized well into adulthood. Because it is often unrecognized, 2008 guidelines for the management of adults with congenital heart disease from the American Heart Association and American College of Cardiology recommend screening for coarctation in both hypertensive children and adults. This includes palpating brachial (or radial) and femoral pulses simultaneously to assess timing and amplitude; looking for a brachial-femoral delay seen in significant aortic coarctation (Fig. 45.4). Further, upper and lower extremity BP measurement should be performed.[46] Typical findings in coarctation of the aorta include elevated SBP in the upper extremities, diminished or delayed femoral pulses, and low or unobtainable arterial BP in the lower extremities with possible manifestation of arterial insufficiency symptoms

such as claudication. The origin of the left subclavian artery and the severity of the luminal narrowing determine the severity of pulse and BP discrepancy. If suspected on physical exam, two-dimensional and Doppler echocardiography is the typical confirmatory study. CT and MRI are complementary imaging modalities that may also help establish the diagnosis.

Management of aortic coarctation includes the initial corrective procedure, and then management of long-term cardiovascular complications. Management of critical coarctation of infants is beyond the scope of this chapter. Based on the aforementioned 2008 guidelines, indications for intervention in adults include a peak-to-peak coarctation gradient greater than or equal to 20 mm Hg, or a gradient less than 20 mm Hg, but with imaging demonstrating significant coarctation and radiologic evidence of substantial collateral flow. Children should be intervened upon if they demonstrate heart failure, a peak pressure gradient across the narrowing of greater than 20 mm Hg, and/or radiologic demonstration of collateral circulation. Surgical repair or percutaneous balloon angioplasty (with or without stent placement) are the general treatment choices. Percutaneous balloon angioplasty and surgical repair are equally effective in reducing the gradient early after intervention, but the risk of recoarctation and aneurysm formation are greater in balloon angioplasty patients than those who were surgically repaired.[47] When percutaneous intervention is chosen, balloon angioplasty with subsequent stent placement is recommended in patients greater than 25 kg and data are emerging that covered stents have similar efficacy to bare metal stents.[48]

BP generally decreases substantially after successful intervention for coarctation, however recurrent hypertension is seen particularly in patients whose repair is performed later in life.[49,50] No specific trials have studied this population for ideal agents to control BP, however reasonable options include diuretics, angiotensin converting enzyme inhibitors, angiotensin receptor blockers, or calcium channel blockers. If aneurysmal disease exists beta-blockers are also a reasonable option.

PERIPHERAL ARTERIAL DISEASE IN HYPERTENSION

As the metabolic syndrome, diabetes mellitus, hypertension, and atherosclerosis become more prevalent, peripheral arterial disease (PAD) is an increasingly recognized contributor to patient morbidity and mortality. What may start as calf pain when ambulating longer distances (intermittent claudication), peripheral arterial disease can progress to critical limb ischemia, necessitating amputation. It is this wide spectrum of disease that makes recognition and control of risk factors for disease progression so important. Primary hypertension coexisting with peripheral arterial is common and there is significant overlap among medications used to treat symptoms and halt disease advancement.

Epidemiology of Peripheral Artery Disease

PAD is a disease process of large arteries in the lower extremities primarily produced by atherosclerotic burden resulting in obstruction of the vascular lumen. This disease process affects approximately 8.5 million Americans over the age of 40, and is often associated with considerable functional limitations.[51] PAD may be diagnosed clinical history/symptoms, using noninvasive methods, and direct angiography of the lower extremity arterial tree. Classically, PAD presents as intermittent claudication (IC), which is defined as pain with exertion in the calf. The thigh or the buttock may also be affected. The pain is often described as a dull ache, cramp, or fatigue and is relieved by rest. However, less than 50% of patients with significant occlusive disease are symptomatic and many symptomatic patients present atypically. Only about 10% of people with PAD have the hallmark symptom of IC.[52]

Detection of subclinical PAD and confirmation of symptomatic PAD can defined by the ankle-brachial index (ABI). To obtain this measurement, SBP in bilateral ankles and arms are gathered. The ratio of the SBP at each ankle to the highest SBP in the two arms delineates the ABI for that leg. Reduction of flow in the lower extremities results in a lowering of the systolic ankle pressure, thus resulting in a decreased ABI. PAD is defined in those patients with an ABI less than 0.90 in either lower extremity. ABIs greater than 1.40 are caused by stiff peripheral arteries, and recent evidence suggests that in as many as half the cases such stiff arteries mask underlying PAD.[53]

Contribution of Hypertension to Peripheral Artery Disease

The major modifiable factors in atherosclerotic cardiovascular disease (ASCVD) include smoking, dyslipidemia, and hypertension (to a lesser but still significant extent.) The prevalence of ASCVD increases with age and men are more commonly affected. Other contributing risk factors include diabetes mellitus, obesity, and physical inactivity. These all likely play a role in PAD, however, cigarette smoking and diabetes mellitus are likely the most important risk factors for the development of PAD. Data exploring how hypertension is associated with PAD development are affected by how PAD is defined (i.e., by the prevalence of IC, abnormal ABI, or by direct angiography).

When one defines PAD based on the presence of IC, this excludes asymptomatic and patients with less severe PAD. Studies on the relationship between hypertension and IC produce inconsistent results. Certain studies demonstrate a positive association, but others do not demonstrate such a relationship. When PAD is defined via ABI (the most common method currently used) studies using the typical definition of an ABI less than 0.9, or more conservative ratios such as less than 0.80, generally demonstrate an association with BP elevations. The Framingham Offspring Study demonstrated a significant trend for increasing prevalence of hypertension with decreasing ABI. Additionally, hypertension was associated with greater than two times the risk for development of PAD (ABI < 0.9) when performing multivariable analysis.[54]

In multiple reports, an association with SBP is stronger than the association with DBP. The Cardiovascular Health Study demonstrated a highly significant inverse relationship between the ABI value and both the percentage of individuals that reported hypertension and the measured SBP. When adjustments for age and gender were performed, as the ABI decreased, the prevalence of persons reporting hypertension, and the relative risk of developing hypertension increased, as did the mean SBP. Conversely, DBP did not differ with varying levels of ABI.[55] In addition, a higher SBP (but not DBP) and hypertension prevalence occurred more often in those with PAD (ABI < 0.90) in a cohort of almost 7000 patients.[56] Similar results were seen in the ATTEST (alteplase versus tenecteplase for thrombolysis after ischemic stroke) study.[57]

Studies exploring the incidence of PAD have the advantage of multiple BP measurements being recorded before an individual develops a diagnosis of PAD. The Multi-Ethnic Study of Atherosclerosis demonstrated that hypertension at baseline, as well as baseline age, presence of diabetes mellitus, and higher levels of smoking were associated with progression from a normal ABI value to less than 0.90.[58] The Cardiovascular Health Study also indicated the presence of baseline hypertension is a significant predictor for the development of PAD.[59]

Hypertension (HTN) and PAD are positively associated in most studies, and typically demonstrate a stronger association for SBP than DBP. Development of PAD is the cardiovascular disease process most strongly associated with widening PP.[37] Results from the limited number of available prospective studies suggest a rather strong relationship between HTN and PAD. Unfortunately, the method to definitively determine if HTN is a causal factor in the development of PAD is a randomized controlled trial. This trial does not exist. Currently available data do not definitively demonstrate that HTN causes PAD, however it is very likely that HTN is an important causal factor in the pathogenesis of PAD.

Hypertension Treatment in Peripheral Artery Disease

Treatment of HTN to reduce cardiovascular events requires careful consideration in patients with PAD. These patients are at increased risk for morbidity and mortality from cardiovascular disease. Regrettably, compared with those with coronary atherosclerosis, individuals with PAD, without evidence of coronary atherosclerosis, are undertreated for cardiovascular disease risk factors including HTN.[60] When a patient is diagnosed with PAD, he or she should be offered aggressive risk factor modification, including measures such as smoking cessation, exercise programs, dietary counseling, and weight reduction. Therapies for hyperlipidemia and antiplatelet therapies as indicated should also be provided.

Systemic cardiovascular disease outcomes respond favorably to management of these risk factors in patients with PAD.[61] Progression of PAD is also affected by SBP. A study published in 1991 prospectively tracked the progression of PAD in diabetics, as defined by the rate of change in the postexercise ABI, over 4 years. It also measured the occurrence of clinical events, such as PAD operations. Upon multivariable analysis, SBP was independently and significantly predictive of PAD progression.[62] Thus, treatment of PAD patients involves two individual but complementary objectives. The primary is the reduction of systemic cardiovascular risk, and the second is improvement in symptoms and walking ability.

For individuals with PAD, the current goal BP is questionable given the results of the SPRINT trial[25] and likely should be more aggressive than previously thought. However, treatment of hypertension in the setting of PAD is complex. Below is a summary of pharmacologic and nonpharmacologic interventions for BP management in patients with PAD.

Nonpharmacologic Treatment: Exercise

Aerobic and endurance exercise programs lower BP in adults with HTN and with normal BP. A meta-analysis published in 2002 demonstrated that SBP is lowered by more than 3 mm Hg and DBP by more than 2 mm Hg in individuals performing aerobic activity.[63] Similarly, a 2013 meta-analysis and systematic review demonstrated exercises' beneficial effects on daytime ambulatory BP (but no nighttime ambulatory BP).[64]

When exercise is performed, peripheral arterial vasodilation occurs distal to sites of arterial obstruction resulting in decreased perfusion pressure, often to levels below those generated in the interstitial tissue by the exercising muscle. It then stands to reason that leg exercise, such as walking, produces IC symptoms in certain individuals with PAD. However, several studies have demonstrated that regular mild-to-moderate intensity exercise improves physical functioning, as well as self-reported health-related quality of life, in those with clinical or subclinical PAD.[65]

Nonpharmacologic Treatment: Diet

A low salt diet and the Dietary Approaches to Stopping Hypertension (DASH) diet[66] lowers BP, however there are no randomized studies on the possible effect of dietary modifications on overall cardiovascular risk, symptoms related to IC, or effect on walking distance in those with PAD.

Pharmacologic Therapy

The number of studies, exploring the effect of pharmacologic therapy for elevated BP in those with PAD with antihypertensive drugs, is limited. In addition none of the trials that were performed include large numbers of subjects. Below is a summary, by drug class and restricted to randomized, placebo-controlled trials, of the available literature on effects of BP therapy for both reduction of systemic cardiovascular risk and on symptoms in PAD patients. A more thorough in-depth analysis can be found in a 2013 Cochrane review entitled "Treatment of hypertension in peripheral arterial disease."[67]

Angiotensin-Converting Enzyme Inhibitors

The Heart Outcomes Prevention Evaluation (HOPE) trial was a large placebo controlled trial of ramipril in 9297 subjects at high risk for cardiovascular events, of which a large percentage had PAD. After an average of approximately 4.5 years of follow-up, treatment with ramipril was associated with a significant risk reduction for the primary composite outcome MI, stroke, and cardiovascular death.[68] The above mentioned Cochrane review obtained unpublished data from the HOPE trial and again demonstrated favorable effects of ramipril treatment in PAD with respect to major adverse cardiovascular events in the subgroup with PAD (approximately 50% of enrolled patients).[67]

The benefit for the primary outcome was, in fact, greater in those with PAD compared with those without. A sub-study of HOPE recruited 38 subjects with PAD performed ambulatory BP monitoring; 24-hour BPs were significantly reduced primarily because of BP-lowering at night.[69]

An older study from 1994 did not demonstrate functional improvement (i.e., change in ABI, walking distance, or symptoms of IC) in 26 subjects treated with perindopril versus 28 provided placebo.[70]

Angiotensin II Receptor Blockers

The most significant data looking at ARB treatment in PAD was published in 2010. It compared 18 patients randomized to telmisartan or placebo. After 12 months of telmisartan the mean walk distance in the intervention group increased significantly, however there was no statistical difference in measured ABI.[71]

Beta-Blockers

Debate about the use of beta-blockers in IC existed as a result of early case reports suggesting they worsen symptoms. This is also based on the physiologic properties of beta-blockers, which compete with catecholamines for binding at sympathetic receptor sites in multiple tissues. Beta-blockers block sympathetic stimulation mediated by beta 2-receptors in vascular smooth muscle resulting in decreased arterial resistance. Consequently, increases in peripheral blood flow occur, unless there is significant obstruction to flow that results in decreased distal flow. Theoretically, in PAD, nonselective beta-blockers would be associated with such a decrease in flow that claudication symptoms could worsen. There is no good evidence to suggest that beta-blockers should not be used in the presence of PAD.

Although no large studies are available, there are some data comparing beta-blockers with other classes of antihypertensive and to other beta-blockers. Nebivolol, when compared with 24 months of hydrochlorothiazide treatment in patients with PAD, demonstrated no statistically significant difference in ABI, and distance walked before onset on IC.[72] Nebivolol was later compared with metoprolol in patients with IC and hypertension. Fifty-two patients received nebivolol and 57 received metoprolol. After 36 weeks of treatment, no difference in outcomes was seen.[73] In 1991, a meta-analysis of the available randomized controlled trials studying beta-blockers in patients with mild to moderate PAD was performed. After pooling 11 available treatment comparisons from 6 trials, the results showed no significant difference in pain-free walking distance.[74]

The unassailable value of beta-blockade in the treatment of hypertension and following MI, in combination with the lack of evidence for worsening PAD symptoms, suggests that the use of this class of drug in hypertensive patients with PAD is acceptable.

Calcium Channel Blockers

Several small studies have been conducted to determine if calcium channel blockers are beneficial in the treatment of PAD. Two randomized studies compared verapamil with placebo in patients with IC. Four weeks of treatment with verapamil resulted in a 7% increase in walking distance despite no change in the ABI.[75] A 1997, randomized, placebo-controlled, double-blind, cross-over trial that also demonstrated no differences in systolic ankle pressure or the ABI when treated with verapamil, but there was a significant increase the mean pain-free and maximum walking distances.[76]

Verapamil was again studied in 1998 when 96 patients, who had undergone peripheral arterial angioplasty, were randomized to placebo versus calcium channel blocker. ABI was not statistically different between the active drug and placebo immediately after angioplasty or at 6 weeks. However, 6 months postangioplasty there was a marginal benefit on ABI measurement in favor of the calcium antagonist.[77]

Combinations of Antihypertensive Agents

A number of trials have examined the effect of antihypertensive class on walking distance in PAD patients with IC. A 1987 study compared placebo with captopril, atenolol, labetalol, and pindolol. Twenty subjects receiving 1 month of beta-blockade demonstrated decreases in claudication free, and maximum walking distances, as well as postexercise calf blood-flow availability. Similar reductions were not seen in the captopril group.[78] No significant differences were seen when comparing amlodipine, chlorthalidone, or lisinopril for hospitalized or treated PAD (a component of a composite secondary endpoint) in the Antihypertensive and Lipid-Lowering to prevent Heart Attack Trial (ALLHAT).[79] Subgroup analysis of the INVEST (international verapamil-trandolapril study) trial, published in 2003, demonstrated that among 2699 PAD patients, no significant differences in the composite endpoints of death, nonfatal MI or nonfatal stroke or death, nonfatal MI or nonfatal stroke, and revascularization were seen between the 1345 patients receiving verapamil sustained-release ± trandolapril compared with 1354 patients receiving atenolol ± hydrochlorothiazide.[67]

SUMMARY

Both peripheral arterial disease and aortic disease lead to significant cardiovascular morbidity and mortality. Hypertension contributes to the development of both, and must be appropriately controlled to prevent disease progression. However, high-level evidence is lacking with respect to appropriate BP goals, and appropriate antihypertensive therapy, for patients with PAD and aortopathies. Future trials directed at studying these questions are needed.

References

1. Hiratzka LF, Bakris GL, Beckman JA, et al. 2010 ACCF/AHA/AATS/ACR/ASA/SCA/SCAI/SIR/STS/SVM Guidelines for the diagnosis and management of patients with thoracic aortic disease. A Report of the American College of Cardiology Foundation/American Heart Association Task Force on Practice Guidelines, American Association for Thoracic Surgery, American College of Radiology,American Stroke Association, Society of Cardiovascular Anesthesiologists, Society for Cardiovascular Angiography and Interventions, Society of Interventional Radiology, Society of Thoracic Surgeons,and Society for Vascular Medicine. *J Am Coll Cardiol.* 2010;55:e27-e129.

2. Lang RM, Badano LP, Mor-Avi V, et al. Recommendations for cardiac chamber quantification by echocardiography in adults: an update from the American Society of Echocardiography and the European Association of Cardiovascular Imaging. *J Am Soc Echocardiogr.* 2015;28:1-39 e14.

3. Howard DP, Banerjee A, Fairhead JF, et al. Population-based study of incidence and outcome of acute aortic dissection and premorbid risk factor control: 10-year results from the Oxford Vascular Study. *Circulation.* 2013;127:2031-2037.

4. Hagan PG, Nienaber CA, Isselbacher EM, et al. The International Registry of Acute Aortic Dissection (IRAD): new insights into an old disease. *JAMA.* 2000;283:897-903.

5. Nienaber CA, Rousseau H, Eggebrecht H, et al. Randomized comparison of strategies for type B aortic dissection: the INvestigation of STEnt Grafts in Aortic Dissection (INSTEAD) trial. *Circulation.* 2009;120:2519-2528.

6. Nienaber CA, Kische S, Rousseau H, et al. Endovascular repair of type B aortic dissection: long-term results of the randomized investigation of stent grafts in aortic dissection trial. *Circ Cardiovasc Interv.* 2013;6:407-416.

7. Lombardi JV, Cambria RP, Nienaber CA, et al. Aortic remodeling after endovascular treatment of complicated type B aortic dissection with the use of a composite device design. *J Vasc Surg.* 2014;59:1544-1554.

8. Booher AM, Isselbacher EM, Nienaber CA, et al. The IRAD classification system for characterizing survival after aortic dissection. *Am J Med.* 2013;126:730:e19-e24.

9. Chan KK, Rabkin SW. Increasing prevalence of hypertension among patients with thoracic aorta dissection: trends over eight decades—a structured meta-analysis. *Am J Hypertens.* 2014;27:907-917.

10. Januzzi JL, Isselbacher EM, Fattori R, et al. Characterizing the young patient with aortic dissection: results from the International Registry of Aortic Dissection (IRAD). *J Am Coll Cardiol.* 2004;43:665-669.

11. Hoff E, Eagle T, Pyeritz RE, et al. Pulse pressure and type A acute aortic dissection in-hospital outcomes (from the International Registry of Acute Aortic Dissection). *Am J Cardiol.* 2014;113:1255-1259.

12. Tsai TT, Bossone E, Isselbacher EM, et al. Clinical characteristics of hypotension in patients with acute aortic dissection. *Am J Cardiol.* 2005;95:48-52.

13. Eggebrecht H, Schmermund A, von Birgelen C, et al. Resistant hypertension in patients with chronic aortic dissection. *J Hum Hypertens.* 2005;19:227-231.

14. Marini CP, Grubbs PE, Toporoff B, et al. Effect of sodium nitroprusside on spinal cord perfusion and paraplegia during aortic cross-clamping. *Ann Thorac Surg.* 1989;47:379-383.

15. Trimarchi S, Eagle KA, Nienaber CA, et al. Importance of refractory pain and hypertension in acute type B aortic dissection: insights from the International Registry of Acute Aortic Dissection (IRAD). *Circulation.* 2010;122:1283-1289.

16. Lederle FA, Powell JT, Nienaber CA. Does intensive medical treatment improve outcomes in aortic dissection? *BMJ.* 2014;349:g5288.

17. Pape LA, Awais M, Woznicki EM, et al. Presentation, diagnosis, and outcomes of acute aortic dissection: 17-year trends from the international registry of acute aortic dissection. *J Am Coll Cardiol.* 2015;66:350-358.

18. Rice RD, Sandhu HK, Leake SS, et al. Is Total Arch Replacement Associated With Worse Outcomes During Repair of Acute Type A Aortic Dissection? *Ann Thorac Surg.* 2015;100:2159-2166.

19. Vallabhajosyula P, Gottret JP, Robb JD, et al. Hemiarch replacement with concomitant antegrade stent grafting of the descending thoracic aorta versus total arch replacement for treatment of acute DeBakey I aortic dissection with arch teardagger. *Eur J Cardiothorac Surg.* 2016;5:156-173.

20. Okita Y. Surgery for thoracic aortic disease in Japan: evolving strategies toward the growing enemies. *Gen Thorac Cardiovasc Surg.* 2015;63:185-196.

21. Tsai TT, Evangelista A, Nienaber CA, et al. Long-term survival in patients presenting with type A acute aortic dissection: insights from the International Registry of Acute Aortic Dissection (IRAD). *Circulation.* 2006;114(1 Suppl):I350-I356.

22. Melby SJ, Zierer A, Damiano RJ Jr., Moon MR. Importance of blood pressure control after repair of acute type a aortic dissection: 25-year follow-up in 252 patients. *J Clin Hypertens (Greenwich).* 2013;15:63-68.

23. Suzuki T, Isselbacher EM, Nienaber CA, et al. Type-selective benefits of medications in treatment of acute aortic dissection (from the International Registry of Acute Aortic Dissection [IRAD]). *Am J Cardiol.* 2012;109:122-127.

24. Nienaber CA, Divchev D, Palisch H, Clough RE, Richartz B. Early and late management of type B aortic dissection. *Heart.* 2014;100:1491-1497.

25. Group SR, Wright JT, Jr., Williamson JD, et al. A Randomized Trial of Intensive versus Standard Blood-Pressure Control. *N Engl J Med.* 2015;373:2103-2116.

26. Chan KK, Lai P, Wright JM. First-line beta-blockers versus other antihypertensive medications for chronic type B aortic dissection. *Cochrane Database Syst Rev.* 2014;2:CD010426.

27. Genoni M, Paul M, Jenni R, Graves K, Seifert B, Turina M. Chronic beta-blocker therapy improves outcome and reduces treatment costs in chronic type B aortic dissection. *Eur J Cardiothorac Surg.* 2001;19:606-610.

28. Clouse WD, Hallett JW Jr., Schaff HV, Gayari MM, Ilstrup DM, Melton LJ 3rd. Improved prognosis of thoracic aortic aneurysms: a population-based study. *JAMA.* 1998;280:1926-1929.

29. Isselbacher EM. Thoracic and abdominal aortic aneurysms. *Circulation.* 2005;111:816-828.

30. Shores J, Berger KR, Murphy EA, Pyeritz RE. Progression of aortic dilatation and the benefit of long-term beta-adrenergic blockade in Marfan's syndrome. *N Engl J Med.* 1994;330:1335-1341.

31. Ahimastos AA, Aggarwal A, D'Orsa KM, et al. Effect of perindopril on large artery stiffness and aortic root diameter in patients with Marfan syndrome: a randomized controlled trial. *JAMA.* 2007;298:1539-1547.

32. Groenink M, den Hartog AW, Franken R, et al. Losartan reduces aortic dilatation rate in adults with Marfan syndrome: a randomized controlled trial. *Eur Heart J.* 2013;34:3491-3500.

33. Lacro RV, Dietz HC, Sleeper LA, et al. Atenolol versus losartan in children and young adults with Marfan's syndrome. *N Engl J Med.* 2014;371:2061-2071.

34. GBD. 2013 Mortality and Causes of Death Collaborators. Global, regional, and national age-sex specific all-cause and cause-specific mortality for 240 causes of death, 1990-2013: a systematic analysis for the Global Burden of Disease Study 2013. *Lancet.* 2015;385:117-171.

35. Kent KC, Zwolak RM, Egorova NN, et al. Analysis of risk factors for abdominal aortic aneurysm in a cohort of more than 3 million individuals. *J Vasc Surg.* 2010;52:539-548.

36. Bhak RH, Wininger M, Johnson GR, et al. Factors associated with small abdominal aortic aneurysm expansion rate. *JAMA Surg.* 2015;150:44-50.

37. Rapsomaniki E, Timmis A, George J, et al. Blood pressure and incidence of twelve cardiovascular diseases: lifetime risks, healthy life-years lost, and age-specific associations in 1.25 million people. *Lancet.* 2014;383:1899-1911.

38. LeFevre ML, Force USPST. Screening for abdominal aortic aneurysm: U.S. Preventive Services Task Force recommendation statement. *Ann Intern Med.* 2014;161:281-290.

39. Filardo G, Powell JT, Martinez MA, Ballard DJ. Surgery for small asymptomatic abdominal aortic aneurysms. *Cochrane Database Syst Rev.* 2015;2:CD001835.

40. Hirsch AT, Haskal ZJ, Hertzer NR, et al. ACC/AHA 2005 Practice guidelines for the management of patients with peripheral arterial disease (lower extremity, renal, mesenteric, and abdominal aortic): a collaborative report from the American Association for Vascular Surgery/Society for Vascular Surgery, Society for Cardiovascular Angiography and Interventions, Society for Vascular Medicine and Biology, Society of Interventional Radiology, and the ACC/AHA Task Force on Practice Guidelines (Writing Committee to Develop Guidelines for the Management of Patients With Peripheral Arterial Disease): endorsed by the American Association of Cardiovascular and Pulmonary Rehabilitation; National Heart, Lung, and Blood Institute; Society for Vascular Nursing; TransAtlantic Inter-Society Consensus; and Vascular Disease Foundation. *Circulation.* 2006;113:e463-e654.

41. Propanolol Aneurysm Trial Investigators. Propranolol for small abdominal aortic aneurysms: results of a randomized trial. *J Vasc Surg.* 2002;35:72-79.

42. Sweeting MJ, Thompson SG, Brown LC, Greenhalgh RM, Powell JT. Use of angiotensin converting enzyme inhibitors is associated with increased growth rate of abdominal aortic aneurysms. *J Vasc Surg.* 2010;52:1-4.

43. Hackam DG, Thiruchelvam D, Redelmeier DA. Angiotensin-converting enzyme inhibitors and aortic rupture: a population-based case-control study. *Lancet.* 2006;368:659-665.

44. Hoffman JI, Kaplan S. The incidence of congenital heart disease. *J Am Coll Cardiol.* 2002;39:1890-1900.

45. Nihoyannopoulos P, Karas S, Sapsford RN, Hallidie-Smith K, Foale R. Accuracy of two-dimensional echocardiography in the diagnosis of aortic arch obstruction. *J Am Coll Cardiol.* 1987;10:1072-1077.

46. Warnes CA, Williams RG, Bashore TM, et al. ACC/AHA 2008 Guidelines for the Management of Adults with Congenital Heart Disease: a report of the American College of Cardiology/American Heart Association Task Force on Practice Guidelines (writing committee to develop guidelines on the management of adults with congenital heart disease). *Circulation.* 2008;118:e714-e833.

47. Cowley CG, Orsmond GS, Feola P, McQuillan L, Shaddy RE. Long-term, randomized comparison of balloon angioplasty and surgery for native coarctation of the aorta in childhood. *Circulation.* 2005;111:3453-3456.

48. Meadows J, Minahan M, McElhinney DB, et al. Intermediate outcomes in the prospective, multicenter coarctation of the aorta stent trial (COAST). *Circulation.* 2015;131:1656-1664.

49. Clarkson PM, Nicholson MR, Barratt-Boyes BG, Neutze JM, Whitlock RM. Results after repair of coarctation of the aorta beyond infancy: a 10 to 28 year follow-up with particular reference to late systemic hypertension. *Am J Cardiol.* 1983;51:1481-1488.

50. Toro-Salazar OH, Steinberger J, Thomas W, Rocchini AP, Carpenter B, Moller JH. Long-term follow-up of patients after coarctation of the aorta repair. *Am J Cardiol.* 2002;89:541-547.

51. McDermott MM, Greenland P, Ferrucci L, et al. Lower extremity performance is associated with daily life physical activity in individuals with and without peripheral arterial disease. *J Am Geriatr Soc.* 2002;50:247-255.

52. Mozaffarian D, Benjamin EJ, Go AS, et al. Heart Disease and Stroke Statistics-2016 Update: A Report From the American Heart Association. *Circulation.* 2016;133:e38-e60.

53. Aboyans V, Ho E, Denenberg JO, Ho LA, Natarajan L, Criqui MH. The association between elevated ankle systolic pressures and peripheral occlusive arterial disease in diabetic and nondiabetic subjects. *J Vasc Surg.* 2008;48:1197-1203.

54. Murabito JM, Evans JC, Nieto K, Larson MG, Levy D, Wilson PW. Prevalence and clinical correlates of peripheral arterial disease in the Framingham Offspring Study. *Am Heart J.* 2002;143:961-965.

55. Newman AB, Siscovick DS, Manolio TA, et al. Ankle-arm index as a marker of atherosclerosis in the Cardiovascular Health Study. Cardiovascular Heart Study (CHS) Collaborative Research Group. *Circulation.* 1993;88:837-845.

56. Diehm C, Schuster A, Allenberg JR, et al. High prevalence of peripheral arterial disease and co-morbidity in 6880 primary care patients: cross-sectional study. *Atherosclerosis.* 2004;172:95-105.

57. Safar ME, Priollet P, Luizy F, et al. Peripheral arterial disease and isolated systolic hypertension: the ATTEST study. *J Hum Hypertens.* 2009;23:182-187.

58. Allison MA, Cushman M, Solomon C, et al. Ethnicity and risk factors for change in the ankle-brachial index: the Multi-Ethnic Study of Atherosclerosis. *J Vasc Surg.* 2009;50:1049-1056.

59. Kennedy M, Solomon C, Manolio TA, et al. Risk factors for declining ankle-brachial index in men and women 65 years or older: the Cardiovascular Health Study. *Arch Intern Med.* 2005;165:1896-1902.

60. Gonzalez-Clemente JM, Pinies JA, Calle-Pascual A, et al. Cardiovascular risk factor management is poorer in diabetic patients with undiagnosed peripheral arterial disease than in those with known coronary heart disease or cerebrovascular disease. Results of a nationwide study in tertiary diabetes centres. *Diabet Med.* 2008;25:427-434.

61. Hackam DG, Sultan NM, Criqui MH. Vascular protection in peripheral artery disease: systematic review and modelling study. *Heart.* 2009;95:1098-1102.

62. Palumbo PJ, O'Fallon WM, Osmundson PJ, Zimmerman BR, Langworthy AL, Kazmier FJ. Progression of peripheral occlusive arterial disease in diabetes mellitus. What factors are predictive? *Arch Intern Med.* 1991;151:717-721.

63. Whelton SP, Chin A, Xin X, He J. Effect of aerobic exercise on blood pressure: a meta-analysis of randomized, controlled trials. *Ann Intern Med.* 2002;136:493-503.

64. Cornelissen VA, Buys R, Smart NA. Endurance exercise beneficially affects ambulatory blood pressure: a systematic review and meta-analysis. *J Hypertens.* 2013;31:639-648.

65. McDermott MM, Ades P, Guralnik JM, et al. Treadmill exercise and resistance training in patients with peripheral arterial disease with and without intermittent claudication: a randomized controlled trial. *JAMA.* 2009;301:165-174.

66. Sacks FM, Svetkey LP, Vollmer WM, et al. Effects on blood pressure of reduced dietary sodium and the Dietary Approaches to Stop Hypertension (DASH) diet. DASH-Sodium Collaborative Research Group. *N Engl J Med.* 2001;344:3-10.

67. Lane DA, Lip GY. Treatment of hypertension in peripheral arterial disease. *Cochrane Database Syst Rev.* 2013;12:CD003075.

68. Yusuf S, Sleight P, Pogue J, Bosch J, Davies R, Dagenais G. Effects of an angiotensin-converting-enzyme inhibitor, ramipril, on cardiovascular events in high-risk patients. The Heart Outcomes Prevention Evaluation Study Investigators. *N Engl J Med.* 2000;342:145-153.

69. Svensson P, de Faire U, Sleight P, Yusuf S, Ostergren J. Comparative effects of ramipril on ambulatory and office blood pressures: a HOPE Substudy. *Hypertension.* 2001;38:E28-E32.

70. Overlack A, Adamczak M, Bachmann W, et al. ACE-inhibition with perindopril in essential hypertensive patients with concomitant diseases. The Perindopril Therapeutic Safety Collaborative Research Group. *Am J Med.* 1994;97:126-134.

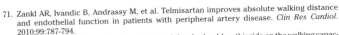
SPECIAL POPULATIONS AND SPECIAL SITUATIONS

71. Zankl AR, Ivandic B, Andrassy M, et al. Telmisartan improves absolute walking distance and endothelial function in patients with peripheral artery disease. *Clin Res Cardiol.* 2010;99:787-794.

72. Diehm C, Pittrow D, Lawall H. Effect of nebivolol vs. hydrochlorothiazide on the walking capacity in hypertensive patients with intermittent claudication. *J Hypertens.* 2011;29:1448-1456.

73. Espinola-Klein C, Weisser G, Jagodzinski A, et al. beta-Blockers in patients with intermittent claudication and arterial hypertension: results from the nebivolol or metoprolol in arterial occlusive disease trial. *Hypertension.* 2011;58:148-154.

74. Radack K, Deck C. Beta-adrenergic blocker therapy does not worsen intermittent claudication in subjects with peripheral arterial disease. A meta-analysis of randomized controlled trials. *Arch Intern Med.* 1991;151:1769-1776.

75. Kimose HH, Bagger JP, Aagaard MT, Paulsen PK. Placebo-controlled, double-blind study of the effect of verapamil in intermittent claudication. *Angiology.* 1990;41:595-598.

76. Bagger JP, Helligsoe P, Randsbaek F, Kimose HH, Jensen BS. Effect of verapamil in intermittent claudication A randomized, double-blind, placebo-controlled, cross-over study after individual dose-response assessment. *Circulation.* 1997;95:411-414.

77. Schweizer J, Kirch W, Koch R, Hellner G, Uhlmann K. Effect of high dose verapamil on restenosis after peripheral angioplasty. *J Am Coll Cardiol.* 1998;31:1299-1305.

78. Roberts DH, Tsao Y, McLoughlin GA, Breckenridge A. Placebo-controlled comparison of captopril, atenolol, labetalol, and pindolol in hypertension complicated by intermittent claudication. *Lancet.* 1987;2:650-653.

79. ALLHAT Officers and Coordinators for the ALLHAT Collaborative Research Group. The Antihypertensive and Lipid-Lowering Treatment to Prevent Heart Attack Trial. Major outcomes in high-risk hypertensive patients randomized to angiotensin-converting enzyme inhibitor or calcium channel blocker vs diuretic: the Antihypertensive and Lipid-Lowering Treatment to Prevent Heart Attack Trial (ALLHAT). *JAMA.* 2002;288:2981-2997.

46 Hypertensive Emergencies and Urgencies

William J. Elliott

High blood pressure (BP), or hypertension, remains a major worldwide public health challenge, despite recent improvements in control rates in many developed nations.[1] because it is a major contributor to cardiovascular disease (CVD), and is increasing in prevalence in developing nations. In the United States, approximately 80 million people had hypertension in 2012[2]; fortunately, true "hypertensive crises" account for less than 1% of health care encounters involving elevated BP. Large U.S. claims databases have suggested that the annual incidence was about 1 to 2 per million population in the late 1990s, and may be decreasing recently, in the U.S. and other developed nations. However, as hypertension becomes more prevalent worldwide, case reports and case series of hypertensive crises continue to be reported.

In 1928, when "malignant hypertension" was first added to the medical lexicon, the prognosis of patients with grade IV hypertensive retinopathy was worse than that of many cancers (17% after 1 year in the 1939 case series, hence the name). About 40% of these deaths occurred from renal failure, with stroke (24%), myocardial infarction (11%), and heart failure (10%) accounting for most of the rest. This situation has markedly changed since the advent of effective chronic oral antihypertensive drug therapy[3]; the diagnoses of "malignant" or "accelerated" hypertension are now used nearly exclusively by coding personnel, and are no longer found in many national or international hypertension guidelines, except to redefine these terms in a more contemporary context.[4]

Traditionally, hypertensive crises are divided into emergencies and urgencies.[5-10] A hypertensive emergency is a very elevated BP in a patient with acute, ongoing target organ damage, and is a true medical emergency, requiring prompt BP reduction (although seldom into the normal range). Of less concern are "hypertensive urgencies" (except for perioperative hypertension, discussed later and in Chapter 44), which may be better termed "major elevations in BP without acute target organ damage." Most patients with this problem are nonadherent to drug therapy or inadequately treated, and often present to the emergency department for other reasons.[11] Such patients require neither hospital admission, nor acute lowering of BP, and can safely be treated in the outpatient setting with any one of a number of appropriate oral medications. It is the distinction between these two types of hypertensive crises that presents the greatest challenge to most physicians. This chapter will discuss the clinical presentation and appropriate evaluation and treatment of the patient with hypertensive crises, and suggest an algorithm to triage patients with major elevations of BP to in-hospital treatment or outpatient management.

Acknowledgments: The author thanks Shakaib U. Rehman, MD, the late Donald G. Vidt, MD, and Jan N. Basile, MD, for their contributions to previous editions of this chapter.

CONTEMPORARY DEFINITIONS

Hypertensive Emergency

A hypertensive emergency is a major and often sudden elevation in BP, associated with progressive, acute target-organ dysfunction. It can present as an acute cerebrovascular event or disordered cerebral function, an acute coronary syndrome with ischemia or infarction, acute pulmonary edema, or acute renal dysfunction (Box 46.1).[5-10] Although the level of BP at presentation is often very high (systolic BP usually >180 mm Hg or diastolic BP > 120 mm Hg), it is not the degree of BP elevation, but rather the clinical status of the patient that defines the emergency.[5-10] For example, a BP of 160/110 mm Hg in a 65-year-old man with an acute aortic dissection or a woman in her third trimester of pregnancy with eclampsia (despite a BP of only 145/95 mm Hg) are true hypertensive emergencies. Such patients almost always should be treated with **parenteral** medications in the intensive care unit or a monitored hospital bed. Risk factors for hypertensive emergencies include: low socioeconomic status, poor access to health care, nonadherence to prescribed antihypertensive drug therapy (including sudden withdrawal from an antihypertensive medicine, e.g., clonidine), substance (particularly cocaine) or alcohol use disorder, oral contraceptive use, and cigarette smoking.[11]

Major Blood Pressure Elevation Without Ongoing Target-Organ Damage (So-Called "Hypertensive Urgencies")

Traditionally, many physicians have been uncomfortable with hypertensive patients who had BP higher than 180/120 mm Hg, simply because such BP levels, if sustained, were first shown to benefit from antihypertensive drug treatment with a reduction in long-term morbidity. To acknowledge this, many older guidelines recognized "hypertensive urgencies:" major elevations in BP without acute, ongoing target organ dysfunction. Examples include major BP elevations associated with severe headache, shortness of breath, mild epistaxis, or severe anxiety. Other sources define a hypertensive urgency as a patient with diastolic BP (DBP) higher than 115 to 120 mm Hg, or systolic BP (SBP) higher than 180 mm Hg. Although such patients may have signs of chronic target organ damage, such as grade II hypertensive retinopathy, left ventricular hypertrophy, or chronic kidney disease with stable proteinuria, the absence of acute or progressively worsening hypertensive target organ damage differentiates these patients from those with hypertensive emergencies. Despite the very high BP, these patients have a low risk of cardiovascular events over the next few months (even if left untreated). Many now-classic case series gathered before antihypertensive drug therapy became available were validated by the first Veterans' Administration Cooperative Trial (published in 1967), in which 70 patients with DBP between 115 and 129 mm Hg randomized to placebo had zero (95% confidence interval [CI] 0 to 5) major CVD or adverse events over the next 2 months.

BOX 46.1 Clinical Situations That Are Usually Hypertensive Emergencies

1. Hypertensive encephalopathy
2. "Malignant hypertension:" elevated blood pressure with papilledema or acute retinal hemorrhages/exudates
3. Intracranial hemorrhage (intracerebral or subarachnoid); ischemic stroke (rarely)
4. Acute coronary syndrome (unstable angina/myocardial infarction)
5. Acute left ventricular failure with pulmonary edema
6. Acute aortic dissection
7. Rapidly progressive renal injury, (e.g., systemic vasculitis, including scleroderma crisis)
8. Eclampsia
9. Life-threatening arterial bleeding
10. Head trauma
11. Less common situations:
    - Pheochromocytoma crisis
    - Tyramine interaction with monoamine oxidase (MAO)-inhibitors
    - Overdose with sympathomimetic drugs, such as phencyclidine, lysergic acid diethylamide (LSD), cocaine, or phenylpropanolamines
    - Rebound hypertension following the sudden withdrawal of antihypertensive agents, such as clonidine or beta-blockers

A descriptive meta-analysis of 86,137 hypertensive subjects in 590 randomized trials collected by the United States Food and Drug Administration (FDA) from 1973 to 2001 showed no significant difference (relative risk [RR]: 1.03, 95% CI: 0.71 to 1.47, $p = 0.86$) regarding short-term "irreversible harm" (a composite of death, stroke, and myocardial infarction [MI]) between subjects randomized to placebo or active drug treatment who dropped out of the trials.[12] There is currently much more evidence showing harm, and little (if any) showing benefit, from acute BP lowering in asymptomatic patients with major BP elevations. Unfortunately, use of the term, "urgency," has led some physicians to over-aggressively treat some patients in emergency departments with one or more parenteral medications, with the object of rapidly normalizing their BP. Although this procedure can impress the patient with the importance of BP-lowering, wild swings in BP have been associated with stroke, MI, and other tragedies. Even oral loading doses of antihypertensive agents can lead to cumulative effects, including hypotension, sometimes following discharge from the emergency department. A now-classic randomized clinical trial by Zeller et al, published in 1989, found no significant difference in BP control at 24 hours between groups of patients who had or had not received clonidine loading before initiation of appropriate chronic oral antihypertensive therapy. This conclusion was recently corroborated by the finding of no significant differences in any outcome for 435 emergency department patients with markedly elevated BPs, but without target-organ damage who received oral antihypertensive therapy, compared with 581 similar patients who received no acute therapy.[13] Many believe that the traditional classification of "hypertensive urgency" needs to be updated (if not abandoned), and that more diagnostic importance should be placed on presenting signs and symptoms, rather than focusing on the BP level. Some have advocated replacing the term, "hypertensive urgency," with "major BP elevation without ongoing target organ damage."

CLINICAL EVALUATION

Early triage of hypertensive emergency versus major BP elevation without ongoing target organ damage should limit the expenditure of scarce health care resources to those who truly need acute care and close monitoring, and reduce their morbidity and mortality.[14] The evaluation of patients presenting with hypertensive crises should include a targeted history, focused physical examination and a limited laboratory examination to differentiate these two conditions. The main purpose of the diagnostic exercise is to assess whether target organ damage is acute and progressive.

The clinical presentation of hypertensive emergencies is most easily classified according to the target organ involved; the prevalence of each type is variable across the large reports. The most common of these include: cerebral infarction (20% to 25%), pulmonary edema (14% to 31%), hypertensive encephalopathy (0% to 16%), acute coronary syndrome (12% to 25%), intracerebral or subarachnoid hemorrhage (4% to 15%), eclampsia (0% to 4%), or aortic dissection (0% to 2%).[3-10,14] A focused history should be obtained, especially regarding headaches, seizures, mental status changes, chest pain, shortness of breath, change in urination, and development of edema. A standardized sphygmomanometer with an appropriately sized cuff should be used to measure BP because many automated BP monitors are inaccurate at very high levels. All patients should have a funduscopic examination by an experienced clinician, looking carefully for hemorrhages, exudates, and/or papilledema. The value of this examination has been questioned[15] because it is neither sensitive nor specific for hypertensive encephalopathy, and interexaminer reliability is low.[16] However, a recent case-series using nonmydriatic ocular fundus photography documented grade III or IV hypertensive retinopathy in 33% of 21 subjects presenting to Emory University Hospital Emergency Department with DBPs 120 mm Hg or higher.[17] A cardiovascular exam should document radial, femoral, and carotid pulses. Pulse deficits should raise the suspicion of aortic dissection. A thorough neurological examination, including mental status, should be conducted.

Few recent studies have determined the prognostic value of abnormal laboratory findings in asymptomatic patients with major elevations in BP, but this is a very valuable method of screening for, and documenting, acute target organ damage. The laboratory evaluation should include a complete blood count, including peripheral smear, to look for schistocytes (indicative of microangiopathic hemolytic anemia[18]), a metabolic profile (blood urea nitrogen, serum creatinine, electrolytes), and a urinalysis. Although proteinuria is important prognostically (particularly if acutely increased, compared with baseline),[19] the most important findings are red blood cells (RBCs) and RBC casts, typical of acute glomerular and/or tubular injury. An electrocardiogram and portable chest radiograph should be performed for patients with chest pain or dyspnea, but not for asymptomatic individuals. For patients with an acute change in mental status or acute neurological signs and symptoms suggestive of cerebral encephalopathy, ischemia or hemorrhage, a computed tomographic (CT) scan of the head should be performed. Antihypertensive drug therapy may need to be initiated before all test results are obtained or the underlying cause of the emergency is determined.

One approach to therapy of hypertensive emergencies stratifies patients according to the patient's plasma renin activity or direct renin level.[20] In most hospitals, the laboratory turnaround time is too long for this strategy to be useful. Until this scheme is prospectively evaluated, empiric treatment for patients with a hypertensive emergency will remain the standard of care.

CLINICAL MANAGEMENT

Because it is no longer ethical to withhold antihypertensive treatment from patients presenting with hypertensive crises, any recent evidence-base for such therapy is lacking.[21,22] Such treatment is, by definition, only provided in the short-term

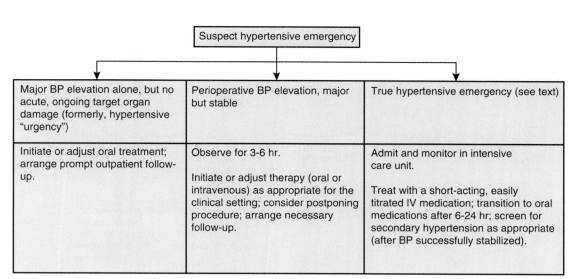

FIG. 46.1 Evaluation of suspected hypertensive emergencies.

(minutes-to-hours), and is routinely followed by conventional oral antihypertensive agents; it is therefore unlikely that long-term CVD outcome differences could be demonstrated.[21,22] No long-term data from randomized clinical trials of different drugs in hypertensive emergencies have been collected; instead, existing data come from long-term cohort studies, comparative trials of acute BP-lowering agents, and expert opinion.[3-10,14,19,21-26] Nonetheless, all authorities agree that therapeutic decisions should be based on the presence of acute, ongoing target-organ damage and not solely on the level of BP. The first priority should be to diagnose each patient who presents with very high BP as shown in Fig. 46.1.

Hypertensive Emergencies

When a hypertensive emergency has been diagnosed, antihypertensive drug therapy should be initiated immediately. This often occurs before the results of all laboratory studies are available. Once the patient is more clinically stable, investigation into the cause of the presentation should be performed.

The primary goal in treating the patient with a hypertensive emergency is to limit target organ damage, by allowing autoregulation to be reestablished in important vascular beds. In most patients with hypertensive emergencies, the BP-flow curve (Fig. 46.2) is shifted, over time, upward and to the right. Lowering BP suddenly, or to a level that would otherwise be considered "normal" (e.g., downward arrow in Fig. 46.2) would leave the patient with an acutely underperfused vascular bed, and may lead to ischemia (cerebral, myocardial, renal, or other). Parenteral therapy is recommended because it can be precisely controlled, and its antihypertensive effect rapidly stopped, should the patient's BP suddenly fall. Although many hospitals have protocols prohibiting the use of short-acting parenteral antihypertensive agents outside of intensive care units, such therapy can be started by a physician at the bedside (even in the Emergency Department), and continued during transfer to a monitored hospital bed. Although there is no clinical trial evidence, experience recommends a reduction in mean arterial pressure to no more than 25% below pretreatment level within the first 2 hours after presentation. Over the next 2 to 6 hours, BP can be reduced slowly toward 160/100 mm Hg. If this level of BP is well tolerated and the patient is clinically stable, further gradual reductions can be implemented in the next 24 to 48 hours. The most notable exceptions to these general targets (see later) are with acute aortic dissection (SBP target: <120 mm Hg over 20 minutes), and acute ischemic stroke-in-evolution (for which no BP lowering

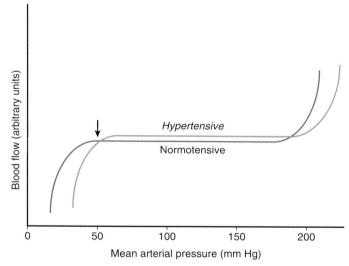

FIG. 46.2 Blood pressure-blood flow relationships in normotensive and chronically hypertensive people. Note that each vascular bed has a different set of usual perfusion pressures, and blood flow is given in arbitrary units. This accounts for why chronically hypertensive people can still maintain reasonable perfusion at very high blood pressures (compared with normotensive people), and for why lowering blood pressure to normal (indicated by the small downward arrow) in chronically hypertensive people leads to hypoperfusion.

is generally recommended in the U.S.). Some of the agents often used in the management of the hypertensive emergencies are listed in Table 46.1. Once BP has been lowered safely for a sufficient period to allow restoration of normal autoregulation (typically 12 to 24 hours), oral agents can be started as the parenteral agent is tapered, thus avoiding rebound hypertension. Typically, patients with hypertensive emergencies are volume depleted, so loop diuretics are not recommended, unless there is evidence of volume overload. The judicious use of diuretics may be necessary after many (typically >12) hours of intravenous vasodilator therapy because, with the exception of fenoldopam,[26] use of these agents is accompanied by sodium and volume retention, and resistance to further BP reduction (so-called "tachyphylaxis").

Much experience, and a recent report[27] indicate that patients with a hypertensive emergency have a higher-than-usual prevalence of secondary hypertension. A 24-hour urine collection that contains levels of catecholamine metabolites within the reference range is strong evidence against pheochromocytoma; screening for renovascular hypertension,

TABLE 46.1 Parenteral Drugs for Hypertensive Emergencies

DRUG	USUAL DOSE	ONSET OF ACTION	DURATION OF ACTION	ADVERSE EFFECTS	SPECIAL FEATURE(S)	SPECIAL CAUTION
Sodium nitroprusside	0.25-8 µg/kg/min (IV)	~20 seconds	1-2 minutes	Nausea, vomiting, muscle spasm	Least expensive to obtain	Cyanide and/or thiocyanate toxicity; contraindicated in pregnancy; shield from light
Nitroglycerin	5-100 µg/min (IV)	2-5 minutes	5-10 minutes	Headache, vomiting, methemoglobinemia, tolerance with prolonged use	Coronary ischemia, acute LV failure, post-CABG	Unpredictable antihypertensive effects; sticks to IV equipment
Fenoldopam mesylate	0.1-1.5 µg/kg/min (IV)	<5 minutes	~20 minutes	Reflex tachycardia, nausea, vomiting, flushing, increased intraocular pressure	Increases several parameters related to renal function, may not require intraarterial line	Caution with glaucoma
Esmolol	250-500 µg/kg/min (IV bolus), then 50-100 µg/kg/min (IV)	1-2 minutes	10-30 minutes	Nausea, first-degree heart block, heart failure	Aortic dissection, myocardial infarction, thyrotoxicosis, post-CABG	Asthma; avoid in cocaine-related hypertension
Enalaprilat	1.25-5 mg IV (q 6 hours)	15-30 minutes	6-12 hours	Acute hypotension not easily reversible; variable response	Acute LV failure, scleroderma renal crisis	Contraindicated with bilateral renal artery stenosis, pregnancy
Labetalol	20-80 mg IV bolus or 0.5-2 mg/min (IV)	5-10 minutes	3-6 hours	Nausea, vomiting, flushing, heart block, orthostatic hypotension	Often used in eclampsia	Contraindicated with heart block, asthma, pregnancy; avoid in acute heart failure
Nicardipine	5-15 mg/hour (IV)	5-10 minutes	1-4 hours	Tachycardia, flushing, headache	Reduces both cardiac and cerebral ischemia; dose not weight-dependent	Avoid in acute heart failure
Clevidipine	1-16 mg/hour	2-4 minutes	5-15 minutes	Headache, nausea, vomiting, reflex tachycardia	Dose not weight-dependent; hydrolyzed by plasma esterases	Given in lipid emulsion through a separate IV line
Hydralazine	10-20 mg (IV); 10-40 mg (IM)	10-20 min (IV); 20-30 min (IM)	1-4 hours (IV); 4-6 hours (IM)	Tachycardia, flushing, headache, vomiting, angina pectoris	Most often used for eclampsia	Contraindicated in coronary heart disease, aortic dissection
Diazoxide	50-100 mg bolus (IV or IM), or 15-30 mg/min (IV)	2-4 minutes	6-12 hours	Nausea, vomiting, precipitous hypotension	Probably obsolete	Sodium/water retention, hyperglycemia, hyperuricemia; contraindicated in coronary heart disease, aortic dissection
Phentolamine	5-15 mg (IV)	1-2 minutes	3-10 minutes	Tachycardia, flushing, headache, orthostatic hypotension	Catecholamine excess states (cocaine, MAO-inhibitor crisis, pheochromocytoma)	Contraindicated in preexisting coronary heart disease

CABG, Coronary-artery bypass graft; *IM,* intramuscular; *IV,* intravenous; *LV,* left ventricular; *MAO,* monoamine oxidase.

sleep apnea, and hyperaldosteronism can be easily and inexpensively performed on the day or so before hospital discharge.

SPECIAL SITUATIONS

Aortic Dissection

The initial aim of medical therapy in patients with acute aortic dissection is to decrease both BP and shear stress on the torn aorta (by decreasing δP/δt and cardiac contractility). Short-acting, easily titratable beta-blockers, such as esmolol and labetalol, are most commonly recommended. If a beta-blocker is contraindicated, diltiazem can be used. Although there are no clinical trial data to prove it, many authorities recommend that patients presenting with an acute aortic dissection should achieve an SBP less than 120 mm Hg within 20 minutes, if tolerated.[28] Generally, nitroprusside is given to achieve this BP target. Direct vasodilators such as diazoxide, hydralazine, and minoxidil should not be used alone, as these drugs increase sympathetic activity, worsen myocardial ischemia, and increase shear stress on the aorta. Surgical consultation should be obtained as soon as possible.

Myocardial Infarction

The primary goal in this setting is to open the offending blocked coronary artery; a variety of medications can be used to lower BP and decrease myocardial oxygen demand. Intravenous beta-blockers and/or nitroglycerin can both be useful.[3-10,14,21,23,24] As with aortic dissection, monotherapy with direct vasodilators should be avoided.

Pulmonary Edema/Heart Failure

Intravenous nitroglycerin or sodium nitroprusside may be used to lower BP.[4-10,23,24] Angiotensin-converting enzyme (ACE) inhibitors have been used extensively because of beneficial effects on both preload and afterload, but can cause precipitous BP lowering that is difficult to reverse. Diuretics may be used as needed for volume control, but a recent placebo controlled trial showed no improvement in dyspnea scores or other outcomes.[29] Furthermore, diuretics can exacerbate pressure natriuresis, further stimulate the renin-angiotensin system, and cause hyponatremia.

Ischemic Stroke

Routine BP-lowering in the setting of an acute ischemic stroke-in-evolution is not currently recommended in the U.S. Although hypertension is very common in this setting, the elevated BP may be a physiological compensatory response, increasing cerebral perfusion to ischemic brain tissue. Lowering BP (especially if rapid or to a great extent) can acutely worsen ischemia and expand the ischemic penumbra. Current U.S. national guidelines recommend labetalol or nicardipine (or another agent, when appropriate) if the patient is a candidate for acute reperfusion therapy, except the BP is higher than 185/110 mm Hg.[30] Otherwise, cautious BP reduction by 15% over the first 24 hours is recommended **only** if the SBP higher than 220 mm Hg or DBP higher than 120 mm Hg.[30] In either case, careful monitoring of patients for neurological deterioration is warranted.[30] Many physicians prefer sodium nitroprusside, or esmolol, because they are very short-acting and can be swiftly discontinued. Calcium channel blockers (CCBs) may increase intracranial pressure, and are generally avoided in patients with acute ischemic stroke.

Hemorrhagic Stroke

Nimodipine, a short-acting dihydropyridine CCB with weak antihypertensive properties, is given orally to patients with subarachnoid hemorrhage to decrease cerebral arterial spasm and rebleeding. Current U.S. stroke guidelines recommend consideration of lowering BP in patients with acute cerebral hemorrhage if SBP higher than 220 mm Hg.[31] For non-American subjects who presented within 6 hours of onset of symptoms of intracranial hemorrhage with BPs between 150 and 220 mm Hg, the Intensive Blood Pressure Reduction in Acute Cerebral Hemorrhage Trial 2 (INTERACT2) showed that lowering SBP to 140 mm Hg was safe, and barely failed to show a significant benefit on death or major disability (*p* = 0.06) at 90 days, although several secondary endpoints did achieve putative statistical significance.[32] Current U.S. stroke guidelines therefore recommend that, for Americans with acute intracranial hemorrhage and SBPs between 150 and 220 mm Hg, antihypertensive therapy may be given if there are no contraindications.[31]

Preeclampsia

Magnesium sulfate, methyldopa, hydralazine, labetalol, and perhaps nifedipine have a long and successful track record in preeclampsia treatment (see Chapter 39). Renin inhibitors, ACE inhibitors, angiotensin receptor blockers, and nitroprusside are contraindicated in pregnancy.

Catecholamine Crisis

Pheochromocytoma, a very rare cause of hypertensive crisis (see Chapter 15), is usually successfully treated intravenously with the nonselective alpha-blocker, phentolamine. A beta-blocker can be added, if needed to control tachycardia. Administration of a beta-blocker alone leaves the alpha-receptors unblocked, and can abruptly increase BP. Treatment failures have been reported with either a selective alpha$_1$-blocker (e.g., doxazosin) or labetalol, an alpha, beta-blocker. Sympathomimetic drugs, such as phenylephrine, cocaine, or methamphetamine can also cause hypertensive crises. Phentolamine, labetalol, or nitroprusside have each been successfully used in this situation.

Perioperative Hypertension

BP elevation during the perioperative period can result from adrenergic stimulation from the surgical event, changes in intravascular volume, or postoperative pain or anxiety (see Chapter 44). With the exception of ACE inhibitors, patients typically take their usual outpatient oral antihypertensive regimen on the day of surgery, and oral agents restarted as soon as possible thereafter. If oral therapy is not possible, other routes of administration (e.g., intravenous clevidipine or labetalol, transdermal clonidine) can be substituted temporarily. Patients with BP levels 180/110 mm Hg or higher either before or immediately after surgery have a greater risk for perioperative cardiac events, and often have their procedure postponed in favor of better BP-lowering over the next 24 hours.

Miscellaneous

In other clinical situations in which major BP elevation is accompanied by gross hematuria, epistaxis, mental status changes, agitation, or severe anxiety, intravenous antihypertensive therapy may be appropriate. Both clonidine and methyldopa should be avoided in hypertensive encephalopathy because of their potential for adverse central nervous system effects.

Major Blood Pressure Elevation Without Ongoing Target Organ Damage (Hypertensive "Urgency")

After ruling out a true hypertensive emergency, a more thorough history should address the duration and severity of hypertension. Most such patients have been diagnosed with hypertension, but are nonadherent to their medications; some have pain or anxiety as their primary problem.[11,13,14] The patient's medication profile should be reviewed, focusing on antihypertensive agents, but including other prescription, alternative, over-the-counter, and recreational drugs (especially cocaine). Intoxication with either alcohol or illicit drugs can elevate BP. Acute withdrawal from some drugs (e.g., clonidine), may cause rebound hypertension. Sympathomimetic medications such as decongestants, anticholinergics, amphetamines, or cocaine may acutely elevate BP.

Serial BP measurements should be obtained before drug therapy is given, as BP often falls spontaneously; 32% of such patients had a "satisfactory response" to 30 minutes of rest in one recent series.[33] The major BP elevation, per se, carries little short-term CVD risk[5-10,12-14,21,22,34]; sometimes, the risk of acute antihypertensive drug treatment is even greater. Nifedipine capsules or intravenous diazoxide can cause precipitous and unpredictable hypotension, and acute stroke or myocardial infarction; these agents are now rarely used. A recent systematic review of therapeutic options for treatment in this setting showed no outcome differences across agents, with slightly better tolerability for ACE inhibitors over CCBs.[35] Most patients with major elevations in BP without acute target organ damage should be treated with at least oral agents, with the intent to decrease their BP over the next 24 to 48 hours. Resuming a previous regimen that the patient tolerated well is a reasonable alternative. Patients may leave the emergency department with an elevated BP as long as there is a definite plan for prompt follow-up for reevaluation and chronic management. Follow-up is very important for all patients with substantial BP elevations, as some patients mistake treatment provided in the emergency situation as a "cure," and do not understand the benefit of long-term BP control. Patients therefore require close clinical follow-up to monitor their adherence to medications and lifestyle modifications, such as tobacco avoidance, physical activity, dietary management, and weight loss. This is an opportunity to improve long-term BP control that should not be lost.

SUMMARY

A hypertensive emergency is a major elevation in BP accompanied by progressive, acute target-organ damage, for example, acute coronary or cerebral ischemia, pulmonary edema, acute kidney injury, aortic dissection, or eclampsia. This condition, if untreated, carries a very high mortality and should be promptly treated with a short-acting, easily titrated, intravenous medication in a monitored setting. Although BP should be reduced within minutes to hours, the initial reduction in mean arterial pressure over the first few hours should be no more than 20% to 25% of baseline BP, to avoid hypoperfusion of vital organs. Once stable, patients should be investigated more thoroughly for a remediable cause of hypertension. Proper education and appropriate follow-up should be arranged to ensure continued and optimal management of hypertension as well as the other cardiovascular risk factors usually present.

Often the result of inadequate treatment of preexisting hypertension, a hypertensive "urgency" is a major elevation of BP without evidence of progressive, acute target-organ damage. Such patients should be treated as outpatients with one or more oral medication(s) to achieve BP control over days. Providing close follow-up in an ambulatory setting to achieve BP control, as well as proper education to avoid future "urgent" presentations is recommended. The major distinguishing feature of the true hypertensive emergency from the "hypertensive urgency" is the presence of ongoing acute target organ damage, not the degree of BP elevation itself.

References

1. Yoon SS, Fryar CD, Carroll MD. Hypertension prevalence and control among adults: United States, 2011-2014. NCHS data brief, no. 220. Hyattsville, MD: National Center for Health Statistics; November, 2015. www.cdc.gov/nchs/data/databriefs/db220.pdf.
2. Mozaffarian D, Benjamin EJ, Go AS, et al. Heart Disease and Stroke Statistics—2016 Update. A report from the American Heart Association. *Circulation.* 2016;133:e38-e60.
3. Cremer A, Amraoui F, Lip GY, et al. From malignant hypertension to hypertension-MOD: a modern definition for an old but still dangerous emergency. *J Hum Hypertens.* 2016;30:463-466.
4. Mancia G, Fagard R, Narkiewicz K, et al. 2013 ESH/ESC guidelines for the management of arterial hypertension: the Task Force for the Management of Arterial Hypertension of the European Society of Hypertension (ESH) and the European Society of Cardiology (ESC). *Eur Heart J.* 2013;34:2159-2219.
5. Muiesan ML, Salvetti M, Amadoro V, et al. for the Working Group on Hypertension, Prevention, Rehabilitation of the Italian Society of Cardiology, the Societa' Italiana dell'Ipertensione Arteriosa. An update on hypertensive emergencies and urgencies. *J Cardiovasc Med (Hagerstown).* 2015;16:372-382.
6. Agabiti-Rosei E, Salvetti M, Farsang C. European Society of Hypertension Scientific Newsletter: treatment of hypertensive urgencies and emergencies. *J Hypertens.* 2006;24:2482-2485 (also available in *Blood Press.* 2006; 15: 255-256).
7. Adebayo O, Rogers RL. Hypertensive emergencies in the emergency department. *Emerg Med Clin North Am.* 2015;33:539-551.
8. Papadopoulos DP, Sanidas EA, Viniou NA, et al. Cardiovascular hypertensive emergencies. *Curr Hypertens Rep.* 2015;17:5.
9. Wolf SJ, Lo B, Shih RD, Smith MD, Fesmire FM. American College of Emergency Physicians Clinical Policies Committee. Clinical Policy: critical issues in the evaluation and management of adult patients in the emergency department with asymptomatic elevated blood pressure. *Ann Emerg Med.* 2013;62:59-68.
10. Pak KJ, Hu T, Fee C, Wang R, Smith M, Bazzano LA. Acute hypertension: a systematic review and appraisal of guidelines. *Ochsner J.* 2014;14:655-663.
11. Saguner AM, Dür S, Perrig M, et al. Risk factors promoting hypertensive crises: evidence from a longitudinal study. *Am J Hypertens.* 2010;23:775-780.
12. DeFelice A, Willard J, Lawrence J, et al. The risks associated with short-term placebo-controlled antihypertensive clinical trials: a descriptive meta-analysis. *J Hum Hypertens.* 2008;22:659-668.
13. Levy PD, Mahn JJ, Miller J, et al. Blood pressure treatment and outcomes in hypertensive patients without acute target organ damage: a retrospective cohort. *Am J Emerg Med.* 2015;33:1219-1224.
14. Goldberg EM, Shah K, Shavne P. An evidence-based approach to managing asymptomatic elevated blood pressure in the emergency department. *Emerg Med Pract.* 2015;17:1-24.
15. van den Born BJ, Hulsman CA, Hoekstra JB, Schlingemann RO, van Montfrans GA. Value of routine funduscopy in patients with hypertension: systematic review. *BMJ.* 2005;331:73-76.
16. Amraoui F, van Montfrans GA, van den Born BJ. Value of retinal examination in hypertensive encephalopathy. *J Hum Hypertens.* 2010;24:274-279.
17. Henderson AD, Biousse V, Newman NJ, Lamirel C, Wright DW, Bruce BB. Grade III or IV hypertensive retinopathy with severely elevated blood pressure. *West J Emerg Med.* 2012;13:529-534.
18. Shavit L, Reinus C, Slotkl I. Severe renal failure and microangiopathic hemolysis induced by malignant hypertension—Case series and review of literature. *Clin Nephrol.* 2010;73:147-152.
19. Gonzàles R, Morales E, Segura J, Ruilope LM, Praga M. Long-term renal survival in malignant hypertension. *Nephrol Dial Transplant.* 2010;25:3266-3272.
20. Blumenfeld JD, Laragh JH. Management of hypertensive crises: the scientific basis for treatment decisions. *Am J Hypertens.* 2001;14:1154-1167.
21. Cherney D, Straus S. Management of patients with hypertensive urgencies and emergencies: a systematic review of the literature. *J Gen Intern Med.* 2002;17:937-945.
22. Vadera R. Does antihypertensive drug therapy decrease morbidity or mortality in patients with a hypertensive emergency? *Ann Emerg Med.* 2011;57:64-65.
23. Perez MI, Musini VM. Pharmacologic interventions for hypertensive emergencies: a Cochrane systematic review. *J Hum Hypertens.* 2008;22:596-607 (also available as *Cochrane Database Syst Rev.* 2008;23:CD003653).
24. Padilla Ramos A, Varon J. Current and newer agents for hypertensive emergencies. *Curr Hypertens Rep.* 2014;16:450.
25. Keating GM. Clevidipine: a review of its use for managing blood pressure in perioperative and intensive care settings. *Drugs.* 2014;74:1947-1960.
26. Murphy MB, Murray C, Shorten GD. Fenoldopam—A selective peripheral dopamine-receptor agonist for the treatment of severe hypertension. *N Engl J Med.* 2001; 345:1548-1555.
27. Börgel J, Springer S, Ghafoor J, et al. Unrecognized secondary causes of hypertension in patients with hypertensive urgency/emergency: prevalence and co-prevalence. *Clin Res Cardiol.* 2010;99:499-506.
28. Hiratzka LF, Bakris GL, Beckman JA, et al. 2010 ACCF/AHA/AATS/ACR/ASA/SCA/SCAI/SIR/STS/SVM guidelines for the diagnosis and management of patients with thoracic aortic disease: a report of the American College of Cardiology Foundation/American Heart Association Task Force on Practice Guidelines, American Association for Thoracic Surgery, American College of Radiology, American Stroke Association, Society of Cardiovascular Anesthesiologists, Society for Cardiovascular Angiography and Interventions, Society of Interventional Radiology, Society of Thoracic Surgeons, and Society for Vascular Medicine. *Circulation.* 2010;121:e266-e369.
29. Holzer-Richling N, Holzer M, Herkner H, et al. Randomized placebo controlled trial of furosemide on subjective perception of dyspnoea in patients with pulmonary oedema because of hypertensive crisis. *Eur J Clin Invest.* 2011;41:627-634.
30. Jauch EC, Saver JL, Adams HP Jr, et al. Guidelines for the early management of patients with acute ischemic stroke: a guideline for healthcare professionals from the American Heart Association/American Stroke Association. *Stroke.* 2013;44:870-947.
31. Hemphill JC III, Greenberg SM, Anderson CS, et al. Guidelines for the management of spontaneous intracerebral hemorrhage: a guideline for healthcare professionals from the American Heart Association/American Stroke Association. *Stroke.* 2015;46:2032-2060.
32. Anderson CS, Heeley E, Huang Y, et al. on behalf of the INTERACT2 Investigators. Rapid blood-pressure lowering in patients with acute intracerebral hemorrhage. *N Engl J Med.* 2013;368:2355-2365.
33. Grassi D, O'Flaherty M, Pellizzari M, et al. for the REHASE Program. Hypertensive urgencies in the emergency department: evaluating blood pressure response to rest and to antihypertensive drugs with different profiles. *J Clin Hypertens (Greenwich).* 2008;10:662-667.
34. Vicek M, Bur A, Woisetschläger C, Herkner H, Laggner AN, Hirschl MM. Association between hypertensive urgencies and subsequent cardiovascular events in patients with hypertension. *J Hypertens.* 2008;26:657-662.
35. Souza LM, Riera R, Saconato H, Demathé A, Atallah AN. Oral drugs for hypertensive urgencies: systematic review and meta-analysis. *Sao Paulo Med J.* 2009;127:366-372.

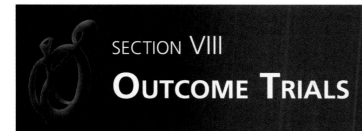

47 Meta-Analyses of Blood Pressure Lowering Trials and the Blood Pressure Lowering Treatment Trialists' Collaboration

Kazem Rahimi and Vlado Perkovic

Over the last few decades, meta-analyses have been central to the advancement of knowledge in a broad range of medical specialties. The "conscientious, explicit and judicious use" of the evidence provided by this technique now underpins much of clinical practice and allows clinicians to make truly informed decisions about how best to deliver care to many different types of patients.[1] In the field of cardiovascular (CV) disease, meta-analyses of the effects of different blood pressure (BP) lowering regimens have allowed for the integrated interpretation of the effects of different therapeutic approaches, and have provided precise estimates of the effects of BP lowering on major CV events, including stroke and coronary heart disease (CHD). As a result, practitioners are now better informed about the implications of their choices of BP-lowering treatment than almost any other mode of therapy to which they have access. For example, meta-analyses have made it possible to determine whether or not important differences exist between drug classes in the protection they afford against different types of serious CV events, and to identify whether the benefits obtained vary according to important characteristics of patients such as risk, age, gender, and the presence or absence of underlying disease. This chapter outlines some key features of meta-analyses and reports the main findings from the most recent, large meta-analyses, including those from the Blood Pressure Lowering Treatment Trialists' Collaboration (BPLTTC).

META-ANALYSES

The term *meta-analysis* describes the statistical procedure whereby the results of several different studies addressing the same or related question are combined in an effort to obtain a more precise and more reliable answer to the question under investigation.[2] The technique may be used for quantitatively summarizing data from a range of different study designs (both observational and interventional), usually through identification of relevant studies in a systematic review of the literature. Meta-analyses of randomized controlled trials have been particularly useful because, although the individual estimates provided by small or modest sized trials may be imprecise, the estimates are usually not biased, as long as the individual trials are properly conducted. Thus the combined result of relevant, high-quality randomized controlled trials should give both a more precise and accurate estimate of the real effect of the intervention under investigation, when compared with the findings from individual trials. In addition to providing a more reliable answer to the original research question posed by individual trials, and by providing clarity in fields where there may be individual studies that may appear to be inconsistent, large meta-analyses often have the statistical power to go beyond those original questions by investigating complementary questions relating to treatment effects in important patient subgroups or on less commonly investigated outcomes.

Ultimately, any meta-analysis will have differences in the characteristics of the included trials; for example, trials addressing the effects of different BP-lowering regimens on major CV events have frequently been combined, but included quite varied participants and markedly different durations of follow-up. Likewise, there are many trials investigating the effects of regimens based on one drug class compared with another, but the specific drugs used and the dosing regimens used vary among them. Whether such differences in trial characteristics ultimately strengthen or weaken meta-analysis findings has been the topic of considerable discussion. On balance, it appears that the availability of multiple different studies with different characteristics probably strengthens, rather than weakens, the conclusions. In particular, exploration of the constancy of treatment effects across different participant subgroups and different trial groupings can be done, if a range of similar but not identical trials is included.

The value of meta-analyses depends on the quality and scope of the individual trials included in them. To obtain unbiased estimates of the treatment effect in a meta-analysis of randomized controlled trials, it is essential that the trials included in the meta-analysis are individually and collectively unbiased. It is well established that trials with inconclusive or unfavorable results are not published as frequently as trials with positive findings (i.e., publication bias), and the systematic exclusion of unpublished neutral or negative trials could result in effect estimates from a meta-analysis being biased toward a positive result.[3] Meta-analyses based solely on published data and done without the cooperation of industry or lead investigators in the field are relatively easy to conduct, but may be especially prone to publication bias. By contrast, more resource-intensive meta-analysis projects conducted by large, well-informed collaborative networks, are less subject to publication bias. Example of such collaborative meta-analyses are those conducted by the Blood Pressure Lowering Treatment Trialists' Collaboration,[4-11] the Cholesterol Treatment Trialists' Collaboration,[12] and the Antithrombotic Treatment Trialists' Collaboration.[13] The prospective and comprehensive nature of such projects limits the potential for bias, because major decisions about analysis and reporting are often specified *before* the results of any of the contributing trials are known or before pooled analyses are conducted, and major efforts by the broad collaborative group ensure that all relevant trials are identified. With strong collaborative arrangements, there is also considerably enhanced scope for the standardization of outcome definitions and the sharing of individual patient-specific datasets with consequent analytic advantages.

The following sections outline the findings from large meta-analyses of different BP-lowering regimens, which have helped shape our knowledge of their effects on major CV events.

THE BLOOD PRESSURE LOWERING TREATMENT TRIALISTS' COLLABORATION

The BPLTTC is an international collaboration involving the principal investigators of large randomized trials of BP-lowering regimens. The collaboration was established in 1995 with the broad aim of providing the most reliable evidence possible about the effects of commonly used BP-lowering drugs on major CV events using prospective meta-analyses of randomized trials. The meta-analyses are all conducted and reported in accordance with protocols[4] that prespecify research questions, trial eligibility criteria, outcomes, main treatment comparisons, and analysis plans.

Trials are eligible for inclusion in the BPLTTC if they satisfy one of the following criteria: (1) random allocation of patients to regimens based on different BP-lowering agents, (2) random allocation of patients to a BP-lowering agent or placebo, or (3) random allocation of patients to various BP goals. In addition, eligible trials must have a (planned) minimum follow-up of 1000 patient-years per treatment arm. Although trials with factorial assignment to other interventions such as cholesterol-lowering treatment are eligible for inclusion, trials in which additional treatments are jointly assigned with BP-lowering treatment are not eligible, as these other treatments act as potential confounders. For the initial cycle of the collaboration, trials could not have published or presented main trial results before the establishment of the Collaboration in 1995. However, more recently the collaboration has widened its scope with the aim of addressing some of the key remaining questions relating to safety and efficacy of blood pressure lowering.

One key feature of the collaboration is that it gathers individual participant level data from each participating trial wherever possible. The three key advantages of such individual participant data meta-analyses are (1) the benefit of

carrying out detailed data checking, (2) the opportunity to better stratify participants into important subgroups using a consistent approach across trials, and (3) the possibility of time-to-event analysis, which increase statistical power, and standard tabular meta-analyses based on aggregate participant data are unable to provide. As per initial agreements, the data requested from investigators included participant characteristics recorded at screening or randomization, selected measurements made during follow-up, and details of the occurrence of all prespecified outcomes during the scheduled follow-up period. In the third cycle of the data collection, which commenced in 2014, all new and existing collaborators were asked to share the full trial dataset, if possible, to facilitate a series of new analyses relating to safety and efficacy of blood pressure lowering.

Since its establishment, the BPLTTC has reported the findings of the overall effects of different BP-lowering regimens in a broad range of patients at risk of CV disease, as well as the effects in specific patient subgroups classified according to patient age, gender, baseline BP, baseline CV risk, and presence or absence of diabetes mellitus (DM). In parallel, there have been other large-scale meta-analyses of BP lowering which have complemented the evidence-base that has been generated by the collaboration.

OVERALL EFFECTS OF BLOOD PRESSURE LOWERING AMONG HIGH-RISK PATIENTS WITH ELEVATED BLOOD PRESSURE

The second cycle of BPLTTC reported updated overall effects of different BP-lowering regimens on major CV events based on data from 29 trials and nearly 160,000 patients. In the majority of trials, patients were selected on the basis of high BP and an additional CV risk factor such as DM, renal disease, or increased age. The overall mean age of participants was 65 years, and just over half (52%) were men. The mean duration of follow-up for contributing trials ranged from 2.0 to 8.4 years, resulting in over 700,000 patient-years of follow-up.

This analysis showed that, compared with placebo, significant reductions in the risk of stroke (28%-38%) and CHD (22%) could be achieved with regimens based on angiotensin-converting enzyme (ACE) inhibitors or calcium channel blockers (CCBs) (Fig. 47.1). In trials that randomized patients to receive either more intensive (lower BP targets) or less intensive BP-lowering regimens, there was also a significant reduction in stroke and a nonsignificant trend toward benefit for CHD with more intensive BP reduction. Heart failure (HF) events were defined as those resulting in death or admission to hospital, and the overviews demonstrated a protective effect against these events from regimens based on ACE inhibitors compared with placebo (18%), a nonsignificant trend toward harm for CCB-based regimens, and a nonsignificant trend toward benefit for regimens targeting lower BP goals.

More than 17,000 major CV events (a composite outcome comprising stroke, CHD, and HF events plus death from any CV cause) contributed to the overview analyses (see Fig. 47.1). There were significant reductions in the risk of this summary outcome measure with active treatment based on either ACE inhibitors (22%) or CCB (18%) compared with placebo, and for more intensive compared with less intensive regimens (14%). For fatal events attributable to CV or all causes, ACE inhibitor–based regimens reduced the risk of death by 20% or 12%, respectively, compared with placebo. There was also a trend toward fewer CV deaths with CCB–based regimens. However, there was no clear evidence of a reduction in risk for fatal CV events or death from any cause with regimens targeting lower BP goals.

These findings from BPLTTC have been confirmed and extended by other large-scale meta-analyses. In a report based on aggregate data from 123 studies with 613,815

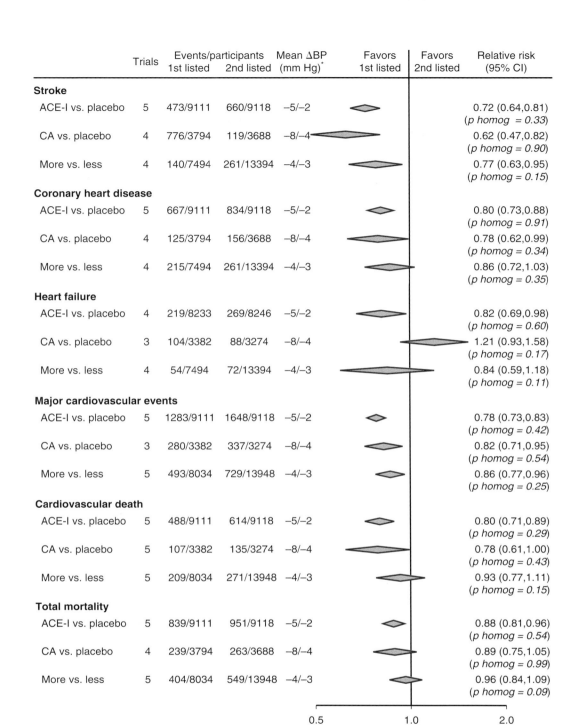

FIG. 47.1 Effects of angiotensin-converting enzyme (ACE) inhibitor and calcium antagonist (CA) compared with placebo and more intensive compared with less intensive blood pressure–lowering regimens on the risks of major vascular outcomes and death. *Overall mean blood pressure difference (systolic/diastolic) during follow-up in the actively treated group compared with the control group, calculated by weighing the difference observed in each contributing trial by the number of individuals in the trial. The negative values indicate lower mean follow-up blood pressure levels in the first-listed treatment groups (i.e., ACE inhibitors, CA, more). *ACE-I,* ACE inhibitor; *CI,* confidence intervals; *more,* more intensive blood pressure–lowering regimen; *less,* less intensive blood pressure lowering regimen. *(Adapted from Blood Pressure Lowering Treatment Trialists' Collaboration. Effects of different blood-pressure-lowering regimens on major cardiovascular events: results of prospectively-designed overviews of randomised trials.* Lancet. *2003;362:1527-1535.)*

randomized participants, relative risk (RR) reductions were proportional to the magnitude of the blood pressure reductions achieved, and every 10 mm Hg reduction in systolic BP significantly reduced the risk of major cardiovascular disease events (RR 0.80, 95% confidence interval [CI] 0.77 to 0.83), coronary heart disease (0.83, 0.78 to 0.88), stroke (0.73, 0.68 to 0.77), and heart failure (0.72, 0.67 to 0.78), which, in the populations studied, led to a significant 13% reduction

in all-cause mortality (0.87, 0.84 to 0.91). However, no clear effect on the risk of developing renal failure was found (0.95, 0.84 to 1.07) (Fig. 47.2)

COMPARISONS OF DIFFERENT DRUG CLASSES

In the BPLTTC, borderline significantly greater protective effects on stroke were seen for regimens based on CCBs,

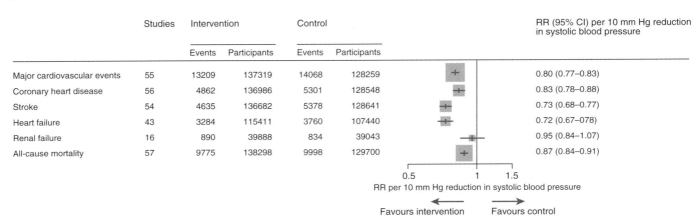

	Studies	Intervention		Control			RR (95% CI) per 10 mm Hg reduction in systolic blood pressure
		Events	Participants	Events	Participants		
Major cardiovascular events	55	13209	137319	14068	128259		0.80 (0.77–0.83)
Coronary heart disease	56	4862	136986	5301	128548		0.83 (0.78–0.88)
Stroke	54	4635	136682	5378	128641		0.73 (0.68–0.77)
Heart failure	43	3284	115411	3760	107440		0.72 (0.67–078)
Renal failure	16	890	39888	834	39043		0.95 (0.84–1.07)
All-cause mortality	57	9775	138298	9998	129700		0.87 (0.84–0.91)

RR per 10 mm Hg reduction in systolic blood pressure

Favours intervention   Favours control

FIG. 47.2 Standardized effects of a 10 mm Hg reduction in systolic blood pressure. *RR,* Relative risk. *(From Ettehad D, Emdin CA, Kiran A, et al. Blood pressure lowering for prevention of cardiovascular disease and death: a systematic review and meta-analysis.* Lancet. *2016;387;957-967.)*

compared with both conventional therapy (diuretic/beta-blockers) and ACE inhibitors, despite minimal BP differences between randomized groups (Fig. 47.3). Although there was a similar borderline greater protective effect on stroke for regimens based on diuretics/beta-blockers compared with ACE inhibitors, the mean 2 mm Hg lower BP in the diuretics/beta-blockers group probably accounted for this.

There was no evidence of any differences between active regimens in the protection afforded against CHD (see Fig. 47.2). There was some heterogeneity across trials contributing to the pooled estimate for the comparison of ACE inhibitors versus CCBs for this outcome. This was attributable to one trial[14] but neither the exclusion of this trial from the fixed-effects model nor the use of a random effects model altered the conclusions for this outcome. These data provide substantial support for prior nonquantitative overviews of the trials,[15,16] thus refuting claims of large increases in coronary risk in hypertensive patients treated with CCBs. However, compared with regimens based on CCBs, those based on diuretics and/or beta-blockers and on ACE inhibitors produced greater reductions in the risk of HF. These differences could not be attributed to different effects of the regimens on BP control and appear to be mediated through some alternative mechanism. Likewise, because HF events were restricted to those that resulted in death or hospitalization, minor side effects of CCBs such as peripheral edema do not account for this finding. Separate analyses of the trials that used dihydropyridine agents and those that used nondihydropyridine agents did not show different effects for this outcome.

There were no significant differences between regimens based on any of the active agents (ACE inhibitors, CCBs, or diuretics and/or beta-blockers) for any of the composite outcomes. The confidence intervals around the estimates of treatment effect were very narrow, reflecting the many thousands of events available for these analyses.

A recent tabular meta-analysis of BP-lowering trials also investigated the comparative effect of different drug classes. Similar to the approach taken by the BPLTTC, the analyses were not standardized for the difference in BP lowering achieved, to account for possible non-BP mediated effects, greater BP lowering potential, or better tolerability of one drug class over others. This study examined possible differences in the effects by each drug class by comparing trials that tested a specific class of drug (ACE inhibitors, ARB, beta-blockers, diuretics, and CCB) against all other classes to which it has

been compared. It showed that different drug classes were of largely comparable effectiveness in preventing the various outcomes (Fig. 47.4).

However, beta-blockers appeared less efficacious than other medications in preventing major cardiovascular disease (CVD) (1.17, 1.11 to 1.24), stroke (1.24, 1.14 to 1.35), and renal failure (1.19, 1.05 to 1.34), with evidence suggestive of less efficacy in prevention of all-cause mortality (1.06, 1.01 to 1.12). CCBs appeared superior to other classes for stroke prevention (0.90, 0.85 to 0.95) but inferior to other classes for heart failure prevention (1.17, 1.11 to 1.24). Diuretics were superior to other classes for heart failure prevention (0.81, 0.75 to 0.88). Although these findings were broadly consistent with BPLTTC, the study lacked access to individual participant data and did not have information about other concurrent BP drugs that may modify treatment effects. Hence, whether or not important class differences among subgroups of patients exist cannot be ruled out and requires further analysis with additional data which the BPLTTC is currently investigating.

BLOOD PRESSURE-DEPENDENT AND BLOOD PRESSURE-INDEPENDENT EFFECTS OF BLOOD PRESSURE TREATMENT

Unbiased, large observational studies have demonstrated the direct and continuous relationship of BP and CV risk; an association that extends to levels of BP traditionally regarded as "normotensive." In the BPLTTC overviews, the weighted mean BP differences between the randomized groups of each treatment comparison plotted against the pooled relative risks for each outcome showed a direct and continuous association between the magnitude of the BP difference and the size of the relative risk reduction (Fig. 47.5). The association was consistent for all CV outcomes, with the exception of HF for which the BPLTTC might have lacked power. A recent tabular meta-regression demonstrated that the relative risk reductions for major CVD, stroke, heart failure, and all-cause mortality were proportional to the magnitude of blood pressure reduction achieved (all $p < 0.05$) (Fig. 47.6).

The meta-regression results were of borderline significance for CHD ($p = 0.058$) and nonsignificant for renal failure ($p = 0.09$).

These analyses were instrumental in demonstrating that BP-lowering per se accounted for a large proportion of the benefit from treatment with commonly used classes of drugs. However, this does not rule out the possibility that different BP-lowering drugs have some relevant benefits beyond

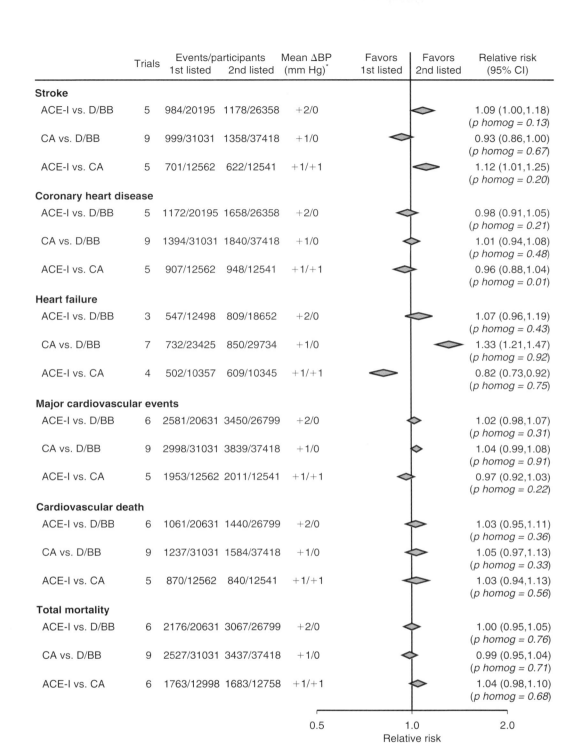

	Trials	Events/participants 1st listed	Events/participants 2nd listed	Mean ΔBP (mm Hg)*	Favors 1st listed	Favors 2nd listed	Relative risk (95% CI)
Stroke							
ACE-I vs. D/BB	5	984/20195	1178/26358	+2/0			1.09 (1.00,1.18) (*p homog = 0.13*)
CA vs. D/BB	9	999/31031	1358/37418	+1/0			0.93 (0.86,1.00) (*p homog = 0.67*)
ACE-I vs. CA	5	701/12562	622/12541	+1/+1			1.12 (1.01,1.25) (*p homog = 0.20*)
Coronary heart disease							
ACE-I vs. D/BB	5	1172/20195	1658/26358	+2/0			0.98 (0.91,1.05) (*p homog = 0.21*)
CA vs. D/BB	9	1394/31031	1840/37418	+1/0			1.01 (0.94,1.08) (*p homog = 0.48*)
ACE-I vs. CA	5	907/12562	948/12541	+1/+1			0.96 (0.88,1.04) (*p homog = 0.01*)
Heart failure							
ACE-I vs. D/BB	3	547/12498	809/18652	+2/0			1.07 (0.96,1.19) (*p homog = 0.43*)
CA vs. D/BB	7	732/23425	850/29734	+1/0			1.33 (1.21,1.47) (*p homog = 0.92*)
ACE-I vs. CA	4	502/10357	609/10345	+1/+1			0.82 (0.73,0.92) (*p homog = 0.75*)
Major cardiovascular events							
ACE-I vs. D/BB	6	2581/20631	3450/26799	+2/0			1.02 (0.98,1.07) (*p homog = 0.31*)
CA vs. D/BB	9	2998/31031	3839/37418	+1/0			1.04 (0.99,1.08) (*p homog = 0.91*)
ACE-I vs. CA	5	1953/12562	2011/12541	+1/+1			0.97 (0.92,1.03) (*p homog = 0.22*)
Cardiovascular death							
ACE-I vs. D/BB	6	1061/20631	1440/26799	+2/0			1.03 (0.95,1.11) (*p homog = 0.36*)
CA vs. D/BB	9	1237/31031	1584/37418	+1/0			1.05 (0.97,1.13) (*p homog = 0.33*)
ACE-I vs. CA	5	870/12562	840/12541	+1/+1			1.03 (0.94,1.13) (*p homog = 0.56*)
Total mortality							
ACE-I vs. D/BB	6	2176/20631	3067/26799	+2/0			1.00 (0.95,1.05) (*p homog = 0.76*)
CA vs. D/BB	9	2527/31031	3437/37418	+1/0			0.99 (0.95,1.04) (*p homog = 0.71*)
ACE-I vs. CA	6	1763/12998	1683/12758	+1/+1			1.04 (0.98,1.10) (*p homog = 0.68*)

0.5   1.0   2.0
Relative risk

FIG. 47.3 Effects of blood pressure–lowering regimens based on different drug classes on the risks of major vascular outcomes and death. *ACE,* Angiotensin-converting enzyme; *ACE-I,* ACE inhibitor; *CA,* calcium antagonist-based regimen; *D/BB,* diuretic- or beta-blocker–based regimen. *Overall, mean blood pressure difference (systolic/diastolic) during follow-up in the group assigned the first-listed treatment compared with the group assigned the second-listed treatment, calculated by weighting the difference observed in each contributing trial by the number of individuals in the trial. The positive values indicate a higher mean follow-up blood pressure in the first-listed treatment group compared with the second-listed treatment group (i.e., for all except diastolic blood pressure in the comparison of calcium antagonists with diuretics/beta-blockers). *(Adapted from Blood Pressure Lowering Treatment Trialists' Collaboration. Effects of different blood-pressure-lowering regimens on major cardiovascular events: results of prospectively-designed overviews of randomised trials.* Lancet. *2003;362:1527-1535.)*

their BP-lowering effects, in particular among certain patient subgroups.

EFFECTS IN IMPORTANT PATIENT SUBGROUPS

Subgroup analyses were designed to investigate whether there were important differences in the effects of different BP-lowering regimens in specific patient groups.

Effects in Patients With Different Baseline Risk of Cardiovascular Disease

The merits of basing treatment decisions for the prevention of CVD on an individual's predicted absolute risk of disease, rather than on the level of a single risk factor, have been discussed for decades. However, the evidence supporting the allocation of BP lowering on predicted absolute risk

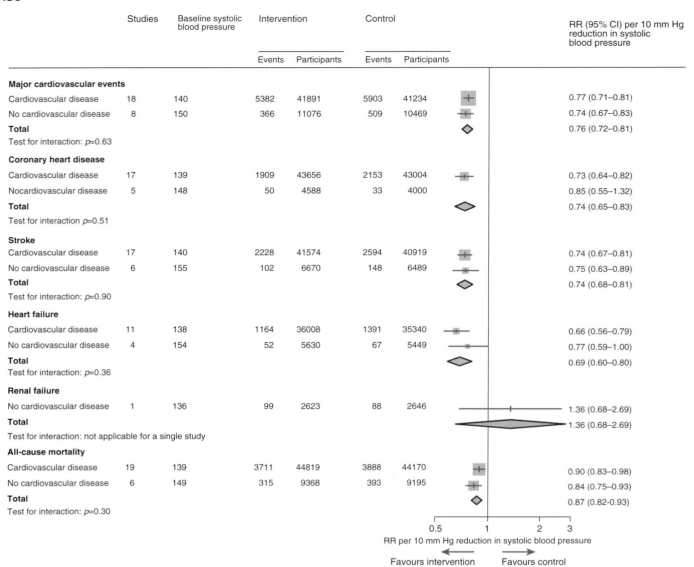

Studies	Baseline systolic blood pressure	Intervention		Control			RR (95% CI) per 10 mm Hg reduction in systolic blood pressure
		Events	Participants	Events	Participants		
Major cardiovascular events							
Cardiovascular disease	18	140	5382	41891	5903	41234	0.77 (0.71–0.81)
No cardiovascular disease	8	150	366	11076	509	10469	0.74 (0.67–0.83)
Total							0.76 (0.72–0.81)
Test for interaction: p=0.63							
Coronary heart disease							
Cardiovascular disease	17	139	1909	43656	2153	43004	0.73 (0.64–0.82)
Nocardiovascular disease	5	148	50	4588	33	4000	0.85 (0.55–1.32)
Total							0.74 (0.65–0.83)
Test for interaction p=0.51							
Stroke							
Cardiovascular disease	17	140	2228	41574	2594	40919	0.74 (0.67–0.81)
No cardiovascular disease	6	155	102	6670	148	6489	0.75 (0.63–0.89)
Total							0.74 (0.68–0.81)
Test for interaction: p=0.90							
Heart failure							
Cardiovascular disease	11	138	1164	36008	1391	35340	0.66 (0.56–0.79)
No cardiovascular disease	4	154	52	5630	67	5449	0.77 (0.59–1.00)
Total							0.69 (0.60–0.80)
Test for interaction: p=0.36							
Renal failure							
No cardiovascular disease	1	136	99	2623	88	2646	1.36 (0.68–2.69)
Total							1.36 (0.68–2.69)
Test for interaction: not applicable for a single study							
All-cause mortality							
Cardiovascular disease	19	139	3711	44819	3888	44170	0.90 (0.83–0.98)
No cardiovascular disease	6	149	315	9368	393	9195	0.84 (0.75–0.93)
Total							0.87 (0.82-0.93)
Test for interaction: p=0.30							

RR per 10 mm Hg reduction in systolic blood pressure

← Favours intervention   Favours control →

FIG. 47.4 Standardised effects of a 10 mm Hg reduction in systolic blood pressure stratified by history of cardiovascular disease. Data are stratified by subgroups in which all (cardiovascular disease) or none (no cardiovascular disease) of the participants had a history of cardiovascular disease at baseline. A cardiovascular disease subgroup is not shown for renal failure because no trial that reported renal failure as an outcome reported an analysis stratified by the presence of cardiovascular disease. *RR,* Relative risk. *(From Ettehad D, Emdin CA, Kiran A, et al. Blood pressure lowering for prevention of cardiovascular disease and death: a systematic review and meta-analysis.* Lancet. *2016;387:957-967.)*

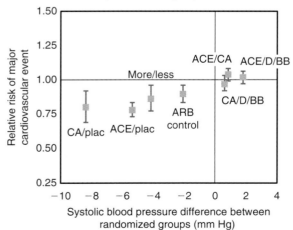

FIG. 47.5 Association of blood pressure differences between randomized groups and the risk of major cardiovascular events. Boxes are plotted at the point estimate of effect for the relative risk of the event and the mean follow-up blood pressure in the first-listed group compared with the second-listed group. The vertical lines represent 95% confidence intervals. *ACE,* Angiotensin-converting enzyme inhibitor-based regimen; *ARB,* angiotensin receptor blocker–based regimen; *CA,* calcium antagonist–based regimen; *D/BB,* diuretic- or beta-blocker–based regimen; *plac,* placebo. *(Adapted from Blood Pressure Lowering Treatment Trialists' Collaboration. Effects of different blood-pressure-lowering regimens on major cardiovascular events: results of prospectively-designed overviews of randomised trials.* Lancet. *2003;362:1527-1535.)*

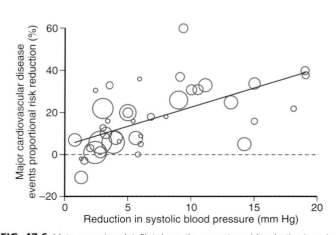

FIG. 47.6 Meta-regression plot. Plot shows the percentage risk reduction in major cardiovascular events regressed against the difference in achieved systolic blood pressure between study treatment groups. *(From Ettehad D, Emdin CA, Kiran A, et al. Blood pressure lowering for prevention of cardiovascular disease and death: a systematic review and meta-analysis.* Lancet. *2016;387:957-967.)*

has been limited. To address this question, the BPLTTC conducted a study to compare the effects of BP-lowering drugs in patient subgroups with different levels of baseline absolute risk of CVD. For the 51,917 patients included in the analysis, pharmacological BP reduction produced significant *relative* risk reductions that were similar across all four risk groups (Fig. 47.7) (*p* = 0.30 for trend). The magnitude of the *absolute* risk reduction, in consequence, increased in a linear fashion from the lowest risk group to the highest risk group (Fig. 47.7) (*p* = 0.04 for trend). These results supported the use of clinical management guidelines that recommend BP-lowering treatment on the basis of predicted risk level, rather than BP levels alone.

Effects in Patients With Different Baseline Blood Pressures

A BPLTTC report defined patient subgroups according to their baseline systolic BP (SBP) (<140, 140 to 159, 160 to 179, and ≥180 mm Hg) and investigated the effect of BP lowering across these strata.[11] For the primary outcome of total major CV events, there was no clear evidence that BP lowering produced proportional reductions in risk that were quantitatively different in patients with a wide range of initial BP levels and different background use of other BP-lowering therapies. The results were similarly consistent when patients were classified according to baseline diastolic BP and in analyses in which baseline BP was fitted as a continuous variable (Fig. 47.6).

The findings from BPLTTC were recently confirmed and extended to patient groups with even lower baseline BP levels. In a tabular meta-analysis, trials were stratified by mean baseline SBP (<130, 130 to 139, 140 to 149, 150 to 159 and ≥160) and the effects of a 10 mm Hg reduction in SBP compared between strata. This showed no evidence for a different effect of BP lowering among the different BP strata for a range of CV outcomes (p_{trend} > 0.05) (Fig. 47.8).

Effects in Patients With and Without Diabetes Mellitus

In analyses of patients with (n = 33,395) and without (n = 125,314) DM, the short-term to medium-term effects (average follow-up times: 2 to 5 years) on major CV events of the BP-lowering regimens studied were highly comparable for most outcomes studied (Fig. 47.9).[7] The few exceptions were the comparisons of ARB-based regimens with others, in which ARBs may provide less protection against stroke among patients with DM compared with those without DM (*p* homogeneity = 0.05); and, conversely, greater protection against HF among patients with DM compared with patients without DM (*p* homogeneity = 0.005). However, whether these differences are real or a consequence of differential BP reductions in the two subgroups or simply the play of chance is unclear.

A more recent systematic review of blood pressure-lowering trials in people with diabetes found that blood pressure lowering clearly reduced the risk of cardiovascular events, myocardial infarction, stroke, new onset albuminuria, and both cardiovascular and all-cause death.[17] The available data suggested that the benefits of BP lowering were less clear among those with baseline systolic BP levels below 140 mm Hg.

Effects in Patients of Different Ages

In analyses of patients classified according to age (<65 versus ≥65 years), there was no clear difference between age groups in the effects of lowering BP or any difference between the effects of the drug classes on major CV events (all *p* ≥ 0.24)

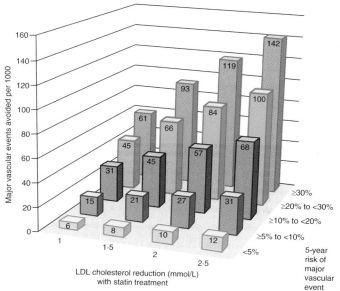

FIG. 47.7 Predicted 5-year benefits of low-density lipoprotein cholesterol reductions with statin treatment at different levels of risk. (*Cholesterol Treatment Trialists' (CTT) Collaborators. The effects of lowering LDL cholesterol with statin therapy in people at low risk of vascular disease: meta-analysis of individual data from 27 randomised trials.* Lancet. *2012;380:581-590.*)

(see Fig. 47.9).[9] Neither was there any significant interaction between age and treatment, when age was fitted as a continuous variable (all *p* > 0.09). The meta-regressions also showed no significant difference in effects between the two age groups for the outcome of major CV events (<65 versus ≥65; *p* = 0.38). In addition, reduction of BP produced similar relative benefits in younger (<65 years) and older (≥65 years) adults alike, with no strong evidence that protection against major vascular events afforded by different drug classes varied substantially with age. The much greater absolute risk in elderly people means that even if proportional reductions were attenuated in this group, the protection afforded would still translate into large numbers of serious CV events prevented.

Effects in Men and Women

In analyses that included 103,268 men and 87,349 women, there was no evidence that levels of protection from BP lowering differed by patient gender or that regimens based on ACE inhibitors, CCBs, ARBs, or diuretics/beta-blockers were more effective in one gender than the other (all *p* homogeneity > 0.08) (see Fig. 47.9).[10]

SUMMARY

Meta-analyses such as those conducted by the BPLTTC provide clinicians and their patients with uniquely accurate and comparative information about the relative benefits and risks of widely used classes of BP-lowering drugs. The results are applicable to a broad population of hypertensive and nonhypertensive individuals at high risk of CV disease.

These overviews show that treatment with any of the commonly used initial therapies reduces the risk of major CV events, and larger reductions in BP produce larger reductions in risk. For some outcomes there are important differences between regimens, which may be independent of BP lowering. The extent to which such differences with be important in management of certain patient subgroups requires even larger and more diverse datasets, and is subject to ongoing investigations by the BPLTTC and others.

	Studies	Intervention		Control			RR (95% CI) per 10 mm Hg reduction in systolic blood pressure	p_{trend}
		Events	Participants	Events	Participants			
Major cardiovascular events								0.22
<130	4	542	4547	530	3881		0.63 (0.50–0.80)	
130-139	17	5375	47103	5856	47167		0.87 (0.82–0.92)	
140-149	7	4365	33333	4694	33062		0.79 (0.72–0.87)	
150-159	13	1289	21290	1257	20088		0.80 (0.71–0.91)	
≥160	14	1638	31045	1731	24060		0.74 (0.69–0.79)	
Total							0.80 (0.77–0.83)	
Coronary heart disease								0.93
<130	5	489	6071	620	5395		0.55 (0.42–0.72)	
130-139	18	2258	47608	2461	47670		0.88 (0.80–0.96)	
140-149	8	1225	34834	1307	34581		0.80 (0.69–0.94)	
150-159	12	409	20386	442	19788		0.84 (0.68–1.05)	
≥160	13	481	28086	471	21113		0.82 (0.73–0.92)	
Total							0.83 (0.78–0.88)	
Stroke								0.98
<130	3	48	3669	47	2984		0.65 (0.27–1.57)	
130-139	18	1191	47608	1403	47670		0.73 (0.62–0.85)	
140-149	7	2130	34166	2381	34347		0.78 (0.70–0.87)	
150-159	11	538	19636	702	19026		0.65 (0.54–0.78)	
≥160	15	728	31603	845	24613		0.70 (0.64–0.78)	
Total							0.73 (0.68–0.77)	
Heart failure								0.27
<130	3	137	3669	138	2984		0.83 (0.41–1.70)	
130-139	15	1493	44029	1778	44104		0.75 (0.66–0.85)	
140-149	6	1121	32665	1207	32828		0.83 (0.70–1.00)	
150-159	7	304	8507	271	7945		0.96 (0.71–1.30)	
≥160	12	229	26541	366	19579		0.61 (0.54–0.70)	
Total							0.72 (0.67–0.78)	
Renal failure								0.52
130-139	5	320	14661	317	14711		1.02 (0.82–1.26)	
140-149	2	76	10945	60	11045		3.23 (0.73–14.30)	
150-159	4	464	7278	428	6755		0.90 (0.76–1.05)	
≥160	5	30	7004	29	6532		0.94 (0.56–1.56)	
Total							0.95 (0.84–1.07)	
All-cause mortality								0.79
<130	7	320	7733	410	7059		0.53 (0.37–0.76)	
130-139	18	3596	47608	3782	47670		0.89 (0.82–0.98)	
140-149	7	3338	34166	3318	34347		0.99 (0.89–1.09)	
150-159	12	1127	20705	1197	19511		0.78 (0.69–0.90)	
≥160	13	1394	28086	1291	21113		0.86 (0.80–0.92)	
Total							0.87 (0.84–0.91)	

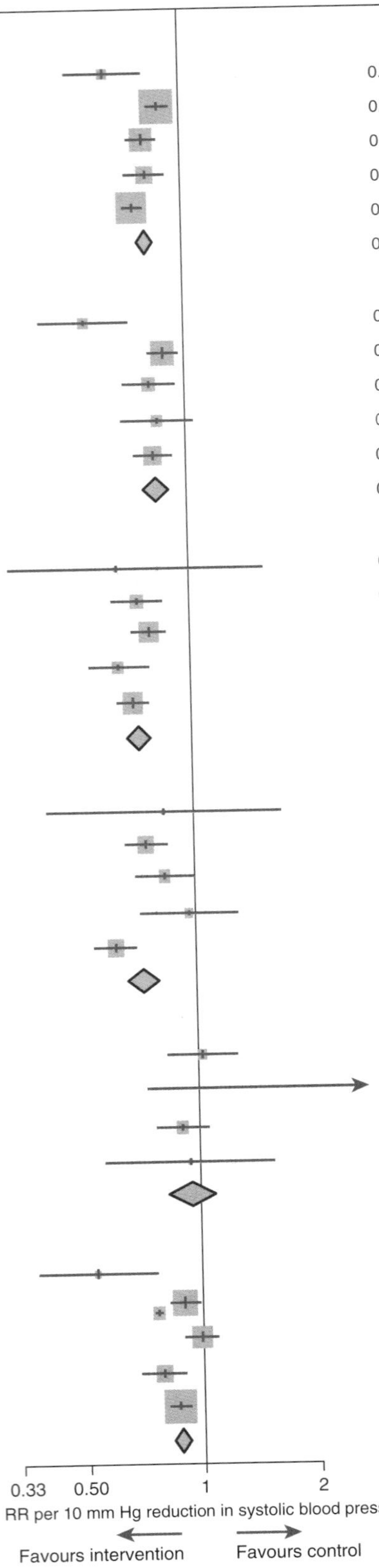

0.33   0.50   1   2

RR per 10 mm Hg reduction in systolic blood pressure

← Favours intervention   Favours control →

FIG. 47.8 Standardized effects of a 10 mm Hg reduction in systolic blood pressure stratified by blood pressure. Blood pressure strata are baseline blood pressure values, not achieved blood pressure after treatment. *RR*, Relative risk. (From Ettehad D, Emdin CA, Kiran A, et al. Blood pressure lowering for prevention of cardiovascular disease and death: a systematic review and meta-analysis. Lancet. 2016;387;957-967.)

	No. of events/patients		SBP/DBP difference	Favors active treatment	Favors placebo	Risk ratio (95% CI)	Phomogeneity
	Active treatment	Placebo					
Male	1701/14920	2135/14990	−4.7/−2.2	◆		0.81 (0.75-0.87)	0.79
Female	536/6129	661/5989	−6.0/−2.5	◆		0.79 (0.68-0.91)	
Age <65	856/10824	1136/10927	−4.9/−2.2	◆		0.78 (0.68-0.89)	0.67
Age ≥65	1381/10225	1660/10052	−5.3/−2.4	◆		0.81 (0.73-0.90)	
Diabetes	549/3246	674/3194	−4.2/−2.2	◆		0.80 (0.71-0.89)	0.54
No diabetes	959/9247	1258/9198	−6.7/−3.0	◆		0.76 (0.70-0.83)	

```
        0.5      1.0      2.0
             Risk ratio
```

FIG. 47.9 Effects of active blood pressure–lowering treatment compared with placebo on major cardiovascular events according to gender, age, and diabetes status. *DBP,* Diastolic blood pressure; *SBP,* systolic blood pressure.

Acknowledgments: The authors would like to thank members of the Blood Pressure Lowering Treatment Trialists' Collaboration: L. Agodoa (National Institute of Diabetes and Digestive and Kidney Diseases, National Institutes of Health, Bethesda, Maryland); C. Anderson, J. Chalmers, S. MacMahon, A. Rodgers, and B. Neal (George Institute, Sydney, Australia); F. W. Asselbergs and W. H. van Gilst (University of Groningen, Groningen and Medical Centre Utrecht, Netherlands); C. Baigent and R. Collins (Clinical Trial Service Unit, University of Oxford, Oxford, United Kingdom); E. Berge and M. Mehlum (Oslo University Hospital, Oslo, Norway); H. Black (New York University School of Medicine, New York); F. Bouwers (University Medical Center Groningen, Groningen, Netherlands); B. Brenner and M. Pfeffer (Brigham and Women's Hospital, Boston, Massachusetts); C. Bulpitt and P. Poole-Wilson (Imperial College, London); R. Byington (Wake Forest University, Winston-Salem, North Carolina); J. Cutler (National Heart, Lung and Blood Institute, Bethesda, Maryland); B. Davis (University of Texas School of Public Health, Houston, Texas); D. de Zeeuw (University Medical Center Groningen, Groningen, Netherlands); J. Dens (University Hospital Gasthuisberg, Leuven, Belgium); R. Estacio (University of Colorado Health Sciences Center, Denver); R. Fagard (University of Leuven, K U Leuven, Belgium); K. Fox (Royal Brompton Hospital and Imperial College, London, United Kingdom); T. Fukui (St. Luke's International Hospital, Tokyo); L. Hansson and R. Holman (Oxford Centre for Diabetes, Endocrinology and Metabolism, University of Oxford, Oxford, United Kingdom); Y. Imai and T. Ohkubo (Tohoku University Graduate School of Pharmaceutical Sciences and Medicine, Sendai, Japan); M. Ishii (Yokohama Seamen's Insurance Hospital, Yokohama, Japan); Y. Kanno and H. Suzuki (Musashino Tokusyukai Hospital, Tokyo, Japan); S. Kjeldsen (Ullevaal University Hospital, Oslo, Norway);

J. Kostis (UMDNJ-Robert Wood Johnson Medical School, New Brunswick, New Jersey); K. Kuramoto (Tokyo Metropolitan Geriatric Hospital, Tokyo); J. Lanke (Lund University, Lund, Sweden); E. Lewis (Rush University Medical Center, Chicago); M. Lièvre (Louis Pradel Hospital Université Claude Bernard-Lyon 1, Lyon, France); L.H. Lindholm (Department of Public Health and Clinical Medicine, Umeå University, Umeå, Sweden); L. Lisheng (Fu Wai Hospital and Cardiovascular Institute, Beijing, China); J. Lubsen (SOCAR Research S.A, Nyon, Switzerland); S. Lueders and J. Schrader (St. Josefs Hospital, Cloppenburg, Germany); E. Malacco (Ospedale L. Sacco, University of Milan, Milan, Italy); G. Mancia (University of Milano-Bicocca, Department of Clinical Medicine and Prevention, San Gerardo Hospital, Milan, Italy); M. Matsuzaki (Yamaguchi University Hospital, Yamaguchi, Japan); S. Nissen (Cleveland Clinic, Cleveland); H. Ogawa (The Heart Institute of Japan, Tokyo Women's Medical University, Tokyo, Japan); T. Ogihara (Osaka University Graduate School of Medicine, Osaka, Japan); T. Ohkubo (Teikyo University, Tokyo Japan); C. Pepine (University of Florida, Gainesville, Florida); B. Pitt (University of Michigan School of Medicine, Ann Arbor, Michigan); M. Rahman (University Hospitals of Cleveland Case Medical Center, Cleveland); H. Rakugi (Osaka University Graduate School of Medicine, Osaka Japan); W. Remme (Sticares Cardiovascular Research Institute, Rhoon, Netherlands); G. Remuzzi and P. Ruggenenti (Mario Negri Institute for Pharmacological Research and Ospedali Riuniti di Bergamo, Bergamo, Italy); T. Saruta (Keio University School of Medicine, Tokyo, Japan); R. Schrier (University of Colorado School of Medicine, Denver); P. Sleight (University of Oxford and John Radcliffe Hospital, Oxford, United Kingdom); J. Staessen (University of Leuven, Leuven, Belgium); K. Teo (McMaster University Medical Centre, Ontario, Canada); L.Thijs (University of Leuven, Leuven Belgium); K. Ueshima (Kyoto University Graduate School of Medicine, Kyoto, Japan); S.Umemoto (Yamaguchi University, Yamaguchi, Japan); P. Verdecchia (Hospital of Assisi, Assisi, Italy); G. Viberti (King's College London, Guy's Hospital, London); J. Wang (Ruijin Hospital, Shanghai); P. Whelton (Loyola University Medical Center, Maywood, Illinois); L. Wing (Flinders University, Adelaide, Australia); Y. Yui (Kyoto University Hospital, Kyoto, Japan); S. Yusuf (Hamilton General Hospital, Ontario, Canada); A. Zanchetti (University of Milan and Instituto Auxologico Italiano, Milan, Italy).

BPLTTC Steering Committee: K. Rahimi–Chair (The George Institute for Global Health UK, University of Oxford, Oxford, United Kingdom); J. Chalmers (The George Institute for Global Health, Sydney Australia), B. Davis (University of Texas School of Public Health, Houston, Texas); C. Pepine (University of Florida, Gainesville, Florida); K. Teo (McMaster University, Ontario, Canada).

References

1. Sackett DL, Rosenberg WM, Gray JA, et al. Evidence based medicine: what it is and what it isn't. *BMJ.* 1996;312:71-72.
2. Egger M, Smith GD, Phillips AN. Meta-analysis: principles and procedures. *BMJ.* 1997;315:1533-1537.
3. Blettner M, Sauerbrei W, Schlehofer B, Scheuchenpflug T, Friedenreich C. Traditional reviews, meta-analyses and pooled analyses in epidemiology. *Int J Epidemiol.* 1999;28:1-9.
4. World Health Organization-International Society of Hypertension Blood Pressure Lowering Treatment Trialists' Collaboration. Protocol for prospective collaborative overviews of major randomized trials of blood-pressure lowering treatments. *J Hypertens.* 1998;16:127-137.
5. Blood Pressure Lowering Treatment Trialists' Collaboration. Effects of ACE inhibitors, calcium antagonists and other blood pressure lowering drugs: results of prospectively designed overviews of randomised trials. *Lancet.* 2000;355:1955-1964.
6. Blood Pressure Lowering Treatment Trialists' Collaboration. Effects of different blood-pressure-lowering regimens on major cardiovascular events: results of prospectively-designed overviews of randomised trials. *Lancet.* 2003;362:1527-1535.
7. Blood Pressure Lowering Treatment Trialists' Collaboration. Effects of different blood pressure-lowering regimens on major cardiovascular events in individuals with and without diabetes mellitus: results of prospectively designed overviews of randomized trials. *Arch Intern Med.* 2005;165:1410-1419.
8. Blood Pressure Lowering Treatment Trialists' Collaboration. Blood pressure-dependent and independent effects of agents that inhibit the renin-angiotensin system. *J Hypertens.* 2007;25:951-958.
9. Blood Pressure Lowering Treatment Trialists' Collaboration. Effects of different regimens to lower blood pressure on major cardiovascular events in older and younger adults: meta-analysis of randomised trials. *BMJ.* 2008;336:1121-1123.
10. Blood Pressure Lowering Treatment Trialists' Collaboration. Do men and women respond differently to blood pressure-lowering treatment? Results of prospectively designed overviews of randomised trials. *Eur Heart J.* 2008;29:2669-2680.
11. Czernichow S, Zanchetti A, Turnbull F, et al. The effects of blood pressure reduction and of different blood pressure-lowering regimens on major cardiovascular events according to baseline blood pressure: meta-analysis of randomized trials. *J Hypertens.* 2011;29:4-16.
12. Cholesterol Treatment Trialists' Collaboration. Efficacy and safety of cholesterol-lowering treatment: prospective meta-analysis of data from 90056 participants in 14 randomised trials of statins. *Lancet.* 2005;366:1267-1278.
13. Antithrombotic Treatment Trialists' Collaboration. Aspirin in the primary and secondary prevention of vascular disease: collaborative meta-analysis of individual participant data from randomised trials. *Lancet.* 2009;373:1849-1860.
14. Estacio R, Jeffers B, Hiatt W, et al. The effect of nisoldipine as compared with enalapril on cardiovascular outcomes in patients with non-insulin dependent diabetes and hypertension. *N Engl J Med.* 1998;338:645-652.
15. Ad Hoc Subcommittee of the Liaison Committee of the World Health Organization and the International Society of Hypertension. Effects of calcium antagonists on the risks of coronary heart disease, cancer and bleeding. *J Hypertens.* 1997;15:105-115.
16. MacMahon S, Collins R, Chalmers J. Reliable and unbiased assessment of the effects of calcium antagonists: importance of minimizing both systematic and random errors. *J Hypertens.* 1997;15:1201-1204.
17. Edmin CA, Rahimi K, Neal B, et al. Blood pressure lowering in type 2 diabetes—A systemic review and meta-analysis. *JAMA.* 2015;313:603-615.

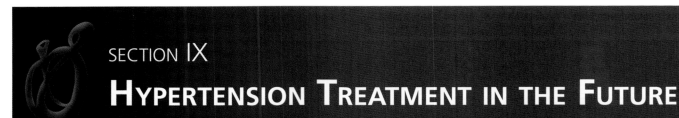

48 Team-Based Care for Hypertension Management

Barry L. Carter

Although blood pressure (BP) control has improved substantially in the last five decades, only half of the United States population with hypertension have adequate BP control.[1] In contrast, BP control in some high-performing health systems is much better and can be as high as 80% to 90%.[2] The strategies used by these high-performing systems may help other providers to improve BP control within their offices or health care settings.

There are many causes for poor BP control besides lifestyle choices, including suboptimal patient medication adherence[3-6] and failure to intensify therapy (clinical inertia) by clinicians.[7,8] Clinical inertia occurs when physicians do not intensify antihypertensives, perhaps because of concern about the predictive value or accuracy of clinic BP measurements, BP that was close to, but not at or below, goal, patient resistance to adding medications, lower home BP measurements, suspected white-coat hypertension, more urgent competing medical problems, or the patient stating they are experiencing more stress on the day of the clinic visit. However, many of these barriers could be overcome if the organizational structure of health care delivery adequately supported physicians and patients (Fig. 48.1).[9-11]

Many quality improvement strategies have been tried to improve BP including patient education, reminders, physician alerts, and others.[12] Most of these had modest effects, with the exception of team-based care, which was the most effective strategy to improve BP.[12-14]

THE PATIENT-CENTERED MEDICAL HOME

The patient-centered medical home (PCMH) has been promoted to minimize episodic care, improve continuity, and provide more comprehensive management of chronic illness and preventive care.[15] The PCMH was developed and endorsed by the American Academy of Family Physicians, American Academy Pediatrics, American College of Physicians, and is now a major component of Accountable Care Organizations within health care reform as a strategy to improve care quality at lower costs.[16-18] The National Committee on Quality Assurance (NCQA) has developed standards and provided formal recognition of health plans and individual providers for many years. NCQA revised the standards to score health systems in 2014 (Table 48.1).[19] Although previous standards supported team-based care, the 2014 standards made team care an essential component of the PCMH by including it as one of the six key standards. Health systems that want to achieve the highest level (level 3, Table 48.1) of PCMH recognition must have well-functioning health care teams because this component is responsible for 20% of the total score. In addition, care management, medication management, care coordination, and coordination of care transitions are all functions typically performed by nonphysicians and make up another 14% of the score (Table 48.1).

The standards also require medication reconciliation across health systems (e.g., between inpatient and primary care) for more than 80% of patients, families, and caregivers, providing information about new prescriptions to more than 80% of patients, assessing medications and barriers to adherence for more than 50% of patients, and documenting over-the-counter medications, herbal therapies, and supplements for more than 50% of patients.[19]

The PCMH emphasizes that care should be organized around the needs of the patient, their relationship with their personal physician, and that physician-led teams assist with care according to the needs of the patient.[9,16] The standards do not dictate who is on the team or how the team functions and communicates. However, the highest performing health systems have nurses, pharmacists, and behavioral health professions (e.g., counselors), and other critical members on this team.[2] The physician delegates responsibility to other members of the team to perform a medication history, identify problems and barriers to achieving disease control, perform counseling on lifestyle modification, and adjust medications following hypertension guidelines. Frequent communication by team members concerning goal-directed therapy allows the physician to address more acute problems and complications. There is early evidence that the PCMH can be used to improve health care outcomes, increase physician satisfaction, and decrease the costs of health care.[20,21] The personal relationship between the patient, physician, and the team has also been used to overcome barriers to care often seen in minorities or other vulnerable populations (see later).[22]

Providers might assume that the PCMH standards apply only to those in typical primary care settings. However, the Referral Tracking and Follow-up standard 5B requires that providers have established agreements and criteria for specialists and the specialist be given the clinical question and type of referral. NCQA maintains a directory of specialists who have been recognized by NCQA as meeting the standards.[19]

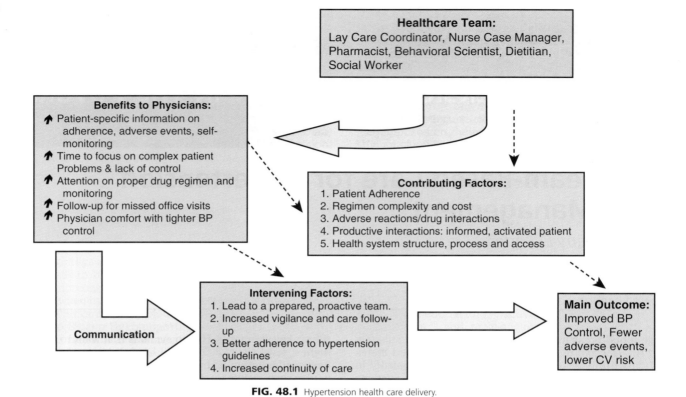

FIG. 48.1 Hypertension health care delivery.

TABLE 48.1 National Center on Quality Assurance Patient-Centered Medical Home 2014 Content and Scoring of Practices on Progress Towards the Patient-Centered Medical Home

Standard 1: Enhance Access and Continuity	Points	Standard 4: Plan and Manage Care	
A. [a]Patient-centered appointment access	4.5	A. Identify patients for care management	4
B. 24/7 Access to Clinical Advice	3.5	B. [a]Care planning and self-care support	4
C. Electronic Access	2	C. Medication management	4
Total points:	10	D. Use electronic prescribing	3
		E. Support self-care and shared decision-making	5
		Total points:	20
Standard 2: Team-Based Care		**Standard 5: Track and Coordinate Care**	
A. Continuity	3	A. Test tracking and follow-up	6
B. Medical home responsibilities	2.5	B. [a]Referral tracking and follow-up	6
C. Culturally and linguistically appropriate services (CLAS)	2.5	C. Coordinate care transitions	6
D. [a]The practice team	4	Total points:	18
Total points:	12		
Standard 3: Population Health Management		**Standard 6: Measure and Improve Performance**	
A. Patient information	3	A. Measure clinical quality performance	3
B. Clinical data	4	B. Measure resource use and care coordination	3
C. Comprehensive health assessment	4	C. Measure patient/family experience	4
D. [a]Use data for population management	5	D. [a]Implement continuous quality improvement	4
E. Implement evidence-based decision-support	4	E. Demonstrate continuous quality improvement	3
Total points:	20	F. Report performance	3
		G. Use certified Electronic Health Record technology	0
		Total points:	20

Scoring Levels
Level 1: 35-59 points
Level 2: 60-84 points
Level 3: 85-100 points

[a]Must pass elements
(Patient Centered Medical Home (PCMH 2014) Standards Training material is reproduced with permission from the National Committee for Quality Assurance (NCQA) website.
Source: http://www.ncqa.org/Programs/Recognition/RelevanttoAllRecognition/RecognitionTraining/PCMH2014Standards.aspx. Last accessed: September 2016.)

Therefore, hypertension specialists and primary care providers who wish to become members of health systems and accountable care organizations will increasingly need to meet these standards.

The challenges of managing chronic conditions have led to strategies to provide care management, previously termed disease-state management. These programs usually focused on a given condition, such as hypertension. The PCMH demands more comprehensive programs that manage multiple conditions such as diabetes, dyslipidemia, hypertension, smoking cessation, and weight management, in an attempt to provide cardiac risk reduction.[23,24] Large health systems may provide population-based strategies to target these patients, identify gaps in care, and guide these patients to programs

TABLE 48.2 Components of Team-Based Care Shown to Improve Blood Pressure

TYPE OF INDIVIDUAL INTERVENTION	MEDIAN REDUCTION IN SYSTOLIC BLOOD PRESSURE (MM HG)	MEDIAN REDUCTION IN DIASTOLIC BLOOD PRESSURE (MM HG)
Pharmacist made treatment recommendation to physician	−9.30[a]	−3.60
Patient education provided	−8.75[b]	−3.60[b]
Pharmacist conducted the medication intervention	−8.44	−3.30
Medication adherence assessed and addressed	−7.90	−3.25
Provided lifestyle modification counseling	−7.59	−3.30
Nurse conducted the medication intervention	−4.80[a]	−3.10

[a]$p < 0.10$ and [b]$p < 0.05$ for Mann-Whitney analysis of reduction in systolic blood pressure and diastolic blood pressure comparing studies with the specific intervention strategy with those without it.
(Data adapted from Carter BL, Rogers M, Daly J, Zheng S, James PA. The potency of team-based care interventions for hypertension: a meta-analysis. Arch Intern Med. 2009;169:1748-1755.)

that improve care.[25] Smaller offices or clinics frequently do not have the resources to provide these comprehensive services because physicians are overworked and the offices do not have resources to hire key team members. Our research team is studying the effect of a centralized cardiovascular risk service in two clinical trials that can provide remote clinical pharmacy services to private physician offices and even patients in rural areas (see later).[26,27]

TEAM-BASED CARE OF HYPERTENSION

Systematic Reviews

Care management within the PCMH emphasizes changes in health care delivery, self-management support, clinical information systems, delivery system redesign, decision support, health care organization, and community resources.[9-11,28,29] One of the most studied areas of system redesign, or organizational change, is the inclusion of pharmacists or nurses as members of the health care team.[13]

Walsh and colleagues evaluated 63 controlled studies using various quality improvement strategies to improve BP control such as patient education, physician reminders, or other approaches.[12] These investigators found that the only statistically significant improvement in BP occurred with organizational change, which included team-based care (37 comparisons), and resulted in a median reduction in systolic BP (SBP) of 9.7 mm Hg and a 21.8% net increase in SBP control. Another meta-analysis of pharmacy based-interventions evaluated 13 studies that included 2200 individuals and found that pharmacists' interventions significantly reduced SBP (10.7 ± 11.6 mm Hg; $p = 0.002$), whereas controls remained unchanged.[30] A meta-analysis evaluated 39 randomized controlled trials in 14,224 patients and found pharmacist interventions reduced SBP by 7.6 mm Hg (95% confidence interval [CI]: −9.0 to −6.3 mm Hg) compared with usual care.[31]

A meta-analysis evaluated 37 controlled clinical trials that involved either pharmacist or nurse case management of hypertension.[13] The type of practitioner and training varied considerably. Although the Pharm.D degree is the only professional degree now awarded in pharmacy, at the time many of these studies were conducted, some pharmacists had a Bachelor of Science degree.[32-38] Most studies that specified qualifications for nurses involved registered nurses (RN)[39,40] or nurse practitioners.[41,42] Nearly all studies involving nurses or pharmacists embedded within clinics provided for dedicated case management activities. Community pharmacists, however, usually had to incorporate the intervention within traditional medication dispensing functions. One goal of this meta-analysis was to evaluate the potency of individual components of team-based care interventions (Table 48.2). The most effective strategies to reduce SBP were when the

TABLE 48.3 Odds Ratios for Controlled Blood Pressure With Team-Based Interventions

TYPE OF CARE MANAGEMENT	ODDS RATIO	95% CONFIDENCE INTERVAL
Interventions by nurses	1.69	1.48-1.93
Interventions by pharmacists within clinics[a]	2.48	2.05-2.99
Interventions by pharmacists within community pharmacies	2.89[a]	1.83-4.55[a]

Adapted from Carter BL, Rogers M, Daly J, Zheng S, James PA. The potency of team-based care interventions for hypertension: a meta-analysis. Arch Intern Med. 2009;169:1748-1755.
[a]Includes an additional study in 410 patients published after the meta-analysis was published from Carter BL, Ardery G, Dawson JD, et al. Physician and pharmacist collaboration to improve blood pressure control. *Arch Intern Med.* 2009;169:1996-2002.

pharmacist made treatment recommendations to the physician (−9.3 mm Hg), the nurse or pharmacist educated the patient about their medications (−8.75 mm Hg), the pharmacists made the medication intervention changes (−8.44 mm Hg), medication adherence was assessed and addressed by the pharmacist or nurse (−7.9 mm Hg), counseling about lifestyle modification was performed (−7.59 mm Hg), or the nurse made the medication intervention changes (−4.8 mm Hg). When we examined the odds ratios for controlled BP with either nurses, pharmacists in clinics, or community pharmacists, all three types of interventions were significant (Table 48.3), although the pharmacy interventions appeared to be more potent.

A meta-analysis of nurse-led interventions with treatment algorithms showed greater reductions in SBP (−8.2 mm Hg, 95% CI −11.5 to −4.9) compared with usual care but no difference in BP control.[43] When results were pooled, nurse interventions significantly lowered SBP compared with usual care in African Americans but there was little difference for other ethnic minority groups.

The Community Prevention Services Task Force conducted a systematic review of team-based care in 2014.[44] The study evaluated 52 international studies involving pharmacists and nurses and 41% of the trials involved a majority of African Americans. BP control was improved by a median of 12 percentage points (interquartile interval [IQI] 3.2, 20.8), SBP 5.4 mm Hg (2.0, 7.2) and diastolic blood pressure (DBP) 1.8 mm Hg (0.7, 3.2). The percent improvement in BP control was "considerably higher" when pharmacists were added (22.0%), compared with nurses (8.5%) or nurses plus pharmacists (16.2%). The improvement was much greater when the team member could make independent changes (17.4%) compared with those that required PCP approval (15.0) or support only (7.9%).

Cost-Effectiveness Analyses

Until recently, few cost-effectiveness studies had been conducted but several studies have now assessed the cost-to-benefit ratio of team-based care. Total costs for the pharmacist-managed group were similar to those in the physician-managed clinic group ($242.46 versus $233.20, p = 0.71), but cost effectiveness ratios were lower in the pharmacist-managed group ($27 versus $193/mm Hg for SBP readings, and $48 versus $151/mm Hg for DBP readings).[36] The authors concluded that pharmacist management was cost effective.

We evaluated the cost of a 6-month intervention by pharmacists embedded within primary care clinics from two clinical trials involving 496 subjects.[45] Total adjusted costs were $775 in the intervention group and $446 in the control group (difference $329.16, p < 0.001). Total costs between the two groups ranged from $224 to $516 with a sensitivity analysis. The cost to lower SBP 1 mm Hg was $36.

We conducted the Collaboration Among Pharmacist and Physicians to Improve Blood Pressure Now (CAPTION) trial that randomized 625 patients from 32 medical offices in 15 states.[46] Each office had an existing clinical pharmacist on staff. Cost-effectiveness ratios were calculated based on changes in BP measurements and hypertension control rates. Thirty-eight percent of patients were African American, 14% were Hispanic, and 49% had annual income less than $25 000. At 9 months, average SBP was 6.1 mm Hg lower (±3.5), DBP was 2.9 mm Hg lower (±1.9) in the intervention group compared with the control group. Total costs for the intervention group were $1462.87 (±132.51) and $1259.94 (±183.30) for the control group, a difference of $202.93. The cost to lower BP by 1 mm Hg was $33.27 for SBP. The cost to increase the rate of hypertension control by 1 percentage point in the study population was $23.

The Community Prevention Services Task Force evaluated costs of team-based care.[47] They determined that the cost to provide either a nurse or pharmacist intervention was $198 per year. The cost to reduce SBP 1 mm Hg was $87 which is much higher than our cost analyses in the two studies above. However, when these authors examined the 20-year cost per quality-adjusted life years (QALY) gained, the cost for the nurse intervention was $16,696 to $24,042 whereas it was $7,114 to $10,244 for pharmacists and "other."

Nurse Case Management of Hypertension

Nurse case management has been an effective strategy to improve cardiovascular risk factors including BP.[48,49] Nurses have assisted physicians by adhering more strictly to treatment algorithms and counseling that busy physicians have difficulty incorporating into an office visit.[13,42,49-54]

One of the earliest studies of nurses was conducted in the work site and compared a nurse-managed group to a control group managed by the patient's family physician.[55] Nurses prescribed and changed drug therapy without physician approval while physicians reviewed the charts of nurse-managed patients on a weekly basis. The study involved 457 subjects and nurse-managed patients were more likely to receive a new antihypertensive (95% versus 63%, p < 0.001), receive two antihypertensives (44% versus 18%, p < 0.001), adhere to the medication regimen (68% versus 49%, p < 0.005), and achieve goal BP at 6 months (49% versus 28%, p < 0.001).

Another study evaluated care of several conditions including hypertension delivered by nurse practitioners compared with physicians.[56] Most patients were Hispanic immigrants and all were enrolled after an emergency department or urgent care visit. Patients were randomized to either a nurse practitioner (n = 806) or a physician (n = 510). BP was slightly better when provided by nurse practitioners compared with physicians (137/82 versus 139/85 mm Hg, p = 0.28 for SBP and p = 0.04 for DBP) following a 12-month intervention.

The use of nurses to provide case management of hypertension has been well described over the past 40 years and has included mobile clinics, home visits, work-based programs, and clinic settings.[42,57] Rudd and colleagues studied nurse case management of hypertension in a randomized controlled trial, in which 76 subjects were managed by their usual physician, and 74 received nurse-based care.[50] At baseline, nurse case managers provided education regarding use of an automated BP device, strategies to improve medication adherence, and identification of adverse drug events. The nurses then conducted telephone interviews at 1 week and at 1, 2, and 4 months, for an average of 10 minutes per telephone call. The nurse independently made medication dosage increases but contacted the physician before initiating new BP medication. Systolic BP declined by 14.2 mm Hg in the intervention group compared only to 5.7 mm Hg in the control group (p < 0.01) after 6 months, and significantly more medications were taken and significantly more medication changes (223 versus 52, p < 0.01) had been made in the intervention group than the control group.

Thus, some studies have found that nurse management can lead to improved BP control whereas others found BP was similar to usual care or that provided by physicians. These seemingly diverse findings are likely explained by important principles indicating the benefits of focused care. Nurse practitioners with a broad scope of practice and who care for a wide variety of patients achieve similar BP control rates as physicians.[56] However, when nurse case managers are carefully integrated into a practice setting, focus on hypertension, are given responsibility for achieving BP goals and making medication modifications, BP control rates can be improved.

Use of Pharmacists in Team-Based Care of Hypertension

Pharmacists now practice in many different settings including physician office practices, academic primary care clinics and Veterans' Affairs Medical Centers (VAMCs), and community pharmacies.[58] Pharmacists in all these environments have assisted physicians with managing patients with hypertension. However, changes in state and federal law, especially the new Medicare prescription drug benefit, have established mechanisms by which pharmacists can bill for services. These changes may increase the ability of group practices to hire clinical pharmacists to assist with managing patients with hypertension.

Community Pharmacy

Community pharmacists have assisted with hypertension management in a number of ways, including screening and referral, education on lifestyle modifications, and monitoring medication adherence. The primary goal of these programs is to assist the physician with monitoring of BP in the patient's community environment. Collaboration between physicians and community pharmacists can be challenging because of distance between providers and limited accessibility of data from medical records to community pharmacists. However, these barriers can be overcome if the physician and pharmacist establish formal policies and procedures regarding patient treatment. These policies and procedures should include goals of therapy, physician preference for the initiation of care plans including whether the pharmacist can initiate new therapies or change dosages, whether medication changes are via protocol or with physician consent, and when to triage or refer patients back to the physician, especially those patients with urgent needs (e.g., new onset of symptoms). These pharmacists need access to coexisting conditions, diagnostic information, and laboratory results. The issue of patient information transfer can be handled several ways. In some cases, patients simply sign a release of medical information and this document is sent to the patient's physician. Pharmacists then frequently communicate with the physician via facsimile and/or with written notes and recommendations mailed to the physician.[59,60] More recently, physicians have provided collaborating pharmacies with access to the electronic medical record (EMR) following appropriate certification including the Health Insurance Portability and Accountability Act (HIPAA) to allow access to their medical record information.[26] In these cases, pharmacists can make recommendations to change medications directly into the EMR, thus making changes occur much more quickly and reliably.

Another classic study was published in *Circulation* in 1973 in 50 patients randomized to traditional pharmacy services or an intervention group.[61] The community pharmacist worked closely with two physicians in an urban health center in Detroit, visited the physician's office to review medical records, and made recommendations for changes in therapy. Patients in the intervention group were seen monthly for 5 months by appointment with the pharmacist in 1 of 3 community pharmacies participating in the study. BP in the physician's office increased in the control group (163/93 versus 166/101 mm Hg) but was lowered in the intervention group (157/99 versus 146/90 mm Hg). The difference between the two groups was significant ($p < 0.001$). Once the intervention was discontinued, BP control and adherence declined in the intervention group.

Zillich et al conducted a randomized trial in 12 community pharmacies that were randomized to a high-intensity (n = 64 patients) versus low-intensity intervention (n = 61 patients). The high-intensity intervention involved four face-to-face visits with a trained community pharmacist who provided patient-specific education about hypertension and recommendations to physicians. Following the first and third visits, patients were given a home BP monitoring device to measure their BP at least once daily for the next month. Home BP readings were used by the pharmacists to develop treatment recommendations for the patient's physician. Recommendations were discussed with the physician and, if approved, implemented by the pharmacist. Patients in the low intervention group had their BP measured by the pharmacists and were then referred to their physician for evaluation if the BP was high. SBP declined 13.4 mm Hg in the high-intensity group and 9.0 mm Hg in the low-intensity group. At the final visit, the difference in SBP/DBP change between the high- and low-intensity groups was –4.5/–3.2 mm Hg ($p = 0.12$ for SBP and $p = 0.03$ for DBP). This is one of the few pharmacy-based studies that found minimal differences between groups. The authors speculated that the large drop in BP in the low-intensity group may have been attributed to the simple act of having the community pharmacists measure the BP and refer patients back to their physician when BP was high. The marked reduction seen in the low intensity group reduced the effect size and power of the trial and led to a lack of statistical significance between groups.

Pharmacists Embedded Within Clinics

Pharmacist-managed hypertension clinics are found in specific settings such as VAMCs or academic health sciences centers. In such settings, pharmacists provide all the patient follow-up and medication changes but any changes were "staffed" with an internist. In other settings with specific protocols and scope of practice descriptions for pharmacists in a VAMC, pharmacists modify medications independently.[62]

A study at Group Health in Seattle enrolled 778 participants aged 25 to 75 years with uncontrolled essential hypertension and Internet access.[25] Participants were randomly assigned to usual care, home BP monitoring, and secure patient Web site training only, or home BP monitoring and secure patient Web site training plus pharmacist care management delivered for 12 months through Web communications. Patients assigned to the home BP monitoring and Web training only group had a nonsignificant increase in the percentage of patients at goal BP (<140/90 mm Hg) compared with usual care (36% [95% CI, 30% to 42%] versus 31% [95% CI, 25% to 37%]; $p = 0.21$). Adding Web-based pharmacist care significantly increased the percentage of patients who were at goal BP (56%; 95% CI, 49% to 62%) compared with usual care (31%; 95% CI, 25% to 37%; $p < 0.001$) and home BP monitoring and Web training only (36%; 95% CI, 30% to 42%; $p < 0.001$). The authors concluded that pharmacist care management was necessary to improve BP control when delivered through a secure website.

Most chronic care management services for hypertension provided by pharmacists are performed in group practices and in close collaboration with physicians.[58,63-65] One study evaluated the effect of a pharmacist working closely with physicians in a medical resident teaching clinic to improve BP control.[65] Patients with uncontrolled hypertension were randomized to either a control (n = 46) or intervention (n = 49) group. SBP decreased 23 mm Hg in the intervention group versus 11 mm Hg in the control group ($p < 0.001$). At the end of the study, 55% in the intervention versus 20% in the control group ($p < 0.001$) were at BP goal.

Borenstein reported on the effect of physician-pharmacist comanagement of hypertension in an integrated health system.[63] Patients were randomized to either usual care (n = 99) or a comanaged group (n = 98), who attended a hypertension clinic run by pharmacists. The pharmacist contacted the patient's physician with an assessment and recommendations based on a previously designed evidence-based algorithm. BP was reduced significantly more in the comanaged group than in the usual care group ($p < 0.01$) at 6, 9 and 12 months (22 versus 9, 25 versus 10 and 22 versus 11 mm Hg, respectively). Significantly more patients in the comanaged group (60%) achieved BP goal than in the usual care group (43%, $p = 0.02$).

We conducted two studies within primary care clinics, most of which included family medicine offices that were randomized to either a control or intervention group in cluster-randomized designs.[38,66] The first study enrolled 179 patients with uncontrolled BP into a 9-month study with BP measurements by a research nurse. The mean adjusted difference in SBP was 8.7 (95% CI: 4.4, 12.9) mm Hg in favor of the intervention group, whereas the difference in DBP was 5.4 (CI: 2.8, 8.0) mm Hg. The 24-hour BP levels showed similar effects, with mean SBP 8.8 (CI: 5.0, 12.6) mm Hg and DBP 4.6 (CI: 2.4, 6.8) mm Hg lower in the intervention group. BP was at goal in 89.1% of patients in the intervention group and 52.9% in the control group (adjusted odds ratio [OR] 8.9; CI: 3.8, 20.7; $p < 0.001$).

The second study involved six family medicine medical offices randomized to either the control or intervention group.[66] The study enrolled 402 patients (mean age 58.3 years) with hypertension not at goal into a 6-month intervention or control group. Clinical pharmacists made drug-therapy recommendations to physicians based on national guidelines. Research nurses performed BP measurements and 24-hour BP monitoring. Mean BP decreased 6.8/4.5 and 20.7/9.7 mm Hg in the control and intervention groups, respectively, ($p < 0.05$ for between-group SBP comparison). The adjusted difference in SBP was –12.0 (95% CI: –24.0, 0.0) mm Hg. The 24-hour BP levels showed similar differences between groups. BP was at goal in 29.9% of patients in the control group and 63.9% in the intervention group (adjusted OR 3.2; CI: 2.0, 5.1; $p < 0.001$).

Most of the studies evaluating team-based care, whether with nurses or pharmacists, were conducted in a small number of medical offices. In contrast, the Collaboration Among Pharmacists and physicians To Improve Outcomes Now (CAPTION) study was a prospective, cluster-randomized trial of 32 primary care offices in 15 U.S. states stratified and randomized to: control, 9-month intervention (brief intervention [BI]), 24-month intervention (sustained intervention [SI]). One goal was to determine the effect of the intervention after it was discontinued (BI) and another was to determine if the intervention was effective in minority populations. We enrolled 625 subjects with uncontrolled hypertension.[67] There were 239 African-American (38%), 89 Hispanic (14%) subjects, and 50% of the total population had diabetes or chronic kidney disease (CKD). BP control (using the Seventh Report of the Joint National Committee on Prevention, Detection, Evaluation, and Treatment of High Blood Pressure [JNC 7]) at 9 months was 43% in intervention offices (n = 401) compared with 34% in the control group (n = 224) (adjusted OR 1.57 [95% CI 0.99 to 2.50], $p = 0.059$). Based on JNC 8, BP control was achieved in 61% of intervention subjects and 45% of control subjects at 9 months (adjusted OR, 2.03 [95% CI 1.29 to 3.22], $p = 0.003$). The adjusted difference in mean SBP/DBP between the intervention and control groups for all subjects at 9 months was –6.1/–2.9 mm Hg ($p = 0.002$ and $p = 0.005$, respectively), and it was –6.4/–2.9 mm Hg ($p = 0.009$ and $p = 0.044$, respectively) in subjects from racial or ethnic minorities. At the 24-month visit, BP control was 63%, 57%, and 46% in the BI, SI, and control groups, respectively. The adjusted OR for the BI compared with the control group was 1.84 [95% CI 0.89 to 3.78], $p = 0.098$) and for the SI with the control group was 1.67 [95% CI 0.86 to 3.26], $p = 0.13$). This is one of the few trials that evaluated what happens when an intervention is stopped. This and other studies[62,68,69] suggest that a pharmacy-based intervention has a sustained effect for at least 18 months after discontinued in most patients. This is also one of the few studies designed to demonstrate that the pharmacy intervention was as effective in underrepresented minority populations as in nonminority subjects.

Svarstad and colleagues enrolled 576 African-American patients for an intervention in community pharmacies.[70] Intervention subjects achieved greater improvements in refill adherence (60% versus 34%, $p < 0.001$), SBP (–12.62 versus –5.31 mm Hg, $p < 0.001$), and BP control (50% versus 36%, $p = 0.01$) compared with controls. Six months after intervention discontinuation, intervention participants showed sustained improvements in refill adherence ($p < 0.001$) and SBP ($p = 0.004$), although the difference in BP control was not significant ($p < 0.05$) compared with control participants. This study demonstrated that the pharmacy-based intervention was very effective in African-American patients.

Telephone Interventions

Bosworth compared two self-management interventions for improving BP control among hypertensive patients (n = 636, 49% African American).[52] Randomized to receive usual care, a behavioral intervention (bimonthly tailored, nurse-administered telephone intervention targeting hypertension-related behaviors), home BP monitoring three times weekly, or the behavioral intervention plus home BP monitoring. At 24 months, improvements in the proportion of patients with BP control relative to the usual care group were 4.3% (95% CI, –4.5% to 12.9%) in the behavioral intervention group, 7.6% (CI, –1.9% to 17.0%) in the home BP monitoring group, and 11.0% (CI, 1.9%, 19.8%) in the combined intervention group. Relative to usual care, the 24-month difference in SBP was 0.6 mm Hg (CI, –2.2 to 3.4 mm Hg) for the behavioral intervention group, –0.6 mm Hg (CI, –3.6 to 2.3 mm Hg) for the BP monitoring group, and –3.9 mm Hg (CI, –6.9 to –0.9 mm Hg) for the combined intervention group; patterns were similar for DBP.

Margolis conducted a cluster, randomized trial in 450 subjects.[71] Compared with the usual care group, SBP decreased more from baseline among patients in the telemonitoring intervention group at 6 months (–10.7 mm Hg [95% CI, –14.3 to –7.3 mm Hg]; $p < 0.001$), at 12 months (–9.7 mm Hg [95% CI, –13.4 to –6.0 mm Hg]; $p < 0.001$), and at 18 months (6 months after discontinuation of the intervention) (–6.6 mm Hg [95% CI, –10.7 to –2.5 mm Hg]; $p = 0.004$). Nearly all of the effect was mediated by two factors: an increase in medication treatment intensity (24%) and increased home BP monitor use (19%).[72]

Artinian offered free BP screenings to African Americans at various community sites and those with uncontrolled BP and a land-line telephone were randomized to enhanced usual care (UC), including education and identifying resources for receiving medications and clinical care, or UC plus home BP monitoring (HBPM), and nurse managed telemetry.[73] At 12 months the telemetry nurse group had significantly decreased SBP compared with enhanced usual care (net difference –5.5 mm Hg ($p = 0.04$). Change in BP control was not reported.

Bosworth randomized patients to either usual care or one of three telephone-based intervention groups: (1) nurse-administered behavioral management, (2) nurse-administered and physician-administered medication management, or (3) a combination of both.[74] Both the behavioral management and medication management alone showed significant improvements in BP control, 12.8% (95% CI: 1.6%, 24.1%) and 12.5% (95% CI: 1.3%, 23.6%), respectively, at 12 months, but there was no difference at 18 months. In a subgroup analyses, among those with poor baseline BP control, SBP decreased in the combined group by 14.8 mm Hg (95% CI: –21.8, –7.8) at 12 months and 8.0 mm Hg (95% CI: –15.5, –0.5) at 18 months, relative to usual care.

Private physician offices often do not have the resources to hire clinical pharmacists to do the interventions described here. We are conducting two trials to address this problem by using a centralized cardiovascular risk service staffed by clinical pharmacists to assist primary care physicians with improving care management. The Improved Cardiovascular Risk Reduction to Enhance Rural Primary Care: (ICARE) trial is being conducted in 12 offices in Iowa and the research pharmacists have obtained EMR access at all intervention offices.[26] Recommendations to physicians are provided directly into the EMR whereas frequent patient contact is done by telephone. We are also conducting another study in 20 medical offices throughout the U.S. that uses a similar intervention.[27] The MEDication Focused Outpatient Care for Underutilization of Secondary Prevention (MEDFOCUS) trial will evaluate a centralized, web-based cardiovascular risk service (CVRS). These studies should help to determine if clinical pharmacists located at a distant site can help improve the management of chronic conditions.

Medicaid and Underserved Populations

Many states have expanded Medicaid following the Affordable Care Act. These patients can have significant socioeconomic issues that make adherence to BP medications a challenge. Most studies do not specifically focus on patients receiving Medicaid so it is difficult to evaluate specific team-based care strategies. However, several studies did examine interventions in low-income, underserved populations.

Hill studied a more intensive nurse intervention with a less intensive educational intervention in 309 urban African-American men. Mean SBP was 7.5 mm Hg lower in the intensive group compared with 3.4 mm Hg higher for the less intensive intervention at 36 months ($p = 0.001$). DBP change from baseline was –10.1 mm Hg for the more intensive group and –3.7 mm Hg for the less intensive group ($p = 0.005$ for between-group differences). The proportion of subjects with controlled BP (<140/90 mm Hg) was 44% in the more intensive group and 31% in the less intensive group ($p = 0.045$).

Ma and colleagues conducted a randomized trial of nurse- and dietitian-led case management for 419 low-income, ethnic minority patients.[75] The study involved managing multiple risk factors but the main effect was improved BP where SBP was lower in the intervention group (–4.2 mm Hg) compared with usual care (+2.6 mm Hg, $p = 0.003$). DBP was also significantly lower in the intervention group compared with usual care (–6.0 versus –3.0 mm Hg, $p = 0.02$).

One study in a Medicaid population found that patients with hypertension commonly receive a large number of other medications with a high probability for potential drug interactions with antihypertensive medications.[76] Two studies of comprehensive pharmacist interventions for multiple problems for patients receiving Medicaid demonstrated improved therapy and reduced costs.[77,78] In our analysis of the CAPTION trial above, we evaluated whether the pharmacist intervention was as effective in subjects receiving different types of insurance. All subjects had uncontrolled BP at baseline. Although these data are as yet unpublished, we found BP control after a 9-month intervention was achieved in 48% of subjects receiving private insurance, 43% receiving Medicare, 38% with no insurance or self-pay, and 36% receiving Medicaid ($p = 0.102$). All of the above studies suggest that more comprehensive strategies will need to be considered to achieve good BP control in patients receiving Medicaid.

AN INTEGRATED MODEL TO PROVIDE HYPERTENSION CARE

Health systems and the Center for Medicare & Medicaid Services (CMS) will continue to implement strategies to improve care at lower costs. The development of these standards will lead health systems to better integrate care through the use of teams to provide chronic care management to improve performance.

The studies discussed above suggest that chronic care management provided by either nurses or pharmacists can improve BP control. Whether a nurse, pharmacist, or both are used to assist the physician will largely be determined by the size and structure of the clinic, office, or health system. The above studies, however, do not help physicians or administrators determine how to most efficiently utilize the blend of professionals required to optimize BP control in large populations cared for by a clinic, health system, or managed care organizations.

Reorganizing the Structure and Process of Care Delivery

The following proposed models require that BP is properly measured and classified as discussed in other chapters of this book. Perhaps the most important aspect of achieving success is for the clinic or health system to have a goal-oriented approach to treating hypertension. Everyone involved with the care of patients with hypertension must understand and have "buy-in" regarding their responsibility to achieve goal BP in each patient. Achieving optimal control rates will likely require a complete change in the structure and process of delivering care to meet the PCMH standards (Table 48.3). The clinic must move from an acute care model to a model for managing chronic conditions proactively and fully engage the patient when possible. For instance, those who schedule patients must understand the requirement for continuity with the hypertension management team. The clinic must institute processes to track patients, remind them of their upcoming office visit, and contact them when they do not show up for an appointment. Patients should have access to schedule their own appointments, send an email to providers, and receive web-based support.

Decision-support tools and evidence-based approaches to managing hypertension that effectively support physicians and other providers are critical to the success of chronic care programs.

Proposed Models for Individual of Team Members

The physician will be responsible for properly diagnosing and evaluating hypertension for potential secondary causes, additional risk factors, and target organ damage. The nurse might provide education and counseling for patients with uncomplicated hypertension taking no antihypertensive medication. This education would include thorough discussions about all lifestyle modifications, smoking cessation, and how to empower the patient to implement these strategies. If the office or health system includes a behavioral counselor or nutritionist, this person might provide the patient with in-depth counseling about diet and weight loss strategies. If these professionals are not available, the nurse who specializes in hypertension management can provide this education. The nurse can then see patients for follow-up at appropriate intervals to evaluate progress. If medication has been prescribed, the nurse might be given responsibility to modify medications and adjust dosages via protocol.[2]

If the clinic employs a pharmacist to assist with care management, the pharmacist should assist with designing a specific drug and monitoring regimen, especially for patients with coexisting conditions, treatment-resistant hypertension, or those at risk for important drug-drug interactions. The pharmacist should be given a clinic schedule and a room to see such patients. The pharmacist could also counsel patients about proper medication use, administration, storage, and adverse reactions that might occur. The best use of a pharmacist may be to provide care and medication titrations for patients who are not at their goal BP. Our data suggest that the pharmacist's medication management needs to occur frequently and medications titrated quickly to achieve the BP goal and work best if the pharmacist is responsible for making the needed medication changes.[38,66,67,79] Once the goal BP is achieved, the pharmacist could refer the patient back to the nurse and physician.

Efficiency can be greatly improved by the use of telephone or the internet for follow-up by the nurse or pharmacist to evaluate medication and diet adherence.[25,80] Monitoring and patient involvement can be further strengthened by the use of home BP monitoring so long as the patient is properly trained and that they reliably and accurately report BP values. It is also critical that the patient and team understand the importance of lower goals for home BP (e.g., <135/85 mm Hg) compared with clinic pressures (<140/90 mm Hg). Again, monitoring may be facilitated by engaging community pharmacists.

An effective chronic care management program must have a mechanism to remind patients of office visits, call patients who do not appear for office visits and, perhaps, include an individual to serve as an initial point of contact when the patient needs assistance. This individual need not be a highly trained professional and, if fact, might be a lay person.[81] Some models include this individual in a care role that includes providing telephone reminders, follow-up scheduling coordination, and initially greeting the patient and placing them in the examination room as a strategy to improve continuity.

The physician should see the patient at appropriate intervals to conduct periodic physical examinations and follow-up assessments for target organ damage. The physician should coordinate the care provided to the patient. If at any point new signs or symptoms develop the physician should evaluate the patient.

Many patients with hypertension will have coexisting conditions, complications, or other drug therapy that may make treatment decisions more difficult. The model described above would generally be effective for these complicated patients with a few modifications except that the physician may need closer follow-up of these more complex patients. In addition, it might be appropriate to more fully engage the clinical pharmacist for such patients.[23,82] In this model the pharmacist would perform a thorough assessment of medications and dosages, evaluate laboratory parameters, adverse reactions, drug-drug interactions, drug-disease interactions, and costs.[23] Depending on the health system, the pharmacist may be delegated responsibility to make medication modifications or dosage adjustments to improve BP control and/or the control of other conditions like diabetes or dyslipidemia. In other settings, the pharmacist would make specific recommendations for changes to the physician. The nurse would continue to see the patient for follow-up visits, but the pharmacist may also see the patient to assist with more complex medication modifications.

This proposed model would obviously require a great deal of communication between the primary care physician, clinical pharmacist, nurse, and any other providers involved with the care of the patient. Accurate and complete medical record documentation is critical. In addition, it would be ideal to establish protocols, policies, and procedures for communication, triage, and referral back to the physician and use of specialists so information transfers are coordinated and complete. Of course, all of the proposed team members should have appropriate skills to manage patients with chronic conditions. Pharmacists can become board certified in pharmacotherapy and there are other certification programs for other professionals. The American Society of Hypertension (ASH) has provided a certification examination for many years for physicians who wish to become hypertension specialists. ASH recently announced that the ASH Certified Hypertension Clinician credentialing examination will be offered to pharmacists, nurses, physician assistants, and primary care physicians in 2016. Certification and credentialing programs will be increasingly important to demonstrate competence in hypertension and other chronic conditions.

SUMMARY

Goal-oriented management of patients with hypertension can be provided by physicians, pharmacists, nurses, and perhaps other professionals. Coordinated and collaborative models that include interdisciplinary management have been superior to care provided by individuals. To optimally provide chronic care for patients with hypertension, the entire delivery system needs to be structured to focus on a chronic care model. Instead of waiting for patients to present to the office or expecting them to come to each scheduled visit, strategies must be implemented to ensure adherence to office visits through reminders and telephone calls for missed appointments. Care needs to be provided at times that are convenient for the patient with minimal waits before being seen. Care and office visits might be coordinated by a lay person who ensures that patients have been reminded of their visits and helps to guide them through the visits with a personal touch. In settings where this interdisciplinary model has been implemented, BP control rates have been markedly improved. Health systems and physician offices should determine how they can incorporate these concepts into the care of patients with chronic conditions, to achieve high levels of performance in the PCMH.

References

1. Egan BM, Zhao Y, Axon RN. US trends in prevalence, awareness, treatment, and control of hypertension, 1988-2008. *JAMA.* 2010;303:2043-2050.
2. Shaw KM, Handler J, Wall HK, Kanter MH. Improving blood pressure control in a large multiethnic California population through changes in health care delivery, 2004-2012. *Prev Chronic Dis.* 2014;11:E191.
3. Hyre AD, Krousel-Wood MA, Muntner P, Kawasaki L, Desalvo KB. Prevalence and predictors of poor antihypertensive medication adherence in an urban health clinic setting. *J Clin Hypertens (Greenwich).* 2007;9:179-186.
4. Kressin NR, Wang F, Long J, et al. Hypertensive patients' race, health beliefs, process of care, and medication adherence. *J Gen Intern Med.* 2007;22:768-774.
5. Ogedegbe G, Harrison M, Robbins L, Mancuso CA, Allegrante JP. Barriers and facilitators of medication adherence in hypertensive African Americans: a qualitative study. *Ethn Dis.* 2004;14:3-12.
6. Christensen AJ, Howren MB, Hillis SL, et al. Patient and physician beliefs about control over health: association of symmetrical beliefs with medication regimen adherence. *J Gen Intern Med.* 2010;25:397-402.
7. O'Connor PJ. Overcome clinical inertia to control systolic blood pressure. *Arch Intern Med.* 2003;163:2677-2678.
8. Okonofua EC, Simpson KN, Jesri A, Rehman SU, Durkalski VL, Egan BM. Therapeutic inertia is an impediment to achieving the Healthy People 2010 blood pressure control goals. *Hypertension.* 2006;47:345-351.
9. Grumbach K, Bodenheimer T. Can health care teams improve primary care practice? *JAMA.* 2004;291:1246-1251.
10. Bodenheimer T, Wagner EH, Grumbach K. Improving primary care for patients with chronic illness. *JAMA.* 2002;288:1775-1779.
11. Wagner EH, Austin BT, Davis C, Hindmarsh M, Schaefer J, Bonomi A. Improving chronic illness care: translating evidence into action. *Health Aff (Millwood).* 2001;20:64-78.
12. Walsh JM, McDonald KM, Shojania KG, et al. Quality improvement strategies for hypertension management: a systematic review. *Med Care.* 2006;44:646-657.
13. Carter BL, Rogers M, Daly J, Zheng S, James PA. The potency of team-based care interventions for hypertension: a meta-analysis. *Arch Intern Med.* 2009;169:1748-1755.
14. Chisholm-Burns MA, Kim Lee J, Spivey CA, et al. US pharmacists' effect as team members on patient care: systematic review and meta-analyses. *Med Care.* 2010;48:923-933.
15. Berenson RA, Hammons T, Gans DN, et al. A house is not a home: keeping patients at the center of practice redesign. *Health Aff (Millwood).* 2008;27:1219-1230.
16. Rosenthal TC. Advancing Medical Homes: evidence-based literature review to inform health policy. www.ahec.buffalo.edu.
17. Kellerman R, Kirk L. Principles of the patient-centered medical home. *Am Fam Physician.* 2007;76:774-775.
18. Rosenthal TC. The medical home: growing evidence to support a new approach to primary care. *J Am Board Fam Med.* 2008;21:427-440.
19. National Committee for Quality Assurance. Patient Centered Medical Home (PCMH 2014) Standards. www.ncqa.org/Programs/Recognition/RelevanttoAllRecognition/RecognitionTraining/PCMH2014Standards.aspx.
20. Reid RJ, Coleman K, Johnson EA, et al. The group health medical home at year two: cost savings, higher patient satisfaction, and less burnout for providers. *Health Aff (Millwood).* 2010;29:835-843.
21. Reid RJ, Fishman PA, Yu O, et al. Patient-centered medical home demonstration: a prospective, quasi-experimental, before and after evaluation. *Am J Manag Care.* 2009;15:e71-e87.
22. Shi L, Forrest CB, Von Schrader S, Ng J. Vulnerability and the patient-practitioner relationship: the roles of gatekeeping and primary care performance. *Am J Public Health.* 2003;93:138-144.
23. Merenich JA, Olson KL, Delate T, Rasmussen J, Helling DK, Ward DG. Mortality reduction benefits of a comprehensive cardiac care program for patients with occlusive coronary artery disease. *Pharmacotherapy.* 2007;27:1370-1378.
24. Smith M, Bates DW, Bodenheimer T, Cleary PD. Why pharmacists belong in the medical home. *Health Aff (Millwood).* 2010;29:906-913.
25. Green BB, Cook AJ, Ralston JD, et al. Effectiveness of home blood pressure monitoring, Web communication, and pharmacist care on hypertension control: a randomized controlled trial. *JAMA.* 2008;299:2857-2867.
26. Carter BL, Levy BT, Gryzlak B, et al. A centralized cardiovascular risk service to improve guideline adherence in private primary care offices. *Contemp Clin Trials.* 2015;43:25-32.
27. Carter BL, Coffey CS, Chrischilles EA, et al. A cluster-randomized trial of a centralized clinical pharmacy cardiovascular risk service to improve guideline adherence. *Pharmacotherapy.* 2015;35:653-662.
28. Wagner EH. The role of patient care teams in chronic disease management. *BMJ.* 2000;320:569-572.
29. Von Korff M, Gruman J, Schaefer J, Curry SJ, Wagner EH. Collaborative management of chronic illness. *Ann Intern Med.* 1997;127:1097-1102.
30. Machado M, Bajcar J, Guzzo GC, Einarson TR. Sensitivity of patient outcomes to pharmacist interventions. Part II: systematic review and meta-analysis in hypertension management. *Ann Pharmacother.* 2007;41:1770-1781.
31. Santschi V, Chiolero A, Colosimo AL, et al. Improving blood pressure control through pharmacist interventions: a meta-analysis of randomized controlled trials. *J Am Heart Assoc.* 2014;3:e000718.
32. Hawkins DW, Fiedler FP, Douglas HL, Eschbach RC. Evaluation of a clinical pharmacist in caring for hypertensive and diabetic patients. *Am J Hosp Pharm.* 1979;36:1321-1325.
33. Schneider PJ, Larrimer JN, Visconti JA, Miller WA. Role effectiveness of a pharmacist in the maintenance of patients with hypertension and congestive heart failure. *Contemp Pharm Pract.* 1982;5:74-79.
34. Erickson SR, Slaughter R, Halapy H. Pharmacists' ability to influence outcomes of hypertension therapy. *Pharmacotherapy.* 1997;17:140-147.
35. Mehos BM, Saseen JJ, MacLaughlin EJ. Effect of pharmacist intervention and initiation of home blood pressure monitoring in patients with uncontrolled hypertension. *Pharmacotherapy.* 2000;20:1384-1389.
36. Okamoto MP, Nakahiro RK. Pharmacoeconomic evaluation of a pharmacist-managed hypertension clinic. *Pharmacotherapy.* 2001;21:1337-1344.
37. Vivian EM. Improving blood pressure control in a pharmacist-managed hypertension clinic. *Pharmacotherapy.* 2002;22:1533-1540.
38. Carter BL, Bergus GR, Dawson JD, et al. A cluster randomized trial to evaluate physician/pharmacist collaboration to improve blood pressure control. *J Clin Hypertens (Greenwich).* 2008;10:260-271.
39. Artinian NT, Washington OG, Templin TN. Effects of home telemonitoring and community-based monitoring on blood pressure control in urban African Americans: a pilot study. *Heart Lung.* 2001;30:191-199.

40. Gabbay RA, Lendel I, Saleem TM, et al. Nurse case management improves blood pressure, emotional distress and diabetes complication screening. *Diabetes Res Clin Pract.* 2006;71:28-35.

41. Curzio JL, Rubin PC, Kennedy SS, Reid JL. A comparison of the management of hypertensive patients by nurse practitioners compared with conventional hospital care. *J Hum Hypertens.* 1990;4:665-670.

42. Hill MN, Han HR, Dennison CR, et al. Hypertension care and control in underserved urban African American men: behavioral and physiologic outcomes at 36 months. *Am J Hypertens.* 2003;16:906-913.

43. Clark CE, Smith LF, Taylor RS, Campbell JL. Nurse led interventions to improve control of blood pressure in people with hypertension: systematic review and meta-analysis. *BMJ.* 2011;341:c3995.

44. Proia KK, Thota AB, Njie GJ, et al. Team-based care and improved blood pressure control: a community guide systematic review. *Am J Prev Med.* 2014;47:86-99.

45. Kulchaitanaroaj P, Brooks JM, Ardery G, Newman D, Carter BL. Incremental costs associated with physician and pharmacist collaboration to improve blood pressure control. *Pharmacotherapy.* 2012;32:772-780.

46. Polgreen LA, Han J, Carter BL, et al. Cost-effectiveness of a physician-pharmacist collaboration intervention to improve blood pressure control. *Hypertension.* 2015;66:1145-1151.

47. Jacob V, Chattopadhyay SK, Thota AB, et al. Economics of team-based care in controlling blood pressure: a community guide systematic review. *Am J Prev Med.* 2015;49:772-783.

48. Allen JK, Dennison CR. Randomized trials of nursing interventions for secondary prevention in patients with coronary artery disease and heart failure: systematic review. *J Cardiovasc Nurs.* 2010;25:207-220.

49. DeBusk RF, Miller NH, Superko HR, et al. A case-management system for coronary risk factor modification after acute myocardial infarction. *Ann Intern Med.* 1994;120:721-729.

50. Rudd P, Miller NH, Kaufman J, et al. Nurse management for hypertension. A systems approach. *Am J Hypertens.* 2004;17:921-927.

51. Bosworth HB, Olsen MK, Dudley T, et al. Patient education and provider decision support to control blood pressure in primary care: a cluster randomized trial. *Am Heart J.* 2009;157:450-456.

52. Bosworth HB, Olsen MK, Grubber JM, et al. Two self-management interventions to improve hypertension control: a randomized trial. *Ann Intern Med.* 2009;151:687-695.

53. Bosworth H, Powers BJ, Olsen MK, et al. Can home blood pressure management improve blood pressure control: results from a randomized controlled trial. *Arch Int Med.* 2011;171:1173-1180.

54. Sikka R, Waters J, Moore W, Sutton DR, Herman WH, Aubert RE. Renal assessment practices and the effect of nurse case management of health maintenance organization patients with diabetes. *Diabetes Care.* 1999;22:1-6.

55. Logan AG, Milne BJ, Achber C, Campbell WP, Haynes RB. Work-site treatment of hypertension by specially trained nurses. A controlled trial. *Lancet.* 1979;2:1175-1178.

56. Mundinger MO, Kane RL, Lenz ER, et al. Primary care outcomes in patients treated by nurse practitioners or physicians: a randomized trial. *JAMA.* 2000;283:59-68.

57. Guerra-Riccio GM, Artigas Giorgi DM, Consolin-Colombo FM, et al. Frequent nurse visits decrease white coat effect in stage III hypertension. *Am J Hypertens.* 2004;17:523-528.

58. Carter BL, Zillich AJ, Elliott WJ. How pharmacists can assist physicians with controlling blood pressure. *J Clin Hypertens.* 2003;5:31-37.

59. Zillich AJ, Sutherland JM, Kumbera PA, Carter BL. Hypertension outcomes through blood pressure monitoring and evaluation by pharmacists (HOME study). *J Gen Intern Med.* 2005;20:1091-1096.

60. Park JJ, Kelly P, Carter BL, Burgess PP. Comprehensive pharmaceutical care in the chain (pharmacy) setting. *J Am Pharm Assoc.* 1996;NS36:443-451.

61. McKenney JM, Slining JM, Henderson HR, Devins D, Barr M. The effect of clinical pharmacy services on patients with essential hypertension. *Circulation.* 1973;48:1104-1111.

62. Parker CP, Cunningham CL, Carter BL, Vander Weg MW, Richardson KK, Rosenthal GE. A mixed-method approach to evaluate a pharmacist intervention for veterans with hypertension. *J Clin Hypertens (Greenwich).* 2014;16:133-140.

63. Borenstein JE, Graber G, Saltiel E, et al. Physician-pharmacist comanagement of hypertension: a randomized, comparative trial. *Pharmacotherapy.* 2003;23:209-216.

64. Bogden PE, Koontz LM, Williamson P, Abbott RD. The physician and pharmacist team. An effective approach to cholesterol reduction. *J Gen Intern Med.* 1997;12:158-164.

65. Bogden PE, Abbott RD, Williamson P, Onopa JK, Koontz LM. Comparing standard care with a physician and pharmacist team approach for uncontrolled hypertension. *J Gen Intern Med.* 1998;13:740-745.

66. Carter BL, Ardery G, Dawson JD, et al. Physician and pharmacist collaboration to improve blood pressure control. *Arch Intern Med.* 2009;169:1996-2002.

67. Carter BL, Coffey CS, Ardery G, et al. Cluster-randomized trial of a physician/pharmacist collaborative model to improve blood pressure control. *Circ Cardiovasc Qual Outcomes.* 2015;8:235-243.

68. Wentzlaff DM, Carter BL, Ardery G, et al. Sustained blood pressure control following discontinuation of a pharmacist intervention. *J Clin Hypertens (Greenwich).* 2011;13:431-437.

69. Carter BL, Doucette WR, Franciscus CL, Ardery G, Kluesner KM, Chrischilles EA. Deterioration of blood pressure control after discontinuation of a physician-pharmacist collaborative intervention. *Pharmacotherapy.* 2010;30:228-235.

70. Svarstad BL, Kotchen JM, Shireman TI, et al. Improving refill adherence and hypertension control in black patients: wisconsin TEAM trial. *J Am Pharm Assoc (2003).* 2013;53:520-529.

71. Margolis KL, Asche SE, Bergdall AR, et al. Effect of home blood pressure telemonitoring and pharmacist management on blood pressure control: a cluster randomized clinical trial. *JAMA.* 2013;310:46-56.

72. Margolis KL, Asche SE, Bergdall AR, et al. A successful multifaceted trial to improve hypertension control in primary care: why did it work? *J Gen Intern Med.* 2015;30:1665-1672.

73. Artinian NT, Flack JM, Nordstrom CK, et al. Effects of nurse-managed telemonitoring on blood pressure at 12-month follow-up among urban African Americans. *Nurs Res.* 2007;56:312-322.

74. Bosworth HB, Powers BJ, Olsen MK, et al. Home blood pressure management and improved blood pressure control: results from a randomized controlled trial. *Arch Int Med.* 2011;171:1173-1180.

75. Carter BL, Lund BC, Hayase N, Chrischilles E. The extent of potential antihypertensive drug interactions in a Medicaid population. *Am J Hypertens.* 2002;15:953-957.

76. Ma J, Berra K, Haskell WL, et al. Case management to reduce risk of cardiovascular disease in a county health care system. *Arch Intern Med.* 2009;169:1988-1995.

77. Smith M, Giuliano MR, Starkowski MP. Connecticut: improving patient medication management in primary care. *Health Aff (Millwood).* 2011;30:646-654.

78. Chrischilles EA, Carter BL, Lund BC, et al. Evaluation of the Iowa Medicaid pharmaceutical case management program. *J Am Pharm Assoc (Wash DC).* 2004;44:337-349.

79. Von Muenster SJ, Carter BL, Weber CA, et al. Description of pharmacist interventions during physician-pharmacist co-management of hypertension. *Pharm World Sci.* 2008;30:128-135.

80. Simon GE, VonKorff M, Rutter C, Wagner E. Randomised trial of monitoring, feedback, and management of care by telephone to improve treatment of depression in primary care. *BMJ.* 2000;320:550-554.

81. Sackett DL, Haynes RB, Gibson ES, et al. Randomised clinical trial of strategies for improving medication compliance in primary hypertension. *Lancet.* 1975;1:1205-1207.

82. Olson KL, Rasmussen J, Sandhoff BG, Merenich JA. Lipid management in patients with coronary artery disease by a clinical pharmacy service in a group model health maintenance organization. *Arch Intern Med.* 2005;165:49-54.

49 Understanding and Improving Medication Adherence

Mary G. George

Disclaimer: The findings and conclusions in this document are those of the author and do not necessarily represent the official position of the Centers for Disease Control and Prevention.

> *"Drugs don't work in patients who don't take them."*
> —C. Everett Koop, M.D.

Medication adherence is a major and growing public health concern. However, adherence to antihypertension medication is crucial to not only hypertension control, but in saving lives.

"High adherence to antihypertensive medication is associated with higher odds of blood pressure control, but nonadherence to cardioprotective medications increases a patient's risk of death from 50% to 80%."[1] Although studies report wide ranges for antihypertensive medication adherence attributed to varying methodologies of estimated nonadherence, one-third to one-half of first prescriptions are never filled, and only 15% to 20% of prescriptions are refilled and continued as prescribed (Fig. 49.1). It is estimated that between one-third and two-thirds of medication-related hospital admissions are as a result of poor adherence.[2] Based on NHANES (National Health and Nutrition Examination Survey) data, 29.3% of adults in the United States have hypertension (2013-2014),[3] 75.6%[4] were on medication (2011-2012), and only 54.0%[3] were controlled (2013-2014). Thus 3 in 10 adults taking medication for hypertension remain uncontrolled.[3,4] Poor adherence to medication is an important reason for not achieving hypertension control.[5]

There are many definitions of medication adherence but most of them refer to two concepts: adherence or compliance, which refers to taking medication as prescribed by their health care provider with respect to timing, dosage, and frequency,[6,7] and persistence, which is continuing to take the medication for the duration that the medication was prescribed (Fig. 49.2).[7,8] Additionally, some people refer to never getting a first prescription filled as primary nonadherence and secondary nonadherence as not taking the medication as prescribed. The World Health Organization defines adherence as the extent to which a person's behavior, in this case taking medication, corresponds with the agreed upon recommendations from a health care provider.[6] Medication adherence involves a complex cluster of behaviors and is affected by multiple factors, including patient-related factors, provider factors, health care system factors, condition-related factors, therapy-related factors, and social/economic factors.[9] Medication adherence has been extensively studied for antihypertensive medications because they are so commonly prescribed and adherence is key to control of hypertension.[10] In a 2004 study, it was estimated that 8.3 million office visits per year for hypertension likely ended with nonadherence to prescribed medication.[10] According to a survey by the National Community

Pharmacists Association,[11] of adults aged 40 years and older, the most commonly prescribed medication for a chronic condition was antihypertensive medication, with 57% of survey respondents reporting taking medication for hypertension.

Effective control of hypertension can significantly reduce the rates of stroke and other cardiovascular diseases, and death.[12] Data from clinical trials, which tend to have high rates of medication adherence, have shown that antihypertensive medication can reduce the risk of stroke by 18% to 40%, the risk of myocardial infarction by 15%, and all-cause mortality up to 60% over an average follow-up of 2 to 3 years.[9,13] Several studies have shown the direct relationship between improved antihypertensive medication adherence and improved rates of blood pressure control.[14-17] Studies looking at short-term levels of medication adherence with disease-related health care costs and hospitalization risk for hypertension, found that in general overall health care costs increased with decreasing quintiles of medication adherence despite increased medication costs with better adherence, and those with lower medication adherence had increasing risk for hospitalization (Fig. 49.3).[18]

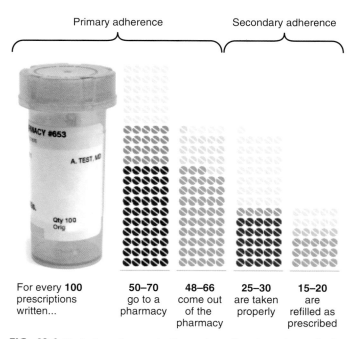

FIG. 49.1 Medication adherence by the numbers. *(From Improving medication adherence among patients with hypertension: a tip sheet for health care professionals. http://millionhearts.hhs.gov and http://millionhearts.hhs.gov/files/TipSheet_HCP_MedAdherence.pdf.)*

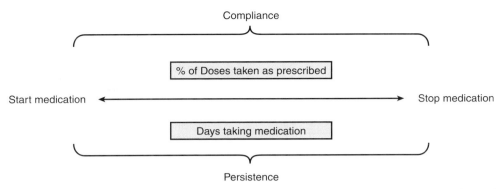

FIG. 49.2 Persistence vs. compliance. *(Adapted from Cramer JA, Roy A, Burrell A, et al. Medication compliance and persistence: Terminology and definitions. Value Health. 2008;11:44-47.)*

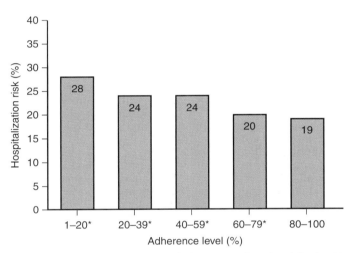

FIG. 49.3 Hospitalization risk by level of adherence. *Indicates hospitalization risk is significantly higher than the risk for the 80% to 100% adherence group (p < 0.05). *(Adapted from Sokol MC, McGuigan KA, Verbrugge RR, Epstein RS. Impact of medication adherence on hospitalization risk and healthcare cost. Med Care. 2005;43:521-530.)*

PREDICTORS OF NONADHERENCE

Medication adherence involves a complex set of behaviors, conditions, and policies that must operate in a coordinated manner and must be individualized for each patient (Box 49.1). More than 100 factors have been identified to be associated with medication adherence.[19] Only half of Americans treated for hypertension are adherent to their long-term therapy. In a recent survey,[11] when asked about nonadherence behaviors, three out of four adult respondents were engaging in at least one of seven nonadherence behaviors (57% had missed doses, 20% did not fill the prescription, and 14% stopped taking the medication). Items identified as strong predictors of medication adherence were connectedness with a pharmacist and always seeing the same doctor, affordability was the second-strongest predictor of adherence, and other predictors were feeling informed about one's health and knowing the importance of taking medication as prescribed. Fischer et al. found that between 26.4% and 28.4% of antihypertensive medication e-prescriptions were never filled the first time the medication was prescribed; yet e-prescriptions for antihypertensives for which the patient had already been taking the medication were more likely to be filled with only 9.8% of antihypertensive e-prescription not being filled.[20,21] They also found that electronic prescriptions sent to a pharmacy were more likely to be filled than printed prescriptions given to the patient, and that e-prescriptions sent directly to a mail-order service were most

BOX 49.1 Predictors of Nonadherence

- Low literacy/limited English language proficiency
- Homelessness
- Depression
- Psychiatric disease
- Substance abuse
- Lower cognitive function or cognitive impairment
- Forgetfulness
- Anger, psychological stress, anxiety
- Lack of insight into illness
- Lack of belief in benefit of treatment
- Belief medications are not important or are harmful
- Complexity of medication regimen
- Tired of taking medications
- Inconvenience of medication regimen
- Side effects or fear of medication side effects
- Cost of medication, copayment, or both
- Barriers to access to care or medications
- Inadequate follow-up or discharge planning missed appointments

(Adapted from Osterberg L, Blaschke T. Adherence to medication. N Engl J Med. 2005;353:487-497; American Society of consultant Pharmacists, American society on Aging. Adult meducation ™ improving medication adherence in older adults. www.adultmeducation.com; Krueger KP, Berger BA, Felkey B. Medication adherence and persistence: A comprehensive review. Adv Ther. 2005;22:313-356.)

likely to be filled, because it required no action on the part of the patient.

REASONS FOR NONADHERENCE

Health care system factors that affect medication adherence include lack of continuity with a care provider or seeing a different care provider each time care is accessed, as can the cost of medication, lack of educational materials about hypertension, and the importance of taking medication as prescribed that are not culturally appropriate or are written at too high of a literacy level (Fig. 49.4). **Provider-related factors** that affect adherence include provider communication skills, lack of positive reinforcement from the provider regarding medication adherence, long wait times at appointments, weak capacity of the provider to educate the patient on their condition, differences between the health beliefs of the provider and the patient, and a less than optimal provider-patient relationship. **Therapy-related factors** include complicated medication regimens or regimens that are inconvenient for the patient, and side effects of the medication. Multiple chronic conditions, especially those that cause the patient to be symptomatic or feel ill, can compete for the patient's attention to medication adherence for a condition such as hypertension,

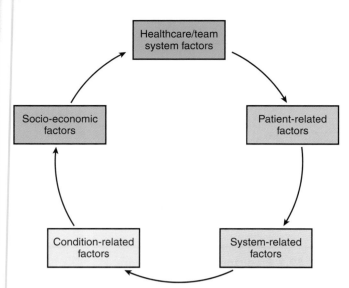

FIG. 49.4 Dimensions of adherence. *(Adapted from World Health Organization. Adherence to long-term therapies: Evidence for action. Geneva. 2003; http://apps.who.int/iris/bitstream/10665/42682/1/9241545992.pdf. Accessed 02/12/2016.)*

BOX 49.2 Predictors of Adherence

1. Connectedness with a pharmacist and always seeing the same doctor
2. Affordability
3. Feeling informed about one's health and knowing the importance of taking medication as prescribed
4. Providers who elicit trust and confidence
5. Involving the patient in decision making
6. Provider understands the patient's problem(s)

(Adapted from Phelan JE ED, Langer G, Holyk G. Medication adherence in America: A national report card. Langer Research Associates for the National Community Pharmacists Association. www.ncpa.co/adherence/AdherenceReportCard_Full.pdf; Ratanawongsa N, Karter AJ, Parker MM, et al. Communication and medication refill adherence: The diabetes study of northern California. JAMA Intern Med. 2013;173:210-218.)

which typically does not have symptoms, conditions such as depression, mental health conditions such as psychosis, and a general lack of symptoms with hypertension can lead to poor adherence. Social and economic-related factors that can hinder medication adherence, including limited English proficiency, medication cost, lack of family support, homelessness, and cultural beliefs about the health care system, illness, or treatment. Lastly, there are **patient-related factors** that contribute to poor adherence, but it is important to recognize that not all of them are controllable by the patient. Impairments such as visual, hearing, cognitive, mobility, or swallowing problems can have an effect on the patient's ability to take the medication as prescribed. Other contributing factors that influence adherence include depression, fear of potential side effects, lack of knowledge about the disease, lack of confidence in their ability to take the medication as prescribed, fear of being stigmatized or labeled as 'having a disease,' lack of belief or confidence in the health care system, expectations or attitudes about the medication that may or may not be unfounded, motivation, forgetfulness, interference with their lifestyle or work schedules, and substance abuse.[2,9,22-24]

A recent consumer survey asked respondents about their reasons for not taking their blood pressure medication as prescribed. Overall, 30.5% admitted to not taking their medication as directed. The most common reasons for nonadherence were forgetting to take it (23.6%), not thinking they need it (27.1%), and not being able to afford it (35.1%).[21] Similarly, when asked about their rationale for nonadherence 39.2% said they were exercising more, 41.9% said they were trying to lose or had lost weight, 42.4% said they were changing their eating habits, and 53.1% said they were cutting down on salt. Adherence was significantly associated with lower income, Hispanic ethnicity, younger age, and depression.[25]

STRATEGIES AND INTERVENTIONS TO IMPROVE ADHERENCE

Strategies to improve medication adherence are based on effective communication, effective interventions, and measuring medication adherence (Box 49.2). A collaborative communication style has been associated with improved medication adherence.[24] Ratanawongsa[26] and colleagues conducted a cross-sectional study within a single health care system of 9377 patients with diabetes on medication

adherence to hypoglycemic agents, lipid-lowering medications, and antihypertensive medications. Patients who offered lower ratings of their health care provider were more likely to have poor medication adherence. Specifically, involving patients in decision making increased medication adherence by 4% (p = 0.04), when the patient thought the provider understood their problem with treatment, adherence increased by 5% (p = 0.02), and patients who felt that the provider displayed confidence and gained the patient's trust improved adherence by 6% (p = 0.03).

Differing attitudes and beliefs towards health affect engagement in positive health behaviors. Understanding a patient's cultural beliefs about a condition such as hypertension is important in gaining patient engagement in hypertension self-management including medication adherence.[27] Motivational interviewing has been used to promote behavior change in various settings such as reducing health-risk behaviors, smoking cessation, and improving medication adherence. It consists of five core principles:

1. Develop discrepancy: assist the patient in identifying the discrepancy between their current behavior and the desired goal of medication adherence.
2. Express empathy: establish and maintain rapport with the patient with engaged listening without judging.
3. Avoid argumentation and the 'righting reflex': instead focus on helping the patient with self-recognition of the problem rather than just trying to 'fix it.'
4. Roll with resistance: involve the patient in problem solving to improve adherence.
5. Support self-efficacy: support and assist the patient in setting realistic strategies and goals to improve adherence.[28,29]

Ogedegbe conducted a trial of motivational interviewing compared with usual care among 190 antihypertensive African Americans. The group that received motivational interviewing had significantly improved rates of adherence compared with usual care and improved reduction in systolic blood pressure.[30]

EFFECTIVE INTERVENTIONS TO REDUCE MEDICATION NONADHERENCE SHOULD BE "SIMPLE"

Using the **SIMPLE** mnemonic can improve patient adherence (Fig. 49.5).[31]

Simplifying the medication regimen can go a long way toward improving medication adherence, such as using a combination antihypertensive or by using a once-a-day regimen, taking into account other medications that the patient is on, and being aware of the patient's activities of daily living that can interfere with medication adherence are extremely important. Inquire as to whether the patient would like to manage his or her medications with daily

SIMPLIFY THE REGIMEN

- Avoid medications with special requirements and adjust timing, frequency, amount, and dosage.
- Match regimen to patient's activities of daily living.

IMPART KNOWLEDGE

- Write down prescription instructions clearly, and reinforce them verbally and patient-provider shared decision making.
- Provide websites for additional reading and information.

MODIFY PATIENTS' BELIEFS AND BEHAVIOR

- Provide positive reinforcement when patients take their medication successfully, and offer incentives if possible.
- Talk to patients to understand and address their concerns or fears.

PROVIDE COMMUNICATION AND TRUST

- Use plain language when speaking with patients.
- Elicit the patient's input on treatment decision and provide support.
- Improve interviewing skills and practice active listening.
- Remind patients to contact your office with any questions.

LEAVE THE BIAS

- Understand the predictors of non-adherence and address them as needed with patients.
- Ask patients specific questions about attitudes, beliefs, and cultural norms related to taking medications.
- Examine self-efficacy regarding care among ethnically and socially diverse populations.

EVALUATE ADHERENCE

- Ask patients about adherence at every visit.
- Use a medication adherence scale—most are available online:
  - Morisky-4 (MMAS-4 or Medication Adherence Questionnaire)
  - Morisky-8 (MMAS-8)
  - Medication Possession Ratio (MPR)
  - Proportion of Days Covered (PDC)

FIG. 49.5 Use the **SIMPLE** method to help improve medication adherence among your patients. (*Adapted from Atreja A, Bellam N, Levy SR. Strategies to enhance patient adherence: making it simple. Med Gen Med. 2005;7:4. http://www.medscape.com/viewarticle/498339_3 [Accessed July 2016]).*

reminders (alarms, electronic reminders, etc.), dose-dispensing units of medication, or pill boxes, because these may all improve adherence. Consider changing the situation to meet the patient's needs rather than changing the patient to fit the regimen. Engage the patient in the discussion of the regimen.

Imparting knowledge about hypertension, that it typically has no symptoms but can still be causing harm, and providing culturally appropriate information that is easy to understand, can improve medication adherence. Again, engaging in provider-patient shared decision making can improve adherence. Keep the care team (physicians, pharmacists, nurses, community health workers) informed of the plan as well as engaging the patient's family or caregiver. Using a team-based approach to hypertension management can reinforce patient-provider discussions, directions for taking medication as well as addressing low-health literacy and cultural competency. Using a teach-back method can also improve the patient's knowledge and understanding of hypertension and the importance of taking their medication. Patients that may be vulnerable to low health literacy include older adults, those with multiple chronic conditions, minority populations, and those with limited English proficiency, the medically underserved. Low health literacy can make it especially challenging to understand medication directions. Familiarize your entire health care team with health literacy resources.[32-36]

Modifying patient beliefs and human behavior by empowering them to self-manage their hypertension can take time but may be very powerful in ensuring good medication adherence. Understanding patient beliefs about

hypertension and medications as well as understanding the patient's confidence in his or her ability to follow through on medication adherence is important. Ensure that patients understand their particular risk if they don't take their medication, and ask them about the consequences of not taking their medication. Use motivational interviewing to understand their beliefs and engaging them to modify their beliefs, especially if they have fears about taking medication or would benefit from rewards for adherence.

Provide communication and trust as identified in the study by Ratanawongsa[26]; providers who put effort into generating trust and confidence results in improved medication adherence. Again, use motivational interviewing to improve your communication skills and be an active listener when communicating with your patient. Provide emotional support to encourage the desired behavior of medication adherence, including using your health care team to provide the right support for each patient. Use plain language that is clear, direct, and thorough, as well as culturally appropriate, and remember to ask for patient input on treatment decisions. Understand if cost is a barrier and provide advice on how to cope with this as well as providing lower-cost generics if appropriate.

Leave the bias. The beliefs a person hold regarding their power to affect situations strongly influences both the power a person actually has to face challenges competently and the choices the person is most likely to make. This is apparent and compelling with regard to health behaviors. Providers should inquire about and understand the patient's attitudes and beliefs about medication therapy as well as their self-efficacy beliefs about their capacity to accomplish a task, such as taking their medication as directed. Motivational interviewing and a team-based approach to hypertension control can improve patients' self-efficacy and allows providers to best tailor interventions to improve medication adherence.

Evaluate adherence. There are many ways to evaluate medication adherence and different ways can contribute important information at the individual patient level as well as at the provider's population level. Self-report is perhaps the simplest but may not be the most accurate for an entire patient population. However, it is important to ask about adherence at each patient visit. The team can review medication containers, or work with the pharmacist to identify late medication refill dates. Some patients may be more likely to respond to a quick survey using any of the validated antihypertensive medication adherence scales. Overall, interventions to improve medication adherence for antihypertensive medications should be patient-tailored to meet the individual's needs, which may be behavior-related (forgetfulness, complicated by other medication regimens, lack of self-efficacy), clinically related (concerns related to harm, fear of potential side-effects, lack of culturally and linguistically appropriate education), as well as cost-related.

MEASURING MEDICATION ADHERENCE

There is no single gold standard for measuring medication adherence, and there are several validated methods for measuring adherence at either the individual patient level or at the provider's or health care organization population level. The benefits of measuring adherence are many, including understanding whether treatment intensification is indicated or whether implementing strategies to improve medication adherence are indicated, understanding patient challenges to adherence, understanding overall adherence of your patient population to identify systemic challenges to adherence. Identify barriers to medication adherence before practice-wide strategies to improve adherence, and ultimately improving the overall health outcomes of your patients.

The following patient questionnaires have been validated for assessing antihypertensive medication adherence:

- The medication adherence scales appropriate for measuring hypertension medication adherence include the Medication Adherence questionnaire, also known as Morisky Medication Adherence Scale (MMAS) 4-item and 8-item scales, the Self-efficacy for Appropriate Medication Use Scale, and the Hill-Bone Compliance Scale. The MMAS was developed for and specifically validated for use in adherence to antihypertensive medications.[37-40]
- The MMAS 8-item has been demonstrated to be reliable with a Cronbach's alpha = 0.83 and significantly associated with blood pressure ($p < 0.05$). It performed well in identifying people with challenges related to medication adherence and low hypertension control (sensitivity 93%), but did less well in identifying patients without issues of medication adherence and who have controlled blood pressure compared with all those with controlled blood pressure. The MMAS 4-item has an Cronbach's alpha = 0.61 and is validated in low-literacy patients but does not assess self-efficacy.[37] This is perhaps the easiest to administer, as it is self-administered and can be filled out at the time of each appointment.
- Self-efficacy for Appropriate Medication Use (SEAMS) has 13 questions, and alpha = 0.89, is validated in low-literacy patients and assesses self-efficacy. This has been validated in chronic disease and coronary artery disease.[41]
- The Hill-Bone Compliance Scale has 14 questions, has a Cronbach's alpha = 0.65, identifies forgetfulness and adverse effects, assesses self-efficacy (9 questions on medication adherence). It is specific to antihypertensive medications. The Hill-Bone Compliance Scale has the added

advantage of assessing behavior related to reduced sodium intake and appointment keeping in additional to antihypertensive medication taking.[41-44]

Other common methods for assessing medication adherence include pill counts, use of electronic monitoring pill container devices, and the use of prescription claims data. Pill counting could be invalid if patients discard but do not take the medication and it does not capture the timing of missed doses between pill counts.[45]

The proportion of days covered (PDC) method uses pharmacy data. The denominator for the calculation is 365 minus the number of days elapsed in the current year to the day of the patient's first fill of the medication. For example, if the medication is first filled on February 2, the denominator would be 332 (365 – 33 = 332). The numerator is defined as the days covered by prescription refills during the denominator period.[46,47] However, there are various modifications of this depending on whether one is accounting for multiple drugs within a drug class to all count as adherence.[48] Using PDC methods, an 'adherent' patient is generally assumed to be one where the PDC is 80% or more.[46] PDC methodology is recommended by the Pharmacist Quality Alliance for measuring adherence for chronic disease medications.[49]

The medication possession ratio (MPR) also uses pharmacy data that estimate the total number of days of medication possessed over a defined time interval. Often, this will be calculated as the number of days of possession between the first fill of a prescription and the last fill of the prescription within the defined time interval, or the number of days from the first fill of a prescription in the measurement period until the last day of the measurement period. This can overestimate adherence in situations where pharmacies put prescriptions on automatic refill and the patient picks up the medication before running out of the medication. Generally, MPR 80% or more is considered good adherence.

SPECIFIC STRATEGIES FOR IMPROVING HYPERTENSION MEDICATION ADHERENCE

Team-Based Care

The Community Preventive Services Task Force recommends team-based care to improve blood pressure control based on strong evidence of effectiveness in improving the proportion of patients with controlled blood pressure. They reviewed evidence from 80 studies of team-based care, which included nurses and pharmacists working in collaborations with primary care providers, patients, and other health care professionals. Implementing team-based care provides multiple opportunities for patients to interact with the health care team, providing education and opportunities for patients to have their specific questions answered and their challenges heard, and improved communication between the patients and provider team. This approach can also make it easier to implement strategies that can address complicated medication regimens for those with multiple chronic diseases, as well as addressing concerns related to cost.[50-52] The Million Hearts® initiative has promoted team-based care to improve medication adherence as a key strategy in its efforts to improve blood pressure control.[1]

"I urge doctors, nurses, nurse practitioners, physician assistants, pharmacists, diabetes educators, community health workers, and others to start a conversation with your patients about the importance of taking medications as directed and to help them overcome the barriers to medication adherence. There is no better time than right now to help our patients with chronic conditions live long and healthy lives."
—Former US Surgeon General Regina Benjamin, MD[53]

The Pharmacist's Role in Collaborative Drug Therapy Management and Medication Therapy Management

Medication therapy management is provided for some enrollees in Medicare Part D.[54,55] Medication therapy management (MTM) provides for pharmacists to review a patient's medications and suggest changes to the prescribing provider for their approval rather than making changes independent of the provider.[55] Collaborative drug therapy management (CDTM) is a team approach where a prescribing provider and pharmacist enter into a collaborative agreement authorizing the pharmacist to initiate, modify, or continue medication therapy or other patient care functions under established guidelines or protocols. States regulate the allowable scope of practice for CDTM. Several studies have shown that these collaborative practice agreements can improve health outcomes and save on health spending.[54,55]

A review of several trials of various interventions from the Agency for Health care Research and Quality (AHRQ)[6] examined different strategies of medication adherence.

Education with behavioral support and e-systems for communication and monitoring—delivered by mail, telephone, video, multicomponent pharmacist led, and case management interventions: several trials showed improvement in adherence during the duration of the trial, but trials were heterogeneous.

Blister packaging: shown to improve both medication adherence and persistence, based on pharmacy refill data.

Electronic monitoring: several solutions exist for using electronic medication monitors that record the time and date when a pill was removed from its container. Several clinical trials have shown benefit in terms of reduction in systolic blood pressure.

Self-measured blood pressure: AHRQ found that there is strong evidence that SMBP plus additional support, including one-on-one counseling with a nurse or pharmacist, web-based or telephonic support, and educational classes, are effective in achieving improved blood pressure control and improving medication adherence. The Community Guide has found strong evidence to support the use of self-measured blood pressure monitoring to improve blood pressure control and engage patients in their care (Box 49.3).[56-58]

SUCCESS STORY

Case Management Intervention

Building on the Health Decision Model, Bosworth et al.[59] included patient characteristics related to medication adherence, as well as social and cultural factors, access to care, and physician communication style, to create a multifaceted, patient-tailored program with nurse case managers to improve medication adherence. The outcome was measured by medication fill rates. The setting of this intervention was a community-based Medicaid network functioning as primary care medical homes. Using this approach, the intervention also incorporated providing tailored information on important lifestyle behaviors important to hypertension control. The intervention incorporated a computerized script that was tailored to patient responses in that certain responses would trigger various additional scripts. Patient contact was by phone at near-monthly intervals over 6 months. They found a near-doubling of the proportion of patients who had a medication possession ratio over 80% and the percent of individuals with a medication possession ratio less than 60% was reduced in half.[59]

BOX 49.3 Actions to Improve Medication Adherence

Encourage patients to use medication reminders.
Promote pill boxes, alarms, vibrating watches, and smartphone applications.
   Provide all prescription instructions clearly in writing and verbally.
- **Limit instruction to 3–4 major points**
- **Use plain, culturally sensitive language**
- **Use written information or pamphlets and verbal education at all encounters**
Ensure patients understand their risks if they do not take medications as directed. Ask patients about these risks, and have patients restate the positive benefits of taking their medications.
   Discuss with patients potential side effects of any medications when initially prescribed and at every office visit thereafter.
   Provide rewards for medication adherence.
- **Praise adherence**
- **Arrange incentives, such as coupons, certificates, and reduced frequency of office visits**
Prescribe medications included in the patient's insurance coverage formulary, when possible.
   Prescribe once-daily regimens or fixed-dose combination pills.
   Assign one staff person the responsibility of managing medication refill requests.
- **Create a refill protocol**
Implement frequent follow-ups (e.g., e-mail, phone calls, text messages) to ensure patients adhere to their medication regimen.
- **Set up an automated telephone system for patient monitoring and counseling**

(From Improving medication adherence among patients with hypertension: a tip sheet for health care professionals. http://millionhearts.hhs.gov and http://millionhearts.hhs.gov/files/TipSheet_HCP_MedAdherence.pdf.)

BOX 49.4 Key Points

1. 20% to 30% of first prescriptions for antihypertensive medications are never filled.
2. Health care system factors, provider-related, treatment-related factors, and patient-related factors all contribute to medication nonadherence.
3. Many successful interventions to improve medication adherence exist, including the use of team-based care.
4. Effective communication is key to medication adherence.

SUMMARY

In conclusion, there are many strategies to improve antihypertension medication adherence, which in turn will reduce patients' risk from stroke, myocardial infarction, and other cardiovascular diseases (Box 49.4). Effective communication with patients, understanding their individual circumstances that interfere with good medication adherence, using team-based care, and engaging the patient in their own care and decision making about their care are critical to improving adherence and patient outcomes. Be willing to partner with your patients to help them help themselves to improve medication adherence.

MEDICATION ADHERENCE TOOLS FOR PROVIDERS

American College of Cardiology—CardioSmart Med Reminder (mobile app) www.cardiosmart.org/Tools/Med-Reminder

National Institute of Health, Nation Heart, Lung, and Blood Institute—Tips to Help You Remember to Take Your Blood Pressure Drugs www.nhlbi.nih.gov/health-pro/resources/heart/hispanic-health-manual/session-4/tips-for-high-blood-pressure-medicine

Script Your Future—Script Your Future Wallet Card www.scriptyourfuture.org/wp-content/uploads/2011/07/i_will_take_my_meds_wallet_card.pdf

NIH Current State of Medication Adherence: Challenges and Solutions (begins 5:10 minutes in) www.youtube.com/watch?v=WquN4Q94EaA

Medicare—The Importance of Medication Adherence www.youtube.com/watch?v=OgqZPEMFQHE

References

1. Improving medication adherence among patients with hypertension: a tip sheet for health care professionals. http://millionhearts.hhs.gov. http://millionhearts.hhs.gov/files/TipSheet_HCP_MedAdherence.pdf.
2. Osterberg L, Blaschke T. Adherence to medication. N Engl J Med. 2005;353:487-497.
3. Yoon SS, Carroll MD, Fryar CD. Hypertension prevalence and control among adults: United States, 2011-2014. NCHS Data Brief. 2015:1-8.
4. Nwankwo T, Yoon SS, Burt V, Gu Q. Hypertension among adults in the United States: National Health and Nutrition Examination Survey, 2011-2012. NCHS Data Brief. 2013:1-8.
5. Krousel-Wood M, Hyre A, Muntner P, Morisky D. Methods to improve medication adherence in patients with hypertension: current status and future directions. Curr Opin Cardiol. 2005;20:296-300.
6. Viswanathan MGC, Jones CD, Ashok M, et al. Medication adherence interventions: comparative effectiveness. Closing the quality gap: revisiting the state of the science. Evidence report no. 208. 2012; 2016.
7. Cramer JA, Roy A, Burrell A, et al. Medication compliance and persistence: terminology and definitions. Value Health. 2008;11:44-47.
8. Ho PM, Bryson CL, Rumsfeld JS. Medication adherence: its importance in cardiovascular outcomes. Circulation. 2009;119:3028-3035.
9. World Health Organization. Adherence to long-term therapies: evidence for action. Geneva. 2003; http://apps.who.int/iris/bitstream/10665/42682/1/9241545992.pdf.
10. DiMatteo MR. Variations in patients' adherence to medical recommendations: a quantitative review of 50 years of research. Med Care. 2004;42:200-209.
11. Phelan JE ED, Langer G, Holyk G. Medication adherence in America: a national report card. Langer Research Associates for the National Community Pharmacists Association. www.ncpa.co/adherence/AdherenceReportCard_Full.pdf.
12. Chobanian AV, Bakris GL, Black HR, et al. Seventh report of the Joint National Committee on Prevention, Detection, Evaluation, and Treatment of High Blood Pressure. Hypertension. 2003;42:1206-1252.
13. Ettehad D, Emdin CA, Kiran A, et al. Blood pressure lowering for prevention of cardiovascular disease and death: a systematic review and meta-analysis. Lancet. 2016;387:957-967.
14. Burnier M. Medication adherence and persistence as the cornerstone of effective antihypertensive therapy. Am J Hypertens. 2006;19:1190-1196.
15. Kettani FZ, Dragomir A, Cote R, et al. Impact of a better adherence to antihypertensive agents on cerebrovascular disease for primary prevention. Stroke. 2009;40:213-220.
16. Esposti LD, Saragoni S, Benemei S, et al. Adherence to antihypertensive medications and health outcomes among newly treated hypertensive patients. ClinicoEcon Outcomes Res. 2011;3:47-54.
17. Kockaya G, Wertheimer A. Can we reduce the cost of illness with more compliant patients? An estimation of the effect of 100% compliance with hypertension treatment. J Pharm Pract. 2011;24:345-350.
18. Sokol MC, McGuigan KA, Verbrugge RR, Epstein RS. Impact of medication adherence on hospitalization risk and healthcare cost. Med Care. 2005;43:521-530.
19. Bosworth HB, Granger BB, Mendys P, et al. Medication adherence: a call for action. Am Heart J. 2011;162:412-424.
20. Fischer MA, Stedman MR, Lii J, et al. Primary medication nonadherence: analysis of 195,930 electronic prescriptions. J Gen Intern Med. 2010;25:284-290.
21. Fischer MA, Choudhry NK, Brill G, et al. Trouble getting started: predictors of primary medication nonadherence. Am J Med. 2011;124:1081 e1089-e1022.
22. American Society of consultant Pharmacists. American society on Aging. Adult meducation™ improving medication adherence in older adults. www.adultmeducation.com.
23. Krueger KP, Berger BA, Felkey B. Medication adherence and persistence: a comprehensive review. Adv Ther. 2005;22:313-356.
24. Schoenthaler A, Chaplin WF, Allegrante JP, et al. Provider communication effects medication adherence in hypertensive african americans. Patient Educ Couns. 2009;75:185-191.
25. Tong XCE, Fang J, Wall HK, Ayala C. Nonadherence to antihypertensive medication among hypertensive adults in the United States—healthstyles, 2010. J Clin Hypertens (Greenwich). 2016. [Epub ahead of print]
26. Ratanawongsa N, Karter AJ, Parker MM, et al. Communication and medication refill adherence: the Diabetes Study of Northern California. JAMA Intern Med. 2013;173:210-218.
27. Centers for Disease Control and Prevention. A closer look at African American men and high blood pressure control: a review of psychosocial factors and systems-level interventions. Atlanta: U.S. Department of Health and Human Services; 2010.
28. Miller W, Rollnick S. Motivational interviewing: preparing people to change. New York: Guilford Press; 2002.
29. Hall K, Gibbie T, Lubman DI. Motivational interviewing techniques—facilitating behaviour change in the general practice setting. Aust Fam Physician. 2012;41:660-667.
30. Ogedegbe G, Chaplin W, Schoenthaler A, et al. A practice-based trial of motivational interviewing and adherence in hypertensive african americans. Am J Hypertens. 2008;21:1137-1143.
31. Atreja A, Bellam N, Levy SR. Strategies to enhance patient adherence: making it simple. Med Gen Med. 2005;7:4.
32. Centers for Disease Control and Prevention. Health literacy for public health professionals. www.cdc.gov/healthliteracy/index.html.
33. AMA Foundation. AMA health literacy. www.youtube.com/watch?v=cGtTZ_vxjyA.
34. Agency for Healthcare Research and Quality. AHRQ health literacy universal precautions toolkit. www.ahrq.gov/professionals/quality-patient-safety/quality-resources/tools/literacy-toolkit/index.html.
35. American College of Physicians. Promoting literacy to increase adherence. www.acpinternist.org/archives/2011/07/literacy.htm.
36. Natioinal Institutes of Health. Clear communication. www.nih.gov/institutes-nih/nih-office-director/office-communications-public-liaison/clear-communication.
37. Morisky DE, Green LW, Levine DM. Concurrent and predictive validity of a self-reported measure of medication adherence. Med Care. 1986;24:67-74.
38. Morisky DE, Ang A, Krousel-Wood M, Ward HJ. Predictive validity of a medication adherence measure in an outpatient setting. J Clin Hypertens (Greenwich). 2008;10:348-354.
39. Morisky DE, DiMatteo MR. Improving the measurement of self-reported medication nonadherence: response to authors. J Clin Epidemiol. 2011;64:255-257; discussion 258-263.
40. Morisky DE, Malotte CK, Choi P, et al. A patient education program to improve adherence rates with antituberculosis drug regimens. Health Educ Q. 1990;17:253-267.
41. Culig J, Leppee M. From morisky to hill-bone; self-reports scales for measuring adherence to medication. Coll Antropol. 2014;38:55-62.
42. Kim MT, Hill MN, Bone LR, Levine DM. Development and testing of the hill-bone compliance to high blood pressure therapy scale. Prog Cardiovasc Nurs. 2000;15:90-96.
43. Lavsa SM, Holzworth A, Ansani NT. Selection of a validated scale for measuring medication adherence. J Am Pharm Assoc (2003). 2011;51:90-94.
44. Krousel-Wood M, Muntner P, Jannu A, Desalvo K, Re RN. Reliability of a medication adherence measure in an outpatient setting. Am J Med Sci. 2005;330:128-133.
45. Krzesinski JM, Leeman M. Practical issues in medication compliance in hypertensive patients. Res Rep Clin Cardiol. 2011;2011:63-70.
46. Leslie RS. Using arrays to calculate medication utilization. Sas paper 043-2007. www2.sas.com/proceedings/forum2007/043-2007.pdf.
47. Benner JS, Glynn RJ, Mogun H, Neumann PJ, Weinstein MC, Avorn J. Long-term persistence in use of statin therapy in elderly patients. JAMA. 2002;288:455-461.
48. Choudhry NK, Shrank WH, Levin RL, et al. Measuring concurrent adherence to multiple related medications. Am J Manag Care. 2009;15:457-464.
49. Pharmacy Quality Alliance. PQA measures used by cms in the star ratings. http://pqaalliance.org/measures/cms.asp.
50. Proia KK, Thota AB, Njie GJ, et al. Team-based care and improved blood pressure control: a community guide systematic review. Am J Prev Med. 2014;47:86-99.
51. Sidney S. Team-based care: a step in the right direction for hypertension control. Am J Prev Med. 2015;49:e81-e82.
52. Community Preventive Services Task Force. Team-based care to improve blood pressure control: recommendation of the community preventive services task force. Am J Prev Med. 2014;47:100-102.
53. National Consumers League. Surgeon general joins Baltimore launch of national script your future campaign to highlight importance of taking medication as directed. 2011. www.natlconsumersleague.org/newsroom/press-releases/582-us-surgeon-general-joins-baltimore-launch-of-national-script-your-future-campaign-to-highlight-importance-of-taking-medication-as-directed.
54. Centers for Disease Control and Prevention. Collaborative practice agreements and pharmacists' patient care services: a resource for pharmacists. Atlanta, GA: U.S. Dept. of Health and Human Services; 2013. www.cdc.gov/dhdsp/pubs/docs/Translational_Tools_Pharmacists.pdf.
55. Snyder ME, Earl TR, Gilchrist S, et al. Collaborative drug therapy management: case studies of three community-based models of care. Prev Chronic Dis. 2015;12:E39.
56. The Community Guide. Self-measured blood pressure monitoring interventions for improved blood pressure control—when comblined with additional support. www.thecommunityguide.org/cvd/SMBP-additional.html.
57. Centers for Disease Control and Prevention. Self-measured blood pressure monitoring: action steps for clinicians. Atlanta (GA): Centers for Disease Control and Prevention, U.S. Department of Health and Human Services; 2014. www.thecommunityguide.org/cvd/SMBP-additional.html.
58. Centers for Disease Control and Prevention. Self-measured blood pressure monitoring: action steps for public health practitioners. Atlanta (GA): Centers for Disease Control and Prevention, U.S. Department of Health and Human Services; 2013. www.thecommunityguide.org/cvd/SMBP-additional.html.
59. Bosworth HB, Dubard CA, Ruppenkamp J, Trygstad T, Hewson DL, Jackson GL. Evaluation of a self-management implementation intervention to improve hypertension control among patients in medicaid. Transl Behav Med. 2011;1:191-199.

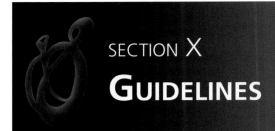

50 | Updated American Heart Association/ American College of Cardiology; European Society of Hypertension/ International Society of Hypertension Guidelines

Raymond R. Townsend and Giuseppe Mancia

UNITED STATES OF AMERICA HYPERTENSION GUIDELINES (PORTION)

Background Story

The groundwork for the first United States hypertension guideline began with the first randomized trial of hypertension treatment in U.S. veterans, which was directed by Dr. Ed Freis, a Veterans Administration Physician. The trial was conducted by the Veterans Administration Cooperative Trial Study Group on Antihypertensive Agents. Two seminal publications resulted from this early effort. The first part of this landmark trial, published in 1967,[1] involved 143 men with diastolic blood pressures (DBP) of 115 to 129 mm Hg of whom 73 were treated with active medication, and 70 received placebos. After about 2 years there were 27 terminating events in the placebo group, and 2 in the active treatment group. This demonstrated for the first time that, although both groups were basically asymptomatic at enrollment, men with significant hypertension benefitted dramatically from antihypertensive drug therapy in a relatively short period of time. Three years later, the second portion of the VA Cooperative Trial was published.[2] This segment randomized men with DBP of 90 to 114 mm Hg of whom 186 were treated with active medication, and 194 received placebos. After about 2 years there were 76 assessable events in the placebo group, and 22 in the active treatment group over the 5 years of the study. Those with DBP of 105 to 114 mm Hg were about twice as likely to benefit, compared with men with similar diastolic pressures in the placebo group, from active treatment when they compared with those within the active treatment group who had diastolic values of 90 to 104 mm Hg at randomization. The trial investigators again stressed the value of antihypertensive therapy, but readers were left with a bit of residual uncertainty over those with DBP in the 90 to 104 mm Hg group.

Despite the dramatic results of these two studies, and their publication in a high profile journal (JAMA), physicians were sluggish to act on these findings and treatment rates remained low (Table 50.1). As a result of this 'inertia' the philanthropist and medical research proponent Mary Lasker, with the lead VA Cooperative Study Group Investigator Dr. Ed Freis, Dr. Thomas Rudeshan, and Deeda Blair (the current Vice President of the Albert and Mary Lasker Foundation) visited Elliot Richardson, who was at that time, Secretary of the Department of Health Education and Welfare. During that meeting Dr. Freis reviewed the VA Cooperative Study data emphasizing the declines in morbidity and mortality from lowering BP with drug treatment. Mr. Richardson's father had been a surgeon at the Massachusetts General Hospital whose career came to an end from a stroke related to his hypertension. Mr. Richardson convinced the Director of the National Heart and Lung Institute (NHLI; this was before 'Blood' was added to the Institute name), Dr. Theodore Cooper, who directed the Institute from 1968 to 1974 to work on a strategy to promote hypertension awareness and treatment. During the Nixon and Ford administrations Dr. Cooper was appointed the Assistant Secretary for Health at the Department of Health, Education, and Welfare (HEW), and he worked in that position, as well as during his Directorship at the National Institutes of Health (NIH), to enable the initiative that became known as the National High Blood Pressure Education Project (NHBPEP). In the beginning, the focus of the NHBPEP was on developing Task Forces to publish papers on aspects such as screenings for blood pressure (BP). Task Force I was devoted to treatment and was chaired by Dr. H. Mitchell Perry Jr. The output of Task Force I was the precursor for the first U.S. guideline. (The author would like to acknowledge the input of Dr. Edward J. Roccella [also from NIH/National Heart, Blood, and Lung Institute {NHLBI}/NHBPEP] in the history covered herein.)

As clamor on the part of patients for more attention to their BP became more audible, the desire to "know your number" and participate in community BP screenings grew. Consequently an early objective of the NHBPEP was to reach consensus on a definition for hypertension. A substantial challenge in this endeavor was to choose between options such as "100 + age" for the 'normal' systolic BP, whereas others favored using only the diastolic BP, and a value such as 105 mm Hg seemed an

TABLE 50.1 United States Hypertension Prevalence, Awareness, Drug Treatment, and Control

	1971-2	1974-5	1976-80	1988-91	1994	2003	2008	2012
U.S. Population[a]	19[b]	23	—	43	50	—	65	70
Aware %	51	64	73 [54]	84 [65]	70	78	81	83
Treated %	36	34	56 [33]	73 [49]	55	62	73	75
At/Below Target Blood Pressure %	16	20	34 [11]	55 [21]	30	41	49	53

[a]United States (U.S.) population with hypertension (in millions). Data extracted from references 82, 83, 84, 85.
[b]Numbers *in italics* represent numbers in millions, or percentages, using the definition of 160/95 mm Hg for hypertension (and below 160/95 mm Hg as controlled); numbers within [brackets], and/or not in italics, represent percentages using 140/90 mm Hg.

TABLE 50.2 Vital Statistics of the Sequential Joint National Committee Reports

	YEAR PUBLISHED/CHAIR	NO. OF PRINT PAGES	STAKEHOLDERS	TABLES	FIGURES	REFERENCES
JNC Report[3]	1977 Marvin Moser	7	9	5	3	1
1980 Report[6]	1980 Iqbal Krishan	6	12	1	0	14
1984 Report[10]	1984 Harriet Dustan	13	15	8	0	40
1988 Report[14]	1988 Aram Chobanian	16	16	10	1	54
JNC V[17]	1993 Ray Gifford	30	43	14	4	117
JNC-VI[86]	1997 Sheldon Sheps	34	45	16	8	254
JNC 7a[18]	2003 Aram Chobanian	13	Many	6	3 ("Boxes")	81
JNC 7b[19]	2003 Aram Chobanian	47	Many	31	17	386
JNC 8d[22]	2014 Paul James & Suzanne Oparil	14	2[c]	6	2 (One Box and one figure)	45

[a]Executive version.
[b]Complete version.
[c]These were the 15 panel members, and the National Institutes of Health (via two additional panel members).
[d]Does not include online supplement information.

attractive cut point based on VA Cooperative data. Detection of hypertension, a key to selecting those who need further evaluation, as well as treatment remained active areas of discussion. The NHBPEP formed a Coordinating Committee to provide guidance on the detection, evaluation, and treatment of hypertension. Stakeholders in this Committee included representatives from the American Academy of Family Practice, American College of Cardiology (ACC), American College of Physicians, American Heart Association (AHA), American Medical Association, the National Kidney Foundation, the National Medical Association, the Veterans Administration, and the United States Public Health Service. The goal was to speak with a single voice about managing hypertension using consensus methodology in the formation of recommendations. The Coordinating Committee was chaired by Dr. Marvin Moser and its publication became the first Joint National Committee (JNC) Report.

A Short History of the United States of America Joint National Committee Guidelines

The first guideline on hypertension was published in the USA in 1977.[3] This first Joint National Committee (JNC) Report spanned seven printed journal pages, made six recommendations, and cited a single reference (Table 50.2). It made the term "stepped-care approach" common parlance in hypertension, and provided guidance on how to evaluate and manage high BP using consensus from input provided by the nine major stakeholder groups cited previously. The Report was accompanied by a half page editorial in the same issue of JAMA, written by William Barclay.[4] In that brief space Barclay makes the following prescient observations:

"Although the report was sponsored by the National Heart and Lung Institute, it is not a government directive on how to practice medicine. The report should be viewed as a useful guide and not as a rigid directive on how to manage high blood pressure. One should be aware that such reports are compromises and do not necessarily reflect the conviction of individual committee members." [4]

In the ensuing decades after the first JNC Report, high BP advanced from fourth place on the World Health Organization (WHO) listing of factors responsible for premature death and disability in 1990, to first place in 2010.[5] In the ensuing decades, new antihypertensive agent classes, new clinical trial results, and redirection in thinking about the importance of systolic pressure have prompted repeated revision of the U.S. hypertension guidelines.

The second JNC Report[6] was issued following the completion of the Hypertension Detection and Follow-up Program (HDFP)[7] and the United States Public Health Service's 10 year intervention trial for hypertension.[8] It introduced a classification system for DBP levels, and was responsible for the terms 'mild' (DBP 90 to 104 mm Hg), 'moderate' (DBP 105 to 114 mm Hg), and 'severe' hypertension (DBP ≥ 115 mm Hg) and recommended initiating antihypertensive therapy with a diuretic because chlorthalidone (a thiazide-type of diuretic) was the initial step in the stepped care (SC) arm of HDFP. Although not often mentioned today, the HDFP made several important contributions in addition to being a major reason for the second JNC Report. First, with an enrollment of 10,940 participants it had enough power to establish the significant benefit of treating diastolic values of 90 to 104 mm Hg in the SC compared with the Referred Care (RC) group, reducing the uncertainty left in the wake of the first JNC Report which did not have enough basis in treatment success to recommend this target. Second, HDFP enrolled participants with preexisting target organ damage and showed there was still benefit in treating their hypertension, but those without prior cardiovascular disease experienced greater benefit, emphasizing the importance of primary over secondary prevention of hypertensive target organ damage. Finally, the HDFP investigators observed that those with a serum creatinine value higher than 1.7 mg/dL at enrollment had more than three-fold greater risk of mortality compared with those who had lower values establishing the importance of kidney disease in hypertensives.[9]

In 1984, the third JNC Report[10] appeared updated based on the results of hypertension trials outside the U.S.[11] and recommended initial therapy with either beta-adrenergic blockade (in younger patients, or those with faster heart rates) or diuretic therapy. The expansion to beta-blocker therapy was driven, in part, because of the emerging findings of reduced death after a myocardial infarction when beta-blockade was employed.[12,13] The classification scheme of BP based on diastolic values remained; however, the 1984 Report introduced the concept of "high normal" blood pressure (DBP 85 to 89 mm Hg) and expanded the classification system to include levels of systolic pressure when the DBP was less than 90 mm Hg.

The fourth JNC Report was published in 1988.[14] The most significant events that transpired between the 1984 and 1988 reports included the growing popularity of two new classes of antihypertensive agents following the approval of the three original calcium channel blockers (verapamil, diltiazem, and nifedipine) in 1981, and the angiotensin-converting enzyme (ACE) inhibitor captopril in 1981, followed by enalapril in 1986. Added to this was the publication of several landmark European trials including the Medical Research Council study[15] and the European Working Party for Hypertension in the Elderly.[16] In a previous understanding of "personalized medicine" the 1988 Report laid emphasis on quality of life, cost of care, and the need to consider ways to prevent hypertension. The main legacies of the 1988 Report were an expansion of the recommendation for treatment to the use of any of the four classes of popular antihypertensives (diuretic, beta-blocker, ACE-inhibitor, or calcium channel blocker), the use of nondrug therapy as foundational to the subsequent drug usage steps, and incorporating mechanisms to step down antihypertensive drug therapy in select cases.

The fifth JNC Report (JNC V) appeared in 1993 and was noteworthy for returning to the emphasis of using a diuretic or a beta-blocker as the initial antihypertensive therapy.[17] The staging system for BP reached its zenith in JNC V which defined stage 1 hypertension as a DBP of 90 to 99 mm Hg or a systolic blood pressure (SBP) of 140 to 159 mm Hg. Stage 2 was defined as a DBP of 100 to 109 mm Hg or an SBP of 160 to 179 mm Hg. Stage 3 hypertension was defined as a DBP of 110 to 119 mm Hg or an SBP of 180 to 219 mm Hg. Stage 4 was defined as a DBP higher than 120 mm Hg or an SBP higher than 220 mm Hg. JNC V emphasized that if the BP fell into discordant categories, such as stage 2 by DBP but a stage 3 by SBP, the higher stage was the category to use in that patient. They also defined an "optimal" category as less than 120/80 mm Hg. The fifth JNC also proposed reasons for doing an Ambulatory Blood Pressure Monitoring (ABPM) test.

JNC VI appeared in 1997 and was noteworthy for its classification of the papers (e.g., "cohort study," "randomized trial," etc.) used in the preparation of the Report, and for simplifying the classification system from four stages to three stages.

The most innovative aspect of JNC VI was the incorporation of nonhypertensive risk factors for cardiovascular disease into the classification system, using a scale ranging from Group A (no cardiovascular [CV] risk factors, target organ damage [TOD], or concomitant cardiovascular disease [CVD]) to Group B which had one or more CV risk factor (not including diabetes mellitus [DM]), but no TOD or concomitant CVD) and designated the highest Risk Group as C defined as the presence of TOD. JNC VI also introduced the term "compelling indications" recommending specific classes of antihypertensive drug therapy in patients with specific comorbidities (e.g., the use of an ACE inhibitor in type 1 diabetes with proteinuria). JNC VI also included the term "Prevention" in the title of the Report for the first time. Drug recommendations per JNC VI continued to recommend diuretic or beta-blocker as initial therapy, and they hinted that low dose combination therapy may be appropriate is some patients.

JNC 7 appeared in 2003 and reduced further the classification system to stage 1 (140 to 159/90 to 99 mm Hg) or stage 2 (≥160/≥ 100 mm Hg). The JNC VI appeared in the Archives of Internal Medicine which allowed the usage of Roman Numerals in the article title. JAMA, the site of initial publication of JNC 7 did not allow the use of Roman Numerals, thus the change to "7." JNC 7 was published in two stages. The first article was published in May 2003,[18] followed about 6 months later by a "Complete Version" published in December in Hypertension.[19] JNC 7 was remarkable for several things. It proposed treatment goals lower than 140/90 mm Hg in diabetes and chronic kidney disease (CKD). One of the most discussion-promoting aspects of JNC 7 was the promotion of a new category of blood pressure called "prehypertension" based on having either an SBP of 120 to 139 mm Hg or a DBP of 80 to 89 mm Hg. This was done to emphasize the opportunity for clinicians to intervene and perhaps prevent the progression to established hypertension through the use of, for example, weight loss and exercise programs that could have greater impact on patients when based upon a label or diagnosis such as *Prehypertension*. JNC 7 also gave concrete recommendations for using combination drug therapy when the starting BP is more than 159/99 mm Hg (either the SBP of the DBP). The next guideline, the Management of Hypertension in Adults (empaneled as JNC 8) took no issue with the classification scheme of JNC 7 and had no reason to update it.

2014 Expert Panel Report

The Report of the group empaneled as JNC 8 appeared in the same journal as the first JNC Report (JAMA), in February 2014. In an ironic fashion the response to this Report was very much predicted in the words of Barclay written almost 4 decades previously.[4] The Expert Panel was careful to point out in the Abstract and the concluding paragraph that guidelines are not a substitute for clinical judgment. When the three panels that were initially commissioned in September 2008 to undertake updates to the lipid (ATP 1-3), obesity (a single prior report in 1998), and the Hypertension guidelines the emphasis placed upon the three panels was principally driven by the Institute of Medicine Report "Crossing the Quality Chasm" which underscored the need to have recommendations for health care based on evidence.[20] When the Expert Panel was empaneled the NHLBI (at that time the sponsor) emphasized strongly the need to produce an evidence-based guideline citing, for example, the experience with the AHA/ACC recommendations in which about 1 in 9 recommendations (11%) made in the management of a variety of cardiovascular disorders had "A" level evidence to support it.[21] Unlike the previous JNC Reports, the Expert Panel Report (JNC 8) was comprised of 18 people, representing a broad range of hypertension expertise, and including two employees of NIH (one from NHLBI and one from the National Institutes of

Diabetes and Digestive and Kidney Diseases [NIDDK]). Early in the process one panel member left academia for Industry and the number was reduced to 17.

The largest hurdle faced by the Expert Panel was the challenge to use evidence in the formulation of "evidence-based recommendations." It was necessary first to construct an evidence base. This required several preparatory steps. The primary focus of the Expert Panel, determined early in the process, was the primary care practitioner. Every evidence statement that was developed, and each of the 9 main recommendations, was crafted with careful attention to the mission of assembling a guidance document that would be useful, and clear, in a primary care practice.

The first step was the development of the critical questions. Initially the panel members identified 23 separate critical questions that were felt to be important for primary care practitioners managing hypertension patients. These were winnowed down to five critical questions, two of which were not addressed in the Expert Panel Report. The fourth critical question asked whether it was better to start with two antihypertensive agents compared with one agent. We could find no data on that question. The fifth question asked whether it mattered where BP was measured (home, office, ABPM, kiosk, or other location). Limitations in time and funding precluded answering critical question five.

Once critical questions were framed it was necessary to develop a search strategy. This meant defining limits on what constituted acceptable "evidence" to include in the evidence base. We used the PICOTSS (population, intervention/exposure, comparison group, outcome, time, setting, and study design) strategy for this as outlined in supplement of the Expert Panel Report.[22] One of the most time-consuming aspects at this stage was defining "important health outcomes." When treating a patient with hypertension using drug therapy, what are the important health benefits? Also, what level of BP reduction does one need to target to achieve these benefits? This area generated controversy after the manuscript first appeared as an e-publication in JAMA. For example, we defined doubling of the serum creatinine concentration, halving of glomerular filtration rate (GFR), or the development of end-stage renal disease as the kidney-related important health outcomes. We did not use the slope of GFR change over time. Consequently, the Expert Panel felt that the original Modification of Diet in Renal Disease (MDRD) study report[23] did not demonstrate a benefit in the more aggressive compared with the standard level of BP in patients with moderate and advanced nondiabetic chronic kidney disease. The MDRD investigators stated as much in their original report, but did note that the *slope* of GFR change was favorably reduced in those in the more aggressive BP target group when the magnitude of urinary protein loss was more than 1 g but less than 3 g a day, and more so if it was more than 3 g a day. After careful review of the African American Trial of Kidney Disease and Hypertension[24] and the Ramipril Efficacy in Nephropathy II[25] trials, both of which compared more intensive to standard BP goals, the Expert Panel agreed that it could not find evidence fitting its definition of an important health outcome in a randomized controlled trial supporting a value lower than 140/90 mm Hg in the management of patients with CKD. This is supported further by a systematic review of BP goals in CKD which reached the same conclusion.[26]

The circumstances underpinning the approach to guideline development become a challenging and confusing issue for practitioners who try to understand, reconcile, and incorporate the various BP targets recommended by different BP guideline writing groups in diverse subsets of hypertensive patients. In the execution of the search strategy the Expert Panel felt it was important to use only prospective randomized clinical trials of antihypertensive therapy that enrolled only hypertensive patients. This excluded trials like the Heart Outcome Prospective Evaluation (HOPE)[27] which, although it was a randomized trial and included hypertensive patients, it also included high cardiovascular risk patients who did *not* have hypertension.

Once the investigations identified by the search criteria were identified it was necessary to have two independent raters categorize the trial as good, fair, or poor using a 14-point set of predefined criteria. After this process, which often reduced 1 to 2000 articles down to about 20 to 25 papers that fit our definition, it was necessary to summarize the data in a fashion that made clear what the benefits were, at what level of BP (systolic and diastolic were treated separately), with what agent(s), and in which subgroups (e.g., general population, self-declared Black, diabetic, or CKD). The Expert Panel did not review the evidence for important health outcomes accrued to patients with preexisting heart disease or stroke from BP management because that was being done in parallel by the American Heart Association/American College of Cardiology (AHA/ACC).[28]

The final steps were the formation of evidence statements which are in the JAMA online supplement, and then crafting recommendations based on the evidence. The recommendations, all 9 of them, are visible within the algorithm in the Expert Panel Report. Equipped with the knowledge of the patient's age (in years), ethnicity (African American, non-African American), diabetic status (Yes/No), and CKD status (Yes/No), the algorithm walks the viewer through what agent to use, what BP target to use, how soon to follow up, and when to refer. After years of poring over the existing evidence, the Expert Panel came to the conclusion that 140/90 mm Hg was the definition of hypertension, and the treatment goal in most patients (with the exception of those over 59 years of age where we recommended <150 mm Hg as the SBP goal). This recommendation, with its Corollary Recommendation, was perhaps the most controversial aspect of the Expert Panel Report. The Expert Panel did not recommend step-down therapy. Moreover it did support continuing therapy even if it achieved a blood pressure substantially lower than 150 mm Hg if therapy was well tolerated.

In the later part of 2015 the AHA and the ACC chose a new hypertension guideline panel. The release of the SPRINT (Systolic blood PRessure INtervention Trial) results in November of 2015[29] provided crucial evidence for managing those over 59 years of age and it is likely that the next guideline will lower the BP target for many hypertension subgroups, including the elderly.

Which Guideline?

High BP is a very common finding in the USA. It is not surprising, then, that several groups have issued guidelines for high BP. What is disconcerting to a practitioner is that despite having access to the same evidence, guideline writing groups can differ in their target BP goals recommendations, particularly within subgroups such as diabetes and chronic kidney disease. Choosing which guideline to follow is a daunting task.

Not Covered in Depth

It would be a disservice to the NHBPEP to leave the reader with the impression that hypertension guidelines via the JNC process was the only impact of the Coordinating Committee for the NHBPEP. Also published, under the auspices of the NHBPEP, were guidelines for managing BP:

- In pregnancy[30]
- In children[31]
- In renovascular disease[32]
- Re: prevalence, awareness, treatment, and control updates[33]
- In the elderly[34]

- Ambulatory blood pressure monitoring[35]
- In chronic kidney disease[36] and
- Primary prevention of hypertension[37]

In the U.S. we owe a large debt of gratitude to the NHBPEP for their unflagging efforts in the area of high BP, particularly the value of screening, the definition of elevated BP, the evaluation of hypertensive patients, and the management of hypertension. Although the profusion of guidelines on hypertension in the last few years generated a great deal of confusion and frustration, there are actually many similarities between the various recommendations made. Given the prevalence of high BP, and the catastrophic nature of hypertensive end-organ damage, it is vital that every practitioner caring for a hypertensive patient has a clear idea of how to measure, evaluate, and manage high BP in their practice.

EUROPEAN GUIDELINES

Background Story

For several decades European physicians involved in the management of hypertension had as reference guidelines those issued by the WHO without or in conjunction with the International Society of Hypertension.[38-40] Several European experts participated in the Task Forces involved in the guidelines elaboration, with the chance to have the European viewpoints on the design and treatment of this condition considered. From the beginning of the year 2000, however, the opinion gained ground that, given the advanced standard of medical practice in Europe, world-focused guidelines that had to adapt to the problems posed by developing countries were not entirely appropriate, and that thus more specific recommendations for European physicians and patients were needed. This led the European Society of Hypertension (ESH) to form an expert committee that prepared a comprehensive document on the diagnostic and treatment aspects of hypertension. The document was approved by the European Society of Cardiology (ESC) via its Working Group on Hypertension and the Heart, and the two Societies eventually published what were the first European guidelines on hypertension in 2003.[41]

The 2003 ESH/ESC guidelines were very well received by the scientific and medical communities, becoming the fifth most widely cited paper in all areas of science (and the first one in health-related sciences) in the following years.[42] This, and the substantial growth of knowledge on hypertension and related diseases, favored a second edition of the guidelines in 2007[43] and a third one in 2013,[44] with in-between a shorter document revisiting some issues of the 2007 recommendations published by the ESH in 2009.[45] In all instances the following procedures were adopted. (1) The Task Force was limited to 20 to 25 members (including two cochairmen and, in 2007 and 2013, representatives of practicing physicians and nurses), half appointed by ESH and half by ESC based on contribution to hypertension research. (2) Members were selected if devoid of major conflicts of interest, their disclosures being made visible in the Societies' websites. (3)A Task Force was allowed about a year to meet, correspond, and complete the text, which then went through three rounds of questions and criticism by more than 60 reviewers, selected because of their expertise on basic and clinical hypertension. (4) The final document was submitted to the ESH and ESC Scientific Councils to be approved for publication in the official Society journals. (5) Expenses for the preparation of the guidelines were covered by the two societies, with no contribution from any external source.

From the very beginning the ESH/ESC guidelines adhered to the following principles. First, guidelines have an educational and not a prescriptive or coercive value because their recommendations largely refer to an average patient, often with a limited (and scientifically weaker) extension to subgroups with different clinical characteristics as well as with a difficult and variable degree of extrapolation to individual patients. In one of the ESH/ESC guidelines this was expressed as follows: ".... guidelines deal with medical conditions in general and therefore their role must be educational and not prescriptive or coercive for the management of individual patients who may differ widely in their personal, medical, and cultural characteristics, thus requiring decisions different from the average ones recommended by guidelines."[43] Second, guidelines must be based on evidence and preferably its highest scientific expression, that is, results from randomized trials. However, randomized trials have limitations and their availability covers only few aspects of daily medical practice. Evidence from other sources (observational studies, case-control investigations, mechanistic data, etc.) thus needs to be also used, including, when necessary, that originating from data interpretation or extrapolation or even from personal clinical experience. Indeed, the recommendations based on the strongest class/level of evidence were no more than 25% of the total in the 2013 ESH/ESC guidelines (Fig. 50.1), those defined as generated by an "Expert Opinion" being 70% of those issued by the USA Expert Panel Report (also known as Joint National Committee or JNC 8) in 2014.[22] Third, in line with its educational purpose, guidelines must explain the reasons behind diagnostic and therapeutic recommendations, which makes the production of a simple and short document difficult. However, to favor guidelines dissemination and use, a compromise between complexity and simplicity is necessary. In the ESH/ESC guidelines this was obtained by having each section reviewing complex scientific evidence followed by boxes with short and simple statements reflecting its implications and transferability to clinical practice.

Classification of Blood Pressure Levels and Definition of Hypertension

In all ESH/ESC guidelines the classification of BP levels as well as the definition of hypertension has been taken from the USA JNC 7 Guidelines published in 2003,[46] which divides subjects based on optimal (<120/80 mm Hg systolic/diastolic), normal (120 to 129 systolic or 80 to 84 mm Hg diastolic), high normal (130 to 139 systolic or 85 to 89 diastolic mm Hg) BP levels, and defines hypertension grades starting from systolic values 140 or higher mm Hg or diastolic values 90 or higher mm Hg. In the European guidelines, however, the term "prehypertension" by which USA guidelines unify subjects with a normal

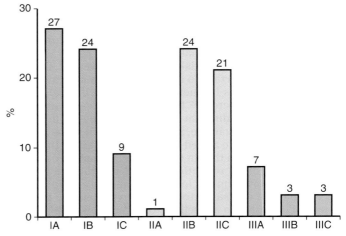

FIG. 50.1 Distribution of combined class and level of evidence in the 2013 European Society of Hypertension/European Society of Cardiology (ESH/ESC) hypertension guidelines. IA corresponds to the highest class (I) and level (A) of evidence, that is, the one obtained by multiple randomized trials.

and a high-normal BP has never been adopted because, as stated in 2007[43] (1) the risk of developing hypertension (i.e., the meaning of the adopted term) is markedly different in the two groups; (2) given the ominous significance of the word "hypertension" for the layman, labelling an individual as "pre-hypertensive" may create anxiety and result in unnecessary medical visits and examinations, and (3) subjects with normal or high-normal BP represent a fraction of the population with markedly different levels of cardiovascular risk[47] that necessitate of widely different treatment-decisions, treatment strategies, and intensity of follow-up.

Another difference between the USA and European guidelines has been the attention devoted to BP measurements other than those conventionally obtained in the office environment. In the European guidelines office BP has always been regarded as the reference one for the classification of BP levels, the identification of hypertension, and the assessment of the BP-lowering efficacy of treatment. However, because of their frequent use in clinical practice, alternative approaches to BP measurement have been always discussed in depth. In the case of "exercise" and "central" BP the conclusion has been that, at present, they do not appear to improve the cardiovascular risk prediction of untreated and treated patients over that provided by office BP, thereby making their use still confined to research. In the case of out-of-office (ambulatory and home) BP, on the other hand, diagnostic advantages such as identification of "white coat" hypertension, masked hypertension, true (rather than "white coat") resistant hypertension, and preeclampsia have been documented. It is also documented that automatic BP measurements over the day and night may detect otherwise unidentifiable conditions of high cardiovascular risk, such as the absence of nocturnal hypotension.[48] Use of out-of-office BP measurements has thus always been regarded by the ESH/ESC guidelines as a source of important clinical information in specific conditions.[41,43,44]

Stratification of Cardiovascular Risk

In the 2003 ESH/ESC guidelines[41] emphasis was placed on the need to complement the diagnosis of hypertension with a stratification of total (or global) cardiovascular risk, which was obtained by identifying four risk categories (average, moderate, high, or very high added risk) depending on the increasing BP levels and the concomitance of 1, 2, 3 or more cardiovascular risk factors, organ damage, diabetes, or an established cardiovascular or renal disease. It was acknowledged that, compared with the classic approaches to risk stratification, that is, those considering cardiovascular risk as a continuous variable,[49,50] categorization might make outcome prediction less accurate. It was nevertheless believed that the simplicity of the new method might increase the presently small percentage of physicians who quantify cardiovascular risk on a regular basis.[51] This was thought to be important to make physicians aware not only that hypertension is frequently accompanied by other cardiovascular risk factors[52] but also that treatment strategies can markedly differ at different risk levels. In grade I hypertension, for example, use of antihypertensive drugs is compelling when the added risk is high or very high but not when it is low, given that in the latter circumstance the beneficial effects of BP reduction are not unequivocally documented.[45,53] Furthermore, in patients at high cardiovascular risk it may be advisable to use antihypertensive drugs at lower BP thresholds as well as to pursue lower BP targets. Finally, antiplatelet treatment may be indicated when cardiovascular risk is high although being unnecessary (and perhaps potentially harmful) when it is low.[54] With few exceptions (e.g., the uncertain relationship between risk levels and threshold and target for BP-lowering treatment)[45]

these considerations have been regarded as valid also by the subsequent ESH/ESC guidelines, which have thus continued to consider global cardiovascular risk stratification as a necessary diagnostic step that helps to take appropriate treatment decisions (Fig. 50.2). To improve the accuracy of risk quantification the ESH/ESC guidelines have also consistently supported the search for asymptomatic organ damage, the role of which is minimized by the classic methods to quantify cardiovascular risk.[49,50] Search for organ damage is strongly supported by the evidence that (1) for any given cardiovascular risk quantification by classic risk factors (age, sex, blood cholesterol, blood sugar, smoking, blood pressure) the presence of asymptomatic organ damage is accompanied by a marked increase of the total cardiovascular risk level, and more so as the number of organs involved increases[55] and (2) in individuals with a BP elevation, organ damage is so common as to make its identification necessary to avoid a widespread underestimation of a high cardiovascular risk condition.[56] Accordingly, in all ESH/ESC guidelines a description of the measures of functional and structural organ derangement with documented prognostic significance has always been provided, together with a list of the recommended instrumental examinations.

Blood Pressure Thresholds and Targets for Drug Treatment

In 2003 the ESH/ESC guidelines[41] advised antihypertensive drugs to be administered at BP values 140 or higher mm Hg systolic or 90 or higher mm Hg diastolic in the general hypertensive population but to start using them in the high normal BP range whenever total cardiovascular risk is defined as high (e.g., patients with diabetes or established cardiovascular or renal disease), the BP target for treatment being less than 140/90 mm Hg and less than 130/80 mm Hg in the two conditions, respectively. These values were recommended also in 2007[43] whereas several conservative modifications were introduced in 2013.[44] Based on a reanalysis of the effects of treatment-induced BP reductions on cardiovascular and renal outcomes in randomized trials[45] the BP threshold for antihypertensive drug administration was set at 140 or higher mm Hg systolic and 90 or higher mm Hg diastolic, regardless of the level of cardiovascular risk, a unified value (<140/90 mm Hg) being recommended also for the BP target for treatment. Based on two randomized trials,[57,58] a somewhat lower DBP target (<85 mm Hg) was advised for diabetic patients, whereas the recommended threshold was made higher for elderly patients in whom the target was placed at an SBP between 140 and 150 mm Hg. Similar threshold and target values were later recommended by the JNC 8 Report,[22] compared with which the ESH/ESC recommendations were, however, somewhat less "trenchant" insofar as the possibility remained to lower systolic BP to (1) less than 140 mm Hg in elderly hypertensives in whom treatment was well tolerated and (2) less than 130 mm Hg in patients with renal disease and proteinuria, based on the observation that BP reductions have an antiproteinuric effect[59] as well as that reducing proteinuria may reflect renal and cardiovascular protection.[60] It was clearly mentioned, however, that these possibilities were supported by "observational" rather than randomized trial data, that is, a less reliable type of evidence. And that the overall value of guidelines recommendations on threshold and target BP values for drug treatment is limited by the unavailability of data in younger patients as well as in patients with a recent incident hypertension and no hypertension-related complications. The possibility exists that under these conditions lower BP targets further decrease outcomes or even that under these circumstances the lower the BP the better it is for the patient, as it has been observed by epidemiological studies in relatively low risk populations.[61]

Other risk factors, asymptomatic organ damage or disease	Blood Pressure (mm Hg)			
	High normal SBP 130–139 or DBP 85–89	Grade 1 HT SBP 140–159 or DBP 90–99	Grade 2 HT SBP 160–179 or DBP 100–109	Grade 3 HT SBP ≥180 or DBP ≥110
No other RF		Low risk	Moderate risk	High risk
1–2 RF	Low risk	Moderate risk	Moderate to high risk	High risk
≥3 RF	Low to moderate risk	Moderate to high risk	High risk	High risk
OD, CKD stage 3 or diabetes	Moderate to high risk	High risk	High risk	High to very high risk
Symptomatic CVD, CKD stage ≥4 or diabetes with OD/RFs	Very high risk	Very high risk	Very high risk	Very high risk

Other risk factors, asymptomatic organ damage or disease	Blood Pressure (mm Hg)			
	High normal SBP 130–139 or DBP 85–89	Grade 1 HT SBP 140–159 or DBP 90–99	Grade 2 HT SBP 160–179 or DBP 100–109	Grade 3 HT SBP ≥180 or DBP ≥110
No other RF	• No BP intervention	• Lifestyle changes for several months • Then add BP drugs targeting <140/90	• Lifestyle changes for several weeks • Then add BP drugs targeting <140/90	• Lifestyle changes • Immediate BP drugs targeting <140/90
1–2 RF	• Lifestyle changes • No BP intervention	• Lifestyle changes for several weeks • Then add BP drugs targeting <140/90	• Lifestyle changes for several weeks • Then add BP drugs targeting <140/90	• Lifestyle changes • Immediate BP drugs targeting <140/90
≥3 RF	• Lifestyle changes • No BP intervention	• Lifestyle changes for several weeks • Then add BP drugs targeting <140/90	• Lifestyle changes • BP drugs targeting <140/90	• Lifestyle changes • Immediate BP drugs targeting <140/90
OD, CKD stage 3 or diabetes	• Lifestyle changes • No BP intervention	• Lifestyle changes • BP drugs targeting <140/90	• Lifestyle changes • BP drugs targeting <140/90	• Lifestyle changes • Immediate BP drugs targeting <140/90
Symptomatic CVD, CKD stage ≥4 or diabetes with OD/RFs	• Lifestyle changes • No BP intervention	• Lifestyle changes • BP drugs targeting <140/90	• Lifestyle changes • BP drugs targeting <140/90	• Lifestyle changes • Immediate BP drugs targeting <140/90

FIG. 50.2 The left part shows the stratification of total cardiovascular risk into the categories of low, moderate, high, and very high, according to the presence of risk factors, organ damage, disease, and blood pressure levels. The right part shows the correspondence of risk stratification to initiation and type of antihypertensive treatment. *BP*, Blood pressure; *CKD*, chronic kidney disease; *CVD*, cardiovascular disease; *DBP*, diastolic blood pressure; *HT*, hypertension; *OD*, organ damage; *RF*, risk factor; *SBP*, systolic blood pressure. (*From Mancia G, Fagard R, Narkiewicz K. 2013 ESH/ESC Guidelines for the management of arterial hypertension. J Hypertens. 2013;31:1281-1357.*)

First Choice Drugs

The ESH/ESC guidelines have never deviated from the principle that because (1) the cardiovascular protection that accompanies BP reductions has been obtained with several drug classes[62-65] and (2) for a given BP reduction different drugs exert an overall similar protective effect,[62-64] the benefit of antihypertensive treatment is largely attributed to BP lowering per se, that is, regardless how it is obtained.[66,67] This has opened the list of drugs believed to be suitable for first choice use to all those showing the ability to effectively lower BP and reduce cardiovascular outcomes in placebo-controlled or comparison trials, obviously with an evidence of a good safety and tolerability profile as well. In 2003 and 2007 the list has included diuretics, beta-blockers, calcium channel blockers (CCBs), ACE inhibitors, and angiotensin receptor blockers. The same drug classes have been confirmed in the first choice position in the 2013 guidelines, which have also made clear that (1) first choice diuretics include thiazides, thiazide-like (chlorthalidone), and indapamide, all of which have evidence of BP-lowering efficacy and outcome protection, without any reliable documentation of a superiority of one versus another and (2) no data support the "a-priori" exclusion of beta-blockers from initial drug use,[68] as done by some guidelines,[58,69] because these drugs reduce the elevated BP values as much as the others.[70] Furthermore, their use has led to cardiovascular outcome reductions in placebo controlled trials, with no consistent differences from other drugs in the degree of the overall protective effect in randomized outcome trials and some large meta-analyses.[63,64]

A peculiar aspect of the 2013 ESH/ESC guidelines[44] has been the criticism of the time-honored concept of all-purpose ranking of antihypertensive drugs into first, second, third choice, and so on. Mention has been made that decades ago this might have been justified by the fact that some agents

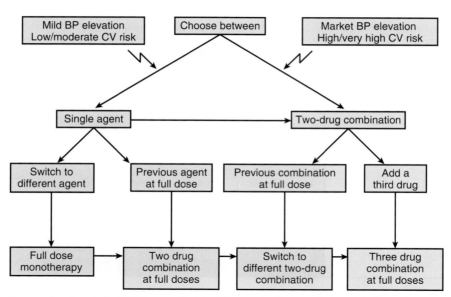

FIG. 50.3 Treatment initiation by one or two drugs in the 2013 European Society of Hypertension/European Society of Cardiology (ESH/ESC) hypertension guidelines. Moving from a less intensive to a more intensive therapeutic strategy should be done whenever blood pressure target is not achieved. *(From Mancia G, Fagard R, Narkiewicz K. 2013 ESH/ESC Guidelines for the management of arterial hypertension.* J Hypertens. *2013;31:1281-1357.)*

could almost never be used alone because their hemodynamic inconveniences made correction by the action of other agents necessary. An example was hydralazine whose sodium-retaining properties required almost invariably the preuse or concomitant use of a diuretic. This is hardly the case today, however, because current treatment of hypertension can count on many drugs employable as initial monotherapy, with no major side effects or other problems. Each drug, however, has pros and cons that make it preferable in some patients but not in others, making no drug always or never suitable as first choice treatment. Thus, the first choice ranking of drugs refers to an average patient that does not exist in real life and offers little practical help to the practicing physician. The opinion of the author (GM) of this chapter is that in future guidelines the "first choice" terminology should be abandoned and replaced with a list of agents that have the basic scientific requirements (see previously) to be recommended for preferential use, no matter if only in in some patient categories.

Choice of Drugs

Because patients responding to one drug class are not superimposable with those responding to another drug class,[71] a large number of drug options has the advantage of increasing the percentage of hypertensives potentially capable of achieving BP control with monotherapy. It has the disadvantage, however, of making the choice of the initial drug more complex. In all ESH/ESC guidelines this has been addressed by laying down the criteria that may help physicians to reach a decision based on evidence as well as, when evidence is not available, clinical and pathophysiological considerations. In the 2013 guidelines these criteria have been (1) the well known compelling or possible contraindications that characterized each antihypertensive drug; (2) the presence and type of asymptomatic organ damage, given that some drugs reduce them more effectively than others[41,43,44]; (3) the presence and type of the clinical events suffered by the patient in his or her medical history; and (4) the clinical condition of the patient, with special reference to his/her metabolic state, that is, lipid abnormalities, diabetes, an impaired fasting glucose state, or a metabolic syndrome. Pregnancy and ethnicity can also offer guidance to drug choice. In contrast, the ESH/ESC guidelines have never listed age as a factor on which to base the selection of drugs to administer because (1) evidence that drugs are differently effective on BP and cardiovascular outcomes in the elderly compared with

younger patients has been regarded as based on small studies when not on unpublished reports[69,72]; (2) in elderly patients the cardiovascular protective effect of antihypertensive treatment has been documented with a variety of drugs[45,73,74]; and (3) the protective effects of antihypertensive drugs for cardiovascular events has been found to remain unmodified by aging in large trial meta-analyses.[73] Thus, according to the European guidelines, although aging does lead to important changes in the management of hypertension (BP measurement in the standing position, use of ambulatory BP monitoring to search for hypotensive episodes, lower initial drug doses, slower titration to final treatment) selection of first choice and subsequent drugs has been regarded as substantially similar in both younger and elderly individuals.

Treatment Strategies

The early guidelines issued by the WHO and the International Society of Hypertension (ISH) have for a long time privileged an antihypertensive treatment strategy based on an increase in the dose of the initially administered drug to try to obtain BP control in patients unresponsive to the ordinary dose. Lately, however, the attitude has changed because of the evidence that increasing drug doses may lead to a greater BP reduction at the price, however, of an even more evident increase in the number and severity of side effects, particularly with drug classes such as diuretics, CCBs, and beta-blockers.[70] This has led more recent guidelines to recommend strategies based on switching from one monotherapy to another or to the addition of other drugs to the initial one.

From the very beginning the ESH/ESC guidelines have strongly supported combination treatment as the most effective strategy to achieve BP control in the hypertensive population. Emphasis has been placed on the fact that (1) sequential monotherapy can be time consuming, leading to patient's frustration that may have unfavorable consequences on long term adherence to treatment; and (2) the multifactorial nature of BP control makes the multiple BP-lowering mechanisms provided by drug combinations much more effective in achieving an adequate reduction of the elevated BP values.[74] The ESH/ESC guidelines, however, have also left the door open to the possible use of two drug combinations as first step treatment in patients with a marked BP elevation or a milder degree of hypertension but a high or very high cardiovascular risk (Fig. 50.3).[44] Although acknowledging that no randomized outcome trial has

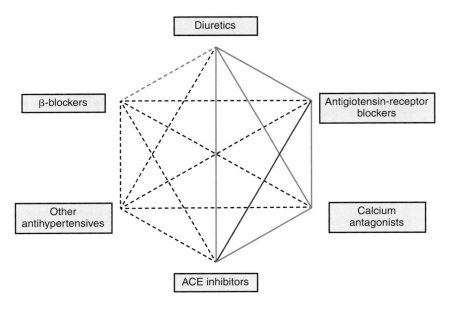

Only dihydropyridines to be combined with β-blockers
(except for verapamil or dilitazem for rate control in AF)
Thiazides + β-blockers increase risk of new onset DM
ACEi + ARB combination discouraged (IIIA)

— preferred
--- useful (with some limitations)
- - - possible but less well tested
— not recommended

FIG. 50.4 Two-drug combinations for antihypertensive treatment in the 2013 European Society of Hypertension/European Society of Cardiology (ESH/ESC) hypertension guidelines. *(From Mancia G, Fagard R, Narkiewicz K. 2013 ESH/ESC Guidelines for the management of arterial hypertension.* J Hypertens. *2013;31:1281-1357.)*

ever compared initial and later combination treatments, the faster BP reduction associated with initial administration of two drugs has been regarded as potentially useful whenever a high cardiovascular risk makes persistence of an uncontrolled BP particularly risky. In the 2013 guidelines this has found support in the "real life" data that, compared with patients starting treatment with two drugs, those in whom combination treatment replaces an initially ineffective monotherapy have a less common BP control up to 1 year,[75,76] possibly because (1) physicians' inertia opposes treatment modifications; and/ or (2) patients under initial monotherapy exhibit a lower long-term adherence to the prescribed treatment regimen compared with patients under initial drug combinations,[77] with a negative impact on cardiovascular protection.[78,79]

The ESH/ESC guidelines have always made use of a geometrical figure to show which combinations, among all those available, may be preferred, also listing the criteria that should guide drug associations.[41,43,44] As shown in Fig. 50.4,[44] in the 2013 guidelines preference has been given to the combination of an ACE inhibitor or an ARB with a diuretic, an ACE inhibitor or an ARB with a CCB or a CCB with a diuretic, based on their large, although nonrandomized, use in outcome trials showing the protective effects of BP-lowering treatment. Despite the recent large trial results,[80] no preference has been given to the combination of a blocker of the renin angiotensin system with a CCB rather than with a diuretic, because the similarity of the protective effects of the two latter drug classes in several comparison trials. Although regarded as less preferable, other combinations have not been banned from use, the only exception being those leading to a double blockade of the renin-angiotensin system (e.g., an ACE inhibitor and an angiotensin receptor blocker) because of the serious inconveniences seen in patients with diabetes and impaired renal function. Given the limited availability of proper outcome comparisons, the 2013 ESH/ESC guidelines have emphasized that recommendations on combination treatment hierarchy are not strongly evidence-based, and that this is an area where future trials are necessary. This is the case also because combination treatment is required for BP control in most hypertensives.[81]

Other Characteristics

The ESH/ESC guidelines have always believed to be necessary to address those aspects of the management of hypertension that, although never explored by or even unsuitable to collection of outcome trial evidence, have great relevance to daily life practice. To this aim they have always included common sense-based recommendations on how to follow treated hypertensive patients, such as, how often to visit them or repeat blood or instrumental examinations. They have given advice on whether and how to treat concomitant risk factors, with focus on lipid lowering, glucose lowering, and antiplatelet or anticoagulant drugs. They have addressed the special treatment problems that may be posed by clinical conditions (18 in the 2013 guidelines) never explored by specifically designed trials. They have always reserved space to discuss how to try to lessen or remove the multifold barriers that make achievement of BP control difficult and maintain hypertension as the first cause of death worldwide. They have in their final part always included mention of gaps of evidence and need of future trials, in the belief that this might be educationally appropriate and prepare physicians to future guidelines changes made necessary by the collection of new evidence.

References

1. Effects of treatment on morbidity in hypertension. Results in patients with diastolic blood pressures averaging 115 through 129 mm Hg. JAMA. 1967;202:1028-1034.
2. Effects of treatment on morbidity in hypertension. II. Results in patients with diastolic blood pressure averaging 90 through 114 mm Hg. JAMA. 1970;213:1143-1152.
3. Report of the Joint National Committee on Detection, Evaluation, and Treatment of High Blood Pressure. A cooperative study. JAMA. 1977;237:255-261.
4. Barclay WR. The report on detection, evaluation, and treatment of high blood pressure. JAMA. 1977;237:267.
5. Murray CJ, Lopez AD. Measuring the global burden of disease. N Engl J Med. 2013;369:448-457.
6. The 1980 report of the Joint National Committee on Detection, Evaluation, and Treatment of High Blood Pressure. Arch Int Med. 1980;140:1280-1285.
7. Anonymous. Five-year findings of the hypertension detection and follow-up program. I. Reduction in mortality of persons with high blood pressure, including mild hypertension. Hypertension Detection and Follow-up Program Cooperative Group. JAMA. 1979;242:2562-2571.
8. Smith WM. Treatment of mild hypertension: results of a ten-year intervention trial. Circ Res. 1977;40:I98-105.
9. Shulman NB, Ford CE, Hall WD, et al. Prognostic value of serum creatinine and effect of treatment of hypertension on renal function. Results from the hypertension detection and follow-up program. The Hypertension Detection and Follow-up Program Cooperative Group. Hypertension. 1989;13:I80-I93.

10. The 1984 Report of the Joint National Committee on Detection, Evaluation, and Treatment of High Blood Pressure. *Arch Int Med.* 1984;144:1045-1057.

11. The Australian therapeutic trial in mild hypertension. Report by the Management Committee. *Lancet.* 1980;1:1261-1267.

12. The beta-blocker heart attack trial. beta-Blocker Heart Attack Study Group. *JAMA.* 1981;246:2073-2074.

13. Timolol-induced reduction in mortality and reinfarction in patients surviving acute myocardial infarction. *N Engl J Med.* 1981;304:801-807.

14. The 1988 report of the Joint National Committee on Detection, Evaluation, and Treatment of High Blood Pressure. *Arch Int Med.* 1988;148:1023-1038.

15. MRC trial of treatment of mild hypertension: principal results. Medical Research Council Working Party. *Br Med J (Clin Res Ed).* 1985;291:97-104.

16. Amery A, Birkenhager W, Brixko P, et al. Mortality and morbidity results from the European Working Party on High Blood Pressure in the Elderly trial. *Lancet.* 1985;1:1349-1354.

17. The fifth report of the Joint National Committee on Detection, Evaluation, and Treatment of High Blood Pressure (JNC V). *Arch Intern Med.* 1993;153:154-183.

18. Chobanian AV, Bakris GL, Black HR, et al. The Seventh Report of the Joint National Committee on Prevention, Detection, Evaluation, and Treatment of High Blood Pressure: the JNC 7 report. *JAMA.* 2003;289:2560-2572.

19. Chobanian AV, Bakris GL, Black HR, et al. Seventh report of the joint national committee on prevention, detection, evaluation, and treatment of high blood pressure. *Hypertension.* 2003;42:1206-1252.

20. Committee on Quality of Health Care in America, Institute of Medicine. *Crossing the Quality Chasm: a New Health System for the 21st Century.* 1st ed. National Academies Press, 2002.

21. Tricoci P, Allen JM, Kramer JM, Califf RM, Smith SC Jr. Scientific evidence underlying the ACC/AHA clinical practice guidelines. *JAMA.* 2009;301:831-841.

22. James PA, Oparil S, Carter BL, et al. 2014 Evidence-Based Guideline for the Management of High Blood Pressure in Adults: report From the Panel Members Appointed to the Eighth Joint National Committee (JNC 8). *JAMA.* 2014;311:507-520.

23. Klahr S, Levey AS, Beck GJ, et al. The effects of dietary protein restriction and blood-pressure control on the progression of chronic renal disease. Modification of Diet in Renal Disease Study Group. *N Engl J Med.* 1994;330:877-884.

24. Wright JT, Jr., Bakris G, Greene T, et al. Effect of blood pressure lowering and antihypertensive drug class on progression of hypertensive kidney disease: results from the AASK trial. *JAMA.* 2002;288:2421-2431.

25. Ruggenenti P, Perna A, Loriga G, et al. Blood-pressure control for renoprotection in patients with non-diabetic chronic renal disease (REIN-2): multicentre, randomised controlled trial. *Lancet.* 2005;365:939-946.

26. Upadhyay A, Earley A, Haynes SM, Uhlig K. Systematic review: blood pressure target in chronic kidney disease and proteinuria as an effect modifier. *Ann Intern Med.* 2011;154:541-548.

27. Yusuf S, Sleight P, Pogue J, Bosch J, Davies R, Dagenais G. Effects of an angiotensin-converting-enzyme inhibitor, ramipril, on cardiovascular events in high-risk patients. The Heart Outcomes Prevention Evaluation Study Investigators. *Clin Nephrol.* 2000;342:145-153.

28. Rosendorff C, Lackland DT, Allison M, et al. Treatment of hypertension in patients with coronary artery disease: a scientific statement from the American Heart Association, American College of Cardiology, and American Society of Hypertension. *Circulation.* 2015;9:453-498.

29. Wright JT, Jr., Williamson JD, Whelton PK, et al. A randomized trial of intensive versus standard blood-pressure control. *N Engl J Med.* 2015;373:2103-2116.

30. Report of the National High Blood Pressure Education Program Working Group on High Blood Pressure in Pregnancy. *Am J Obstet Gynecol.* 2000;183:S1-S22.

31. The fourth report on the diagnosis, evaluation, and treatment of high blood pressure in children and adolescents. *Pediatrics.* 2004;114:555-576.

32. NHLBI workshop on renovascular disease. Summary report and recommendations. *Hypertension.* 1985;7:452-456.

33. Hypertension prevalence and the status of awareness, treatment, and control in the United States. Final report of the Subcommittee on Definition and Prevalence of the 1984 Joint National Committee. *Hypertension.* 1985;7:457-468.

34. National High Blood Pressure Education Program Working Group Report on Hypertension in the Elderly. National High Blood Pressure Education Program Working Group. *Hypertension.* 1994;23:275-285.

35. National High Blood Pressure Education Program (NHBEP). Working Group Report on Ambulatory Blood Pressure Monitoring. *NIH PUblication no 92-3028*; 1992.

36. National High Blood Pressure Education Program. National high blood pressure education program working group report on hypertension and chronic renal failure. *Arch Intern Med.* 1991;151:1280-1287.

37. National High Blood Pressure Education Working Group. National High Blood Pressure Education Program Working Group Report on Primary Prevention of Hypertension. *Arch Intern Med.* 1993;153:186-208.

38. 1993 guidelines for the management of mild hypertension: memorandum from a World Health Organization/International Society of Hypertension meeting. Guidelines Sub-Committee. *J Hypertens.* 1993;11:905-918.

39. WHO Expert Hypertension Control Committee. WHO Technical Report Sewries no 862. *World Health Organization* [serial online] 1996; Available from: WHO.

40. 1999 World Health Organization-International Society of Hypertension Guidelines for the Management of Hypertension. Guidelines Subcommittee. *J Hypertens.* 1999;17:151-183.

41. 2003 European Society of Hypertension-European Society of Cardiology guidelines for the management of arterial hypertension. *J Hypertens.* 2003;21:1011-1053.

42. Anonymous. Top ten papers published. *The Scientist.* 2005;19:26.

43. Mancia G, De Backer G, Dominiczak A, et al. 2007 Guidelines for the Management of Arterial Hypertension: the Task Force for the Management of Arterial Hypertension of the European Society of Hypertension (ESH) and of the European Society of Cardiology (ESC). *J Hypertens.* 2007;25:1105-1187.

44. Mancia G, Fagard R, Narkiewicz K, et al. 2013 ESH/ESC Guidelines for the management of arterial hypertension: the Task Force for the management of arterial hypertension of the European Society of Hypertension (ESH) and of the European Society of Cardiology (ESC). *J Hypertens.* 2013;31:1281-1357.

45. Mancia G, Laurent S, Agabiti-Rosei E, et al. Reappraisal of European guidelines on hypertension management: a European Society of Hypertension Task Force document. *J Hypertens.* 2009;27:2121-2158.

46. Chobanian AV, Bakris GL, Black HR, et al. Seventh report of the Joint National Committee on Prevention, Detection, Evaluation, and Treatment of High Blood Pressure. *Hypertension.* 2003;42:1206-1252.

47. Vasan RS, Larson MG, Leip EP, et al. Impact of high-normal blood pressure on the risk of cardiovascular disease. *Clinical Nephrology.* 2001;345:1291-1297.

48. Mancia G, Verdecchia P. Clinical value of ambulatory blood pressure: evidence and limits. *Circ Res.* 2015;116:1034-1045.

49. Kannel WB. Risk stratification in hypertension: new insights from the Framingham Study. *Am J Hypertens.* 2000;13:3S-10S.

50. Conroy RM, Pyorala K, Fitzgerald AP, et al. Estimation of ten-year risk of fatal cardiovascular disease in Europe: the SCORE project. *Eur Heart J.* 2003;24:987-1003.

51. Hobbs FD, Erhardt L. Acceptance of guideline recommendations and perceived implementation of coronary heart disease prevention among primary care physicians in five European countries: the Reassessing European Attitudes about Cardiovascular Treatment (REACT) survey. *Fam Pract.* 2002;19:596-604.

52. Mancia G, Facchetti R, Bombelli M, et al. Relationship of office, home, and ambulatory blood pressure to blood glucose and lipid variables in the PAMELA population. *Hypertension.* 2005;45:1072-1077.

53. Sundstrom J, Arima H, Woodward M, et al. Blood pressure-lowering treatment based on cardiovascular risk: a meta-analysis of individual patient data. *Lancet.* 2014;384:591-598.

54. Baigent C, Blackwell L, Collins R, et al. Aspirin in the primary and secondary prevention of vascular disease: collaborative meta-analysis of individual participant data from randomised trials. *Lancet.* 2009;373:1849-1860.

55. Sehestedt T, Jeppesen J, Hansen TW, et al. Risk prediction is improved by adding markers of subclinical organ damage to SCORE. *Eur Heart J.* 2010;31:883-891.

56. Cuspidi C, Ambrosioni E, Mancia G, Pessina AC, Trimarco B, Zanchetti A. Role of echocardiography and carotid ultrasonography in stratifying risk in patients with essential hypertension: the Assessment of Prognostic Risk Observational Survey. *J Hypertens.* 2002;20:1307-1314.

57. Hansson L, Zanchetti A, Carruthers SG, et al. Effects of intensive blood-pressure lowering and low-dose aspirin in patients with hypertension: principal results of the Hypertension Optimal Treatment (HOT) randomised trial. HOT Study Group [see comments]. *Lancet.* 1998;351:1755-1762.

58. Intensive blood-glucose control with sulphonylureas or insulin compared with conventional treatment and risk of complications in patients with type 2 diabetes (UKPDS 33). UK Prospective Diabetes Study (UKPDS) Group. *Lancet.* 1998;352:837-853.

59. Mancia G, Schumacher H, Redon J, et al. Blood pressure targets recommended by guidelines and incidence of cardiovascular and renal events in the Ongoing Telmisartan Alone and in Combination With Ramipril Global Endpoint Trial (ONTARGET). *Circulation.* 2011;124:1727-1736.

60. Schmieder RE, Mann JF, Schumacher H, et al. Changes in albuminuria predict mortality and morbidity in patients with vascular disease. *J Am Soc Nephrol.* 2011;22:1353-1364.

61. Lewington S, Clarke R, Qizilbash N, Peto R, Collins R. Age-specific relevance of usual blood pressure to vascular mortality: a meta-analysis of individual data for one million adults in 61 prospective studies. *Lancet.* 2002;360:1903-1913.

62. Law MR, Morris JK, Wald NJ. Use of blood pressure lowering drugs in the prevention of cardiovascular disease: meta-analysis of 147 randomised trials in the context of expectations from prospective epidemiological studies. *BMJ.* 2009;338: b1665.

63. Turnbull F, Neal B, Algert C, et al. Effects of different blood pressure-lowering regimens on major cardiovascular events in individuals with and without diabetes mellitus: results of prospectively designed overviews of randomized trials. *Arch Intern Med.* 2005;165:1410-1419.

64. Thomopoulos C, Parati G, Zanchetti A. Effects of blood pressure-lowering on outcome incidence in hypertension: 5. Head-to-head comparisons of various classes of antihypertensive drugs—overview and meta-analyses. *J Hypertens.* 2015;33:1321-1341.

65. Ettehad D, Emdin CA, Kiran A, et al. Blood pressure lowering for prevention of cardiovascular disease and death: a systematic review and meta-analysis. *Lancet.* 2016;387:957-967.

66. Turnbull F. Effects of different blood-pressure-lowering regimens on major cardiovascular events: results of prospectively-designed overviews of randomised trials. *Lancet.* 2003;362:1527-1535.

67. Reboldi G, Gentile G, Angeli F, Ambrosio G, Mancia G. Verdecchia P. Effects of intensive blood pressure reduction on myocardial infarction and stroke in diabetes: a meta-analysis in 73,913 patients. *J Hypertens.* 2011;29:1253-1269.

68. Mancia G, Zanchetti A. Choice of antihypertensive drugs in the European Society of Hypertension-European Society of Cardiology guidelines: specific indications rather than ranking for general usage. *J Hypertens.* 2008;26:164-168.

69. www.nice.org.uk/guidance/cg127. www.nice.org.uk/guidance/cg127. 2014.

70. Law MR, Wald NJ, Morris JK, Jordan RE. Value of low dose combination treatment with blood pressure lowering drugs: analysis of 354 randomised trials. *BMJ.* 2003;326:1427.

71. Mancia G, Grassi G. Individualization of antihypertensive drug treatment. *Diabetes Care.* 2013;36(Suppl 2):S301-S306.

72. Dickerson JE, Hingorani AD, Ashby MJ, Palmer CR, Brown MJ. Optimisation of antihypertensive treatment by crossover rotation of four major classes. *Lancet.* 1999;353:2008-2013.

73. Turnbull F, Neal B, Ninomiya T, et al. Effects of different regimens to lower blood pressure on major cardiovascular events in older and younger adults: meta-analysis of randomised trials. *BMJ.* 2008;336:1121-1123.

74. Zanchetti A, Mancia G. Longing for clinical excellence: a critical outlook into the NICE recommendations on hypertension management—is nice always good? *J Hypertens.* 2012;30:660-668.

75. Gradman AH, Parise H, Lefebvre P, Falvey H, Lafeuille MH, Duh MS. Initial combination therapy reduces the risk of cardiovascular events in hypertensive patients: a matched cohort study. *Hypertension.* 2013;61:309-318.

76. Egan BM, Bandyopadhyay D, Shaftman SR, Wagner CS, Zhao Y, Yu-Isenberg KS. Initial monotherapy and combination therapy and hypertension control the first year. *Hypertension.* 2012;59:1124-1131.

77. Mancia G, Zambon A, Soranna D, Merlino L, Corrao G. Factors involved in the discontinuation of antihypertensive drug therapy: an analysis from real life data. *J Hypertension.* 2014;32:1708-1715.

78. Corrao G, Nicotra F, Parodi A, et al. Cardiovascular protection by initial and subsequent combination of antihypertensive drugs in daily life practice. *Hypertension.* 2011;58:566-572.

79. Corrao G, Rea F, Ghirardi A, Soranna D, Merlino L, Mancia G. Adherence with antihypertensive drug therapy and the risk of heart failure in clinical practice. *Hypertension.* 2015;66:742-749.

80. Jamerson K, Weber MA, Bakris GL, et al. Benazepril plus amlodipine or hydrochlorothiazide for hypertension in high-risk patients. *N Engl J Med.* 2008;359:2417-2428.

81. Bakris GL, Williams M, Dworkin L, et al. Preserving renal function in adults with hypertension and diabetes: a consensus approach. National Kidney Foundation Hypertension and Diabetes Executive Committees Working Group. *Am J Kidney Dis.* 2000;36:646-661.

82. Rocella EJ, Burt V, Horan MJ, Cutler J. Changes in hypertension awareness, treatment, and control rates. 20-year trend data. *Ann Epidemiol.* 1993;3:547-549.

83. Fields LE, Burt VL, Cutler JA, Hughes J, Roccella EJ, Sorlie P. The burden of adult hypertension in the United States 1999 to 2000: a rising tide. *Hypertension.* 2004;44:398-404.

84. Egan BM, Zhao Y, Axon RN. US trends in prevalence, awareness, treatment, and control of hypertension, 1988-2008. *JAMA.* 2010;303:2043-2050.

85. Yoon SS, Gu Q, Nwankwo T, Wright JD, Hong Y, Burt V. Trends in blood pressure among adults with hypertension: United States, 2003 to 2012. *Hypertension.* 2015;65:54-61.

86. The sixth report of the Joint National Committee on prevention, detection, evaluation, and treatment of high blood pressure. *Arch Intern Med.* 1997;157:2413-2446.

51 Putting All Guidelines Into Perspective

George L. Bakris and Bryan Williams

BACKGROUND

The term "guideline" needs to be defined before any meaningful discussion can occur about their need and more importantly, interpretation. "Guideline" was originally defined as "a cord or rope to aid a passer over a difficult point or to permit retracing a course."[1] In medicine a guideline is a document that should influence decisions and provide criteria regarding diagnosis, management, and treatment in specific areas of health care. Such documents have been in use over the entire history of medicine. However, in contrast to previous approaches, often based on tradition or authority, modern medical guidelines are based on an examination of current evidence within the paradigm of evidence-based medicine.[2-4]

Modern clinical guidelines identify, summarize, and evaluate the highest quality evidence and most current data about prevention, diagnosis, prognosis, therapy including dosage of medications, risk/benefit, and cost-effectiveness. Prior and some current guidelines include consensus statements on best practice for a given disease, like hypertension, where evidence is lacking in some areas. Some recent guideline committees like the Expert Panel Report, also known as the JNC 8 (Eighth Joint National Committee) were instructed to stick purely to evidence and minimize expert opinion when designing the latest, now former NIH (National Institutes of Health) guidelines.[5] This approach leads to other shortcomings as will be noted later in the chapter. A health care provider is expected to know the medical guidelines for his or her area of medicine, and decide whether the recommendations are appropriate for an individual patient.

Additional objectives of clinical guidelines are to standardize medical care, raise quality of care, and reduce several kinds of risk (to the patient, health care provider, medical insurers, and health plans or government). Put simply, "what is the most cost-effective way of getting the correct diagnosis or treatment for the patient and payer?"

Guidelines are usually produced at national or international levels by medical associations or governmental bodies, such as the United States Agency for Healthcare Research and Quality or formally the National Institute of Health Heart Lung and Blood Institute now given to the American Heart Association/American College of Cardiology Societies (ACC/AHA guidelines). In the United Kingdom the National Institute for Health and Care Excellence (NICE) carries out guideline development across all areas of medicine and the European Society of Hypertension (ESH) has its own set of guidelines as do most individual nations around the world.

Although guidelines are useful in many settings, recently some payers in the United States and certain government agencies have established them more as "edicts of performance" rather than true guidelines. Guidelines change based on the most recent evidence, as is illustrated by changes in blood pressure goals since the inception of blood pressure guidelines in 1977 (Fig. 51.1). Certain insurers provide grades and basically elevate guidelines to some 'holy grail' status of practice, in a way not justified or expected by anyone who has written such guidance. Thus, what was meant as a meaningful

informative guide for physicians is increasingly used to mandate performance and judge outcomes.

This edict of exclusively evidence-based guidelines emerged around 2008 in the United States when the American Heart Association produced a report noting that there was a 48% increase in the number of recommendations, however, the majority had class 2 level of evidence.[6] Only 9% (245/2711) were based on the highest standard of evidence, that is class I and level A evidence.[6] Thus, it was concluded by almost all guideline development groups that recommendations should be restricted to those supported by high quality evidence. Unfortunately, in some important areas of medicine, rigid application of this policy would severely limit recommendations needed in routine clinical practice.

Guideline developers are aware of this limitation and try to balance the high quality evidence with common sense, experience and pragmatism. As a result, guidelines may have both methodological problems and limitations based on the limitations of the evidence. Another concern has been potential conflicts of interest.[4,7-10] It has been concluded, without good justification, that guideline developers must always be unduly influenced by pharmaceutical companies to bias statements favoring certain products. In many cases intellectual conflicts of interest, more than industry-based conflicts, are apparent among guideline development groups Hence, it is impossible to eliminate conflicts of interest based only on monetary remuneration. This and other partially unjustified edicts have resulted in guidelines that have a very limited scope, as a result of lack of evidence in key areas and committee members who have limited experience in the areas under discussion.

The key is to publish clear methodology for guideline development so that readers have a clear understanding of the process of how the evidence has been used to frame the recommendations. Thus, guidelines from countries that require evidence-based guidelines interpreted by professionals who are experienced clinicians in a respective area may be more reasonable as compared with the more draconian approach where people with knowledge of methodology but no experience in the topic area in question or who lack patient interaction experience are interpreting the evidence.

Some simple clinical practice guidelines are not routinely followed to the extent they might be and that providing a nurse or other health care professional with a checklist of recommended procedures can result in the attending physician being reminded, in a timely manner, regarding procedures that might have been overlooked.[11,12] This illustrates that a team approach is needed for guideline implementation and translation to improved medical care.

This chapter will focus on the development of hypertension guidelines through the years in the United States, United Kingdom, and Europe and provide a perspective on where we came from and where we are today.

UNITED STATES GUIDELINES

The major organization producing guidelines for management of hypertension until 2011 was the Heart Lung and Blood Institute

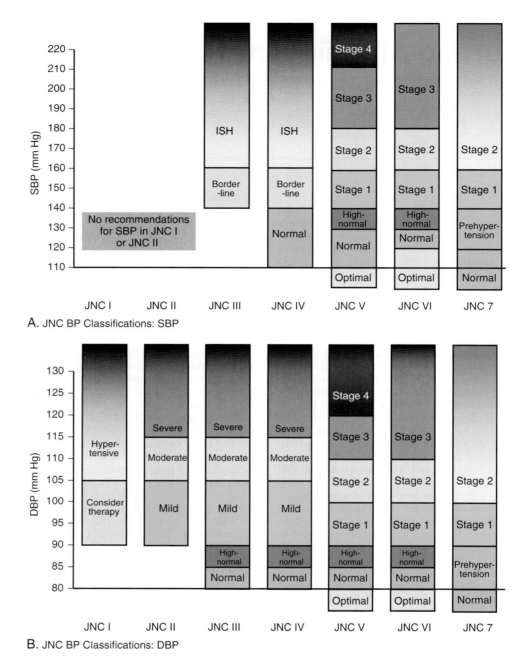

FIG. 51.1 History of Joint National Committee Guidelines since their inception. To simplify the classification of hypertension, the seventh report of the Joint National Committee on Prevention, Detection, Evaluation, and Treatment of High Blood Pressure (JNC 7) has reclassified stages 2 and 3 hypertension as outlined in JNC VI as "stage 2" hypertension. JNC 7 also introduces a new term, "prehypertension" to include individuals with blood pressure (BP) measurements between 120 and 139 mm Hg systolic BP among those requiring intervention. Background: Simplification of the classification of hypertension was one of the three main goals of the JNC 7 report. The other two goals were to include recently published clinical trials in the recommendations and to urgently provide updated hypertension guidelines. The inclusion of the new class "prehypertension" recognizes that the risk of vascular morbidity and mortality becomes evident at BP levels as low as 115/75 mm Hg in adult patients. *(From Chobanian AV, Bakris GL, Black HR, et al. The Seventh Report of the Joint National Committee on Prevention, Detection, Evaluation, and Treatment of High Blood Pressure: The JNC 7 Report. JAMA. 2003;289:2560-2571.)*

of the NIH. This is the group that produced the Joint National Committee Reports I-7 and commissioned what is known as the Expert Panel Report (Fig. 51.1). This effort started shortly after some of the first Framingham data were published in the 1960s. The Framingham Heart Study, a longitudinal study begun in 1949, reported a strong correlation between elevated blood pressure (BP) and heart attacks, heart failure, stroke, and kidney damage. In addition to this data, one of the first clinical outcome trials, developed by Ed Freis, the Veterans Administration (VA) Cooperative Study was published in 1970. This trial demonstrated that lowering BP with the available medications in male patients with severe hypertension dramatically improved their outcome when compared with placebo.[13]

Based on epidemiological and treatment data available, the National High Blood Pressure Education Program was born in 1973, with the goal of enlightening health care professionals and the public on the dangers of hypertension and the lifesaving benefits of treatment.[14,15] It was apparent that the Federal Government, industry, organized medicine, volunteer groups, physicians, nurses, and other professionals could work together effectively with a Coordinating Committee of the National High Blood Pressure Education Program to control a major disease.

In 1977, the First Joint National Committee on Detection, Evaluation, and Treatment of High Blood Pressure established guidelines for management and introduced the stepped-care approach to hypertension treatment. Since then, guidelines have been revised approximately every 4 to 5 years in 1980, 1984, 1988, 1993, 1997, 2003[16-22] (Fig. 51.1). The exception to this was the Expert Panel Report (JNC 8), which was commissioned in 2008 but published 11 years after JNC 7.[5]

The guideline committees that originally consisted of 10 individuals chosen from national organizations by the National Heart, Lung and Blood Institute (NHLBI) to review and evaluate available data on diagnostic and treatment approaches and to publish their conclusions, had grown to 50 consultants from a diverse group of organizations (Box 51.1). These organizations approved all JNC reports except JNC 8, a document reviewed by only 25 national experts.

From the six-page report in JAMA in 1977, the reports expanded considerably to a 47-page report in 2003, but regressed back to a 13-page document in JNC 8. Over the years, the guidelines have stressed a scientifically acceptable but relatively simple diagnostic evaluation and encouraged approaches to treatment which, although not suitable for all patients, had been proven effective.

The JNC reports have been criticized by some investigators as being too simple or too complicated, not workable, or too concerned with cost considerations. In general, however, they have stood the test of time and have evolved as a standard guideline for the management of most hypertensive patients.

All guidelines were evidence based and up until the Expert Panel Report, writers had the freedom and ability to work on research projects with industry but all the while being true to the evidence available to them to make solid general clinical decisions. Interestingly, the Expert Panel Report, which was considered pristine because it excluded people who consult for industry, had only minimal changes to what was put forth in JNC 7 regarding management approaches. Hence, there needs to be a reevaluation of the draconian approach to guidelines and to get people involved who have produced and are familiar with the literature as well as see patients, rather than social and population scientists familiar only with methodology and statistics.

Other guidelines from around the world have similar recommendations to the U.S guidelines, given they all are reviewing similar data. The highlights of some of the commonalties and differences are shown in Table 51.1.

UNITED STATES GUIDANCE VERSUS NATIONAL INSTITUTE FOR HEALTH AND CARE EXCELLENCE AND EUROPEAN GUIDANCE

The NICE guideline development process involves a number of stages and in many ways, the JNC 8 process replicated some of the features of the NICE guideline development process. Before discussing the key features of the current NICE guidance on hypertension, it is worth reflecting on the process for guideline development. The hypertension guideline was last updated in 2011 (NICE CG 127).

The NICE guideline updating process is generally on a 5-year cycle. The process begins with surveillance of published research since the cut-off for the previous guideline review, to determine if there are any areas of the existing guideline that might warrant an update based on new evidence. If there is new evidence, this frames "the proposed scope" of the guideline update. An important feature of the NICE guidance process is engagement with a range of stakeholders as part of the consultation on the proposed scope for any guideline update. These stakeholders range from specialist medical societies, patient groups, health care providers, and the pharmaceutical industry. Comments from the scoping process and the basis for subsequent decisions on the final scope for the guideline are posted online for full transparency. Indeed, transparency and wider consultation are key features of the NICE guideline process.

The Chair and members of the guideline development group are appointed via an application process and all potential conflicts of interest are declared and published. Once the scope for the guideline update has been decided, an evidence review is commissioned by NICE and this is undertaken by one of a number of organizations that are experienced in undertaking a full systematic review of the evidence. This may also include a cost effectiveness analysis if major changes in recommendations are contemplated. The guideline development group then reviews the outputs of the evidence review and decides whether or not changes to the existing guidance are needed and what the changes should be. The "evidence-to-recommendations" section of the guideline describes how the thinking around the recommendations evolved and the strength of the evidence grading. Before the final guideline is published, a further round of stakeholder consultations takes place.

In the most recent NICE guideline update (2011), NICE made a number of key recommendations that changed clinical practice. First, the process of diagnosis of hypertension was reviewed and it was concluded that to eliminate "white coat

TABLE 51.1 Summary of Different International Guideline Statements

CATEGORIES	NICE[a] 2011	ESH/ESC 2013	ASH/ISH 2014	AHA/ACC/CDC 2013	JNC 8[a] 2014
Definition of hypertension	≥140/90 and daytime ABPM (or home BP) ≥ 135/85	≥140/90	≥140/90	≥140/90	Not addressed
Drug therapy/low-risk patients after nonpharm treatment	≥160/100 or daytime ABPM ≥ 150/95	≥140/90	≥140/90	≥140/90	<60 years of age ≥140/90; ≥60 years of age ≥150/90
Beta-blockers: first line drug	No	Yes	No	No	No
Diuretic	Chlorthalidone, indapamide	Thiazides, chlorthalidone, indapamide	Thiazides, chlorthalidone, indapamide	Thiazides	Thiazides, chlorthalidone, indapamide
Initial single pill combo Rx	Not mentioned	Markedly elevated BP	≥160/100	≥160/100	≥160/100
Blood pressure targets	<140/90 ≥80 years of age; <150/90	<140/90; <80 years of age, SBP 140-150; SBP < 140 in fit patients. Elderly ≥80 years of age, SBP 140-150.	<140/90 ≥80 years of age; <150/90	<140/90 Lower targets may be appropriate in some patients including the elderly	<60 years of age <140/90; ≥60 years of age <150/90
Blood pressure target in diabetes	Not addressed	<140/85	<140/90	<140/90 Consider lower targets	<140/90

[a]Expert panel report.

AHA/ACC/CDC, American Heart Association/American College of Cardiology/Centers for Disease Control and Prevention; *ASH/ISH*, American Society of Hypertension/International Society of Hypertension; *ABPM*, ambulatory blood pressure monitoring; *BP*, blood pressure; *ESH/ESC*, European Society of Hypertension/European Society of Cardiology; *JNC*, Joint National Committee; *NICE*, National Institute for Health and Care Excellence; *Rx*, to take; *SBP*, systolic blood pressure.

hypertension," it would be cost-effective to use ambulatory BP monitoring (ABPM), based on a daytime average threshold of 135/85 or higher mm Hg which would be equivalent to a seated clinic BP threshold of 140/90 mm Hg. The proposal was to encourage *wider use of home BP monitoring or ABPM*. With regard to treatment thresholds, it was recognized that the data for the drug treatment of low risk stage 1 hypertension (i.e., generally younger people with 10 years cardiovascular risk lower than 20%, without diabetes, chronic kidney disease, or target organ damage) were inadequate and the benefits of treatment were uncertain. This contrasts with most international guidelines which recommend treatment of all hypertension when BP is greater than 140/90 mm Hg. In this regard, the recommendations of the JNC 8 committee are particularly strange in that they recommend treating at 140/90 mm Hg in lower risk younger people but adopted a higher threshold of 150/90 mm Hg for people over the age of 60 years; because age is a major risk factor, such patients would be at manifestly higher risk than the younger people with a more aggressive treatment threshold.

Consistent with the European Society of Cardiology/European Society of Hypertension (ESC/ESH) guidelines, NICE recommended a higher systolic treatment threshold of higher than 160 mm Hg (i.e., stage 2 hypertension, equivalent to >150 mm Hg using ABPM daytime or home BP averages) in the "very elderly" that is, aged 80 years or older, for people not yet treated and reaching this age. Thus, outside of the U.S. Expert Panel Report, international guidelines in Europe advocate a more aggressive treatment threshold for people aged 60 to 80 years.

With regard to treatment targets, NICE recommended a treatment clinic BP target of less than 140/90 mm Hg, which is consistent with the ESC/ESH recommendations, with the caveat in both guidelines that a more relaxed target of lower than 150/90 mm Hg would be appropriate for people aged 80 years or more. The recommendations for people aged 80 years or more were largely based on the findings of the HYVET (HYpertension in the Very Elderly Trial) study. In contrast, the JNC 8 guidance has adopted this less aggressive BP goal for people aged 60 years or more, which was and remains surprising.

An interesting feature of guideline recommendations on BP goals is that they identify the target but don't really define "how low to go." Perhaps a more useful recommendation would be to recommend a "range" such as below 140 and aiming for 130 to 135 mm Hg. As it stands the recommendations on BP goals are open-ended. It will be curious to see how NICE and ESC/ESH guidance respond to the recently published data from the SPRINT (Systolic blood PRessure INtervention Trial) study in the U.S. which demonstrated a significant reduction in the risk of major cardiovascular events and all-cause mortality in patients randomized to a systolic BP (SBP) target of less than 120 mm Hg versus the current target of less than 140 mm Hg. This treatment benefit on clinical outcomes was associated with increased adverse effects in the more intensively treated group, which suggests that a more personalized approach to BP targets is needed, individualized to the patient's tolerability of lower BP targets.

An interesting feature of all guidelines is their convergence with regard to optimal treatment strategies and in particular optimal drug combinations. NICE has used the nomenclature ACD, where A is an angiotensin-converting enzyme (ACE) inhibitor or angiotensin II receptor blocker (ARB), C is a calcium-channel blocker (CCB), and D is a thiazide-type diuretic (Fig. 51.2). NICE, JNC 8, ESC/ESH, and the American Society of Hypertension/International Society of Hypertension (ASH/ISH) guidance all concur that there should be wider use of combinations of drug therapy and that the optimal two-drug combination would be A+C or A+D, with NICE giving a stronger steer than the other guidance towards A+C (this was largely as a resut of NICE's cost-effectiveness analysis mitigating against the preferred use of thiazide because of the cost of the increased risk of developing diabetes). Preferred three-drug combinations for all guidance was A+C+D.

With regard to initial therapy, NICE uses an age and ethnic group stratification, arguing that for younger people (aged <55 years) an A drug would usually produce the most effective BP lowering, whereas for those over 55 years of age and those of African origin at any age, a CCB would generally be preferred as initial treatment. The U.S. JNC 8 guidance is less prescriptive and suggests any of A, C, or D are suitable as initial therapies, (Fig. 51.3).

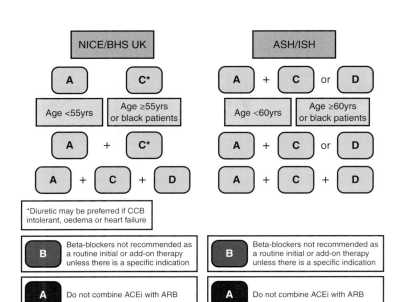

FIG. 51.2 National Institute for Health and Care Excellence (NICE) Guideline treatment algorithms for hypertension. *A*, Angiotensin-converting enzyme (ACE) inhibitor or angiotensin II receptor blocker (ARB); *C*, calcium-channel blocker (CCB); *D*, thiazide-type diuretic. *(From Krause T, Lovibond K, Caulfield M, et al. Management of hypertension: summary of NICE guidance. BMJ. 2011;343:d4891.)*

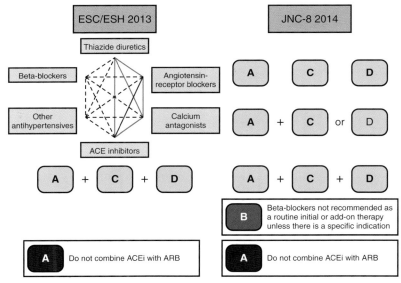

FIG. 51.3 Comparison of Approaches from European and United States guideline. *A*, Angiotensin-converting enzyme (ACE) inhibitor or angiotensin II receptor blocker (ARB); *C*, calcium-channel blocker (CCB); *D*, thiazide-type diuretic. *(From Reference 5 and Mancia G, Fagard R, Narkiewicz K, et al. 2013 ESH/ESC Guidelines for the management of arterial hypertension: the Task Force for the management of arterial hypertension of the European Society of Hypertension (ESH) and of the European Society of Cardiology (ESC). J Hypertens. 2013;31(7):1281-1357.)*

The ESC/ESH guidance differs most with regard to initial therapy, suggesting A, C, D, beta-blocker, or other treatments would all be potential initial therapy options, the decision based on the patient profile and specific indications and contraindications for each drug, (Fig. 51.3). This is somewhat difficult to reconcile when one considers the preferred combinations of treatment according to the ESC/ESH guidance, which are A+C or D, or C+D, in others words, does not strongly recommend the other drugs as part of optimal combination therapy which the guideline notes most people will need. Thus, aside from a few minor differences, all guidance from the U.S., ESC/ESH, and NICE have converged towards A, C and D being the commonly recommended drug treatments, combined as A+C+D and then A+C+D.

Finally, all guidelines recommend that lifestyle advice should be offered to all patients with hypertension, whether they are treated or not. If effectively deployed, this may alleviate the need for drug treatment in patients with prehypertension or stage 1 hypertension and will usually increase the efficacy of concomitant drug therapy when needed. The lifestyle guidance has remained consistent in recommending strategies that may assist in BP lowering such as maintaining a healthy body weight, partaking in regular aerobic exercise, moderating the daily sodium intake, and avoiding excessive alcohol intake. Many of which, along with smoking cessation and eating a balanced and health diet, will help reduce cardiovascular disease risk as well.

In summary, there are now many more points of convergence versus divergence in international hypertension guidelines. Although the evidence base is the same for all, some divergence is to be expected based on a region's ability to fund and thus endorse specific guideline recommendations, and whether cost-effectiveness rather than just effectiveness is factored into the analysis. It is worth reflecting of the fact that seemingly subtle shifts in BP thresholds or targets can have a major impact on the numbers of people treated country-wide and how much treatment they receive, all of which has a huge impact on the "cost of the recommendation." That said, NICE, in its cost-effectiveness analysis in 2011, demonstrated that treating hypertension was very cost-effective and that the least cost-effective option for the health-care system was "no treatment," as the cost of the resulting increase in cardiovascular morbidity and mortality outweighs the cost of prevention.

References

1. www merriam-webster com/dictionary/guideline, 2015 www.merriam-webster.com/dictionary/guideline.
2. Burgers JS, Grol R, Klazinga NS, Makela M, Zaat J. Towards evidence-based clinical practice: an international survey of 18 clinical guideline programs. *Int J Qual Health Care*. 2003;15:31-45.
3. Development and validation of an international appraisal instrument for assessing the quality of clinical practice guidelines: the AGREE project. *Qual Saf Health Care*. 2003;12:18-23.
4. Institute of Medicine Report. 2011. Ref Type: Pamphlet
5. James PA, Oparil S, Carter BL, et al. 2014 evidence-based guideline for the management of high blood pressure in adults: report from the panel members appointed to the Eighth Joint National Committee (JNC 8). *JAMA*. 2014;311:507-520.
6. Tricoci P, Allen JM, Kramer JM, Califf RM, Smith SC Jr. Scientific evidence underlying the ACC/AHA clinical practice guidelines. *JAMA*. 2009;301:831-841.
7. Akl EA, El-Hachem P, Abou-Haidar H, Neumann I, Schunemann HJ, Guyatt GH. Considering intellectual, in addition to financial, conflicts of interest proved important in a clinical practice guideline: a descriptive study. *J Clin Epidemiol*. 2014;67:1222-1228.
8. Minter RM, Angelos P, Coimbra R, et al. Ethical management of conflict of interest: proposed standards for academic surgical societies. *J Am Coll Surg*. 2011;213:677-682.
9. Reames BN, Krell RW, Ponto SN, Wong SL. Critical evaluation of oncology clinical practice guidelines. *J Clin Oncol*. 2013;31:2563-2568.
10. Williams MJ, Kevat DA, Loff B. Conflict of interest guidelines for clinical guidelines. *Med J Aust*. 2011;195:442-445.
11. Berra K. Does nurse case management improve implementation of guidelines for cardiovascular disease risk reduction? *J Cardiovasc Nurs*. 2011;26:145-167.
12. Tra J, van dW, I, Appelman Y, de Bruijne MC, Wagner C. Adherence to guidelines for the prescription of secondary prevention medication at hospital discharge after acute coronary syndrome: a multicentre study. *Neth Heart J*. 2015;23:214-221.
13. Effects of treatment on morbidity in hypertension. II. Results in patients with diastolic blood pressure averaging 90 through 114 mm Hg. *JAMA*. 1970;213:1143-1152.
14. Moser M. Evolution of the treatment of hypertension from the 1940s to JNC V. *Am J Hypertens*. 1997;10:2S-8S.
15. Moser M. From JNC I to JNC 7—what have we learned? *Prog Cardiovasc Dis*. 2006;48:303-315.
16. Report of the Joint National Committee on Detection, Evaluation, and Treatment of High Blood Pressure. A cooperative study. *JAMA*. 1977;237:255-261.
17. The 1980 report of the Joint National Committee on Detection, Evaluation, and Treatment of High Blood Pressure. *Arch Intern Med*. 1980;140:1280-1285.
18. The 1984 Report of the Joint National Committee on Detection, Evaluation, and Treatment of High Blood Pressure. *Arch Intern Med*. 1984;144:1045-1057.
19. The 1988 report of the Joint National Committee on Detection, Evaluation, and Treatment of High Blood Pressure. *Arch Intern Med*. 1988;148:1023-1038.
20. The fifth report of the Joint National Committee on Detection, Evaluation, and Treatment of High Blood Pressure (JNC V). *Arch Intern Med*. 1993;153:154-183.
21. The sixth report of the Joint National Committee on prevention, detection, evaluation, and treatment of high blood pressure. *Arch Intern Med*. 1997;157:2413-2446.
22. Chobanian AV, Bakris GL, Black HR, et al. Seventh report of the Joint National Committee on Prevention, Detection, Evaluation, and Treatment of High Blood Pressure. *Hypertension*. 2003;42:1206-1252.

Index

Note: Page numbers followed by f, t, and b indicate figures, tables, and boxes, respectively.

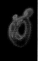

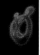

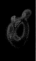

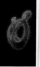